W9-BSC-744

A Massage Therapist's Guide to Pathology

Fourth Edition

A Massage Therapist's Guide to Pathology

FOURTH EDITION

Ruth Werner, LMP, NCTMB

Wolters Kluwer Health | Lippincott Williams & Wilkins

Acquisitions Editor: John Goucher
Managing Editor: Linda G. Francis
Marketing Manager: Nancy Bradshaw
Production Editor: John Larkin
Creative Director: Doug Smock
Designer: Candice M. Carta-Myers
Compositor: Maryland Composition

Fourth Edition

351 West Camden Street
Baltimore, MD 21201

530 Walnut Street
Philadelphia, PA 19106

Printed in China

9 8 7 6 5 4

Library of Congress Cataloging-in-Publication Data

Werner, Ruth (Ruth A.)
A massage therapist's guide to pathology / Ruth Werner. — 4th ed.
p. ; cm. — (LWW massage therapy & bodywork educational series)
Includes bibliographical references and index.
ISBN-13: 978-0-7817-6919-8
ISBN-10: 0-7817-6919-1
1. Massage therapy. 2. Physiology, Pathological. 3. Diseases. I. Title. II. Series.
[DNLM: 1. Massage. 2. Diagnosis, Differential. WB 537 W494m 2009]
RM721.M366 2009
615.8'22--dc22

2007026173

DISCLAIMER

Care has been taken to confirm the accuracy of the information present and to describe generally accepted practices. However, the authors, editors, and publisher are not responsible for errors or omissions or for any consequences from application of the information in this book and make no warranty, expressed or implied, with respect to the currency, completeness, or accuracy of the contents of the publication. Application of this information in a particular situation remains the professional responsibility of the practitioner; the clinical treatments described and recommended may not be considered absolute and universal recommendations.

The authors, editors, and publisher have exerted every effort to ensure that drug selection and dosage set forth in this text are in accordance with the current recommendations and practice at the time of publication. However, in view of ongoing research, changes in government regulations, and the constant flow of information relating to drug therapy and drug reactions, the reader is urged to check the package insert for each drug for any change in indications and dosage and for added warnings and precautions. This is particularly important when the recommended agent is a new or infrequently employed drug.

Some drugs and medical devices presented in this publication have Food and Drug Administration (FDA) clearance for limited use in restricted research settings. It is the responsibility of the health care provider to ascertain the FDA status of each drug or device planned for use in their clinical practice.

The publishers have made every effort to trace the copyright holders for borrowed material. If they have inadvertently overlooked any, they will be pleased to make the necessary arrangements at the first opportunity.

To purchase additional copies of this book, call our customer service department at **(800) 638-3030** or fax orders to **(301) 223-2320**. International customers should call **(301) 223-2300**.

Visit Lippincott Williams & Wilkins on the Internet: http://www.lww.com. Lippincott Williams & Wilkins customer service representatives are available from 8:30 am to 6:00 pm, EST.

RRS1006

*This book is and will forever be dedicated
to the memory of my grandmother,
Dora Charak Beckhard,
who probably never
got a massage in her life—but she
sure could have used one.*

The Pathologies

Abortion, spontaneous and elective, p. 610
Acne rosacea, p. 50
Acne vulgaris, p. 52
Acromegaly, p. 560
Acute bronchitis, p. 443
Addison disease, p. 562
Allergic reactions, p. 418
Alzheimer disease, p. 223
Amyotrophic lateral sclerosis, p. 226
Anemia, p. 341
Ankylosing spondylitis, p. 124
Anxiety disorders, p. 254
Aortic aneurysm, p. 368
Asthma, p. 462
Atherosclerosis, p. 371
Attention deficit hyperactivity disorder, p. 259
Autism spectrum disorders, p. 261
Avascular osteonecrosis, p. 110
Baker cysts, p. 168
Bell palsy, p. 283
Benign prostatic hypertrophy, p. 641
Bladder cancer, p. 597
Boils, p. 26
Breast cancer, p. 627
Bunions, p. 169
Burns, p. 74
Bursitis, p. 172
Cancer, general, p. 671
Candidiasis, p. 548
Carpal tunnel syndrome, p. 200
Celiac disease, p. 486
Cellulitis, p. 28
Cerebral palsy, p. 286
Cervical cancer, p. 612
Chemical dependency, p. 265
Chronic bronchitis, p. 465
Chronic fatigue syndrome, p. 421
Cirrhosis, p. 525
Colorectal cancer, p. 511
Common cold, p. 445
Complex regional pain syndrome, p. 289
Crohn disease, p. 489
Cushing syndrome, p. 564
Cystic fibrosis, p. 472
Decubitus ulcers, p. 77
Depression, p. 270
Dermatitis/Eczema, p. 56
Diabetes mellitus, p. 567
Disc disease, p. 204
Dislocations, p. 127
Diverticular disease, p. 516
Dupuytren contracture, p. 174
Dysmenorrhea, p. 616
Dystonia, p. 236
Eating disorders, p. 277
Edema, p. 407
Ehlers-Danlos syndrome, p. 158
Embolism, thrombus, p. 345
Emphysema, p. 469
Encephalitis, p. 244
Endometriosis, p. 618
Esophageal cancer, p. 494
Fever, p. 425
Fibroid tumors, p. 621
Fibromyalgia, p. 90
Fractures, p. 112
Fungal infections, p. 30
Gallstones, p. 530
Ganglion cysts, p. 177
Gastroenteritis, p. 497
Gastroesophageal reflux disease, p. 500
Gout, p. 129
Guillain-Barré syndrome, p. 313
Headaches, p. 316
Heart attack, p. 388
Heart failure, p. 395
Hematoma, p. 348
Hemophilia, p. 350
Hepatitis, p. 534
Hernia, p. 178
Herpes simplex, p. 34
Herpes zoster, p. 246
HIV/AIDS, p. 427
Hives, p. 60
Hypertension, p. 378
Hyperthyroidism, p. 573
Hypothyroidism, p. 576
Impetigo, p. 38
Inflammation, p. 13

Influenza, p. 447
Interstitial cystitis, p. 601
Irritable bowel syndrome, p. 520
Kidney stones, p. 589
Leukemia, p. 352
Lice and mites, p. 40
Liver cancer, p. 539
Lung cancer, p. 475
Lupus, p. 433
Lyme disease, p. 133
Lymphangitis, p. 410
Lymphoma, p. 412
Malaria, p. 356
Marfan syndrome, p. 161
Ménière disease, p. 321
Meningitis, p. 249
Menopause, p. 652
Metabolic syndrome, p. 579
Mononucleosis, p. 415
Multiple sclerosis, p. 230
Muscular dystrophy, p. 163
Myasthenia gravis, p. 209
Myeloma, p. 359
Myofascial pain syndrome, p. 96
Myositis ossificans, p. 100
Osgood-Schlatter disease, p. 181
Osteoarthritis, p. 137
Osteogenesis imperfecta, p. 166
Osteoporosis, p. 114
Ovarian cancer, p. 634
Ovarian cysts, p. 637
Paget disease, p. 119
Pancreatic cancer, p. 543
Pancreatitis, p. 546
Parkinson disease, p. 239
Patellofemoral syndrome, p. 141
Peptic ulcers, p. 504
Peripheral neuropathy, p. 235
Peritonitis, p. 551
Pes planus, Pes cavus, p. 183
Plantar fasciitis, p. 186
Pneumonia, p. 451
Polio, postpolio syndrome, p. 251
Postural deviations, p. 121
Pregnancy, p. 655
Premenstrual syndrome, p. 659
Prostate cancer, p. 643
Prostatitis, p. 646
Psoriasis, p. 62
Pyelonephritis, p. 592
Raynaud syndrome, p. 382
Renal failure, p. 594
Rheumatoid arthritis, p. 144
Scar tissue, p. 79
Scleroderma, p. 189
Seizure disorders, p. 323
Sexually transmitted diseases, p. 661
Shin splints, p. 102
Sickle cell disease, p. 361
Sinusitis, p. 454
Skin cancer, p. 66
Sleep disorders, p. 326
Spasms, Cramps, p. 105
Spina bifida, p. 293
Spinal cord injury, p. 297
Spondylosis, p. 147
Sprains, p. 151
Stomach cancer, p. 508
Strains, p. 107
Stroke, p. 302
Temporomandibular joint disorders, p. 154
Tendinopathies, p. 191
Tenosynovitis, p. 193
Testicular cancer, p. 650
Thoracic outlet syndrome, p. 211
Thrombophlebitis, deep vein thrombosis, p. 364
Thyroid cancer, p. 581
Traumatic brain injury, p. 308
Tremor, p. 243
Trigeminal neuralgia, p. 310
Tuberculosis, p. 458
Ulcerative colitis, p. 523
Urinary tract infection, p. 603
Uterine cancer, p. 623
Varicose veins, p. 385
Vestibular balance disorders, p. 331
Warts, p. 47
Whiplash, p. 196

FOREWORD

The field of massage has seen a dramatic transformation in the past several decades. Its use as a personal care service in spas, cruise ships, and private practice settings for general relaxation has become commonplace. Along with the rapid rise of massage as a personal care service has been its equally important emergence as a powerful health care practice. With increasing frequency, articles are appearing in the popular press as well as the scientific literature depicting the beneficial effects of massage for addressing numerous adverse health conditions.

In the United States many are describing a breakdown in our health care system. Costs are skyrocketing, and despite the impressive advances in technology, many people are unable to find effective treatments for conditions that afflict them. It is these rising costs and the ineffectiveness of modern medicine that have driven the explosive interest in complementary and alternative medicine approaches such as massage therapy.

Many people have found relief from various ailments in the effective application of massage therapy. Clients seek it for many purposes, from relief of general aches and pains related to exercise and occupational stress to palliative care and pain management in life-threatening conditions. The scientific research community has begun to take interest in this therapy. Initial studies show beneficial outcomes in a wide variety of applications, from the structural and mechanical perspective, such as low back and neck pain, to the psychosomatic realm, including reduction of anxiety and depression.

Massage is not benign, and it can have adverse effects. In less severe cases it may not cause harm but simply be ineffective. The use of massage to address any compromised health condition must be based on sound physiological principles. For the massage practitioner an understanding of pathology is a necessary first step to using this approach in a positive therapeutic context.

Since it first appeared on the scene a number of years ago, Ruth Werner's book, *A Massage Therapists' Guide to Pathology*, has been a foundational text, one that every practitioner should have on the shelf. Over the years our understanding of massage has expanded, and so has the need for expanding the information in this text. While its solid foundation of valuable information remains, the new features in this text are a welcome adjunct that continues to enhance its value.

The material presented in the new introductory chapter helps establish a more solid grounding for understanding each of the pathological conditions described throughout the book. A number of myths and inaccuracies continue to pervade our profession in such areas as infectious agents, hygiene, and cancer. The principles in this chapter should help each practitioner better understand these topics and how they relate to numerous pathological conditions.

A valuable new addition in this text is the inclusion of recommendations for how several modalities of massage should or should not be used with each condition. While these recommendations should not be taken as strict rules, their inclusion is a helpful step toward understanding a condition and making sound clinical decisions about the appropriateness of treatment.

Research and education are the foundation for continued growth in our profession. Massage practitioners who are going to work with people who have compromised health should stay abreast of new developments and published findings in our field. However, research literacy is still in its infancy as a subject in many initial massage training programs. Werner's inclusion of an appendix addressing the topic of research literacy as well as resource materials for instructors teaching the topic in the classroom is a valuable addition to the new text as well.

As our profession grows, an increasing number of resources are available for students and practitioners. However, certain foundation texts that have a long track record of valuable contributions to the field should remain in every practitioner's library. I was impressed with this text when it first came out, and each successive edition has improved on the state of knowledge and reflected new and current research. Werner's many years as an educator have helped her design a text that is user friendly, graphically interesting, and most important, well organized and easily accessible. I am certain this book will continue to move us forward as it once again raises the bar in our professional literature.

Whitney Lowe
Sisters, Oregon
2007

PREFACE

It's hard to believe that the first edition of *A Massage Therapist's Guide to Pathology* was written more than 10 years ago. I wrote it to answer a specific need in our field. With the expansion of our profession that need has grown, and the book has grown with it. At the same time, the use of massage as a therapeutic intervention for people struggling with health issues has grown as well. This means massage therapists *must* be well informed about pathology, and if they encounter a client with a problem they've never heard of, they had better be able to find good information fast.

Ultimately, the study of massage in the context of pathology can be reduced to some basic concepts:

- How does the human body work when it is healthy?
- How does a disease or condition influence that process?
- Where does massage or bodywork best enter that dance?

The last question shows that the role of massage therapy for people who live with diseases or disorders simply *cannot* be rubber stamped to say one condition always indicates massage and another always contraindicates it. The answer to "Is massage safe for this person?" is *always* "It depends." It is the therapist's job to determine what it depends *on*. What are the variables in any given situation? One way to do that is to answer these questions:

- What are the best possible benefits massage can offer this person?
- What are the possible risks?
- How can the therapist tip the scales to get the best benefits while avoiding the risks?

A Massage Therapist's Guide to Pathology aims to help students and practitioners to make safe and productive decisions about bodywork in a wide variety of circumstances. Over the years we have worked hard to provide information in a complete but accessible and user-friendly form, and this edition continues with that purpose in mind.

WHAT'S NEW WITH THIS EDITION?

Several exciting features have been added to the fourth edition:

General Features

Alphabetized List

A full list of all the conditions in this text and their page numbers can be found on pages vi–vii.

Reorganization

The book has been extensively reorganized to include an introductory chapter with fundamental concepts, and a concluding chapter dedicated solely to principles of cancer.

New Articles

New articles have been added, including myeloma, sickle cell disease, autism spectrum disorders, and many others.

New Appendix: Research Literacy

This addresses the role of massage therapists in evaluating and conducting credible research in this field.

Modality Recommendation Charts

Ever since the first edition, readers of *A Massage Therapist's Guide to Pathology* have requested more specific guidelines or advice about what kinds of modalities to pursue or avoid in various circumstances. I resisted addressing this for several reasons, but mainly because I thought that the moment one modality was mentioned over another, people would be justifiably upset at being excluded from the discussion.

Many years of encouragement finally convinced me that it *is* possible to answer this need, and in this edition we have added a new feature that is, to my knowledge, unique in texts of this kind. I have invited eight leading subject matter experts to render their opinions about how their specialty might be applied in the context of the conditions being discussed. Their input is found at the end of each pathology in the form of modality recommendation charts. While many classes of bodywork have been represented here, some inevitably have been left out. This is due to restrictions on time and space, not to any lack of respect or appreciation for other techniques.

The Contributors

Our modality recommendation contributors are brave souls who said yes to a project that, because we were trying something entirely new, was a mystery in size and scope. They saw it through with great aplomb, even when I kept changing the rules. I hope readers appreciate their work as much as I do.

Deep Tissue/Myofascial Release

Jonathan Martine is a Certified Advanced Rolfer®, Rolf movement practitioner, registered movement therapist (ISMETTA), Pilates instructor, and certified massage therapist. Since 1990, Jonathan has practiced with doctors, chiropractors, and physical therapists offering structural integration, manual therapy, and rehabilitative exercise. His training in biodynamic craniosacral therapy, visceral manipulation, rehabilitative exercise, joint mobilization, and manual therapy complements his extensive study in Rolfing® Structural Integration. His clients present the gift of witnessing the adaptability of the human form, the innate wisdom of the body, and the resilience of the spirit.

He is presently the chair of the faculty at the Rolf Institute, life sciences instructor, and a teacher in their certification program. In addition to teaching with the Rolf Institute, he offers continuing education classes for structural integrators and massage therapists. For more information on CE offerings, Jonathan can be contacted at jsmartine@aol.com.

Lymphatic Drainage

Charlotte Michael Versagi, LMT, NCTMB, is a regular contributor to both massage and oncology national publications, is a national speaker on oncology massage and lymphedema, and specializes in treatment and consulting on oncology patients at risk for lymphedema. As a pathophysiology instructor, she brings this knowledge combined with her decade of experience in oncology massage to her 100-hour hospital-based oncology massage program. Her training in lymphedema was with Joe Zuther's Academy of Lymphatic Studies, and she regularly serves as an expert in lymphedema as related to the care of cancer patients.

Polarity Therapy and Reiki Therapy

Carol Ann Lucia, RPP, RPE, LMT, is a certified psychosynthesist, registered polarity practitioner, Reiki master, and nationally certified and licensed massage therapist specializing in energy medicine. Carol Ann helps individuals uncover their inherent healing wisdom by integrating the principles of psychosynthesis and energy healing, including polarity therapy, Reiki, craniosacral therapy, meditation, and regression therapy. Since 1984, she has maintained a private practice offering individual sessions, educational classes, and workshops. She is an instructor at the Connecticut Institute for Psychosynthesis and Connecticut Center for Massage Therapy and has offered classes at Western Connecticut State University and University of Connecticut. She has also served on the American Polarity Therapy Association Ethics Committee. Carol Ann was one of the original members to be named a Registered Polarity Educator by the American Polarity Therapy Association, and she offers a 675-hour approved polarity therapy training course. She is a member of the Association for the Advancement of Psychosynthesis, American Polarity Therapy Association, and Lotus—The Educational Center for Integrative Healing and Wellness, and she has served as coordinator introducing complementary care to the Harold Leever Cancer Center. Carol Ann can be reached at the Energy Healing and Polarity Therapy Center or at Elements4Wellness.com.

Proprioceptive Neuromuscular Facilitation

Bob McAtee, NCTMB, CSCS, is the author of *Facilitated Stretching*, a how-to book about PNF stretching published by Human Kinetics. The book has sold over 70,000 copies since its release in 1994 and has been translated into Spanish, Italian, Portuguese, and Japanese.

Bob is also a sports massage therapist with more than 25 years of experience. He owns and operates Pro-Active Massage Therapy in Colorado Springs, Colorado. He regularly presents workshops on facilitated stretching, massage therapy, and injury care nationally and internationally. Bob is nationally certified in therapeutic massage and bodywork (1992), is a certified strength and conditioning specialist (1998), and is a personal trainer certified by the American Council on Exercise (2006). For more information, you can contact him at www.stretchman.com.

Reflexology

Janene Jaynes has been a licensed massage therapist since 1994. She specializes in teaching nutrition, yoga, kinesiology, reflexology, imagery, and business, and she has taught a variety of other classes. She is adding to her career by finishing her physical education for teaching education degree with an emphasis on personal training and nutrition. Janene serves as chairperson of the Utah Department of Public Licensing Massage Education Review Board, helping to determine curriculum guidelines for massage schools all over the state.

When Janene opened her business in 1998, she realized that many of her clients had temporomandibular joint (TMJ) disorders, a condition Janene had had most of her life. She tried reflexology to help her clients deal with this chronic condition and was amazed at how simple, painless, and efficient this modality was.

Janene's clientele grew as word quickly spread of how effective her treatments were. Soon her clinic was filled with clients who had fibromyalgia, irritable bowl syndrome, gallstones, and many other conditions, and reflexology was the key to their recovery. Janene especially appreciates reflexology for how well it supports other modalities and how adaptable it is for her clients to use at home with their loved ones.

Shiatsu

Lindy Ferrigno, CI (AOBTA®), Dipl. ABT (NCCAOM), LMT, has developed certified shiatsu programs in schools and colleges in five states since 1977. With colleagues across the United States, she spearheaded the founding of the American Association for Bodywork Therapies of Asia (AOBTA). She established national criteria for the education and practice of Asian bodywork through committee work with the National Commission for the Certification of Acupuncture and Oriental Medicine (NCCAOM). In addition to her ongoing studies in shiatsu, she has apprenticed with osteopaths, chiropractors, and indigenous healers on three continents over 30 years of private practice. She teaches workshops across the United States designed to lead bodyworkers beyond their rudimentary knowledge base to the art of healing.

Swedish Massage

Meade Steadman is a licensed massage practitioner and aesthetician in Salt Lake City, Utah. He has been on the faculty of the Myotherapy College of Utah and the Myotherapy Institute of Massage since 1997, where he teaches Swedish massage, sports massage, acutherapy, practice building and professional ethics, hydrotherapy, spa techniques, geriatric massage, hot stone massage, and several other courses. He is also the featured expert in the multiple-award-winning videos by Aesthetic Video Source: *The Art & Practice of Stone Massage*; *The Ultimate Face, Scalp, Neck & Shoulder Massage*; *The Complete Guide to Full Body Chair Massage*; *Comprehensive Reflexology & Massage: The Hand*; *Comprehensive Reflexology & Massage: The Foot*; and *Essentials of Swedish Massage*. In addition, Meade regularly performs 45 hours of massage each week. He can be reached at www.tranquiltouch.com.

Trigger Point Therapy

Joseph (Joe) Muscolino, DC, is author of five publications: *The Muscular System Manual: The Skeletal Muscles of the Human Body*; *Kinesiology: The Skeletal System and Muscle Function*; *The Musculoskeletal Anatomy Coloring Book*; *Musculoskeletal Anatomy Flashcards*; and *Flashcards for Bones, Joints, and Actions of the Human Body*. All of Joe's books and student resources are published by Mosby of Elsevier Science and are used by massage and bodywork schools across the United States and Canada. He also writes a regular column for *Massage Therapy Journal* entitled "Body Mechanics."

Joe has been an instructor at the Connecticut Center for Massage Therapy for more than 20 years. He is an approved provider of continuing education credit by the National Certification Board for Therapeutic Massage and Bodywork and provides continuing education courses for massage therapists and bodyworkers across the country as well as in-services for instructors of massage therapy. For more information or to contact Joe, visit: www.learnmuscles.com.

Fully Revised and Updated Student Resource CD

The student resource CD has been fully updated, and several new features have been added. In addition to an audio glossary, a full set of quiz questions for each chapter, and answers to the Chapter Objective and Chapter Review questions, the student resource CD contains the following:

- **Animations and film clips.** Pathology animations and film clips, including some from the acclaimed *Acland's DVD Atlas of Human Anatomy*.
- **Bibliography.** The full bibliography from the text. Cited references are still at the conclusion of each chapter in the print text.
- **Client endangerments.** Users of previous editions will recognize this appendix, which has been moved to the Student Resource CD.

- **Taking a Client History with printable forms.** This has also been moved from print text to the CD, and it appears now with printable forms from *Hands Heal: Communication, Documentation, and Insurance Billing for Manual Therapists*, Third Edition (Lippincott, Williams & Wilkins, 2005).
- **Quick reference charts.** These charts, which are composed of all of the In Brief boxes from the text in alphabetical order, can now be found on the student resource CD in an easily printable format.
- **Printable flash cards.** Students will appreciate these valuable study aids, which are based on the quick reference charts. Another set of printable flash cards are based on the Greek and Latin word roots discussed in Chapter 1 of the text.
- **Games.** Student activities in the form of word searches, hangman games, and crossword puzzles will help to solidify key concepts.

Fully Revised and Updated Instructor Resource CD

The instructor resource CD has also been revised and updated. It includes the following:

- **Lecture notes for each chapter** can be adapted and printed for instructor or student use.
- **PowerPoint slides** are based on lecture notes, with incorporated art and animations.
- **Illustrations** from the fourth edition.
- **Sample syllabi** for 40- and 60-hour pathology courses, along with a curriculum development guide.
- **A full test bank** and test generator software.

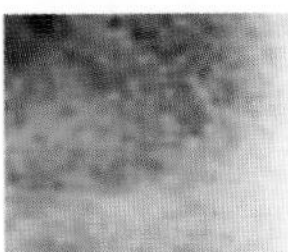

What Are We Bringing from the Third Edition?

The structure and features that constitute the heart of this book have been preserved and improved.

Chapter Structure

Chapter 1 is an introduction to basic concepts in pathology, and Chapter 12 focuses only on cancer. Chapters 2 to 11 are dedicated to specific body systems, as in previous editions. Each chapter opens with Chapter Objective questions (answers are provided on the Student Resource CD) and a brief review of the structure and function of the system under discussion. Topics are grouped by type, so that conditions with similar etiologies are found close together in the text. Chapters then conclude with review questions (also found with answers on the Student Resource CD).

Article Structure

Each article is discussed in an organized and predictable format. *In Brief* boxes provide a thumbnail sketch of the condition under discussion. Then each topic is addressed with the following headings: *Definition*, *Etiology*, *Signs and Symptoms*, *Implications for Massage*, and *Modality Recommendations*. Additional headings include *Demographics*, *Complications*, *Prevention*, *Treatment*, and others as necessary. All of the articles have been thoroughly updated for this edition.

Other Features

Several other features enrich the core material. *Sniglets* give background or history of some terminology. *Sidebars* discuss peripheral issues relating to conditions or give more detailed information about cancer staging. *Compare and Contrast* charts lay out aspects of similar conditions side by side, so that readers may better understand where they overlap and where they diverge. *Case histories* share the stories of people who live with various diseases and disorders so that readers may appreciate how these abstract ideas lead to concrete realities.

Where Are We Going?

There has never been a better time to be a massage therapist. Our field is growing in numbers, in public acceptance, and in professionalism. Entry-level massage therapists know *so much more* than some of us old-timers did when we first got started. While it is certainly true that massage education continues to have room for improvement, we can all take heart in the fact that the range of learning resources for massage students has never been better.

One especially exciting shift I have seen is a new interest in the role of research about massage. From anecdotes to formal case reports to randomized controlled trials, information is finally being generated that challenges, in the best possible ways, much of the best-guessing folklore that has been the backbone of massage theory. Some of what we're finding validates what we have always thought, and some has yielded very surprising results.

Appendix B, **Research Literacy**, was developed in recognition of this movement. This is a brief introduction to the research process, and it would not exist without the generous effort of Ravensara Travillian, whose upcoming book, *Massage Therapy: A Guide to Reading the Research Literature*, will be an invaluable resource to anyone interested in the fascinating subject of research for massage therapy. The future of our profession lies in our ability to document how massage affects function in health and in illness. We are just beginning to dip our toes in this massive ocean, and I hope that by demystifying some of the language around research, we can help make this process accessible to more people, whether they are students, instructors, or practitioners.

In this context, it is appropriate to acknowledge the work of the Massage Therapy Foundation for its dedication to funding and promoting international research in massage. It is my honor to work with this organization, and I encourage all readers to become familiar with and support the foundation. For more information, visit it at http://www.massagetherapyfoundation.org/.

Finally, my traditional closing words: I invite you to read this with joy. Do more research in what interests you, and share your findings with others. Remember that some of the questions dealt with here will probably never be completely answered. And what we think we know today may be revised or proved wrong tomorrow. Isn't that terrific?

Many thanks and many blessings,
Ruth Werner
Layton, UT
Summer 2007

How to Use This Book

 User's Guide

A Massage Therapist's Guide to Pathology gives you the tools to make informed decisions about bodywork for clients who live with a wide variety of diseases and conditions. This user's guide shows how to put the book's features to work for you.

 Alphabetical List of Conditions

Every condition in the book is listed in alphabetical order with page numbers, starting on page vi.

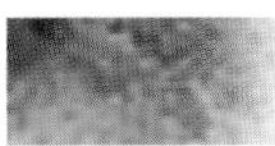 Chapter Objectives

These begin every chapter, alerting the reader to important pieces of information that follow and providing a framework for independent study. Answers to the Chapter Objective questions are provided on the Student Resource CD.

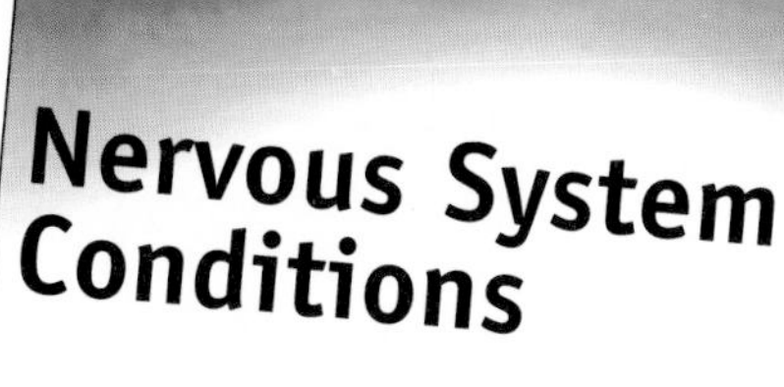

4

Nervous System Conditions

Chapter Objectives

After reading this chapter, you should be able to . . .

- Name three diseases that could be confused with multiple sclerosis.
- Name two movement disorders in addition to tremor.
- Name the causative agent of herpes zoster.
- Name three types of depression.
- Name three types of anxiety disorders.
- Name the most subtle type of autism spectrum disorder.
- Name two types of stroke.
- Name the nerve involved in Bell palsy.
- Name three complications of spinal cord injury.
- Name two signs that a headache could be a medical emergency.
- Name the four classic symptoms of Ménière disease.
- Name three major cautions for massage in the context of nervous system disorders.

Introduction

By the time most massage therapists finish their training, they probably know more about the nervous system than they ever suspected existed, and they'll probably still feel like rank amateurs on the subject. That feeling is common to most people who study this topic. Fortunately, only a passing familiarity with the structure and function of this system is needed to make educated decisions about massage and many nervous system disorders. Most of the conditions considered here affect the peripheral nerves rather than the central nervous system (CNS), so this introductory discussion focuses mainly on the structure and function of the parts of the nervous system massage therapists can touch—which, not coincidentally, are also the parts of the system that are most vulnerable to injury.

Function and Structure

Nerves are bundles of individual neurons, fibrous cells capable of transmitting electrical impulses from one place to another. At their most basic level, the function of neurons is to transmit information from the body to the brain (sensation) and responses from the brain to the body (motor control). Interconnecting neurons in the brain also provide

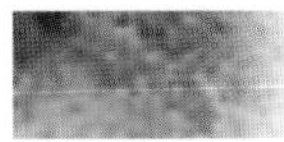 Introductory Chapter

New with this edition, Chapter 1 introduces key concepts on which the study of pathology is built. Terminology, infectious agents, hygienic methods, and the inflammatory process are discussed here. This chapter also gives background on the modalities that are represented in the new modality recommendation charts.

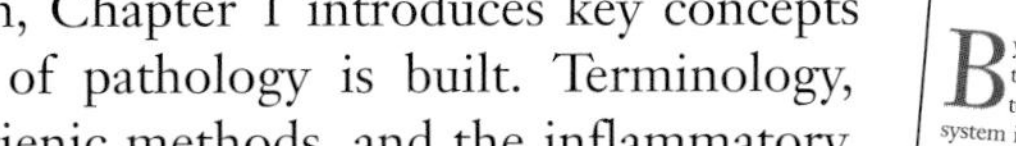

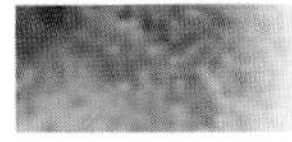 Body System Overviews

Chapters 2 to 11 open with a brief review of the body system under discussion, with special emphasis on processes that may be interrupted by conditions that change the way we function.

Modality Recommendation Charts

New with this edition, these conclude each discussion and offer input from eight experts on the role of their specialties in the context of each condition.

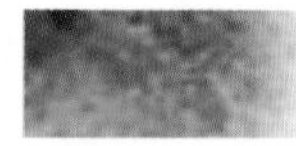

In Brief Boxes

These give a synopsis of the definition, signs and symptoms, and guidelines for bodywork for each condition discussed. All the In Brief Boxes are then repeated alphabetically in Appendix E to provide a printable *Quick Reference Guide* on the Student Resource CD.

If a client is comatose, massage or other stroking techniques may be performed to help preserve the health of the tissues and prevent complications such as decubitus ulcers, but these must be performed with caution, since the client cannot give feedback to manage the risk of overtreatment.

In either case, TBI is a complicated, serious problem with many long-term problems that affect many aspects of health. Any TBI survivor who receives massage as part of a rehabilitative process should do so as part of integrated health care management, incorporating massage with other therapies for the best result.

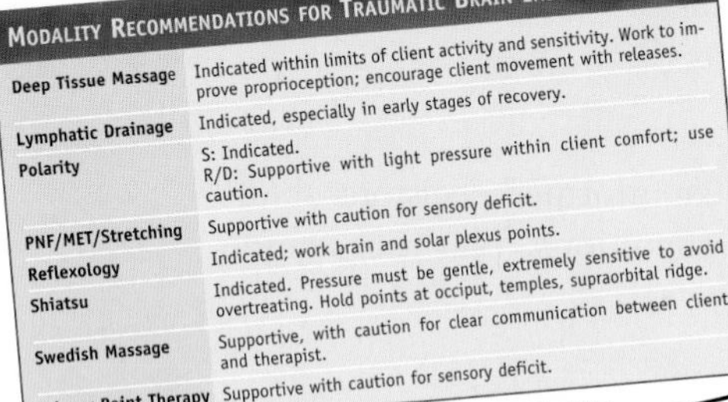

Modality Recommendations for Traumatic Brain Injury

Modality	Recommendation
Deep Tissue Massage	Indicated within limits of client activity and sensitivity. Work to improve proprioception; encourage client movement with releases.
Lymphatic Drainage	Indicated, especially in early stages of recovery.
Polarity	S: Indicated. R/D: Supportive with light pressure within client comfort; use caution.
PNF/MET/Stretching	Supportive with caution for sensory deficit.
Reflexology	Indicated; work brain and solar plexus points.
Shiatsu	Indicated. Pressure must be gentle, extremely sensitive to avoid overtreating. Hold points at occiput, temples, supraorbital ridge.
Swedish Massage	Supportive, with caution for clear communication between client and therapist.
Trigger Point Therapy	Supportive with caution for sensory deficit.

See Chapter 1 for a brief description of each modality, including definitions of abbreviations.

Trigeminal Neuralgia in Brief

Pronunciation: try-JEM-ih-nul nur-AL-je-ah

What is it?
Trigeminal neuralgia (TN) is a condition involving sharp electrical or stabbing pain along one or more branches of the trigeminal nerve (CN V), usually in the lower face and jaw.

How is it recognized?
The pain of TN is very sharp and severe. Patients report stabbing, electrical, or burning sensations that occur in brief episodes but that repeat with or without identifiable triggers. A muscle tic is often present as well.

Is massage indicated or contraindicated?
Trigeminal neuralgia is intensely painful, and even very light touch may trigger an attack. It therefore contraindicates massage on the face unless the client specifically guides the therapist into what feels safe and comfortable. Massage elsewhere on the body is appropriate, although clients with TN may prefer not to be face down.

Trigeminal Neuralgia

Definition: What Is It?

Trigeminal neuralgia (TN) is *neuro-algia* ("nerve pain") along one or more of the three branches of Cranial Nerve V, the trigeminal nerve (Figure 4.16) It is also called *tic douloureux*, which is French for *painful spasm* or *unhappy twitch*.

Demographics: Who Gets It?

TN is a relatively rare disorder; it affects about 40,000 people in the United States. Women have it more often than men, with a ratio of about 3 to 2. The average patient is 60 to 70 years old, although it has been documented among all ages. When it occurs in younger people, it is most likely to be a complication of an underlying problem such as MS or a tumor.

Etiology: What Happens?

TN is usually classified as primary or secondary. In either case, the trigeminal nerve is irritated, and the result is brief, repeating episodes of sharp, electrical, burning, or stabbing pain on one side of the face.

Sidebars

These present information that is important but peripheral to the core discussion. Disease histories, some statistics, and specific cancer staging protocols are provided in the sidebars.

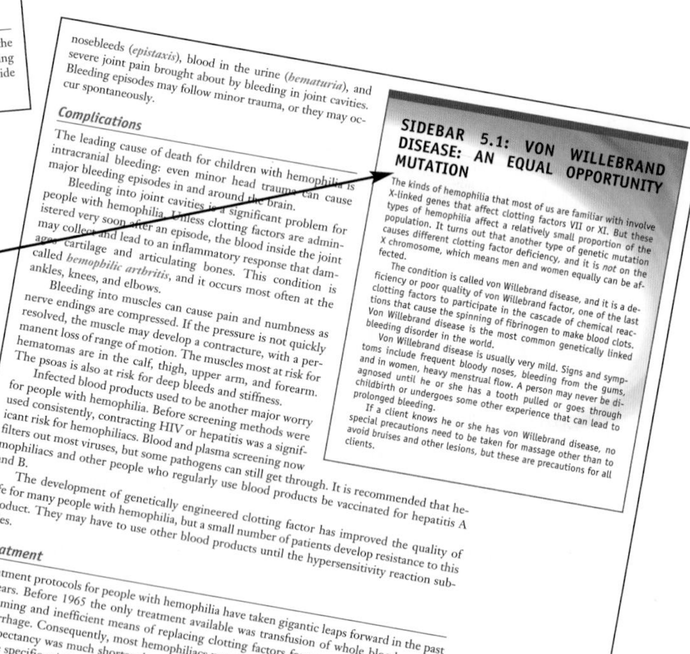

nosebleeds (*epistaxis*), blood in the urine (*hematuria*), and severe joint pain brought about by bleeding in joint cavities. Bleeding episodes may follow minor trauma, or they may occur spontaneously.

Complications

The leading cause of death for children with hemophilia is intracranial bleeding: even minor head trauma can cause major bleeding episodes in and around the brain.

Bleeding into joint cavities is a significant problem for people with hemophilia. Unless clotting factors are administered very soon after an episode, the blood inside the joint may collect and lead to an inflammatory response that damages cartilage and articulating bones. This condition is called *hemophilic arthritis*, and it occurs most often at the ankles, knees, and elbows.

Bleeding into muscles can cause pain and numbness as nerve endings are compressed. If the pressure is not quickly resolved, the muscle may develop a contracture, with a permanent loss of range of motion. The muscles most at risk for hematomas are in the calf, thigh, upper arm, and forearm. The psoas is also at risk for deep bleeds and stiffness.

Infected blood products used to be another major worry for people with hemophilia. Before screening methods were used consistently, contracting HIV or hepatitis was a significant risk for hemophiliacs. Blood and plasma screening now filters out most viruses, but some pathogens can still get through. It is recommended that hemophiliacs and other people who regularly use blood products be vaccinated for hepatitis A and B.

The development of genetically engineered clotting factor has improved the quality of life for many people with hemophilia, but a small number of patients develop resistance to this product. They may have to use other blood products until the hypersensitivity reaction subsides.

Sidebar 5.1: Von Willebrand Disease: An Equal Opportunity Mutation

The kinds of hemophilia that most of us are familiar with involve X-linked genes that affect clotting factors VII or XI. But these types of hemophilia affect a relatively small proportion of the population. It turns out that another type of genetic mutation causes different clotting factor deficiency, and it is *not* on the X chromosome, which means men and women equally can be affected.

The condition is called von Willebrand disease, and it is a deficiency or poor quality of von Willebrand factor, one of the last clotting factors to participate in the cascade of chemical reactions that cause the spinning of fibrinogen to make blood clots. Von Willebrand disease is the most common genetically linked bleeding disorder in the world.

Von Willebrand disease is usually very mild. Signs and symptoms include frequent bloody noses, bleeding from the gums, and in women, heavy menstrual flow. A person may never be diagnosed until he or she has a tooth pulled or goes through childbirth or undergoes some other experience that can lead to prolonged bleeding.

If a client knows he or she has von Willebrand disease, no special precautions need to be taken for massage other than to avoid bruises and other lesions, but these are precautions for all clients.

Treatment

Treatment protocols for people with hemophilia have taken gigantic leaps forward in the past 30 years. Before 1965 the only treatment available was transfusion of whole blood, a time-consuming and inefficient means of replacing clotting factors for someone with an internal hemorrhage. Consequently, most hemophiliacs were in wheelchairs by their teens, and their life expectancy was much shorter than the norm. In 1965 techniques were developed to isolate the specific missing clotting factors, allowing a much more efficient treatment.

More recently, clotting factors have been manufactured in a form that can be stored at home and self-administered. These recombinant factors radically increase a hemophiliac's independence and ability to work and travel.

Synthetic or blood-based clotting factors can be administered after an injury takes place to limit bleeding into a joint or between muscles. They can also be taken prophylactically, before a surgical or dental procedure, for instance, to limit anticipated bleeding.

People with mild hemophilia A can also treat themselves with an injected or inhaled form of the hormone *desmopressin*, which stimulates production of extra clotting factor in response to an injury.

In addition to managing bleeding, people with hemophilia are counseled to exercise (although they must obviously avoid contact sports) and to keep their weight under control; both

SNIGLETS

These give extra tidbits of information about word derivations, the people who first named or documented various diseases, and other fascinating details.

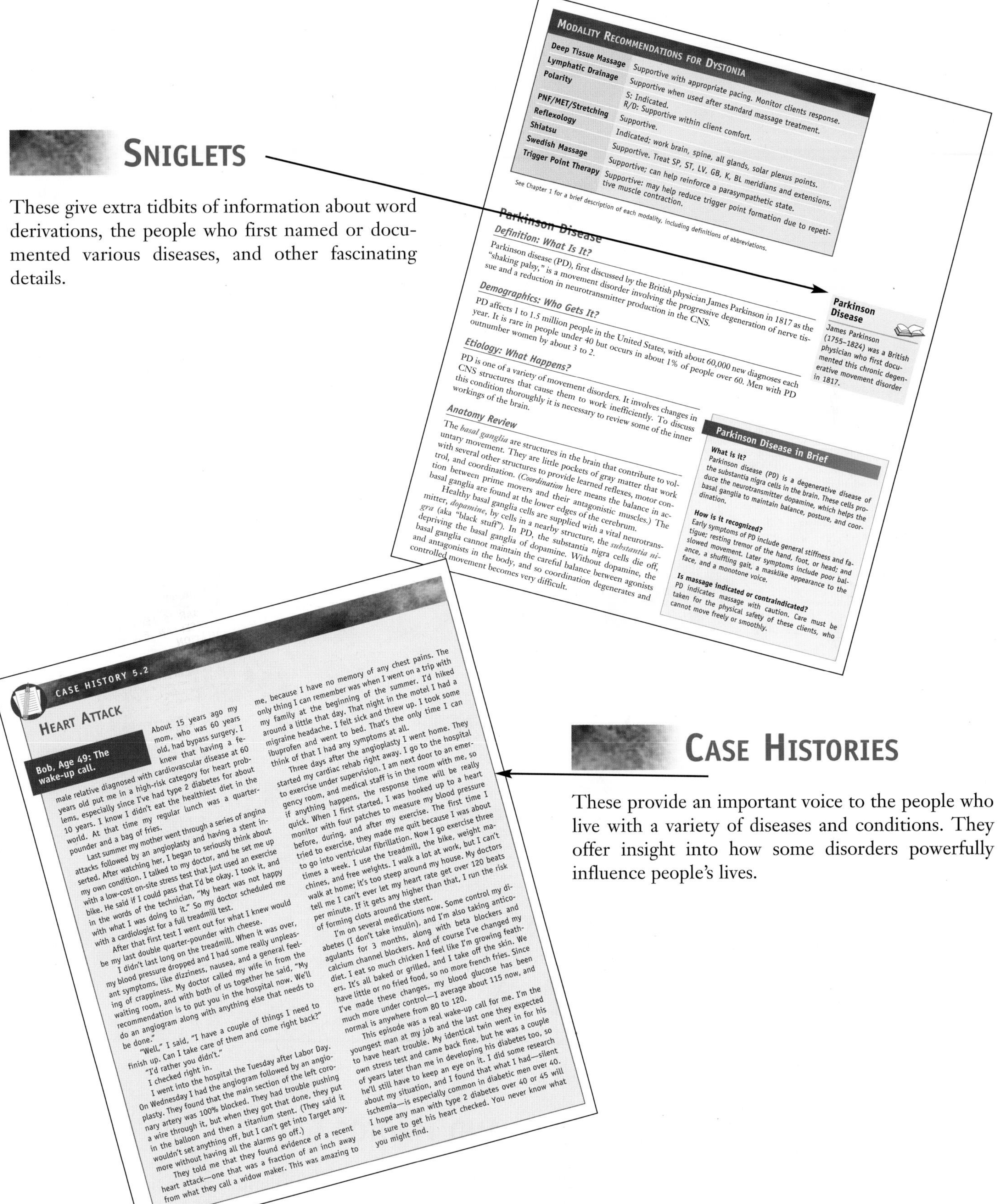

MODALITY RECOMMENDATIONS FOR DYSTONIA

Deep Tissue Massage	Supportive with appropriate pacing. Monitor clients response.
Lymphatic Drainage	Supportive when used after standard massage treatment.
Polarity	S: Indicated. R/D: Supportive within client comfort.
PNF/MET/Stretching	Supportive.
Reflexology	Indicated; work brain, spine, all glands, solar plexus points.
Shiatsu	Supportive. Treat SP, ST, LV, GB, K, BL meridians and extensions.
Swedish Massage	Supportive; can help reinforce a parasympathetic state.
Trigger Point Therapy	Supportive; may help reduce trigger point formation due to repetitive muscle contraction.

See Chapter 1 for a brief description of each modality, including definitions of abbreviations.

Parkinson Disease

Definition: What Is It?

Parkinson disease (PD), first discussed by the British physician James Parkinson in 1817 as the "shaking palsy," is a movement disorder involving the progressive degeneration of nerve tissue and a reduction in neurotransmitter production in the CNS.

Demographics: Who Gets It?

PD affects 1 to 1.5 million people in the United States, with about 60,000 new diagnoses each year. It is rare in people under 40 but occurs in about 1% of people over 60. Men with PD outnumber women by about 3 to 2.

Etiology: What Happens?

PD is one of a variety of movement disorders. It involves changes in CNS structures that cause them to work inefficiently. To discuss this condition thoroughly it is necessary to review some of the inner workings of the brain.

Anatomy Review

The *basal ganglia* are structures in the brain that contribute to voluntary movement. They are little pockets of gray matter that work with several other structures to provide learned reflexes, motor control, and coordination. (*Coordination* here means the balance in action between prime movers and their antagonistic muscles.) The basal ganglia are found at the lower edges of the cerebrum.

Healthy basal ganglia cells are supplied with a vital neurotransmitter, *dopamine*, by cells in a nearby structure, the *substantia nigra* (aka "black stuff"). In PD, the substantia nigra cells die off, depriving the basal ganglia of dopamine. Without dopamine, the basal ganglia cannot maintain the careful balance between agonists and antagonists in the body, and so coordination degenerates and controlled movement becomes very difficult.

Parkinson Disease

James Parkinson (1755–1824) was a British physician who first documented this chronic degenerative movement disorder in 1817.

Parkinson Disease in Brief

What is it?
Parkinson disease (PD) is a degenerative disease of the substantia nigra cells in the brain. These cells produce the neurotransmitter dopamine, which helps the basal ganglia to maintain balance, posture, and coordination.

How is it recognized?
Early symptoms of PD include general stiffness and fatigue; resting tremor of the hand, foot, or head; and slowed movement. Later symptoms include poor balance, a shuffling gait, a masklike appearance to the face, and a monotone voice.

Is massage indicated or contraindicated?
PD indicates massage with caution. Care must be taken for the physical safety of these clients, who cannot move freely or smoothly.

CASE HISTORY 5.2

HEART ATTACK

Bob, Age 49: The wake-up call.

About 15 years ago my mom, who was 60 years old, had bypass surgery. I knew that having a female relative diagnosed with cardiovascular disease at 60 years old put me in a high-risk category for heart problems, especially since I've had type 2 diabetes for about 10 years. I know I didn't eat the healthiest diet in the world. At that time my regular lunch was a quarter-pounder and a bag of fries.

Last summer my mother went through a series of angina attacks followed by an angioplasty and having a stent inserted. After watching her, I began to seriously think about my own condition. I talked to my doctor, and he set me up with a low-cost on-site stress test that just used an exercise bike. He said if I could pass that I'd be okay. I took it, and in the words of the technician, "My heart was not happy with what I was doing to it." So my doctor scheduled me with a cardiologist for a full treadmill test.

After that first test I went out for what I knew would be my last double quarter-pounder with cheese.

I didn't last long on the treadmill. When it was over, my blood pressure dropped and I had some really unpleasant symptoms, like dizziness, nausea, and a general feeling of crappiness. My doctor called my wife in from the waiting room, and with both of us together he said, "My recommendation is to put you in the hospital now. We'll do an angiogram along with anything else that needs to be done."

"Well," I said, "I have a couple of things I need to finish up. Can I take care of them and come right back?"

"I'd rather you didn't."

I checked right in.

I went into the hospital the Tuesday after Labor Day. On Wednesday I had the angiogram followed by an angioplasty. They found that the main section of the left coronary artery was 100% blocked. They had trouble pushing a wire through it, but when they got that done, they put in the balloon and then a titanium stent. (They said it wouldn't set anything off, but I can't get into Target anymore without having all the alarms go off.)

They told me that they found evidence of a recent heart attack—one that was a fraction of an inch away from what they call a widow maker. This was amazing to me, because I have no memory of any chest pains. The only thing I can remember was when I went on a trip with my family at the beginning of the summer. I'd hiked around a little that day. That night in the motel I had a migraine headache. I felt sick and threw up. I took some ibuprofen and went to bed. That's the only time I can think of that I had any symptoms at all.

Three days after the angioplasty I went home. They started my cardiac rehab right away. I go to the hospital to exercise under supervision. I am next door to an emergency room, and medical staff is in the room with me, so if anything happens, the response time will be really quick. When I first started, I was hooked up to a heart monitor with four patches to measure my blood pressure before, during, and after my exercise. The first time I tried to exercise, they made me quit because I was about to go into ventricular fibrillation. Now I go exercise three times a week. I use the treadmill, the bike, weight machines, and free weights. I walk a lot at work, but I can't walk at home; it's too steep around my house. My doctors tell me I can't ever let my heart rate get over 120 beats per minute. If it gets any higher than that, I run the risk of forming clots around the stent.

I'm on several medications now. Some control my diabetes (I don't take insulin), and I'm also taking anticoagulants for 3 months, along with beta blockers and calcium channel blockers. And of course I've changed my diet. I eat so much chicken I feel like I'm growing feathers. It's all baked or grilled, and I take off the skin. We have little or no fried food, so no more french fries. Since I've made these changes, my blood glucose has been much more under control—I average about 115 now, and normal is anywhere from 80 to 120.

This episode was a real wake-up call for me. I'm the youngest man at my job and the last one they expected to have heart trouble. My identical twin went in for his own stress test and came back fine, but he was a couple of years later than me in developing his diabetes too, so he'll still have to keep an eye on it. I did some research about my situation, and I found that what I had—silent ischemia—is especially common in diabetic men over 40. I hope any man with type 2 diabetes over 40 or 45 will be sure to get his heart checked. You never know what you might find.

CASE HISTORIES

These provide an important voice to the people who live with a variety of diseases and conditions. They offer insight into how some disorders powerfully influence people's lives.

Compare and Contrast 7.1:
Is it a Cold? Is it the Flu? Does It Matter?

Colds and flu are both caused by viral attacks on cells in the respiratory tract. They have similar symptoms, and they carry similar cautions about working with clients who have these infections. Still, flu can be much worse than a cold. Flu is more contagious, and it can linger in the body much longer. Therefore, it's useful to have a clear idea of which pathogen a client is battling.

Presentation	Common Cold	Influenza
Duration	Usually less than a week.	Could be 10 days or more.
Fever	Usually low (under 102°F, 38.9°C) and short-term (resolves within 48 hours).	Usually high (over 102°F, 38.9°C) and long-term (may persist for 3 days or more).
	Symptoms strictly in upper respiratory tract.	Possible systemic muscle and joint pain, inflamed lymph nodes, debilitating fatigue.
Location		
Complications	Complications usually involve sinus or ear infection.	Complications affect the lower respiratory tract as bronchitis or pneumonia.
Communicability	Usually spread by hands touching contaminated surfaces. Contagious, but not usually epidemic.	Usually spread by inhalation of airborne virus. Often highly virulent; may infect high proportion of population.
Resolution	Quickly eliminated; when symptoms are over, no longer contagious.	May linger several days after symptoms abate, still communicable.

Some antiviral medications are finding use among flu patients. *Amantadine* can reduce the duration of symptoms of flu caused by a type A virus, but it is associated with central nervous system side effects, including sleeplessness, restlessness, and confusion, especially among elderly patients. A closely related medication, rimantadine, usually has fewer side effects. Neither amantadine nor rimantadine is effective against type B or C virus, and both medications have been seen to allow the mutation of flu virus into more dangerous drug-resistant strains. Further, they must be administered within 2 days of exposure to have any efficacy.

Another class of drugs, called *neuraminidase* inhibitors, includes the name brands Tamiflu and Relenza. These drugs have some advantages in that they tend to cause fewer side effects than amantadine and rimantadine. However, they are expensive and not suitable for use in children. Tamiflu in particular is associated with resistance in avian flu virus.[7,8]

Every year the Food and Drug Administration distributes a vaccine to fight a combination of type A and type B viruses. These vaccines are formulated about 9 months ahead of flu season (November through March). Consequently, the vaccine may or may not be fully effective against the viruses that are circulating when it's administered. Furthermore, because viruses mutate quickly, flu vaccines must be updated every year. Nonetheless, flu vaccines are recommended for high-risk populations to avoid complications and to avoid a new risk: the possible reassortment of avian flu virus with human flu virus (Sidebar 7.2).

Massage?

A person with flu who receives circulatory body... a much more serious infection than otherwise. ... tion has peaked and is on the mend may recove... mind, however. One is that squeezing several d... client feel sick again; he or she should know th... son who is recovering from the flu may still be... pist at risk for getting sick.

Compare and Contrast Boxes

These put key features of closely connected disorders side by side for a point-by-point comparison of similarities and differences.

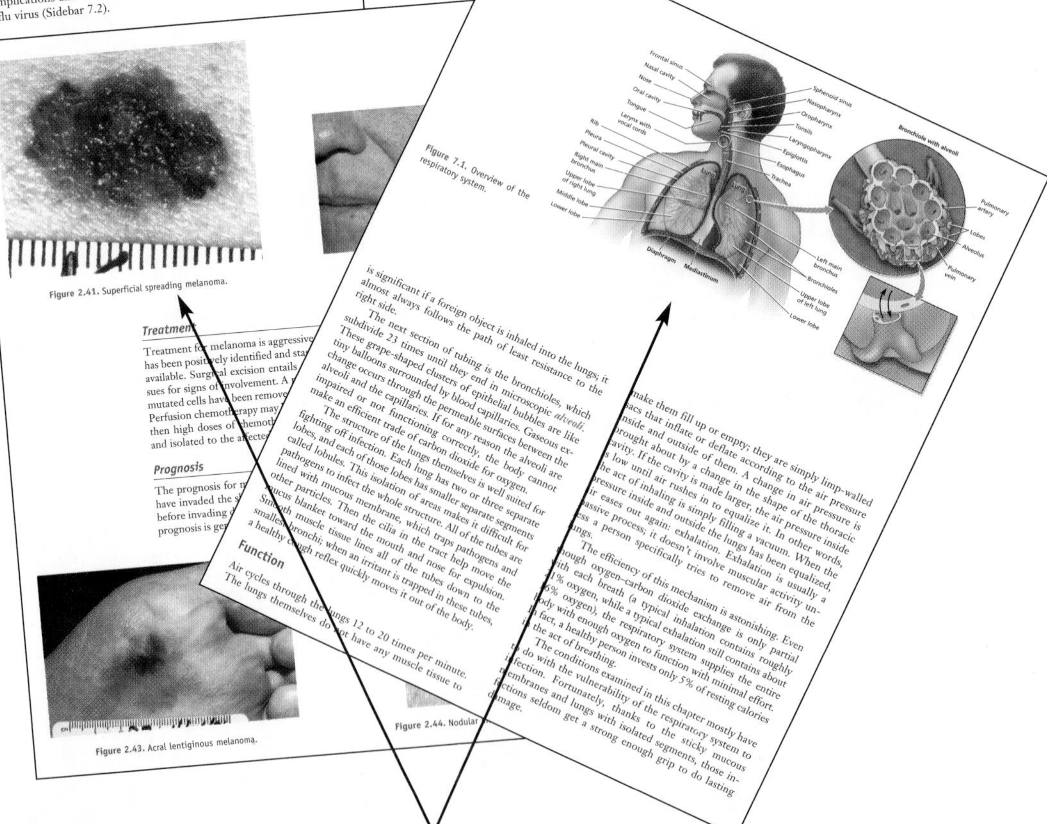

Artwork and Photos

These are rendered in full color throughout the book help to illustrate key points. They provide a valuable resource to help readers recognize a wide range of skin conditions in various stages of severity.

Chapter Review Questions

These require critical thinking skills and the ability to use information to draw conclusions about the safe practice of bodywork in complicated situations. Answers to the Chapter Review questions are provided on the Student Resource CD.

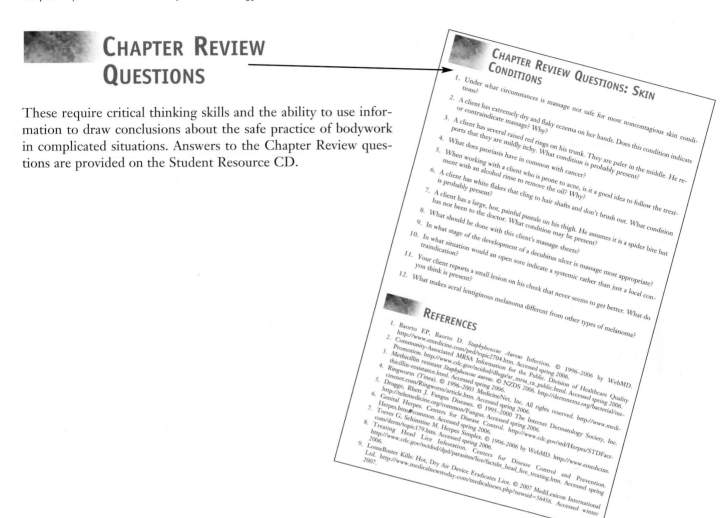

Chapter Review Questions: Skin Conditions

1. Under what circumstances is massage not safe for most noncontagious skin conditions?
2. A client has extremely dry and flaky eczema on her hands. Does this condition indicate or contraindicate massage? Why?
3. A client has several raised red rings on his trunk. They are paler in the middle. He reports that they are mildly itchy. What condition is probably present?
4. What does psoriasis have in common with cancer?
5. When working with a client who is prone to acne, is it a good idea to follow the treatment with an alcohol rinse to remove the oil? Why?
6. A client has white flakes that cling to hair shafts and don't brush out. What condition is probably present?
7. A client has a large, hot, painful pustule on his thigh. He assumes it is a spider bite but has not been to the doctor. What condition may be present?
8. What should be done with this client's massage sheets?
9. In what stage of the development of a decubitus ulcer is massage most appropriate?
10. In what situation would an open sore indicate a systemic rather than just a local contraindication?
11. Your client reports a small lesion on his cheek that never seems to get better. What do you think is present?
12. What makes acral lentiginous melanoma different from other types of melanoma?

References

1. Baorto EP, Baorto D. *Staphylococcus Aureus* Infection. © 1996–2006 by WebMD. http://www.emedicine.com/ped/topic2704.htm. Accessed spring 2006.
2. Community-Associated MRSA Information for the Public. Division of Healthcare Quality Promotion. http://www.cdc.gov/ncidod/dhqp/ar_mrsa_ca_public.html. Accessed spring 2006.
3. Methicillin resistant *Staphylococcus aureus*. © NZDS 2006. http://dermnetnz.org/bacterial/methicillin-resistance.html. Accessed spring 2006.
4. Ringworm (Tinea). © 1996–2003 MedicineNet, Inc. All rights reserved. http://www.medicinenet.com/Ringworm/article.htm. Accessed spring 2006.
5. Drugge, Rhett J. Fungus Diseases. © 1995–2000 The Internet Dermatology Society, Inc. http://telemedicine.org/common/Fungus. Accessed spring 2006.
6. Genital Herpes. Centers for Disease Control. http://www.cdc.gov/std/Herpes/STDFact-Herpes.htm#common. Accessed spring 2006.
7. Torres G, Schinstine M. Herpes Simplex. © 1996-2006 by WebMD. http://www.emedicine.com/derm/topic179.htm. Accessed spring 2006.
8. Treating Head Lice Infestation. Centers for Disease Control and Prevention. http://www.cdc.gov/ncidod/dpd/parasites/lice/factsht_head_lice_treating.htm. Accessed spring 2006.
9. LouseBuster Kills: Hot, Dry Air Device Eradicates Lice. © 2007 MediLexicon International Ltd. http://www.medicalnewstoday.com/medicalnews.php?newsid=56456. Accessed winter 2007.

Appendices

This text has two valuable appendices to take readers deeper into pathology studies; additional appendices are included on the Student Resource CD.

- **Medications and Massage.** Updated for this edition, this appendix addresses the role of bodywork when clients use medications to treat or manage their conditions.
- **Research Literacy.** This new appendix introduces concepts in research literacy so that therapists may become familiar with the skills of reading, interpreting, and possibly even conducting research projects about massage therapy.

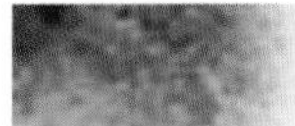

Glossary

A full glossary with pronunciations and definitions is provided in the text.

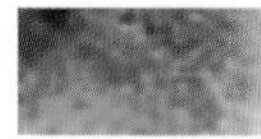

Student Resource CD

This has several features to support students through learning pathology:

- All of the answers to the Chapter Objective and Chapter Review questions
- Additional practice quiz questions and answers, arranged by chapter
- Animations and video clips to demonstrate several anatomical features or disease processes
- An audio pronunciation guide of glossary terms found in *Stedman's Medical Dictionary for the Health Profession and Nursing*

New on the Student Resource CD with this edition:

- **Flash cards** reinforce key concepts from In Brief boxes and Greek and Latin roots and their English equivalents.
- **Games**, including crossword puzzles, hangman, and other activities, help build familiarity with important ideas.
- **Client endangerment sites** are fully illustrated and annotated.
- **Taking a Client History** provides information on how to gather a full picture of each client's health history, with **printable intake forms.**
- **Full bibliography**, including the print and electronic resources used to gather information for the text, are listed here to point the way for further research.

Items in the text that refer to the Student Resource CD-ROM have this icon:

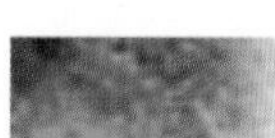

Instructor's Resource CD

Pathology instructors who use this text will get their own ancillary CD, containing the following items:

- **Pathology curriculum guidelines.** This document is based on many years of experience. It provides suggestions for how to customize a pathology course to individual needs, including how to choose content, how to use quizzes and examinations, examples of student projects, and much more.
- **Syllabi.** These suggested syllabi for 40- and 60-hour pathology courses have schedules, grading guidelines, and suggested timing for quizzes and examinations.
- **Lecture notes.** These printable outlines of the text can be used for teaching notes, student handouts, or both. As PowerPoint slides they can project content outlines with images and animations embedded in the appropriate places.
- **Lecture notes in printable form**. These outlines of the text can be used for teaching notes, student handouts, or both.
- **Lecture notes as PowerPoint slides.** These can project content outlines with images, film clips, and animations embedded in the appropriate places.
- **Images.** All of the art from the text is available in an easily downloadable format.
- **Test bank.** More than 1,000 new multiple-choice questions for the new edition have been compiled in a Brownstone test generator. These can be used for quizzes, tests, or homework assignments.

ACKNOWLEDGMENTS

With every edition of *A Massage Therapist's Guide to Pathology* the list of people to whom I am grateful grows. A work of this scope can never be done alone, nor should it be. Reader, you hold in your hand the effort of hundreds who have knowingly or unknowingly contributed to the final product. Here is the short list:

As always, Brian Utting, my first and most influential massage teacher, and Suzanne Carlson, who introduced me to the concept of massage for people who aren't perfectly healthy: Your seeds continue to grow in this project. See what you've started?

Students from all of the schools I have called home (the Brian Utting School of Massage, the Ogden Institute of Massage Therapy, and the Myotherapy College of Utah): Thank you for continually reminding me that to be a good teacher means to be a good listener.

Workshop participants: You have shared your stories and deepened my understanding of how illness and healing live together and how we can enter that dance with respect, grace, and thanksgiving. That richness of experience feeds everything I do, including this text. Thank you.

My friends and colleagues at Lippincott Williams & Wilkins: I am proud to work with a group so clearly dedicated to excellence. A special recognition to Linda Francis, my (no-longer-associate) managing editor: It has been an outstanding pleasure to work with you. Your gentle guidance has helped to materially improve this project. I'm glad we have more work to do together.

Contributors: Eight subject matter experts undertook to offer complicated input in a minimum of space, and they did it with great skill. They are listed individually in the preface. Other contributors include Ravensara Travillian, who wrote the Research Literacy appendix, and Diana Thompson, who generously contributed her client history form to the Student Resource CD. Many people will benefit from your generosity and wisdom. Thank you with all my heart.

Carrie and Robert Bateman: You compiled the material on which this is based; it wouldn't have happened without you. I hope you win many fans with your flash cards and student activities to reinforce key concepts. Both of you made this book and the ancillaries possible with your support, advice, invaluable feedback, and grueling, tedious, mind-numbingly boring labor. I can hardly wait to start on the fifth edition!

Other people have helped me along the way. You know who you are (Tracy, Roger . . .), and I hope you know how grateful I am to each of you.

And of course, to my ever-evolving family:

Curtis (can we go to the beach?)

Nathan ("trauma junkie") and

Lily Anne Rose (Renaissance woman)

You are my heroes. Words fail; love triumphs. All the time, every minute, no matter what.

R. Werner
Winter 2007

What a beautiful gift working with Ruth has been, and what a fun ride. I couldn't have done my part without the help and support of my wonderful husband, Robert. To my beautiful children, thank you for your joy and energy. I wish so much love and peace to my family and friends for supporting me when I wasn't sure how I could manage it all.

I love you all. Thank you.

Carrie Bateman
Winter 2007

Reviewers

Suzie Goggin, BA, CMT, CNMT
Rising Spirit Institute of Natural Health
Conyers, Georgia

Antonella Sena, DC
Academy of Massage Therapy
Hackensack, New Jersey

Heather Cooperstein, BS (Exercise Science)
Kessler Institute for Rehabilitation
Piscataway, New Jersey

Donna Dillon, LMT
Tallahassee, Florida

Paula Keefe, MA, CNMT, NCTMB, LMT
Roane State Community College
Oak Ridge, Tennessee

Micah Soyka Dobush, BS, CPE, RPP
Ashland Institute of Massage and Heartwood Institute
Mount Shasta, California

Lloyd Mills, CMT
Massage Therapy Institute of Colorado
Denver, Colorado

CONTENTS

Chapter 1: **Fundamental Concepts in Pathology** 1

Chapter 2: **Integumentary System Conditions** 23

Chapter 3: **Musculoskeletal System Conditions** 85

Chapter 4: **Nervous System Conditions** 219

Chapter 5: **Circulatory System Conditions** 337

Chapter 6: **Lymph and Immune System Conditions** 403

Chapter 7: **Respiratory System Conditions** 441

Chapter 8: **Digestive System Conditions** 483

Chapter 9: **Endocrine System Conditions** 557

Chapter 10: **Urinary System Conditions** 587

Chapter 11: **Reproductive System Conditions** 607

Chapter 12: **Principles of Cancer** 671

Appendix A: **Medications** 683

Appendix B: **Research Literacy, Research Capacity** 701

Appendix C: **Client Endangerments**

Appendix D: **Taking a Client History**

Appendix E: **Pathologies in Brief**

Full Bibliography

Glossary 711

Illustration Credits 743

Index 749

1

Fundamental Concepts in Pathology

Chapter Objectives

After reading this chapter, you should be able to . . .

- Identify the meaning of the following words based on their word roots: hyperglycemia, diarrhea, cardiomegaly, dermatitis, thrombolysis, arthritis.
- Define *complication* and give an example.
- Name three types of bacteria.
- Name two viruses of particular concern for health care professionals.
- Name three animal parasites.
- Define *antisepsis, disinfection*, and *sterilization*.
- Name three components of inflammation.
- Name two proinflammatory chemicals.
- Name one dangerous outcome for chronic inflammation in the gastrointestinal tract.
- Name the cardinal signs of inflammation.

To undertake the study of diseases and disorders in the context of massage therapy can feel like an overwhelming task to students and practitioners. Some consider that the subject is irrelevant, either because they doubt massage has much impact on the health and disease process or because they plan to work only with healthy clients. Many massage therapists are intimidated by the thought of all the things that can go wrong with the human body. They may find medical writing confusing and obscure or be squeamish about looking at pictures of sick people.

The wonderful thing about studying pathology, though, is the discovery that much of the time, even after a serious illness, *people get better*. The reparative capacity of the human body is awe inspiring, and the study of pathology illuminates that process. And for people who don't recover—for those who live with chronic diseases that can be managed but not eradicated or those whose condition marks the end of life—those people too have much to teach us about living in grace and extracting power, pleasure, and fullness from every moment. It is a deep and important privilege for a massage therapist to be invited into that process.

This chapter lays out some of the starting principles for the study of pathology for massage therapists. Being familiar with key concepts will help the reader integrate and mentally organize the rest of the material in this text. This chapter introduces terminology for pathology discussions and looks at common infectious agents, hygienic practices, and the inflammatory process.

Finally, this chapter introduces a feature new to this edition: the role of selected bodywork modalities in the context of the conditions under discussion. Previous editions of this text have elicited calls for more specific guidelines for what types of bodywork might be most effective in some cases or should be avoided in others. In this edition eight subject matter experts have been called upon to render their opinions about where and when their specialties are appropriate. Descriptions of these modalities appear in the final section of this chapter.

Terminology

Many people who are new to the field of massage are surprised to find that the study of anatomy, physiology, and pathology requires learning a new language. It doesn't take much, but a smattering of Greek and Latin not only can help to demystify anatomical terminology but can even make it fun. Knowing that *vermiform appendix* really means *hanging thing that looks like a worm* can add tremendous satisfaction to learning new ways to describe the body.

Much of medical terminology seems steeped in tradition and a desire to confuse people rather than being a tool to understand and appreciate the glories of the human body. Rules about when to use which word elements can seem frustrating and arbitrary. For instance, it can be difficult to work out when to use *syn-*, *sym-*, *con-*, or *com-*, since they all mean the same thing. Other patterns are easier to track, since they are linked to the presence or absence of vowels. Thus we say ***an***algesic to refer to a painkilling drug but ***amenorrhea*** to refer to the absence of a menstrual cycle, because *a-* and *an-* mean the same thing: without. Fortunately it is not our job to determine which word roots to use; all we have to do is identify their meaning when we find them.

The list in Table 1.1 includes the Greek and Latin fragments that are most useful in the study of pathology. This is not a comprehensive or exhaustive list, and it omits many of the terms that turn up in beginning anatomy courses. It *does* include most of the roots for terms that are used in this book, however. Familiarity with these word fragments will make the study of pathology much simpler and even possibly enjoyable. In addition to Greek and Latin word roots that form the basis for much medical terminology, it is important to define some central ideas. Some terms are used in many pathophysiology discussions, but their meanings are not always consistent. Table 1.2 provides basic definitions for key concepts in this text.

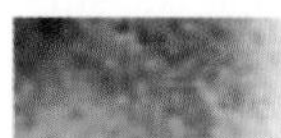

Infectious Agents

A pathogen is any disease-causing organism. The many thousands of pathogens that can threaten human health have been categorized into five basic types: prions, viruses, bacteria, fungi, and animal parasites. These organisms are the causes of many diseases, some of which are communicable. However, any individual's ability to resist pathogenic invasion may be at least partly determined by other factors. That is to say, a person who exercises carefully and eats well, who gets plenty of good sleep, and who has a generally positive attitude toward life is often better equipped to fight off many of the pathogenic threats listed here. A legitimate argument can be made that while viruses cause colds, other factors like nutrition, sleep, and stress may influence immune system activity, which can add to or subtract from a person's ability to resist getting sick.

TABLE 1.1 Greek and Latin Word Parts

Word Parts	Meaning	Example
a-, an-	Without	Malignant melanoma lesions may show as **a**symmetrical discolorations on the skin.
acro-	Extremity	**Acral** lentiginous melanoma usually begins on the fingers or toes.
adeno-	Glandular	**Adeno**carcinoma is cancer that begins in glands.
-algia	Pain	An an**alg**esic is a painkiller.
angio-	Blood or lymph vessels	**Angio**genesis is the production of new blood vessels.
arthr-	Joint	**Arthro**plasty is surgical implantation of an artificial joint, often to treat osteo**arthr**itis.
brady-	Slow	**Brady**cardia means slow heartbeat.
carcin-	Crab (cancer)	A **carcin**ogen is a cancer-triggering agent.
cardio-	Heart	**Cardio**myopathy refers to damaged heart muscle.
cervi-, cervico-	Neck	**Cervi**cal cancer originates in cells found in the neck of the uterus.
-cele	Swelling, hernia	In spina bifida meningo**cele**, the dura mater and arachnoid protrude through an incompletely closed vertebral arch.
cep-, ceph-	Head, brain	En**ceph**alitis refers to inflammation of the brain.
chole	Bile	**Chole**cyst is another term for gallbladder.
com-, con-	With, together	A **con**centric muscle **con**traction brings the bony attachments closer together.
contra-	Against	A coup-**contre**coup head injury occurs when the brain hits the opposite side of the cranium from the direction of the original blow.
cyst	Hollow organ	Chole**cyst**itis is inflammation of the gallbladder.
demo-	People	**Demo**graphics is recorded information about a specific group of people.
derm-	Skin	**Derm**atophytosis is the condition of having plants (in this case fungi) growing on the skin.
dia-	Through	**Dia**betes mellitus means *sweetness flowing through,* referring to excessive production of urine that is high in sugar.
dys-	Difficulty	**Dys**phagia is difficulty with swallowing or eating.
ecto-, -ectomy	Outside, removal	An append**ectomy** is the removal of the appendix.
-emia	Blood	Septic**emia** is a type of infection of the blood.
endo-	Inside	An **endo**scopy is a test to examine the lining of the gastrointestinal tract.
epi-	Upon	An **epi**demic is a contagious disease that affects a lot of people. (Literally this word means *upon the people.*)
erythr-	Red	**Erythr**opoietin is a hormone that stimulates production of red blood cells.
ex-	Out of	**Ex**ophthalmos is a condition in which the eyes bulge out of their usual position.
-gen	Beginning, producing	An aller**gen** is an allergy-producing substance.
glyco-	Relating to sugar	Hypo**glyc**emia is another term for low blood sugar.
-graphy	Recording, writing	Veno**graphy** is a test to measure blood flow through veins.

continued

TABLE 1.1 Greek and Latin Word Parts *continued*

Word Parts	Meaning	Example
hemi-	Half	**Hemi**plegic cerebral palsy affects half of the body.
hemo-	Blood	**Hemo**rrhage means *flowing blood*.
hepat-	Liver	**Hepat**itis is inflammation of the liver.
hydro-	Water	**Hydro**cephalus is a condition involving too much cerebrospinal fluid.
hyper-	Above, too much	**Hyper**uricemia describes having too much uric acid in the blood.
hypo-	Below, too little	**Hypo**tension is another term for low blood pressure.
-itis	Inflammation	Arthr**itis** is inflammation of a joint.
-lepsis	Seizure	Epi**lepsy** is a type of seizure disorder.
leuko-	White	**Leuk**emia is a cancer involving overproduction of white blood cells.
lipo-	Fat	Hyper**lip**idemia describes high levels of fat in the blood.
litho-	Rock	The presence of a kidney stone is nephro**lith**iasis.
-logy	Study	Patho**logy** is the study of disease.
-lysis, -lyso	Destruction	Para**lysis** is the loss of normal function.
mega-	Large	Spleno**mega**ly (enlarged spleen) is a potential complication of mononucleosis.
meno-	Month	**Men**struation is the monthly detachment and expulsion of the uterine lining.
metr-	Mother (uterus)	The endo**metr**ium is the inner lining of the uterus.
micro-	Small	**Micro**graphia (shrinking of handwriting) is a possible symptom of Parkinson disease.
myco-	Fungus	**Myco**sis is any disease caused by a yeast or a fungus.
mye-	Marrow or spinal cord	A **mye**locele is a protrusion of the spinal cord, seen with some types of spina bifida.
myo-	Muscle	Fibro**my**algia is fiber muscle pain.
narco-	Stupor	**Narco**lepsy means *sleep seizure*.
necro-	Death	**Necro**sis is the condition of tissue death.
neo-	New	A **neo**plasm is a *new formation*; it sometimes refers to a cancerous growth.
nephro-	Kidney	**Neph**ritis is the inflammation of a kidney.
neuro-	Nerve	Peripheral **neuro**pathy is a complication of untreated diabetes mellitus.
-oid	Resembles	The sigm**oid** colon looks like an S.
-oma	Tumor	A lip**oma** is a benign fatty tumor.
onco-	Tumor	An **onco**logist is a doctor who specializes in cancer.
orchi-	Testes	**Orch**itis is inflammation of the testicles.
-osis	Pathologic condition	Hyperkyph**osis** is the condition of having an accentuated kyphotic curve.
osteo-	Bone	**Osteo**porosis is the condition of developing porous bones.

continued

TABLE 1.1 Greek and Latin Word Parts *continued*

Word Parts	Meaning	Example
para-	Alongside, near	The **para**spinal muscles run **para**llel to the spine.
peri-	Around	The **peri**cardium wraps around the heart.
phagia-	Eating	Poly**phagia**, or constant hunger, is a symptom of diabetes mellitus.
-philia	Affinity	Hemo**philia** is a blood clotting disorder.
phleb-	Vein	Thrombo**phleb**itis is inflammation of a vein because of a clot.
phyto-	Plants	Dermato**phyto**sis is another term for fungal infection of the skin.
-plasia	Growth	Hyper**plasia** means too much growth.
-plasm, -plasma	Formed	A wart is a type of neo**plasm**.
patho-	Disease state	A **patho**gen is a disease-causing organism.
physio-	Nature	**Physio**logy is the study of normal life functions.
pseudo-	False	**Pseudo**-gout involves different chemical deposits from those seen with acute gouty arthritis.
psych-	The mind, mental	**Psych**ogenic tremor develops in stressful situations.
ren-	Kidney	The ad**ren**al glands are on top of the kidneys.
-rrhagia, -rrhea	Flowing	Rhino**rrhagia** is a runny nose.
rhino-	Nose	A **rhino**plasty is a nose job.
sarco-	Flesh	Kaposi s**arco**ma is a type of cancer.
sclero-	Hardness, scarring	**Sclero**derma is a disease involving the hardening of the skin.
spondy-	Spine	**Spondy**losis is osteoarthritis in the spine.
-stasis	Stagnation, standing still	**Stasis** dermatitis is related to poor circulation.
stoma-	An opening; mouth	**Stoma**titis is the development of inflamed lesions at the corners of the mouth.
syn-, sym-	With	The two pubic bones come together at the **sym**physis pubis.
thrombo-	Clot	Deep vein **thrombo**sis is a risk factor for pulmonary embolism.
therm-	Temperature	Hypo**therm**ia is the state of getting too cold.
-trophy, -trophic	Nutrition, growth	Muscular dys**trophy** is a condition in which muscles degenerate.
vaso-	Blood vessel	Raynaud syndrome involves severe **vaso**spasm in the extremities

Prions

Prions are unique among pathogens: although they are composed of proteins, they contain neither DNA nor RNA. They begin as slightly malformed proteins in neurons that essentially get in the way of normal neuronal activity. For reasons that aren't yet clear, prions cause the infected cells to produce *more* prions (similarly to how viruses work). They spread via contaminated transplant tissue, contaminated surgical instruments, or consumption of infected meat products.

Prions are the causative agents for bovine spongiform encephalopathy (also called mad cow disease) and the human variant of this disorder, Creutzfeldt-Jakob disease (CJD); kuru, a disease that used to be seen among human cannibals; scrapie in sheep; and a few other rare diseases. All prion diseases affect the nervous system, and all are eventually fatal.

TABLE 1.2 Pathology Terms

Term	Definition
Acute	Rapid onset, brief, can be severe
Chronic	Prolonged, long-term, can be low intensity
Complication	A process or event that occurs during the course of a disease that is not an essential part of that disease
Contraindicated	Describing an intervention that may have a negative outcome in a given condition
Demographic	An identified group of people about which information is gathered
Diagnosis	The determination of the nature of a disease, injury, or defect
Endemic	A pattern of disease incidence that is limited to a particular population or area
Epidemic	Widespread outbreak of a contagious disease
Idiopathic	A disease of unknown origin
Incidence	The number of new cases of people falling ill with a specified disease during a specific period within a specific population
Indication	The basis for an intervention that is likely to have a positive outcome in a given condition
Lesion	A pathologic change in tissue
Morbidity	A diseased state; the ratio of sick to well people within a population
Mortality	Death rate from a specific disease
Pandemic	A contagious disease affecting the global population
Prevalence	The number of cases of a disease existing in a given population during a specific period or at a particular moment; the proportion of people affected
Prognosis	Expected outcome of a disease or disorder
Sign	An objectively observable indication of a disease or disorder
Stenosis	A stricture or abnormal narrowing of any canal or orifice
Subacute	Between acute and chronic; a stage in healing or tissue repair
Symptom	A subjective experience relating to a disease or disorder
Syndrome	A collection of signs and symptoms associated with a specific disease process
Systemic	Describing a whole-body contraindication for massage, as opposed to a local contraindication.
Trauma	Any physical or mental injury

Viruses

Viruses are packets of DNA or RNA wrapped in a protein coat. They can't replicate outside of a host; instead, they use the machinery of their target cells to make more viruses. The infected cell eventually releases many copies of the virus, which may invade other nearby cells. Every virus that affects humans has at least one specific target cell type, although some viruses have multiple levels of infectious activity. Poliovirus, for example, first invades cells in the gastrointestinal tract and then migrates to motor neurons in the spinal cord.

Outside of a host many viruses are fragile and disintegrate quickly. Some, however, are extremely stable and can remain infectious for long periods. The most common stable viruses that massage therapists are likely to encounter include herpes simplex, hepatitis B, and hepatitis C. For more information on these infections, see Chapters 2 and 8 respectively.

Bacteria

Bacteria are single-celled microorganisms that can survive outside of a host. Not all bacteria are pathogenic; some are necessary for good health. But others can cause serious illnesses, either by invading healthy tissues or by releasing enzymes or toxins that destroy healthy cells.

Antibiotics are a group of drugs that interfere with bacterial reproduction. Aggressive bacterial infections with a high replication rate often respond to antibiotic therapy better than slow-growing infections. Another feature that helps to determine the virulence of a bacterium is whether it develops a tough waxy coat that protects it from the environment. Coated bacteria, sometimes called spores, can survive for extended periods outside a host. Tuberculosis, tetanus, and anthrax are infections caused by bacteria that form resistant spores.

Bacteria come in several basic forms, although some species show an ability to change their shape depending on environmental factors.

- *Cocci* are spherical bacteria that appear in predictable patterns.
  - *Diplococci* are paired cocci. These bacteria are associated with a type of pneumonia (Figure 1.1).
  - *Staphylococci* clump together in groups that resemble bunches of grapes (Figure 1.2). Staph infections of the skin are usually (but not always) local to a specific area. Some varieties of staph have become resistant to common antibiotics and can be difficult to treat. One example is methicillin-resistant *Staphylococcus aureus*, or MRSA, which is discussed in the section on boils in Chapter 2.
  - *Streptococci* cling together in chains. (Figure 1.3). They tend to cause systemic infections such as strep throat or rheumatic fever. Necrotizing fasciitis, or "flesh-eating bacteria," is often a strep infection, although some other agents have been seen with this as well.
- *Bacilli* are elongated, rod-shaped bacteria. These are the most capable of forming spores.
- *Spirochetes* are spiral bacteria. Technically they are greatly elongated bacilli, with filaments that wind around the cell wall, pulling them into a spiral. Infections caused by spirochetes include syphilis *(Treponema pallidum)* and Lyme disease *(Borrelia burgdorferi)* (Figure 1.4).
- *Mycoplasma* are very tiny bacteria that cause some sexually transmitted infections and a common type of pneumonia.

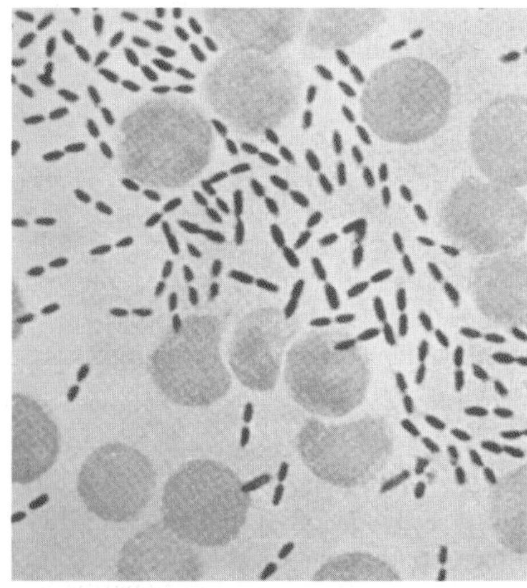

Figure 1.1. Diplococci.

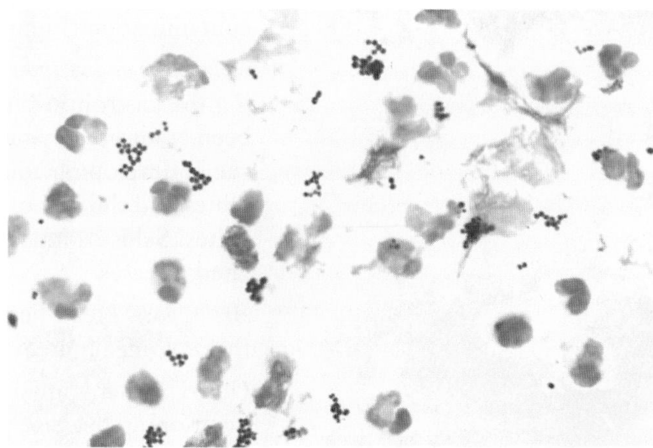

Figure 1.2. Staphylococci.

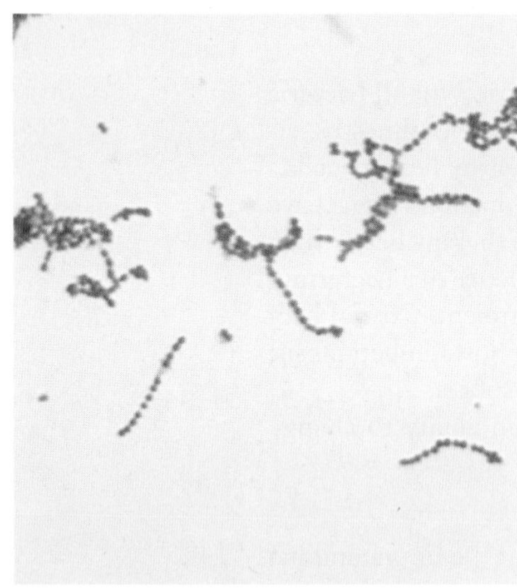

Figure 1.3. Streptococci.

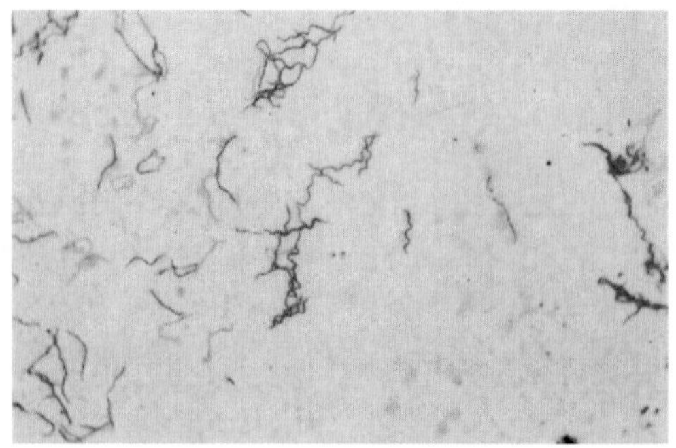

Figure 1.4. Spirochetes.

Fungi

Fungi are a group of organisms that includes both yeasts and molds. Most internal fungal infections are indications of imbalances that allow normal yeasts to replicate uncontrollably; candidiasis is an example. Other fungal infections are usually limited to the skin. Ringworm, athlete's foot, and jock itch are superficial fungal infections.

Animal Parasites

Animal parasites can be unicellular or multicellular. The parasites listed here are animals that live on or in a host rather than those that visit one host after another. Animal parasites are annoying in their own right, but they can also function as vectors for other contagious diseases.

- *Protozoa.* These single-celled organisms cause diseases that include giardiasis, malaria, and amebic dysentery. The protozoan associated with malaria is vector borne through mosquitoes, but giardiasis and amebic dysentery are transmitted through oral-fecal contamination (Figure 1.5).
- *Helminths and roundworms.* Parasitic worms colonize various places in the body, including the gastrointestinal tract, the liver, and the urinary bladder. Most helminths have been eradicated from the United States, but they are still a significant public health issue in developing countries. Roundworms are still common infestations in the United States and the rest of the world, although they tend to be most prevalent in warm climates. Schistosomiasis, which can cause bladder cancer, and trichinosis are worm-related diseases.
- *Arthropods.* Head lice, crab lice, and the mites that cause scabies are animal parasites that colonize human skin. They are all bloodsuckers, discussed in detail in Chapter 2.
- *Others.* Other animal parasites don't necessarily live on or in a host, but they are worth mentioning because they can spread other pathogens through the blood. Mosquitoes (malaria, West Nile virus), ticks (Lyme disease, Rocky Mountain spotted fever), and fleas (bubonic plague) are common disease vectors (Figures 1.6 to 1.8).

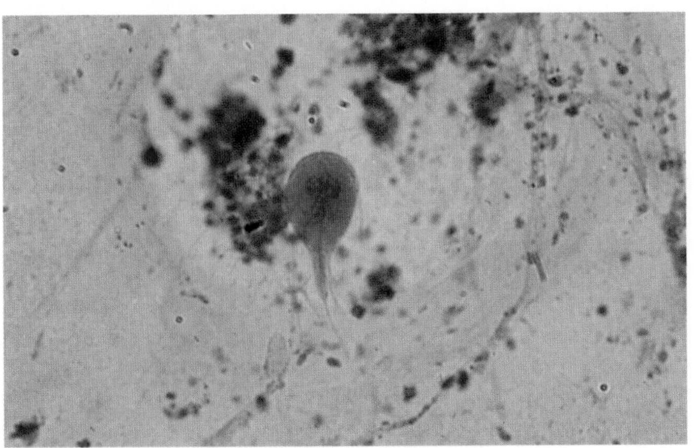

Figure 1.5. Protozoa: vector for *Giardia*.

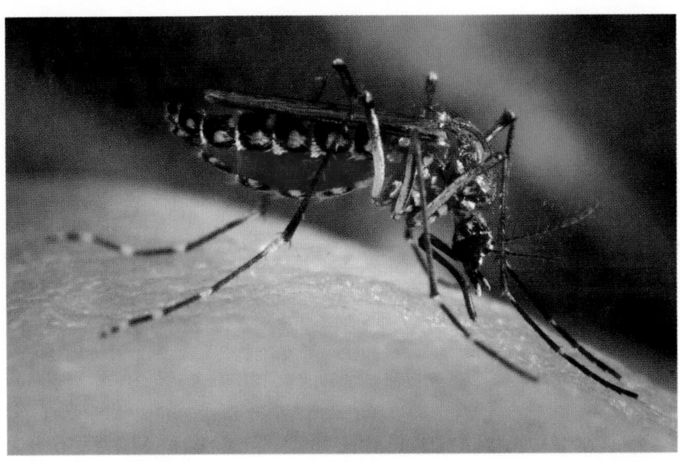

Figure 1.6. Mosquito: vector for West Nile virus.

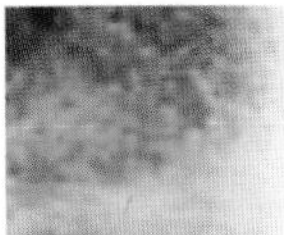

Hygienic Practices for Massage Therapists

Massage therapists work with a physical intimacy unmatched by practically any other health care profession. How many health professionals, outside of nurses, surgeons, dentists, and dental hygienists, spend an hour or more devoting the total of their concentration and focus, as well as their touch, to the well-being of their clients? This kind of prolonged close contact puts both therapists and clients at risk for sharing pathogens.

The hygienic practice guidelines provided here are drawn from recommendations by the Centers for Disease Control and other resources for health care professionals in hospital and dental settings. Individual states may also have specific guidelines for massage therapists. The recommendations suggested here are probably more elaborate than most practicing massage therapists observe. Massage is a quickly growing profession, however, and massage therapists

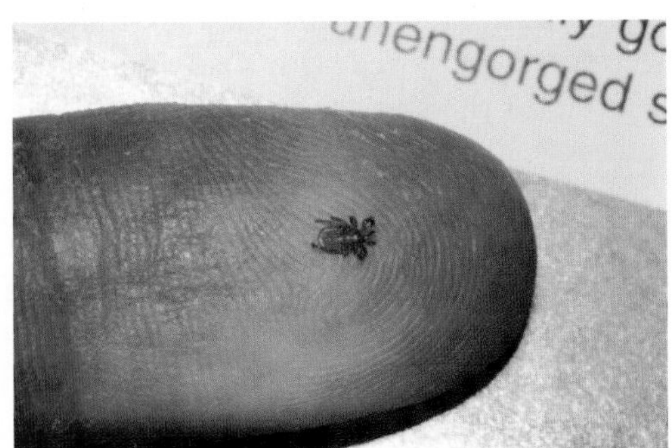

Figure 1.7. Deer tick: vector for Lyme disease.

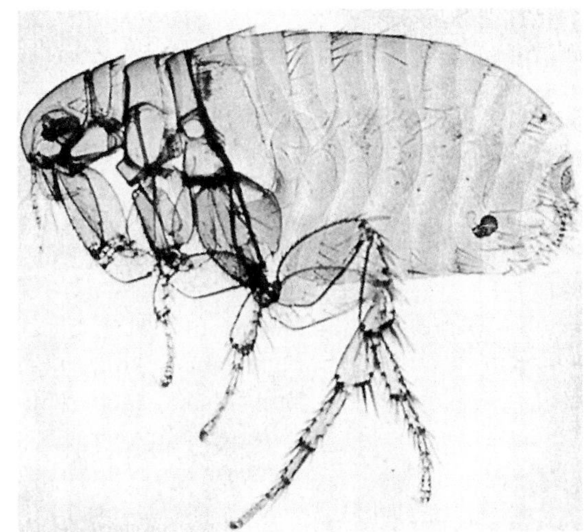

Figure 1.8. Flea: vector for bubonic plague.

are increasingly at risk for professional liability if stringent standards of cleanliness and professionalism are not followed.

Definition of Terms

- *Antisepsis* is prevention of infection by inhibiting the growth of infectious agents.
- *Disinfection* is destruction of pathogenic microorganisms or their toxins by direct exposure to chemical or physical agents. Disinfectants are described as low level (not effective against stable viruses or spores), intermediate level (not effective against spores), and high level (effective against some spores and all other bacteria, fungi, and viruses).
- *Sterilization* is destruction of all microorganisms in a given field. It is accomplished with baking, steam under pressure, or chemicals under pressure.
- *Sanitation* is use of measures designed to promote health and prevent disease; it usually refers to creating a clean environment but does not specify the level of cleanliness.
- *Plain soap* is any detergent that contains no antimicrobial products or only small amounts of antimicrobial products to act as preservatives.
- *Antimicrobial soap* is a detergent that contains antimicrobial substances.
- *Alcohol-based hand rub* contains 60% to 95% alcohol (usually ethanol, isopropanol, or both).
- *Universal and standard precautions* are a set of protocols that were introduced in 1987 to create some uniformity in how medical professionals, especially dentists, should limit contact with body fluids in the working environment. Standard precautions were added to universal precautions to include guidelines on how to avoid all potentially harmful body fluids. The following fluids are specifically mentioned in standard precautions as potentially infectious: semen, vaginal secretions, breast milk, cerebrospinal fluid, synovial fluid, pleural fluid, pericardial fluid, amniotic fluid, blood, blood-tinged saliva, and vomit (emesis). Sweat is described as a noninfectious fluid.[1]

Applications for Massage Therapists

Hand Washing

Healthy skin is composed of several layers of cells that are manufactured deep in the epidermis. As they mature, new cells underneath push older cells toward the surface. By the time they reach the outside of the body, they are no longer living and their cytoplasm has been filled with keratin to create a tough, waterproof covering. A layer of intercellular lipid anchors the epidermis. This lipid layer, with the stratum corneum of the epidermis, forms an impermeable barrier between the inside and the outside of the body.

Various types of bacteria colonize the epidermis. Transient bacteria are found in the superficial layers of the skin; these microbes are easily removed with soap and water or other friction. Resident bacteria colonize deeper layers of the skin, and they are more difficult to remove. Fortunately, they also tend to be less aggressive and less likely to cause serious infections.

Hand washing with soap and water removes new dirt and some transient bacteria, at least temporarily. Depending on the temperature of the water and the nature of the soap, frequent hand washing can also interfere with the function of the lipid layer: hot water and some detergents can reduce intercellular lipids and increase cell proliferation. This can interfere with the uptake of essential fatty acids that help to preserve the impermeability of the skin. In other words, too-frequent hand washing with hot water and harsh soap can actually make the skin *more* vulnerable to infection by compromising the shield.

After extensive research comparing the benefits and risks of frequent hand washing with plain soap and water, antimicrobial soap, and alcohol-based gels, the CDC released findings and recommendations for normal use and for health care workers.[2] It was found that running warm water (not hot water, which raises the risk of skin irritation) plus plain soap for 30 seconds is adequate for most everyday use. This method is also recommended to remove any visible or palpable dirt. It is preferable to dispense soap in liquid form, because bacteria can colonize bar soap.

Alcohol-based gel, used according to manufacturers' directions (which means using the amount prescribed and rubbing until the skin is dry) is often faster and more convenient than washing with soap and water, and it is an effective antibacterial and antiviral mechanism, although it is not effective against spore-forming bacteria. Alcohol-soaked towelettes are *not* recommended because their alcohol concentration isn't high enough to be effective.

Washing hands with water and antimicrobial soap is effective but carries a higher level of risk of negative reactions in the form of allergies or contact dermatitis than does washing with plain soap. Concerns that use of antimicrobial soaps may accelerate the mutation of drug-resistant forms of bacteria have not yet been borne out, but this issue is being carefully watched.

For people whose skin is very sensitive, it is important to choose a soap with no or minimal dyes or perfumes. These substances raise the risk of developing allergic contact dermatitis. In addition, using an emollient that is likewise free of dye or perfume can help support a healthy lipid layer while minimizing the risk of an allergic reaction. One benefit of alcohol gels is a relatively low risk of allergic reactions, although skin drying must be counteracted by the use of moisturizing lotion.

Other Hand Care

In addition to keeping hands clean, massage therapists must be vigilant about the risk of open lesions. Hangnails that peel and fray can become portals of entry for serious infections. Hangnails must be kept short and controlled; a good pair of cuticle scissors and appropriate lotion can help with this.

Any other open lesions on the hands must be covered during a massage. This can be done with a simple bandage, if it is in a place that doesn't come in direct contact with a client and is changed with each session; a liquid bandage (which can be washed with regular hand washing); or a finger cot, a small latex sheath that must be replaced for every session. Fingernails must be kept short, of course, and artificial nails should be avoided. Astonishing assortments of bacteria and fungi have been cultured from under the long fingernails of health care workers.[2] Imagine getting a massage from someone with long nails, knowing what could be growing under there... how relaxing could that be?

Care of Surfaces and Equipment

In a massage therapy office or clinic, it is a good goal to create an environment where nothing that one client touches directly or indirectly is touched by another client before it is cleaned. This means isolating table linens and other fabrics and cleaning massage furniture, massage tools, lubricant and lubricant dispensers, and any other items that might come into use during a session.

Fabrics The fabrics that clients directly contact include linens on the massage table, face cradle covers, bolster and pillow covers, and the therapist's clothing. Any fabric item that a client contacts should be laundered before another client touches it. Similarly, any item that a massage therapist touches during a session with one client should be cleaned or re-covered before it is used again. For instance, even if a knee bolster is inserted under the bottom sheet (i.e., not touching the client), if the therapist puts it there with her oily hands, it is contaminated, so the bolster cover should be cleaned or replaced for the next client.

Therapists have some choices about their own clothing. Some wear aprons that can be changed with every appointment; this is appropriate as long as the client does not directly contact other articles of clothing. It is also possible to own several uniform shirts that can be changed between sessions. Aprons, uniform shirts, and other clothing items can be laundered with linens.

Guidelines for laundering are not universally agreed upon, but here are some important facts:[3]

- Professional laundering services use water that is 160°F or above, with a minimum of 25 minutes of agitation to reduce microbial populations.
- Good antimicrobial effect is found with temperatures between 71°F and 77°F, if the detergent is strong and used according to manufacturers' directions.
- If bleach is added to the wash, it becomes most active at temperatures above 135°F to 145°F. The recommended amount is a ratio of 50 to 150 ppm (parts per million).
- Bleached laundry must be thoroughly rinsed to minimize irritation to users.
- Laundry must not be left damp for any significant length of time.
- All laundry must be dried on high heat. Ironing adds extra antimicrobial action, but this is probably not a practical suggestion for most massage therapists.
- Clean laundry must be packaged to keep it clean until its next use. It could be wrapped in plastic or stored in a closed, freshly disinfected container.

Therapists who use a professional laundry service will probably rent their sheets from the service. This means the therapist has no control over the quality, texture, color, or newness of the linens. Also, all items except sheets must be laundered by the therapist. This includes towels, face cradle covers, bolster covers, pillow cases, and clothing.

Therapists who do their own laundry should be aware that adding bleach will shorten the life of their fabrics, and of course it is impractical for colored sheets or clothing. Washing with strong detergent and drying on high heat are sufficient for most situations, however.

Other fabric items include mattress pads, bolsters, pillows, blankets, and heating pad covers. Any of these should be laundered if a client touched it directly, but if the contact was through some other covering (i.e., a mattress pad that is *always* covered by a sheet), then laundering for every session is unnecessary. The exception to this rule is when there are signs of contamination (i.e., bleeding or other fluid seepage) that may penetrate through the protective layer of fabric.

Other Equipment Massage tables and chairs can be swabbed with disinfectant between clients. This is especially important for face cradles, of course. Therapists may choose which product they prefer, but it should be at least an intermediate-level disinfectant. The CDC recommends a 10% bleach solution for surfaces[3]; this is inexpensive and easily available. It is important to mix fresh solution frequently, however, as bleach solutions lose potency if they are not used promptly. Alcohol is specifically *not* recommended for cleaning surfaces because it evaporates too quickly; it works best with prolonged contact against targeted pathogens.

Massage lubricants must be kept free from the risk of cross-contamination. Lubricants that are solid at room temperature (e.g., beeswax, coconut oil) must be dispensed into individual containers and leftovers discarded so that double-dipping never occurs. Liquid lubricants must be dispensed in bottles that are washed between every session. Bottles should be kept away from possibly contaminated surfaces, such as desktops or the floor.

Hot or cold rocks and crystals may be the only massage tools that lend themselves to full sterilization. Depending on their composition, these may be boiled or baked between uses to ensure removal of all pathogens. Items that are not disposable, such as massage tools, vibrators, and hot and cold packs, must have their contacting surfaces disinfected every time they are used.

The Massage Environment Research indicates that fabrics such as curtains, carpeting, and upholstery are not significant sites of transmission for infectious agents, but they may harbor pet hair or dander that could cause an allergic reaction. For this reason, upholstery and carpets should be vacuumed frequently.[3] Vinyl upholstery can be swabbed with disinfectant. Any carpeting that gets wet can harbor bacteria and fungi; it should be replaced if it isn't completely dry within a few hours. Hard floors can be washed regularly with detergent, but no particular benefit has been found in washing frequently with high-level disinfectants.

Other surfaces that clients and therapists contact should also be cleaned frequently. These include doorknobs, bathroom fixtures, switch plates, telephones, and coat rack or hooks. If a therapist uses a computer, the keyboard may provide a rich growth medium for pathogens. This can be ameliorated with antiseptic-soaked towelettes or keyboard covers that can be washed in the sink. Also, cash is not called filthy lucre for nothing; it is typically handled by numerous dirty hands and is an excellent vector for contamination.

The guidelines suggested here are probably more stringent than those most massage therapists use, and they may seem unnecessarily alarmist. However, as more people seek massage and as new forms of pathogens develop, it becomes increasingly important for massage therapists in any setting to create the most professional and safest environment possible.

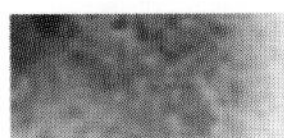

THE INFLAMMATORY PROCESS

What Is Inflammation?

Inflammation is a tissue response to damage or the threat of invasion by *antigens*: bits of non-self. It is typically caused by physical injury (trauma, chemical burn, hypothermia), invasion with foreign bodies (pathogens, splinter, shrapnel), hormonal changes, or autoimmune activity. The inflammatory response is expressed through cellular and vascular functions that are coordinated by chemical mediators.

The purpose of inflammation is to protect the body from pathogenic invasion, to limit the range of contamination, and to prepare damaged tissue for healing. Once an acute inflammatory response has begun, it has only a few possible courses: complete resolution with no significant tissue changes, accumulation of scar tissue, formation of cysts or abscesses, or chronic inflammation.

The Language of Inflammation

Massage therapists are well trained to recognize the basic signs of inflammation: pain, heat, redness, swelling, sometimes loss of function. This litany has a long and venerable history beginning with the earliest practitioners of the healing arts. The traditional names for signs of inflammation come from Latin:

Dolor (pain)
Calor (heat)
Rubor (redness)
Tumor (swelling)
Functio laesa (loss of function)

Components of Inflammation: Vascular Activity

The vascular component of inflammation comes into play when tissue is damaged by trauma or other factors. For the sake of simplicity, consider a basic laceration or puncture wound as a model, although the same principles hold true for any kind of local injury (Figure 1.9). In the first moments, vasoconstriction occurs. This is easily observable on scratching the skin: a white wheal is followed by a red mark within a few seconds. The vasoconstrictive stage is over within moments for a minor injury and several minutes for a more serious one.

Vasodilation is the next step in vascular activity. Damaged endothelial cells and mast cells release a host of chemicals that increase the permeability of blood vessel walls, reinforce capillary dilation, attract platelets, and slow blood flow away from the area, limiting the risk of deeper penetration of pathogens.

Vasodilation is immediate and short-lived with minor injuries, but it may last for several days with more severe injuries. In some situations the vascular reaction to tissue damage is delayed for several hours; this is the case with sunburns, for instance.

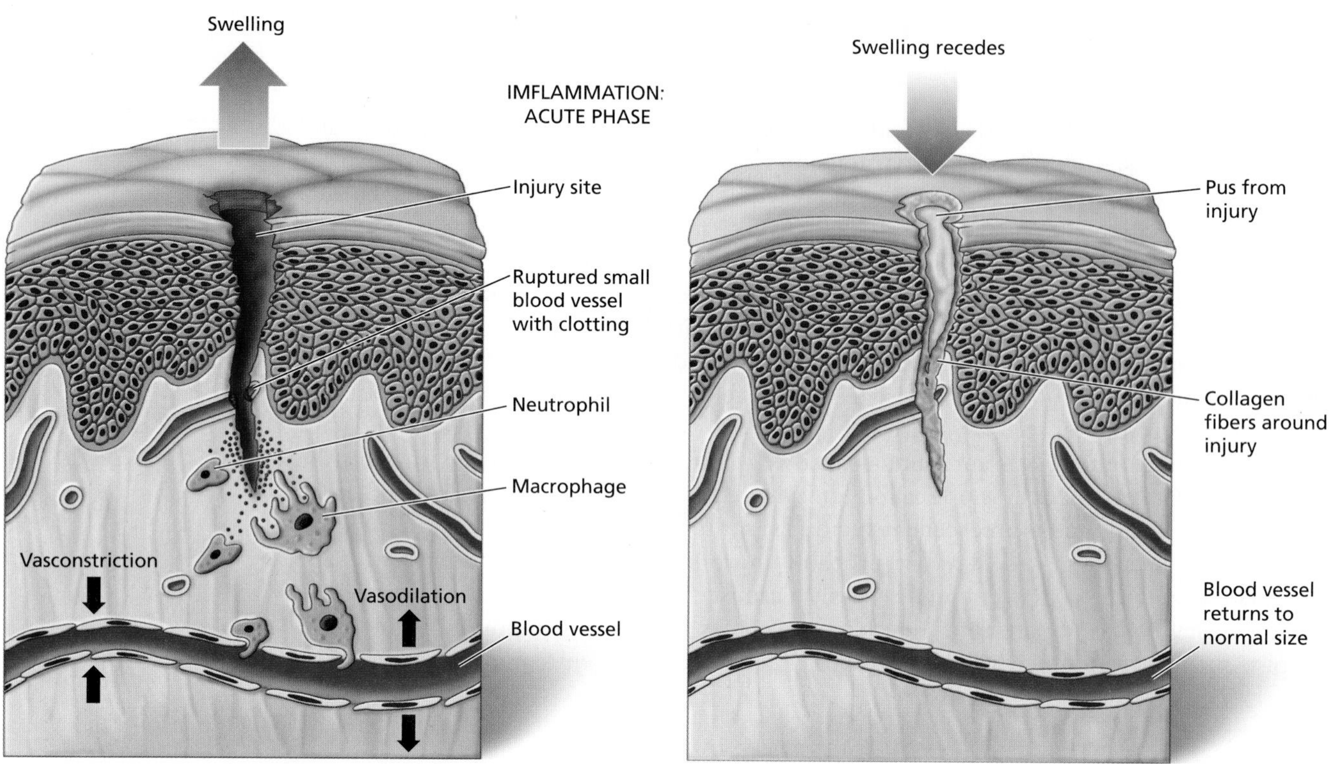

Figure 1.9. Many cellular changes happen with the inflammatory response to protect the body from infection and prepare the area for healing.

Components of Inflammation: Cellular Activity

Many cells are recruited to manage tissue damage and contamination risk with injury:

- *Endothelial cells.* The endothelial cells of damaged blood vessels release chemicals that activate platelets and allow white blood cells to escape their boundaries. These cells are also sensitive to chemical signals to proliferate: in later stages of healing, endothelial cells build capillaries to supply new tissue growth.
- *Platelets.* When platelets are stimulated, they become jagged and sticky, and they release several chemicals that help to create the net of fibrin that catches passing red blood cells to form a blood clot.
- *White blood cells.* Several types of white blood cells participate in the inflammatory process. Which types depends on how long the injury has been present and what types of pathogens are involved.
  - *Granulocytes.* Granulocytes are the smallest, fastest white blood cells. They are called granulocytes because when they are isolated and stained, they appear to have tiny granules in them. Neutrophils are the most common type of granulocyte to be involved in early stages of inflammation. These tiny white blood cells are associated with bacterial infection and musculoskeletal injury. Other granulocytes include eosinophils (associated with allergic reactions and parasites) and basophils (associated with allergies and histamine release).
  - *Mast cells.* Mast cells are found in tissues most vulnerable to damage: skin, the respiratory tract, and gastrointestinal tract. When they are activated, they release histamine and other chemicals that reinforce and prolong the inflammatory response.
  - *Monocytes and macrophages.* Monocytes are large, mobile white blood cells. They are sensitive to chemical signals that call them to sites of injury or potential infection. Monocytes can become permanently fixed macrophages. They are typically in-

volved in later stages of inflammation: they help clean up cellular debris to prepare the area for healing.

  - *Lymphocytes.* Some lymphocytes are involved in the resolution of inflammation. They work with macrophages to clean up dead and damaged cells and to help form scar tissue and new blood vessels.
- *Fibroblasts.* Fibroblasts produce collagen and other components of extracellular matrix. They also respond to chemical signals that call them to the site of injury or invasion. They typically begin by migrating to local blood clots and may proliferate to create more scar tissue if necessary.

Chemical Mediators

All cells involved in inflammation are coordinated by chemical messages that tell them what to do. Some of these chemicals are suspended in plasma (clotting factors, complement, and a group of chemicals called ***kinins*** that increase pain sensation and the permeability of capillaries). Platelets, mast cells, and basophils release histamine and serotonin, which also increase vasodilation and capillary permeability. Injured cell membranes release platelet-activating factors and arachidonic acid metabolites that are used to form prostaglandins and leukotrienes—other inflammatory chemicals. One inflammation indicator that has been drawing attention recently is C-reactive protein. This substance is associated with long-term inflammation, and it has been examined as a possible predictive factor for atherosclerosis and Alzheimer disease.

Stages of Healing

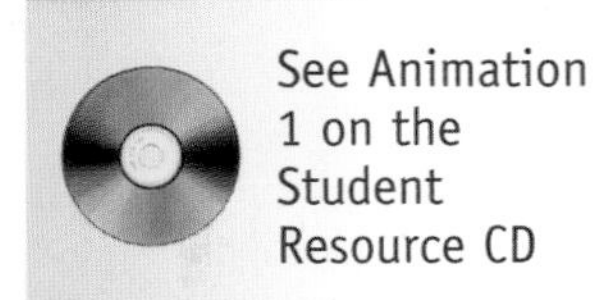

See Animation 1 on the Student Resource CD

The process of healing from injury or infection is extremely complex. It requires the highly coordinated interaction of vascular, cellular, and chemical components to come to a successful resolution. Healing typically happens in three stages.

- *Acute stage.* In this initial inflammatory phase, damaged cells release their chemicals, causing vasoconstriction and dilation, the accumulation of fluid between cells (edema), and the attraction of platelets and fast-moving white blood cells. Tissue exudate begins to form: this can take the shape of the fluid that fills blisters, pus, or other material that indicates immune system activity. Depending on the severity of the injury, the acute stage may last 1 to 3 days or longer.
- *Subacute stage.* Also called the proliferative stage, this is the phase when specific cells accumulate and work to fill in damaged tissue. Endothelial cells grow into new capillaries to supply granulation tissue, the framework for new cells. If the damage affects deeper layers, fibroblasts spin new collagen fibers. At the same time, slower-moving white blood cells are active during this time to clean up dead pathogens and other cellular debris. The subacute stage may last for 2 to 3 weeks, depending on the severity and depth of the injury and the healing capacity of the person who has been injured.
- *Postacute stage.* Also called the maturation stage, this is when new collagen undergoes changes: it is remodeled and reshaped, and it becomes denser and aligns according to force. In other words, if a muscle, tendon, or ligament is injured and accumulates scar tissue, and if that structure is stretched and exercised carefully, those new collagen fibers eventually lie down in alignment with uninjured fibers.

Chronic Inflammation

Occasionally the inflammatory process is not wholly successful. Pathogens or irritants are not removed from the body, the immune system continually attacks some type of tissue, or musculoskeletal structures never fully regain full function. When this happens, the result is called chronic inflammation. This is different from standard inflammation, involving different types of cells and holding a different prognosis.

When chronic inflammation is connected to an infection or an autoimmune process, several things can happen. Pus that is never reabsorbed is surrounded by a cyst: this is an abscess. It carries a risk of rupture and dangerous infection. Persistent signals to fibroblasts can cause a dangerous accumulation of scar tissue. This can interfere with organ function, as seen with cirrhosis of the liver. Scar tissue can also block the digestive tract or other passageways. The body sometimes attempts to build new "exit routes" when tubes are otherwise blocked. When these drain into the skin, they are called *sinuses*; when they connect to other hollow organs they are called *fistulae*. Sinuses and fistulae are possible complications of chronic conditions such as ulcerative colitis, Crohn disease, and others. Sometimes chronic inflammation leads to the formation of granulomas, or clusters of macrophages. Granulomas can stimulate the formation of connective tissue cysts, as in tuberculosis, or damage to other tissues, such as the kidney damage often seen with lupus.

The inflammatory process can also run into problems in musculoskeletal tissues. Under normal circumstances, when a fibrous structure like a muscle, tendon, or ligament is injured, it undergoes a typical inflammatory response: neutrophils arrive to scout the area for potential invaders. Monocytes and fibroblasts follow afterward to clean up the debris and lay down the framework for new collagen fibers. But sometimes the quality of the new collagen is never well established, and the injured structure never satisfactorily heals. While inflammation itself subsides, pain and limitation may continue. This situation, called *tendinosis* when it affects tendons, is discussed further in the section on *tendinopathies* in Chapter 3.

Finally, when inflammation and the formation of scar tissue are overactive with skin injuries, the resulting lesion can be large and difficult to resolve. This situation is called keloid scarring.

Signs and Symptoms

Every massage therapist should know this litany: the symptoms of inflammation are pain, heat, redness, swelling, and sometimes loss of function. In some cases itching, clotting, and pus formation can be added to the list.

The sources of these symptoms are easy to identify. Vasodilation brings about the redness, heat, and swelling by drawing extra blood to a small area. Pain and itching can be the result of several factors: edematous pressure, damaged nerve endings, irritating pathogenic toxins, and inflammatory chemicals that increase pain sensation. If the inflammation limits movement, the injured or invaded area loses function. Clotting and pus formation have already been discussed. Not all of these symptoms are present in all cases of inflammation.

Treatment

The typical treatment for inflammation is no surprise; a wide variety of anti-inflammatory drugs have been developed to interfere with pain perception at various steps along the pathway. Several of these medications are discussed in detail in Appendix A. Regardless of their chemical effect on the body, anti-inflammatories have significant effects on massage decisions, because they may hide the results of overtreatment, raising the risk that massage can cause injury. If a client takes anti-inflammatories for a condition that does *not* contraindicate massage, it is wise to try to do the massage when the drug is at its lowest activity. In this way it is possible to get the most accurate feedback from the client's tissues about the effects of the massage.

Massage?

Acute local infections at very least locally contraindicate circulatory massage. Thickened fascial walls and local edema can help to isolate the invasion to a certain extent, but working anywhere around an acute infection may help pathogens to invade the system further. If the infection is systemic and contagious, as in influenza, most types of bodywork are contraindicated, at least in the acute stage.

Lymph drainage techniques are well suited to control edema and improve the quality of healing when inflammation without infection is present. Any pathogen-related problem, however, should be avoided until the infection has cleared entirely.

Bodywork may be helpful in flushing out debris and improving sluggish and congested circulation in the postacute stages of infection and inflammation.

Modality Recommendations for Inflammation

MODALITY	RECOMMENDATION
Deep tissue massage	May be supportive if not acute and not infectious. Avoid local work when tissue is compromised; work away from the area may be helpful to address compensation patterns.
Lymphatic drainage	Contraindicated while acute; otherwise indicated if no infection is present.
Polarity therapy	S: Indicated. R/D: Locally contraindicated while acute; supportive above and below injury site.
PNF/MET/stretching	Locally contraindicated while acute; otherwise supportive.
Reflexology	Indicated; work lymphatic system, lungs, diaphragm, and heart points.
Shiatsu	Indicated with caution for edematous or pitting areas. Focus on K, SP, TH meridians, all meridians at site of injury.
Swedish massage	Indicated with caution when inflammation is related to injury, not infection or disease.
Trigger point therapy	Locally contraindicated while acute; otherwise supportive.

A brief description of each modality, including definitions of abbreviations, follows.

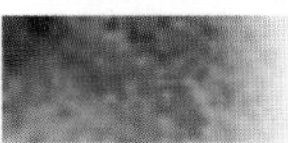

Bodywork Modalities

In this chapter the discussion of inflammation concludes with a modality recommendation table. These tables, which conclude the discussion of every condition in the book, provide opinions from eight subject matter experts about how their specialties apply in various circumstances.

In these charts *contraindicated* means that the modality should be avoided locally or for the whole body: the term for this is *systemically contraindicated. Supportive* means that the modality may have no direct impact on the condition under discussion, but it can certainly support the health and well-being of the person with the condition. And *indicated* means that the modality may temporarily or permanently improve the experience or outcome of the condition.

Please note: *this is not a technique book*! The purpose of these modality recommendations is to provide readers with a launching point from which to develop their own strategies to work with their clients, *not* to provide recipes or protocols for treatment sessions. And as always, nothing in this book is offered as a substitute for professional medical advice.

Finally, the modalities that are represented here have been chosen because they encompass a wide range of classes of bodywork that many readers will be able to identify with. They were *not* selected because the author thinks they are more valid than any others.

Information about the contributing experts can be found in the preface. Their descriptions of the represented modalities follow.

Deep Tissue Massage/Myofascial Release

Connective tissue and fascia play a vital role in the support of the body, since they surround and attach to all structures. Connective tissue invests the muscles (myofascia); thickens to attach muscle to bone (tendon); secures bone to bone as a ligament; and wraps the organs, nerves, tubes, and vessels. Connective tissues even provide structure to each cell in the form of its cytoskeleton. This web forms a supportive continuity for the transfer of tension and stresses throughout the body. When this system is healthy and balanced, the connective tissue can stretch and adapt as a person moves. When trauma, injury, repetitive motion, or more severe pathology occurs, connective tissue can become compromised. This compensation may result in thickening, fibrosity, adhesions, and other structural change to these tissues. When the structure and adaptability change in these tissues, the function of the adjoining tissue, organ, nerve, or vessel can also be altered. When applying deep tissue techniques or myofascial release, it is important to "listen" for the release or melting of the fascia and resist pushing or forcing a change. These are part of refined techniques like structural integration but also are appropriate for the relaxation-based or palliative approaches. Remember that the deeper you work, the more slowly you must proceed and the more you must listen and wait for the softening and release. Especially when working with tissue that is compromised or challenged by pathology, it is crucial to work with pacing that is respectful of the client's needs and tolerance. Listen to the body and support its natural intelligence and wisdom.

Slow, gradual application of pressure and attentive waiting for release require patience, communication with the client, and a sense of safety and trust that is gained through respect and rapport. Slow pressure invites a parasympathetic response, which is the primary goal for most clients with pathology.

—*Jonathan Martine*

Lymphatic Drainage

Lymphatic drainage is a gentle pumping and stimulation of the exquisitely fragile lymphatic system. These manual techniques (not appropriately called massage) are used alone or in combination with wrapping and exercises, depending upon the extent of the therapist's training and the condition being treated.

Used alone to pump the axillary, inguinal, or submandibular lymph nodes followed by gentle, wavelike hand movements on the skin (always in the appropriate direction), lymphatic drainage is used postoperatively to help flush anesthesia from the body and in the early phases of flu and colds to help stimulate and flush the body's defenses. It is also used extensively post plastic surgery and post injury to relieve the body's natural swelling after insult. Used as part of a complicated therapy called complete decongestive therapy and manual lymphatic drainage, special techniques are used and combined with graduated wrapping of upper and lower extremities, a regimen of skin care and exercise, with manual lymphatic drainage playing one part in the overall regimen.

For the average massage therapist, beginning lymphatic techniques can be taught in a weekend workshop.

—*Charlotte Michael Versagi*

Polarity Therapy

This modality was developed by Randolph Stone, DC, DO. Bodywork is one aspect of Stone's holistic system and encompasses caring intention and three levels of touch, the primary principles of motion as Satva, Rajas, and Tamas:

- Soft (S)—soft, gentle, still, balancing, relaxing, and nonreactive (Satva)
- Rocking (R)—directive, stimulating (Rajas)
- Dispersing (D)—heavier and more strongly reactive (Tamas)

Based on the idea that we are fields of pulsating life energy, polarity therapy offers techniques to balance our elemental frequencies of ether, air, fire, water, and earth. Pathology is seen as the manifestation of blocked or restricted energy flow. Through assessment, touch, presence, and creating a safe place for clients to experience feelings, practitioners sense/feel the restrictions *and* the wellness, the free-flowing energy of the body. My experience is that polarity therapy addresses the whole person through bodywork, nutrition, physical exercise, and clarity of mind and is indicated in all aspects of pathology. It also helps to reduce negative side effects, such as those from chemotherapy, surgery, and invasive procedures. Exceptions are acute medical emergencies and/or risk to practitioner, as in active tuberculosis.

The 2006 minimum requirement for certification as a registered polarity practitioner is 675 hours.

—*Carol Ann Lucia*

Reiki

Reiki is a Japanese word for universal life energy and is a gentle laying on of hands that can occur on or off the body. Mikao Usui taught and attuned Reiki masters in Japan, and Hawayo Takata brought Reiki from Japan to the West. Although spiritual in nature, Reiki has no dogma and does not conflict with any religious beliefs. Indications for the use of Reiki are the same as the soft (S) touch in polarity therapy, and the modality is beneficial for all aspects of pathology. Reiki also helps to reduce negative side effects, such as those from chemotherapy, surgery, and invasive procedures. Exceptions are acute medical emergencies and/or risk to practitioner, as in active tuberculosis.

—*Carol Ann Lucia*

Proprioceptive Neuromuscular Facilitation/Muscle Energy Technique/Stretching

PNF (proprioceptive neuromuscular facilitation) stretching, and MET (muscle energy technique) are similar modalities that seek to improve flexibility and range of motion by incorporating an isometric contraction by the client/patient prior to attempting to move farther in the desired direction. The exact protocols for each technique differ in the details, but both are safe to use as long as the isometric contraction and the movements are performed without pain or discomfort.

—*Bob McAtee*

Reflexology

Reflexology is a holistic supportive modality that involves pressure and massage of the reflex points found on the hands, feet, ears, and head. If a reflex area is blocked, the energy (chi/ki) of the corresponding body part becomes stagnant. This also affects nerves, blood, and lymph, decreasing the nutrition and vitality of the body part in question. While many professional reflexologists use deep pressure to treat the reflex zones of the body, gentler, lighter pressure can be equally effective and is definitely more comfortable for the client.

—*Janene Jaynes*

Shiatsu

Shiatsu is a discipline of massage/bodywork from Japan that uses thumbs and/or fingers, palms, forearms, and in some methods, feet to apply pressure along the meridians and points seen on acupuncture charts. Literally translated, *shi* means *finger* and *atsu* means *pressure*. There are several styles of shiatsu, each with its preferred method of applying technique and assessing the energetic meridian structure. The most widely practiced in the United States is Zen shiatsu. For that reason two of the distinguishing features of that system, namely the assessment areas of the *hara* (abdomen) and back and the meridian extensions that are characteristic of Zen shiatsu are included here.

Shiatsu is based on the Asian, rather than the Western, medical model. This means that illnesses and their signs and symptoms may fall into different categories from the ones used here. However, given the information in this text, it is possible to correlate one medicine with

TABLE 1.3 Abbreviations for the Organs and Meridians in the Modality Recommendation Charts in This Text (Shiatsu Row)

Organ/Meridian	Abbreviation
Bladder (urinary)	BL
Conception vessel	CV
Gallbladder	GB
Governing vessel	GV
Heart	H
Kidney	K
Large intestine	LI
Liver	LV
Lung	L
Pericardium	PC
Small intestine	SI
Spleen	SP
Stomach	ST
Triple heater	TH

the other and formulate general treatment strategies based on symptoms. Of course, trained shiatsu practitioners always assess the client's energetic system before treatment. Therefore, they may find it necessary to adjust the recommendations given here according to the unique condition of the client at the time of treatment. The suggestions offered here are meant as guidelines for the general attention and intention of the shiatsu session. However, the entire treatment or treatment plan may well include more or less than what is mentioned.

Some pathologies respond well to a multipronged approach. For instance, just as Western treatment solutions may include drugs along with physical therapy, Asian medicine may recommend herbs along with bodywork. Practitioners of Asian bodywork therapy (ABT) receive their national certification from the National Commission for the Certification of Acupuncture and Oriental Medicine (NCCAOM), which provides certification in Chinese herbology as well. Many topical herbal preparations fall under the ABT certification, but practitioners who hold both certifications qualify to prescribe ingestible herbs as part of their client's treatment plan. Those who do not may find it beneficial to incorporate a qualified practitioner of Chinese herbs in combination with shiatsu for best results. In my opinion, this is true especially with conditions of the integumentary system. Digestive and reproductive system complaints also respond well to this combination.

Abbreviations for the zang/fu (organs) and meridians vary from text to text. The ones used in this text are shown in Table 1.3.

—*Lindy Ferrigno*

Swedish Massage

Per Henrick Ling systematically incorporated *effleurage*, *pétrissage*, *friction*, *tapotement*, and *vibration* into a style he called the Swedish movement cure, or Swedish massage. The intention in this text is to provide guidelines for deciding whether a Swedish massage in its pure form may be indicated or contraindicated for particular conditions.

An educated, experienced massage therapist will know that depending on the client's activity restrictions, we can match *some* of these strokes to those physical limitations for the benefit of each individual. For example, *superficial* gliding (effleurage), when properly applied, may not have a mechanical or secondary effect on circulation and would therefore be appropriate even for someone with circulatory issues. Another example is gentle rocking or vibration, which has no more physical effect than normal respiration, but the nurturing component is unmistakably positive.

Because this takes knowledge, good judgment, and a lot of experience, recommendations given here tend to be conservative. Further, because Swedish massage is a systematic application of the classic five strokes, if the therapist leaves any of them out, technically the procedure no longer constitutes a Swedish massage.

—*Meade Steadman*

Trigger Point Therapy

A trigger point (TrP) is a focal area of hypertonicity, usually found within a muscle. In lay terms, TrPs are called muscle knots. Although research is continuing, it seems fairly certain that a TrP is caused by an insufficient supply of energy (supplied by adenosine triphosphate [ATP] molecules) in the region of the TrP as a result of local ischemia. This local ischemia is usually caused by a sustained contraction of the muscle that houses the TrP. Therefore, a vicious cycle develops in which the muscular TrP causes local ischemia, which perpetuates the TrP.

For decades, manual TrP treatment was termed *ischemic compression* (now called *sustained pressure*). It consisted of holding very deep, often painful, pressure upon the TrP for a sustained period. The premise was that when the pressure was released, blood would be drawn into the area, breaking the cycle. However, if the pathomechanism of a TrP is ischemia, then causing *further* ischemia for a sustained period has little or no rationale. For this reason, ischemic compression, or sustained pressure, has come under criticism. If the benefit is derived from the release after the application of sustained pressure, why not press more gently but more frequently, up to 30 to 60 times a minute? This would result in 30 to 60 releases, causing much more circulation to enter the region of the TrP, which more effectively reduces the ischemia. For this reason, *deep stroking massage* is now the preferred method of TrP treatment.

TrP treatment should be considered when formulating the care plan for any client whose primary complaint is a musculoskeletal condition or who has any pathologic condition that has musculoskeletal sequelae.

—*Joseph (Joe) Muscolino*

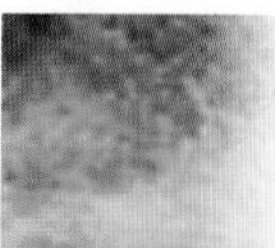

Chapter Review Questions: Fundamental Concepts in Pathology

1. Define the following terms: sign, symptom, syndrome.
2. What is an epidemic?
3. Name five classes of infectious agents.
4. What is the purpose of universal or standard precautions?
5. What are the risks of repeated hand washing with hot water and harsh soap?
6. What is the recommended handwashing protocol if warm running water and soap are not available?
7. What is the purpose of inflammation?
8. What are three possible outcomes for the inflammatory process?
9. Describe what happens during the postacute, or maturation, phase of inflammation.
10. What adjustments must be made if a client takes anti-inflammatory medication shortly before a massage session?

References

1. (Lack of) Universal Precautions. Occupational Safety & Health Administration. http://www.osha.gov/SLTC/etools/hospital/hazards/univprec/univ.html.
2. Guideline for Hand Hygiene in Health-Care Settings. Recommendations of the Healthcare Infection Control Practices Advisory Committee and the HICPAC/SHEA/APIC/IDSA Hand Hygiene Task Force. http://www.cdc.gov/mmwr/preview/mmwrhtml/rr5116a1.htm#top.
3. CDC Guidelines for Environmental Infection Control in Health Care Facilities. Centers for Disease Control and Prevention. http://www.cdc.gov/ncidod/dhqp/gl_environinfection.html.

2

Integumentary System Conditions

Chapter Objectives

After reading this chapter you should be able to . . .

- Explain why broken skin contraindicates massage.
- Name three differences between acne and boils.
- Name three variations on fungal infections of the skin.
- Name what kinds of bacteria are associated with boils.
- Name what kinds of bacteria are associated with cellulitis.
- Name two dangers associated with widespread burns.
- Name three dangers associated with the long-term use of corticosteroid creams.
- Name the ABCDE's of malignant melanoma.
- Name the cardinal sign of skin cancer other than melanoma.
- Name a feature that distinguishes plantar warts from callus.

Introduction: Function and Construction of the Skin

Massage practitioners speak in a language of touch. The messages practitioners give are invitations to a number of different possibilities: to enjoy a state of well-being, to heal and repair what is broken, to reacquaint a client with his or her own body. All this happens through the skin, a medium equipped like no other tissue in the body to take in information and respond to it, largely on a subconscious level. The goal of massage practitioners is to anticipate these reactions and set the stage for them in a way that is most beneficial for their clients.

Functions of the Skin

A student once said that the purpose of skin is to keep our insides from falling out. That's true, but that's not all skin does; its functions are manifold. Among them are several devices to keep the body healthy and safe, all wrapped up in one tidy 18- to 30-lb package.

Protection

The skin keeps pathogens *out* of the body, just by being intact, and it discourages their growth on its surface by secreting the acidic lubricants otherwise needed for keeping hair shafts lubricated. Furthermore, by constantly sloughing off dead cells, it sloughs off potential invaders too.

The skin is the first line of defense against invasion, and the superficial fascia is especially well supplied with immune system cells that are constantly on the lookout for potential sources of infection. These mast cells and other nonspecific white blood cells respond to injury or the threat of invasion quickly. When these defense mechanisms become hyperactive, they can cause certain types of rashes and other skin problems. For more details on hypersensitivity reactions, see the introduction to Chapter 6.

Homeostasis

The skin protects us from fluid loss, a top homeostatic priority, and one of the most dangerous functions to lose when the skin is damaged. The skin is the membrane that connects inner bodies to the outside world. It helps to maintain a constant internal temperature in spite of what's happening outside, because blood supply to the skin far exceeds the need for local nutrition: capillaries will dilate or constrict according to what is needed at the time. The fat in the subcutaneous layer also acts as insulation.

Sensory Envelope

With as many as 19,000 sensory receptors in every square inch of skin, it's obvious that this is the organ (or tissue, or membrane, or system—depending on the source of information) that tells us the most about our environment. Eyes and ears appear to be indispensable, but look how far Helen Keller got with just her skin to take in information. Massage therapists must develop the skill of becoming *conscious* of the subtle information their hands pick up when they touch their clients and must understand that every sensation on a client's skin is also causing ripples of reactions all through the client's body.

Absorption and Excretion

The skin can be recruited as an organ of absorption and excretion, but only under certain circumstances. The skin does not typically absorb topical substances into the bloodstream unless they are administered with a chemical that allows for transcutaneous absorption; this is the mechanism behind nicotine patches and birth control patches.

The skin can excrete metabolic wastes, but it does so only as a last-ditch option. When the liver, colon, or kidneys are so congested that they can't handle any more waste products, sweat can carry noxious chemicals out of the body.

Construction of the Skin

Skin varies from being very thin (on the lips) to remarkably thick (on the heels). It remodels according to stresses put upon it. *Callus* is an example of this phenomenon: extra-thick, extra-hard epidermis on places that really take a beating.

The construction of the skin is important, because it has relevance for how disease occurs and how easily it can spread. Three basic layers of tissue define the skin, and within those layers are more layers (Figure 2.1). The subcutaneous tissue is probably familiar: it is also called superficial fascia. The dermis, or "true skin," is the location of hair shafts, oil and sweat glands, and some nerve endings. The outermost layer of dermis, the basal layer, lies just deep to the epidermis and has the best capillary supply. This is where new skin cells arise. It is also the site of pigment cells (called *melanocytes*), which protect people from harmful ultraviolet (UV) rays. Some of the worst diseases begin here too, for reasons described later in this chapter.

New cells, called keratinocytes, are cloned near the base of the epidermis and migrate toward the top, dying of starvation and becoming waterproof and scaly in the process, which takes about a month. By the time they reach the surface they are long dead and are eventually sloughed off to become the major ingredient of household dust. Bacteria colonize these layers of keratinocytes. Transient bacteria, which tend to be more aggressive, are found in the superficial layers. They are removed with friction and running water but are easily replaced. Resident bacteria, which tend to be less aggressive, colonize deeper layers of the epidermis. They are difficult to get rid of and come back quickly.

Epithelium heals faster than any other type of tissue, which is good because no other tissue is as vulnerable to damage as skin. It would be nice if the central nervous system healed as readily as the skin does, but compare the number of neurological traumas a person is likely to experience with the number of cuts, scrapes, scratches, tears, and punctures he will endure: it makes sense that skin should be equipped to replace itself quickly and easily. Nevertheless, healing quickly has its disadvantages. Cells that have instructions to replicate at the drop of a hat sometimes replicate *without* the hat dropping, which causes trouble.

Rules for Massage

Skin conditions have a special relevance for massage therapists because we are in a position to notice lesions and blemishes that clients often don't know are present. This is why it is especially important to be able to recognize most common skin conditions, at least to recommend that

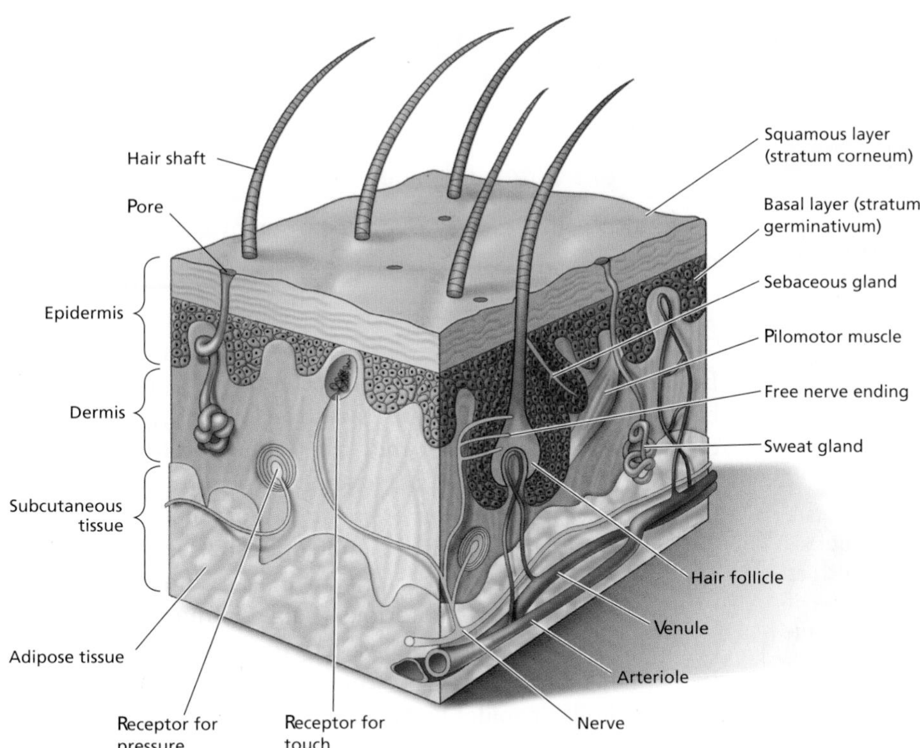

Figure 2.1. Cross-section of the skin.

clients investigate further with their own doctor. Many skin conditions contraindicate massage because they might be contagious. But beyond that danger, the one cardinal rule for skin conditions and massage is this: *if the intactness of the skin has been compromised in any way, the client is a walking invitation to infection.* Open skin, broken skin, scabbed skin, oozing skin, or any skin that allows access to the blood vessels inside is a red flag for massage practitioners.

Many technical terms describe the ways skin can be injured. Here is a list of common skin lesions:

- Lacerations (rips and tears)
- Incisions (cuts)
- Excoriations (scratches)
- Fissures (cracks)
- Papules (firm raised areas, like pimples)
- Vesicles (blisters)
- Pustules (vesicles filled with pus, like whiteheads)
- Punctures (any kind of hole)
- Avulsions (something has been ripped off, like a finger or an ear)
- Abrasions (scrapes)
- Ulcers (sores with dead tissue that don't go through a normal healing process)

Knowing this vocabulary is important, but it is not as important as knowing that hands-on massage is inappropriate for any condition in which skin is not entirely intact.

Integumentary System Conditions

Contagious Skin Disorders

Boils
Cellulitis
Fungal infections
Herpes simplex
Impetigo
Lice and mites
Warts

Noncontagious Inflammatory Skin Disorders

Acne vulgaris
Acne rosacea
Dermatitis, eczema
Hives

Neoplastic Skin Disorders

Psoriasis
Skin cancer

Skin Injuries

Burns
Decubitus ulcers
Scar tissue

Contagious Skin Disorders

Boils in Brief

What are they?
Boils are local bacterial infections of the skin. The causative agent is usually *Staphylococcus aureus.*

How are they recognized?
Boils form painful, hot, red pustules on the skin. They may occur singly, in groups called folliculitis, or in interconnected clusters called carbuncles.

Is massage indicated or contraindicated?
Boils contraindicate massage at least locally, and care should be taken to make sure the infection is not systemic (screen the client for other symptoms, such as swelling, fever, or discomfort other than at the site of the lesion). The bacteria that cause boils can be virulent and communicable. The sheets of a client with boils should be isolated from the rest of the laundry and disinfected.

Boils

Definition: What Are They?

Boils, also called *furuncles,* are local staphylococcal infections of the skin.

Etiology: What Happens?

Boils are staphylococcus (staph) infections. They often occur at sebaceous glands or hair shafts that are clogged by dirt, dead skin cells, or other debris, but they can begin wherever the skin has been compromised by a cut, scrape, or friction. They have much in common with acne, but *S. aureus* is a particularly virulent, aggressive variety (see Compare and Contrast 2.1). Staph A is resistant to temperatures up to 45°C (113°F), salt, and drying.[2]

Staphylococci are notoriously able to mutate to adapt to changing environments. One variety that is demanding attention is methicillin-resistant *S. aureus* (MRSA). These infections can look like boils or spider bites, but they require different antibiotics from those for standard staph infections. MRSA has been identified in about 12% of boils outside of hospital settings.[3] For more information about *S. aureus,* see Sidebar 2.1.

Boils usually occur in areas where hair follicles are numerous, and where friction, in combination with sweat, can irritate or injure skin. They are most common in the axilla or groin, where if they are recurrent they may be referred to as *hidradenitis suppurativa.* A specific type of boil, *pilonidal cysts,* occurs around the buttocks.

Signs and Symptoms

Boils are large and painful infections. They usually occur one at a time (Figure 2.2). A cluster of boils connected by channels under the skin is called a *carbuncle* (Figure 2.3). Tiny infections in many hair shafts close together are called *folliculitis* (Figure 2.4).

A boil typically begins as a hard, painful, red or pinkish bump that develops over a day or two. For the next several days it increases in size, and the center of the abscess fills with pus: bacteria and leukocytes. It may grow to the size of a golf ball during this time. Finally, unless it is surgically drained, the boil spontaneously ruptures and resolves. Large infections that penetrate into deep layers of the skin may leave a permanent scar.

Treatment

Conservative treatment for boils begins with topical antibiotic ointment and hot compresses. If this is not sufficient, a physician may lance and drain the infection. Oral antibiotics are sometimes prescribed, but they tend to be slow acting

SIDEBAR 2.1: *STAPHYLOCOCCUS AUREUS*: A MOVING TARGET

Staphylococcus aureus (named *staphyle,* Greek for grapes, and *aureus* for its yellow color under a microscope) is a group of bacteria known for colonizing human skin and nasal passages. It has two mechanisms to cause damage to humans: active tissue invasion through the building of abscesses and the release of potentially corrosive toxins that can kill skin cells.

Most people have colonies of staphylococcal (staph) bacteria on their skin or in their nasal passages. While these pathogens can be transmitted through person-to-person contact or via contaminated surfaces, they can also be transmitted from one area to another. In other words, if a person wipes his nose and then scratches his scabbed knee, the knee injury could develop a staph infection. Further, once such an infection is established, it is possible for the bacteria to travel through the bloodstream to set up infections elsewhere. Pneumonia, bone and joint infections, heart valve damage, and varieties of toxic shock syndrome are all possible complications of superficial staph infections. These are particular risks for people who are already immunocompromised.

To add more risk to an already risky situation, staphylococci are capable of mutations that make them resistant to antibiotic treatment. *Methicillin-resistant S. aureus* (MRSA) has been recognized in hospital settings since the 1950s and has recently been tracked outside of health care facilities. MRSA is resistant to several antibiotics, including methicillin, penicillin, amoxicillin, and others. It is sensitive to vancomycin, but vancomycin-resistant bacteria have been observed in some settings, and the crossover from MRSA to vancomycin-resistant staph is a distinct possibility.[1] This makes observing hygienic practices even more important for any person who comes in close contact with other people.

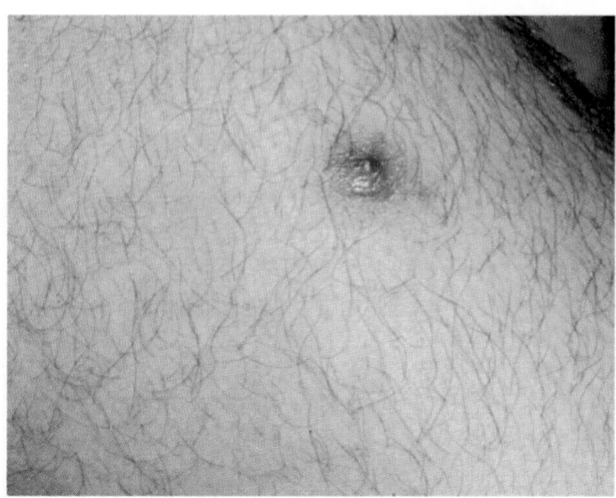

Figure 2.2. Single boil.

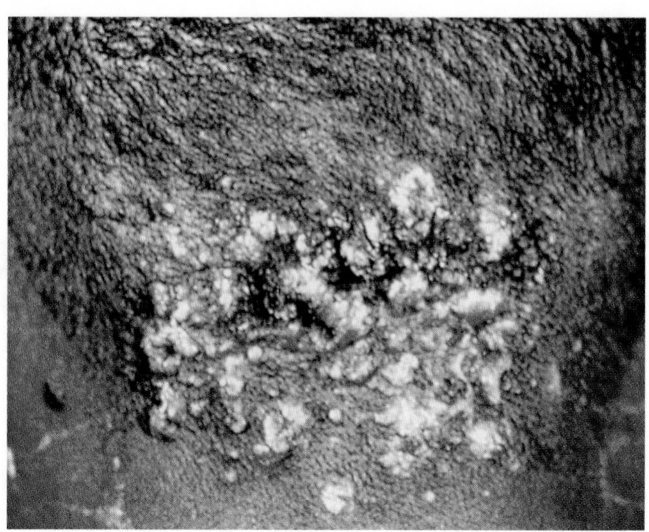

Figure 2.3. A group of interconnected boils is called a carbuncle.

and have the best effect for people who have a recurring problem. If a boil is unresponsive to topical or oral antibiotics, MRSA may be the culprit. A different course of antibiotics is then prescribed.

It is important never to try to squeeze or pop a boil. It could force the infection deeper into tissues or spread the bacteria over the surface of the skin. Boils also carry a risk of complications brought about by invasion of other parts of the body, including the lungs, heart, kidneys, bones, joints, and gastrointestinal tract.

Prevention

The increasing appearance of antibiotic-resistant bacteria outside of hospitals means that people need to be especially careful to limit their risk of developing boils or other skin infections. Consistent hand washing is the first level of defense, along with being careful to cover any open lesions on the skin. It is also recommended that people *not* share personal items like towels or razors to prevent the spread of bacteria.

Massage?

A boil is a superficial infection with virulent, hardy bacteria that can spread deeper into the body or from one person to another. A client who has a boil with no signs of systemic infec-

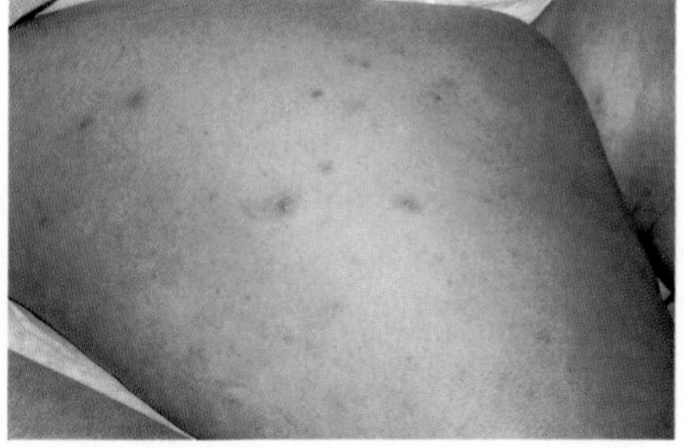

Figure 2.4. Folliculitis: boils in multiple hair shafts.

tion may receive massage, but not on or near the lesion. If signs of systemic infection (fever, swelling at nearby lymph nodes, discomfort anywhere other than the site of the boil) are present, it is necessary to reschedule the massage.

The sheets of a client with a boil must have special treatment: isolate them and wash them at high temperature with extra bleach to ensure that any bacteria are eradicated.

Modality Recommendations for Boils

MODALITY	RECOMMENDATION
Deep tissue massage	Locally contraindicated; otherwise supportive.
Lymphatic drainage	Systemically contraindicated.
Polarity therapy	S: Indicated within client comfort; work off site of infection. R/D: Locally contraindicated while acute.
PNF/MET/stretching	Locally contraindicated while acute; otherwise supportive.
Reflexology	Locally contraindicated; work intestine, liver, kidney points.
Shiatsu	Locally contraindicated when contagious or acute; otherwise supportive, especially with Chinese herbs. Use L/LI for skin, K/SP/TH for immune function.
Swedish massage	Locally contraindicated unless systemic symptoms are present.
Trigger point therapy	Locally contraindicated while acute; otherwise supportive.

See Chapter 1 for a brief description of each modality, including definitions of abbreviations.

Cellulitis

Definition: What Is It?

Cellulitis is a streptococcal infection of the cells in the skin. It usually involves one of the group A class of bacteria, which are also causative factors for strep throat, impetigo, toxic shock syndrome, and necrotizing fasciitis ("flesh-eating bacteria"). One variety of cellulitis, called *erysipelas,* is also known as St. Anthony's fire.

Cellulitis in Brief

Pronunciation: sel-yu-LY-tis

What is it?
Cellulitis is a bacterial infection leading to painful inflammation of the skin. The infectious agent is usually one of the group A streptococci. Cellulitis usually occurs on the lower leg.

How is it recognized?
Cellulitis is marked by redness and tenderness at the initial site of infection, along with fever, headache, malaise, and other signs of systemic infection.

Is massage indicated or contraindicated?
Cellulitis is a bacterial infection that can invade both the lymph and circulatory systems. Cellulitis systemically contraindicates hands-on bodywork until the infection has completely passed.

Etiology: What Happens?

It is virtually impossible to remove all of the bacteria from a living person's skin; colonies of organisms are always growing on our surface. Bacteria colonize both superficial and deep layers of the epidermis. Pathogens may be dislodged temporarily with washing, but they are quickly replaced. When they get *inside* the skin through some breach in the defenses, the enzymes they produce break down healthy cells. In this way a local infection may become systemic quickly, involving first the lymphatic and then the circulatory systems.

Streptococcal bacteria must gain access to the body through some portal of entry. In many cases it can be difficult to identify exactly where the bacteria got in, but sometimes the infection can be traced to a specific cut or scratch, athlete's foot (see the section on ringworm, later in the chapter), an insect bite, surgery, or some other skin injury.

Signs and Symptoms

Sometimes signs of systemic infection precede an obvious skin infection with cellulitis, but it often begins with a tender, red, swollen area (Figure 2.5). The wound soon shows signs of infection, which may include red streaks running toward the nearest set of lymph nodes. This is also a sign of lymphangitis. If the infection starts on the face, a raised, hot, tender, red area may spread across the bridge of the nose. One hallmark of erysipelas, a subtype of cellulitis, is a sharp margin between involved and uninvolved skin; the red edges are usually very clear (Figure 2.6). Other forms of cellulitis have less distinct borders.

When the infection has thoroughly engaged the lymph system, symptoms include fever, chills, and systemic discomfort. Facial infections are particularly dangerous because of the risk of intracranial spreading through lymphatic capillaries. If cellulitis is left untreated, the bacteria may get past the lymph system and enter the circulatory system, leading quickly and perhaps fatally to septicemia, or blood poisoning.

Treatment

Most of the bacteria associated with cellulitis are sensitive to antibiotics. If the infection is well contained, oral antibiotics are generally recommended. If the infection has penetrated to the lymph or circulatory system, aggressive treatment with intravenous antibiotics is probably called for.

Massage?

Here is a condition involving skin damage, a highly contagious bacterial infection, and the risk of blood poisoning if the infection should spread into the circulatory system. Cellulitis systemically contraindicates massage until all signs of infection have passed.

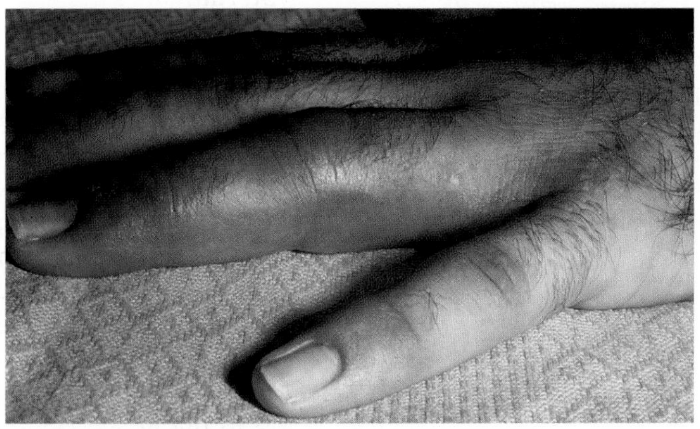

Figure 2.5. Cellulitis: a streptococcal infection of the skin.

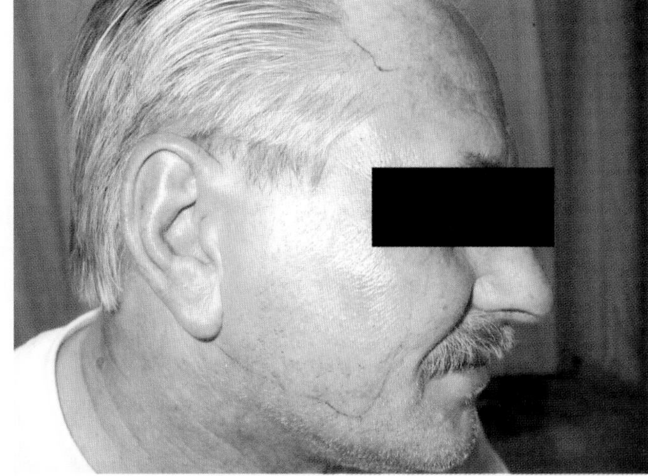

Figure 2.6. Erysipelas: note the clear delineation between involved and uninvolved skin.

Modality Recommendations for Cellulitis

MODALITY	RECOMMENDATION
Deep tissue massage	Systemically contraindicated.
Lymphatic drainage	Systemically contraindicated during whole course of condition.
Polarity therapy	S: Indicated within client comfort; work off site of infection. R/D: Contraindicated until infection is resolved.
PNF/MET/stretching	Contraindicated while acute; otherwise supportive.
Reflexology	Contraindicated while acute; later work lymphatic system points.
Shiatsu	Locally contraindicated when contagious or acute; otherwise supportive, especially with Chinese herbs. Use L/LI for skin, K/SP/TH for immune function.
Swedish massage	Systemically contraindicated until infection has resolved.
Trigger point therapy	Locally contraindicated while acute; otherwise supportive.

See Chapter 1 for a brief description of each modality, including definitions of abbreviations.

Fungal Infections in Brief

What are they?
Fungal infections of human skin, also called *mycoses,* are caused by fungi called *dermatophytes.* The characteristic lesions caused by dermatophytes are called *tinea.* Several types of dermatophytes cause tinea in different areas; they are typically named by location.

How is it recognized?
Most tinea lesions begin as one reddened circular itchy patch. Scratching the lesions spreads the fungi to other parts of the body. As the lesions grow, they tend to clear in the middle and keep a red ring around the edges. Athlete's foot, another type of mycosis, produces oozing blisters and cracking between the toes. Fungal infections of toenails or fingernails produce thickened, pitted, discolored nails that may detach.

Is massage indicated or contraindicated?
Fungal infections locally contraindicate massage in all stages. If the affected areas are very limited, such as only the feet or only one or two small, covered lesions on the body, massage may be administered elsewhere. If a large area is affected, and especially if the infection is acute (i.e., not yet responding to treatment) then it systemically contraindicates massage.

Fungal Infections

Definition: What Is It?

The nomenclature for the range of superficial fungal infections is dizzying. Fungal infections of human skin, also called *mycoses*, can be caused by several different types of fungi (*dermatophytes*). *Dermatophytosis*, then, is another term for *mycosis*. The lesions the infections create are called *tinea*. And to top it all off, the generic term *ringworm*, although it is misleading because there are no worms, is frequently used to refer to several types of tinea.

Etiology: What Happens?

Dermatophytes live on dead skin cells. They thrive in warm, moist places like skin folds between toes or around the groin. They tend to infect people with depressed or sluggish immune systems. Fungal infections are transmitted via touch: either skin to skin or skin to anything that has some fungus on it, like massage sheets, locker room benches, or the family hairbrush. Dogs and cats can also transmit fungal infections to humans. It takes anywhere from 4 to 14 days for lesions to appear, and during that time the carrier is infectious, which makes this condition very hard to control.

Several types of dermatophytes may create tinea lesions. Most cases of ringworm are related to colonies of *Trichophyton*, *Epidermophyton*, or *Microsporum* fungi.

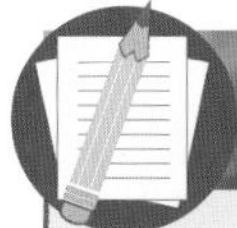

CASE HISTORY 2.1

Ringworm, Delores G

Delores G: "It wasn't until I remembered petting the kittens that I realized where they came from."

In June 1994, I was working hard in massage school. I was living in a house where some stray kittens were close by. I wanted to pet them, so I brought them some food. They came out, and I got to pet them while they were eating.

I was sitting down next to them with my knees up. I had shorts on. I was petting them with my left hand, and then I held my legs with the same hand when I was done. I also folded my arms, so my left hand touched my right biceps.

About 9 days later there were specific round red spots, the size of a half-dollar, on my left calf, and then on my right arm. It wasn't until I remembered petting the kittens that I realized where they came from. About a week after the spots appeared, they started really burning and keeping me awake.

Having ringworm was awful. It turns out that I had massaged only two people between being exposed and being diagnosed, so it didn't spread through the class, but I had to wait until I was cleared up before I could work again. I sat out of practices, which was really depressing, *plus* it was spreading all over me, from my right arm to my right breast, and on my other calf.

I treated it by showering and then putting tea tree oil and antifungal vaginal cream all over me. I did that for 2 or 3 weeks before it started clearing up. I was all cleared up in about 4 weeks. I waited an extra week just to be sure, so I missed a total of 3 weeks of massage.

When I got ringworm I was extremely run down from school, which probably made me susceptible. My teacher said it was interesting that my body chose ringworm as the thing that would slow me down, but it worked!

Signs and Symptoms

Tinea infections vary considerably depending on the causative agent and where they appear. Several varieties of tinea affect humans; here are descriptions of the most common ones.

- *Tinea corporis,* or *body ringworm,* is relatively common and very contagious, so it deserves special attention. It generally begins as one small round, red, scaly, itchy patch of skin on the trunk. Scratching spreads the fungus to other parts of the body, and so other lesions appear. They heal from the center first, and they soon take on the appearance of red circles or rings with a scaly edge that may gradually increase in size as the fungus spreads out for new food sources (Figure 2.7). The causative agent for tinea corporis is usually some variety of *Trichophyton.*

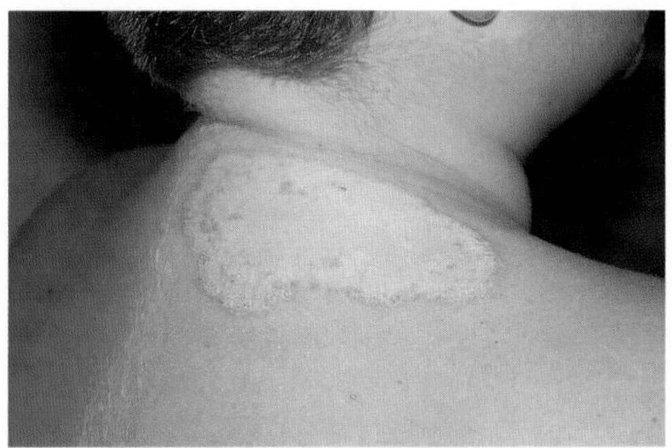

Figure 2.7. Tinea corporis: body ringworm.

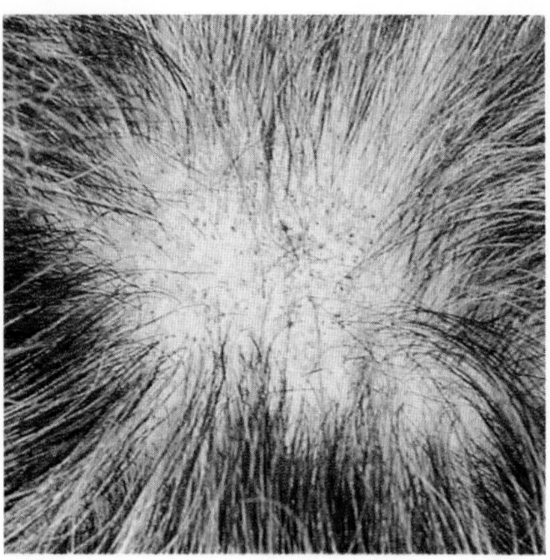

Figure 2.8. Tinea capitis: head ringworm.

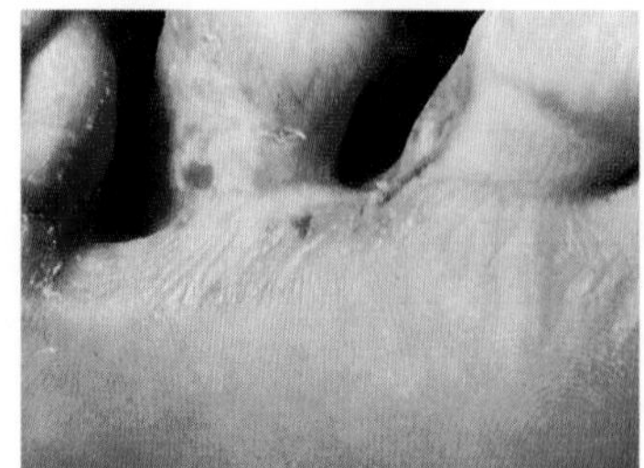

Figure 2.9. Tinea pedis: athlete's foot.

Tinea corporis looks like nummular eczema. It is important to know the source of the rash because treatment options are very different, and while ringworm is communicable, eczema is not.

- *Tinea capitis*, or *head ringworm*, inhabits the scalp. Lesions here result in itchiness and flaking (like bad dandruff), and if scratching and secondary infection result in scar tissue, temporary or permanent hair loss may occur (Figure 2.8). This variety, most common in children, is highly contagious. *Trichophyton tonsurans* is a common agent in this condition, but if it is a *Microsporum* or *Epidermophyton* infection, the fungi fluoresce under black light: this is a common diagnostic tool.
- *Tinea pedis*, or *athlete's foot*, is caused by *Trichophyton mentagrophytes* when it occurs between the toes. It usually starts between the third and fourth digits (Figure 2.9). This condition is the most common and the most stubborn of all fungal infections.[4] It burns and itches, and it carries the additional complication of weeping blisters, cracking, peeling skin, and the possibility of infection; athlete's foot can even lead to a potentially dangerous infection, like lymphangitis or cellulitis. One variety of athlete's foot fungus presents as dry, scaly, itchy lesions on the heel and sole of the foot. This is called a moccasin distribution, and the causative agent is usually *Trichophyton rubrum*. (Figure 2.10)

  People with athlete's foot who handle their feet frequently are at risk for a secondary infection of the hand called *tinea manus*. Fungi on the foot or hand can become established under the nailbed, in which case it is called *tinea unguium*, or *onychomycosis*. Infections here are difficult to treat and may require a long course of oral antifungal medication.

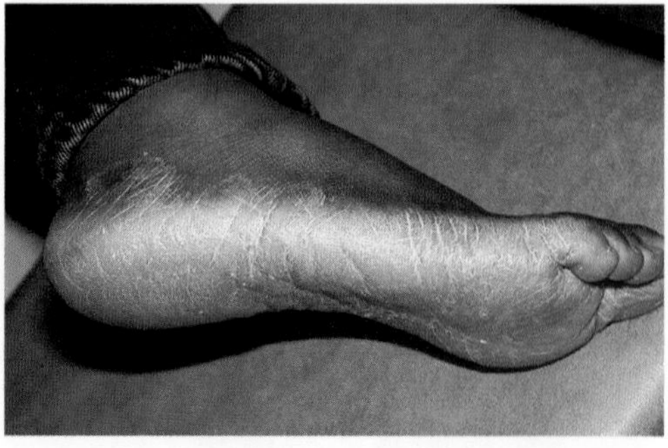

Figure 2.10. Tinea pedis: moccasin distribution.

- ***Tinea cruris***, or *jock itch*, doesn't stay exclusively in the groin. It can also be found on the upper thigh and buttocks, and the client may have lesions and be unaware of them, but massage therapists must avoid them carefully (Figure 2.11). Some controversy exists over the relationship between tinea cruris and candidiasis, a yeast infection of the gastrointestinal tract. Some resources suggest that when jock itch involves the scrotum as well as skin around the groin, it is likely to be an external manifestation of an internal yeast imbalance. When the scrotum is spared, the causative agent is more likely to be a type of *Trichophyton*, *Epidermophyton*, or *Microsporum*.[5]
- **Other varieties of tinea** include ***tinea barbae***, and ***tinea versicolor***. Tinea barbae affects the bearded area of the face; it closely resembles bacterial folliculitis, a variety of boils. Tinea versicolor is a condition frequently picked up from the sand on Caribbean beaches. It creates variegated pigmentation on the skin.

Treatment

Treating fungal infections can be frustrating. Dermatophytes can be resistant to standard fungicides, and when they grow under toenails or fingernails, they can be difficult to reach. Topical applications of fungicidal cream or powder is the normal treatment, but oral medications are recommended for stubborn or hard-to-reach infections.

Athlete's foot thrives in the growth medium provided by closed shoes. If a person has athlete's foot, it is especially important to make sure his feet and shoes are always as dry as possible, since these fungi thrive in warm, dark, moist places. In addition, persons with athlete's foot should treat their shoes as well as their feet with antifungal powder.

Prevention

Where any kind of dermatophytosis is concerned, an ounce of prevention is worth a pound of cure. Using footwear in public settings like pools or steam rooms is often recommended. People are counseled to avoid sharing towels or wearing clothes that have been exposed to fungi for long periods.

The best way for massage therapists to avoid picking up ringworm is to know what it looks like and to stay away from it. It's also particularly important to maintain one's own health. This gives the body every chance of fighting off any fungal attack.

Massage?

Fungal infections locally contraindicate massage in every phase (including the invisible gestation period, which can be challenging). But a small infestation (just one or two lesions) can be considered safe to work with as long as the lesions are treated and covered. For clients with athlete's foot that shows blistering or weepy skin, the feet are a local contraindication.

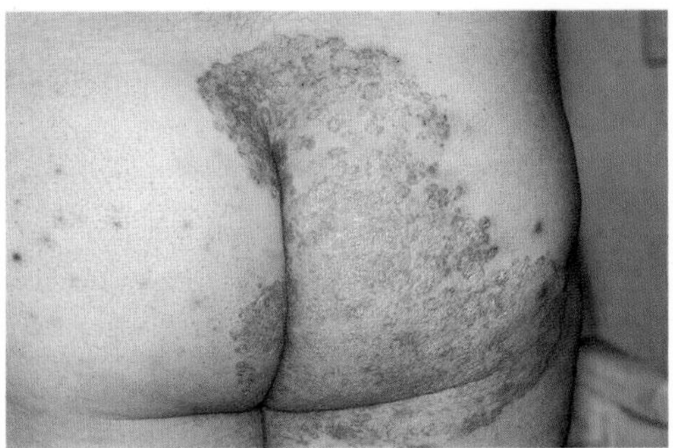

Figure 2.11. Tinea cruris: jock itch.

The decision might also depend on the therapist's own state of health; if the therapist is feeling run down and vulnerable, this may not be the week to work on someone with ringworm.

Modality Recommendations for Fungal Infections

MODALITY	RECOMMENDATION
Deep tissue massage	Systemically contraindicated.
Lymphatic drainage	Systemically contraindicated.
Polarity therapy	S: Indicated within client comfort; work off site of infection. R/D: Contraindicated while acute.
PNF/MET/stretching	Locally contraindicated while acute; otherwise supportive.
Reflexology	Locally contraindicated while acute; otherwise supportive.
Shiatsu	Locally contraindicated when contagious or acute; otherwise supportive, especially with Chinese herbs. Use L/LI for skin, K/SP/TH for immune function.
Swedish massage	Locally contraindicated while acute; otherwise supportive.
Trigger point therapy	Locally contraindicated while acute; otherwise supportive.

See Chapter 1 for a brief description of each modality, including definitions of abbreviations.

Herpes Simplex in Brief

Pronunciation: HUR-peze SIM-pleks

What is it?
Herpes simplex is a viral infection resulting in painful blisters on a red base that develop around the mouth, genitals, or other areas.

How is it recognized?
Herpes outbreaks are often preceded by a prodromic stage: 2 or 3 days of tingling, itching, or pain. Then blisters appear gathered around a red base. The blisters gradually crust and disappear, usually within 2 weeks.

Is massage indicated or contraindicated?
Herpes simplex of any kind locally contraindicates massage during the acute stage. Because live virus may be shed during the prodromic stage, any client who knows he or she may be developing a lesion should be encouraged to reschedule the massage appointment. The linens of a client with an active herpes lesion should be isolated and washed with bleach.

Herpes Simplex

Definition: What Is It?

Among the several viruses in the herpes family that affect humans, herpes simplex viruses are especially common. Herpesvirus type 1 (HSV-1) is typically associated with lesions that appear around the mouth, while herpesvirus type 2 (HSV-2) is associated with genital herpes. More broadly, any herpes lesions that appear above the waist are most likely to be HSV-1, while lesions that appear below the waist are likely to be HSV-2. Exceptions to this rule are increasingly common, however, and because the treatment options for type 1 and type 2 are identical, the distinction between them is less important than it used to be.

Demographics: Who Gets It?

Estimates about the prevalence of herpes vary. The Centers for Disease Control suggest that 20% to 25% of American adults and teens are infected with HSV-2, and women are infected slightly more commonly than men.[6] Estimates for infection with HSV-1 are higher, ranging from around 60% to 80% of the adult population.[7]

Etiology: What Happens?

Oral herpes is transmitted through oral or respiratory secretions. Genital herpes is transmitted through mucous secretions during sexual contact. In either case, a person's first outbreak, which usually occurs 2 to 20 days after exposure, is called *primary* herpes. All subsequent outbreaks are called *recurrent* herpes.

A primary herpes outbreak may be very severe or almost unnoticeable. Most cases of oral herpes are picked up during childhood, and the new carrier may never be aware of his or her infection. In extreme cases, the primary infection may be accompanied by fever, swollen glands, and many painful sores that may last 2 to 6 weeks.

One of the distinguishing features of all herpesviruses is that they are never fully expelled from the body. After the primary outbreak, the HSV goes into hiding in the dorsal root ganglia of the spine or the cranial nerves. There it waits for an appropriate trigger, which could be a fever, a systemic infection, a sunburn, stress, a menstrual period, or some other stimulus that may never be identified. When the virus reactivates, a recurrent outbreak occurs, usually at or near the site of the original infection.

Communicability

Herpes simplex is famous for its communicability. Unlike many pathogens, herpes simplex can remain infectious outside of a host body for hours at a time; exactly how long is a matter of some debate. This means that the face pad that an infected client used can pass the virus to another client. Face cloths and towels also may be infectious. Even leaving aside the possibility of infecting other people, herpes can spread to other parts of the body. Touching a cold sore and then touching the eye can result in a painful and dangerous herpetic infection of the cornea.

One of the most dangerous aspects of a herpes infection is that a person can shed the virus even from skin that has no visible lesion; this is especially likely during the prodromic stage. This means that all it takes to catch herpes from another person is skin-to-skin contact with live virus: the carrier need *not* have an active lesion to spread the virus to other people.

While these features of the virus seem alarming, it should be remembered that most adults in the United States have probably already been exposed to some form of herpes simplex virus. The presence of HSV antibodies provides significant protection from infections in new areas. This protection isn't foolproof, but it does mean that not all contact with HSV inevitably leads to new infections.

Signs and Symptoms

Whether type 1 or type 2, herpes simplex usually presents in the same way: the affected area may have some pain or tingling a few days before an outbreak (the *prodromic* stage); then a blister or cluster of blisters appears on a red base. The blisters erupt and ooze virus-rich liquid all around the area (Figure 2.12). The blisters scab over after a week or 10 days, ending the most contagious phase of the disease. Altogether the outbreak lasts about 2 to 3 weeks.

Types of herpes

- *Oral herpes* tends to erupt when immunity is otherwise depressed (lesions are called cold sores or fever blisters because they often occur when a person is fighting off some other infection); during hormonal changes, as in pregnancy or menstruation; after prolonged exposure to sunlight; or following any emotional stress. They appear most often on the lips and on the skin around the mouth. They may be a lifelong problem.
- *Genital herpes* outbreaks also correspond to depressed immunity and general stress levels, but they run a course of appearing with less and less frequency until finally they

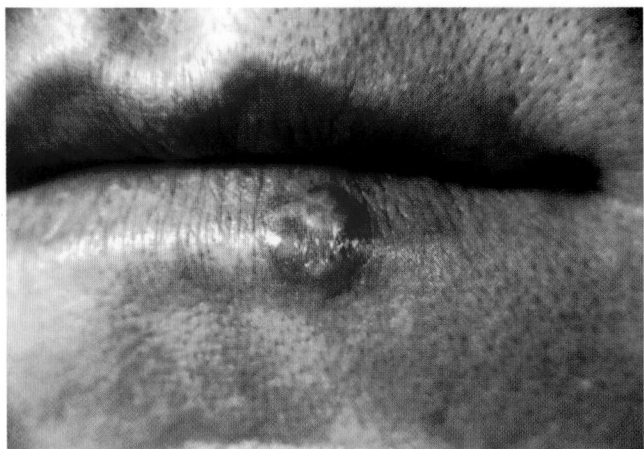

Figure 2.12. Oral herpes.

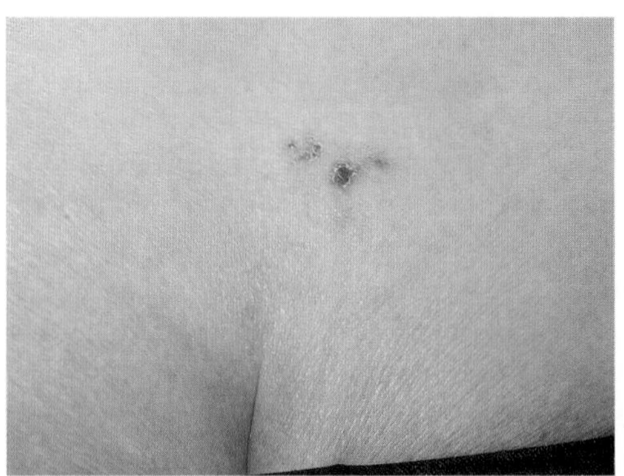

Figure 2.13. Genital herpes.

simply never come back. These blisters may appear on the genitals, but they can also be found on the thighs, buttocks, and on the skin over the sacrum (Figure 2.13). People who have herpes and are immunosuppressed tend to have outbreaks over larger areas of the body than others. The lesions are usually quite painful, but if they are inside the vaginal canal, a woman may be unaware of them, which has important implications for communicability. Genital herpes outbreaks are sometimes accompanied by systemic symptoms: fever, muscular aches, swelling in the inguinal lymph nodes, and difficult or painful urination.

- *Herpes whitlow* is an outbreak of lesions around the nail beds of the hands. This condition has traditionally been associated with children who suck their thumbs, and before the days of consistent glove use, with health care workers, especially dental hygienists (Figure 2.14). Because massage therapists usually work without gloves, they may be at

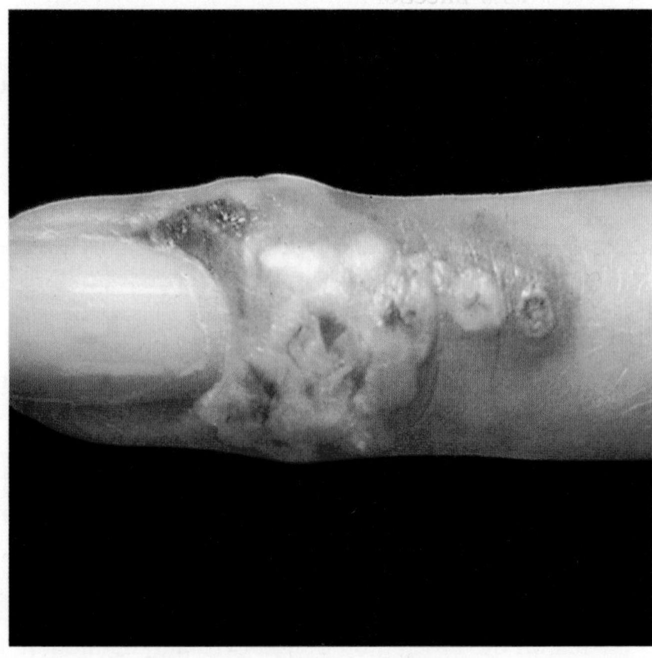

Figure 2.14. Herpes whitlow.

risk for herpes whitlow if clients are shedding virus from any accessible herpes lesion.

- *Herpes gladiatorum* occurs on the trunk and extremities of wrestlers and other athletes who share skin-to-skin contact. In this situation vesicles often rupture through physical contact, so the presentation may look more like painful ulcers than blisters on a red base.
- *Herpetic sycosis* is a condition in which multiple herpes lesions develop over the beard area. It is the result of repeated shaving while a lesion is active: this allows the virus to spread into tiny cuts in new areas on the face.
- *Eczema herpeticum* is a condition in which herpes simplex is associated with atopic dermatitis, a type of eczema. It is most common in children and produces a widespread outbreak of herpes lesions.

SIDEBAR 2.2: WHEN IS A MOUTH SORE NOT HERPES?

Oral herpes causes the familiar lesions we call fever blisters or cold sores, but not all sores around the mouth are caused by herpesvirus.

Angular stomatitis is a condition involving painful irritated cracks around the corners of the mouth. This is often associated with denture wearers, who may drool while they sleep. The accumulation of saliva around the corners of the mouth provides a rich growth medium for the yeast that causes these lesions.

Aphthae, or *"canker sores,"* are lesions *inside* the mouth, often on the gums and cheeks. These are small, painful ulcers whose cause is unknown. Aphthae may be viral, but they are not contagious.

Complications

Secondary bacterial infection is a common complication of herpes lesions. Immunosuppressed people are especially susceptible to secondary infections. People who are co-infected with HIV and genital herpes have a greater risk of communicating HIV to sexual partners. Herpes has also been seen to accelerate the progression of HIV to AIDS.[7] Vaginally delivered newborns of mothers with active genital herpes may develop blindness, pneumonia, or brain damage.

Treatment

Herpes is a viral infection, so antibiotics are ineffective. No vaccine against herpes has yet been developed. Antiviral drugs suppress viral activity and shorten the duration of an infection, but they don't prevent future outbreaks. Prevention is the main thrust of treatment for this condition; this means isolating towels, bedding, and clothing and avoiding sexual contact while lesions are present. Keeping as healthy as possible between outbreaks is an important way to reduce the frequency and severity of herpes episodes.

Massage?

Obviously, acute herpes outbreaks at least locally contraindicate massage. If a client has a history of herpes, it's important to explain why it's a bad idea to receive a massage during an outbreak and request that she reschedule if she has prodromic symptoms or blisters on her appointment day. Even after a lesion has scabbed over, herpes is a local contraindication. Because this virus can survive outside of a host for hours at a time, isolate the linens of a client with an active infection in a closed container and either have them professionally sterilized or add extra bleach to their wash cycle.

Massage therapists who have active oral herpes outbreaks also must respect their clients' health by not exposing them to the virus. Cold sores are often painful or itchy. Bodyworkers need to take special care not to brush their face with their sleeves, wrists, or hands and then touch their client. Some massage therapists suggest that one way to minimize the transfer of herpes simplex from the client to the practitioner is to avoid working on the face and hands when the client has an active lesion.

Modality Recommendations for Herpes Simplex

MODALITY	RECOMMENDATION
Deep tissue massage	Systemically contraindicated while acute; otherwise supportive.
Lymphatic drainage	Systemically contraindicated while acute; otherwise supportive.
Polarity therapy	S: Locally contraindicated while acute; otherwise indicated. R/D: Contraindicated while acute, otherwise supportive within client comfort.
PNF/MET/stretching	Locally contraindicated while acute; otherwise supportive.
Reflexology	Locally contraindicated while acute; otherwise supportive.
Shiatsu	Locally contraindicated when contagious or acute; otherwise supportive, especially with Chinese herbs. Use L/LI for skin, K/SP/TH for immune function.
Swedish massage	Locally contraindicated while acute; otherwise supportive.
Trigger point therapy	Locally contraindicated while acute; otherwise supportive.

See Chapter 1 for a brief description of each modality, including definitions of abbreviations.

Impetigo in Brief

Pronunciation: im-peh-TY-go

What is it?
Impetigo is a bacterial (staphylococcal or streptococcal) infection of the skin. It is usually seen in infants and young children.

How is it recognized?
Sores that scab with a yellow-brown crust are the most common sign of impetigo, but other forms may involve large blisters or ulcers.

Is massage indicated or contraindicated?
Until the lesions have completely healed, this highly contagious condition systemically contraindicates massage.

Impetigo

Definition: What Is It?

Impetigo is an infection of the skin, usually with some of the staphylococci or streptococci that normally colonize superficial layers of the epidermis. It occurs mostly among children, although adults can get it too. Lesions usually occur around the nose and mouth, sometimes inside the nostrils or ear canals. Although it often begins on the head, impetigo can infect the skin anywhere on the body.

Signs and Symptoms

Impetigo has three presentations:

- *Impetigo contagiosa* is the most common form. This is the result of an infection with *Streptococcus pyogenes*. In this form, red sores with small blisters appear, typically around the mouth or nose. The sores are itchy but not painful. The blisters rupture and ooze liquid, and a characteristic yellow-brown crust that resembles honey develops. Left untreated, these sores heal in 2 to 3 weeks, leaving no scars (Figure 2.15).
- *Bullous impetigo* occurs most often in children under 2 years old. It is an infection with *Staphylococcus aureus* that leads to large, painless blisters on the trunk, arms, and legs. Unlike impetigo contagiosa, bullous impetigo is accompanied by fever, diarrhea, and general weakness in the infant.
- *Ecthyma* is a form of impetigo related to chronic skin inflammation or poor circulation. It produces painful, pus-filled blisters on the legs and feet, along with malaise and

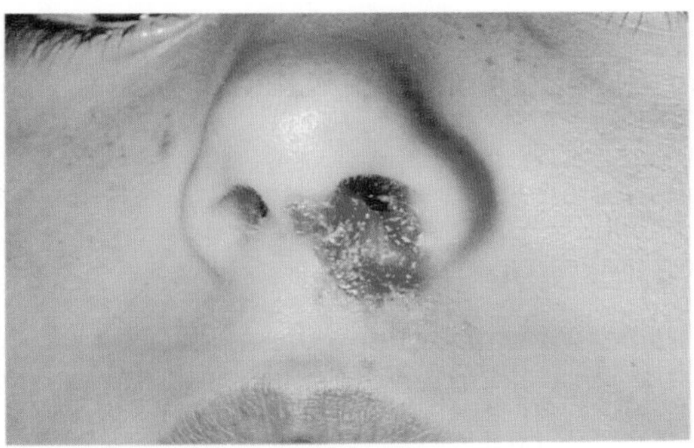

Figure 2.15. Impetigo contagiosa.

swollen lymph nodes. Unlike the other two forms of impetigo, ecthyma can leave permanent scars because the infection penetrates to deep layers of the skin. It is a particular risk for people with atopic dermatitis or diabetes.

Treatment

Mild impetigo can be treated with topical antibiotic cream. But if the blisters have spread over much of the body and especially if there are other signs of systemic infection (i.e., fever and chills), oral antibiotics are prescribed. Impetigo can have serious complications, including renal failure, meningitis, and cellulitis, if it isn't treated carefully.

Prevention

Impetigo often appears where the skin has been damaged: scabbed-over mosquito bites, chapped lips or noses, cuts, and sores. The first step in prevention is to stop any kind of infection from developing at these sites. Chapped skin should be treated with lubricant to prevent damage. All other wounds should be cleaned thoroughly, treated with antibacterial ointment, and covered.

This is an extremely contagious condition, and since it is both very itchy and most common in children, special precautions are recommended to prevent its spread. First, the patient must be discouraged from touching or scratching the lesions; impetigo can easily be spread to other parts of the body this way. The lesions must be kept clean and dry and crusts removed as soon as possible because the moistness underneath the crusts harbors bacteria. Doctors suggest soaking the scabbed area in a weak vinegar solution to help loosen the crusts. The patient's bedding and towels must be strictly isolated during the infection. Children with impetigo are encouraged to stay home from school and avoid contact with other children for at least 24 hours after they begin treatment.

Massage?

Impetigo is a contagious bacterial infection of the skin involving virulent pathogens that can be drug resistant. It systemically contraindicates massage until the lesions have healed completely .

Modality Recommendations for Impetigo

MODALITY	RECOMMENDATION
Deep tissue massage	Systemically contraindicated.
Lymphatic drainage	Systemically contraindicated.
Polarity therapy	S: Locally contraindicated while acute; otherwise indicated. R/D: Locally contraindicated; otherwise supportive.
PNF/MET/stretching	Locally contraindicated while acute; otherwise supportive.
Reflexology	Systemically contraindicated until all symptoms are resolved.
Shiatsu	Locally contraindicated when contagious or acute; otherwise supportive, especially with Chinese herbs. Use L/LI for skin and K/SP/TH for immune function.
Swedish massage	Systemically contraindicated until all symptoms are resolved.
Trigger point therapy	Locally contraindicated while acute; otherwise supportive.

See Chapter 1 for a brief description of each modality, including definitions of abbreviations.

Lice and Mites in Brief

What are they?
Lice and mites are tiny parasites that drink blood. They spread primarily through close contact with skin or infested sheets or clothing.

How are they recognized?

- **Mites** that cause scabies are too small to see, but they leave itchy trails or nodules where they burrow under the skin. They prefer warm, moist places, such as the axillae or between fingers.
- **Head lice** are easy to see, but they can hide. A more dependable sign is their eggs: nits are small, rice-shaped flecks that cling strongly to hair shafts.
- **Body lice** look very similar to head lice, but they live primarily in clothing and only visit the host for blood meals.
- **Pubic lice** look like tiny white crabs in pubic and coarse body hair.

All of these parasites create a lot of itching through allergic reactions to the toxins they produce.

Is massage indicated or contraindicated?
All four parasite infestations contraindicate massage until they have been eradicated. If a massage therapist is exposed to any of these parasites, every client he or she works on subsequently may also be exposed even before the therapist shows any symptoms.

Lice and Mites

Parasitic infestations are something every massage therapist fears, because bodyworkers are so vulnerable to whatever is crawling around on their clients' skins. But here, as in all things fearful, the best defense is information.

Mites

Definition: What Are They?

Tiny mites called ***Sarcoptes scabiei*** are arachnids that cause the skin lesions called scabies (Figure 2.16). Juvenile mites mature on the surface of the skin; mating takes place here too. After mating, the males die. The females burrow into the epidermis in warm, moist spots where they drink blood, defecate and urinate, and lay eggs so the next generation can carry on. The average life cycle of a female mite is 30 to 60 days. As an adult, she lays approximately three eggs per day, although only a small percentage of them hatch.

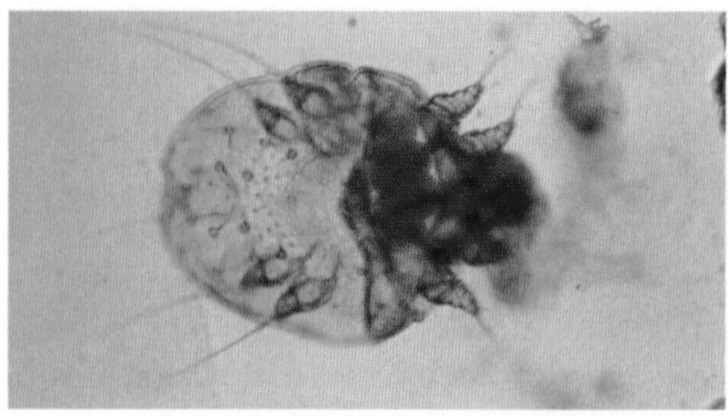

Figure 2.16. Scabies mite.

Newly hatched mites migrate to the surface of the skin, where it takes about 14 days for them to achieve maturity.

The mites' waste is highly irritating, causing an itchy allergic reaction in most hosts. If scratching damages the skin, the risk of secondary infection is high.

One type of scabies, called crusting or Norwegian scabies, is caused by a different parasite. Where a typical mite infestation might involve a dozen parasites, crusting scabies can involve thousands or even millions of mites. The lesions cover large areas and develop dry, flaky scabs, but they tend not to itch. Crusting scabies is a relatively rare condition except among immunocompromised people and those living in overcrowded institutions.

How Do They Spread?

Mites spread readily through skin-to-skin contact or through contact with something someone else has worn or lain on, including massage sheets. Depending on local conditions, scabies mites can live for several hours or several days without a host.

Signs and Symptoms

Scabies mites are too small to see with the naked eye, so a visual diagnosis is based on the trails they leave behind. Sometimes their burrows are visible: these look like reddish or grayish lines around the areas the mites favor: the groin, axilla, elbows, belt line, or between fingers. Other signs of mite infestation are secondary bacterial infection and the irritated blisters and nodules that arise from allergic reactions to their waste (Figure 2.17).

This condition is itchiest at night, when the mites are most active, but many skin irritations seem to itch more at night, simply because a person who is trying to sleep has few distractions. The itching caused by mites, however, has a distinctive unrelenting quality. Where eczema or mosquito bites might itch intermittently and then subside, scabies itching gets worse and worse.

Diagnosis

Scabies lesions can be tricky to diagnose if a parasite isn't isolated and identified. A typical test involves treating an area with sterile mineral oil and then taking a skin scraping to look for evidence of the parasites. Sometimes a felt tip marker is rubbed around a suspected scabies track and then excess ink is removed with alcohol: the remaining ink sinks into any openings in the skin to mark the track.

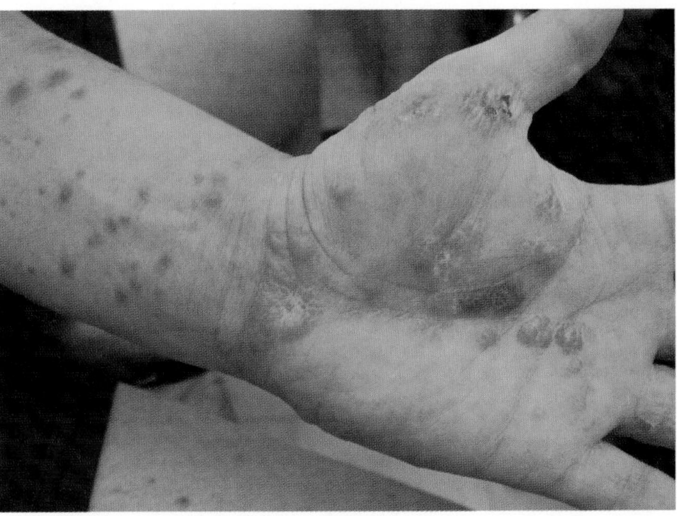

Figure 2.17. Scabies lesions.

Scabies can resemble psoriasis, eczema, and several other skin conditions, so it is important to get an accurate diagnosis. Missing the correct diagnosis increases the risk of further spread and secondary infection; a false-positive diagnosis means a person may be exposed to potentially toxic material unnecessarily.

Treatment

Mites, like other parasitic infestations, are treated by bathing with pesticidal soap. This treatment can be highly toxic and so must be used carefully. Washing and then isolating bedding, towels, and clothing is important to prevent further outbreaks. It is not necessary to fumigate the home, because mites don't stray far from their hosts.

One danger associated with scabies treatment is that the itching can outlast the infestation by days or weeks. It is easy for a person to assume that the infection is still present and to re-treat unnecessarily. Repeated exposure to scabicides is potentially toxic.

Massage?

Direct contact with a person who has scabies mites is not safe. A massage therapist who might have been exposed to mites by accident should consider those sheets hot (isolate them from other sheets and wash them with extra bleach) and see a doctor about treatment right away. The symptoms of scabies sometimes don't show up for 4 weeks or more; it takes that long to build up enough toxins to be irritating. But the therapist is certainly contagious the whole time; anyone she works on could become infested too.

Head Lice

Definition: What Are They?

Head lice are wingless insects *(Pediculus humanus capitis)* that live in head hair and suck blood from the scalp. Infestation with lice is sometimes called pediculosis. Lice are quite a bit larger than mites and can easily be seen without a microscope (Figure 2.18). Their saliva is very irritating, causing itching and possibly infection. Lice gestate in the egg for 7 to 16 days (depending on ambient temperature). When they hatch, they go through three molts and live an average of 2-3 weeks. Their life consists mainly of taking blood meals, mating, and laying eggs.

Historically, head lice and body lice have been vectors of diseases that include typhus, ricketts, and trench fever. While no longer considered a health threat in developed countries,

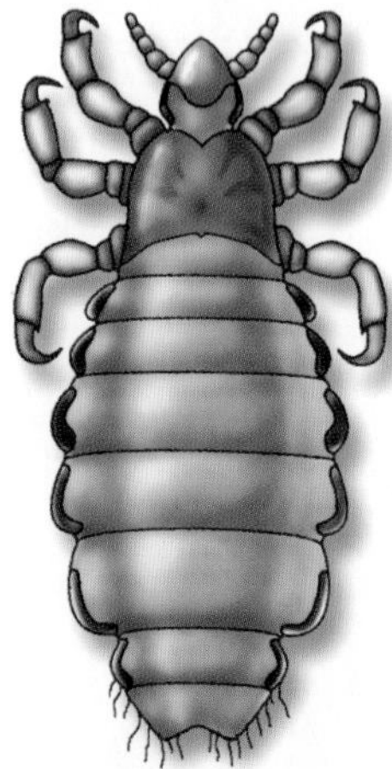

Figure 2.18. Head louse.

these diseases are still spread by lice in refugee camps and other areas where people live in close contact and where good hygiene is difficult.

How Do They Spread?

Head lice spread most easily through direct contact: human heat allows them to move quickly from scalp to scalp during sports, camping trips, and other close-contact events. When they are separated from a host, they tend to be more sluggish.

Lice can also use hats and scarves to travel from one host to another. They may live in batters' helmets that are shared by Little League teams, hairbrushes that are shared by best friends, and car seats that are shared by carpool buddies. While this is not the most efficient way to spread lice throughout an environment, it is certainly a possible way.

Signs and Symptoms

If a client has lice, the actual insects may or may not be obvious; when they are warm, they move fast and can hide. But they lay eggs called *nits*. (This is the source of the word *nitpicky*.) Nits are glued to hair shafts and look like tiny grains of rice (Figure 2.19). They hatch after about a week. Dark nits may not yet have hatched. White nits are usually the empty eggshells that are still sticking to the hair. Nits are a prime diagnostic feature for pediculosis; anything else of that size and color (like dandruff) would brush out easily.

Lice lay their eggs right at the base of the hair shaft, mostly behind the ears and along the back of the head near the hairline. One way to determine how long an infestation has been present is to observe how far the nits have grown away from the scalp. Any nit less than one-quarter of an inch (about 1 month's growth of hair) from the scalp indicates an active infestation.[8]

A person with lice has itchiness and the sensation of movement on the scalp. Rigorous scratching can damage the skin and open the door to secondary infection.

Treatment

Repeated applications of pesticidal shampoo to kill adults and eggs is the first step in treating lice. Controversy has developed over the best choices in pediculicides. Options are limited: most products use lindane (now outlawed as a toxic substance in some states), malathion (flammable and malodorous), or pyrethrum (highly irritating to some patients, especially children with asthma). Furthermore, some types of lice have become resistant to the standard pesticides, so it is now recommended that applications of the medicine be followed by systematically combing every section of hair with a very fine-toothed comb to dislodge adult animals and nits.

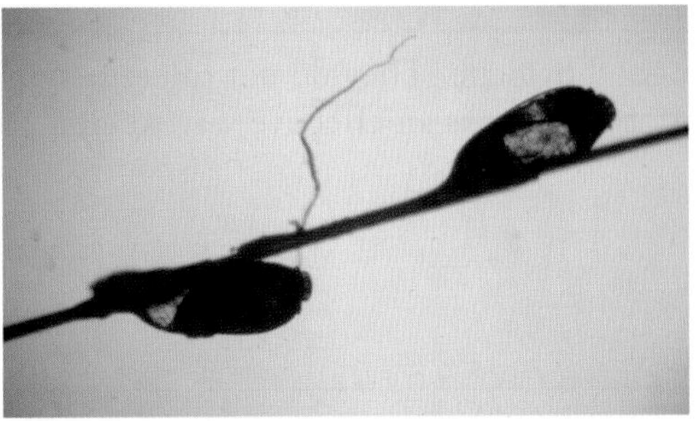

Figure 2.19. Nits attached to a hair shaft.

Persons averse to using pesticides may choose to smother the lice with petroleum jelly, oil, or mayonnaise. These treatment options are less effective than medicated shampoos, so it is especially important to combine them with systematic use of a nit comb.

One new treatment option that is still in development shows a lot of promise. It is a modified hair dryer that essentially dehydrates the adult lice and eggs without chemicals or the risk of increasing resistance.[9]

Washing bedding, towels, and clothing is also an important part of head lice treatment, as is thoroughly cleaning hats, hairbrushes, combs, and anything else that comes in contact with the head. Washing items at 130°F and drying them on high heat for 20 minutes is considered sufficient. Dry cleaning is also effective. Anything else that might harbor lice (e.g., pillows, stuffed animals, soft toys) should be tied in a dry cleaning bag or other plastic sheeting and isolated for 2 weeks.[8]

Massage?

A client who knows he or she has head lice should not receive massage. If a therapist suspects that she has been exposed in a work setting, precautionary measures should be taken at once: clothing should be laundered, carpets and upholstery should be vacuumed, and the therapist should be examined for head lice as quickly as possible.

Body Lice

Definition: What Are They?

Body lice (***Pediculus humanus***) are closely related to head lice, but they have different living and feeding patterns. Body lice tend not to live directly on their host but in the host's clothing, especially in the seams. They are about the same size as head lice, and they also take blood meals, causing an itchy reaction.

Body lice are fairly rare except among homeless and transient populations who have limited access to laundry facilities and so spend a lot of time in unwashed clothing. Like head lice, body lice are potential vectors of communicable diseases.

How Do They Spread?

Body lice live in clothing, so sharing unwashed clothing is the most efficient way for them to spread from one host to another. They may also crawl from infested clothing to other clothing in a laundry basket or other close proximity.

Signs and Symptoms

The primary sign of body lice is an itchy rash that gets worse. The insects seldom live directly on the skin, and they usually lay eggs in clothing, so unless the clothing is examined, a live body louse may not be found.

Treatment

Body lice are treated most effectively with good hygiene. They do not tolerate high temperatures, so frequent bathing and laundering of clothing is an effective way to eradicate an infestation.

Pubic Lice

Definition: What Are They?

Pubic lice (*Pthirus pubis*) are tiny animals that look a lot like their nickname, crabs (Figure 2.20). Crabs are a bit less discerning in their tastes; they like pubic hair in the groin best, but

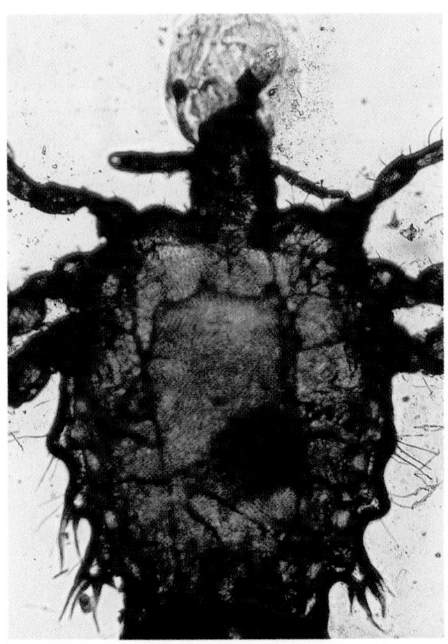

Figure 2.20. Pubic (crab) louse.

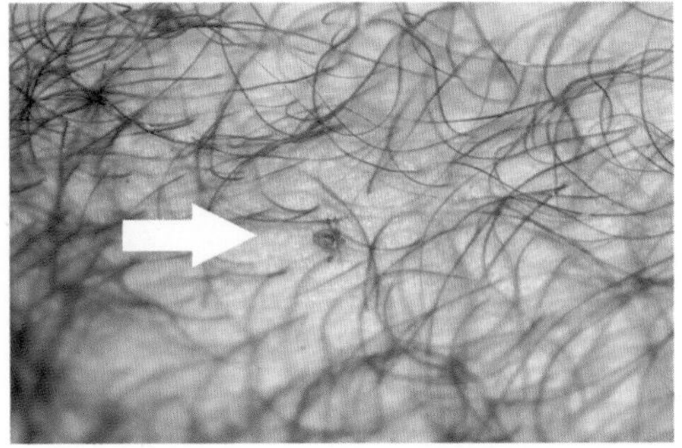

Figure 2.21. Pubic louse in body hair (arrow).

they also live in armpit hair and other coarse body hair (Figure 2.21). They may also be found in mustaches, beards, eyebrows, and eyelashes.

How Do They Spread?

Pubic lice are usually spread through sexual contact, but infested clothing, linens, or massage sheets can spread them, too.

Signs and Symptoms

Pubic lice look like tiny white crabs about 1 mm across. They also leave nits, but they are so small they are barely visible without magnification. Like all of the infestations being discussed, the primary symptom is itching.

Treatment

Crab lice carriers must follow the same protocols as head lice carriers. The sheets of any massage client suspected of a crab infestation should be isolated from all others and disinfected as soon as possible.

Massage?

Infestations of pubic lice, body lice, head lice, mites, and any other parasitic infestation of the skin contraindicate massage.

Parasitic infestation carries a powerful social stigma that is negatively (and inaccurately) associated with poverty and poor hygiene. *Anybody* (including massage therapists) can have this problem, and people in touch professions are in a position to cause a lot more damage with it than anyone else. So be respectful and remember that it could happen to anyone.

Modality Recommendations for Lice and Mites

MODALITY	RECOMMENDATION
Deep tissue massage	Systemically contraindicated while acute; otherwise supportive.
Lymphatic drainage	Supportive.
Polarity therapy	S: Locally contraindicated until infestation is resolved. R/D: Supportive after infestation is resolved.
PNF/MET/stretching	Locally contraindicated; otherwise supportive.
Reflexology	Locally contraindicated; otherwise supportive.
Shiatsu	Locally contraindicated when contagious or acute; otherwise supportive, especially with Chinese herbs.
Swedish massage	Systemically contraindicated until infestation is resolved.
Trigger point therapy	Locally contraindicated while acute; otherwise supportive.

See Chapter 1 for a brief description of each modality, including definitions of abbreviations.

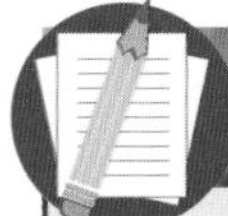

CASE HISTORY 2.2

Scabies, Valerie

Valerie: "Mystery rash."

Valerie was a massage student. She worked with a variety of people, including fellow students, friends, and her student internship group, people with AIDS.

One day Valerie noted that she had some areas on the outsides of her elbows that were slightly but persistently itchy during the day. They gradually developed red bumps. Ironically, this occurred while Valerie was studying skin conditions in her massage course. "It's natural to convince yourself that you have symptoms of a lot of things. I knew something was going on, and it seemed like it *could* be scabies, but my symptoms were different from anything I'd seen described," she said. The itching was not particularly worse at night and there were no tracks or typical signs of infestation. Even the site of the infestation was unusual: scabies mites usually go for warm, moist, protected areas like skin folds on the *insides* of elbows, but not the outsides.

Eventually Valerie went to her general practitioner, who pronounced her condition a "mystery rash" and suggested a corticosteroid cream to limit the itchiness. In a way, Valerie was relieved by this diagnosis. "You never want to think you have scabies," she said. When her husband also developed symptoms, however, he went straight to a dermatologist, who immediately diagnosed scabies and prescribed enough pesticidal soap for both of them.

The cream was applied all over the body up to the chin; evidently scabies do not infest the head or face. "That night after I washed off the cream, I was really, really, *really* itchy, and then for 4 or 5 weeks my skin was raw and uncomfortable." The cream itself can cause symptoms that mimic a scabies infestation for weeks at a time. This can lead to **scabiosis,** in which a person is convinced of the need to medicate for scabies again and again, although the infestation is gone. Scabiosis can become a life-threatening condition if the person repeatedly self-medicates.

Six to eight weeks passed between the onset of Valerie's symptoms and a final diagnosis. During this time Valerie continued to work on friends and clients and to receive massage from other students. Two other classmates were infested and finally diagnosed. "The first few days [after we knew it was scabies] were full of panic and fear. Within a couple of days of people getting over their fear and paranoia there was a lot of support. People had the attitude that this is just one of the things that can happen when you're a bodyworker."

Warts

Definition: What Are They?

Warts are small, benign growths caused by varieties of *human papillomavirus* (HPV) that invade keratinocytes. These infected protein-making cells produce a lot of extra keratin, which is the material that makes epithelial cells hard and scaly. The result is *verruca vulgaris*, or common warts.

Demographics: Who Gets Them?

Warts affect young children occasionally, adults rarely, and teenagers mercilessly. Adults who get lots of warts are probably somehow immunosuppressed. It is estimated that warts affect 7 to 12% of the population overall and up to 20% of teens.[10]

Warts in Brief

What are they?
Warts are growths caused by slow-growing viral infections of keratinocytes in the epidermis.

How are they recognized?
The most common warts (verruca vulgaris) look like hard, cauliflower-shaped lumps. They usually occur on the hands or knees. They can affect anyone, but children and teenagers are especially prone to them.

Is massage indicated or contraindicated?
Warts are a local contraindication for massage. The virus is contained in the blood and shedding skin cells, and while it is unlikely, it is not impossible to get warts from another person.

Etiology: What Happens?

HPV is a group of over 100 pathogens that have been associated with several types of human warts. These viruses spread when someone with compromised skin directly touches a wart or through indirect contact, when a new host picks up the virus from a surface or contaminated item. Warts don't spread easily, though; it may take repeated exposures to start an infection. After exposure the virus grows extremely slowly. It may incubate anywhere from a month to 3 years before symptoms develop.

When a person who has a wart picks at it or damages skin nearby (like picking at hangnails or biting fingernails near a wart), the virus can spread. The same caution exists for trying to clip or cut away warts: the blood from these growths may carry the virus to cause new infections nearby.

Signs and Symptoms

Warts look like hard, cauliflower-shaped growths on the skin (Figure 2.22). They are usually just a nuisance, but when they occur on the bottom of the feet, they can make it difficult to

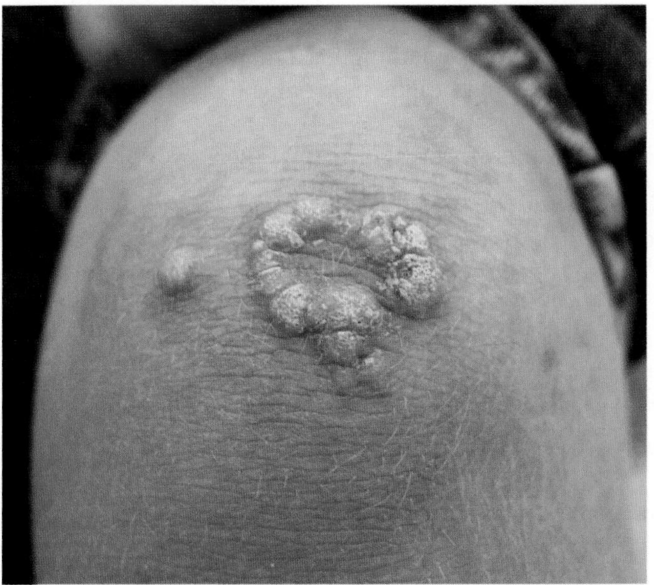

Figure 2.22. Warts on a Knee.

Compare and Contrast 2.1
PLANTAR WARTS VERSUS CALLUSES

Plantar warts often look like simple calluses: the thick skin that grows on areas of the feet subject to a lot of wear and tear. The problem is that while people may file or snip off their calluses with no ill effects, to do the same with a plantar wart is to risk having that wart virus spread all over the foot and lead to more growths until it becomes difficult to walk.

Massage therapists are in a unique position to observe their clients' feet and notice the subtle differences between plantar warts and callus. They may be able to give clients guidance about getting the right kind of care.

CHARACTERISTICS	PLANTAR WARTS	CALLUS
Location	Anywhere on plantar surface of foot. Usually *not* bilateral.	Appears in areas of wear and tear, especially back of heels and lateral aspect of feet. Callus usually grows in a similar pattern on both feet.
Appearance	May be white, but with darker speckling under thickened skin—capillary supply for wart.	Thick, white skin.
Sensation	Very hard and unyielding, like stepping on a stone.	No particular sensation.

walk. In this case (and sometimes when they occur on the palm of the hands) the warts grow *inward*, creating a sensation of always stepping on something hard that never goes away. It is important to distinguish between plantar warts and callus to avoid the risk of making a bad situation worse (see Compare and Contrast 2.1).

Verruca vulgaris is the most common kind of wart, but many other types of warts have been identified; only a few are discussed here.

- *Deep palmoplantar warts*, also called ***myrmecia***, are plantar warts that grow on the soles of the feet (Figure 2.23). When they occur on the hands, they are often around or under the fingernails. Plantar warts are sometimes (but not always) caused by the same subtype of HPV as verruca vulgaris. Very rarely, an HPV that causes plantar warts becomes malignant. Called *verrucous carcinoma*, it is classified as a type of squamous cell carcinoma. It doesn't tend to metastasize, but it can cause extensive local damage.
- *Cystic warts* usually occur on the sole of the foot, but unlike plantar warts, they are smooth and soft. When they are excised, a cheesy substance can be squeezed out. Cystic warts are not well understood, but some researchers suggest that they may involve blocked sweat glands or an attempt to encyst the original viral infection.
- *Butcher's warts* are associated with meat handling. They look like common warts but are caused by a different variety of HPV.

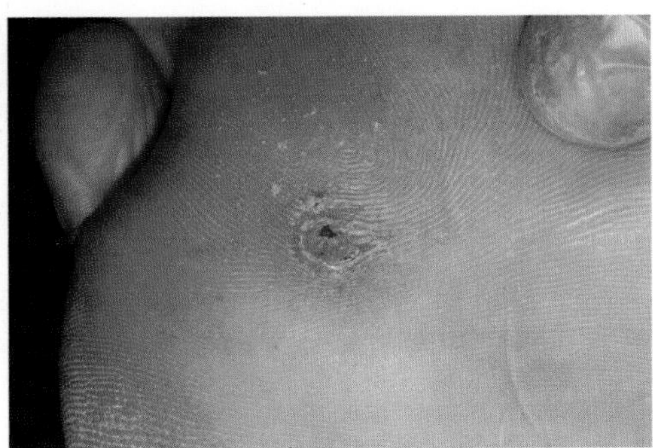

Figure 2.23. Plantar warts.

- *Plane or flat warts* are small, brown, smooth warts. They can grow a few at a time or with hundreds spread over a large area. They appear most often on the hands, face, and shins. Plane warts on the face may spread to other nicks and cuts during shaving.
- *Molluscum contagiosum* is usually a children's malady involving small white lumps. The pathogen is not HPV; it is from the pox family. Molluscum contagiosum in adults can be a sexually transmitted disease.
- *Genital warts* are a sexually transmitted disease brought about by any of several varieties of HPV. Most genital warts come and go with no symptoms, but others may become cancerous. HPV is a causative agent for cervical cancer, discussed in Chapter 11.

Treatment

If warts are left alone (*benign neglect*), most of them spontaneously resolve within 2 years, leaving no scar. Some people are unwilling to wait through this process, however, and so seek treatment options. Any drugstore carries preparations that claim to be effective, but they must be used with caution to avoid damage to surrounding tissues. The common ingredient in most of these products is salicylic acid.

Other remedies include rubbing garlic (which has antiviral properties) on the lesion, using duct tape to cover and slightly irritate it, or employing one of the most interesting aspects of warts: the link between expectation and immune system activity. If a person believes that a treatment will work, it likely to be successful. This has led to some interesting approaches to wart management. One of the best came from a student who said, "Take a potato and cut it in six pieces. Bury each of the pieces in a different place, and *don't tell anyone where you hid them*. The wart will go away in a couple of weeks. Mine did."

Medical intervention for warts often begins with liquid nitrogen to freeze them off. Other options include electrosurgery, lasers, painting the warts with a medication derived from blister beetles, injecting them with drugs that improve immune system sensitivity, and cutting them out. Any of these options can work, but they don't prevent other warts from growing, and they all carry possible side effects or complications.

Massage?

Warts are a local contraindication. A massage therapist is unlikely to pick up a new infection, but it is inappropriate to rub on or irritate these growths. As stated previously, the virus is found in the shedding skin cells around the lesion. Further, warts are often caught and torn around the edges, and if the skin is not intact, the client may be vulnerable to a secondary infection.

Modality Recommendations for Warts

MODALITY	RECOMMENDATION
Deep tissue massage	Locally contraindicated; otherwise supportive.
Lymphatic drainage	Supportive.
Polarity therapy	S/R/D: Locally contraindicated; can work off site of infection.
PNF/MET/stretching	Locally contraindicated; otherwise supportive.
Reflexology	Locally contraindicated; otherwise supportive.
Shiatsu	Locally contraindicated when contagious or acute; otherwise supportive, especially with Chinese herbs. Use L/LI for skin, K/SP/TH for immune function.
Swedish massage	Locally contraindicated; otherwise supportive,
Trigger point therapy	Locally contraindicated; otherwise supportive,

See Chapter 1 for a brief description of each modality, including definitions of abbreviations.

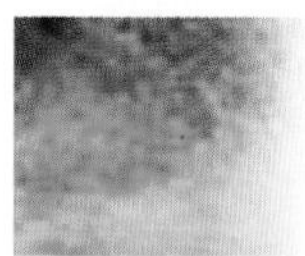

Noncontagious Inflammatory Skin Disorders

Acne Rosacea

Definition: What Is It?

Acne rosacea is an idiopathic chronic skin condition seen mostly in fair-skinned people between 30 and 60 years old. It primarily affects the skin of the face, especially the nose and cheeks. It can also affect the conjunctiva of the eyes and the eyelids. Acne rosacea seldom develops elsewhere on the body.

Acne Rosacea in Brief
Pronunciation: AK-ne ro-SAY-shuh

What is it?
Acne rosacea is a chronic inflammatory condition involving facial skin, eyes, and eyelids.

How is it recognized?
Acne rosacea occurs in stages of severity, starting with occasional flushing and continuing through general inflammation of the face and eyes, the formation of papules and pustules, and finally permanent thickening and distortion of facial skin, especially around the nose.

Is massage indicated or contraindicated?
Acne rosacea may be exacerbated by local massage, and some clients may be sensitive to some lubricants.

Etiology: What Happens?

The pathophysiology of acne rosacea is not well understood. It may be inherited, but no gene has been specifically identified with this condition.

The symptoms of acne rosacea may come and go in the early stages but ultimately may become permanent. Triggers for flare-ups are fairly predictable. They may include exposure to sunlight, wind, and cold temperatures; drinking hot liquids or alcohol; eating spicy food; menopause; the use of steroidal anti-inflammatories on the face; and emotional stress.

Signs and Symptoms

Acne rosacea tends to progress through predictable stages. Not all patients have it severely, but it can create permanent changes in the quality of the delicate skin on the face. Four stages have been identified to mark the progression of this condition:

- *Facial flushing.* In this stage the patient may experience frequent flushing, usually in the center of the face. The skin may feel hot or stinging, but it doesn't usually itch.
- *Vascular rosacea.* Skin is red, especially on the nose and cheeks. Small blood vessels may become permanently dilated and visible in a condition called *telangiectasia*. About half of all rosacea patients also have chronic inflammation and irritation of the eyes and eyelids.
- *Inflammatory rosacea.* If the condition progresses to this point, papules and pustules may develop. (Figure 2.24)
- *Rhinophyma.* This is the damage to the skin on the nose seen in people with chronic, very severe acne rosacea. The skin becomes thick, bumpy, distorted, and permanently reddened. Men develop this condition more often than women (Figure 2.25).

Complications

Acne rosacea can lead to a number of other disorders. When it affects the eyes, it may lead to rosacea keratitis, which may eventually damage the cornea. Perhaps the greatest issue with acne rosacea is its consequences on self-esteem and public perception. Persons with this disorder are very likely to develop depression or anxiety disorders, as they perceive being judged by the appearance of their skin. Furthermore, a traditional but incorrect association between the bulbous nose seen with advanced acne rosacea and alcoholism can lead to social stigmas that are difficult to challenge.

Treatment

Acne rosacea has no permanent cure and so is treated palliatively. Patients are taught to recognize their specific triggers and to avoid them when possible. Topical or oral antibiotics may be prescribed for pustules, but they are ineffective for the permanent redness seen with this

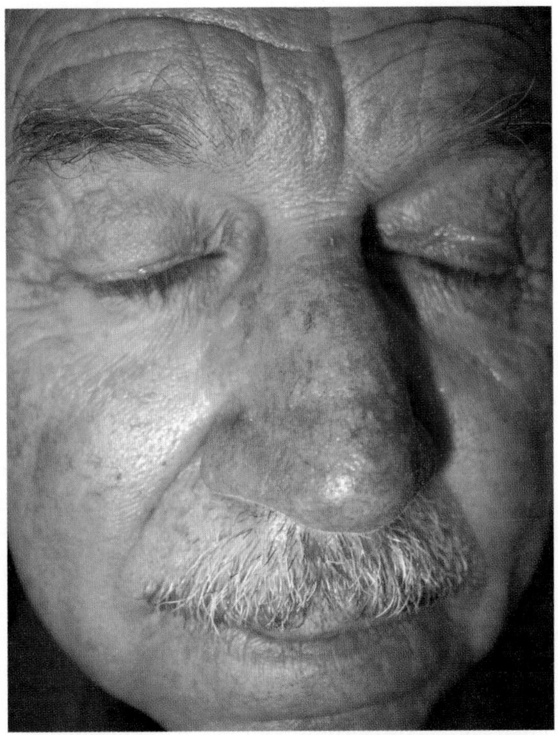

Figure 2.24. Acne rosacea: inflammatory rosacea.

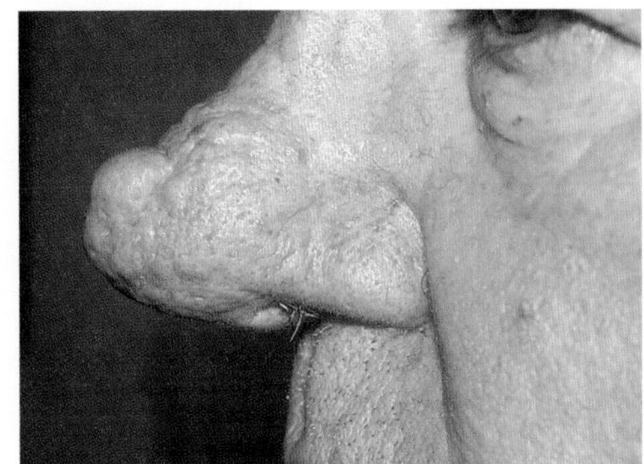

Figure 2.25. Acne rosacea: rhinophyma.

condition. Laser surgery or dermabrasion may help the appearance of the skin and mask telangiectasias. Plastic surgery may be considered for a person with advanced rhinophyma.

Massage?

Acne rosacea may be exacerbated with stimulation of facial skin. Further, some clients may be sensitive to substances in the massage lubricant. Bodywork elsewhere is safe and appropriate.

Modality Recommendations for Acne Rosacea

MODALITY	RECOMMENDATION
Deep tissue massage	Locally contraindicated; otherwise supportive.
Lymphatic drainage	Supportive.
Polarity therapy	S/R/D: Locally contraindicated; otherwise indicated.
PNF/MET/stretching	Supportive.
Reflexology	Indicated.
Shiatsu	Indicated. Use L/LI for skin, K/SP/TH for inflammation.
Swedish massage	Locally contraindicated while acute; otherwise supportive.
Trigger point therapy	Locally contraindicated while acute; otherwise supportive.

See Chapter 1 for a brief description of each modality, including definitions of abbreviations.

Acne Vulgaris

Definition: What Is It?

Acne is a condition in which a person becomes susceptible to small, localized skin infections. They usually appear on the face, neck, and upper back.

Acne Vulgaris in Brief
Pronunciation: AK-ne vul-GAR-is

What is it?
Acne vulgaris is a bacterial infection of sebaceous glands usually found on the face, neck, and upper back. It is closely associated with adolescence or liver dysfunction that results in excess testosterone.

How is it recognized?
It looks like raised, inflamed pustules on the skin, sometimes with white or black tips.

Is massage indicated or contraindicated?
Acne locally contraindicates massage because of the risk of infection, causing pain, and exacerbating the symptoms with the application of an oily lubricant.

Demographics: Who Gets It?

Many people have painful, awkward memories of adolescence thanks to this condition. When individuals make the transition from childhood to adulthood, the body starts to secrete the hormones (some estrogen but mostly testosterone) that are responsible for more than sexual maturity; they also sponsor mood swings, teenage rebellion, proliferation of certain keratinocytes, and excess sebum production. This change in hormone levels along with some other issues account for the high incidence of acne among teenagers. Adults can get acne too, although not necessarily because of excessive testosterone production.

About 85% of Americans have acne at one time or another. During adolescence boys with acne outnumber girls, but during early adulthood women with acne outnumber men. After about age 45, the prevalence of acne is about 5% for both men and women.[11]

Etiology: What Happens?

The process of developing acne is complicated, with many contributing factors. This is a condition often associated with puberty, but it isn't exclusive to teens. The key factors that lead to acne include the following.

Factor 1: Testosterone production When a person enters puberty, one of the changes that occurs is the sudden secretion of high levels of androgens, male hormones that are secreted by both boys and girls. High levels of testosterone cause sebaceous glands, the oil glands that lubricate hair shafts, to shift into high gear. At this point it is especially important that sebaceous ducts to the surface of the skin stay clear. If any tiny particle, such as a bit of duct lining or a flake of dead skin, obstructs the duct, sebum rapidly accumulates behind the blockage. Unfortunately, keratinocytes in hair shafts are also sensitive to testosterone. When they hyperproliferate, the risk of a clogged sebaceous gland is very high.

Factor 2: Bacterial activity The pooling of oil in hair shafts is an invitation to the colonies of bacteria that grow on the skin. Most lesions are due to *Propionibacterium acnes*, which produces enzymes that exacerbate inflammation and cause bacteria to clump together. This leads to more colonization of the sebaceous ducts. Soon a localized infection leads to a pustule, a pimple, or some other acne lesion. These blemishes usually appear on the face, upper neck, and upper back.

Factor 3: Stress Stress can upset endocrine balance and slow the activity of immune system cells. (Stress and adolescence are also practically synonymous.) If the macrophages in the superficial fascia are sluggish, they don't fight off the bacteria that colonize the sebaceous glands. Furthermore, once the infection has subsided, those same suppressed macrophages are slower to consume the residual dead bacteria and white blood cells, so it takes longer for pimples to fade. Stress doesn't necessarily cause acne, but it can exacerbate it and slow the healing process.

Factor 4: Liver congestion When acne affects adults, it is often because liver congestion makes it difficult to neutralize the normal amounts of testosterone in the system. This leads to excess sebum production, bacterial colonization of sebaceous glands, and all the signs of acne. Causes of liver congestion vary from person to person, but high-fat diets, smoking, drugs, and chemical pollutants are the most common culprits.

Factor 5: Hormonal imbalance Hormonal changes that accompany the menstrual cycle or the beginning or ending of birth control pill prescriptions will often contribute to acne in women. Once an infection has become established in a sebaceous gland, the resultant inflammation and destructive enzymes may destroy the walls of the structure. This causes a more extreme inflammatory response and provides a better chance for the bacteria to invade more skin.

Signs and Symptoms

The symptoms of acne are probably familiar to most people. It can be locally painful, but it is not usually associated with systemic infection (Figure 2.26). An exception to this rule is a rare form called *acne fulminans*: this condition involves fever, joint pain, and general illness.

Bacterial infections of the skin can cause several different types of acne lesions:

- *Pimples* are infections trapped below the surface of the skin; they are raised, red, painful bumps or papules.
- *Cysts* are infections trapped deep in the dermis. They can protrude into the subcutaneous layer. Cysts may or may not be inflamed.

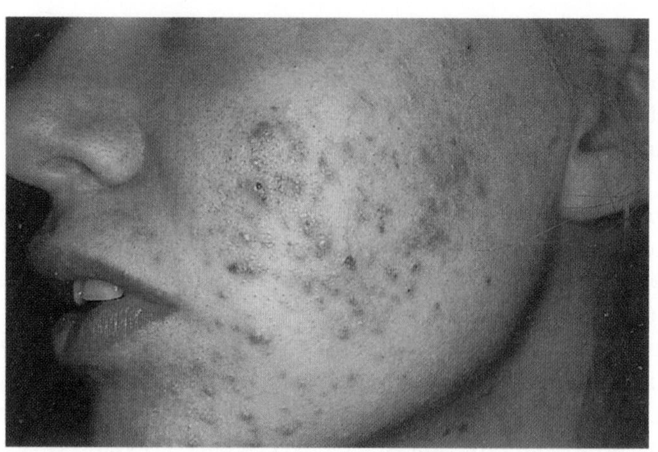

Figure 2.26. Acne vulgaris.

- *Open comedones* are also called blackheads. These infections are superficial, and the passage into the hair follicle is open to the air. This allows the trapped sebum to oxidize and turn dark. Blackheads are not, as popular belief would have it, trapped particles of dirt.
- *Closed comedones* are also called whiteheads, or pustules. They are superficial infections that are covered with a thin layer of epithelium that traps the sebum and pus.

Compare and Contrast 2.2
ACNE VERSUS BOILS

Boils and acne have some characteristics in common: they are both bacterial infections that may begin at hair follicles. But boils are far more serious than acne and require different precautions for massage therapists. Here are some differentiating features:

CHARACTERISTICS	BOILS	ACNE
Pattern of appearance	One lesion at a time or a small interconnected group of pustules.	Spread over large areas (face, back, neck)
Virulence	Aggressive bacteria; attack living tissue.	Less aggressive bacteria; take advantage of hospitable growth medium.
Symptoms	Extremely painful.	Mildly painful.
Communicability	Highly communicable.	Only with prolonged contact.
Special precautions	Local contraindication; may be systemic if signs of general infection are present. Isolate and bleach sheets.	Local contraindication; no other precautions necessary.

Treatment

For teenagers with acne the best advice is the most difficult to follow: *don't touch the face*. Touching, scratching, and popping acne lesions does little except to spread the bacteria and open the possibility of permanent scarring.

Washing the face twice daily with gentle soap and warm water is generally recommended before trying other interventions. Harsh soaps or scrubbing pads can make this condition much worse. Over-the-counter preparations usually use benzoyl peroxide or other similar substances to limit the activity of *P. acnes*.

When medical help is requested for acne, interventions usually involve topical or oral antibiotics, steroidal anti-inflammatories, or a group of drugs called *retinoins*. Retinoins can be used topically or as an oral medication. They are contraindicated if the patient may be pregnant during treatment, because they can cause birth defects.

Treatment options for acne-related scars are numerous. They include laser surgery, dermabrasion, and filling pockmarks with fat to smooth out their appearance.

Working with diet and other life habits to cleanse the liver and make its filtering job easier often results in clearer skin and a host of other benefits. Massage of the abdomen and liver may support this process, but it's erroneous to claim that massage clears up acne; too many other factors influence this process.

Massage?

Massage directly on acne lesions is obviously inappropriate. Pimples are infections, and they are associated with a compromised shield: the skin is no longer intact, which means massage can make the infection worse. Lesions can be locally painful. And finally, the lubricant can block sebaceous glands, further aggravating an already irritable situation. If just a few lesions are present, they can be locally avoided. But if the whole face, back, or neck is affected by acne, these areas may have to be skipped until the skin is healthier.

Wiping an acne-prone client with alcohol after an oily treatment would seem to make some sense because alcohol can remove *all* of the oil from the skin. But the sebaceous glands then work overtime to replace all the natural oils the alcohol just removed. If a client is concerned about the lubricant, the best options are to use a water-based lotion instead of oil or to recommend that the client shower with an astringent soap as soon as possible after treatment.

Modality Recommendations for Acne Vulgaris

MODALITY	RECOMMENDATION
Deep tissue massage	Locally contraindicated; otherwise supportive.
Lymphatic drainage	Supportive.
Polarity therapy	S/R/D: Locally contraindicated; otherwise indicated.
PNF/MET/stretching	Supportive.
Reflexology	Locally contraindicated; work intestines, liver, endocrine system, kidney points.
Shiatsu	Indicated. Use L/LI for skin, K/SP/TH for inflammation.
Swedish massage	Locally contraindicated while acute; otherwise supportive.
Trigger point therapy	Locally contraindicated while acute; otherwise supportive.

See Chapter 1 for a brief description of each modality, including definitions of abbreviations.

Dermatitis and Eczema in Brief

Pronunciation: dur-mah-TY-tis, EK-zeh-muh

What are they?

Dermatitis is an umbrella term for inflammation of the skin. Eczema is a noncontagious skin rash brought about by a hypersensitivity reaction. Contact dermatitis is an inflammation brought about by irritation or allergic responses on the skin.

How are they recognized?

Allergic or contact dermatitis presents in various ways, depending on what type of skin reactions are elicited. Exposure to poison oak or poison ivy results in large inflamed wheals; metal allergies tend to be less inflamed and more isolated in area.

Eczema may appear as very dry and flaky skin, coin-shaped lesions, yellowish oily patches, or blistered, weepy skin.

Is massage indicated or contraindicated?

The appropriateness of massage depends completely on the source of the problem and the condition of the skin. If the skin is very inflamed or has blisters or other lesions, massage is at least locally contraindicated until the acute stage has passed. If a rash could spread (i.e., poison oak), massage is systemically contraindicated while the irritation is present. If the skin is not itchy and the affected area is highly isolated, as with a metal allergy to a watchband or earrings, massage is only locally contraindicated.

Dermatitis and Eczema

Definition: What Is It?

Dermatitis is an umbrella term meaning skin inflammation, which is stunningly nonspecific. Many of the conditions in this chapter could be called dermatitis, although by convention the term *dermatitis* is reserved for disorders that are not infectious. This section focuses on eczema and contact dermatitis, with some brief discussions of other types of skin inflammation.

Contact dermatitis is a skin inflammation caused by an externally applied irritant or allergen. *Eczema* is a condition connected to immune dysfunction and hypersensitivity reactions expressed in the skin.

Demographics: Who Gets It?

Statistics on contact dermatitis are unavailable, since this is a general kind of problem and can accompany many other disorders. Eczema is common, affecting anywhere from 10% to 20% of infants. Most people grow out of it, but it continues to affect a small percentage of adults. Estimates suggest that about 15 million adults in the United States have eczema. While some of those people developed eczema as adults, about 95% of them first developed symptoms before age 5.[12]

Etiology: What Happens?

Many types of dermatitis are brought about by an overreaction in the immune system to some irritating substance. This is discussed in detail in the section on hypersensitivity reactions in Chapter 6, but it's useful to look at an encapsulated version here.

The two types of hypersensitivity reactions that create skin symptoms are type I allergic reactions and type IV delayed reactions.

Eczema is a type I reaction. These are systemic immune system responses to nonthreatening stimuli. In this situation mast cells release vasodilating chemicals, including histamine, which create an inflammatory response. Someone with eczema almost certainly has family members who live with hay fever or asthma, and about 75% of eczema patients develop these conditions themselves.[13]

Allergic contact dermatitis is a type IV reaction mediated by a complex organization of immune system agents. Poison oak, poison ivy, and local skin reactions to metals, soaps, dyes, and latex are examples of allergic contact dermatitis. With this type of reaction symptoms typically develop 12 to 48 hours after exposure.

Causes of Eczema

Research into the causes of eczema is proceeding, but no single factor has been identified. Contributing factors to eczema include the following:

- **A deficiency in certain fatty acids.** The lipid layer in the stratum corneum of the epidermis requires the correct nutrients to stay strong and intact. Without them it is weak, and any irritant or contaminant can stimulate an extreme reaction.
- **T-cell imbalance and dysfunction.** Some helper T cells are in short supply, while others are overly abundant in the skin of eczema patients. This alters the secretion of immunoregulating chemicals, especially inflammation-stimulating interleukin-4 (IL-4).

- **Elevated immunoglobulin-E (IgE).** These allergy-related antibodies cause excessive secretion of histamine. Histamine reinforces many inflammatory reactions, including capillary dilation, red skin, and itching.

Although it seems clear that eczema is connected to an immune system dysfunction, flares can be triggered by local irritations such as rough textures, detergents, harsh chemicals, extreme temperatures, and excessive sweating.

Causes of Contact Dermatitis

Contact dermatitis can arise from simple irritation or from an allergic reaction. Irritant contact dermatitis usually arises from prolonged contact with some substance that would eventually be irritating to *anyone*; this distinguishes it from allergic contact dermatitis. Irritants that can reliably bring about a reaction include working in water, harsh cleansers, acids and alkalis, and ongoing friction. These stimuli eventually damage even the healthiest skin, but removal from the irritation results in a cessation of symptoms.

Allergic contact dermatitis differs from irritant contact dermatitis because the causative factors create a specific type of allergic response in the skin of the affected person. Some common allergens associated with allergic contact dermatitis include nickel (found in watchbands, snaps, the buttons on jeans, and earrings), preservatives used in lotions, the adhesive used in many medical bandages, some perfumes and dyes, and latex. Allergic contact dermatitis tends to develop several hours after exposure to the trigger.

Signs and Symptoms of Eczema

Signs and symptoms of eczema vary according to what type is present.

- *Atopic dermatitis* is the most common variety. Atopic dermatitis is usually red, flaky and dry, occurring in the creases on the sides of the nose and other skin creases, such as knees, elbows, ankles, and hands (Figure 2.27). The skin may thicken and feel rough: this is called *lichenification*. As long as the skin is dry, intact, and not puffy or itchy, atopic dermatitis indicates massage. Therapists should be cautious, though, to make sure no breaks in the skin are present, and they should use a hypoallergenic lubricant that won't exacerbate the situation.

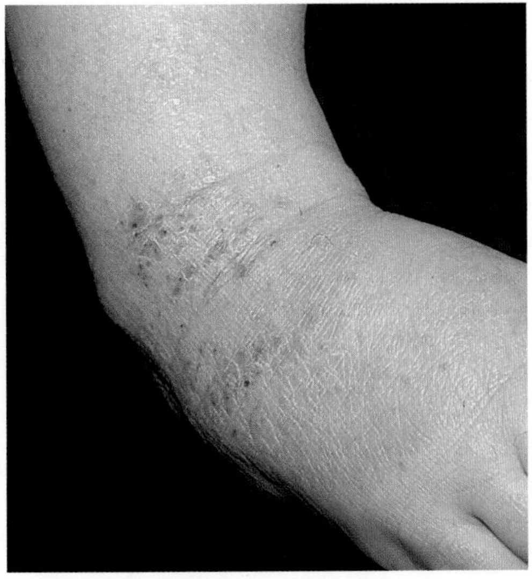

Figure 2.27. Atopic dermatitis.

- *Seborrheic eczema* produces yellowish, oily patches, usually in the skin folds around the nose or on the scalp.
- *Dyshidrosis* produces blisters filled with fluid that appear mostly on hands and feet. It is sometimes described as looking like a combination of fungal infection and a contact allergy (Figure 2.28). It often occurs in response to hot weather or emotional stress. Dyshidrosis can be difficult to treat and sometimes necessitates systemic steroids. Like atopic dermatitis, dyshidrosis is not contagious, but *unlike* the dry presentation of eczema, this one has seeping wounds, which exposes the client to infection. It is therefore a local contraindication for massage.
- *Nummular eczema* appears in small circular lesions, often on the legs and buttocks (Figure 2.29). It can resemble ringworm and be intensely itchy.

Signs and Symptoms of Contact Dermatitis

The symptoms of contact dermatitis vary according to the causative factors. Acute situations are typically locally red, swollen, and itchy or tender, showing exactly where the irritation took place (Figure 2.30). Long-lasting, low-grade reactions may not show signs of inflammation, although mild itchiness is common. Contact dermatitis locally contraindicates massage.

Other types of dermatitis show specific patterns but are not related to irritation or contact with allergenic substances:

- *Stasis dermatitis* usually appears on the lower legs in association with poor circulation, as seen with diabetes or heart failure. Stasis dermatitis is red or purplish and may occur with small ulcers where the skin has been deprived of nutrition. It often resembles erysipelas, a bacterial infection of the skin. Stasis dermatitis implies severe problems with blood flow and therefore contraindicates vigorous massage.
- *Neurodermatitis* involves a small injury, such as a mosquito bite, that creates an enormous inflammatory response and localized scaly patches of skin. It locally contraindicates massage until the inflammation has subsided.

Complications

Both contact dermatitis and eczema can begin a process by which a mildly irritating skin problem becomes a debilitating problem. When a person with dermatitis scratches the mildly itchy

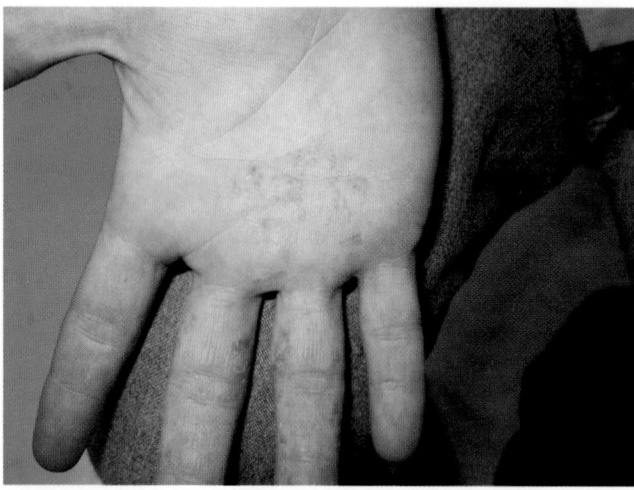

Figure 2.28. Dyshidrosis.

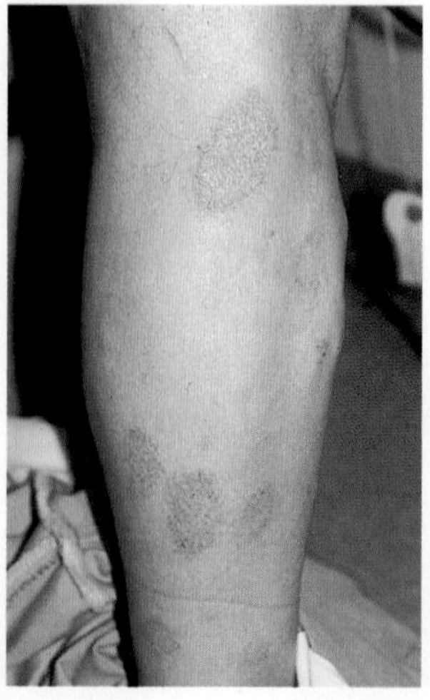

Figure 2.29. Nummular eczema.

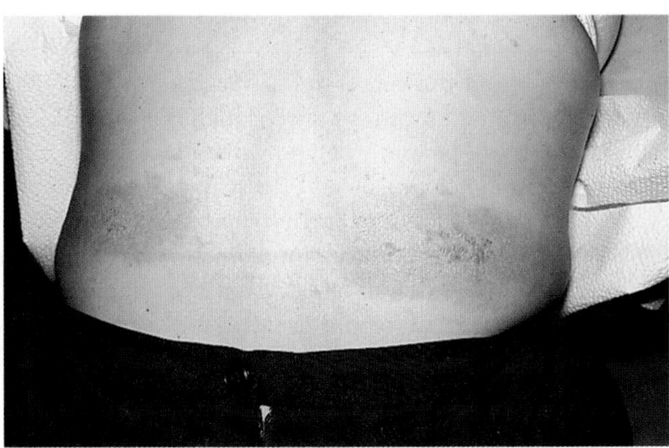

Figure 2.30. Contact allergic dermatitis.

lesions, the lesions are stimulated and become much itchier. This leads to more scratching, more itchiness, and a vicious circle called the itch-scratch cycle.

Persons with dermatitis or eczema are particularly susceptible to secondary infection because their skin may be delicate and easy to invade. Impetigo, herpes simplex, fungal infections, and warts are common complications of dermatitis and eczema.

Treatment

Self-help measures for people with contact dermatitis and eczema begin with trying to isolate the substances that irritate them and then avoiding them carefully. Persons with eczema must also try to maintain adequate hydration of the skin. This means finding a moisturizer or emollient that doesn't contain any irritating substances and applying it while the skin is still wet from bathing. Essential fatty acid supplements that help to strengthen the lipid layer in the skin may also be recommended.

Medical interventions for eczema and other skin problems include several options. Topical immunomodulators are creams that suppress immune system hyperactivity without the risks of long-term corticosteroids. These show good results for several inflammatory skin disorders, but they are associated with a low risk of cancer when used on children, so they are being watched carefully for long-term complications.

Antihistamines can sometimes quell an inflammatory response enough to stop the itch-scratch cycle and allow the skin to heal.

The traditional treatment for eczema is corticosteroids, which may be administered topically or orally. Cortisol is a powerful anti-inflammatory (Sidebar 2.3), but corticosteroid creams must be used *exactly* as prescribed because the risk of side effects is high. Corticosteroid creams can cause thinning skin, stretch marks, and an increased risk of skin infections. Orally administered steroids are also powerful anti-inflammatories, but they are associated with thinning bones, high blood pressure, high blood sugar, an increased risk of infection, cataracts, and other complications, so they are used only when no other options have been successful.

SIDEBAR 2.3: STRESS, ALLERGIES, AND CORTISOL

Stress can ripple through the body in a number of chemical ways. Massage therapists study some of these effects because they too have some influence over what chemicals are being released, and that influence should be informed and intentional.

For people who are prone to allergies, long-term stress creates some special problems. Cortisol is the hormone that is specifically related to long-term stress. When it is secreted over a long time, cortisol can damage the body by systemically weakening the connective tissues. But cortisol has one quality that makes it very, *very* useful: it is a powerful anti-inflammatory agent. When people undergo long-term stress, their cortisol supplies can be depleted. When cortisol is depleted, limited resources are available within the body to quell the inflammatory reaction. And for individuals subject to allergies, this means that they have a difficult time reducing the inflammation from immune system attacks against nonthreatening stimuli such as wheat, pollen, cat dander, and other irritants. If an immune reaction takes the form of a skin rash, it may be called dermatitis or eczema.

This is not to suggest that stress is the only cause of allergies or even the most important one; it's just to point out that long-term stress and cortisol depletion can often make allergies *worse*.

Massage?

The appropriateness of massage depends entirely on the causes and severity of a client's dermatitis. If the skin is red, hot, puffy, and itchy from a morning walk through poison oak, massage is *not* appropriate. First, the inflammation would be exacerbated by extra blood flow to the area, and second, the irritating substance (the poison oak oils) can be distributed over more of the body surface, and possibly to the therapist as well. Massage for this person and all other persons with acute dermatitis is systemically contraindicated until the inflammation has subsided.

If, on the other hand, a client displays a small, slightly reddened, flaky circular area on the back of the left wrist (about the place where a wristwatch would usually rest), it may be possible to pursue a line of questioning to determine that there is no danger of massage aggravating or spreading the irritation, which is probably being caused by an allergy to nickel.

The appropriateness of massage for eczema depends on the type and whether or not the skin has been compromised to point where there is danger of infection. For more details, see the individual descriptions earlier in the chapter.

Modality Recommendations for Dermatitis/Eczema

MODALITY	RECOMMENDATION
Deep tissue massage	Locally contraindicated; otherwise supportive.
Lymphatic drainage	Supportive.
Polarity therapy	S/R/D: Locally contraindicated; otherwise indicated.
PNF/MET/stretching	Locally contraindicated while acute; otherwise supportive.
Reflexology	Indicated: work liver, endocrine glands, lymphatic system, intestines, kidneys.
Shiatsu	Indicated. Use L/LI for skin, K/SP/TH for inflammation.
Swedish massage	Locally contraindicated while acute; otherwise supportive.
Trigger point therapy	Locally contraindicated while acute; otherwise supportive.

See Chapter 1 for a brief description of each modality, including definitions of abbreviations.

Hives in Brief

What are they?
Hives are an inflammatory skin reaction to a variety of triggers.

How are they recognized?
Hives range from small red spots to large wheals, which are pink to red, warm to the touch, and itchy. Individual lesions generally subside within a few hours, but successive hives may appear; the cycle can continue for several weeks.

Is massage indicated or contraindicated?
Hives contraindicate most types of massage during the acute stage. Hands-on bodywork would bring even more circulation to the skin, making a bad situation worse.

Hives

Definition: What Are They?

Hives, also called *urticaria*, are the result of emotional stress, an allergy, or some other stimulus. They are areas of intense heat, swelling, and itchiness on the skin. Hives are very common; it is estimated that 15% to 20% of people have them at some point.[14]

Etiology: What Happens?

Consider someone who is allergic to shellfish. Somehow a shrimp finds its way into his lemon grass soup. Within moments his immune system cells launch a full-scale attack—but they don't quite know where to go. In the confusion, specialized cells called mast cells freely distributed in the superficial fascia release histamine and a host of other inflammatory chemicals. This causes local capillary dilation, extra cell permeability, and edema.

Triggers for hives vary from one individual to another. Sometimes hives are an allergic reaction, but others seem to be related to physical or emotional stress. Some allergy immunologists have organized hives into these classifications:

- *Acute hives* are short-lived (lasting from minutes to up to 6 weeks). They can be set off by an allergic reaction; an infection with strep throat, a common cold, or mononucleosis; an insect bite or sting; or triggers that are never fully identified.
- *Cholinergic hives* typically appear as hundreds of tiny wheals that appear with rapid changes in temperature. Exercise, especially in cold temperatures that is followed by rapid heating, can elicit these. Swimming in cold water may trigger them in sensitive people. Other people may develop them with too much exposure to the sun or excessive sweating. Cholinergic hives can be extreme and may require medical treatment.
- *Physical hives* appear in response to a physical trigger, like scraping or constant pressure on the skin. They are large, hot, and slow to subside. *Dermographia* (skin writing) is the term used to describe hives that arise after mild scratches to the skin.
- *Chronic hives* is a rarer presentation that involves lesions that may persist for 6 weeks or more. They are often idiopathic, but a small percentage of people with chronic hives can trace them to thyroid problems, autoimmune diseases, liver dysfunction, or viral infection.

Signs and Symptoms

Histamine release in the skin causes a localized inflammatory response (redness), and the edema presses on nerve endings (itching). Hives begin as small, raised, reddened areas called wheals that may join to become larger irregular patches (Figure 2.31). The lesions are red around the outside and are sometimes paler in the middle. They are often hot to the touch. They are not contagious but are usually brought about by a food allergy, an insect bite or sting, a reaction to medication, emotional stress, or environmental changes.

Individual hives usually clear within a few hours, but they may be replaced by other hives, sometimes in other locations. It is common for a person to have ongoing hives for days or weeks at a time.

Treatment

Hives are always annoying but seldom serious. If they require treatment, it is usually in the form of an antihistamine to quell histamine release. Even chronic urticaria is treated this way. Antihistamines for hives are usually prescribed in heavy doses to undo all the work of the mast cells. This can be problematic, as high doses of antihistamines often have a sedative effect. If antihistamines are unsuccessful, topical or systemic doses of steroidal anti-inflammatories may be recommended.

Angioedema is a variation on hives that can be a medical emergency. These hives involve deeper layers of the skin, usually around the face and throat. The tissue can swell to the point that

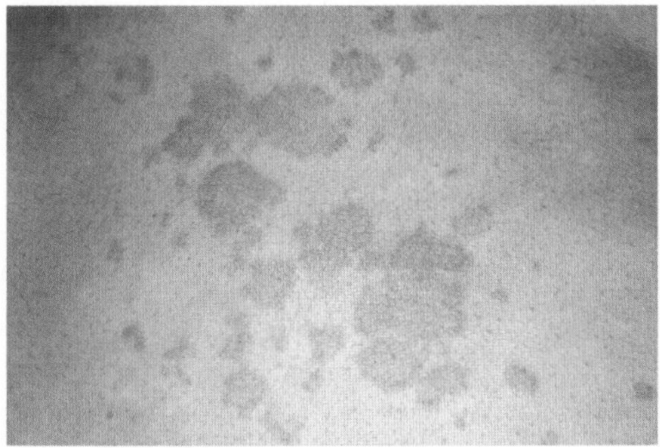

Figure 2.31. Hives.

breathing becomes difficult. It is rare, but angioedema can be life threatening, requiring an immediate injection of steroids to bring down the swelling and restore ease of breathing. Angioedema is discussed in more detail in the section on allergic reactions in Chapter 6.

Massage?

Most types of bodywork tend to exacerbate hives by pulling more blood flow to areas that are already hyperactive. If a treatment can be devised to quell or cool an irritated area, that would be an appropriate intervention. Clients with a tendency toward hives may require therapists to use hypoallergenic lubricants to avoid creating a trigger.

Modality Recommendations for Hives

MODALITY	RECOMMENDATION
Deep tissue massage	Locally contraindicated; otherwise supportive.
Lymphatic drainage	Systemically contraindicated.
Polarity therapy	S/R: Indicated within client comfort. D: Contraindicated while acute; otherwise supportive.
PNF/MET/stretching	Contraindicated while acute; otherwise supportive.
Reflexology	Contraindicated while acute; once cleared, work lymphatic system points.
Shiatsu	Indicated. Use L/LI for skin, fire element meridians for stress.
Swedish massage	Locally contraindicated while acute; otherwise supportive.
Trigger point therapy	Locally contraindicated while acute; otherwise supportive.

See Chapter 1 for a brief description of each modality, including definitions of abbreviations.

Psoriasis in Brief
Pronunciation: so-RY-uh-sis

What is it?
Psoriasis is a noncontagious chronic skin disease involving the excessive production of new skin cells that pile up into isolated or connected lesions.

How is it recognized?
The most common variety of psoriasis looks like pink or reddish patches, sometimes with a silvery scale on top. It occurs most frequently on elbows and knees, but it can develop anywhere. Other types of psoriasis look like pustules, small red circles, or shiny reddened skin.

Is massage indicated or contraindicated?
Psoriasis locally contraindicates mechanical massage during the acute stage, because the extra stimulation and circulation massage provides can make a bad situation worse. But in subacute stages, as long as the skin is intact, massage is safe and appropriate.

Neoplastic Skin Disorders

Psoriasis

Definition: What Is It?

The introduction to this chapter discusses how the readiness of epithelium to repair itself is a two-edged sword. On the one hand, the body can heal quickly and thoroughly from most insults to the skin. On the other hand, sometimes the ease of replication in skin cells can cause problems, as with this condition. ***Psoriasis*** is a chronic skin disease with occasional acute episodes in which epithelial cells in isolated patches replicate too rapidly. Where normal skin cells replace themselves every 28 to 32 days, psoriatic skin cells divide every 2-4 days. The result is a pileup of excess cells that are itchy, red or pink, and scaly. This condition comes and goes, and at present no permanent cure is available.

Demographics: Who Gets It?

Statistics on psoriasis vary. It probably affects 6 to 7 million Americans and is most common in whites. About 150,000 new cases are diagnosed every year. Some cases have a genetic link. It is most commonly diagnosed in middle years, but it has been seen on tiny babies as well as quite elderly people. Psoriasis occurs in a range of severity. Most people have it in a mild form; only about 20% report their psoriasis as moderate to severe.[15]

Etiology: What Happens?

The mysteries of psoriasis are slowly being solved. It seems clear now that this disease is related to an immune system dysfunction involving overactive T cells and the chemical signals they release. These chemicals trigger inflammation and proliferation of new skin cells. These insights have led to new treatment options for psoriasis that have been more successful than past efforts.

Signs and Symptoms

Plaque psoriasis is a very common condition; most people have at least seen it. It usually takes the form of raised red or pink patches that over a long time develop a white or silvery scale on top (Figure 2.32). Plaques have well-defined edges. They may be itchy, but they are seldom very uncomfortable unless they are in an acute stage, when they can itch and burn severely. Most plaques are on the knees or elbows, but they can be found on the scalp, trunk, palms and soles, inside the mouth, and around the genitals. Some patients develop psoriatic plaques over much of their skin (Figure 2.33). Psoriasis can also get under fingernails and toenails, where it can cause pitting, infection, and sometimes loss of the nail altogether, a condition called *onycholysis.*

Psoriasis often occurs in cycles of acute flares followed by periods of remission; this is a pattern seen with many diseases involving immune system dysfunction. Psoriatic flares can be triggered by a number of things: physical or emotional trauma, skin damage, sunburn, hormonal changes, prescription drugs for high blood pressure and depression, or a state of immunosuppression.

In its subacute or inactive phase, a slight discoloration may remain on the skin where the lesions tend to appear. This is true especially on the trunk.

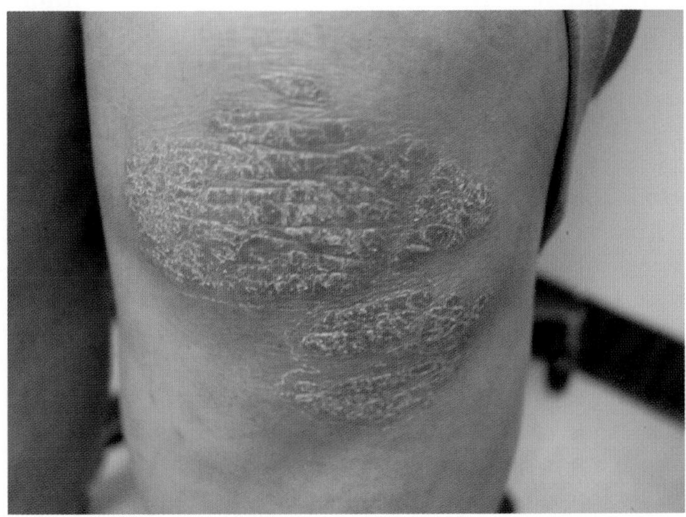

Figure 2.32. Psoriasis.

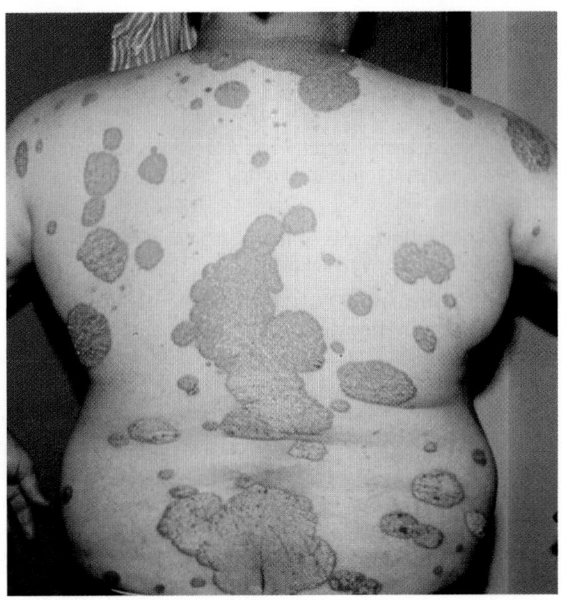

Figure 2.33. Severe psoriasis.

Other varieties of psoriasis are less common than plaque psoriasis but can be more serious. They include the following:

- *Guttate psoriasis* is usually triggered by a viral or bacterial infection of the respiratory tract. It looks like small circular lesions spread over large areas. It resembles plaque psoriasis, but the lesions tend to be smaller and shallower.
- *Pustular psoriasis* involves small, noninfectious pustules in the affected areas. It is triggered by some medications, topical irritants, too much exposure to UV radiation, and pregnancy. It often occurs on the palms and soles.
- *Inverse psoriasis* appears at skin folds under the breasts, in the armpits, and around the genitals. The skin becomes red and shiny and is vulnerable to secondary infection with yeast or fungus.
- *Erythrodermic psoriasis* is triggered by sunburn and steroidal anti-inflammatories (or by a sudden *stop* in the use of steroidal anti-inflammatories). It covers large areas of skin in a bright red, hot, painful rash. The extensive fluid loss and exfoliation that can occur with an acute episode of erythrodermic psoriasis can be a medical emergency.

Complications

Psoriasis is rarely a life-threatening condition, although it can be extreme and uncomfortable in the acute stages. In severe cases profound drying and cracking of the skin can lead to infection, fluid loss, and shock.

Another complication of psoriasis is *psoriatic arthritis*. This is a type of joint inflammation that affects about 10% to 30% of psoriasis patients.[16] It occurs in several subtypes (Sidebar 2.4) but follows the typical flare-and-remission cycle as other autoimmune disorders. The guidelines for massage and psoriatic arthritis are the same as those for rheumatoid arthritis, discussed in Chapter 3.

SIDEBAR 2.4: PSORIATIC ARTHRITIS

Between 6 and 7 million people in the United States have psoriasis, and somewhere between 10% and 30% of them are at risk for developing a serious related condition called psoriatic arthritis.[15] This joint disease occurs in several subtypes, in varying degrees of severity.

- **Symmetric arthritis** resembles rheumatoid arthritis, although it is less severe. As its name implies, it appears in a symmetric pattern.
- **Asymmetric arthritis** may affect few or several joints, especially in the hands and feet. Fingers and toes may swell significantly with this disorder; this is called *dactylitis*, or sausage digit.
- **DIP arthritis** means *distal interphalangeal predominant*. This affects the distal joints at the fingers and toes and may also damage the nail.
- **Spondylitis** affects the spine. In many ways this condition resembles ankylosing spondylitis.
- **Arthritis mutilans** is the most severe form of psoriatic arthritis, and it affects fewer than 5% of all patients. It can be severely crippling, damaging joints in the hands, feet, neck, and low back.

Flares of psoriatic arthritis are usually preceded by an outbreak of skin psoriasis. This condition is easily confused with gout, rheumatoid arthritis, and reactive arthritis (joint inflammation related to an infection or reaction to medication), so getting an accurate diagnosis is important, because psoriatic arthritis requires a different treatment from that of most other types of joint inflammation.

Treatment

Psoriasis has no permanent cure, but recent insights into the mechanism of the disease have led to the discovery of new options for treating this stubborn condition. Traditionally the three main avenues pursued with psoriasis treatments include topical medications, phototherapy, and systemic medications.

Topical medications vary from coal tar (popular because it carries a minimum of side effects but problematic because it smells bad and stains clothing) to vitamin D ointments to steroid creams of various strengths. Other topical treatments include salicylic acid (which is also used to remove warts) to help dissolve and remove plaques, and oatmeal or Epsom salt baths.

Phototherapy includes limited exposure to sunshine or carefully regulated doses of exposure to UVA or UVB lights. UV exposure stimulates vitamin D production, which in turn inhibits skin cell replication. Too much UV exposure can exacerbate symptoms though, so this therapy must be used cautiously.

Systemic medications may be steroidal drugs, retinoids to limit sebaceous secretions, or cytotoxic drugs (as in chemotherapy) to limit the activity of those skin cells that have run amok.

Topical and systemic therapies are often combined with phototherapy. PUVA is a common example: this is a combination of a systemic medication (psoralen) and UVA light exposure. PUVA is often successful. Unfortunately, it is also linked to increased chances of contracting squamous cell carcinoma as well as some other serious side effects.

A new strategy in the treatment of psoriasis involves a group of drugs called TNF blockers. TNF (tumor necrosis factor) is an immune system mediator associated with inflammation. Blocking its activity keeps the inflammatory process (and accompanying proliferation of extra skin cells) under control. Other biological therapies are in development as well.

Although many types of treatment for psoriasis have been developed, none of them has shown to be a permanent solution. Patients with very severe cases of psoriasis must frequently change strategies as their skin builds up resistance to treatment.

Massage?

In ancient Greece, massage with olive oil was the prescribed treatment for psoriasis. It is now recognized that massage *on* the lesions during an acute outbreak may aggravate the situation by stimulating circulation in an area where too much activity is already taking place. Psoriasis is a local contraindication when it itches or hurts, but otherwise massage is appropriate. (Of course, it is necessary to ensure that no cracking of the skin could make the client vulnerable to secondary infection.)

Psoriasis isn't spread by massage, it isn't contagious, and massage may be able indirectly to help deal with some of the internal and external stress factors that can stimulate an outbreak. Furthermore, people with psoriasis may have issues with self-image that massage—nonjudgmental, welcomed, educated touch—can help to address.

Modality Recommendations for Psoriasis

MODALITY	RECOMMENDATION
Deep tissue massage	Locally contraindicated; otherwise supportive.
Lymphatic drainage	Supportive.
Polarity therapy	S: Indicated within client comfort. R: Supportive, within client comfort. D: Locally contraindicated; indicated elsewhere.
PNF/MET/stretching	Supportive.
Reflexology	Indicated: work liver, endocrine glands, lymphatic system, kidney points.
Shiatsu	Supportive.
Swedish massage	Locally contraindicated; elsewhere highly indicated for parasympathetic activity.
Trigger point therapy	Locally contraindicated while acute; otherwise supportive.

See Chapter 1 for a brief description of each modality, including definitions of abbreviations.

Skin Cancer

Definition: What Is It?

Cancer is the uncontrolled replication of cells into tumors. These tumors can invade surrounding tissues, can spread throughout the body, and are sometimes fatal. The tissues that are most vulnerable to cancer are those that tolerate a lot of wear and tear: skin cells, the epithelium of the lungs, and the inner layer of the colon are some good examples. These cells heal easily and rapidly, but sometimes that feature backfires and cells that have endured a lifetime of abuse start "healing" in a way that can quite possibly kill.

Skin Cancer in Brief

What is it?
Skin cancer is cancer in the stratum basale of the epidermis (basal cell carcinoma, or BCC); cancer of the keratinocytes in the epidermis (squamous cell carcinoma, or SCC); or cancer of the melanocytes (pigment cells) of the epidermis (malignant melanoma).

How is it recognized?
For BCC and SCC, look for the giveaway sign: sores that never heal or that consistently come and go in the same place. These sores can resemble blisters, warts, pimples, scars, or simple unexplained bumps and abrasions. They are usually painless but may bleed or be slightly itchy as the cells become active. For malignant melanoma, look for a molelike lesion that exhibits the ABCDE signs of melanoma or that looks significantly different from all other moles on the person.

Is massage indicated or contraindicated?
For BCC, which does not metastasize, massage is a local contraindication as long as a dermatologist has diagnosed the lesion. SCC and malignant melanoma carry the risk of metastasis. Therefore any decisions about massage must be made according to stage at diagnosis and the treatments the client undergoes.

Demographics: Who Gets It?

Some people wish that sleep could be cumulative: that a person could sleep an extra 14 hours on a weekend and then not be tired for all of the following week. Well, in a certain way, *sunlight* is cumulative. Picture a person playing on the monkey bars when he's 5, rollerblading when he's 10, hiking in the mountains when he's 15, sailing when he's 40, and snorkeling when he's 50. His skin cells are keeping accurate records of exactly how much and how often he's insulted them with too much sun. And one day, those skin cells may respond to all that exposure by going into overactive production. This is a particular risk with these additional factors:

- Multiple severe sunburns in childhood
- Living in the South or at high elevation
- Immunosuppression
- Any previous history of any kind of skin cancer
- Multiple or atypical moles
- History of exposure to coal tar, creosote, arsenic compounds, or radium.[17]

Skin cancer is the most common variety of cancer in humans; it accounts for almost half of cancer diagnoses in the United States.[18] The American Academy of Dermatology estimates that 1 in 5 American adults will have skin cancer at some time. About 1 million Americans are diagnosed with cancer each year. Of those diagnoses, approximately 110,000 are for malignant melanoma and 890,000 are for other skin cancer.[19]

{AU}

Skin cancer kills about 11,000 people per year: 7,900 die of malignant melanoma and 2,800 of other skin cancer. The mortality rate of skin cancer has risen 165% over the past 50 years; this is probably related to longer life spans and an increasing population of elderly people, who are most at risk for developing this disease.[19]

Etiology: What Happens?

Three basic types of skin cancer and one precancerous condition are the most common forms of this disease; each is discussed in detail.

Actinic Keratosis: Precancerous Lesions

Definition: What Is It?

Also called solar keratosis, *actinic keratosis* (AK) can lead to squamous cell carcinoma (SCC). Some authorities describe AK as a cancer that develops in the deepest layers of the epidermis; others maintain that it is a precancerous condition. Several subtypes of AK include *actinic*

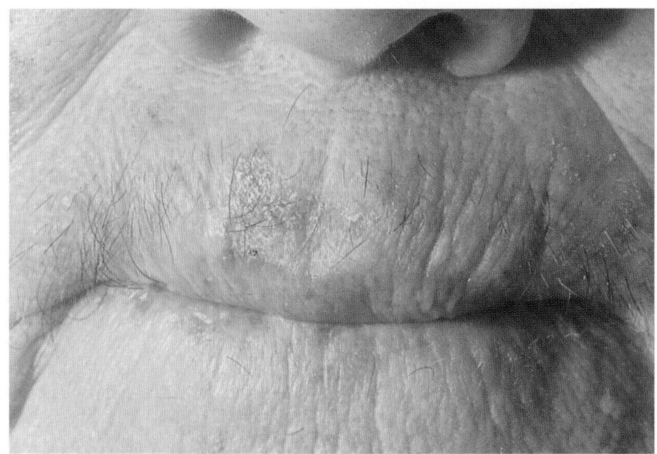

Figure 2.34. Actinic keratosis: lips.

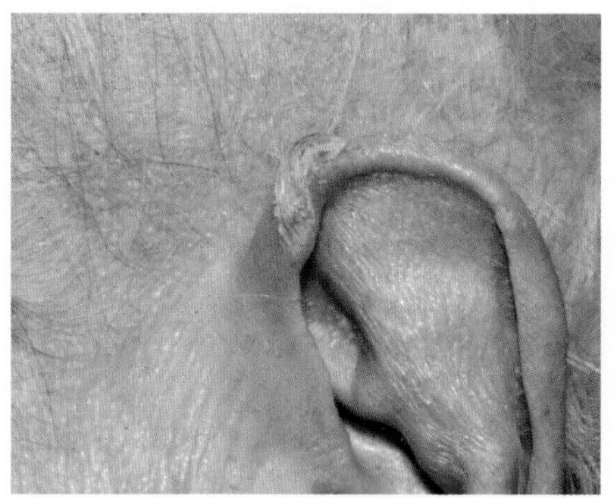

Figure 2.35. Actinic keratosis: ear.

cheilitis (an aggressive form of AK lesions that appear on the lips), *leukoplakia* (white patches on the tongue or inside the cheek), and *Bowen's disease,* a form of in situ squamous cell carcinoma.

Signs and Symptoms

Brown or red scaly lesions usually appear on the forehead, tops of ears, hands, or other areas subject to a lot of sun exposure (Figures 2.34 and 2.35). People often report that the lesions have a rough or gritty texture. About 5% to 20% of all untreated AK lesions have the potential to develop into SCC, which is a potentially dangerous disease.[20]

Treatment

AK lesions are usually frozen off with liquid nitrogen. They may also be injected with medication, or a topical ointment may be applied. Very large lesions may be excised.

Massage?

AK is usually considered a precancerous condition and therefore does not contraindicate massage. However, a client who has AK lesions should consider having them removed promptly. If he has a history of AK but nothing more serious has developed, massage is appropriate. All undiagnosed skin lesions are a caution for massage therapists, who should recommend that their clients consult their doctor as soon as possible.

Basal Cell Carcinoma

Definition: What Is It?

BCC is by far the most common type of skin cancer; it accounts for about 75% to 90% of all skin cancer cases.[21] It is a slow-growing tumor of epithelial cells in the stratum basale of the epidermis. It does not metastasize and is not usually dangerous, although if the tumor is left untreated it can become threatening because of the other tissues that are eroded by the tumor's growth: nearby arteries or nerves, for example.

The risk of BCC is related to long-term, low-grade exposure to UV radiation as opposed to occasional severe sunburns. Other contributing factors include exposure to other forms of radiation, high levels of arsenic in the drinking water, and a rare genetic disease *(xeroderma pigmentosum)* that makes it difficult to recover from UV radiation damage.

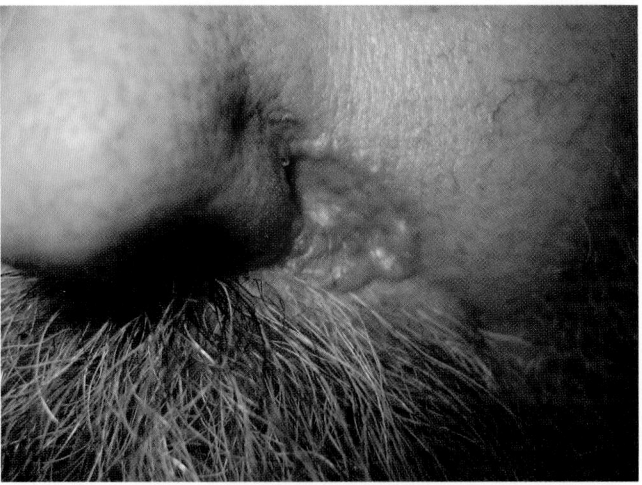

Figure 2.36. Basal cell carcinoma.

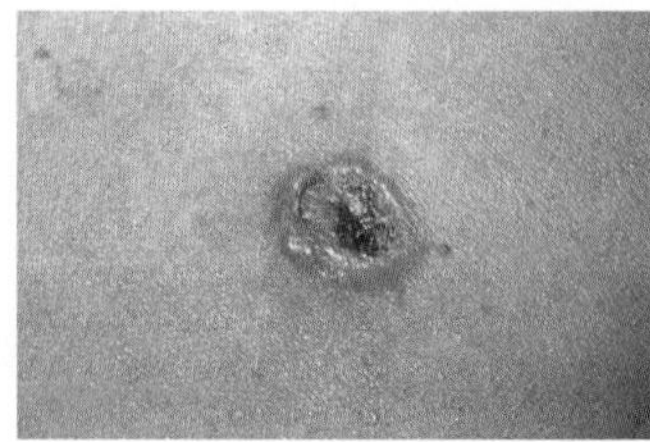

Figure 2.37. Basal cell carcinoma.

Signs and Symptoms

BCC can be difficult to describe because it has several presentations (Figures 2.36–2.38). The most common versions of BCC include the following:

- *Nodular BCC* is the most common form. Typically it appears on the head, neck, or back. It looks like a small, hard lump, with rounded edges and a soft, sunken middle. It may have visible tiny blood vessels, called telangiectasias. The borders are usually well defined, with a pearly sheen. BCC tends to bleed easily and form crusts. The scab may fall off and reform, but the lesion never permanently heals. This pattern is the single most important sign of skin cancer other than melanoma: it usually shows as a sore that doesn't heal or that comes and goes in the same place.
- *Pigmented BCC* looks like nodular BCC, but the lesions tend to be dark brown or black. They appear most often on people with dark skin.
- *Superficial BCC* can resemble eczema or psoriasis. It often appears on the trunk in pink or reddish-brown patches. It tends not to be aggressive, affecting only the superficial layers of the skin. Multiple lesions may indicate a history of exposure to arsenic.
- *Micronodular BCC* can be aggressive, showing multiple small, well-defined, yellowish-white lesions.

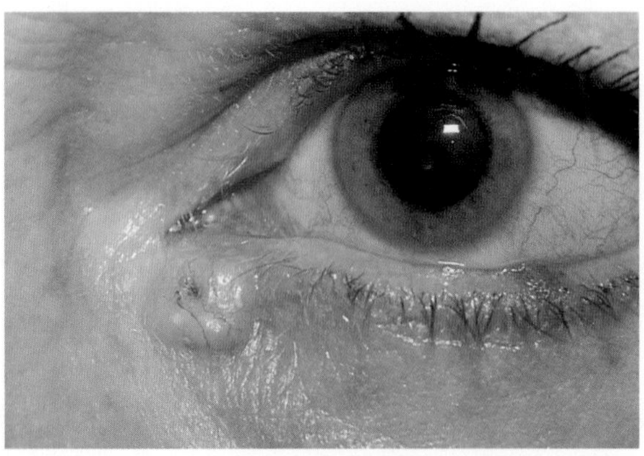

Figure 2.38. Basal cell carcinoma.

- *Morpheaform or infiltrating BCC* often looks like scar tissue on the surface of the skin (in a place where no trauma has taken place). It can be aggressive and can invade deep tissues while showing only a small mark on the surface of the skin.

Treatment

BCC has an extremely high survival rate if lesions are removed before they invade deep tissues. It is usually excised: cut out with a curette (a scoop-shaped blade) or a laser. The tumor-producing cells can also be killed off with liquid nitrogen or with radiation. BCC frequently recurs: about half of patients have another lesion within 5 years of the first one. Furthermore, a history of BCC increases the risk of developing malignant melanoma later in life, so it is important to be vigilant about any skin changes.

Massage?

Any tumor is a local contraindication, of course. BCC doesn't spread through the body, so the risk of making the situation worse is nonexistent. Because massage therapists often see more of a client's skin than the client can, they are in an excellent position to point out anomalies early that may lead to a successful diagnosis and treatment.

Squamous Cell Carcinoma

Definition: What Is It?

SCC is a malignancy of keratinocytes in the middle layers of the epidermis. It's incidence is about 105 cases per 100,00 people in the United States.[22]

SCC can develop anywhere in epidermis cells: it is usually found on the external skin, but occasionally it develops in mucous membranes too. It is especially common on ears, hands, and lower lips, but it can also grow *inside* the mouth, often as a response to pipe smoking or chewing tobacco and the constant irritation that those habits incur. SCC that grows on the penis or vaginal walls is associated with a history of genital warts.

Most cases of SCC are related to long-term sun exposure: it has been found that chronic exposure to UVB radiation (mid-range UV light) can lead to inactivation of an important tumor suppressor gene. Chronic skin inflammation, as seen with decubitus ulcers, repeating boils, or draining sores, can also increase the risk of SCC. Immunosuppression is another contributing factor: SCC is 18 to 36 times more common in transplant recipients who take medication to prevent tissue rejection than in the general population.[22]

SCC is potentially more dangerous than BCC, because in 2% to 6% of cases it metastasizes through the lymph system. Close to 3,000 people die of SCC every year in the United States.[22]

Signs and Symptoms

SCC tumors often appear on preexisting lesions and on sun-exposed skin or in places where the skin has a long history of damage and repair. The sores appear and *don't heal*: the cardinal sign of non-melanoma skin cancer. The borders of SCCs are often less distinct than those of the more self-contained basal cell tumors (Figures 2.39 and 2.40). Some but not all SCC lesions begin as actinic keratosis. They may appear as hard, firm lumps that look like a wart. They may be tender and bleed easily. Some tumors invade nearby nerves and may interfere with sensation or motor control.

Treatment

SCC lesions are typically frozen with liquid nitrogen, carefully shaved in thin layers with examination for a clear border of healthy cells (this is called Mohs micrographic surgery, or

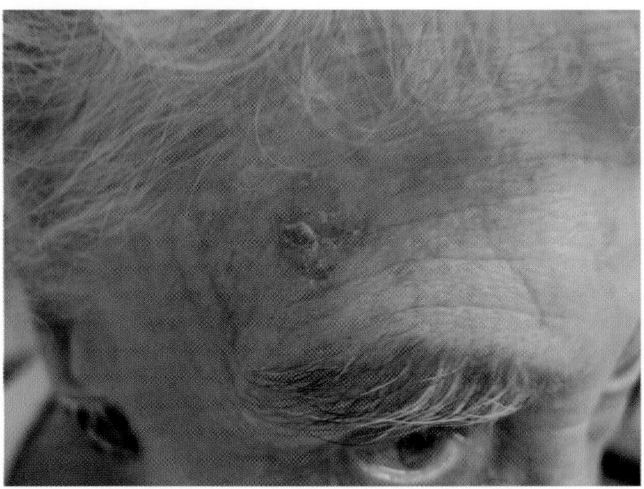

Figure 2.39. Squamous cell carcinoma.

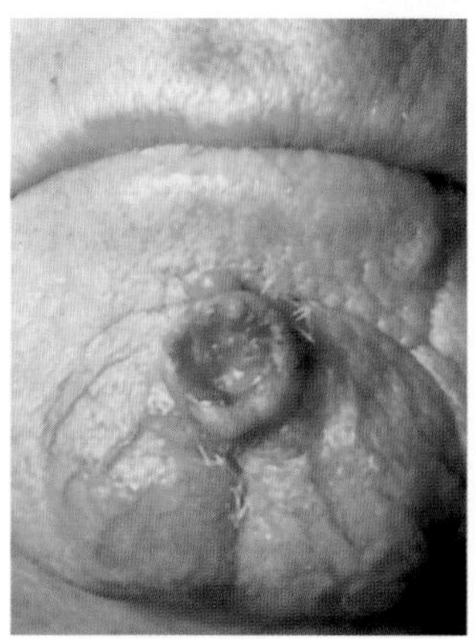

Figure 2.40. Squamous cell carcinoma.

MMS), or excised. With SCC it is especially important to be sure that *all* of the affected tissue is removed, because if any cells find their way into the lymph system, the cancer could spread elsewhere in the body. Therefore, excess tissue is often also taken, which may require postoperative skin grafts. The area may also then be irradiated to make doubly sure all of the cancer-causing cells are dead.

Massage?

SCC is not always aggressive, but it can be. People in treatment may undergo surgery, skin grafts, irradiation, chemotherapy, or any combination thereof. These treatments carry specific cautions for massage that are outlined in the article on cancer in Chapter 12. Massage can be appropriate for people who are fighting cancer, but the therapist must make sure the client and the health care team are fully informed and design a treatment that delivers maximum benefit with a minimum of risk.

Malignant Melanoma

Definition: What Is It?

Melanocytes are the pigment cells that give skin its color. They are deep in the epidermis, but they are also found in the eye, the gastrointestinal and reproductive tracts, and a few other locations in the body. Melanin in the skin protects us, as much as it can, from harmful UV radiation from the sun. As in the other cancers discussed here, if melanocytes get *too much* stimulation, they may undergo a genetic mutation that signals them to replicate without control. This is malignant melanoma.

Although a history of exposure to sunlight (especially with extreme, blistering sunburns) is a leading risk factor for malignant melanoma, it *can* develop in areas that are not usually exposed to the sun. It can even grow in internal melanocytes: mucous membranes of the respiratory, digestive, reproductive, and urinary tract may all develop malignant melanoma.

Demographics: Who Gets It?

Melanoma is the leading cause of death from skin diseases and the cause of about 72% of deaths from skin cancer. The incidence of malignant melanoma is rising quickly; numbers of people diagnosed with this disease rise by 5% to 9% each year.[23]

While this disease can affect adults of any age, gender, or racial background, it is most common in elderly white men. It is the fifth most commonly diagnosed cancer in men and the seventh most common cancer diagnosis among women.[19]

Signs and Symptoms

Melanoma often starts from a preexisting mole that one day begins to change; it lightens, darkens, thickens, and may become elevated. Sometimes it itches or bleeds around the edges. In later stages its texture may change. Melanoma doesn't always start from a mole, however, nor does it always begin in areas that have been exposed to the sun.

Here is a simple mnemonic to remember the key features for melanoma:

- *A: Asymmetrical.* Most benign moles are circular or oval. A melanoma has an indeterminate shape.
- *B: Border.* The borders of melanomas are irregular and may be indistinct as it blends into the skin.
- *C: Color.* The colors of most moles are consistent: they are brown or black but not both. Melanomas are typically multicolored, with brown, black, and even purple all mixed together.
- *D: Diameter.* Melanomas are large. Any mole that is bigger than 6 mm across should be examined by a dermatologist.
- *E: Elevated.* Melanomas are usually at least partly elevated from the skin. They may even be big enough to snag on things and bleed.

Elevation is not a consistent sign with melanoma, so any lesion that exhibits the ABCD signs should be investigated.

Men most often get melanoma on the trunk, neck or head. Women tend to get it on the arms or legs.

Four specific types of malignant melanoma have been identified:

- *Superficial spreading melanoma* is the most common variety. It spreads along the surface before invading the deeper tissues. It may be multicolored and slightly elevated (Figure 2.41).
- *Lentigo melanoma* also begins as a superficial discoloration, usually very flat, in varying shades of brown (Figure 2.42). Lesions often show a marked notch.
- *Acral lentiginous melanoma* is the variety that is as common in nonwhite people as in whites. It is also the most common among young adults. It usually appears on the hands or feet, between the fingers or toes, or under the nails (Figure 2.43).
- *Nodular melanoma* is the most aggressive and dangerous type of skin cancer; it exhibits significant elevation from the skin, and the lesions often invade deeper tissues early in development (Figure 2.44). It tends to be small in diameter and firm to the touch, and it grows rapidly: people typically report seeing changes within several weeks.

SIDEBAR 2.5: SKIN PIGMENTATIONS

Age and the uneven distribution of melanin in the skin can give rise to several types of skin patches. Because massage therapists work closely with the skin, it is important to be familiar with the most common types of marks clients carry.

Moles

Moles, or *nevi,* are benign neoplasms: areas where melanocytes replicate on site without threatening to invade surrounding tissues. The melanocytes produce excessive melanin, the coloring agent for skin. Most moles are small, symmetrical, and one color (brown, black, purple, blue, or reddish), with clearly defined borders. When moles begin to change or if new ones develop (especially in adulthood) that display other characteristics, they should be examined by a dermatologist.

Port Wine Stains

A variety of moles that affect blood vessels near the surface of the skin cause port wine stains. They are often quite large and are harmless.

Freckles

Freckles are simple concentrations of melanin in the skin. They can range from light tan to red but are always darker than the surrounding skin. Most freckles are about the size of a nail-head, although when several blend together they can seem much larger. Fair-skinned people are more susceptible to freckles than others. Freckles often darken when they are exposed to sunlight and fade when they are protected from UV radiation.

Lentigines

Lentigines (singular *lentigo*) are similar to freckles, but they usually appear on older people, and they are often much larger than freckles. They are often mistakenly referred to as liver spots, but they have nothing to do with liver function.

Seborrheic keratosis

Seborrheic keratoses are skin lesions that are very common in older people. They are benign growths on the skin that have a waxy, pasted-on appearance. They often develop a warty appearance when they have been present for a long while. Seborrheic keratosis blemishes can appear singly or in groups. The chest, back, and face are most often affected; they rarely appear below the waist. When seborrheic keratoses are very dark, they can look like malignant melanoma, although these growths are entirely benign.

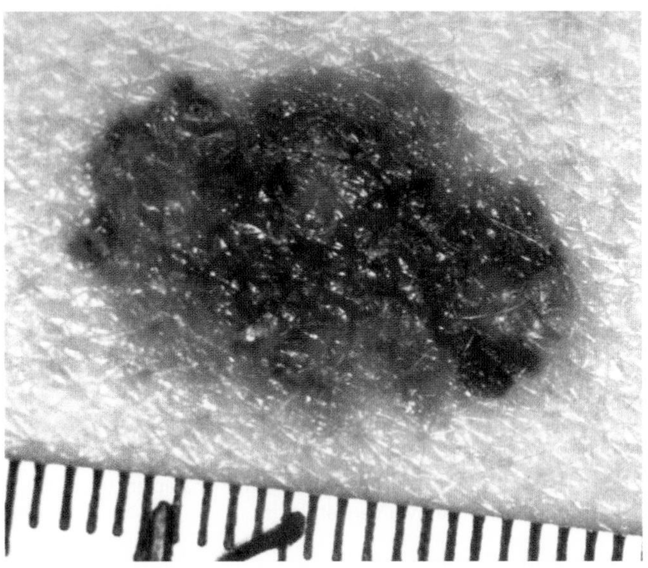

Figure 2.41. Superficial spreading melanoma.

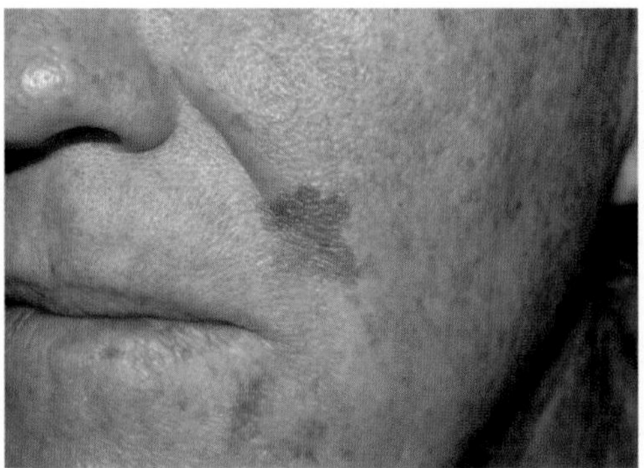

Figure 2.42. Lentigo melanoma.

Treatment

Treatment for melanoma is aggressive because this cancer spreads very rapidly. Once a lesion has been positively identified and staged (Sidebar 2.6), it is usually attacked with every weapon available. Surgical excision entails removing the growth and examining the surrounding tissues for signs of involvement. A margin of healthy tissue is taken as well, to be sure all of the mutated cells have been removed. Irradiation and examination of nearby lymph nodes follows. Perfusion chemotherapy may be employed: the affected limb is tied off with a tourniquet, and then high doses of chemotherapeutic drugs (sometimes heated for extra effect) are injected and isolated to the affected area.

Prognosis

The prognosis for malignant melanoma is determined largely by how far the cancerous cells have invaded the skin. Melanoma usually begins by spreading shallowly across the epidermis before invading deeper tissues. If it is caught and removed before it is about 0.7 mm deep, the prognosis is generally hopeful. If it gets up to 4 mm deep, it will probably have invaded nearby

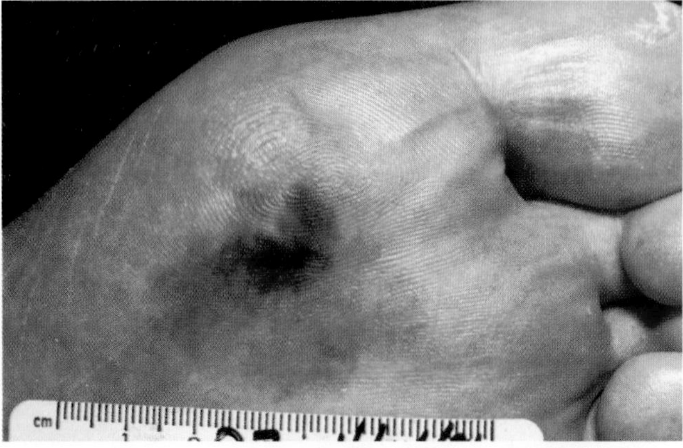

Figure 2.43. Acral lentiginous melanoma.

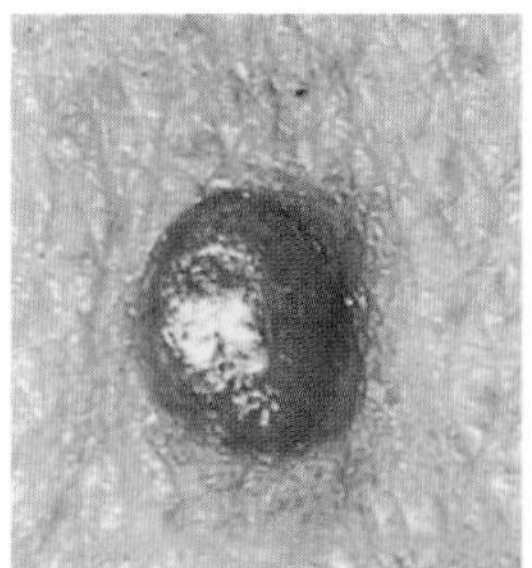

Figure 2.44. Nodular melanoma.

SIDEBAR 2.6: MALIGNANT MELANOMA STAGING

Malignant melanoma is staged based on how thick the lesions are, whether they are ulcerated, and how far the cancer has invaded lymph nodes and other tissues. Staging of melanoma is complicated, using both the TNM and stages 0 to IV classifications; a simplified version follows:[23]

TNM classification is assigned according to these criteria:

Tumor	Definition
Tx	Tumor cannot be evaluated
T0	No evidence of a primary tumor
Tis	In situ: the tumor has not spread to nearby tissue
T1 A/B	Lesion is <1 mm
T2 A/B	Lesion is 1.01-2 mm
T3 A/B	Lesion is 2.01-4 mm
T4 A/B	Lesion >4 mm

A, not ulcerated; B, ulcerated.

Node	Definition
Nx	Node involvement cannot be evaluated.
N0	No cancer found in nearby nodes.
N1 A/B	One node is involved.
N2 A/B	2-3 nearby nodes are involved.
N3 A/B	4 or more nodes are involved *or* distant nodes are involved

A, melanocytes are microscopic; B, melanocytes are visible without magnification.

Metastasis	Definition
Mx	Metastasis cannot be evaluated.
M0	No distant metastasis found.
M1	Distant metastasis found.
M1A	Metastasis involves subcutaneous tissues or distant lymph nodes.
M1B	Metastasis involves lungs.
M1C	Metastasis involves other organs.

Stages for malignant melanoma are assigned according to the following criteria:

Stage	Definition
0	Tis; N0; M0
IA	T1A; N0; M0
IB	T1B *or* T2A; N0; M0
IIA	T2B *or* T3A; N0; M0
IIB	T3B *or* T4A; N0; M0
IIC	T4B; N0; M0
III	T-any; N1-3; M0
IV	T-any; N-any; M1

Staging is used to identify the best possible treatment options. Staging also corresponds to survival rates.[23] The survival rates for malignant melanoma are based on staging as follows:

Stage at diagnosis	5-year survival, no node involvement (%)	5-year survival, node involvement (%)
0	97	
I	90-95	75
IIA	85	65
IIB	72-75	50-60
IIC	53	44
III	45	Nodes are always involved
IV	10	Nodes are always involved

lymph nodes and metastasized through the body. In this case the prognosis is generally poor; 5-year survival rates for melanoma in various stages are listed in the sidebar.

Prevention

Skin cancer is usually preventable. The single most important step in limiting this disease is avoiding the sun when UV radiation is most intense. In most latitudes that means staying out of direct sunlight between 10 A.M. and 4 P.M. Some experts suggest following the shadow rule: stay out of the sun when your shadow is shorter than you are. Other recommendations include the following:[17]

- Cover up with tightly woven clothing.
- Make sure that hats cover the ears and the back of the neck.
- Use sunscreen with a minimum of SPF 15 and reapply after swimming or perspiring.
- Use UV-absorbing sunglasses.

Observe these precautions even on hazy or cloudy days, since UV radiation can travel through clouds.

Massage?

Melanoma is an aggressive form of cancer that spreads through the lymph system. Persons undergoing treatment for melanoma may be receiving high doses of chemotherapy or radiation or dealing with surgery and skin grafts. Cautions for massage revolve around circulatory impact and the side effects of cancer treatments.

If a cancer patient is dying, massage can be a valuable part of comfort care. In hospices, if the patient is aware of the risks and is more interested in the quality of life than quantity, massage may performed or taught to family members and friends who are caring for the dying person.

MODALITY RECOMMENDATIONS FOR SKIN CANCER

MODALITY	RECOMMENDATION
Deep tissue massage	Locally contraindicated; otherwise supportive.
Lymphatic drainage	Locally contraindicated; otherwise supportive.
Polarity therapy	S: Indicated within client comfort. R/D: Locally contraindicated; otherwise supportive.
PNF/MET/stretching	Supportive as part of health care team; match to activity levels.
Reflexology	Locally contraindicated; work lymphatic system and pituitary points.
Shiatsu	Supportive.
Swedish massage	Can be supportive; stay within the client's activity restrictions.
Trigger point therapy	Locally contraindicated while acute; otherwise supportive.

See Chapter 1 for a brief description of each modality, including definitions of abbreviations.

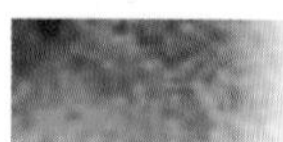

SKIN INJURIES

Burns

Definition: What Are They?

Many people think about burns in the context of touching a hot iron or brushing a hand across a broiler rack, but the world of burns goes far beyond household appliances. A person can sustain burn damage from dry heat, wet heat such as hot liquids or steam, electricity, radiation, and corrosive chemicals. Any one of these can destroy the proteins in the exposed skin cells, which causes the cells to die. If a significant amount of skin is affected, it is unable to accomplish its protective tasks: it can't provide a shield from microbial invasion, it can't help to maintain a stable temperature, and it can't provide protection from fluid loss. The massive loss of water, plasma, and plasma proteins that seep out of capillaries around the injury may lead to shock.

The skin is not the only tissue to sustain damage from burns. The respiratory tract can be burned if a person inhales air that is too hot; and the mouth, esophagus, and stomach can be damaged by hot liquids or by the ingestion of corrosive chemicals.

Etiology: What Happens?

The severity of burns is determined by how deep they go, how much surface area they cover, and what part of the body has been affected. Losing more than 15% of skin function can put a person at risk for infection, shock, and circulatory collapse. Burns to the face and neck are more serious than to other areas because the resulting inflammation can block breathing passages.

Burns are graded in three levels of depth:

- **First-degree burn** is sometimes quite painful but a relatively mild irritation of the superficial epidermis characterized by redness but no blistering. Mild sunburn is perhaps the most common example of a first-degree burn. Overexposure to the sun damages cells in the epithelium, setting up an inflammatory response. This leads to pain, heat, redness, and swelling (Figure 2.45). Sunburns generally heal in 2 to 3 days, sometimes with flaking and peeling.
- **Second-degree burn** is damage that involves all layers of the epidermis and possibly some of the dermis too. Symptoms include redness, blisters that appear instantly, edema, and pain (Figure 2.46). Second-degree burns often leave a permanent scar.

Burns in Brief

What are they?
Burns are caused by damage to the skin that kills cells. They can be caused by heat, radiation, corrosive chemicals, and electricity.

How are they recognized?
First-degree burns produce mild inflammation. Second-degree burns also cause blistering and damage at the deeper levels of the epidermis. Third-degree burns go down into the dermis itself and beyond. They often show white or black charred edges. In the postacute stage, serious burns often produce shrunken, contracted scar tissue over the affected skin.

Is massage indicated or contraindicated?
All burns (except mild sunburns) contraindicate massage in the acute stage. In the subacute and postacute stages, massage may be performed around the damaged area within pain tolerance of the client. After a burn has healed, judgments about bodywork are based on the sensitivity of the client.

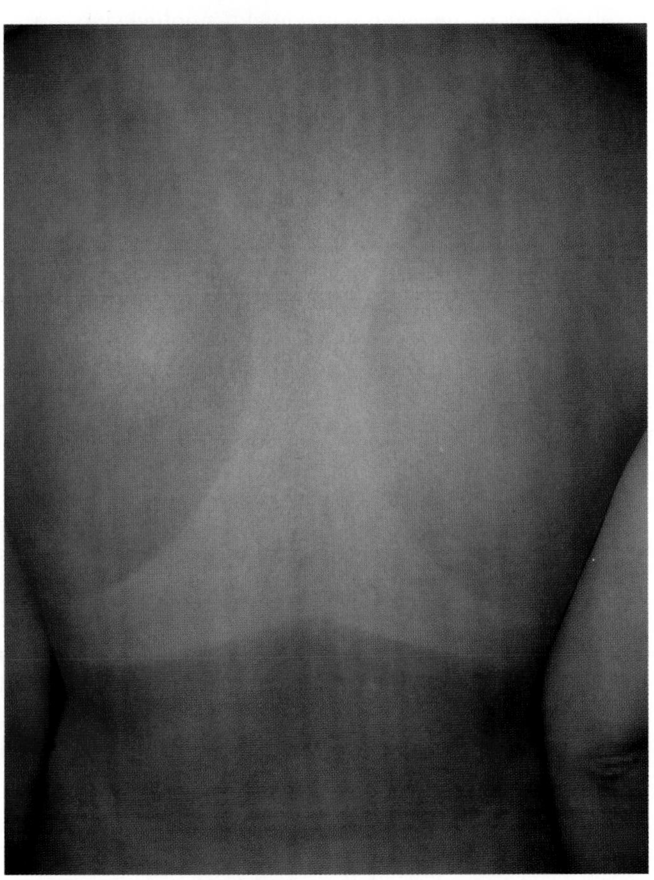

Figure 2.45. First-degree burn.

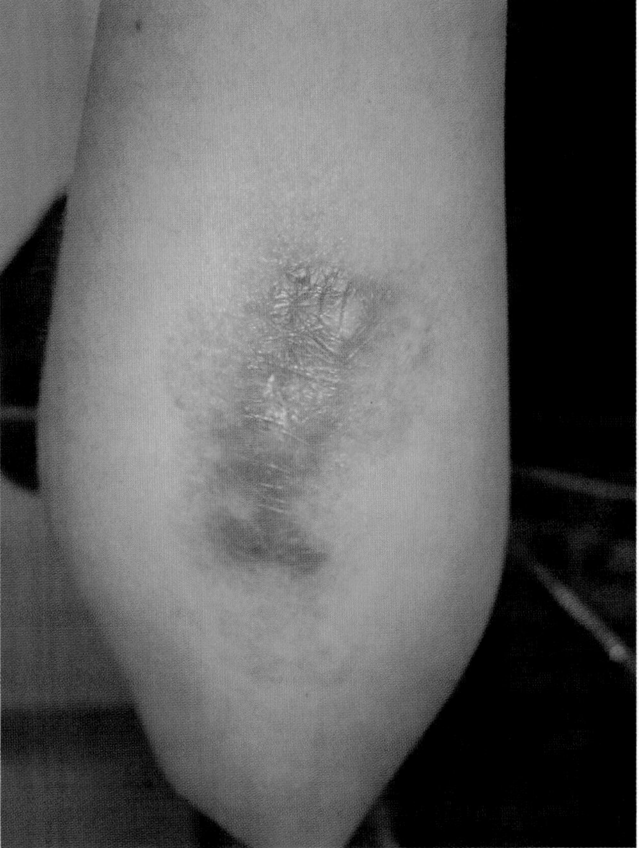

Figure 2.46. Second-degree burn.

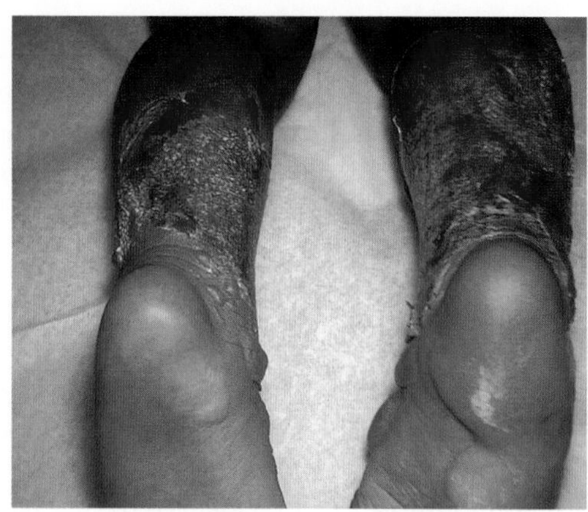

Figure 2.47. Third-degree burn.

- **Third-degree burn** goes through the dermis or beyond, destroying hair shafts, sebaceous glands, erector pilae muscles, sweat glands, and even nerve endings, which paradoxically makes third-degree burns less painful than second-degree burns. Symptoms include whiteness and/or charring and a leathery texture of the skin in the affected area (Figure 2.47). Third-degree burns are dangerous for the reasons mentioned earlier: risk of infection, fluid loss and shock, especially if a significant percentage of the body surface has been affected. If they affect deep tissues, muscle damage may lead to a dangerous accumulation of toxins in the blood that contributes to kidney failure. In addition, one of the special problems with third-degree burns is that they tend to contract rapidly, forming a confining web of scar tissue, even with quickly applied skin grafts.

Signs and Symptoms

The symptoms of burn damage depend on what level of skin has been affected. Details on symptoms by degree of damage are listed with each description.

Treatment

First- and second-degree burns are seldom treated with anything more than soothing lotion and possibly antibiotic cream if the skin has been damaged to the point of not providing protection from infectious agents. Third-degree burns, however, must be treated with more care to minimize the accumulation of binding scar tissue. This often means wound cleansing and debridement (aggressive skin brushing to remove debris), as well as skin grafts and plastic surgery.

Untreated severe burns tend to develop tightly restrictive tissue contractures. These can be so severe that they interfere with blood flow and may lead to the loss of healthy cells through starvation. In addition, the epithelium that grows over the burned area is often delicate and easily torn, even months or years after the trauma. Skin grafts reduce contractures and provide a healthier covering for the injured tissues.

Massage?

The only kind of burn that is appropriate for hands-on massage in the acute stage is a very mild sunburn, and of course even then one must work within pain tolerance. Massage may speed the healing process along by helping to slough off dead cells, but this is not something to do without a client's permission.

More severe burns may be approached in the subacute stage as a local contraindication; it is appropriate to work around the edges within pain tolerance to improve elasticity and minimize scar tissue, as long as the risk of infection is minimized. In this situation it is important to be working with a health care team to establish when the burn is in a subacute stage and to rule out any other tissue trauma that may contraindicate massage. Finally, if burns are obviously long past the acute and subacute stages, that is, no pain remains and only residual scar tissue is left, massage is safe as long as sensation is intact.

Relaxation techniques can help maintain the quality of tissues around the edges of a healing burn. Furthermore, massage has been used successfully to reduce the stress associated with treatment for third-degree burns. The pain of debriding damaged skin tissue is often described as worse than the burn itself. When patients receive massage prior to their wound care sessions, they report lower levels of anxiety, pain, and depression, and their levels of stress-related hormones and pulse rates are appreciably decreased. These benefits set the stage for a less painful, more efficient healing process.[24]

Modality Recommendations for Burns

MODALITY	RECOMMENDATION
Deep tissue massage	Indicated when postacute: work slowly with feedback to help return elasticity to area and adjacent tissue.
Lymphatic drainage	Indicated in acute and subacute stages.
Polarity therapy	S/R/D: Indicated for work off site of injury within client comfort.
PNF/MET/ stretching	Locally contraindicated while acute; otherwise supportive.
Reflexology	Locally contraindicated while acute; otherwise supportive.
Shiatsu	Indicated. Use SI for trauma, TH/K/SP for inflammation systemically. Avoid burn site.
Swedish massage	Locally contraindicated; otherwise very supportive.
Trigger point therapy	Locally contraindicated while acute; otherwise supportive.

See Chapter 1 for a brief description of each modality, including definitions of abbreviations.

Decubitus Ulcers

Definition: What Are They?

Decubitus ulcers, also known as *bedsores*, *pressure sores*, and *trophic ulcers*, are problems massage therapists are most likely to see when working in a hospital, a nursing home, or some other setting with bedridden patients. They stem from inadequate blood flow to the skin that stretches over bony or otherwise prominent areas. They almost always occur in some area that has had constant contact with a surface: usually a bed, sometimes a stretcher, a cast, or a splint.

Demographics: Who Gets Them?

The persons most at risk for developing *decubitus ulcers* are elderly, underweight, male, unable to walk, and incontinent. Most patients with bedsores are 70 years of age or older. Also, 17% to 28% of residents in extended care facilities develop bedsores. This does not

Decubitus Ulcers in Brief

Pronunciation: de-KYU-bih-tus UL-surz

What are they?

Decubitus ulcers, also called bedsores, are lesions caused by impaired circulation to the skin. Lack of blood supply leads to tissue death and a high risk of infection.

How are they recognized?

Unlike other sores, ulcers don't crust over; they remain open wounds that may penetrate to deep layers of tissue.

Is massage indicated or contraindicated?

Bedsores indicate massage only *before* they happen. Once the tissue has been damaged, the risk of infection is so high that the area must be avoided until the ulcer has healed.

preclude other people from developing them, however; anyone who is immobile even for just a few hours can develop pressure sores.[25]

Etiology: What Happens?

Imagine looking microscopically into the skin of an immobilized person. Nothing stimulates his circulation. Capillaries are squeezed between bone and bed, and new epithelial cells are starving for nutrition. The cells close to the surface of the skin died long ago, but now the cells in the deeper layers of the epidermis are dying too. Although the damage to deep layers of the skin may be extensive, only small lesions appear at the surface. Bacteria take advantage of the opportunity, and they begin to attack the weakened skin cells, exposing more of the damaged tissues. Capillaries are too narrow to let anything through, including the white blood cells that would otherwise limit the intruders. Gradually the surface tissue dies, and along with it the possibility of regeneration. Left unchecked, the ulcer can destroy the epidermis, the dermis, and the superficial fascia and can erode tissues down to the bone (Figure 2.48). Secondary infection of the open wound can lead to blood poisoning and death.

Bedsores can start in a surprisingly short amount of time. They can be a significant danger for people with spinal injuries, who may have to travel for hours strapped to a backboard, or for people undergoing long surgeries. Bedsores, along with joint and muscle degeneration, are the main reason immobilized patients are turned at least every 2 hours. Heels, buttocks, the sacrum, and elbows are the most common places for bedsores to appear.

Signs and Symptoms

The first stage of decubitus ulcers shows a marked change in skin temperature (it can become cooler or warmer than the surrounding area). Localized reddening becomes visible on pale skin, while on dark skin the discoloration may appear to be red, purple, or bluish. Pain and itching accompany these changes. The skin doesn't break, and if circulation is restored, the lesion may reverse.

In later stages the lesions turn purple, and then necrosis (tissue death) begins. Sores may extend into deep layers of the skin or into fascia, tendons, and down to the bone. Bacteria may invade the damaged tissue, which results in local or systemic infection.

Ulcers on the skin (and anywhere else on the body) differ from other types of sores because they don't go through a normal healing process. Where most injuries stimulate the production of new epithelial cells and connective tissue fibers to replace the damaged tissues, the poor circulation that causes decubitus ulcers prevents this from happening. Eventually they *can* heal, but not in a normal way; when circulation to the affected area is finally restored, the

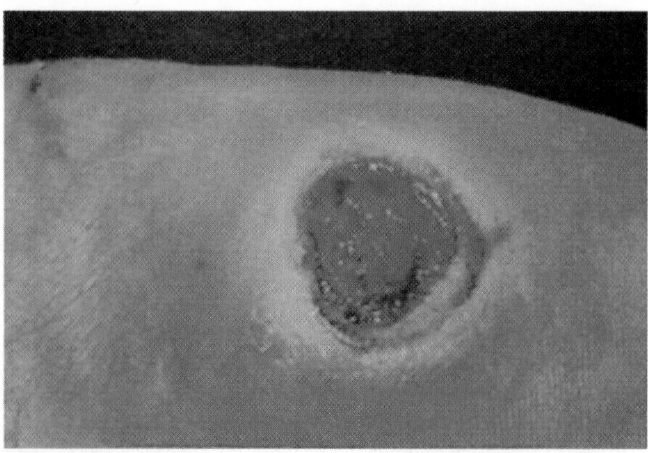

Figure 2.48. Decubitus ulcer.

lesion closes by having scar tissue grow over the area, but a permanent dip remains where the dead tissue never grows back.

Treatment

Treatment for pressure sores depends on their stage and location. Topical antibiotics and dressings can be effective for some lesions, while bigger, more advanced sores may require debridement and plastic surgery. Dressings treated with hydrocolloids support the manufacture of healthy new cells.

The biggest danger for someone with bedsores is the possibility of infection, which can be life-threatening for someone who is bedridden and immunosuppressed already. Furthermore, chronic inflammation and infection contribute to the risk of aggressive SCC.

Massage?

Bedsores develop because circulation to a specific area is interrupted long enough that cells starve to death. While opinions vary about the width of the margin around a decubitus ulcer that should be left untouched, it is obvious that massage is at least locally contraindicated for these patients. Massage is a much better preventive measure than treatment option for bedsores.

MODALITY RECOMMENDATIONS FOR DECUBITUS ULCER

MODALITY	RECOMMENDATION
Deep tissue massage	Locally contraindicated; otherwise supportive.
Lymphatic drainage	Supportive, especially if local swelling is present.
Polarity therapy	S/R/D: Indicated for work off site of injury within client comfort.
PNF/MET/stretching	Locally contraindicated while acute; otherwise supportive
Reflexology	Locally contraindicated in acute and subacute stages; work liver and lymphatic system if possible
Shiatsu	Indicated except at local site. Use PC for circulation, TH/SP for lymph.
Swedish massage	Locally contraindicated while acute; otherwise supportive.
Trigger point therapy	Locally contraindicated while acute; otherwise supportive.

See Chapter 1 for a brief description of each modality, including definitions of abbreviations.

Scar Tissue

Definition: What Is It?

Scar tissue is the development of new material to repair damage from some kind of trauma. During this amazing process, the new material knits damaged tissue back together.

This discussion is limited to the regenerative capacities of the skin. For information on scar tissue associated with musculoskeletal injuries, see the section on tendinopathies in Chapter 3.

Scar Tissue in Brief

What is it?
Scar tissue is new skin or connective tissue that grows after an injury, infection, or surgery.

How is it recognized?
Scar tissue on the skin often lacks pigmentation, hair follicles, and sweat glands.

Is massage indicated or contraindicated?
Massage is contraindicated during the acute stage of any injury in which the skin has been damaged. In the subacute stage massage may improve the quality of the healing process.

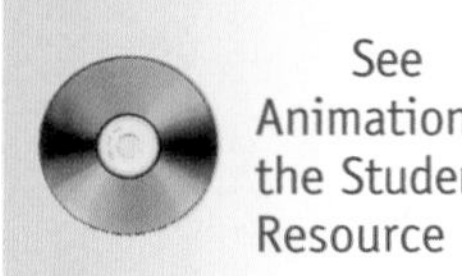

See Animation 6 on the Student Resource CD

Etiology: What Happens?

Skin cells, because they are subject to such a lot of wear and tear, are particularly ready to reproduce. Imagine a scrape or abrasion: clotting mechanisms allow a scab to begin to form within a few minutes of the trauma. Under the new scab, basal cells detach from the basement membrane and begin to migrate in a single-layered sheet across the wound. When they reach the other side and touch other epithelial cells, an internal code makes them stop moving. (It is the absence of this internal code, called *contact inhibition*, which makes cancer cells so dangerous; nothing ever tells them to ***stop***.)

Back at the original site, stationary basal cells duplicate to build up the ranks of migrating cells. When the whole wound has been covered, the new sheet of basal cells begins dividing to form new strata. Finally the superficial cells become keratinized, and the scab falls off. Then the wound is healed; the blood supply is protected from the outside world, and it is no longer vulnerable to infection. The whole process can take place within 24 hours to several days, depending on the size and location of the injury.

If the damage goes deeper than the dermis or if the wound is complicated by any inflammatory risk factor such as an infection or a foreign body, the healing process is more complicated. Fibroblasts in the area are summoned to the site, so beneath all that basal cell activity collagen and other extracellular matrices are growing. This fill-in connective tissue is called *granulation tissue*. Eventually it changes to become an accumulation of collagenous scar tissue, meant to knit up the fascia, but it may intrude on the superficial layers as well. Collagenous scar tissue differs from normal scar tissue in some important ways: the collagen fibers are thicker, they don't lie down in the same patterns as uninjured tissue, and the surface is usually missing hair follicles, normal skin glands, and possibly even sensory neurons.

Signs and Symptoms

If the scar tissue bulges at the boundaries of the original injury, it is called *hypertrophic* scar. Hypertrophic scars usually form within a month of the injury and then stabilize or regress.

Sometimes the fibroblasts get much too active and produce significantly more collagen than is necessary. The scar overflows the injury, resulting in a permanently raised mass of tissue. This is called ***keloid scar*** (Figure 2.49). Keloid scar can be a very annoying complication of surgery or any kind of deep wound healing, but it is seldom a debilitating problem. Keloids

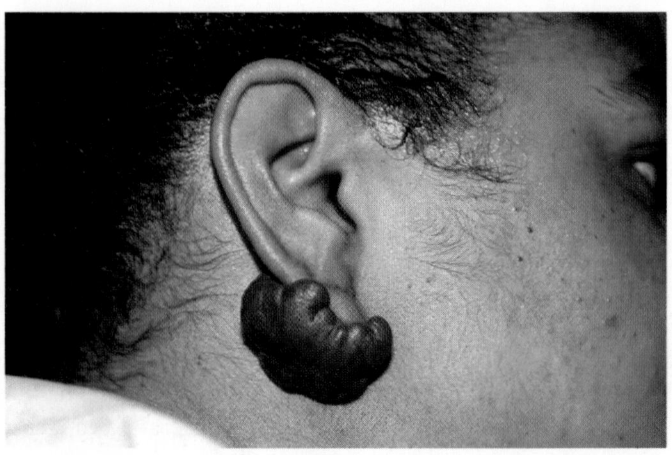

Figure 2.49. Keloid scar.

typically form where skin tension is high: on the chest, shoulders, and neck. They also form where chronic irritation and inflammation occur—at the site of piercings, for example. They usually form within a year of the injury, and they don't regress without intervention. Keloids are most common in people with dark complexions. People of African or Chinese descent have the highest rate of keloid development.

Treatment

Several treatment options have been developed to minimize the appearance of scar tissue on the skin, but none of them can eradicate the scars themselves. Scarred areas that dip into underlying tissues may be injected with collagen or fat to help them fill out their normal area. Other options include dermabrasion (the skin is buffed to remove excess epithelium), chemical peels (the top layers of epithelium are chemically treated and removed to create more even texture and coloring), punch grafts (small pieces of normal skin are surgically implanted to replace localized scars such as old acne lesions), and laser resurfacing.

Hypertrophic scar tissue may be injected with cortisone, which dissolves the excess collagen. Keloids may be treated with any combination of liquid nitrogen, injection with cortisone or other substances, silicone gel packs, or pressure bandages, but they may still recur.

When a large area of skin has been damaged, it is important to control the amount of scar tissue that accumulates, because masses of scar can contract into uncomfortable and unsightly areas. Skin grafts can control the accumulation of new scar tissue for the best possible long-term results.

Massage?

Obviously, massage is appropriate only in the postacute stage of skin healing, because if the skin is not intact, the client is a walking invitation to infection. If someone is healing from a deep wound such as a surgery, he/she may benefit from work *around* the area, which can keep the skin supple and may inhibit the buildup of hypertrophic scar tissue. If a client has old, deep scar tissue on the skin, sensation in those areas may be reduced. In such a case, massage therapists should be careful to elicit client feedback.

Modality Recommendations for Scar Tissue

MODALITY	RECOMMENDATION
Deep tissue massage	Indicated in postacute phase: work slowly with feedback to help return elasticity to area and adjacent tissue.
Lymphatic drainage	Indicated in acute and subacute stages after appropriate scar work is performed.
Polarity therapy	S: Indicated. R/D: Indicated if skin is intact, within client comfort.
PNF/MET/ stretching	Indicated during subacute stage, to client's tolerance.
Reflexology	Indicated.
Shiatsu	Indicated.
Swedish massage	Indicated as long as skin is intact.
Trigger point therapy	Indicated during subacute and chronic stages.

See Chapter 1 for a brief description of each modality, including definitions of abbreviations.

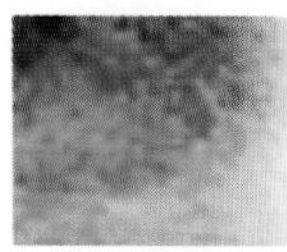

Chapter Review Questions: Skin Conditions

1. Under what circumstances is massage not safe for most noncontagious skin conditions?
2. A client has extremely dry and flaky eczema on her hands. Does this condition indicate or contraindicate massage? Why?
3. A client has several raised red rings on his trunk. They are paler in the middle. He reports that they are mildly itchy. What condition is probably present?
4. What does psoriasis have in common with cancer?
5. When working with a client who is prone to acne, is it a good idea to follow the treatment with an alcohol rinse to remove the oil? Why?
6. A client has white flakes that cling to hair shafts and don't brush out. What condition is probably present?
7. A client has a large, hot, painful pustule on his thigh. He assumes it is a spider bite but has not been to the doctor. What condition may be present?
8. What should be done with this client's massage sheets?
9. In what stage of the development of a decubitus ulcer is massage most appropriate?
10. In what situation would an open sore indicate a systemic rather than just a local contraindication?
11. Your client reports a small lesion on his cheek that never seems to get better. What do you think is present?
12. What makes acral lentiginous melanoma different from other types of melanoma?

References

1. Baorto EP, Baorto D. *Staphylococcus Aureus* Infection. © 1996–2006 by WebMD. http://www.emedicine.com/ped/topic2704.htm. Accessed spring 2006.
2. Community-Associated MRSA Information for the Public. Division of Healthcare Quality Promotion. http://www.cdc.gov/ncidod/dhqp/ar_mrsa_ca_public.html. Accessed spring 2006.
3. Methicillin resistant *Staphylococcus aureus*. © NZDS 2006. http://dermnetnz.org/bacterial/methicillin-resistance.html. Accessed spring 2006.
4. Ringworm (Tinea). © 1996–2003 MedicineNet, Inc. All rights reserved. http://www.medicinenet.com/Ringworm/article.htm. Accessed spring 2006.
5. Drugge, Rhett J. Fungus Diseases. © 1995–2000 The Internet Dermatology Society, Inc. http://telemedicine.org/common/Fungus. Accessed spring 2006.
6. Genital Herpes. Centers for Disease Control. http://www.cdc.gov/std/Herpes/STDFact-Herpes.htm#common. Accessed spring 2006.
7. Torres G, Schinstine M. Herpes Simplex. © 1996-2006 by WebMD. http://www.emedicine.com/derm/topic179.htm. Accessed spring 2006.
8. Treating Head Lice Infestation. Centers for Disease Control and Prevention. http://www.cdc.gov/ncidod/dpd/parasites/lice/factsht_head_lice_treating.htm. Accessed spring 2006.
9. LouseBuster Kills: Hot, Dry Air Device Eradicates Lice. © 2007 MediLexicon International Ltd. http://www.medicalnewstoday.com/medicalnews.php?newsid=56456. Accessed winter 2007.

10. Rinker M. Warts, Nongenital. © 1996–2006 by WebMD. http://www.emedicine.com/derm/topic457.htm. Accessed spring 2006.
11. Harper JC, Fulton J Jr. Acne Vulgaris. © 1996-2006 by WebMD. http://www.emedicine.com/derm/topic2.htm. Accessed spring 2006.
12. Krafchik BR. Atopic Dermatitis. © 1996-2006 by WebMD. http://emedicine.com/derm/topic38.htm. Accessed spring 2006.
13. What is Eczema? © American Academy of Dermatology, 2005 All rights reserved. http://www.skincarephysicians.com/eczemanet/whatis.html. Accessed spring 2006.
14. Crawford MB. Urticaria. © 1996-2006 by WebMD. http://www.emedicine.com/emerg/topic628.htm. Accessed spring 2006.
15. What is Psoriasis? © American Academy of Dermatology, 2005. http://www.skincarephysicians.com/psoriasisnet/whatis.html. Accessed spring 2006.
16. Psoriatic arthritis. ©2006 National Psoriasis Foundation/USA. http://www.psoriasis.org/about/psa/, http://www.psoriasis.org/treatment/psa/. Accessed spring 2006.
17. Introduction. National Cancer Institute. http://www.cancer.gov/cancertopics/wyntk/skin/allpages. Accessed spring 2006.
18. Skin cancer epidemic underway in the US. Copyright © 2006 by Reuters Limited. http://www.nlm.nih.gov/medlineplus/news/fullstory_32435.html. Accessed spring 2006.
19. 2006 Skin Cancer Fact Sheet. © 2006 American Academy of Dermatology. http://www.aad.org/aad/Newsroom/2005+Skin+Cancer+Fact+Sheet.htm. Accessed spring 2006.
20. McGovern T, Lefell D. Actinic Keratoses and Non-Melanoma Skin Cancer. Copyright © 2006 American Academy of Dermatology. http://www.aad.org/professionals/Residents/MedStud CoreCurr/DCActinicKer-NoMelCancer.htm. Accessed spring 2006.
21. Ramsey M. Basal Cell Carcinoma. © 1996–2006 by WebMD. http://www.emedicine.com/derm/topic47.htm. Accessed spring 2006.
22. Goldman G. Squamous Cell Carcinoma. © 1996–2006 by WebMD. http://www.emedicine.com/DERM/topic401.htm. Accessed spring 2006.
23. Heistein J, Ruberg RL. Skin Malignancies, Melanoma. © 1996–2006 by WebMD. http://www.emedicine.com/plastic/topic456.htm. Accessed spring 2006.
24. 2006 Skin Cancer Fact Sheet. © 2006 American Academy of Dermatology. http://www.aad.org/aad/Newsroom/2005+Skin+Cancer+Fact+Sheet.htm. Accessed spring 2006.
25. Field T. Touch Therapy. © Tiffany Field 2000. Churchill Livingstone. pp 53–58.
26. Revis, Don R Jr. Decubitus Ulcers. © 1996-2006 by WebMD. http://www.emedicine.com/med/topic2709.htm. Accessed spring 2006.

3

Musculoskeletal System Conditions

Chapter Objectives

After reading this chapter, you should be able to . . .

- Describe a trigger point "energy crisis"
- Name the role of dystrophin in normal muscle function.
- Name three causative factors for muscle spasm.
- Name three factors that can accelerate calcium loss.
- Name what feature Paget disease and osteoporosis have in common.
- Identify the causative agent for Lyme disease.
- Name the difference between strains and sprains.
- Name the difference between patellofemoral syndrome and patellar tendinitis.
- Define tendinosis.
- Name three differences between osteoarthritis and rheumatoid arthritis.
- Name the feature that Ehlers-Danlos syndrome, Marfan syndrome, muscular dystrophy, and osteogenesis imperfecta all share.
- Name three muscles and bones that may help to pin or trap the structures damaged with thoracic outlet syndrome.

Introduction

This chapter addresses disorders and injuries of muscles, bones, and joint structures: ligaments, tendons, tendinous sheaths, and bursae. Together these structures are the tools that provide humans with shape, strength, and movement. They are composed almost entirely of the material that binds people together and permeates every part of the body: connective tissue.

Injury to any of the connective tissue structures (except bone and sometimes cartilage) can be difficult for many medical professionals to identify. Magnetic resonance imaging (MRI) can be useful, but at present the ability to identify soft tissue damage is extremely limited. A thorough clinical examination still yields the most comprehensive information about injury to muscles, tendons, ligaments, and other connective tissues. Massage therapists, with their in-depth understanding of the musculoskeletal system, particularly with the formation of adhesions and scar tissue, are in a unique position to be able to help individuals with these types of injuries.

Bones

Bone Structure

The arrangement of living and nonliving material in bone is elegant and efficient. The collagen matrix on which solid bone is built is arranged as circles within circles. Calcium and phosphorus deposits accumulate on this scaffolding in a similarly circular pattern, leaving holes for blood vessels. In addition, most long bones in the body grow in a slight spiral, much like evergreen tree trunks. The shaft, or *diaphysis,* of long bones is hollow, filled with red marrow in youth and yellow marrow in adulthood. All of these design features give bone some remarkable properties: terrific resilience, support, and weight-bearing capacity combined with a lightweight construction.

The commands to move the rocklike calcium and phosphorus salts around the collagen matrix are carried out by specialized cells. *Osteoblasts,* or ***b**one **b**uilders*, help to lay new deposits, while **osteoclasts**, or bone *c*learers, break them down. These cells are located both in the periosteum, around the outside of the bone, and the *endosteum,* which lines the central cavity. They can alter the shape of the bones from interior and exterior aspects.

Osteoblasts and osteoclasts are controlled by hormones. *Calcitonin,* from the thyroid, *lowers* blood calcium by telling osteoblasts to pull calcium out of the blood and put it wherever the bones need it most. Parathyroid hormone (PTH) *raises* blood calcium by telling the osteoclasts to dismantle calcium deposits and put the valuable mineral back into the bloodstream. There it is available to help with muscle contractions, nerve transmission, blood clotting, and maintenance of the appropriate pH balance in the blood and tissues. Consequently, the health and shape of the bones depend not only on a person's physical activity but also on whatever other chemical demands the body may make on its calcium banks. This is, in essence, Wolff's law: "Every change in the form and the function of a bone, or in its function alone, is followed by certain definite changes in its internal architecture and secondary alterations in its external conformation."[1] In other words, bone is living tissue that remodels according to the stresses that are placed upon it.

Bone Function

The skeleton provides a bony framework, protection for vulnerable organs, and leverage for movement. It also produces new red blood cells and stores calcium and phosphorus for future use. For young people, bone is not a mass of stonelike inert material; in fact, osteoblasts and osteoclasts quickly remodel bone to accommodate whatever stresses are put on it. The younger the body, the higher a percentage of living material exists within bones. Gradually the ratio of inert material to living material shifts; in elderly people bone has little remaining living tissue, and the density of its mineral stores has decreased, hence its brittleness and slowness to heal.

Muscles

Muscle Structure

Muscles are composed of specialized threadlike cells that with electrical and chemical stimulation have the power to contract while bearing weight. These cells, or *myofibers,* run the full length of the muscle, and each one is encased in a connective tissue envelope, the *endomysium.* Packets of wrapped myofibers are bound in another connective tissue envelope, creating bundles called *fascicles.* Fascicles are bound together by yet another connective tissue membrane, the *perimysium* (Figure 3.1). Finally, some large muscle groups are further bound by an external connective tissue membrane *(epimysium),* which blends into the subcutaneous layer of the skin, the superficial fascia (which is—surprise!—another connective tissue membrane).

Muscle Function

When muscles work, they consume fuel and produce both energy (the pulling together of their bony attachments) and wastes. What kinds of wastes are produced depends on how much work is done, how fast it goes, how long it takes, and what kind of fuel is available to do it. Muscles that work when adequate supplies of oxygen are easily accessible burn very cleanly (*aerobic metabolism*): the waste products they produce are carbon dioxide and water. But when they work without adequate oxygen (*anaerobic metabolism*), a variety of other wastes are produced. Among these is lactic acid, a byproduct of anaerobic combustion that is also a nerve irritant.

This raises the question: what causes muscle soreness? Delayed-onset muscle soreness is the subject of ongoing debate. One factor is probably the accumulation of lactic acid, which irritates nerve endings in overused muscles. Another theory is that some calcium leakage from *sarcomeres* (segments of myofibrils where chemical reactions take place) occurs. This leakage can cause microspasms. Soreness may also arise from microscopic tears of myofibers. Even with microscopic injuries like these, tiny pockets of inflammation accompany them. Swelling and tearing stimulate *nociceptors* (nerve endings that transmit messages about tissue damage), which give the brain information about pain and injury. Massage can influence the processing of chemical residues and minor inflammations by moving fresh, highly oxygenated blood into sore areas while flushing old, toxic, stagnant interstitial fluid out. Imagine a person rinsing an old, dirty, smelly sponge in a stream of clean running water. Every time she squeezes, dirty, discolored liquid flows out of the sponge. Each time

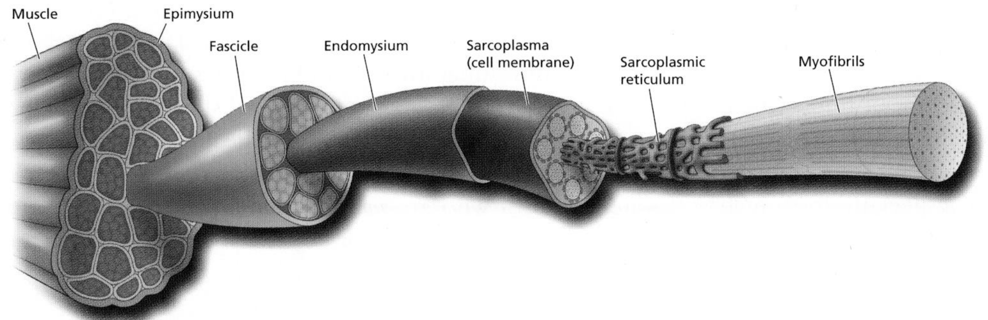

Figure 3.1. Muscles are composed of bundles within bundles, all enveloped by connective tissue membranes.

she releases, clean, fresh water fills it up again. This is what vigorous, well-applied circulatory massage does for muscles that are sore, tired and suffused with waste products.

Joints

The joints in the body have been organized into three classes: ***synarthroses*** ("immovable" joints, such as those between the cranial bones—although even these joints aren't *completely* immovable), ***amphiarthroses*** (slightly movable joints, such as those between the bodies of the vertebrae), and ***diarthroses*** (freely movable joints). Of these classes of joints, the diarthrotic, or synovial, joints are by far the most vulnerable to injury. For this reason, it is worth briefly reviewing synovial joints in preparation for a discussion of what happens when they're injured.

Joint Structure

As shown in Figure 3.2, synovial joints are constructed so that no rough surfaces ever touch, even in joints that bear an enormous amount of weight, such as the knees and ankles. Articular cartilage, made of collagen fibers densely arranged around ***chondroitin sulfate*** (very slippery material) and water, caps the ends of bones where they meet. Maintaining the slickness of that cartilage is key to maintaining the health of the joint. Fortunately, each synovial joint has a synovial membrane, which produces synovial fluid, creating a generally slick, eggy environment (*synovial* means *with egg*). As long as the membrane and cartilage stay moist and smooth, the joint stays healthy. It takes only a very small amount of synovial fluid to lubricate the inside of a joint space.

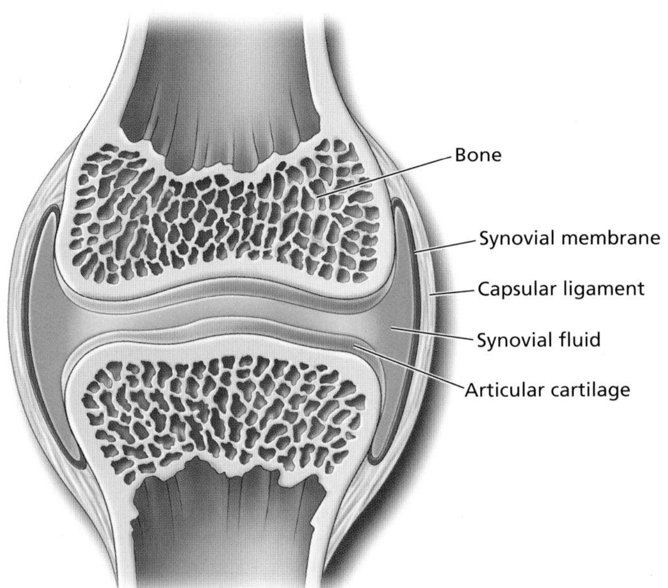

Figure 3.2. Synovial joint.

Joint Function

This isn't a kinesiology text, so the naming of synovial joint movements isn't discussed here. Suffice it to say that the function of synovial joints is to allow movement between bones, providing the fulcrum that bones can use for leverage.

Joints, like most other structures in the body, are designed for use. With healthy use, the joint structures stay smooth, slick, and well lubricated. Movement of the joint capsule stimulates the production of synovial fluid, which circulates through the joint space for the health of all joint components. Lack of movement results in a shortage of synovial fluid; too much movement, especially too much *irritating* movement, can damage articular cartilage or cause the bones of the joint to change shape in such a way that smooth surfaces are made rough, thus opening the door to irreversible arthritis. Other factors that can influence joint health include trauma, hydration, calcium metabolism, nutrition, and autoimmune disease.

Other Connective Tissues

Structures outside of the joint capsule (tendons, tendinous sheaths, ligaments, bursae) are also susceptible to damage. Tendons connect muscle to bone, and they are an early line of defense when a joint undergoes traumatic stress. Depending on the force of the trauma, ligaments are also quick to accrue injury. The medial and lateral stabilizers outside the joint capsule and the internal stabilizers are generally damaged before the specialized capsular ligament that comprises the joint capsule itself. Bursae, fluid-filled sacs that cushion areas where two bones might otherwise knock heads or allow tendons to slide over sharp corners, tend to get irritated with repetitive stress. The body grows new bursae anywhere it needs a little extra protection, and these new bursae can also become irritated and painful.

Connective Tissue Problems in General

Every part of the body is supported by connective tissue. It wraps around muscle cells and neurons; it supports blood vessels and the tubes of the digestive tract. It is the framework on which bones grow. Connective tissue provides the scaffolding for the functioning cells of most organs. It gives strength and elasticity to most of the body's membranes. Indeed, connective tissue is such a large proportion of the human body, it can be said that a person's general health can be determined by the strength, resiliency, and power of the connective tissues.

What happens when a person's connective tissues become systemically weak? Most people know someone who seems to get injured at the drop of a hat. She twists her ankle getting out of the car; he wrenches his back when he picks up a basket of laundry. It seems pain and injury follow them wherever they go. Very often the culprit in situations like this is a complicated interconnected problem involving long-term stress, poor nutrition, high levels of chronic muscle contraction, elevated cortisol levels in the blood, sleep disorders, and incomplete healing.

The hormone most closely linked to long-term stress is cortisol. This is an important beneficial chemical that helps to limit inflammation and redirects metabolism away from fast-burning glucose and toward slower-burning proteins. This is a fine mechanism for dealing with the threat of long-term hunger, but it means that people with elevated cortisol who are *not* experiencing a life-threatening food shortage are at risk for cortisol to weaken all types of connective tissue. It is clear then, how this increases the chances for injury and ongoing pain.

When injury occurs, long-term stress coupled with pain interferes with sleep cycles to the point that secretions of ***somatotropin*** (growth hormone) are significantly inhibited, as are the neurotransmitters that moderate pain sensation. This makes it difficult to heal from simple injuries and reinforces a pain-stress-sleeplessness cycle that is similar to the pain-spasm-ischemia cycle seen with many muscular problems.

SIDEBAR 3.1: CONNECTIVE TISSUE FIBERS

Connective tissue comes in all shapes and forms. It can be difficult to accept that the loose, jiggly deposits of fat in the subcutaneous layer of the skin are technically in the same class of tissues as bones, but it's true. The unifying feature in all types of connective tissue (except blood and lymph) is the presence of particular types of protein fibers. The two discussed here are collagen and elastin.

Elastin is a protein fiber that lives up to its name. It is stretchy and has good potential for rebound; in other words, it snaps back to its original size after being stretched. However, elastin and other similar connective tissue protein fibers are low in tensile strength; it is relatively easy to break these fibers to pieces.

Collagen is quite different in most qualities from elastin. It has little ability to stretch and poor rebound potential; once collagen has been stretched, it tends to stay loose rather than go back to its original length. Collagen does have tremendous tensile strength: it takes a great deal of force to stretch collagen and even more force to tear or fray the fibers.

One other property of collagen is that in certain circumstances it can tend to bind things together. If general circulation to an area is impaired, the collagen-based connective tissue membranes that are intended to be slick and slippery for freedom of movement instead become thick and gluey. Collagen fibers from one structure may even fuse with fibers from a neighboring structure. This can happen at any level within muscle groups or individual muscles. Muscle sheaths can stick to each other so that individual muscles can no longer contract independently. Fascicles can stick together within muscle bellies. Even individual myofibers can stick together. These sticky places, or ***adhesions***, can greatly reduce mobility and flexibility while increasing the chances for injury when they are stretched to the point of tearing.

The point of all this is that contrary to how many people view the body, it is not made of a series of interchangeable parts. When a car has a tire that keeps going flat, the owner replaces the tire and the problem is solved. But when a person has an ankle that is repeatedly sprained or a back that is so fragile he can't pick up his child or headaches that interfere with her day-to-day functioning, the answer isn't just in the ankle or the back or the neck muscles. It's in the totality of how mental and emotional states are echoed in the physical body. It's in how eating habits support or don't support healing. It's in whether a person gets adequate amounts of high-quality sleep. Massage therapists who specialize in helping people with musculoskeletal problems should address all of these issues when clients have recurring, ongoing, or stubborn injuries that don't follow what is usually considered a normal healing process.

The convenient feature in musculoskeletal problems, as far as massage therapists are concerned, is that most are *not* related to an infectious agent. A massage therapist can't catch or distribute an epidemic of sprained ankles. Nor do these injuries usually lead to permanent damage that massage can make worse. Increasing circulation does *not* spread tendon injuries throughout the body. But skillful, careful, knowledgeably applied massage administered in the appropriate stage of healing can help many musculoskeletal conditions to improve. Sometimes that improvement is just a temporary cessation of pain (which is a fine purpose in itself), but often this work can bring about the lasting changes that make structural massage an important factor in the healing process.

Musculoskeletal System Conditions

Muscular Disorders

- Fibromyalgia
- Myofascial pain syndrome
- Myositis ossificans
- Shin splints
- Spasms, cramps
- Strains

Bone Disorders

- Avascular osteonecrosis
- Fractures
- Osteoporosis
- Paget disease
- Postural deviations

Joint Disorders

- Ankylosing spondylitis
- Dislocations
- Gout
- Lyme disease
- Osteoarthritis
- Patellofemoral syndrome
- Rheumatoid arthritis
- Spondylosis
- Sprains
- Temporomandibular joint disorders

Genetic Musculoskeletal Disorders

- Ehlers-Danlos syndrome
- Marfan syndrome
- Muscular dystrophy
- Osteogenesis imperfecta

Other Connective Tissue Disorders

- Baker cyst
- Bunions
- Bursitis
- Dupuytren contracture
- Ganglion cysts
- Hernia
- Osgood-Schlatter disease
- Pes planus, pes cavus
- Plantar fasciitis
- Scleroderma
- Tendinopathies
- Tenosynovitis
- Whiplash

Neuromuscular Disorders

- Carpal tunnel syndrome
- Disc disease
- Myasthenia gravis
- Thoracic outlet syndrome

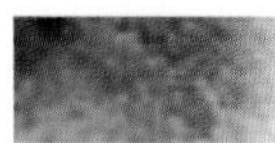

Muscular Disorders

Fibromyalgia

Definition: What Is It?

Fibromyalgia is a group of signs and symptoms that include chronic pain in muscles, tendons, ligaments, and other soft tissues. It is one of a collection of chronic disorders that often go hand in hand. Fibromyalgia syndrome (FMS) is frequently seen with chronic fatigue syndrome, irritable bowel syndrome, migraine headaches, sleep disorders, and several other chronic conditions.

Fibromyalgia in Brief
Pronunciation: fy-bro-my-AL-je-ah

What is it?
Fibromyalgia syndrome (FMS) is a chronic pain syndrome involving sleep disorders and the development of a predictable pattern of tender points in muscles and other soft tissues.

How is it recognized?
Fibromyalgia syndrome is diagnosed when other diseases have been ruled out and when 11 active tender points are found distributed among all quadrants of the body, along with fatigue, morning stiffness, and poor quality sleep.

Is massage indicated or contraindicated?
FMS indicates massage. Care must be taken not to overtreat, however, because clients are extremely sensitive to pain and may have accumulations of waste products in the tissues that are difficult to flush out adequately.

Demographics: Who Gets It?

FMS affects 2% to 3% of the U.S. population. Women account for 85% to 90% of diagnoses, but that number may be misleading, because men may be less likely to seek medical intervention for its symptoms. Fibromyalgia has been seen in all ages and economic groups, but its incidence seems to increase with age.[2]

Etiology: What Happens?

This is a very different disorder from most other muscle problems. It is not a viral or bacterial or fungal infection; it is not an autoimmune mistake, nor is it often a direct result of injury. Rather, it is a complicated combination of a sleep problem, neuroendocrine imbalances, and emotional state. Indeed, FMS may eventually be reclassified as a central nervous system disorder, but because muscle pain is among its most obvious symptoms, it continues to be discussed as a musculoskeletal disorder.

While the etiology of FMS is not well understood, several issues are consistent among people who meet the diagnostic criteria for this disorder:

- **Sleep disorder.** Sleep studies of persons with FMS reveal that they seldom or never enter the deepest level of sleep, stage IV. It is in this stage that adults secrete growth hormone, which stimulates the production of new cells and collagen for healing and recovery. Furthermore, not getting adequate high-quality sleep reduces serotonin levels. Among other things, serotonin helps to modulate pain sensation. Without adequate secretion of this important neurotransmitter, everything hurts *more*. So here is a particularly vicious circle: a person is in stress and/or chronic pain. This makes it difficult to sleep. Sleeplessness exacerbates the pain, which further limits the ability to sleep, and so on. Fibromyalgia patients often report getting 8 hours or more of sleep a night, but they also reliably report waking up feeling unrefreshed, as though they'd been working all night long. Studies in which volunteers who were deprived of stage IV sleep rapidly developed symptoms of FMS indicate that this is a significant issue in this disorder.[3]
- **Fatigue.** The fatigue FMS patients report may be caused by more than poor sleep. Some researchers suggest that FMS is related to a problem in mitochondrial function: phosphates accumulate in muscle cells rather than attaching to adenosine to form adenosine triphosphate (ATP). The phosphate attracts calcium ions to preserve pH balance. This leads to problems with energy production and with calcium reabsorption. The result is inefficient muscle contractions and debilitating fatigue.
- **Pain.** The origin of the debilitating pain is one of the most mysterious aspects of this syndrome. Current studies suggest that the pain is *not* in fact generated in the muscles,

as the name implies. Instead, examinations of the cerebrospinal fluid of FMS patients reveal pathologically high levels of two neurotransmitters, **substance P** and **nerve growth factor**. These substances are believed to initiate nerve activity, cause vasodilation, and increase pain sensation.

- **Tender points.** Fibromyalgia patients eventually develop tender points that are distributed all over the body (Figure 3.3) but that concentrate around the neck, shoulders, and low back. Tender points themselves are not well understood. Histological studies of affected tissue have yielded no useful information about how these areas develop.
- **Other Issues.** Fibromyalgia has become the focus for an enormous amount of research in the allopathic and complementary medical communities. Factors that have been explored include a vast array of possibilities including oxidative stress and free radical activity; an inefficient hypothalamus-pituitary-adrenal axis (this is a major issue in chronic fatigue syndrome and various types of depression as well); aspartame use and other issues.

SIDEBAR 3.2: HISTORY OF A DISEASE

The history of the documentation of FMS is a fascinating study of how information that stretches across the globe and over nearly 200 years has been gathered to create a picture of what is still a very mysterious disorder but also the second most common musculoskeletal diagnosis in the United States today.

- **1816.** Dr. William Balfour, a physician, first documents a chronic pain syndrome involving sore muscles, stiffness, and fatigue.
- **1904.** Sir William Gowers, a physician from Britain, first uses the word *fibrositis* in relation to this disorder. This name implies an inflammatory reaction in muscle or connective tissue fibers.
- **1940.** The word *fibrositis* first finds usage in North American medical texts.
- **1979.** A Canadian group of physicians matches the symptoms of muscle achiness to chronic fatigue and sleep disorders.
- **1981.** Research on this condition reveals that it does *not* after all involve inflammation of muscle or other tissues. Muhummad Yunus, an Illinois rheumatologist, coined the term *fibromyalgia* to refer to connective tissue, muscle tissue, and the pain that plagues them both.
- **1987.** The American Medical Association officially recognizes that FMS, which affects up to 3% of the American population, does indeed exist.
- **1990.** The American College of Rheumatology creates a set of standardized diagnostic criteria for FMS.
- **1993.** The World Health Organization officially recognizes FMS as a disorder.

Signs and Symptoms

The signs and symptoms of FMS include the following:

- Widespread pain in shifting locations that is extremely difficult to pin down. The intensity of the pain may vary widely (in other words, patients have good days and bad days). The pain can range from a deep ache to burning and tingling.
- Tender points. Nine predictable pairs of these are distributed among all quadrants of the body. When FMS is triggered by a specific trauma, extra tender points may develop in the area around the injury.
- Stiffness after rest.
- Poor stamina.
- Sensitivity amplification and low pain tolerance. All kinds of sensation become more intense and likely to cause pain. This includes light and sound, but is true especially of cold, texture, and pressure.

Diagnosis

No objective diagnostic test has been developed for FMS. It is typically diagnosed after ruling out all other diseases with similar signs and symptoms, including Lyme disease, multiple sclerosis, rheumatoid arthritis, lupus, and several others. Several of these diagnostic differentials are *also* made by ruling out similar-looking conditions. Obviously, this can be a long, expensive, and frustrating process.

Fibromyalgia is particularly challenging because most people who meet the diagnostic criteria for this problem may also have a host of other disorders. Such a close correlation exists between FMS, irritable bowel syndrome, and chronic fatigue syndrome that many experts

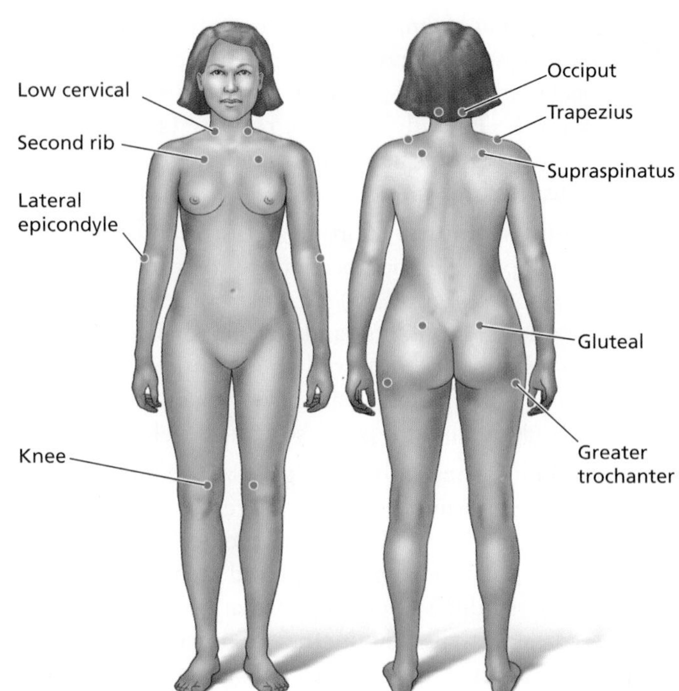

Figure 3.3. Fibromyalgia tender point map.

believe these may all be different manifestations of a single problem. People with FMS often also have migraine headaches, temporomandibular joint disorders, and restless leg syndrome. Furthermore, mild hypothyroidism, low-grade celiac disease, multiple chemical sensitivity syndrome, and candidiasis may present similar symptoms, but when these conditions aren't extreme, they are often under the radar of the mainstream medical community. Finally, a long history of confusion between FMS *tender* points and myofascial pain syndrome (MPS) *trigger* points continues to cloud the issue. A side-by-side comparison is provided in the table in Compare and Contrast 3.1.

The American College of Rheumatology, along with the Second World Congress on Fibromyalgia and Myofascial Pain, have defined a set of diagnostic criteria for FMS[4]:

- The patient reports chronic pain for a minimum of 3 months.
- The patient shows at least 11 of 18 mapped tender points to be active (that is, they must elicit significant diffuse pain with digital pressure of about 4 kg—enough to blanch a thumbnail).
- The active tender points are widely distributed, with some from each quadrant of the body.
- The patient reports persistent fatigue.
- The patient reports non-refreshing sleep, and awakens with morning stiffness.

The average FMS patient spends about 5 years and consults at least five health care specialists before arriving at a diagnosis. This is a remarkable figure, considering that this problem is the second most commonly diagnosed musculoskeletal problem in the United States (the first being osteoarthritis).

Complications

While FMS is not a life-threatening disease, it certainly threatens quality of life. The pain it causes is "invisible" pain; that is, no recognizable outward signs of a problem are perceptible.

Compare and Contrast 3.1
FIBROMYALGIA VERSUS MYOFASCIAL PAIN SYNDROME

Chronic pain disorders are identified more and more frequently as our understanding of them improves. Two such disorders that share many qualities are FMS and MPS. It is certainly possible for these two conditions to occur simultaneously, but they have some differing characteristics that require different treatment choices.

CHARACTERISTICS	FIBROMYALGIA SYNDROME	MYOFASCIAL PAIN SYNDROME
Prevalence	Up to 3% of U.S. population.	Unknown.
Demographics	85% women.	Women and men equally affected.
Prognosis	Life-long problem; can be managed, but may never be eradicated.	Can be a short-term problem that is permanently resolved.
Primary symptom	Tender points: predictable areas; light pressure yields intense, diffuse pain. Tender points are often hypotonic, and are not always in muscle tissue.	Trigger points: predictable areas in individual muscles, microtraumatized areas of hypertonicity. May be nodular or appear as a taut band that generates a twitch response. Manual pressure on active trigger point elicits pain locally, and also in predictable patterns of referral.
Implications for massage	Massage can help, but manual pressure exacerbates tender points.	Responds well to massage; rhythmic pressure can break through pain-spasm cycle to eradicate trigger points.

Nothing shows up on imaging tests; no signs of this disorder are readily visible. No blood test reveals specific markers for this problem. A person with this syndrome may be discounted as a faker or malingerer by doctors, employers, even friends and family. By the time a patient has reached a definitive diagnosis, the experience with the medical community has often been frustrating and overwhelmingly negative.

Consider what it would be like to live in chronic pain: pain all the time, pain that never stops, pain that no one else can see or understand. A person who lives in pain, especially when that pain makes it difficult to sleep, may tend to lose perspective about many things. Time ceases to have any real meaning. She hurts now; she's been hurting for a long time; she will always, *always*, ***always*** hurt. And ultimately, that pain begins to define what she can do, what she can eat, where she can go, and in a fundamental way, *who she is*. In other words, a person can become dependent on pain to tell her she's alive. Take away that pain, and what's left?

It is not surprising, then, that depression is a common and dependable complication of FMS. It is clear that depression doesn't *cause* FMS, but it can exacerbate symptoms, as it disrupts sleep and tends to cause people to isolate themselves from support givers.

Treatment

For most people FMS is a lifelong condition. Treatment then focuses on finding ways to *manage* the disorder so that the patient may lead as normal a life as possible.

What seems to work best is a course of therapy that gives the patient control of her own healing process. The first priority is to educate her as completely as possible about her condition, emphasizing that though she may feel incapacitated, this is not a progressive or life-threatening disease.

Second, the responsibility for managing the condition must be put entirely in the patient's hands, through nutrition, sleep, exercise, stretching, and reducing emotional stress. Daily exercise is an important therapy for many FMS patients. Some specialists recommend supplementing guaifenesin, a substance that helps to flush phosphate deposits out of cells to promote more efficient ATP production. Mild tricyclic antidepressants are often prescribed both to reduce levels of depression and to improve the quality of sleep. Painkilling drugs are generally avoided, because they interfere with sleep and can be habit forming. One new avenue in pharmacological approaches to FMS follows a recent discovery about restless leg syndrome: this disorder, which has a significant overlap with FMS, is related to a problem with dopamine production and uptake. Drugs that were developed for Parkinson disease are finding success with patients who have restless leg syndrome, and those drugs are now being studied for patients who have FMS.

Among the obstacles to FMS management is the fact that it takes an enormous investment of time, effort, money, and energy to find the right strategies for each individual. If a person lives in a body that feels painful and tired virtually all the time, it is especially difficult to make the energetic investment that FMS requires.

Massage?

Fibromyalgia patients live in pain. Some moments are more severe than others, but a constant, ongoing, uninterrupted bodywide ache is a hallmark of this condition. Their tissues are drowning in irritating chemicals, and they lack the neurotransmitters that block some of the pain transmission. In other words, these people are extremely hypersensitive and very easy to overtreat.

With that consideration, gentle massage is very appropriate for clients with FMS. Research on massage and FMS patients shows that massage reduces reported levels of pain, anxiety, and depression.[5] Massage may be best used to relax the client and aid with toxic flushing, a little with each session. Fibromyalgia contraindicates the use of ice or ice massage; any kind of cold can exacerbate symptoms. FMS patients may have myofascial trigger points along

Modality Recommendations for Fibromyalgia

MODALITY	RECOMMENDATION
Deep Tissue Massage	Indicated within client tolerance. Treatment can have inconsistent response, so approach each session individually.
Lymphatic drainage	Indicated when subacute.
Polarity	S: Indicated. R/D: Indicated lightly within client comfort.
PNF/MET/stretching	Indicated within client tolerance during acute and subacute stages; can have inconsistent response, so treat each session individually.
Reflexology	Indicated; use light technique with short, frequent sessions: focus on lymphatic system, thalamus, solar plexus points.
Shiatsu	Indicated, for calming and promoting sleep. Use light pressure on GB/LV for joints; avoid ROM.
Swedish massage	Indicated with caution to stay within pain tolerance.
Trigger point therapy	Gentle work is supportive when symptoms are not acute.

See Chapter 1 for a brief description of each modality, including definitions of abbreviations.

CASE HISTORY 3.1

Fibromyalgia Syndrome, Kim

Kim, aged 48: "I'm NOT a hypochondriac, I'm not, I'm NOT!"

Kim was a graphic artist, writer, and creative developer at a children's museum. She was working with the museum at its opening, just having left an extremely stressful job in another city. It was at this time that she first began to have new physical symptoms, powerful tingling sensations in her left arm. The sensations felt like an electrical current running up and down her arm. Eventually they spread into her right arm as well. In the beginning, the sensations came and went quickly, but eventually the episodes came in waves, leaving her arms numb and useless for hours at a time.

At first, she thought she was having a ministroke or even a heart attack because the initial symptoms were in her left arm. She went to a general practitioner, who began to look for signs of stroke or heart attack with an electrocardiogram (ECG), computed tomography (CT), and MRI of her neck and head. Since none of these tests was positive, her doctor suggested that she had herniated a disc and recommended that she consult a neurosurgeon.

The neurosurgeon found no signs of a herniated disc and recommended that Kim consult a neurologist to look for signs of multiple sclerosis.

The neurologist found no signs of multiple sclerosis but felt strongly that Kim was dealing with FMS and referred her to a rheumatologist.

The rheumatologist confirmed this finding. Kim reported that when her tender points were palpated, "It felt like somebody hit me with a baseball bat."

Kim, like so many other FMS patients, endured many tests, examinations, and doctor visits before a final diagnosis was made. Because FMS is an invisible condition, she suffered many remarks from friends and coworkers about it all being in her head.

Kim's other symptoms are less dramatic but in many ways just as debilitating as the numbness and tingling in her arms. She has difficulty sleeping and takes a sleeping aid. She wakes up feeling foggy and extremely stiff. She reports that her pain is worst in the morning, but her neck, shoulders, and sternum hurt "all the time." Her hands and feet are constantly tingling, although this is not as extreme as her initial symptoms.

She has recently developed irritable bowel syndrome, with bloating, cramping, gas, and alternating diarrhea and constipation. These symptoms are becoming worse, and although she can control some of them with diet, they still interfere significantly with her life.

Kim also deals with chronic headaches, probably a result of FMS, in combination with arthritis in her neck and ongoing sinus problems. Her vision has been affected; she reports seeing "specky things." Her balance is inconsistent. She has to keep a finger on the wall as she walks along a hall or she veers off course. Mentally Kim is frustrated (and often amused) by new problems with language. She flips words when she's speaking or writing and frequently accidentally substitutes one word for another when she's typing or even listening to other people. For example, she was once attempting to type "try your hand at bartering for products from Nepal," and she typed "try your hand at bartending . . . "

Kim's FMS is part of a complicated health picture. She is a recovering alcohol and drug abuser and has dealt with depression intermittently for 30 years. She has been treated for posttraumatic stress disorder since leaving her previous job. She has arthritis in her neck, bursitis in her hip, and plantar fasciitis. Her job involves a great deal of sitting, and she feels stiff and painful whenever she stands and moves. Her knees and hips make popping, crackling noises. All of these disorders together exacerbate her sleeping problems, which may in turn exacerbate her FMS.

Management of Kim's condition is challenging. She takes a course of vitamin and mineral supplements recommended by an FMS specialist. She recently began taking yoga classes, and they seem to be providing significant relief. She also still spends plenty of time on a full-length massage mat that her mother sent her immediately after finally getting a diagnosis for her problems. She receives chiropractic care for her neck and lots of pet therapy from her two cats. Despite her many obstacles, Kim keeps a positive attitude toward life. She says that although the physical aspects of her condition are taxing, the mental twists and turns it provides are vastly entertaining.

with tender points. With these clients more than anyone, it is important not to treat trigger points with aggressive deep pressure. Shorter, pulsing, gentler pressure is much more appropriate for this population.

It usually takes a long time to become incapacitated by FMS; it can also take a long time to find ways to cope with this condition. But a client who can be pain free, even for a short time after each massage, will feel more able to take control of her own healing process, which is the most important step toward recovery.

Myofascial Pain Syndrome

Definition: What Is It?

Myofascial pain syndrome (MPS) is identified when a person develops many trigger points: irritable spots in muscles that are palpable as knots or taut bands within muscles.

Demographics: Who Gets It?

MPS affects men and women more or less equally. MPS is seen in people of all ages, although its prevalence seems to taper off with advancing age. Sedentary people are vulnerable to this condition, as are physically active people.

The incidence of MPS is difficult to estimate. Among one group of patients with chronic pain, 35% of them had active trigger points.[6] Other researchers suggest that up to 23 million people in the United States have chronic musculoskeletal pain that involves trigger points.[7] But even people with no symptoms can show signs of latent trigger points, which may develop into active MPS with little provocation.

Myofascial Pain Syndrome in Brief
MY-o-fash-al pane SIN-drome

What is it?
MPS is a collection of signs and symptoms associated with the development of myofascial trigger points in muscles.

How is it recognized?
MPS is recognized mainly by the trigger points in predictable locations in affected muscles. Active trigger points are tight and painful; the pain may refer to distant locations. Latent trigger points may not generate pain until they are irritated.

Is massage indicated or contraindicated?
MPS indicates massage, which can interrupt the cycle of ischemia and tightness and help to drain off the irritating metabolic wastes that accumulate around trigger points.

Etiology: What Happens?

Our understanding of myofascial trigger points continues to evolve. Traditionally it was thought that they began as microscopic injuries to individual muscle fibers; these fibers descended into a pain-spasm-ischemia cycle. This may be the situation with some trigger points, but current thinking suggests that they are more closely related to problems with the synapse between the motor neuron and the motor end plate of the myofiber than to an initiating injury.

The center of the trigger point phenomenon is a sustained, involuntary contraction of an isolated group of sarcomeres (the overlapping units of myofibrils that create the striations associated with skeletal muscles). When this occurs close to the neuromuscular junction, it is called a *central trigger point.* Contractions that develop close to the tenoperiosteal junction may also involve folded and dehydrated collagen fibers; these are called *attachment trigger points.*

When a microscopic contraction pulls on the rest of the myofiber, it creates a taut band; this gives rise to two simultaneous problems: an *increased* need for fuel and a *decreased* supply of blood due to local ischemia. This situation is sometimes called an *ATP energy crisis.* Chemicals that increase sensitivity and pain are released, including prostaglandins, bradykinin, serotonin, substance P, and others: this helps to a generate pain sensation. In response to pain, the muscle attempts to tighten further, causing more secretion of acetylcholine (ACh). Poor local circulation limits the availability of ACh-neutralizing enzymes, and it inhibits the movement of calcium back into channels in the cell membrane. The consequence: a tiny, involuntary, but prolonged and painful contraction of one part of a muscle cell.

Prolonged immersion in pain-causing chemicals carries a toll for local sensory neurons. Some research suggests that the neurons become locally demyelinated, which may contribute to the unique referred pain pattern seen with trigger points[8] (Figure 3.4).

Satellite points Satellite points are trigger points that form as secondary issue to primary trigger points. They may develop in areas where referred pain is perceived, in areas where muscle fibers are overloaded because of compensation patterns to protect a primary trigger point, in the antagonists to muscles with active trigger points, or in muscles that are referred pain areas for the heart or other organs.

Active and latent trigger points Trigger points that are not irritated may become latent: they are not painful, nor do they refer pain. Latent trigger points are associated with restricted range of motion and muscle weakness, however. Further, very little stimulus can turn a latent trigger point into an active one, which is locally and distantly painful even when the muscle is at rest. These sore spots have palpable knots or taut bands that send pain shooting in predictable directions.

It is clear that trigger points form at areas under stress due to postural habits, poor ergonomics, and repetitive motion. But trigger points can also be a complication of more standard types of injuries, when a person accommodates to the pain and/or limited range of motion that might be the result of an automobile accident, a sports injury, or any other kind of damage.

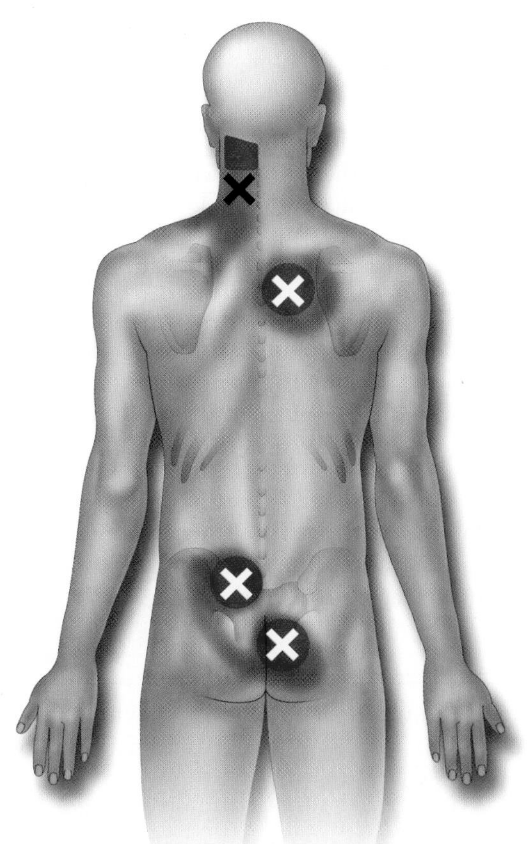

Figure 3.4. Myofascial pain syndrome: trigger points and referred pain pathways.

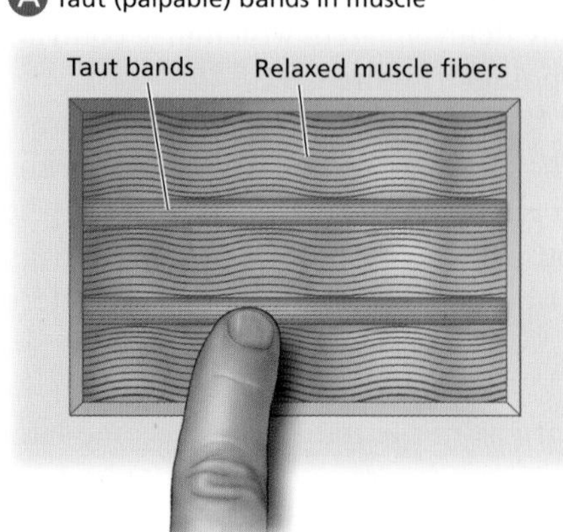

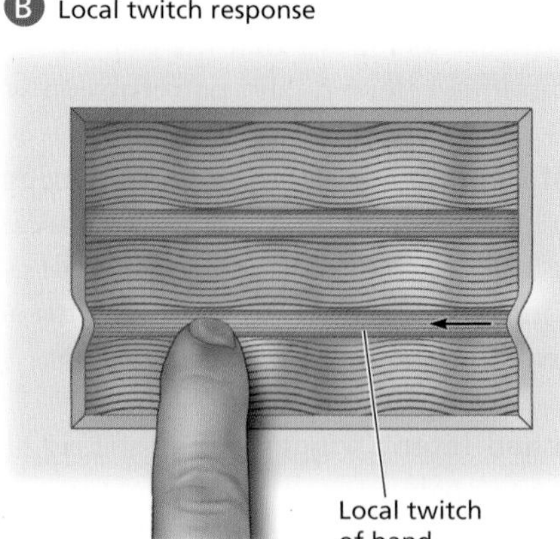

Figure 3.5. Myofascial pain syndrome: twitch response.

Signs and Symptoms

MPS is recognized by the accumulation of active trigger points. These trigger points have some qualities that make them unique among muscle disorders.

- *Taut bands or nodules.* Trigger points can be palpated in muscle tissue as taut, hypertonic bands of fibers within a mass of muscle that is less tight (Figure 3.5) or as small nodules that dissipate under static pressure. A muscle flicker, or twitch response, is often seen when a trigger point is palpated.
- *Predictable trigger point map.* Each skeletal muscle in the body has an area or group of areas where trigger points are most likely to form. These areas have been extensively mapped.[9]
- *Referred pain pattern.* Active trigger points are always locally painful under digital pressure, but they often refer pain to other areas in the body as well. Their referred pain patterns are consistent from person to person. However, they don't follow patterns understood in the context of nerve pathways, energy meridians, or other pathways of flow through the body. Referred pain patterns of trigger points have been documented along with the maps of where they occur.
- *Regional pain.* MPS is seldom a whole-body dysfunction. More often, trigger points flare up in specific regions, often around the neck and shoulders. Jaw muscles are notorious for developing trigger points, which refer pain all over the face and head. This variety of MPS is often discussed in the context of temporomandibular joint disorders.

Other symptoms of MPS are less predictable than trigger point development. Sleep disorders occur occasionally but not consistently. Depression and anxiety are also possible, especially when a person has little success in getting an accurate diagnosis and effective treatment.

Diagnosis

At this point no specific criteria have been agreed upon for a definitive diagnosis of MPS. A diagnosis is usually arrived at after a thorough pain history, physical examination, movement and postural analysis, and palpation of active trigger points.

One complicating factor that interferes with getting a clear picture of this disorder is that most people have trigger points. They may be latent, that is, not actively causing pain, but only moderate stimulus may cause them to become active. The line between a person with some active trigger points and a person with MPS is vague indeed.

Treatment

Perhaps the best news about MPS is that it is a chronic pain disorder with an excellent prognosis. The top priority for MPS treatment, of course, is to eradicate trigger points. This is accomplished in a number of ways, including the use of vapo-coolant spray, local injections of anesthetics, dry needling, and acupuncture. Injections of ***botulinum*** toxin type A have been explored to block ACh release at the neuromuscular junction. All of these approaches work to interrupt the pain-spasm cycle or the ATP energy crisis, allowing the tight fibers to relax while the muscle is stretched.

Bodywork in several forms has been seen to have success in the resolution of trigger points. Prolonged ischemic pressure has been the traditional strategy, but new approaches to trigger points indicate that pulsing pressure that follows the taut band of the muscle may be even more effective while being far less painful.

Because MPS often develops out of chronic overuse or poor ergonomics, the patient's movement and work habits are often examined and adjusted so that perpetuating factors may be eliminated.

Massage?

MPS indicates massage, both for its effectiveness at improving myofiber function and for its ability to help clean up the debris left behind from chronic muscle tightness. When muscle cells are working, they can't exchange nutrients for waste products. Irritating metabolic wastes accumulate in the tissues, perpetuating soreness and fatigue. Massage is an excellent mechanism to help flush the waste away, with the precaution that someone in this condition is easy to overtreat.

Modality Recommendations for Myofascial Pain Syndrome

MODALITY	RECOMMENDATION
Deep tissue massage	Indicated within client tolerance. Work around contracture with slow gradual pressure; avoid forcing tissue.
Lymphatic drainage	Supportive.
Polarity	S/R/D: Indicated within client comfort.
PNF/MET/stretching	Indicated in acute and subacute (active and latent) stages.
Reflexology	Indicated; work adrenals and lymphatic system points.
Shiatsu	Indicated. Treat BL, SI, GB, ST, SP meridians and extensions systemically and all meridians and points at affected local areas.
Swedish massage	Indicated; facilitates body's search for homeostasis.
Trigger point therapy	Indicated in acute and subacute (active and latent) stages.

See Chapter 1 for a brief description of each modality, including definitions of abbreviations.

Myositis Ossificans in Brief
Pronunciation: my-o-SY-tis os-IF-ih-kanz

What is it?
This is the growth of a bony deposit in soft tissues. It usually follows trauma that involves significant leakage of blood between fascial sheaths.

How is it recognized?
Radiography is the best way to see this problem, but it is palpable as a dense mass where no such mass should be.

Is massage indicated or contraindicated?
Myositis ossificans locally contraindicates most types of massage, but work around the edges of the area may stimulate reabsorption of the bone tissue without doing further damage.

Myositis Ossificans

Definition: What Is It?

Myositis ossificans means *muscle inflammation with bone formation.* This is a bit of a misnomer, because it can happen in any type of soft tissue and it doesn't always involve inflammation. Its synonym, *heterotopic ossification,* is closer to the mark; this describes an abnormal placement of some part of the body, specifically bone tissue. This condition most often affects adolescents and young adults, and it usually occurs in the quadriceps group or the brachialis.

Etiology: What Happens?

The most common variety of myositis ossificans, called *myositis ossificans traumatica,* follows a blunt injury with bleeding into the muscle belly or between fascial sheets. For reasons that are not entirely clear, this kind of injury may leave behind a formation that looks and feels like a bone embedded in soft tissue (Figure 3.6).

Myositis ossificans can occur freely within muscle or other soft tissue, but in many cases the growth is attached continuously or by a stalk to nearby periosteum. It typically hardens from the periphery of the growth and stays soft and disorganized in the center. This pattern helps to distinguish myositis ossificans from other conditions (such as varieties of bone cancer) that can give rise to similar symptoms.

Theories about the calcification process of myositis ossificans traumatica vary. Some propose that in the original trauma some osteoblasts are released from the damaged periosteum, and they stimulate the deposition of calcium in the soft tissues. Another possibility is that in the proliferation of cells that occurs with a deep muscle injury, some stem cells are triggered to become osteoblasts, and they lay down new bone tissue.

In the long run the body usually recognizes that the calcium deposits don't belong there, and it eventually breaks down and reabsorbs this bony anomaly. This can take months or years, but in most people the lesion finally just goes away.

Other forms of myositis ossificans are associated with disorders that either limit mobility or involve excessive growth of bone tissue. Spinal cord injury, traumatic brain injury, ankylosing spondylitis (AS), Paget disease, and some autoimmune disorders carry an increased risk for developing associated heterotopic ossification. Hip replacement surgery also carries a significant risk of developing bony deposits in surrounding soft tissues.

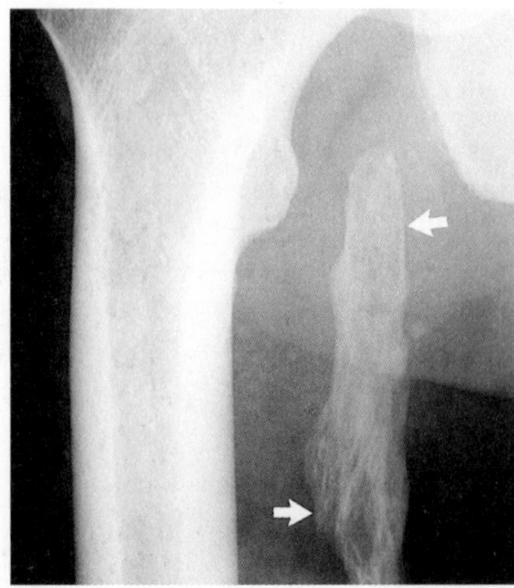

Figure 3.6. Myositis ossificans (arrows).

Signs and Symptoms

In the acute stage of trauma-based myositis ossificans, the area feels bruised; within a few days it may feel hard and locally very tender. The range of motion in the nearby joint is limited: if it occurs in the brachialis, the elbow doesn't fully extend, and when it occurs in the quadriceps, the knee can't fully flex. Eventually little or no local pain may be present, but a dense, unyielding mass develops where nothing hard should be.

Treatment

Treatment for myositis ossificans traumatica tends to be conservative. Patients are recommended to rest and isolate the injured area in the acute stage to limit further bleeding. In the subacute stage passive stretching is employed to restore range of motion, followed by exercises to restore normal muscle strength. Athletes in particular are counseled to pad the injured area carefully to prevent a repeat injury.

If a fully mature and calcified mass interferes with muscle or tendon function, it can be surgically removed. This kind of surgery is avoided if possible, however, because many patients have a postsurgical recurrence of the growth.

Massage?

Myositis ossificans is always a local contraindication. If the injury is acute, it is unwise to increase the bleeding or impair the healing process by stimulating and stretching the affected tissue. If the leakage has begun to coagulate but has not yet calcified, massage can be instrumental in stimulating reabsorption, but it is still important to work just around the edges of the injury because working in the middle can aggravate it and lead to more bleeding. If the injury is old, it is *still* a local contraindication; massage may compress soft tissues against the bony growth and cause more internal bleeding. Working within tolerance around the edges, however, may stimulate the body's own mechanisms to reabsorb this old, useless deposit.

Modality Recommendations for Myositis Ossificans

MODALITY	RECOMMENDATION
Deep tissue massage	Locally contraindicated; otherwise supportive.
Lymphatic drainage	Supportive.
Polarity	S: Indicated. R/D: Locally contraindicated; otherwise supportive within client comfort.
PNF/MET/stretching	Locally contraindicated; otherwise supportive.
Reflexology	Locally contraindicated; otherwise supportive.
Shiatsu	Indicated. Treat BL, K, LV, SP, SI systemically. Use light pressure at and around local site.
Swedish massage	Locally contraindicated; work around the area can aid in reabsorbing the deposits.
Trigger point therapy	Locally contraindicated; otherwise supportive.

See Chapter 1 for a brief description of each modality, including definitions of abbreviations.

Shin Splints in Brief

What are they?
Shin splints are a collection of lower leg injuries including compartment syndromes, muscle tears, periostitis, hairline fractures, and other problems. They are usually brought about by overuse and/or misalignment at the ankle.

How are they recognized?
Pain along the tibia may be superficial or deep, mild or severe. The pattern of pain differs with the specific structures that are injured.

Is massage indicated or contraindicated?
Muscle injuries indicate massage, but periostitis or stress fractures require more caution. Massage may be useful for chronic compartment syndrome, but it is inappropriate for acute compartment syndrome, which is a medical emergency.

Shin Splints

Definition: What Is It?

Shin splints is an umbrella term used to describe a variety of lower leg problems. Medial tibial stress syndrome is the injury most commonly associated with shin splints, but closely related problems include *periostitis,* stress fractures, and chronic or acute compartment syndrome.

Etiology: What Happens?

Several features make the lower leg susceptible to certain injuries. Before discussing what goes wrong here, it is worthwhile to take a brief look at the construction of the lower leg and foot.

Anatomy review Many muscles in the body are almost entirely separate from their attaching bones, touching only at the ends of their tendons. Tibialis anterior and posterior muscles, however, attach to the tibia from beginning to end and almost along the entire length of the muscle bellies. The tibialis anterior fascia blends directly into the periosteum along the whole bone (Figure 3.7). The tibialis posterior attaches to the posterior aspect of the tibia in a similar way; the endomysial sheaths blend directly into the periosteum and interosseous ligament of the tibia and fibula. The soleus also has a long attachment on the periosteum of the medial tibia.

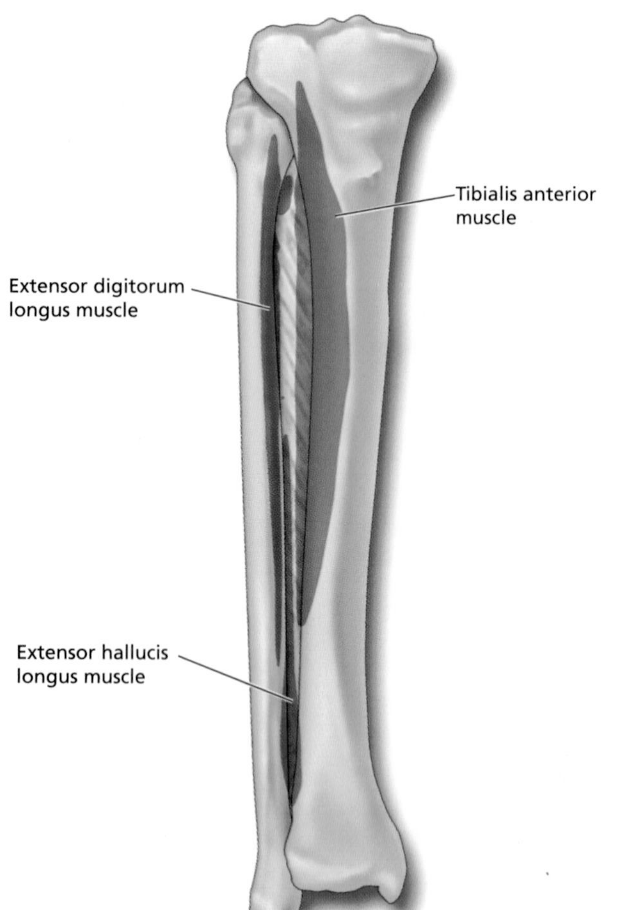

Figure 3.7. Shin splints: the anterior compartment muscles blend into the tibial periosteum.

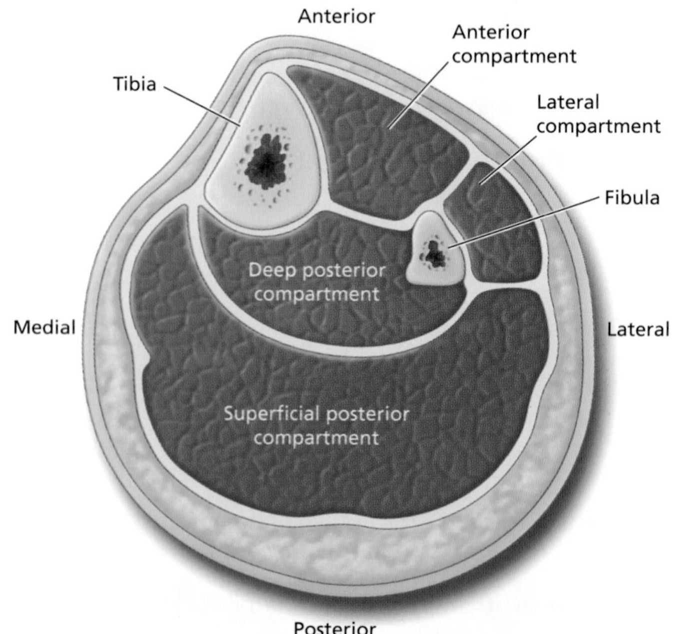

Figure 3.8. Four fascial compartments in the lower leg.

The musculature of the lower leg is contained in four tough fascial compartments (Figure 3.8). Each compartment has its own motor nerve supply. The fascia that wraps around these compartments is so dense and unyielding that if fluid accumulates beyond a certain point, it can interfere with normal lymphatic and venous drainage. This traps the excess fluid inside the fascial sheath. The pressure this causes can be very painful and can damage muscle tissue and nerves.

The other key piece to lower leg function is the shock-absorbing capacity of the feet. Feet are designed to spread out and rebound with each step. If the foot has inadequate shock absorption—because of flat feet or jammed arches (pes planus or pes cavus, respectively), worn-out shoes, hard surfaces, or any combination thereof—the tibia and the muscles in the lower leg, especially the soleus, tibialis anterior, and tibialis posterior, absorb a disproportionate amount of the shock. They are not designed for this job, and ongoing stress causes the periosteum to become irritated, the bone to crack, and the muscles to fray and become inflamed.

Chronic overuse or misalignment may cause the lower leg muscles to accrue internal microtearing along with general inflammation. The periosteum of the injured tibia may do the same. The difficulty with inflammation in this area is that those fascial sheaths simply have no room for excess fluid. Even a small amount of edema puts pressure on nerve endings and limits blood flow, which in a typical vicious circle makes it hard for excess fluid to leave the area.

Causes of inflammation in the lower leg include exercising with inadequate foot support or on bad surfaces; unusual amounts of exercise followed by a period of rest (continued gentle movement helps the fluid to keep moving out of the area); a sudden change in an exercise routine, or running mostly uphill, downhill, or on uneven surfaces.

Not all cases of lower leg injuries are brought about by overuse. Trauma to the lower leg (including fractured tibia), snakebite, and ruptured Baker cyst are all possible contributors to shin splints and associated problems.

Signs and Symptoms

Pain from shin splints can be mild or severe, and the location varies according to which of the structures has been damaged. It gets worse with whatever actions the affected muscles do: dorsiflexion, inversion, or plantarflexion. Simple muscle injuries are rarely visibly or palpably inflamed. If the tibia is red, hot, and puffy, suspect a more severe injury than muscle damage to the lower leg.

Lower Leg Injuries

Muscle strains are the first step in a series of lower leg injuries. The following lists associated problems, and the serious complications that may follow if they are not treated.

- *Tibialis anterior, tibialis posterior injury.* The pain associated with these injuries may be familiar to many people. The ache often runs most of the length of the tibia on the lateral side (for tibialis anterior) or deep in the back of the calf (for tibialis posterior).
- *Medial tibial stress syndrome.* This muscular injury on the medial side of the tibia usually involves the soleus and tibialis anterior. It is typically painful at the distal third segment of the medial tibia.
- *Periostitis.* This inflammation of the periosteum may happen with damage to the soleus, the anterior tibialis, or posterior tibialis muscles. That seamless connection of membranes begins to rip apart, and the fibers of the muscles pull away from the bone. This condition may sometimes leave the bone feeling bumpy or pitted; that's where scar tissue has knitted the connective tissue membranes back together.
- *Stress fractures.* These hairline fractures of the tibia are extremely painful, and nothing heals them except time. They are frequently the result of "running through the pain." They are best diagnosed by bone scan, which looks for areas of increased circulatory activity. Stress fractures of the tibia often don't show up well on radiographs.

- *Chronic compartment syndrome.* This is caused by production of excessive fluid in any of the four compartments of the lower leg. Local pressure from blood and lymph, which is normally increased with exercise, puts mechanical pressure on local nerves, causing pain and inflammation. These symptoms are relieved by rest but recur in a predictable pattern with activity.
- *Acute compartment syndrome.* This is a culmination of that vicious circle of local edema, which limits blood flow, which in turn limits the exit of excess fluid. Because the fascia on the lower leg is such a tough container, the swelling can actually cause tissue death if it's not resolved naturally or with surgical intervention. Acute compartment syndrome is an emergency and should be treated as quickly as possible.

Treatment

The typical approach to mild shin splints is to reduce activity and to alternate applications of heat and cold to the affected area. If the situation (i.e., becomes chronic or acute compartment syndrome) steroid injections may be suggested, or surgery may be performed to split the fascia and allow room for those compressed blood vessels that were unable to do their jobs. This surgery is followed by physical therapy to limit the accumulation of scar tissue that could bind up the compartments even more tightly than before.

Massage?

As long as the problem is not too advanced, shin splints indicate massage. The lower leg muscles are impossible to stretch out thoroughly and clean up with exercise alone, but massage can give them a luxurious inch-by-inch compression and broadening that cleanses the tissues more efficiently than anything else. In fact, massage is an excellent way to *prevent* shin splints and periostitis from complicating into compartment syndrome.

For palpably hot, inflamed, painful cases, however, it is necessary to wait until the pain and inflammation have subsided. Obviously, if too much fluid has accumulated in a closed area, the last thing the person needs is massage to exacerbate it. What this person really needs is to see a doctor. Stress fractures and compartment syndrome are serious problems that require medical attention.

Modality Recommendations for Shin Splints

MODALITY	RECOMMENDATION
Deep tissue massage	Indicated when subacute: work with crural fascia and compartments, then muscles and tendons to the foot. Use ROM at ankle and toes.
Lymphatic drainage	Supportive.
Polarity	S: Indicated. R/D: indicated within client comfort.
PNF/MET/stretching	Indicated in acute or subacute stages.
Reflexology	Locally contraindicated; otherwise supportive.
Shiatsu	Indicated. Treat ST meridian, TH extension in lower leg.
Swedish massage	Contraindicated while acute; rule out compartment syndrome. Can be useful when subacute. Stay within pain tolerance.
Trigger point therapy	Locally contraindicated for compartment syndrome; indicated when subacute.

See Chapter 1 for a brief description of each modality, including definitions of abbreviations.

Spasms, Cramps

Definition: What Are They?

A spasm or cramp is an involuntary contraction of a voluntary muscle. The difference between *spasms* and *cramps* is somewhat arbitrary; cramps are strong, painful, usually short-lived spasms. One could say that chronically tight, painful paraspinals are in *spasm*, while a gastrocnemius with a charley horse is a *cramp*. The severity of these episodes depends on how much of the muscle is involved.

The terms "spasms" and "cramps" are sometimes used in reference to visceral muscle too (i.e., *spastic constipation*), but this discussion is restricted to the involuntary contraction of skeletal, or so-called voluntary muscle.

Spasms, Cramps in Brief

What are they?
Spasms and cramps are involuntary contractions of skeletal muscle. Spasms are considered to be low-grade, long-lasting contractions, while cramps are short-lived, very acute contractions.

How are they recognized?
Cramps are extremely painful, with visible shortening of muscle fibers. Long-term spasms are painful and may cause inefficient movement but may not have acute symptoms.

Is massage indicated or contraindicated?
Acutely cramping muscle bellies do not invite massage, though stretching and origin or insertion work can trick the proprioceptors into letting go. Muscles that have been in spasm or cramp respond well to massage, which can reduce residual pain and clean up chemical wastes. Underlying cramp-causing pathologies must be ruled out before massage is applied. Long-term spasm indicates massage because it can break through the ischemia-spasm-pain cycle to reintroduce circulation to the area and to reduce muscle tone and flush out toxins.

Etiology: What Happens?

Four of the most common situations are addressed here.

Nutrition Calcium and magnesium deficiencies, in addition to causing all sorts of problems later in life, can make one prone to cramping, especially in the feet.

Ischemia When a muscle or part of a muscle is suddenly or gradually deprived of oxygen, it can't function properly. Rather than becoming loose and weak, it becomes tighter and tighter. Often this is a gradual process, but sometimes it is a sudden and violent reaction to oxygen shortage.

Anything that impedes blood flow into the affected areas can cause a local oxygen shortage. Consider a typical tight, painful iliocostalis, one of the paraspinal muscles that holds the back erect. Here is a muscle that is tight, hard, a little achy, but most of all, *overworked*. The fibers are shortened and thickened with the effort of keeping the spine upright, and this makes it harder for the supplying capillaries to deliver oxygen. In protest, the iliocostalis draws up even tighter. This further inhibits the influx of oxygen, starting a vicious circle of ischemia causing spasm, causing pain, which leads to spasm, and so on. Furthermore, muscles that are forced to work without oxygen accumulate the chemical byproducts of anaerobic combustion. These metabolic wastes irritate nerve fibers and reinforce the spasm. The whole picture is complicated by the fact that as postural habits develop, the brain comes to interpret these sensations as being normal. The proprioceptors eventually reinforce the patterns that cause the problem. This situation can go on for years at a time without any real relief until the circle of ischemia-spasm-pain is interrupted (Figure 3.9).

Pregnancy can be another cause of ischemic cramping. As the fetus lies on the femoral artery (just where it splits off from the abdominal branch), it can interfere with blood flow into the leg, prompting a violent contraction of the gastrocnemius. This is a classic example of an acute cramp, or charley horse. Other kinds of circulatory interruptions or nervous system problems can cause them too, so in a decision about whether massage is appropriate, it's important that no underlying pathology, such as cardiac weakness, is creating an oxygen deficiency.

Exercise-associated muscle cramping Athletes often report problems with muscles cramping at or near the end of vigorous workouts. Dehydration, electrolyte imbalance, and hyperthermia may all be contributing factors, but these cramps may be primarily due to a neurological abnormality that overexcites muscle spindles (the proprioceptors involved in tightening) while inhibiting the activity of Golgi tendon organs (the proprioceptors that al-

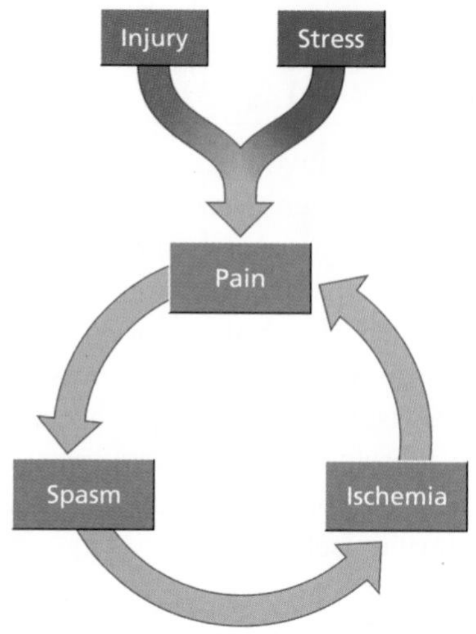

Figure 3.9. Pain-spasm-ischemia cycle.

low muscles to let go). The target muscles usually cross two joints, and they cramp when they are contracted from a shortened position. Stretching the muscles and manipulating the tendons limit these cramps, but they tend to recur if the athlete is inadequately warmed up or stretched out before beginning to exercise.

Splinting This is a reflexive reaction against injury. Consider an acute whiplash: the supraspinous and intertransverse ligaments have been severely wrenched, and the body senses a potentially dangerous instability in the cervical spine. Of course the postural neck muscles contract; as far as they're concerned, they are keeping the head from falling off. This kind of spasm is an important protective mechanism. It prevents movements that could cause further injury. The muscles create an effective splint; the range of motion of affected joints is generally very small. The proprioceptors say, "You can move this far, no farther."

Massage?

Ischemic or exercise-related cramps indicate massage, as long as the ischemia isn't related to a contraindicating condition. But even when underlying pathology has been ruled out, massage must be used with caution. If a therapist tries to fluff up a cramping gastrocnemius, the fibers may be damaged. A better strategy is to stretch the tendons and antagonists of the affected muscle to persuade the proprioceptors, gently but quickly, that they may safely allow the muscle to let go. Alternatively, reciprocal inhibition (actively contracting the antagonists of the cramping muscle) can be effective. When the problem has moved out of the acute stage, it is possible to go back and clean up some of the toxic waste left behind, always at the tolerance of the client.

When tight muscles splint a newly injured area, massage therapists should not interfere with this protective mechanism. If they do, the client may get up off the table with newly loosened scalenes, but those muscles will clamp right back down, maybe even more tightly than before.

In time the ligaments will be ready to take on some weight-bearing stress, but the muscles may no longer be able to let go spontaneously: the proprioceptors have become accustomed to an inefficient level of tension. *Now* massage can do some real good. By working to soften the hardened muscle tissue, massage can reset tension levels, reduce toxicity, improve blood flow, and speed healing. Spasm as a splinting mechanism is to be highly respected. When the injury moves into a subacute stage, massage is indicated and can contribute to healing with a minimum of scar tissue, fibrosis, and permanent shortening.

Modality Recommendations for Spasms and Cramps

MODALITY	RECOMMENDATION
Deep tissue massage	Indicated; use passive ROM. May use active client movement if well tolerated.
Lymphatic drainage	Supportive following standard massage.
Polarity	S/R/D: Indicated within client comfort.
PNF/MET/stretching	Indicated in acute and subacute stages when injury, other contraindications ruled out.
Reflexology	Indicated.
Shiatsu	Indicated. Hold joints in opposite direction of cramped position; apply pressure directly to area of spasm according to pain tolerance.
Swedish massage	Indicated when injury, other contraindications are ruled out. Direct compression, reciprocal inhibition, approximation, and stretching are good strategies.
Trigger point therapy	Locally contraindicated for muscles in acute spasm; otherwise indicated.

Strains

Strains in Brief

What are they?
Strains are torn muscle fibers.

How are they recognized?
Pain, stiffness, and occasionally palpable heat and swelling are all signs of muscle strain. Pain may be exacerbated by passive stretching or resisted contraction of the affected muscle.

Is massage indicated or contraindicated?
Muscle strains indicate massage, which can powerfully influence the production of useful scar tissue, reduce adhesions and edema, and reestablish range of motion.

Definition: What Are They?

Strains are a subject of semantic debate. Some people say the word *strain* refers to tendon tears; others insist it refers only to muscle tears. In this text strain refers to an injury to the muscle-tendon unit, with an emphasis on muscles. Tendon injuries are covered in the section on tendinopathies, later in the chapter.

Etiology: What Happens?

Muscle strains and other soft tissue injuries may arise from trauma, but they appear more often in the context of chronic, cumulative overuse patterns with no specific onset.

When a muscle is injured, myofibers are torn, the inflammatory process begins, and fibroblasts flood the area with collagen to knit the injury back together. Like ligament injuries, strains are graded by severity. First-degree strains are mildly painful but don't seriously impede function, while third-degree strains involve ruptured muscles and possibly avulsed bony attachment sites.

Signs and Symptoms

Symptoms of muscle strain are mild or intense local pain, stiffness, and pain on resisted movement or passive stretching. Unless it is a very bad tear, no palpable heat or swelling is usually present. Muscles, unlike tendons and ligaments, are not made exclusively of connective tissue, and while this is a good thing in terms of blood supply, an accumulation of excess scar tissue in muscles has different implications than it does in tendons and ligaments:

Impaired contractility Scar tissue can seriously impede the contractility of uninjured muscle fibers. When the muscle tries to contract, it bears the weight not only of its bony insertion but also of the fibers that are disabled by the mass of collagen that binds them up. This significantly increases the load on uninjured fibers and the chance of repeated injury, more scar tissue, and further weakening of the muscle.

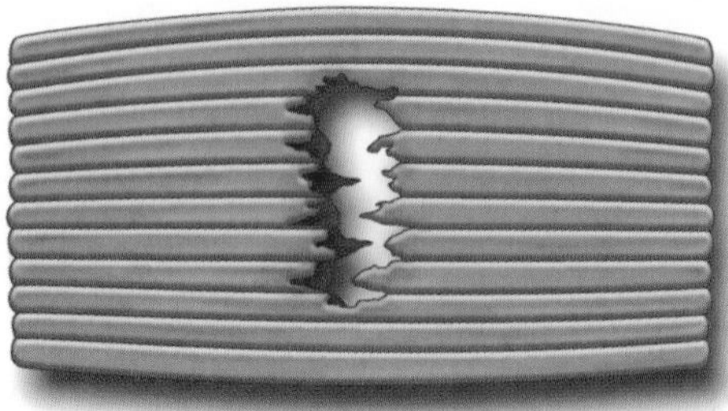

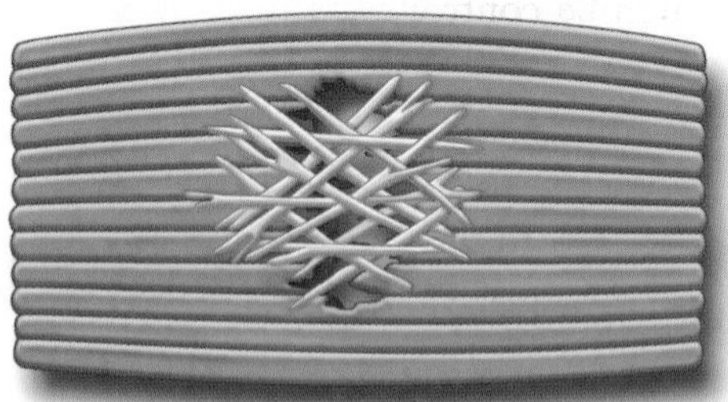

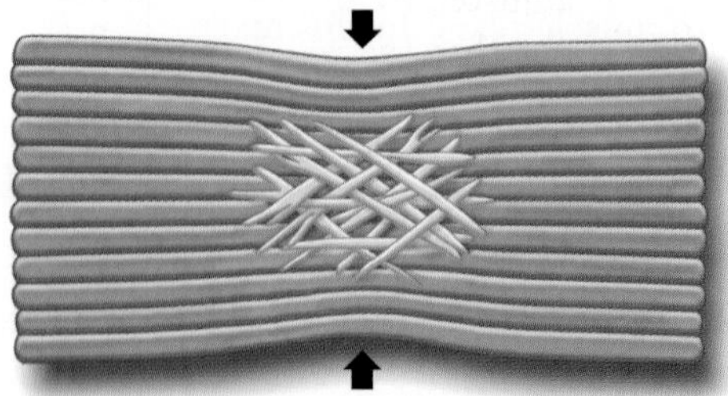

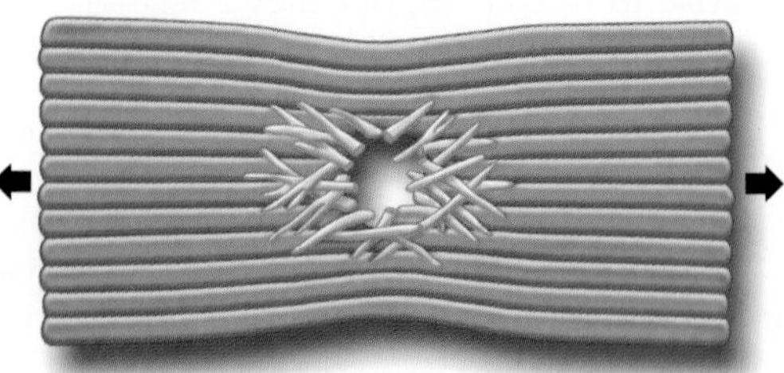

Figure 3.10. Strains, sprains, and tendinitis: the injury-reinjury cycle.

Adhesions Collagen that is manufactured around an injury isn't laid down in perfect alignment with the muscle fibers; instead it is deposited quickly but in haphazard form. Randomly arranged collagen fibers tend to bind up different layers of tissue that are designed to be separate: these are adhesions. Adhesions can occur wherever layers of connective tissue come in contact with each other. They may occur *within* the muscle, as is frequently seen with the paraspinals, or *between* muscles, when muscle sheaths stick to other muscle sheaths. Hamstrings are a common place for this phenomenon. Wherever they occur, adhesions limit mobility and increase the chance of injury (Figure 3.10).

Treatment

The management of muscle injuries has taken some giant steps forward in recent years. While at one time an injured person would be given a prescription for anti-inflammatories and painkillers, it is now recognized that early intervention in the healing process can powerfully affect the long-term quality of the healed tissue.

Although individual specialists approach musculoskeletal injuries with different tactics, some of their procedures are consistent:

- *Get an accurate diagnosis.* Evaluating muscular injuries requires a thorough patient history and a skilled clinical examination. Other diagnostic procedures (e.g., radiographs, bone scans, CT, MRI) may be recommended as well.
- *Control inflammation.* Inflammation is a valuable tool in dealing with acute injuries, but it can outlive its usefulness and end up causing more harm than good. Inflammation can often be controlled by RICE (rest, ice, compression, elevation), but some physicians now use the PRICES protocol, which adds protection and support to the list.
- *Rehabilitate damaged tissues.* This part of the treatment involves exercises that add incremental amounts of weight-bearing stress to the injured muscle to help the scar tissue realign with the original fibers and to gradually increase strength and fitness. This may be the most vulnerable time in the process, as athletes who are eager to resume training may try to go too fast and get injured again, and others may neglect the need to exercise and allow scar tissue to accumulate to inefficient levels.
- *Prevent further injury.* Most chronic muscle injuries are related to controllable factors that can be adjusted to help prevent future problems. These include dealing with muscle imbalances that make one area weaker while another may be tighter, improving technique in specific sports, making sure that equipment is appropriate and in good repair, adjusting training schedules so that changes are incorporated slowly, taping or bracing vulnerable areas, and being careful about good warmup and cool-down procedures.

Massage?

Skillful, knowledgeable massage can make the difference between a one-time muscle strain that takes a few weeks to resolve and a painful, limiting, chronically recurring condition that makes it impossible to do some activity a client used to love.

Once a therapist has a clear picture of what structure or structures have been injured, various kinds of lymphatic drainage techniques can help to limit edema. Cross-fiber and linear friction can influence the way old scar tissue matures and new scar tissue is laid down. Passive stretches of healing muscles can also influence the correct alignment of collagen. When massage therapists apply their skills to the proper formation of scar tissue, reduction of edema, limiting of adhesions, and improvement of circulation and mobility, they can help turn an irritating muscle tear into a trivial event.

Modality Recommendations for Strains

MODALITY	RECOMMENDATION
Deep tissue massage	Indicated; use passive ROM with release within tolerance to influence direction of fiber repair.
Lymphatic drainage	Indicated in acute and subacute stages, following standard massage.
Polarity	S: Indicated. R/D: Light locally within client comfort.
PNF/MET/stretching	Locally contraindicated while acute; indicated in subacute stage.
Reflexology	Locally contraindicated; otherwise supportive.
Shiatsu	Indicated. When acute and inflamed, use TH, SP, K systemically, light pressure at local site. Add more pressure in subacute stages.
Swedish massage	Locally contraindicated while acute; superior centripedal flushing can decrease swelling. Supportive when subacute.
Trigger point therapy	Locally contraindicated while acute; indicated in subacute stage.

See Chapter 1 for a brief description of each modality, including definitions of abbreviations.

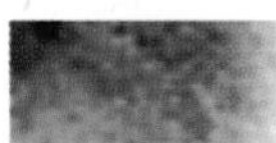

Bone Disorders

Avascular Osteonecrosis

Definition: What Is It?

Avascular necrosis (AVN) is a condition in which blood supply to a bone is impeded by some combination of factors. Bone tissue and blood vessels disintegrate and are never fully replaced. The resulting weakness leads to a high risk of fractures, arthritis, and joint collapse.

> **Avascular Osteonecrosis in Brief**
> Pronunciation: a-VAS-kyu-lar os-te-o-nek-RO-sis
>
> **What is it?**
> Avascular osteonecrosis (AVN) is a condition in which blood supply to an area of bone is interrupted and the bone tissue consequently dies. It occurs most frequently at the head of the femur.
>
> **How is it recognized?**
> Depending on the cause of the disorder, AVN may be silent in early stages. Later stages show pain at the affected area, along with signs of arthritis and the risk of total joint collapse if the damage is near an articulation.
>
> **Is massage indicated or contraindicated?**
> AVN can be brought about by any of several underlying disorders. Decisions about the appropriateness of massage must be made according to contributing factors. Generally speaking, massage may exacerbate pain and damage local to the affected area, but it may be appropriate elsewhere.

Demographics: Who Gets It?

AVN is diagnosed most frequently in people between 30 and 50 years of age. It is rare in elderly people, because of changes in the construction of bone tissue that occur with age. AVN is diagnosed about 10,000 to 20,000 times a year in the United States and is the reason for about 50,000 total hip replacement surgeries per year.[10]

One type of this disease, *Legg-Calvé-Perthes disease,* is almost exclusive to boys between 3 and 12 years of age.[11]

Etiology: What Happens?

Several factors may work together to interrupt blood flow to a bone. The head of the femur, because of its peculiar shape and the concentration of weight that it bears, is particularly vulnerable. The presence of tiny emboli of blood clots, fat cells, or nitrogen bubbles may block arterial capillaries in the femoral head, leading to the death of bone tissue (Figure 3.11). Congestion on the venous side of circulatory turnover may also lead to damage.

Decompression sickness (the bends) is one contributor to AVN. It occurs when nitrogen bubbles in the bloodstream. Fat cells in yellow marrow of the femoral head take up nitrogen readily and expand rapidly. They can then interfere with the movement of blood into or out of surrounding bone tissue.

AVN frequently accompanies lupus and other autoimmune diseases. Vasculitis and Raynaud syndrome frequently accompany these disorders, and autoimmune disease patients often take steroidal anti-inflammatories for long periods. These drugs can contribute to blood flow problems in the femoral head. Pancreatitis can lead to AVN because fat-dissolving enzymes from the pancreas may induce fatty bone marrow to form tiny plugs of fat globules in the bloodstream. Hemophilia and sickle cell disease can lead to blockages in blood supply. Alcoholism is also associated with this disorder.

Signs and Symptoms

Early AVN is often silent and difficult to detect without intrusive tests. It may begin with joint pain just during movement, but the pain worsens and becomes prevalent even during rest. In later stages it shows all the signs of osteoarthritis. Eventually it may lead to total collapse of the joint.

Diagnosis

AVN is difficult to diagnose in early stages. Radiographs, bone scans, and CT scans are most useful in later stages of the disease. An MRI may show pathological changes early, but the most definitive diagnosis involves biopsies and a bone stress test that must be conducted surgically.

Treatment

Treatment options for AVN are determined by the age of the patient, the stage of the disorder, the underlying causes, and the severity of the damage. Nonsurgical treatments, such as use of braces or crutches to temporarily relieve weight-bearing stress, are frequently used. Electrical stimulation of the bone may be recommended to stimulate healthy new growth. These strategies are most successful if the condition is caught early, but even with early intervention AVN is frequently progressive and difficult to control.

Most AVN patients eventually undergo some kind of surgery to decompress the medullary canal, to remove dead tissue, to reshape the bone for better strength, or to rebuild a ruined joint.

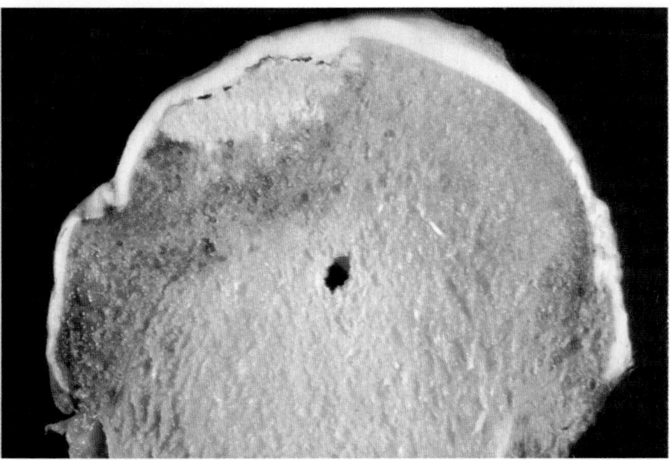

Figure 3.11. Avascular necrosis: the death of tissue in the femoral head.

Massage?

AVN is associated with problems with blood flow and fragile, damaged bones. It locally contraindicates massage where symptoms could be exacerbated, but bodywork could be useful in coping with postural and movement problems that may arise because of damage to the hip joint.

Underlying conditions that may contribute to AVN must be accommodated in any decisions about bodywork.

Modality Recommendations for Avascular Necrosis

MODALITY	RECOMMENDATION
Deep tissue massage	Locally contraindicated; work elsewhere to balance fascias in legs and feet to address compensations.
Lymphatic drainage	Supportive.
Polarity	S: Indicated. R/D: Locally contraindicated; otherwise supportive.
PNF/MET/stretching	Supportive.
Reflexology	Locally contraindicated; work all circulatory and glandular system points.
Shiatsu	Supportive.
Swedish massage	Locally contraindicated if area is fragile or sensitive; otherwise supportive.
Trigger point therapy	Locally contraindicated; otherwise supportive.

See Chapter 1 for a brief description of each modality, including definitions of abbreviations.

Fractures in Brief

What are they?
A fracture is any kind of broken or cracked bone.

How are they recognized?
Most fractures are painful and involve loss of function at the nearest joints, but some may be difficult to diagnose without radiography, bone scan, or other imaging techniques.

Is massage indicated or contraindicated?
Acute fractures locally contraindicate massage, but work done on the rest of the body can yield reflexive benefits. Massage is indicated for people in later stages of recovery from fractures.

Fractures

Definition: What Are They?

Fractures are any variety of broken bone, from a hairline crack to a complete break with protrusion through the skin.

Fractures come in all shapes and sizes. The three basic classes are as follows: In *simple fractures*, the bone is completely broken but little or no damage has occurred to the surrounding soft tissues. In *incomplete fractures*, the bone is cracked but not completely broken. In *compound fractures*, the bone is completely broken and a great deal of soft tissue damage has occurred—in fact, the bone protrudes through the skin and is susceptible to infection. Several variations on these themes are possible, including *stress fractures* and *compression fractures;* a variety called a *march fracture* occurs in the metatarsals. *Greenstick fractures* involve bending and partial breakage of the bone. *Comminuted fractures* involve shattering of the broken bone. *An impacted fracture* is a broken bone with one end wedged into the other (Figure 3.12). *Compression fractures* involve collapsed vertebral bodies. These are often associated with osteopenia, or loss of bone density, as seen with osteoporosis and osteogenesis im-

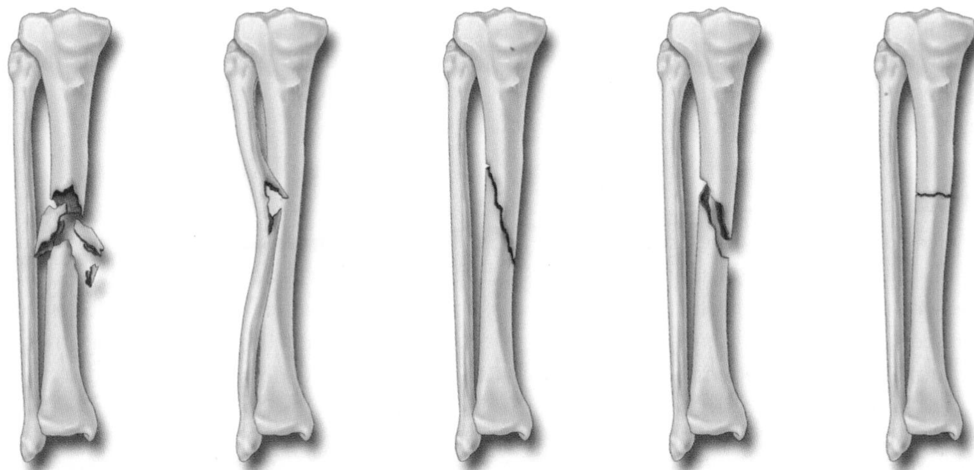

Figure 3.12. Varieties of fractures.

perfecta. *Malunion fractures* heal in a nonanatomical position. Many other types of fractures have been named for the doctors who first described them or the special joints they affect, but they are not discussed here.

Demographics: Who Gets Them?

It is difficult to estimate how many people have broken bones. Children are affected more often than others because they engage in the risky behaviors that invite that sort of accident. But children's bones have a much higher proportion of living cells and flexible cartilage to inert mass than adults' bones do. Children also have more growth hormone, which allows them a faster and more complete recovery than most adults can hope for. Elderly people, while not doing much tree climbing and skateboarding, have bones that are more brittle and less resilient than young peoples', and it takes much less stress to fracture them.

Signs and Symptoms

Big bone breaks are usually obvious: they are painful, they usually follow a specific traumatic event, and they severely limit the function of the affected joints. But some fractures can be difficult to identify without radiography or bone scan, particularly if they are accompanied by a lot of soft tissue trauma. Sprained ankles and shin splints are two conditions that frequently hide bone fractures.

Treatment

Most fractures heal well if the bones are immobilized with a cast or other device. Fibroblasts immediately infiltrate the area and build a framework of collagen. These are followed by osteoblasts laying down the framework for bone tissue, which quickly becomes dense and hard.

Some fractures need more support than a standard cast can offer, especially if the break involves a joint, as in the wrist or ankle. Pins or plates may be introduced to further stabilize the joint, but these carry the risk of introducing infection to the site. Other fractures, especially those involving the femoral neck or head, may require reparative surgery before they heal satisfactorily.

Several grafting procedures have been developed to speed the healing of broken bones. Autologous grafts are insertions of the patient's own bone tissue (usually harvested from the ilium) to provide the scaffolding on which new material may grow. Cadaverous bone has also been used with success, although the replacement process is slower than with an autologous graft. Various types of bone paste may be applied or injected into a fractured area. Electrical stimulation may be applied to slowly healing fractures. All of these interventions help bone to heal faster than it would on its own, but none of them is usually strong enough to support the lesion without some kind of fixative device: pins, plates, or screws.

Massage?

The rules for working with fractures are guided by common sense: acute or unset broken bones obviously contraindicate massage. Casted fractures may result in stasis and edema that can be very much improved by massage if access is available. Even if access to a broken leg is limited, reflexive benefits may be gained by working on the other limb. In addition, massage can minimize how movement compensation patterns may affect the rest of the body.

MODALITY RECOMMENDATIONS FOR FRACTURES

MODALITY	RECOMMENDATION
Deep tissue massage	Contraindicated while acute. Supportive during recovery, once weight bearing or free of cast. Work with compensatory patterns.
Lymphatic drainage	Indicated immediately following injury and throughout the course of healing.
Polarity	S: Indicated. R/D: Locally contraindicated while acute; otherwise indicated.
PNF/MET/stretching	Locally contraindicated; otherwise supportive.
Reflexology	Locally contraindicated; work parathyroid points.
Shiatsu	Indicated. Avoid deep pressure locally during acute stage.
Swedish massage	Locally contraindicated until no risk of thrombus; then supportive.
Trigger point therapy	Locally contraindicated while acute; otherwise supportive. Indicated when bone is healed.

Osteoporosis

Definition: What Is It?

Osteoporosis literally means *porous bones*. In this condition calcium is pulled off the bones faster than it is replaced, leaving them thin, brittle, chalky, and prone to injury.

Demographics: Who Gets It?

This disease affects about 10 million Americans (8 million women and 2 million men). It is estimated that up to 34 million more have *osteopenia* (significant bone thinning) but are unaware of their risk. It affects women more often than men for several reasons: Women have lower bone density to begin with; they bear children—an enormous drain on calcium reserves; and at menopause women undergo rapid changes in hormone levels that have great influence on how much calcium is added to bone mass. Small-boned, thin women get osteoporosis more than others. Women who are postmenopausal and/or have a history of eating disorders are at especially high risk. White and Asian women are most likely to develop this condition, but African American and Hispanic women also are subject to it.[12]

> **Osteoporosis in Brief**
> Pronunciation: os-te-o-por-O-sis
>
> **What is it?**
> Osteoporosis is loss of bone mass and density brought about by endocrine imbalances and poor metabolism of calcium.
>
> **How is it recognized?**
> Osteoporosis in the early stages is virtually silent. In later stages compression or spontaneous fractures of the vertebrae, ribs, wrists, or hips may occur. Hyperkyphosis brought about by compression fractures of the thoracic vertebrae is a frequent indicator of osteoporosis.
>
> **Is massage indicated or contraindicated?**
> Gentle massage is appropriate for persons with osteoporosis, with extra caution for the comfort and safety of the client. Massage does not affect the progression of the disease once it is present, but may significantly reduce associated pain. Acute fractures, however, contraindicate massage.

Etiology: What Happens?

In general, people accumulate most of their bone density by about age 20, but small gains are made until around age 30. After that point either bone density is maintained at a stable level, or withdrawals are made from the "calcium bank". Osteoporosis develops when calcium is withdrawn from bones faster than it is deposited.

Logically, high calcium consumption should lead to high bone density, and high bone density should be linked to a low risk of osteoporosis and bone fractures. Long-range studies on these questions yield inconsistent answers, however.[15,16] Many factors beyond calcium consumption influence bone health, including other vitamins and minerals, exercise habits, pH balance in the blood (especially as it is influenced by meat-based proteins), other diseases, medications, and even mood.[17]

Calcium absorption Calcium requires an acidic environment in the stomach to be absorbed into the body. If calcium enters the body in a form that impedes its contact with hydrochloric acid (for instance, in dairy products), the body has only limited access to this mineral. Similarly, if natural secretions of hydrochloric acid are reduced, as in older women and men, it becomes harder to absorb whatever calcium is consumed.

Some vitamins influence how the body uses calcium. Vitamin D controls absorption and retention of this important mineral. The body synthesizes adequate amounts of vitamin D in response to direct sunlight (it takes about 15 minutes of exposure per day, depending on latitude), but vitamin D can also be easily supplemented. Vitamin K, found in many dark, leafy greens, also supports calcium absorption. Preformed vitamin A, however, can *increase* the risk of fractures if it is consumed in high quantities.

Calcium loss Calcium is constantly lost in sweat and urine. Some substances, specifically meat-based proteins, cause higher levels of calcium to be excreted in urine. So a person who takes in ample amounts of dietary calcium but who eats a lot of meat also tends to lose a lot of calcium. This may help to explain why, although the United States is a leading consumer of dairy products, it also has higher numbers of spontaneous fractures than other countries where diets are lower in both calcium and animal proteins.[18]

Several other factors can lead to calcium loss. High caffeine consumption (more than three or four cups of coffee or servings of caffeinated soda per day) has been seen to have a negative impact, although the exact mechanism is not fully understood. Other factors include medications (chemotherapeutic agents, corticosteroids, some diuretics, anticonvulsant drugs); hyperthyroidism; heavy alcohol use; smoking; inflammatory bowel disease (Crohn disease, ulcerative colitis); a history of eating disorders; and endocrine disorders, including Cushing disease, low testosterone, and low estrogen.

Maintaining bone density The shape and density of bones are determined by the activity of osteoclasts and osteoblasts. These cells work to remodel bones according to the commands of calcitonin, parathyroid hormone, estrogen, and progesterone. If hormones tell the osteoclasts to work faster than the osteoblasts, bone density declines. Osteoclasts pull calcium off bones to respond to immediate needs as they arise. Osteoclasts and osteoblasts are most active in spongy, or trabecular, bone, which is found in epiphyses of long bones and vertebral bodies. The loss of key struts of calcium deposits in these areas can cause bones to collapse.

Bones are not the only part of the body that needs calcium. They happen to be a convenient storage medium, but calcium is consumed in nearly every chemical reaction that results in muscle contraction and nerve transmission. Calcium is essential to blood clotting and nerve transmission, and it works as a buffer to help maintain the proper pH balance. These are very important functions, and the body has a strict priority system: chemical reactions that are crucial to moment-to-moment survival are more important than maintaining the density of the vertebrae or femoral neck.

When a person develops osteoporosis, it is usually because the balancing act between calcium absorption, calcium loss, and bone density maintenance is upset. The calcium stored in the bones is pulled off faster than it is replaced (Figures 3.13, 3.14). The bones, especially in the spine and femur, get progressively thinner, leaving the person vulnerable to the primary complications of osteoporosis: spinal or hip fractures.

SIDEBAR 3.3: OSTEOPOROSIS STATISTICS

The statistics surrounding osteoporosis are among the most startling of all musculoskeletal diseases. This silent disease is responsible for drastic life changes and extraordinary medical costs.

Incidence

Osteoporosis is fully developed in 10 million Americans and is a future threat for approximately 34 million more.[12]

Eighty percent of osteoporosis diagnoses are in women. Of women over 50, 1 in 2 will probably have an osteoporosis-related fracture. Of men over 50, 1 in 8 will have a fracture.

Osteoporosis and Fractures

Osteoporosis is directly responsible for 1.5 million fractures in the United States every year. This is three times the number of heart attacks diagnosed in the same period.[13] Osteoporosis-related fractures lead to 37,000 deaths each year. A rough breakdown of osteoporosis-related fractures looks like this:

- 700,000 vertebral fractures
- 300,000 hip fractures
- 250,000 wrist fractures
- 300,000 other fractures

A woman's risk of hip fracture is equal to her *combined* risk of developing breast, uterine, or ovarian cancer. Women are two to three times as likely to fracture a hip as men, but men are twice as likely to die of complications related to hip fractures.

Osteoporosis and Medical Costs

The direct costs of treating osteoporosis and related fractures (this is treatment only, not lost work hours or death costs) amounts to $14 billion per year, or more than ***$38 million per day***, and those costs are rising.[14]

Signs and Symptoms

Osteoporosis has no symptoms in its early stages. People who are at particularly high risk may undergo testing to try to identify it early, but it is often missed until complications, namely fractures, develop.

Symptoms of osteoporosis center on pathologically weak bones. Thinned or collapsed vertebrae lead to a loss of height and the characteristic rounded "widow's hump" of hyperkyphosis. Chronic and/or acute back pain appears in this stage as the vertebrae continue to degenerate.

Complications

People with osteoporosis are prone to fractures with little or no cause; these are called spontaneous or pathological frac-

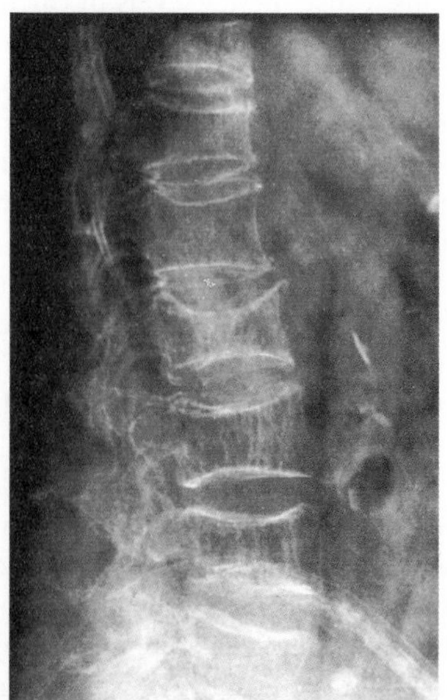

Figure 3.13. Demonstrable bone loss with osteoporosis (compare Fig. 3.15).

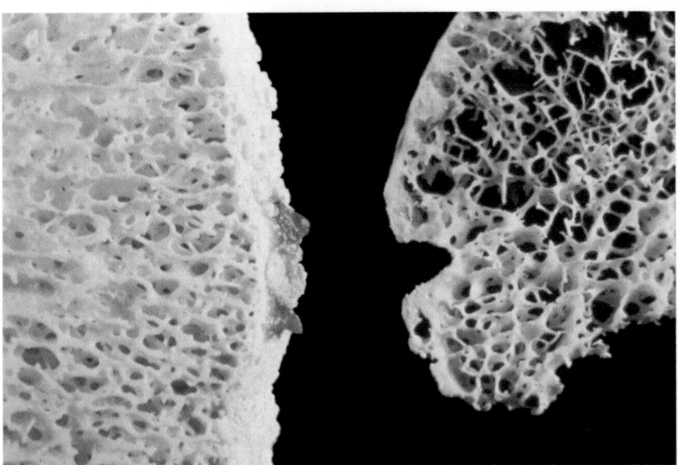

Figure 3.14. Loss of bone density with osteoporosis.

tures. Hips (usually the femoral neck rather than the ilium), vertebrae, and wrists are particularly vulnerable to breakage. Brittle ribs are often associated with corticosteroid use. And since in advanced age people are naturally low on both living osteocytes and growth hormone to support the healing process, it is particularly difficult to recover from any injury of this severity. Fewer than one-third of people who break a hip return to prefracture levels of activity.[19]

Diagnosis

Early identification of osteoporosis is challenging. The gold standard is a test called DEXA (dual x-ray absorptiometry). This is performed at key bone loss sites—hips, wrists, ribs, and the spine—to look for signs of density loss. Other tests may include ultrasound or CT, but osteoporosis frequently isn't identified until a fracture occurs.

Treatment

Once osteoporosis has been recognized, a number of treatment options are available to keep it from getting worse. Among these is hormone replacement therapy (HRT). Estrogen influences calcium absorption. Postmenopausal women secrete this hormone only in small amounts, so replacing it should improve calcium uptake. Unfortunately, estrogen supplements are also associated with breast and uterine cancers and an increased risk of some cardiovascular diseases. Furthermore, it has been found that estrogen supplementation promotes bone density maintenance in the short run, but benefits are lost if a person stops taking the hormone.

A group of medications called ***bisphosphonates*** are often recommended. These inhibit resorption of calcium and work to keep bone density high. Calcitonin, a synthetic version of the hormone that stimulates osteoblasts, is another treatment option. Finally, a group of drugs that are also used to reduce the risk of recurrent cancer have been found to be effective; these are called SERMs (selective estrogen receptor modulators).

Exercise is almost always a part of the osteoporosis treatment strategy. Since bone remodels according to the stresses placed on it, weight-bearing stress ensures that maintaining healthy mass is a high priority. For someone with this condition, gentle weight training or walking is more beneficial than cardiovascular exercises such as swimming or cycling.

Diet also plays an important part in dealing with osteoporosis. Specific vitamins and other substances may improve calcium uptake, even for postmenopausal women, but that subject is outside the scope of this book.

Prevention

It is possible to prevent osteoporosis, feasible to slow it down or halt it, and difficult or impossible to reverse it. The causes are many and varied, but they center on one main theme: the time to build up calcium reserves is in youth and early adulthood. The skeleton grows in height until about age 20, but it continues to accumulate density until about age 30. After that point it either stays stable or progressively demineralizes. Studies show that today many Americans get only half or less of the recommended daily allowance of calcium; this, combined with our dismal rates of getting exercise, doesn't bode well for future osteoporosis statistics.

Four main steps have been recommended to achieve and maintain optimal bone density and avoid osteoporosis:

- *Get dietary calcium from absorbable sources.* Dairy products are abundant and convenient, but not the most efficient source for all people. Other recommended calcium sources include beans and greens: legumes and most green leafy vegetables. (Spinach and chard, while rich in calcium and other nutrients, also have substances that limit calcium absorption.) Calcium supplements vary in absorbability; calcium carbonate, calcium phosphate, and calcium citrate are generally recognized to have good accessibility.
- *Exercise.* Weight-bearing stress makes it necessary for the body to maintain healthy bone density.
- *Get vitamin D.* The RDA for vitamin D is 200 units, or 5 μg, per day. This can be ingested in supplement form or naturally synthesized by exposure to sunlight.
- *Avoid substances and behaviors that pull calcium off bones.* Salt, animal proteins, caffeine, and alcohol all require calcium to be processed by the body. Cigarette smoking has also been associated with low bone density.

Massage?

In the treatment of clients with osteoporosis, the appropriateness of massage differs from person to person. The only way massage can worsen the situation is to exert undue mechanical force, which could lead to the possibility of fractures. On the other hand, consider the condition of the muscles of someone with osteoporosis; massage can offer symptomatic relief, even if it can't reverse the degeneration of the bone tissue. In any case, caution is the key with this condition. Don't look for miracles; taking someone out of the pain for a few hours is miracle enough.

Modality Recommendations for Osteoporosis

Modality	Recommendation
Deep tissue massage	Supportive, with caution to avoid excessive pressure, especially at the ribs. Use oblique angle of contact and work slowly.
Lymphatic drainage	Supportive.
Polarity	S: Indicated. R/D: Light work is supportive, depending of level of bone mass.
PNF/MET/stretching	Supportive.
Reflexology	Locally contraindicated; work all endocrine system points.
Shiatsu	Indicated. If condition is very advanced, avoid deep compression.
Swedish massage	Indicated with caution for the client's resilience.
Trigger point therapy	Supportive with gentle work only.

See Chapter 1 for a brief description of each modality, including definitions of abbreviations.

Paget Disease

Definition: What Is It?

Paget disease is a condition in which normal bone is reabsorbed up to 50 times faster than normal. It is replaced with disorganized fibrous connective tissue, which never completely matures. This leaves the affected bones weakened and distorted. Another name for Paget disease is *osteitis deformans.*

Paget Disease in Brief
PAJ-et dih-ZEZE

What is it?
Paget disease is a chronic bone disorder in which healthy bone is rapidly reabsorbed and replaced with fibrous connective tissue that never fully calcifies.

How is it recognized?
Paget disease is often silent. When it does cause symptoms, they usually include deep bone pain, local heat, and sometimes visible deformation of the affected bones. The risk of arthritis and fractures is high.

Is massage indicated or contraindicated?
Paget disease is often treated with exercise and physical therapy to maintain flexibility. Massage may fit into this context as well, with caution for the extreme fragility of the affected bones.

Demographics: Who Gets It?

This is one of the most common metabolic bone diseases, second only to osteoporosis. About 1 million people have been diagnosed with this disease in this country.[20] Men have Paget disease more often then women, and though African Americans can have it, it is especially prevalent in whites from northwestern Europe. It is very rare in Asians.[21]

Although no specific site of genetic mutation has been found, Paget disease clearly runs in families. A person who has a first-degree relative (a sibling, parent, or child) with Paget disease has a seven times greater chance of developing this disease than someone with no family history.[21]

Etiology: What Happens?

Every day, on a microscopic level, small amounts of calcium in the bones are dissolved into the bloodstream, to be replaced by new supplies. The osteoclasts, which break down bone, and osteoblasts, which build it up, keep each other in balance. In Paget disease, the osteoclasts become huge (up to five times larger than normal) and hyperactive. Osteoblasts also increase activity, although they don't change in size or form. The result is that bony tissue is broken down and replaced at an accelerated pace. (Figures 3.15 and 3.16)

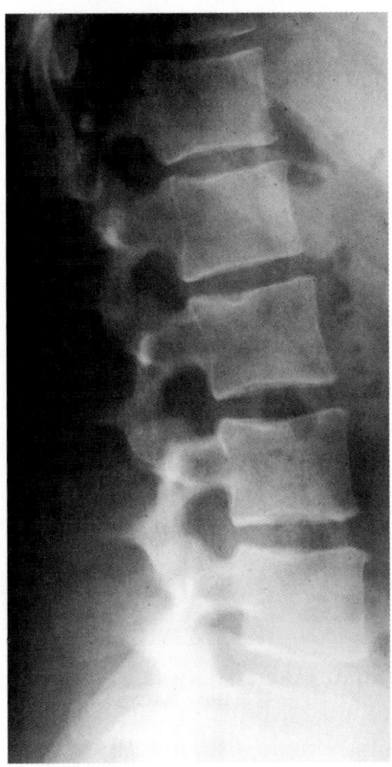

Figure 3.15. Normal spine.

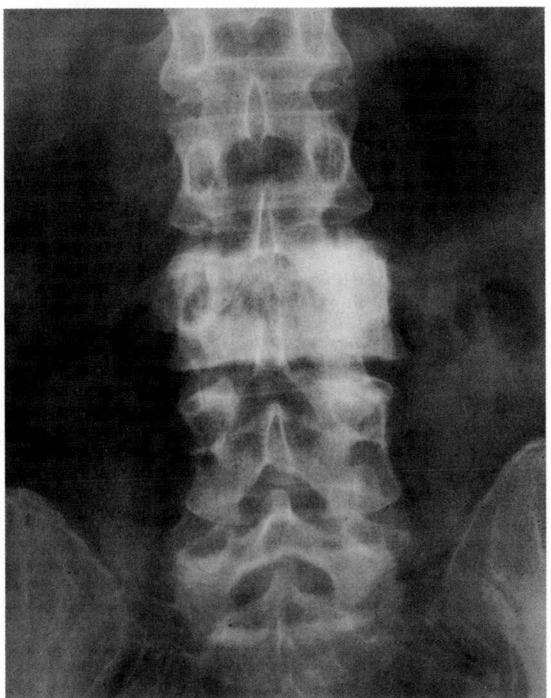

Figure 3.16. Overgrowth of the vertebral body at L3 in patient with Paget disease; compare Fig. 3.15.

Most people with Paget disease have it in only one bone, but some have it in two or more. The skull, vertebrae, pelvis, and legs are affected most often. It does not seem to spread from one bone to another, however.

The cause of Paget disease is unknown, but research is leaning toward the idea of a very slow-acting virus, which may exist in the system for years before causing any damage. A genetic component is probable, since Paget disease often runs in families, but this may simply indicate a susceptibility to the particular virus involved.

Signs and Symptoms

Paget disease usually has no symptoms until it is advanced enough to cause visible changes to the affected bones. When it is found early, it is often because a person has a radiograph or blood test taken for some other reason.

Later signs and symptoms of Paget disease include deep bone pain, palpable heat where the bones are affected, and problems related to a change in bone shape in the affected areas. These can include a loss of hearing and chronic headaches if the skull is affected, pinched nerves and vertebral fractures if the disease is in the spine, and a visible change in bone shape. The long bones of the femur and lower leg may become bowed and distorted.

Complications

Paget disease has several serious complications brought about by changes in bone size and strength. The most common complication is arthritis, or fractures in the affected bones. If the cranial bones press on parts of the central nervous system, deafness, headaches, or vision problems could develop. Teeth can loosen if the disease distorts the mandible. Congestive heart failure may occur because the heart must pump blood through whole massive networks of vessels in the new, useless fibrous tissue.

Approximately 1% of Paget disease patients develop a rare but aggressive form of bone cancer.

Diagnosis

Paget disease is diagnosed primarily by radiography or bone scan. A blood test to look for *alkaline phosphatase* (an enzyme produced by overactive osteoblasts) may confirm the diagnosis.

Because this disease has a clear genetic link, family members of Paget disease patients may be recommended to have blood tests for heightened levels of alkaline phosphatase every few years after they turn 40. This may allow for early diagnosis and more effective treatment of the disease.

Treatment

Treatment for Paget disease is surprisingly similar to that for osteoporosis; the unwanted breakdown of healthy bone tissue is a feature common to both disorders. The first recommendations are exercise and physical therapy to maintain function and healthy bone mass as long as possible. Aspirin and anti-inflammatories may be suggested for pain relief. Finally, calcitonin or bisphosphonates may be prescribed to inhibit osteoclast activity.

Surgery may become necessary to repair fractures or replace joint surfaces when the bones become badly distorted.

Massage?

Paget disease is accompanied by inflammation, impaired circulation, and weakened bones. All of these issues require caution from massage therapists. But if a Paget disease patient is engaging in exercise and physical therapy to maintain bone health, massage could be a useful adjunct to this effort, as long as the client's health care team is informed.

Modality Recommendations for Paget Disease

MODALITY	RECOMMENDATION
Deep tissue massage	Contraindicated unless working with the rest of the health care team.
Lymphatic drainage	Supportive.
Polarity	S: Indicated. R/D: Supportive, depending on level of disease.
PNF/MET/stretching	Locally contraindicated; otherwise supportive.
Reflexology	Locally contraindicated; work all endocrine system points.
Shiatsu	Supportive.
Swedish massage	Supportive if no other contraindications are present.
Trigger point therapy	Locally contraindicated for deep pressure; otherwise supportive.

See Chapter 1 for a brief description of each modality, including definitions of abbreviations.

Postural Deviations

Definition: What Is It?

Although it is tempting to think about the spine in terms of a ship's mast, a column, or a tent pole held erect by muscular tension, it is actually much stronger than any of those. The curves in the cervical, thoracic, and lumbar regions give the spine many times the resistance it would have if it were straight. Sometimes, though, these natural curves are overdeveloped, which reduces resiliency and strength rather than enhancing it. Hyperkyphosis (humpback), hyperlordosis (swayback), and scoliosis (S, C, or reverse-C curve) are the specific postural deviations addressed here (Figure 3.17).

Etiology: What Happens?

It is sometimes convenient to think about the spine in only two dimensions. In other words, scoliosis would be simply an S-shaped curve from left to right, and hyperlordosis and hyperkyphosis would be exaggerated forward and backward curves. The truth is not nearly so simple. With any imbalance in the stacking of the vertebrae, rotations in one direction or another complicate the issue. Thus scoliosis is not merely a left-right aberration but a spiral twisting of the vertebral column as well. This is sometimes referred to as **rotoscoliosis.** Similar lateral imbalances are observable with most cases of hyperlordosis and hyperkyphosis.

One important thing to identify with postural deviations is the difference between a functional problem and a structural one. In the early stages of any of these conditions, it may be that soft tissues pull the spine out of alignment: a functional problem. Functional deviations are often identified if observable curves disappear or are significantly reduced when the patient goes into trunk flexion or side flexion. The condition is most treatable at this point: muscles, tendons, and ligaments can be exercised, stretched, and manipulated into new holding and movement patterns.

Postural Deviations in Brief

What are they?
Postural deviations are overdeveloped thoracic or lumbar curves (hyperkyphosis and hyperlordosis) or a lateral curve in the spine (scoliosis).

How are they recognized?
Extreme curvatures are easily visible, although radiography is used to pinpoint exactly where the problems begin and end.

Is massage indicated or contraindicated?
All postural deviations indicate massage as long as other underlying pathologies have been ruled out. Bodywork may or may not be able to reverse any damage, but it can certainly provide relief for the muscular stress that accompanies spinal changes.

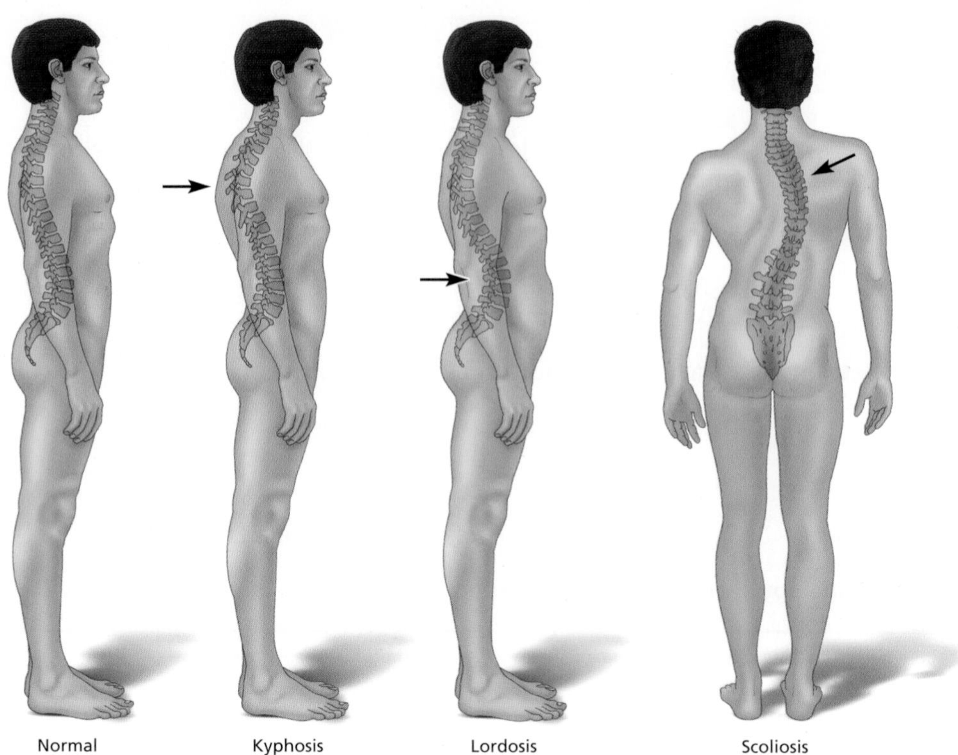

Figure 3.17. Postural deviations.

Functional deviations can also be brought about by structural problems elsewhere in the body: unequal leg length, for instance, or a sacrum that isn't level. These are correctable, but if the soft tissues are left untreated and the bones are constantly pulled in one direction or another, they eventually change shape to adapt to those stressors. Vertebral bodies and discs adopt a wedge shape, and the facet joints may become distorted. At this point the condition becomes a structural dysfunction, which is much harder to reverse.

Most cases of postural deviations are idiopathic, that is, of unknown origin. However, a small percentage of structural problems in the spine can be related to congenital or neuromuscular problems such as cerebral palsy, polio, muscular dystrophy, osteogenesis imperfecta, or spina bifida. These contributing factors must be addressed before any attempt is made to correct the postural deviations they produce.

Signs and Symptoms

Postural deviations range from being painfully obvious to quite subtle. A visual examination yields a lot of information about hyperkyphosis and hyperlordosis, and even mild scoliosis may be visible with a forward-bending test. Patients often report muscular tension and sometimes nerve impairment along with chronic ache and loss of range of motion. If the condition is very advanced, movement of the ribs may be impaired, leaving the patient vulnerable to breathing problems, lung infections, and even problems with heart function.

- *Scoliosis* is a problem for approximately 1% to 2% of teenagers. It affects girls seven times more frequently than boys and almost always involves a bend to the right.[22] It usually appears during the rapid-growth years of late childhood and early adolescence. Mild scoliosis, which is any curve less than 30 to 40 degrees, is treated, if at all, with exercise, chiropractic, a corrective brace, and/or electromuscular stimulation. If the scoliosis appears at over 40 degrees in childhood, the chances that it will worsen are significant. It typically progresses at 1 degree every year.[23] Complications of scoliosis include nerve irritation as misshapen bones press on nerve roots, spondylosis, and serious heart and lung problems arising from a severely restricted rib cage. Surgery for scoliosis involves inserting rods that straighten and fuse the affected vertebrae. This limits spinal mobility but can definitely improve the quality of life for people with a threatening and debilitating situation.

- *Hyperkyphosis* is an overdeveloped thoracic curve. In young people it is very often a result of muscular imbalance and may be treated with physical therapy. Scheuermann disease is a type of idiopathic hyperkyphosis that affects young men. It is usually painless and is treated with physical therapy and/or bracing. Hyperkyphosis in older people may be due to muscular imbalance, but it can also be a complication of osteoporosis or ankylosing spondylitis. A kyphotic curve of 20 to 40 degrees is considered normal. Surgical intervention isn't usually suggested for anything under a 75-degree curvature.
- *Hyperlordosis,* or swayback, is an overpronounced lumbar curve. The architecture and musculature of the low back makes it particularly vulnerable to this kind of imbalance. It can often be much improved by exercise and physical therapy (including massage). Hyperlordosis, although not dangerous in itself, can lead to serious low back pain.

Treatment

Treatment options for different kinds of postural deviations are outlined in the preceding descriptions.

Massage?

As long as no underlying pathology contributes to spinal problems, all kinds of postural deviations indicate massage. In the early stages of these diseases, chronic soft tissue (that is, muscular, tendinous, and ligamentous) stresses pull on the bones and change the architecture of the spine. Caught early enough, many inefficient postural habits can be reversed without permanent damage. It is often suggested to focus special attention to the concave side of a scoliotic curve to support chronically tight muscles that may atrophy in a shortened position.[24]

Massage certainly won't make any of these conditions any worse, and may well offer relief by simply reducing some of the tension that both causes and accompanies spinal imbalance. If a therapist is very skilled and the circumstances are just right, massage may set the stage for a permanent change in bony alignment.

Modality Recommendations for Postural Deviations

MODALITY	RECOMMENDATION
Deep tissue massage	Indicated to reduce compensation. Work with client movement and breathing to restore appropriate length in fascias; work in all three dimensions.
Lymphatic drainage	Supportive.
Polarity	S/R/D: Indicated.
PNF/MET/stretching	Indicated to help reduce compensation and restore muscle balance.
Reflexology	Indicated; work endocrine system, spine, and hip points.
Shiatsu	Indicated; treat BL, SI systemically and all local areas of discomfort and compensation. Use meridian stretches, ROM.
Swedish massage	Supportive if no other contraindications are present.
Trigger point therapy	Indicated in all stages.

See Chapter 1 for a brief description of each modality, including definitions of abbreviations.

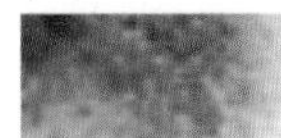

Joint Disorders

Ankylosing Spondylitis

Ankylosing Spondylitis in Brief

Pronunciation: ang-kih-LO-sing spon-dih-LY-tis

What is it?
Ankylosing spondylitis (AS) is a progressive inflammatory arthritis of the spine.

How is it recognized?
AS generally begins as stiffness and pain around the sacrum, with occasional referred pain down the back of the buttocks and into the legs. It has acute and subacute episodes. In advanced AS the vertebrae fuse in flexion or lateral flexion. Signs and symptoms may also include inflammation of the iris, inflammatory bowel disease, and other issues.

Is massage indicated or contraindicated?
The subacute stage of AS indicates hands-on bodywork, where along with exercise and physical therapy it may be useful in maintaining flexibility.

Definition: What Is It?

Ankylosing spondylitis (AS) is spinal inflammation (*spondylitis*) leading to stiff joints (*ankylosis*). This means really stiff: the joints between and around vertebrae can become permanently fused. AS is a progressive inflammatory arthritis of the spine. It is sometimes called *rheumatoid spondylitis*.

Demographics: Who Gets It?

AS is an inherited disorder that most often affects men between 16 and 35 years of age. A genetic marker (HLA-B27) has been identified that seems to increase the tendency to develop this disease, but it is not a definitive factor; the incidence among people who have this marker and another relative with AS is about 20%. About 1% of people in the United States have some degree of AS; males outnumber females by about 3 to 1.[25]

Etiology: What Happens?

The precise cause of AS is not entirely clear, but many consider it to be autoimmune, perhaps triggered by a bacterial infection. It is unique among autoimmune conditions, however, because the blood of people with AS shows no sign of the antinuclear antibodies (ANA) that are typical of other autoimmune diseases. For this reason it is classified as a *seronegative spondyloarthropathy*. Other seronegative autoimmune diseases include inflammatory bowel disease (Crohn disease and ulcerative colitis), psoriasis, and psoriatic arthritis. Interestingly, these conditions are frequently seen in people with AS or in the family members of AS patients.

AS typically begins with chronic inflammation at the sacroiliac joint on one or both sides. Although it is usually limited to intervertebral and costal joints, the hips, shoulders, toes, and sternoclavicular joints may be affected too. The affected joints become inflamed in the acute or flare stage, and their cartilage begins to deteriorate. The articular cartilage thickens, cartilaginous discs ossify, and bony deformation leads to the squaring of vertebral bodies. These fusions are called *syndesmophytes*. Surrounding ligaments and tendons may also become inflamed and ossified.

The pattern of inflammation and damage proceeds up the spine, leaving in its wake a trail of injured vertebrae that may eventually fuse in slight or sometimes extreme flexion (Figures 3.18 and 3.19). If the progression reaches all the way up to the neck, the cervical vertebrae may fuse with the head in a permanently flexed position as well. Fusions may also occur at the vertebrocostal joints, resulting in a locked rib cage and difficulty breathing.

Signs and Symptoms

AS usually starts as chronic low back pain. Often pain is felt in the buttocks, sometimes all the way down into the heels. This can sometimes lead to a misdiagnosis of herniated disc. The spine and hips feel stiff and immobile; this is usually much worse in the morning or after prolonged immobility.

This condition has acute and subacute stages. During acute episodes a general feeling of illness and a slight fever may be present. The eyes may become dry, red, and uncomfortable; this is called *iritis*. Pain and stiffness gradually spread higher and higher up the spine. When

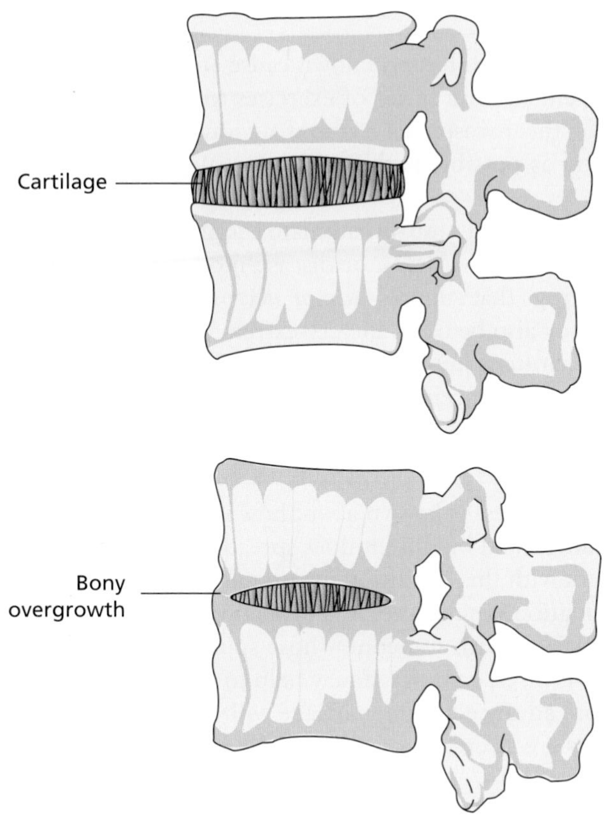

Figure 3.18. Ankylosing spondylitis: spinal fusions.

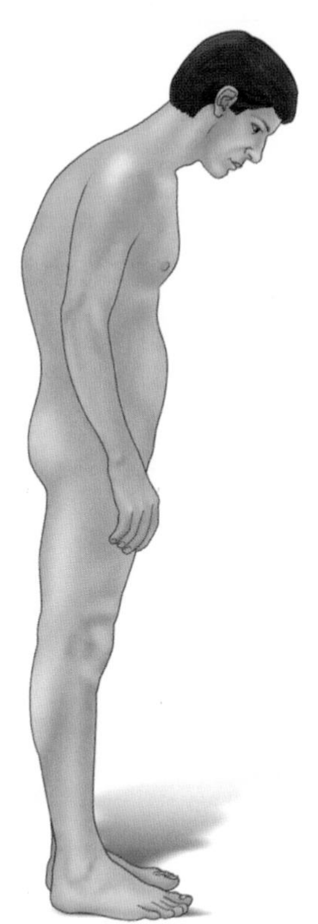

Figure 3.19. Ankylosing spondylitis.

the inflammation subsides the fever and acute pain are resolved, but stiffness and pain may continue to be present. Usually the disease is limited to the low back, but occasionally it progresses up into the neck or other joints in the body.

Complications

This condition carries a high risk of vertebral fracture. As the spine fuses and loses mobility, it becomes more vulnerable to shearing forces. Poor support from damaged ligaments means a greater chance of peripheral nerve pressure or cauda equina syndrome (loss of bowel and bladder control due to pressure on the cauda equina).

Loss of lung capacity is another complication of AS. If a person's ribs can't expand, it is difficult to get an adequate supply of oxygen into the body or to get carbon dioxide and air contaminants out. This results in constant shortness of breath, low stamina, and reduced resistance to chest infections such as pneumonia, from which, depending on posture, it can be very difficult to recover. In rare cases, the lungs may develop fibrosis and hollow areas that resemble tuberculosis infections. These cavitations are especially vulnerable to fungal infections.

The inflammation may involve other organs as well, including the eyes, heart, aorta, and kidneys.

Diagnosis

AS is diagnosed through observable symptoms, blood tests, and radiography. It can be difficult to identify in the early stages, since many disorders can cause diffuse back pain and stiffness. It sometimes takes years to confirm a diagnosis of AS. This is true especially when the condition is present in women, for whom the initial symptoms tend to be less predictable.

Treatment

The first, best option for dealing with AS (which has no known cause and therefore no cure) is exercise. Physical therapy is recommended for a series of exercises to preserve the suppleness of the spine and the strength of the paraspinals without aggravating the condition. Maintaining correct posture for as long as possible is the primary goal, since the vertebrae tend to fuse in a flexed position.

If exercise alone doesn't help, painkillers and anti-inflammatories are usually prescribed. Drugs that suppress immune system activity (DMARDs, or disease-modifying antirheumatic drugs) might be recommended. Other drugs that suppress *tumor necrosis factor* (a proinflammatory cytokine present in active AS) may also be used. In very extreme cases surgery may be suggested: an *osteotomy* is a procedure that fuses joints in a straightened position. If the knees, shoulders, or hips have been impaired, joint replacement surgery may also be suggested.

Massage?

Little is well understood about AS, and even less is known about how massage might affect it. But because it is an inflammatory condition and because it does spread, massage practitioners must proceed with caution. Always work with this condition in conjunction with a health care team, and only work when the inflammation is subacute; it is probably best to reschedule an appointment rather than working intensively with someone whose spinal joints are inflamed.

If a client is in the early stages of this disease, massage may help to preserve precious mobility of the spine. If a client is in a more advanced stage, massage will probably have little effect except pain relief, since the muscles are stretched over immobile joints.

Modality Recommendations for Ankylosing Spondylitis

MODALITY	RECOMMENDATION
Deep tissue massage	Contraindicated unless working with the health care team.
Lymphatic drainage	Supportive.
Polarity	S: Indicated. R/D: Supportive within client comfort.
PNF/MET/stretching	Supportive.
Reflexology	Indicated; work endocrine system, lymphatic system, spine points.
Shiatsu	Indicated. Deep pressure as within client tolerance relieves pain and discomfort.
Swedish massage	Supportive if not in flare.
Trigger point therapy	Locally contraindicated while acute; otherwise supportive.

See Chapter 1 for a brief description of each modality, including definitions of abbreviations.

Dislocations

Definition: What Are They?

When the bones in a joint are separated so that they no longer articulate, the joint is said to be dislocated. It's hard to imagine that happening without damage to most of the surrounding tissues as well: muscles, tendons, blood vessels and nerves are generally also injured in a traumatic dislocation (Figure 3.20). Nearby bursae often become inflamed as well. Dislocations are most often due to trauma, but some are brought about by congenital weakness of the ligaments, malformations of the joint, or a disease such as rheumatoid arthritis, Marfan syndrome, or Ehlers-Danlos syndrome.

Dislocations in Brief

What are they?
Dislocations are injuries to joints in which the articulating bones are forcefully separated.

How are they recognized?
Acute (new) dislocations are extremely painful. The bones may be visibly separated, and the joint loses all function.

Is massage indicated or contraindicated?
Dislocations indicate massage in the subacute stage, as long as work is conducted within pain tolerance. As the area heals, massage may be useful for managing scar tissue accumulation and muscle spasm around the affected joint.

Etiology: What Happens?

Most of the joints in the body do not dislocate without significant force, as seen with sports injuries or other traumas. The shoulder, because of the shallowness of the glenoid fossa, and the fingers are most at risk for dislocation (Figure 3.21). The jaw and elbow are other frequent sites for this kind of injury.

One subtype of dislocation is ***hip dysplasia***. This is a congenital condition that occurs about 4 times in every 1000 live births. A baby may be born with a dislocated hip, or the femur may dislocate with minimal force or stress. Hip dysplasia is generally painless in childhood, but it is associated with a high risk of painful osteoarthritis in adulthood.

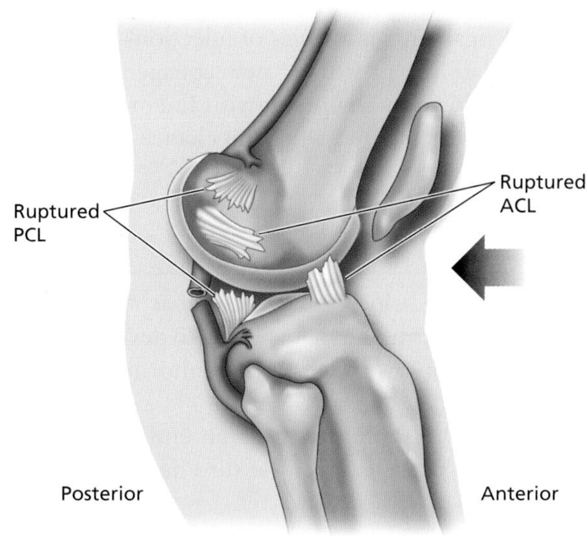

Figure 3.20. Synovial joint.

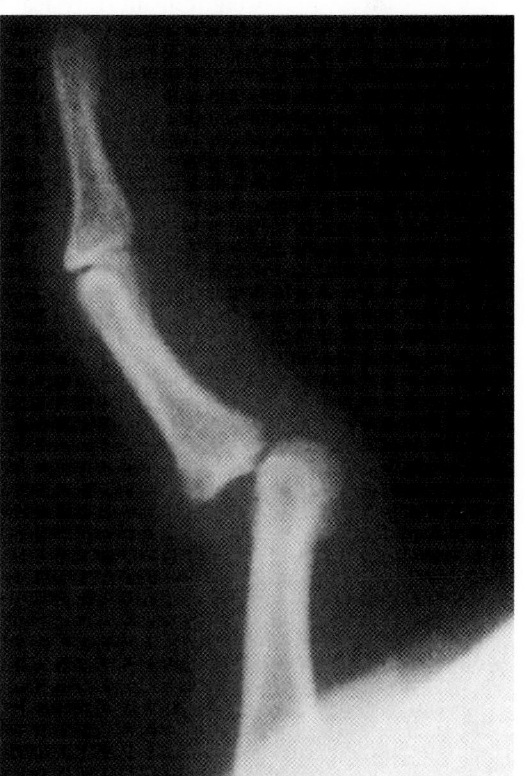

Figure 3.21. Dislocations often are accompanied by extensive soft tissue damage.

Signs and Symptoms

Symptoms of a newly dislocated joint include swelling, discoloration, loss of function, and, most obviously, a lot of pain.

Complications

Uncomplicated traumatic dislocations are painful and take a long time to heal, but they are not usually serious. Fibrosis and excessive scarring of the surrounding soft tissues may develop after prolonged splinting. Occasionally a nerve or blood vessel is severely damaged by the trauma, but this is the exception rather than the rule.

If, however, the ligaments supporting the damaged joint are stretched, they may lose some of their ability to do their job. The ligaments may even rupture and detach from the bone altogether. When ligaments are permanently damaged, the joint may become unstable and prone to reinjury: subluxation if the bones move out of alignment, spontaneous dislocation if the bones completely separate. These mishaps are especially common in the shoulder and jaw. The muscles that cross over these unstable joints are likely to be much tighter than is ideal, because the ligaments aren't doing their job. This can lead to MPS or tendinosis. The most serious long-term consequence of ligament laxity is the possibility of developing osteoarthritis.

Treatment

Acute dislocations require immediate attention. If large joint dislocations are not reduced within about 15 minutes, the tissues swell and the muscles contract so tightly that it is difficult to move the joint without a general anesthetic. After the joint is reduced, a radiograph is usually taken to rule out the possibility of a fracture. The joint is then splinted for 2 or 3 weeks, until the capsular ligament and other supportive ligaments are ready to carry their weight again. Physical therapy is prescribed to strengthen and retrain the muscles surrounding the joint.

If the ligaments have ruptured or are simply too lax to support the joint capsule, surgery may be recommended. Typically this involves shortening and/or reattaching the damaged ligaments to the bone using stitches or staples. Arthroscopic surgery for dislocated shoulders may be able to improve joint function without the complications of major surgery. ***Thermal capsulorraphy*** is a type of arthroscopic surgery designed to improve ligament stability. A thermal probe heats up specific areas of the joint capsule. This causes the collagen fibers to shrink, tightening the capsular ligament.

An alternative to surgery for chronically lax ligaments is a series of injections with proliferants. ***Proliferant*** therapy is designed to stimulate the growth of new collagen fibers that, with appropriate stretching and exercise, are laid down in alignment with the original fibers. This procedure can tighten stretched-out ligaments, thus reducing the chance of future injury.

Massage?

Obviously, massage is out of the question for an acute dislocation. In the subacute stage massage may help untangle the muscular and tendinous scar tissue that is likely to develop, as long as basic rules about working within tolerance, following with ice, and monitoring results are followed.

If a client has an old dislocation that occasionally subluxates or even entirely dislocates without trauma, massage will do no harm as long as care is taken be sure he or she is positioned in a way that feels safe and comfortable.

Modality Recommendations for Dislocations

MODALITY	RECOMMENDATION
Deep tissue massage	Contraindicated while acute. Supportive during recovery to minimize compensation.
Lymphatic drainage	Indicated in all stages.
Polarity	S: Indicated. R/D: Locally contraindicated while acute; otherwise supportive.
PNF/MET/stretching	Locally contraindicated; otherwise supportive.
Reflexology	Locally contraindicated; otherwise supportive.
Shiatsu	Locally contraindicated; otherwise indicated to reduce swelling and speed healing.
Swedish massage	Locally contraindicated while acute; otherwise supportive.
Trigger point therapy	Locally contraindicated while acute; indicated when subacute.

See Chapter 1 for a brief description of each modality, including definitions of abbreviations.

Gout

Definition: What Is It?

Gout is one of the oldest diseases in recorded medical history. In 580 A.D., Alexander of Tralles wrote, "Gout sufferers should eat little meat, drink no alcohol and eat the underground stems of calcium" (autumn crocus).[26]

One of the drugs in use today for the treatment of gout is *colchicine*, a synthetic version of autumn crocus.

Gout has been known as the disease of kings, associated with rich diet and decadent living. This is witnessed by a list of some of gout's most famous victims: Alexander the Great, Henry VIII of England, Charles V of Spain, his son Philip II, Dr. Samuel Johnson, Wolfgang von Goethe, and Benjamin Franklin. Rich diet is not the only risk factor for this disease, however.

Gout is a type of inflammatory arthritis. It is unique among the arthritides because it has a chemical cause rather than arising from wear and tear or immune system mistakes.

Gout in Brief

What is it?
Gout is an inflammatory arthritis caused by deposits of sodium urate (uric acid) in and around joints, especially in the feet.

How is it recognized?
Acute gout causes joints to become red, hot, swollen, shiny, and extremely painful. It usually has a sudden onset.

Is massage indicated or contraindicated?
Gout systemically contraindicates massage when it is acute. Gouty joints locally contraindicate massage at all times.

Demographics: Who Gets It?

Gout affects men more than women by a wide margin: 90% of gout patients are men; of the 10% who are women, most are postmenopausal.[27] More than 1 million gout patients have been diagnosed in the United States.[28]

Etiology: What Happens?

Uric acid is a naturally occurring byproduct of protein digestion. Under normal circumstances it is extracted from the blood by the kidneys. If the kidneys are unable to perform this function, either because too much uric acid is present or because they are otherwise impaired, ***hyperuricemia*** develops: this is the state of having higher than normal levels of uric acid in the blood. Hyperuricemia is a risk factor for gout.

Under normal circumstances, the kidneys should extract uric acid from the blood. This is where the problems may start.

- *Metabolic gout.* The kidneys may be functioning normally, but the body produces too much uric acid for them to keep up. This is the case for someone with a particularly high protein and/or alcohol intake.
- *Renal gout.* The uric acid load may be normal, but the kidneys aren't functioning well. They can't handle the job of excreting all the uric acid, and so it ends up in the bloodstream and eventually in the feet. This kind of kidney insufficiency may be hereditary or related to other problems, such as diabetes or lead poisoning.
- *Both.* The kidneys are compromised *and* the purine intake is high. This is gout, waiting to happen.

The transition from hyperuricemia to an acute gouty attack is often precipitated by some specific event: binge eating or drinking, surgery, sudden weight loss, or a systemic infection. All of these things alter fluid levels in the body. When uric acid consolidates, it forms sharp, needlelike crystals that accumulate in and around the joint capsule, grinding on and irritating synovial membranes, bursae, tendons, and other tissues (Figure 3.22). The crystals attract neutrophils, and these white blood cells initiate an extreme inflammatory response. This can happen in a short period: typically a person goes to bed feeling fine and wakes in the night with a foot that is red, throbbing, and painful.

The joint between the first metatarsal and proximal phalanx of the great toe may be the primary target for uric acid crystals because of gravity, but it may also have to do with the lower temperature found in extremities that aids in the crystallization process.

In later stages of the disease, deposits of sodium urate called ***tophi*** may develop inside and around joints. These tophi erode the joint structures, leading to a complete loss of function. Tophi also grow along tendons and in subcutaneous tissues. They have been found in myocardium, pericardium, aortic valves, and even the pinna of the ear!

Risk Factors

Uric acid is a waste product from the metabolism of a component of nucleic acids called *purines.* A diet that is high in purines tends to produce more uric acid in the body than a diet that is not. Foods that are particularly high in purines include red meat, organ meats, shellfish, alcohol, lentils, mushrooms, and some vegetables: peas, asparagus, and spinach. It has been found that vegetable-sourced purines carry a lower risk of leading to hyperuricemia, however.

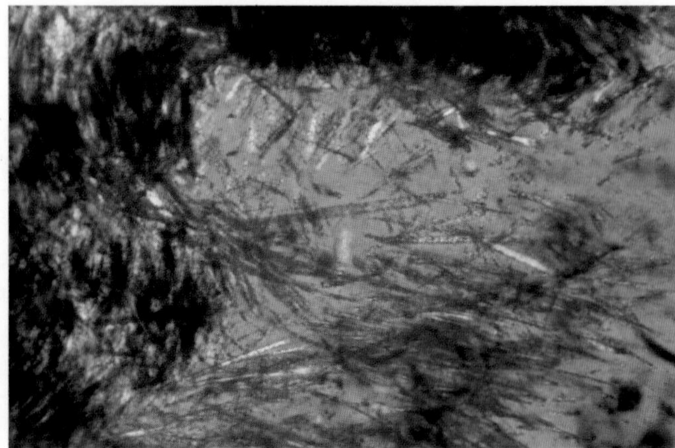

Figure 3.22. Gout: crystals erode joint capsules.

Hyperuricemia is clearly connected to gout, but the two things are not always identical. Many people have hyperuricemia without ever having gout. Conversely, some people with gout show normal or even below-normal levels of uric acid in the blood.

Other risk factors for gout include obesity, sudden weight gain or loss, moderate to high alcohol consumption, high blood pressure, and certain disorders that can raise uric acid levels, including lymphoma, leukemia, psoriasis, and Down syndrome.

Sometimes a person has just one attack of gout and then is never bothered by it again. If a second attack occurs, it comes several years later. The third attack happens after a shorter interval, and the fourth one, shorter still. Each event resolves itself in a few days or weeks. After 10 to 20 years a patient may end up with almost constant acute attacks of this disease, but often by that time the associated problems of this condition may make toe pain the least of his worries.

Signs and Symptoms

Acute gouty arthritis has some very predictable patterns. It has a sudden onset and almost always happens in the feet first, especially at the joints of the great toe. Cumulative damage creates a characteristic punched-out pattern of bony erosion (Figure 3.23). Gout may also appear in the instep, around the Achilles tendon, and in later stages, in the knees and elbows.

An acute gouty joint shows all of the signs of extreme inflammation. The joint may swell so much that the skin is hot, red, dry, shiny and exquisitely painful. This phase of inflammation is often accompanied by a moderate fever (up to 101°F, or 38.3°C) and chills.

Compare and Contrast 3.2
Gout versus Pseudogout

Gout is a variety of arthritis brought about by the accumulation of uric acid crystals in and around joint capsules, especially in the feet. It is a manageable disorder as long as the person keeps a close watch on his uric acid levels. Calcium pyrophosphate dihydrate deposition, or **pseudogout**, has a very similar presentation, but since it doesn't involve uric acid or hyperuricemia, it requires a different treatment plan. Massage therapists are not required to be able to tell the difference between gout and pseudogout, but we can certainly counsel our clients to explore options if the treatment they receive doesn't seem to meet their needs.

CHARACTERISTICS	GOUT	CPDD (PSEUDOGOUT)
Prevalence	100:100,000.	Unknown.
Demographics	90% men over 40; most women postmenopausal.	Women and men equally affected; most over 60.
Primary symptom	Exquisitely painful inflammation, usually around great toe, also in instep and heel. Occasionally affects other joints in later stages, but foot usually affected first.	Exquisitely painful inflammation, usually at knee or wrist.
Implications for massage	Most patients have some hyperuricemia, carry risk of kidney stones, other urinary system disorders. These need to be ruled out for circulatory massage.	Idiopathic disease; may or may not be related to other underlying problems. Clients must be screened for other contributing factors, but none may be present.

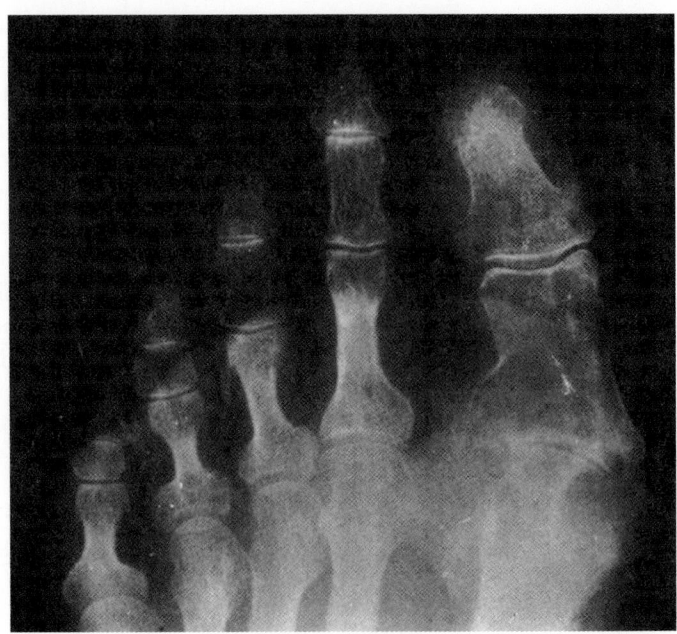

Figure 3.23. Gout: note the punched-out pattern of erosion.

Complications

The complications of gout are complications of having too much uric acid in the bloodstream, which indicates kidneys that are not functioning at adequate levels. Uric acid crystals don't just cause gout; they can also cause kidney stones. If the kidneys become sufficiently clogged by kidney stones, the result is renal failure. Impaired kidneys can't process fluid adequately. This stresses the rest of the circulatory system, causing high blood pressure, the end result of which can be atherosclerosis or stroke. All of these problems—hyperuricemia, kidney insufficiency, gout, high blood pressure, and cardiovascular disease—are closely related.

Diagnosis

Gout is usually easily recognized by its specific pain profile: sudden onset in the feet with long intervals between attacks. However, it sometimes mimics a few other conditions, including rheumatoid arthritis, septic arthritis, psoriatic arthritis, or pseudogout, another chemically based arthritis in which crystals of an entirely different type are deposited in and around joints. The only conclusive diagnosis for gout is an examination of aspirated fluid from an affected joint to look for uric acid crystals.

Treatment

A standard medical approach to gout has three prongs: pain relief (with analgesics *other* than aspirin, which inhibits uric acid excretion); anti-inflammatory drugs, and finally, drugs that modify metabolism and uric acid management. Preventive measures include increasing fluid intake (other than caffeine or alcohol, which act as diuretics), losing weight, and limiting purine-rich foods.

Massage?

Gout is at very least a local contraindication for painful gouty joints. The last thing this client needs is to have someone grind those crystals any deeper into his flesh.

In the acute stage gout is a systemic contraindication, but it's unlikely that anyone in a full-blown attack would try to keep a massage appointment. Ice is likewise contraindicated, since lowering the temperature of the area promotes crystal formation. Any client who is prone to gout is a good candidate for other circulatory or excretory problems; this possibility should weigh into any decisions about modalities.

Modality Recommendations for Gout

MODALITY	RECOMMENDATION
Deep tissue massage	Contraindicated while acute.
Lymphatic drainage	Indicated locally; very effective working proximally.
Polarity	S: Indicated. R/D: Locally contraindicated; otherwise supportive.
PNF/MET/stretching	Locally contraindicated while acute; otherwise supportive.
Reflexology	Locally contraindicated; work endocrine system, kidneys, colon, ureter, bladder, lymphatic system points.
Shiatsu	Indicated. Treat GB, LV, K systemically; gently in local area.
Swedish massage	Locally contraindicated while acute; otherwise supportive.
Trigger point therapy	Locally contraindicated; otherwise supportive.

See Chapter 1 for a brief description of each modality, including definitions of abbreviations.

Lyme Disease

Definition: What Is It?

Lyme disease is an infection with a spirochetal bacterium called ***Borrelia burgdorferi.*** This pathogen spreads by the bite of two species of ticks: deer ticks (***Ixodes** scapularis*) and Western black-legged ticks (*Ixodes pacificus*). These ticks are very small, especially in the nymph stage, when they most frequently affect humans. This can make it difficult to find them on the skin. An unfed deer tick nymph is slightly larger than the period at the end of this sentence (Figure 3.24).

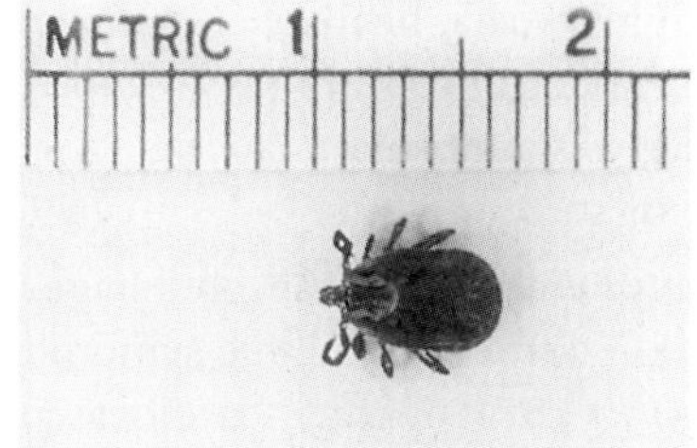

Figure 3.24. Lyme disease: deer tick.

Lyme Disease in Brief

What is it?
Lyme disease is a bacterial infection spread by the bites of certain species of ticks. The immune response to the bacteria causes inflammation of large joints and neurological and cardiovascular symptoms.

How is it recognized?
The hallmark early symptom of Lyme disease is a circular bull's-eye rash at the site of the tick bite. The skin is red, itchy, and hot but not usually raised. The rash may be accompanied by fever, fatigue, and joint pain. Later symptoms may include acute intermittent inflammation of one or more large joints, numbness, poor coordination, Bell palsy, and an irregular heartbeat.

Is massage indicated or contraindicated?
The inflammation associated with Lyme disease runs in acute and subacute phases. During subacute phases, massage may be appropriate to maintain joint function and relieve pain. In this situation it is important to be working as part of a health care team for the maximum benefit and minimum risk to the infected person.

Demographics: Who Gets It?

Lyme disease has been reported in 49 states and the District of Columbia. (Montana is the only state that has no report of Lyme disease as of 2004.) However, 90% of cases were found in the Northeast and mid-Atlantic states, along with Wisconsin and Minnesota. Smaller concentrations of the disease have been noted in northwestern California.

Persons most at risk for Lyme disease are those who work or play outside in grassy or wooded areas; the ticks don't thrive in sunny or arid environments. Overall, approximately 20,000 cases of Lyme disease are reported every year in this country. It has also been reported across Europe and Asia.[29]

Etiology: What Happens?

The life cycle of the deer tick and Western black-legged tick lasts about 2 years. Adult ticks spend fall and winter mating and taking blood meals from warm-blooded hosts. In the spring, females detach from their hosts and fall onto the ground to lay eggs. The eggs hatch, and the larvae spend summer and fall taking meals from mice, birds, and large mammals, especially white-tailed deer. Dormant in the winter, the larvae molt into the nymph stage the following spring. They climb onto grass or bush stems and wait for a warm-blooded host to brush close by. This is the stage of development during which the animals most often find their way to human hosts. The final molt to the adult tick occurs in the insect's second summer, and the cycle begins again.

Ticks pick up the spiral bacterium *B. burgdorferi* from the blood of their animal hosts, especially mice. If an infected tick then bites a human, that bacterium may be transmitted to the human host. The bacterial invasion can cause several reactions, depending on the severity and the stage of the infection.

B. burgdorferi is a slow-growing bacterium. This creates several problems, including a delayed immune response and difficulties in getting accurate information from blood tests. So far three subspecies of the bacterium have been found, and up to 100 different strains are active in the United States.

SIDEBAR 3.4: HISTORY OF LYME DISEASE

Although Lyme disease was only definitively identified and named in 1982, it has probably been present for much longer.

In the early 20th century, doctors made note of target-shaped red rashes, which were named **erythema migrans.** People who developed these rashes seemed to have a high incidence of arthritis, but if they were treated with penicillin, their chances of developing arthritis were significantly lessened.

Then in 1974 a group of children in Lyme, Connecticut, were diagnosed with juvenile rheumatoid arthritis. Parents became suspicious of having such a high concentration of a disease that was not supposed to be in any way communicable. This led to intensive research, during which a scientist named Burgdorfer isolated the spirochete now called *B. burgdorferi.* He found it in highest concentrations in the midgut of deer ticks.

Burgdorfer's discovery in 1982 began a process of surveillance that continues today. The incidence of Lyme disease rises yearly; it causes about 12,500 new infections annually.

B. burgdorferi did not make its first appearance with human infections; it probably has been around for ages. As the human population expanded into undeveloped areas, this bacterium suddenly had access to human hosts. It remains to be seen what other kinds of illnesses may be encountered as we continue to expand into previously undeveloped areas.

Signs and Symptoms

Lyme disease moves in stages, with signs and symptoms particular to each.

- *Early localized disease* is the first stage of a Lyme disease infection. Ticks are slow feeders, so it may take several days for the bacteria to enter the body and some days after that for symptoms to appear. Early symptoms generally appear 7 to 30 days after an initial tick bite. They include a circular red rash (a bull's-eye rash) that is hot and itchy but not raised from the skin (Figure 3.25), accompanied by high fever, fatigue, night sweats, headache, stiff neck, and swollen lymph nodes. If no rash appears (as in more than 50% of cases), these early symptoms may be mistaken for flu, mononucleosis, or meningitis.
- *Early disseminated disease* is the second stage, during which the infected person develops systemic symptoms of infection with *B. burgdorferi.* These include cardiovascular symptoms

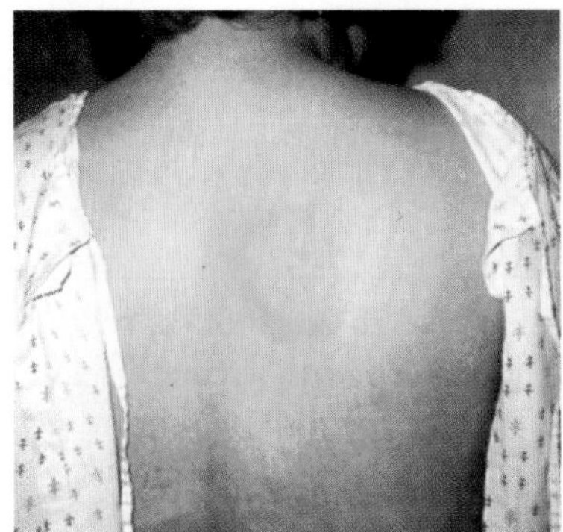

Figure 3.25. Lyme disease: bull's-eye rash.

(especially irregular heartbeat and dizziness), neurological symptoms (chronic headaches, Bell palsy, numbness, tingling, forgetfulness, and poor coordination), along with more general problems, including debilitating fatigue.

- *Late disease* is the final outcome of a Lyme disease infection. It is associated with extreme inflammation of one or more large joints. The knees are the most commonly affected area, but elbows and shoulders are often inflamed as well. Most patients don't have the infection in more than three joints at a time. The inflammation can be extreme enough to damage the joint permanently, especially if it is left untreated.

The tendency for Lyme disease to affect joints is what classifies it as an arthritic condition. In fact, the first cases of Lyme disease ever identified were among a group of children who were all initially misdiagnosed with juvenile rheumatoid arthritis.

Most people with Lyme disease have symptoms for several weeks or months, and then they subside. A small number develop a chronic condition, which can progressively get worse. It is unclear whether these patients have a continuing chronic infection or develop an autoimmune response that is originally triggered by the bacterial infection.

Diagnosis

The accurate diagnosis of Lyme disease is one of the most contentious issues surrounding this condition. Blood tests that identify antibodies are unreliable: they frequently miss the presence of bacteria, leading to a false-negative result, or they show the presence of antibodies but cannot distinguish whether the infection is active or part of a person's immune system history, leading to false-positive results. To make matters more complicated, other tickborne diseases can occur simultaneously with Lyme disease, but they interfere with successful treatment. (See Sidebar 3.5)

This leaves the description of symptoms and the observation of signs as the primary means to diagnose Lyme disease. Unfortunately, many patients have no memory of a tick bite or a rash, so doctors must depend on the signs of fever, fatigue, swollen lymph nodes, and headache to make an early diagnosis. All of these symptoms can be associated with several other diseases, including mononucleosis, flu, meningitis, and several others. Doctors are now counseled to consider Lyme disease when investigating conditions like FMS, chronic fatigue syndrome, and multiple chemical sensitivity syndrome.

At this point it is unclear whether Lyme disease is overdiagnosed or underdiagnosed. What is clear is that more accurate tests are needed to identify this infection. Some of these are in development. They will show not only the evidence of a bacterial infection but whether that infection is current or in the past.

Treatment

B. burgdorferi is sensitive to antibiotics, so the outlook for someone who is diagnosed with Lyme disease in the early stages is often hopeful. Lyme disease requires a much longer course of antibiotics than most other bacterial infections, however. It is fairly common for a person to take medication for 6 weeks or more; relapse rates for those who try shorter courses of medication are high. When Lyme disease becomes a chronic problem, antibiotics may be prescribed for 12 months or even more.

Prevention

The best protection against Lyme disease is protection from disease-bearing ticks. This means wearing long sleeves and long pants when working or playing in areas where tick infestation is high. Tucking pants into socks or boots may make it harder for ticks to gain access to skin. Wearing light-colored clothing is recommended, to make it easier to find and remove ticks. Using insect repellants can also reduce the risk of tick bites.

Examining the skin after being in a high-risk area is another important preventive measure. Ticks prefer to occupy warm, protected areas such as the groin, axilla, backs of knees, and insides of elbows. If a tick is found, it should be carefully removed with tweezers to keep the mouth parts intact, and then the person should report being bitten and take the tick to the doctor. If the tick is found and removed within 24 hours, the risk of infection is very low.

Vaccines against Lyme disease are no longer available.

SIDEBAR 3.5: IS IT JUST LYME DISEASE?

Lyme disease is caused by tickborne bacteria that infect joints and cause debilitating arthritis. Some Lyme disease patients live with pain and progressive inflammation for years, in spite of antibiotics that should provide relief. It turns out that some of these patients may have more than Lyme disease alone: deer ticks can carry two other pathogens that affect humans:

- **Ehrlichiosis** is a tickborne bacterial infection that can easily coexist with Lyme disease. Consequences of ehrlichiosis infection include low white blood cell and platelet counts. This infection can be cleared with antibiotics from the tetracycline family, but this is a different class of antibiotics from that usually used for Lyme disease alone. Ehrlichiosis is less common than Lyme disease, so some patients may live with this infection for a long time before it is discovered.
- **Babesiosis** is a parasite similar to the protozoan that causes malaria. It can also coexist with Lyme disease. Babesiosis can cause anemia and an enlarged spleen, as well as other serious problems, especially for immunosuppressed people. Babesiosis responds well to quinine *if* it is identified as an infection separate from Lyme disease.

To complicate matters further, two other tickborne illnesses may also be confused with Lyme disease:

- **Southern tick-associated rash illness** (**STARI**) is a condition endemic to southeast and southcentral states. It is spread by the Lone Star tick, which carries the spirochete *Borrelia lonestari*. STARI also causes a bull's-eye rash and is treatable with antibiotics.
- **Rocky Mountain spotted fever** (**RMSF**) is an infection with the bacterium *Rickettsia rickettsii*, spread by hard ticks all over the western United States. Early symptoms include fever, headache, muscle pain, and malaise, followed by a spotty rash (as opposed to a bull's-eye rash). Although RMSF is treatable with antibiotics, it is a potentially life-threatening infection that can affect blood and blood vessels all over the body, leading to serious long-term consequences.

Massage?

The arthritic phase of Lyme disease involves intermittently severe inflammation of joints that is acutely painful. This contraindicates massage when inflammation is acute. At other times, as long as sensation is present and the client is comfortable, a person with Lyme disease may derive significant benefits from massage. But because this disease can affect the nervous and circulatory systems and because treatment can take a long time to take effect, it is important for massage therapists to operate as part of a client's health care team.

Massage therapists who live and work in areas where Lyme disease is especially common should be aware of what deer ticks and Western black-legged ticks look like so that if they find these parasites during a session, they can counsel clients to receive appropriate medical care.

MODALITY RECOMMENDATIONS FOR LYME DISEASE	
MODALITY	RECOMMENDATION
Deep tissue massage	Contraindicated while acute; otherwise supportive when working with the health care team.
Lymphatic drainage	Supportive.
Polarity	S: Indicated. R/D: Carefully, within client comfort.
PNF/MET/stretching	Supportive while subacute, within client tolerance.
Reflexology	Indicated; for severe inflammation, work lymphatic system points.
Shiatsu	Supportive. Treat immune system via TH, SP.
Swedish massage	Supportive while subacute, within client tolerance.
Trigger point therapy	Indicated in subacute stage for musculoskeletal effects.

See Chapter 1 for a brief description of each modality, including definitions of abbreviations.

Osteoarthritis

Definition: What Is It?

Also called *degenerative joint disease*, osteoarthritis is a condition in which synovial joints, especially weight-bearing joints, lose healthy cartilage. This condition is distinguished from other types of arthritis by being directly related to age and wear and tear of the joint structures.

Demographics: Who Gets It?

This is by far the most common type of arthritis in the world. Statistics vary, but most report that osteoarthritis affects 20 to 40 million Americans. Men and women are affected in equal numbers, but women tend to develop it earlier and be affected more severely. More than half of people over 75 years old have been diagnosed with osteoarthritis in at least one joint. Besides age, the single leading risk factor for osteoarthritis is being overweight. Clinically obese people (those with a body mass index over 30) are four times more likely to develop osteoarthritis than the rest of the population.[30,31]

Osteoarthritis is also an occupational hazard for massage therapists, who may get it at the saddle joint (between the trapezium and first metacarpal), because it is easy put too much pressure on this joint if good body mechanics aren't employed.

Etiology: What Happens?

Joints, especially knees and hips, put up with tremendous weight-bearing stress and repetitive movements; their design is a marvel of efficiency and durability. But the environment inside a joint capsule is precarious. Any imbalance can have cumulative destructive impact. This can take the

Osteoarthritis in Brief
Pronunciation: os-te-o-arth-RY-tis

What is it?
Osteoarthritis is joint inflammation brought about by wear and tear causing cumulative damage to articular cartilage.

How is it recognized?
Affected joints are stiff, painful, and occasionally palpably inflamed. Bony deformation may be easily visible or palpable. Osteoarthritis most often affects knees, hips, and distal joints of the fingers.

Is massage indicated or contraindicated?
Arthritis contraindicates massage if it is acutely inflamed. It indicates massage in the subacute stage, when bodywork can contribute to muscular relaxation and mobility of the affected joint.

shape of excessive stress on a healthy joint or normal stress on a joint that has already been compromised. Once the path toward arthritis has begun, it may be possible to stop it, but capacity for regeneration and repair is limited at best (Figure 3.26).

The environment within the cartilage turns out to be the key feature in the development of osteoarthritis. Hyaline or articular cartilage is constructed of a relatively small number of living chondrocytes that produce collagen (mostly type II fibers), along with proteoglycans: large negatively charged molecules that attract water. The cells, protein fibers, and molecules of fluid are arranged in slightly different patterns, depending on whether they are superficial, intermediate, or attached directly to the chondral surface of the articulating bone. This gives layers of cartilage the ability to resist both shearing and compressive forces.

Chondrocytes remain active all through life, constantly replacing and rebuilding the cartilage surface, but they don't migrate to damaged areas. When the delicate balance in the articular cartilage is upset, chondrocytes make less fluid and collagen, and cartilage degrades. This stimulates osteocytes in the epiphyses of the affected bones to become more active: the condyle of the bone may become enlarged, osteophytes (bone spurs) may develop, and in some cases cystlike cavities develop under the cartilage of the affected bone.

Causes

Many changes in the body may trigger joint degeneration. Age alone changes the quality of articular cartilage, making it drier and more prone to injury. Being overweight adds stress to knees and hips. If the ligaments that surround joints are chronically lax, the joint can become unstable, raising the risk of arthritis; this can be a long-term problem with joints that have been dislocated. A history of trauma or surgery (to remove pieces of the meniscus, for instance) is another predisposing factor. Repetitive pounding stress, such as running or jump-

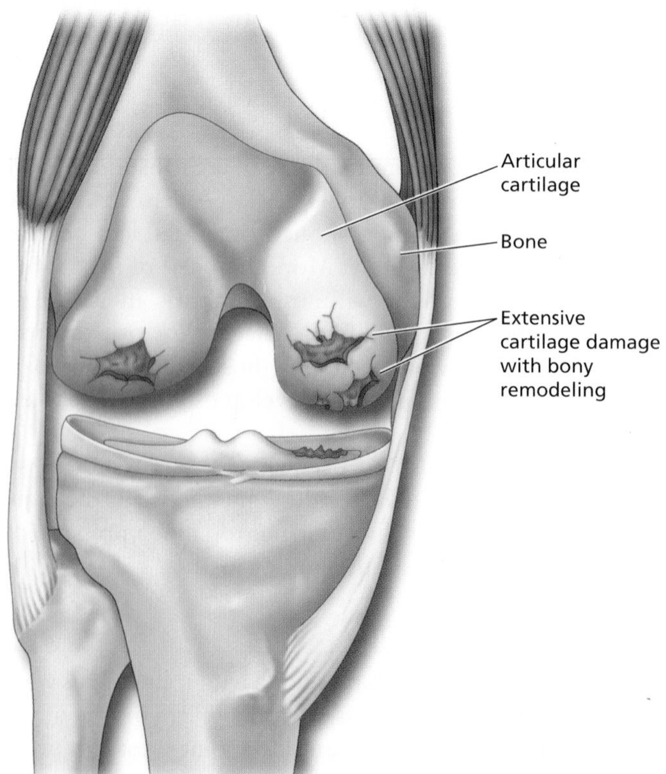

Figure 3.26. Osteoarthritis.

Compare and Contrast 3.3
Osteoarthritis versus Rheumatoid Arthritis

Of the 100 conditions that cause painful inflammation of joints, the two most common are osteoarthritis and rheumatoid arthritis. Osteoarthritis is a wear-and-tear disorder that could possibly be exacerbated by overenthusiastic bodywork but can't be spread through the body. Rheumatoid arthritis is an autoimmune disorder that *can* spread from joint to joint and must be avoided by bodyworkers in the acute, or flare, stage.

It is important for clients to know the source of their joint pain. Massage therapists are not equipped to tell the difference between the two conditions—and of course it's a perfectly reasonable possibility that a client could have both simultaneously. Still, it can be difficult to come to a conclusive diagnosis for joint pain. The following is a brief list of the most common patterns seen with osteoarthritis compared with rheumatoid arthritis.

CHARACTERISTICS	OSTEOARTHRITIS	RHEUMATOID ARTHRITIS
Prevalence	Radiographs show bony deformation in 33%–90% of people over 65.	Up to 1.5% of the population.
Demographics	Most common in people over 40. Men and women affected equally.	Women affected two to three times as often as men; men more likely to have systemic symptoms. May affect children.
Pain patterns	Spine, knees, hips most frequently affected. Distal finger joints, saddle joint (trapezium, first metacarpal) also at risk.	Proximal joints in hands and feet, ankles, wrists usually affected. Extreme distortion of joint capsules can cause joints to be visibly misshapen. Pain appears in flare and remission stages.
Other symptoms	None	In early stages and acute episodes, fever, malaise, lack of appetite, muscle pain may be present.
Implications for massage	Can be useful to maintain range of motion and relieve pain in muscles that cross over affected joints, as long as inflammation is not acute.	Can be useful for joint function during remission. During acute stages, avoid circulatory massage.

ing with inadequate support, can also open the door to problems. Hormonal imbalances and nutritional deficiencies, including dehydration, inadequate calcium metabolism, and foods that trigger inflammatory responses, may compromise the health of joint structures.

Signs and Symptoms

The symptoms of osteoarthritis all revolve around irritation of the joint structures. Osteoarthritis is seldom hot, painful, and swollen. More often it lingers in a chronic stage in which the joints have ongoing deep pain and stiffness, especially when they are not warmed up or when they have been overused. Osteoarthritis can be crippling when it occurs at the hip or knee, because the pain and limitation are badly exacerbated by walking.

When osteoarthritis develops in the fingers, characteristic thickening of the phalangeal epiphyses is present. Bulges at the distal interphalangeal joints (DIPs) are called **Heberden nodes**. When they appear at the proximal interphalangeal joints (PIPs), they are called **Bouchard nodes**.

Diagnosis

Osteoarthritis is identified by physical examination and history. Tests may be conducted to rule out other conditions, but no blood test definitively identifies osteoarthritis. Even radiographs can be misleading. They may be used to confirm a diagnosis, but a surprisingly high percentage of people who show osteoarthritis-like bony deformations on radiography have no pain at all.[32]

Treatment

Treatment options for osteoarthritis have improved considerably in recent years. The goals of treatment are to reduce pain and inflammation and to limit or reverse the damage to the joint structures. These goals are accomplished in a number of different ways, depending on how advanced the condition is.

- *Nonsteroidal anti-inflammatory drugs.* These are the usually the first recourse to deal with arthritis pain. Some patients don't tolerate them well, and alternatives that were developed to preserve the stomach have since been seen to increase the risk of cardiovascular problems, so some have been withdrawn from the market.
- *Topical applications.* Counterirritants like camphor and menthol are the ingredients that make some creams feel cold or hot. These sensations can mitigate some of the pain associated with arthritis. Capsaicin, the chemical that puts the heat in hot peppers, has also been used in skin creams for chronically painful conditions.
- *Exercise.* Osteoarthritis patients are advised to exercise within pain tolerance to achieve three goals: to improve and maintain healthy range of motion, to increase stamina and lose weight, and to improve the strength of muscles surrounding affected joints.
- *Nutritional supplements.* ***Glucosamine*** and ***chondroitin sulfate*** are two substances that may not only limit the progression of arthritis damage but may be able to reverse it. Research on how (or whether) taking supplements of these naturally occurring connective tissue building blocks helps to repair damaged cartilage is still ongoing. Current data suggest that these supplements are most useful to people with moderate to severe arthritis.[33] Although public interest in these supplements is high, they are unregulated by the FDA, and so potency and dosages may vary from one brand to another. These supplements are not without risk. Glucosamine may affect insulin levels in diabetic patients, and it is made from the shells of shellfish, so people with allergies should watch for reactions. Chondroitin may affect blood clotting, so patients who also take blood thinners should consult their primary care providers about this risk.[34]
- *Arthroscopic procedures.* Various approaches to manipulating the joint environment are used with osteoarthritis. Proliferants (substances that promote the creation of new ligament fibers) may be injected into lax cruciate ligaments of the knee: this has the goal of tightening the joint and reducing the risk of progression of arthritis. Corticosteroids may be introduced to reduce pain and inflammation, but this can be done only two or three times per year. Synovial fluid may be withdrawn to reduce pressure. Joint ***lavage*** and ***debridement*** work to remove loose bits of cartilage (these are sometimes called "joint mice") and to smooth articulating surfaces.
- *Joint replacement surgery.* A last resort for debilitating osteoarthritis is to replace the surfaces of the affected joint with artificial cartilage. Joint replacement surgery for knees and hips has become a commonplace intervention, and the expected recovery time from such surgery is a matter of weeks. About 256,000 knee replacements and 117,000 hip replacements are performed each year in this country.[31] It is important to delay this surgery as long as possible, however, because the lifespan of a typical joint replacement is only about 10 years, and subsequent surgeries tend to be less successful.

- *Procedures in development.* The high incidence of osteoarthritis, along with an aging population in this country, have made finding ways to support the rebuilding of cartilage a high priority. Numerous strategies are in development, including the creation of a cartilage paste that can be injected into damaged areas, surgery to drill into the epiphysis of the affected bone in a way to stimulate the building of new cartilage, transplanting osteochondral plugs from non–weight-bearing areas into the damaged surface, and others.

Massage?

Most osteoarthritis patients seldom have acute swelling with pain, heat, and redness. This is good news for massage therapists, who want to avoid exacerbating acute inflammation. Chronic osteoarthritis indicates massage to reduce pain through release of the muscles surrounding the affected joints and to maintain range of motion through gentle stretching and passive range of motion exercises.

Modality Recommendations for Osteoarthritis

MODALITY	RECOMMENDATION
Deep tissue massage	Indicated to release fascias that cross affected joint. Use gentle active movements to assist release.
Lymphatic drainage	Locally indicated when acute; supportive during normal course of condition.
Polarity	S: Indicated. R/D: Indicated within client comfort.
PNF/MET/stretching	Locally contraindicated while acute; indicated while subacute.
Reflexology	Locally contraindicated; work all glands, kidney, lymphatic system points.
Shiatsu	Indicated to reduce pain and swelling locally. Treat GB, TH, SP systemically.
Swedish massage	Supportive while subacute, within client tolerance.
Trigger point therapy	Indicated while subacute.

See Chapter 1 for a brief description of each modality, including definitions of abbreviations.

Patellofemoral Syndrome

Definition: What Is It?

Patellofemoral syndrome (PFS) is a condition in which the patellar cartilage becomes irritated as it contacts the femoral cartilage. This situation can be a precursor of osteoarthritis.

PFS is almost always associated with overloading or overuse of the patellofemoral joint, although it may be precipitated by a specific injury or trauma. For a long while the term *patellofemoral syndrome* was used interchangeably with ***chondromalacia patellae***. The term chondromalacia is now reserved for fraying and chipping of the patellar cartilage. More current synonyms for PFS include *jumper's knee*, *movie-goer's knee*, *anterior knee pain syndrome*, and *over utilization syndrome*.

Patellofemoral Syndrome in Brief

Pronunciation: pah-tel-o-FEM-or-al sin-drome

What is it?

Patellofemoral syndrome (PFS) is an overuse disorder that can lead to damage of the patellar cartilage.

How is it recognized?

PFS causes pain at the knee, stiffness after immobility, and discomfort in walking down stairs.

Is massage indicated or contraindicated?

PFS indicates massage, as long as the knee is not acutely inflamed. Massage may or may not be useful to correct this problem, but it will certainly do no harm and can address issues of muscle tightness and imbalance.

Etiology: What Happens?

When the knee is bent, whether or not it is bearing weight, the femur and the patella press together. Furthermore, the range of motion for the patella is broader than most people understand. This bone moves superiorly and inferiorly, but it can also move medially and laterally, and it can rotate or tip in any direction. If pressure is not evenly distributed across the back of the patella, disruptions to the patellar cartilage can occur. While this condition can be stopped or even reversed if it is caught early, long-term irritation can ultimately lead to permanent cartilage damage and osteoarthritis at the knee.

Two main issues have been identified as contributors to PFS: overuse or overloading, and poor alignment. Overuse can be a result of percussive activities, especially with twisting and jumping. Overloading of the joint can occur even without repetitive percussive activity if the person is overweight.

Inefficient alignment at the knee can take many forms. Poor footwear or running on uneven surfaces can change how force moves up the leg into the knee. Flat feet, jammed arches, or problems in how the foot hits the ground can do the same thing. Unequal development of the medial and lateral quadriceps muscles is frequently identified; PFS almost always involves a lateral pull on the patella. Muscular imbalances between the quadriceps, hamstrings, and iliotibial band are factors. An exaggerated *Q angle* is sometimes suggested as a cause of PFS, but studies of female athletes fail to reveal any incidence of this disorder that correlates to the degree of the Q angle.

Signs and Symptoms

Symptoms of PFS include pain that is usually felt on the anterior aspect of the knee, stiffness after long immobility, difficulty walking down stairs, and a characteristic crackling, grinding noise on movement called *crepitus*.

Diagnosis

PFS can be difficult to diagnose, especially in the early stages, before visible damage to the bones has occurred. The problem is that what is often called PFS may actually be another condition, *patellar tendinitis*. This is significant because while PFS is largely unaffected by massage, patellar tendinitis responds beautifully, and can have a virtually pain-free resolution. Consequently, it is important to have a clear idea of what a client really has. One clue that is sometimes useful is that patellar tendinitis often hurts going *up* stairs (resisted extension of the leg) while PFS may hurt more going *down* stairs (the weight of the femur pushing on the patella). However, these two conditions can certainly be present simultaneously. Ultimately only a doctor with imaging techniques can give a definitive diagnosis.

Treatment

The long-term prognosis for a person with PFS depends entirely on what he or she does with it. Although damage to the patellar cartilage may set the stage for osteoarthritis in the knee, PFS doesn't always get to the point of requiring a joint replacement. But this condition is badly irritated by jarring, jouncing, bouncing kinds of exercise. If one kind of activity becomes prohibitive (running and aerobics are not great choices for someone with PFS), it can probably be replaced with something else, such as swimming, walking, cycling, or skating. Patients may have to experiment under a doctor's supervision to find the exercise activities that work best.

Physical therapy for PFS often includes exercises to strengthen and balance tension in the muscles that cross the knee and that influence knee alignment. The quadriceps, hamstrings, tensor fascia latae, and deep lateral rotators are often addressed in the challenge to improve alignment and stop the progression of damage that PFS can cause.

Other interventions include ice, nonsteroidal anti-inflammatories for pain management, orthotics to improve alignment in the feet, and improved footwear. Some orthopedists recommend the use of a knee brace to stabilize the patella or special taping of the knee for the same purpose: these are only for times when activities may stress the knee.

With careful exercise and attention to correct alignment an athlete with PFS may be able to return to previous activities.

Massage?

PFS is usually a chronic, low-level irritation that interferes with normal activity. Because the irritation occurs inside the joint capsule, it is doubtful whether massage can be instrumental in improving the situation. Certainly bodywork can address the stiffness, tension, and chronic pain experienced in muscle-tendon units that cross the knee joint. If a treatment strategy is developed to retrain the knee extensors to track the patella appropriately over the joint, massage may be a useful part of an effort to slow down or stop permanent cartilage damage.

Modality Recommendations for Patellofemoral Syndrome

MODALITY	RECOMMENDATION
Deep tissue massage	Supportive to balance fascias across joint. Often involves lateral side of leg and IT band.
Lymphatic drainage	Supportive.
Polarity	S: Indicated. R/D: Indicated while subacute.
PNF/MET/stretching	Indicated in all stages. Releasing quadriceps tension can decrease pain and irritation.
Reflexology	Indicated.
Shiatsu	Indicated. Treat ST, SP systemically and locally.
Swedish massage	Indicated while subacute; releasing quadriceps tension can decrease pain, irritation.
Trigger point therapy	Supportive.

See Chapter 1 for a brief description of each modality, including definitions of abbreviations.

Rheumatoid Arthritis in Brief

Pronunciation: RUE-mah-toyd arth-RY-tis

What is it?

Rheumatoid arthritis is an autoimmune disease in which immune system agents attack synovial membranes, particularly of the joints in the hands and feet. Other structures, such as muscles, tendons, and blood vessels, as well as serous membranes, may also be affected.

How is it recognized?

In the acute phase affected joints are red, swollen, hot, and painful. They often become gnarled and distorted. It tends to affect the body symmetrically, and it is not determined by age.

Is massage indicated or contraindicated?

Hands-on bodywork is indicated in the subacute or remission stages of rheumatoid arthritis only. At that point it may be used to reestablish mobility and to reduce the stresses that can trigger another flare.

Rheumatoid Arthritis

Definition: What Is It?

Rheumatoid arthritis is an autoimmune condition in which the synovial membranes of various joints are attacked by immune system cells. Unlike many other forms of arthritis, rheumatoid arthritis can also involve inflammation of tissues outside the musculoskeletal system.

Demographics: Who Gets It?

This disease affects 3.1 million people, or about 1% of Americans. Women are affected about three times more frequently than men. Statistics indicate that it is most common among 20- to 50-year-olds, but it can strike anyone, including children and adolescents.[35]

Etiology: What Happens?

The etiology of rheumatoid arthritis is not well understood, but most researchers consider it to be an autoimmune disease: the immune system attacks parts of the body. The primary target in rheumatoid arthritis is synovial membranes of certain joints, but other areas (blood vessels, serous membranes, the skin, eyes, lungs, liver, and heart) may also be affected.

When a synovial membrane is under attack, all of the signs of inflammation develop: heat, pain, redness, swelling, and loss of function. Studies of joint tissues show that B cells, T cells, antibodies, and many other inflammatory chemicals are present during a flare. In response, the synovial membrane thickens and swells. Fluid accumulates inside the joint capsule, which causes pressure and pain. The inflamed tissues release enzymes that erode cartilage, eventually all the way down to the bone. This is the process that causes the telltale deformation of the joint capsules and gnarled appearance of rheumatoid arthritis (Figure 3.27).

Signs and Symptoms

Symptoms of rheumatoid arthritis vary considerably at the onset of the disease. Many people have a period of weeks or months with a general feeling of illness: lack of energy, lack of ap-

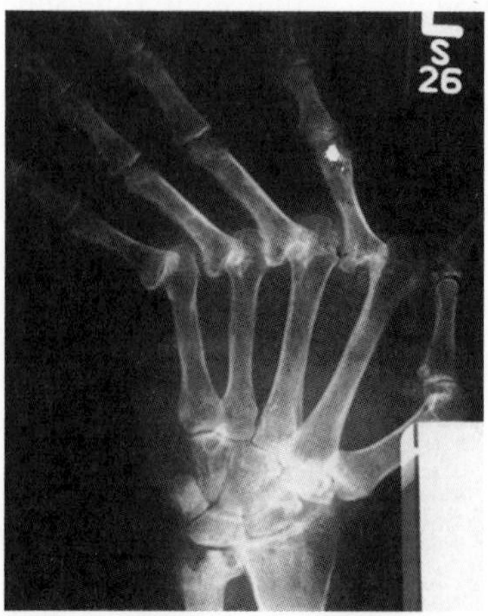

Figure 3.27. Rheumatoid arthritis.

petite, low-grade fever, and vague muscle pain, which gradually becomes sharp, specific joint pain. Some patients have a sudden onset with joint pain alone. Rheumatic nodules, small, painless bumps that appear around fingers, elbows, and other pressure-bearing areas, are also common indicators of the disease.

In the acute stage the affected joints are red, hot, painful, and stiff, although they improve considerably with moderate amounts of movement and stretching. The joints rheumatoid arthritis most often attacks are the knuckles in hands and toes. It frequently develops in ankles and wrists; knees are less common. One of the most serious places to get it is in the neck, where it can lead to dangerous instability. It generally affects the body bilaterally, although it is sometimes worse on one side than the other.

Like many autoimmune diseases, rheumatoid arthritis appears in cycles of flare followed by periods of remission. Some patients have only a few flares in their life and are never affected again. Moderate cases involve cycles of flare and remission up to several times a year. Severe rheumatoid arthritis involves chronic inflammation that never fully subsides.

Complications

If someone has rheumatoid arthritis, it means her immune system is confused about what it should be fighting off. Synovial membranes are just one of the types of tissue that may be attacked. Other possibilities include:

- Rheumatic nodules on the sclera (whites) of the eyes.
- *Sjögren syndrome* (pathologically dry eyes and mouth).
- Pleuritis, which makes breathing painful and increases vulnerability to lung infection.
- Carditis or pericarditis, that is, inflammation of the heart or pericardial sac.
- Hepatitis, or inflammation of the liver.
- Vasculitis, or inflammation of blood vessels. This complication carries another set of risks: Raynaud syndrome, skin ulcers, bleeding intestinal ulcers, and internal hemorrhaging.
- Bursitis and anemia, especially when onset of the disease occurs in childhood.

Advanced structural damage brings a different set of complications. Deformed and bone-damaged joints may dislocate or even collapse, rendering them useless. The tendons that cross over distorted joints sometimes become so stretched that they snap. If the disease is at the C1-C2 joint and the joint collapses, the resultant injury to the spinal column may even result in paralysis.

Diagnosis

Rheumatoid arthritis can be difficult to diagnose because its early symptoms are often subtle; they vary greatly from one person to another; and a long list of diseases with similar symptoms must be ruled out before a diagnosis can be conclusive. A sense of urgency exists around a conclusive diagnosis however, because it has been found that cartilage and bone damage may occur as early as the first or second year of the disease process, and if treatment can be administered earlier, this damage can be averted.

Rheumatoid arthritis is typically diagnosed through a description of symptoms, radiography, and a blood test to check for rheumatoid factor, a substance that is present in most but not all cases. An erythrocyte sedimentation test may be conducted to look for signs of general inflammation, and the blood is also examined for signs of anemia. Even when all signs are positive, the diagnosis is sometimes not considered conclusive until the patient has been under observation for a long while.

A set of diagnostic criteria has been provided by the American Rheumatology Association.[21] When four of these seven signs are present, a diagnosis of rheumatoid arthritis can be made:

- Morning stiffness that lasts at least 1 hour
- Arthritis in three or more joints
- Involvement of the proximal interphalangeal joints (PIPs), distal interphalangeal joints (DIPs), or wrist
- Bilateral distribution
- Positive serum rheumatoid factor
- Rheumatoid nodules
- Radiographic (x-ray) evidence

Treatment

Once the diagnosis of rheumatoid arthritis has been confirmed, the goals of treatment are to reduce pain, limit inflammation, halt joint damage, and improve function. Medications that help to achieve these goals are divided into first-line and second-line drugs.

First-line drugs include nonsteroidal anti-inflammatories, corticosteroids, and cyclo-oxygenase (COX)-2 inhibitors to limit inflammation and pain. These are often used along with exercise, hydrotherapy, physical therapy, and occupational therapy in the hopes that progression can be limited without further intervention.

Second-line drugs attempt to interfere with the disease process. These include biological response modifiers and immunosuppressant drugs. They often give significant relief, but they also carry a long list of serious side effects and sometimes cannot be used for long-term care.

Nonmedical intervention for rheumatoid arthritis can include adjustments to diet, exercise, and stress reduction techniques (including massage). Research is being conducted into the use of some alternative and complementary strategies for symptom management, including botanicals, t'ai chi, and meditation.[36]

Surgery can be a successful option for rheumatoid arthritis patients, if the disease has affected joints that can be easily treated. Joint replacement is sometimes an option, along with surgery to rebuild damaged or ruptured tendons and to remove portions of affected synovial membranes. The synovial membranes grow back, however, so this surgery is a temporary measure.

Massage?

In its acute (flare) phase, rheumatoid arthritis is an inflammatory condition caused by agents in the circulatory system. Any type of massage that promotes circulation is probably not appropriate at this time.

In its subacute phase, rheumatoid arthritis leaves the joints stiff but not inflamed, and the muscles and tendons around them are stressed and tight from chronic pain. Rheumatoid arthritis indicates massage in the subacute stage. Massage can improve mobility and the health of the soft tissues surrounding the joints. In addition to the structural benefits it offers, massage can also be an important part of the prevention strategy of keeping healthy and stress free. If bodywork can help to balance the autonomic nervous system, it may also help to reduce the incidence of attack.

Modality Recommendations for Rheumatoid Arthritis

MODALITY	RECOMMENDATION
Deep tissue massage	Contraindicated while acute. Supportive when subacute: work surrounding areas to decompress joint.
Lymphatic drainage	Locally contraindicated while acute; indicated while subacute.
Polarity	S: Indicated. R/D: Supportive while subacute, depending on client comfort.
PNF/MET/stretching	Locally contraindicated while acute; indicated while subacute.
Reflexology	Locally contraindicated; work all glands, kidneys, solar plexus points. During flare, work lymphatic system points.
Shiatsu	Indicated. Treat immune system via TH/SP/K and pain, stiffness via GB/LV.
Swedish massage	Supportive while subacute, within client tolerance.
Trigger point therapy	Locally contraindicated while acute; indicated while subacute.

See Chapter 1 for a brief description of each modality, including definitions of abbreviations.

Spondylosis

Definition: What Is It?

Spondylosis is a term sometimes used as a synonym for osteoarthritis in the spine, but not all specialists agree with this usage. It describes age-related changes of the vertebrae, discs, joints, and ligaments of the spine.

Spondylosis in Brief

Pronunciation: spon-dih-LO-sis

What is it?

Spondylosis is degeneration of the bones and discs in the spine. It is sometimes referred to as osteoarthritis in the spine.

How is it recognized?

It is identifiable by radiography, which shows a characteristic thickening of the affected vertebral bodies, facets, and ligamentum flava. Symptoms are present only if pressure is exerted on nerve roots, causing pain, numbness, paresthesia, and specific muscle weakness. Otherwise, the only sign of spondylosis may be slow, progressive loss of range of motion in the spine.

Is massage indicated or contraindicated?

Spondylosis indicates massage with caution. If any signs of nerve impingement are present, the client should be positioned in a way to reduce nerve pressure.

Etiology: What Happens?

The key feature with spondylosis is the development of osteophytes on the vertebrae. These usually appear on the anterior or lateral aspects of the vertebral bodies but occasionally grow on the facets or in a place to put pressure on the nerve roots or spinal cord itself.

Although the intervertebral discs are not synovial joints, in this location they are prone to some of the same problems that freely movable joints can develop. It can be a useful analogy to think of the vertebral bodies as articulating bones, the tough annulus fibrosus as a capsular ligament, and the softer gelatinous nucleus pulposus as the synovial fluid inside a joint. As the spine ages, especially if the connecting ligaments are lax or if the vertebrae are out of optimal alignment, shearing and compressive stresses can affect the cartilaginous joint. The disc thins, and bone spurs may develop around the vertebral body or on the facet joints (Figures 3.28 and 3.29).

Not all osteophytes cause pain. Indeed, a large proportion of people over 50 years of age have radiographic evidence of bone spurs with no pain at all. Back and neck pain with spondylosis happens only when the growths put mechanical pressure on nerve roots, and this occurs only when the foramen is less than 30% of its normal size.[37]

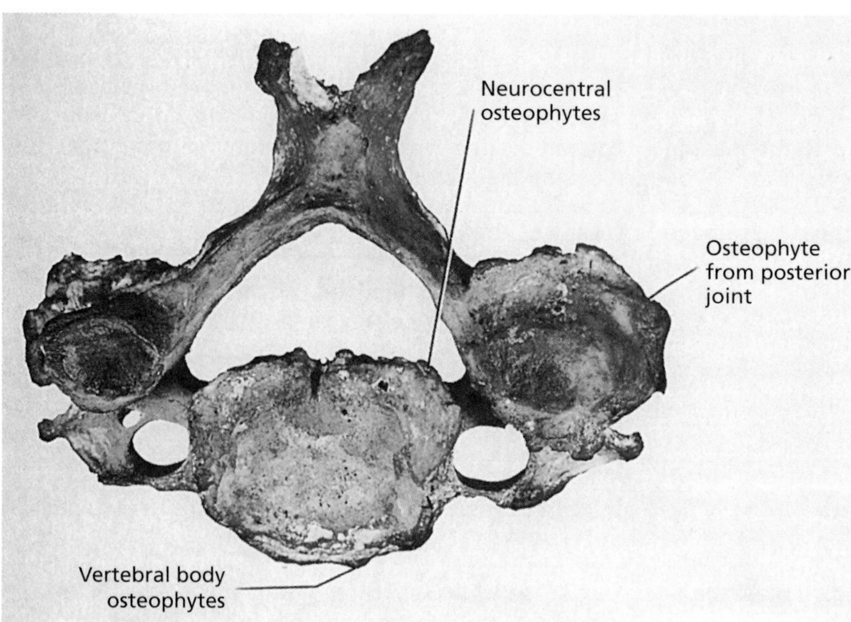

Figure 3.28. Osteophytic growths with spondylosis.

In addition to excessive calcium deposits on vertebrae, advanced age may contribute to the ossification of the long vertical ligaments that stabilize the spine. The anterior longitudinal ligament runs on the anterior aspect of the vertebral bodies. ***Diffuse idiopathic skeletal hyperostosis*** is a common condition involving calcium deposits along this structure. This may be a major contributor to the gradual painless loss of range of motion that is frequently reported with spondylosis. The posterior longitudinal ligament runs along the posterior aspect of the vertebral bodies (on the anterior side of the spinal canal). Ossification may occur here as well; this carries a higher risk of spinal cord pressure. Finally, the ***ligamentum flavum,*** which runs on the posterior aspect of the spinal canal, often thickens with age; this can contribute to stenosis too.

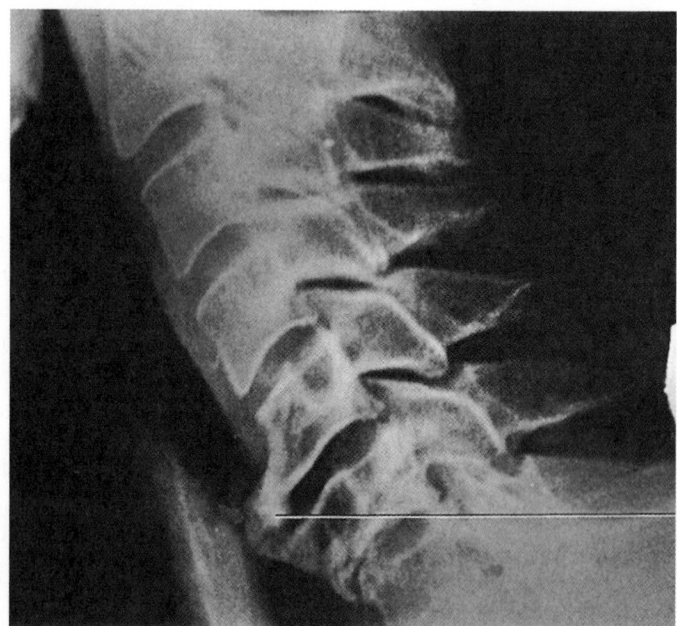

Figure 3.29. Fusion of vertebral bodies with spondylosis.

More typical presentations of osteoarthritis may occur at the facet joints between the vertebrae, at the sacroiliac joints, or at the costovertebral joints. In these areas one may see the typical osteoarthritis-related changes: cartilage damage, bony adaptation, and muscle splinting in response to pain.

Signs and Symptoms

Often spondylosis has no symptoms whatever. If the bony changes do *not* press on nerve roots but grow somewhere that impedes movement, the main symptom is slow, painless, but irreversible stiffening of the spine.

When the osteophytes *do* press on nerve roots, the symptoms include shooting pain, tingling, pins and needles, numbness, and muscle weakness only in muscles supplied by the affected nerve. If the pressure is on the spinal cord, symptoms are bilateral and may include loss of bladder or bowel control.

One distinguishing feature of nerve pressure from osteophytes is that the pain is absolutely consistent; if the bone spurs are in a place to create pain when a person is in a certain position or posture, that pain is predictable and tends to get worse over time instead of better.

Complications

Spondylosis is a slowly progressing condition that mostly affects middle-aged and elderly people. Usually it is not dangerous, but it can have some serious complications.

- *Spreading problems in the spine.* This is not a progressive disease that travels through the blood, but if two vertebrae become fused through bony remodeling, that puts much more stress on the joints above and below the fusion to provide mobility. Those joints can become unstable, develop arthritis, and undergo the same bony remodeling that created the first problem. Or the stress of hypermobility may cause disc problems. Disc disease can be both a predisposing factor and a complication of spondylosis.
- *Nerve pain.* This is the consequence of having osteophytes grow where they can put pressure on nerve roots in the foramina.
- *Secondary spasm.* This accompanies nerve pain. Muscle spasm may be confined to the paraspinals, where it exacerbates the problem by compressing the affected joints, or it may follow the path of referred pain. Muscles may also go into spasm to protect the spine from movement that would otherwise be excruciatingly painful.
- *Blood vessel pressure.* Osteophytes in the neck sometimes press on the vertebral arteries as they go up the transverse foramina. If the head is turned or extended in a certain position, the patient may feel dizzy or have headaches or double vision from impaired blood flow into the head.
- *Spinal cord pressure.* This is an extremely serious complication of spondylosis in the neck. In 5% to 10% of patients with spondylosis symptoms, osteophytes grow in a place to put pressure not on the nerve roots but in the spinal cord itself, a condition called ***cervical spondylitic myelopathy.*** This is felt as progressive weakening down the body, possible loss of bladder and bowel control, and even eventual paralysis. The surgery for this condition involves creating a larger foramen for the spinal cord to pass through, and permanently fusing the involved vertebrae.

Diagnosis

The characteristic thickening or hypertrophy of the vertebral bodies that accompanies spondylosis is easily identified by radiography, but MRI is considered more accurate for identifying sources of nerve pressure.

SIDEBAR 3.6: SPONDYLO-TONGUE TWISTERS

The terminology used in the discussion of arthritis and stenosis in the spine can be puzzling. Here is a brief look at some of the most confusing terms:

- *Spondylosis*. A general term for any degenerative condition of the vertebrae. This comes from the Greek root *spondylo-*, for *vertebra*.
- *Spondylolysis*. A specific defect in vertebrae, usually in the lumbar spine, that impairs the weight-bearing capacity of the bone. The word roots are *spondylo-* and *lysis*, or *loosening*.
- *Spondylolisthesis*. An anterior displacement of the body of a lumbar vertebra onto its inferior vertebra or onto the sacrum. This is a combination of *spondylo-* and *olisthesis*, Greek for a *slipping and falling*.

All three of these conditions can contribute to ***stenosis***, or a narrowing of the spinal canal.

Treatment

Treatment for spondylosis depends on which (if any) complications are present. Anti-inflammatories are the usual first recourse. Movement and exercise can limit progression once the damage has begun. Massage, acupuncture, and hydrotherapy are often recommended before more intrusive steps are tried.

If noninvasive measures are insufficient, local injections of steroids can provide temporary relief. A variety of surgeries can create more space for nerve roots or the spinal cord. These often involve spinal fusions, however, and they work best for younger patients who have not been having arthritic symptoms for a long time or in more than one joint.

Massage?

Massage for spondylosis is appropriate with caution. If bone spurs are irritating nerves, the surrounding muscles tend to splint them against painful movement. This splinting mechanism is important and must be respected by massage therapists. For this reason and because of the other serious complications of spondylosis, in this situation it is highly recommended to work with a primary caregiver who has a complete set of MRIs or radiographs.

MODALITY RECOMMENDATIONS FOR SPONDYLOSIS

MODALITY	RECOMMENDATION
Deep tissue massage	Contraindicated unless working with health care team.
Lymphatic drainage	Supportive.
Polarity	S: Indicated. R/D: Indicated while subacute, depending on client comfort.
PNF/MET/stretching	Supportive while subacute, within client tolerance.
Reflexology	Indicated; work spine and gland points.
Shiatsu	Indicated. Treat BL meridian; K, SI extensions on back. Treat GB, LV, SP, ST meridians systemically.
Swedish massage	Supportive while subacute, within client tolerance.
Trigger point therapy	Indicated while subacute.

See Chapter 1 for a brief description of each modality, including definitions of abbreviations.

Sprains

Definition: What Are They?

Sprains are tears to ligaments, the connective tissue strapping tape that links bone to bone throughout the body.

Etiology: What Happens?

Sprains, strains, and tendinopathies are all injuries to structures that are composed largely of connective tissue fibers arranged in linear patterns. They have a lot in common in the way of symptoms, healing mechanisms, and treatment protocols. Thus much of the information in this segment is applicable to all three conditions. Their differences are emphasized here, as are guidelines for how they may be seen in the same light.

Linear structures like muscles, tendons, and ligaments are injured when some of their fibers are ripped. The severity of the injury depends on what percentage of the fibers is affected. First-degree injuries involve just a few fibers; second-degree injuries are much worse, and third-degree injuries are ruptures: the entire structure has been ripped through and no longer attaches to the bone.

Repairing muscle, tendon, or ligament tears involves the laying down of new collagen fibers, *not* in alignment with the injured structure but whichever way the fibroblasts happen to deposit them. The perfect combination of movement, stretching, and weight-bearing stress in the maturation phase of recovery helps to reorient the fibers in alignment with the uninjured structure. If this happens in the best possible way, the new scar tissue actually becomes part of the muscle fascia, tendon, or ligament. But if a new injury is immobilized, the scar tissue becomes dense and contracted, pulling on all the uninjured fibers nearby and significantly hampering the weight-bearing capacity of the ligament (Figure 3.10).

Sprains in Brief

What are they?
Sprains are injured ligaments. Injuries can range from a few traumatized fibers to a complete rupture.

How are they recognized?
In the acute stage pain, redness, heat, swelling, and loss of joint function are evident. In the subacute stage these symptoms are less extreme, although perhaps not entirely absent. Passive stretching of the affected ligament is painful until all inflammation has subsided.

Is massage indicated or contraindicated?
Subacute sprains indicate massage. Bodywork can influence the healthy development of scar tissue and reduce the swelling and damage due to edematous ischemia. Therapists must take care to rule out bone fractures or other injuries that sprains may temporarily mask.

Distinguishing Features A few things distinguish sprains from strains and tendon injuries, which are discussed in other sections.

- *Sprains are injured ligaments, not muscles or tendons.* Ligaments are the connectors that hold the bones together. Structurally they are slightly different from tendons: the dense linear arrangement of collagen fibers affords little stretch and almost no rebound. If a ligament is stressed enough to become injured, it tends to tear before it stretches. If it does get stretched, it doesn't rebound to its original length, and it cannot stabilize the joint as well as it did before the injury. This ligament laxity is also seen with chronic injury-reinjury situations and is a contributor to the risk of osteoarthritis.
- *Sprains are more serious than strains and tendinosis.* Because tendons and muscles tend to be more elastic and less densely arranged than ligaments, they stretch before a ligament does. Furthermore, ligaments don't have the same rich blood supply as muscles, and they are denser than tendons. Consequently, they don't have the same access to circulation, which makes them slower to heal than muscles or tendons.
- *Sprains tend to swell.* With a few exceptions, acute sprains swell much more than muscle strains or tendinosis; this is one way to differentiate between injuries. Swelling is a protective measure that recruits the body's healing resources and limits movement, which prevents further injury. Ligaments are often contiguous with the joint capsules of the joints they cross over, so an injury to them may signal the joint to swell too. Ligaments that are *not* attached to joint capsules swell much less than those that are.

SIDEBAR 3.7: COMMON ORTHOPEDIC INJURIES

Injuries of muscles, tendons, and ligaments are among the most common complaints clients may carry, and they are among the most satisfying things massage therapists can work with. Cross-fiber friction, linear friction, proprioceptive neuromuscular facilitation, lymph drainage, and dozens of other modalities have been developed to help create a healing process that is efficient and long lasting.

The purpose of this text is to provide information about the appropriateness of massage in the context of many diseases and disorders but *not* to give specific recipes about exactly what modalities to use when and in what circumstances; that judgment must be made by the individual therapist, depending on his or her own skills and the needs of the client. For this reason, many orthopedic injuries are not specifically addressed in the body of the text, since they fit into the broader headings of strains, sprains, and tendinopathies.

Nonetheless, it is useful to list some of the most common orthopedic injuries and make some reference to where they may fit in the context of massage.

Soft tissue injuries can often be identified with carefully isolated resisted contractions or passive stretches, but injuries seldom happen in a vacuum; they often appear in combination with other damage. This is why it is important to accompany a massage therapist's informed opinion with a thorough diagnosis conducted by a medical professional.

Common Tendon Injuries

Rotator Cuff Injuries

Rotator cuff injuries can affect any combination of the rotator cuff muscles of the shoulder. One of the trickiest things about rotator cuff injuries is that they can refer pain down the arm or even into the wrist and hand. This can make it difficult to get a clear diagnosis. Rotator cuff injuries often respond well to friction and rehabilitative exercise.

Patellar Tendinitis

Patellar tendinitis is an injury to the quadriceps attachment somewhere around the patella or distally in the patellar tendon on the way to the tibia. Most cases are probably tendinosis rather than tendinitis, however. Several things make patellar tendon injuries difficult to pin down: The quadriceps are so strong that they often aren't painful with resisted contractions unless they are already fatigued; the patellar tendon is large and thick, and it can be difficult to isolate exactly where the lesion has developed; and this injury is frequently misdiagnosed as PFS, which can be problematic, as PFS implies damage *inside* the joint capsule, while this condition involves irritation *outside* the joint.

Patellar tendon injury often arises in conjunction with muscular imbalances and overuse. It responds well to massage, both at the site of injury and generally around the lower extremity as the injured person works to create better balance.

Epicondylitis

Epicondylitis refers to irritation of either the extensors or flexors of the forearm. Golfer's elbow refers to flexor problems, while tennis elbow refers to extensor injuries. These injuries respond very well to friction and carefully gauged exercise, but they *do not* improve if the massage is applied to the wrong area. The greatest challenge with both flexor and extensor injuries is to isolate the damaged structure and the exact site of injury.

Common Ligament Injuries

Ankle Sprains

Most ankle injuries involve rolling outward and stressing structures on the lateral side of the foot. The most commonly injured ligament in the body is the anterior talofibular ligament, which is almost always a part of lateral ankle sprains.

Ligaments are not contractile structures, so they are not isolated by muscle contractions and are not rehabilitated by exercise. Rather, friction, stretching, and gradually increasing weight-bearing stress are the interventions that work best for most ankle sprains.

If a ligament ruptures, it cannot stabilize its joint. Surgery may be necessary to reattach the ligament and restore its ability to function.

Cruciate Ligament Sprains or Ruptures

The anterior and posterior cruciate ligaments (ACL and PCL) inside the knee joint capsule are responsible for most of the anteroposterior stability of this massive weight-bearing joint. When they are injured, the whole joint becomes unstable and susceptible to further injury.

Cruciate ligament sprains break the pattern of most orthopedic injuries: they do not benefit from immediate mobilization, and they are not accessible for friction or other hands-on therapies. Instead, arthroscopic surgery is often necessary to repair the damage, followed by physical therapy to limit scar tissue and restore function. Massage can be useful in the postsurgical recovery period but has no access to an untreated cruciate ligament injury.

Common Joint Injuries

Meniscus Tears

The menisci are mobile pieces of cartilage that help track the femur on top of the tibia. Occasionally they crack, tear, fragment, or otherwise sustain damage. This situation requires arthroscopic surgery to remove loose bits of cartilage before joint surfaces become rough and arthritic. Because they are inside the joint capsule, massage therapists have no access to meniscus injuries. Massage can be a beneficial part of the postsurgical recovery period, however.

Acromioclavicular (AC) Joint

The joint where the clavicle meets the acromion of the scapula is a vulnerable spot because it is subject to bumps, falls, and other trauma. When the joint is inflamed, movement at the shoulder is limited and painful. AC joint problems often respond well to friction followed by ice to limit inflammation.

Frozen Shoulder (Adhesive Capsulitis)

Adhesive capsulitis affects the synovial joint capsule at the glenohumeral joint. It is often precipitated by some other inflammatory problem (bursitis or tendinitis). The joint capsule gradually adheres to the anterior head of the humerus, causing pain, inflammation, and loss of range of motion. The onset is usually gradual, and without intervention it often spontaneously resolves, although it may leave a permanent loss of range of motion at the joint. Physical therapy to minimize and reverse the adhesive process is often recommended for persons with frozen shoulder; massage can fit into this context as well.

Signs and Symptoms

Acute stage Acute sprains show the usual signs of inflammation: pain, heat, redness, and swelling, with the bonus of loss of function because the rapid swelling splints the unstable joint and makes it extremely painful to move. Inflamed ligaments are especially painful with passive stretches of the structure.

Sprains can happen at almost any synovial joint, but the anterior talofibular ligament of the ankle is the most commonly sprained ligament in the body. Ligaments overlying the sacroiliac joint are also very commonly injured, as are various ligaments around the knees and fingers.

Subacute stage In the subacute stage, signs of inflammation may still be present, but the joint has begun to regain some function. The physiological processes are no longer geared toward blood clotting and damage control; they have shifted toward clearing out debris and rebuilding torn fibers. The amount of time that passes between acute and subacute stages varies with the severity of the injury, but the 24- to 48-hour rule is usually dependable. However, some injuries waver back and forth between acute and subacute, especially in response to certain kinds of activity or massage.

Complications

Injured ligaments occasionally lead to more serious problems. Sprains are such a common injury that it is important for massage therapists to be familiar with all their repercussions.

- *Masking symptoms.* An acute sprain may mask the symptoms of a bone fracture, especially in the foot. It is important to have clients undergo radiography to rule out fracture before beginning to work with a sprained ankle.
- *Repeated injury.* Internal scar tissue (scar tissue that accumulates within a specific structure) that never remodels can interfere with the function of undamaged fibers. It can weaken the integrity of the whole structure, which along with the increase in ligament laxity, makes repeated injury a very common complication of sprains. This pattern is present with strains and tendinitis too.
- *Ligament laxity.* A ligament that has been injured, in addition to having torn some fibers, is often looser than uninjured ligaments. This is because it has been asked to stretch farther than it could go, and ligaments have almost no rebound capability. When a joint becomes unstable because of loose, lax ligaments, excessive movement of the bones becomes possible. The bones may rock around and knock together, causing osteoarthritis.

Treatment

Once upon a time the recommendations for sprains included hot soaks and total immobilization. Clearly, both of these strategies were counterproductive: heat increases edema and the accumulation of scar tissue, while immobilization prevents the new fibers from aligning with the rest of the structure.

These days RICE therapy (rest, ice, compression, elevation) is considered the norm, with an emphasis on moving the joint within range of pain tolerance absolutely as soon as possible. The potential benefits are clear: ice keeps edema at bay, limiting further tissue damage from ischemia. Compression does the same. Elevation also encourages lymph flow *out* of an already impacted area.

Orthopedic specialists sometimes recommend this mnemonic for sprain management: PRICEMMM. This stands for protection (with taping or a brace), rest, ice, compression, elevation, medication (analgesics for pain management), mobility (begin to move the structure as tolerated as soon as possible), and modalities (including ultrasound, exercise, and proprioceptive training).[38] Clearly, carefully applied massage has a place here too.

Massage?

Massage is *great* for sprains. It can reduce adhesions and influence the direction of new collagen fibers. It can address edema and toxic accumulations from secondary muscle spasm. Massage also helps with stiffness from the temporary loss of joint function. But most massage must be done *after* the acute stage. Modalities in lymph drainage for dealing with acute sprains are effective, but it's a highly technical field and not for casual experimentation.

Modality Recommendations for Sprains

MODALITY	RECOMMENDATION
Deep tissue massage	Contraindicated while acute. Indicated when subacute: use passive ROM to influence fiber repair; stay within client tolerance.
Lymphatic drainage	Indicated in all stages, especially acute.
Polarity	S: Indicated. R/D: Locally contraindicated when acute; otherwise indicated.
PNF/MET/stretching	Locally contraindicated while acute; indicated when subacute.
Reflexology	Locally contraindicated; otherwise supportive.
Shiatsu	Indicated. When acute and inflamed use TH, SP, K systemically, with light pressure at local site. Add more pressure in subacute stages.
Swedish massage	Locally contraindicated when acute; proximal flushing can decrease swelling. Supportive when subacute.
Trigger point therapy	Locally contraindicated while acute; indicated when subacute.

See Chapter 1 for a brief description of each modality, including definitions of abbreviations.

Temporomandibular Joint Disorders

Definition: What Are They?

The term *temporomandibular joint disorders* can mean a multitude of problems in and around the jaw. This collection of signs and symptoms is usually associated with ***malocclusion*** (a dysfunctional bite), ***bruxism*** (teeth grinding), and loose ligaments surrounding the jaw that allow excessive movement between the bones, damage to the internal cartilage, and possible dislocation of the joint. TMJ disorders are also referred to as *TMD*, for **t**emporo**m**andibular joint **d**isorders.

Demographics: Who Gets It?

It is difficult to pin down exact numbers of people who live with jaw pain. Some estimates suggest that up to 10 million people in the U.S. population have some degree of TMJ disorders, but only a small fraction may ever seek help. Of those who do, women outnumber men significantly.

Etiology: What Happens?

When chronic misalignment, trauma, or muscle tension affects the highly specialized joints at the jaw, a person may find it difficult to open or close the mouth without pain. Chewing and swallowing become problematic, and pain in the jaw can reverberate systemically throughout the body. The construction of the jaw is delicate, and it is easy for structures to become injured or improperly balanced.

The TMJ is like no other in the body. Far from being a simple hinge joint, the TMJ moves up, down, forward, back, and side to side. The jaw is unusually mobile, as the joint actually stretches with the position of the mouth (Figure 3.30). A fibrocartilage disc cushions the two bones (the temporal bone and the condyle of the mandible) but this disc is sometimes pulled awry or injured, which can lead to problems in the joint.

Furthermore, the muscles that work together to control chewing and jaw movement during speech are particularly prone to developing trigger points, which can refer pain into the jaw, the face, over the head, and into the neck. The tension in the muscles of mastication (the masseter, the medial and lateral pterygoids, and the temporalis, among others) can be both a symptom and trigger of TMJ disorders.

Temporomandibular Joint Disorders in Brief

Pronunciation: tem-por-o-man-DIB-u-lar joint dis-OR-durz

What are they?
Temporomandibular joint (TMJ) disorders are any problem that causes pain and loss of function at the TMJ.

How are they recognized?
Symptoms of TMJ disorders include pain in the head, neck, shoulder, ear, and/or mouth; clicking or locking in the jaw; and loss of range of motion of the jaw.

Is massage indicated or contraindicated?
Massage can be useful for TMJ problems if intervention is begun before bony deformation begins. However, this condition can be difficult to diagnose, so it's important to be working with other medical professionals in these situations.

See Video Clip 1 on the Student Resource CD.

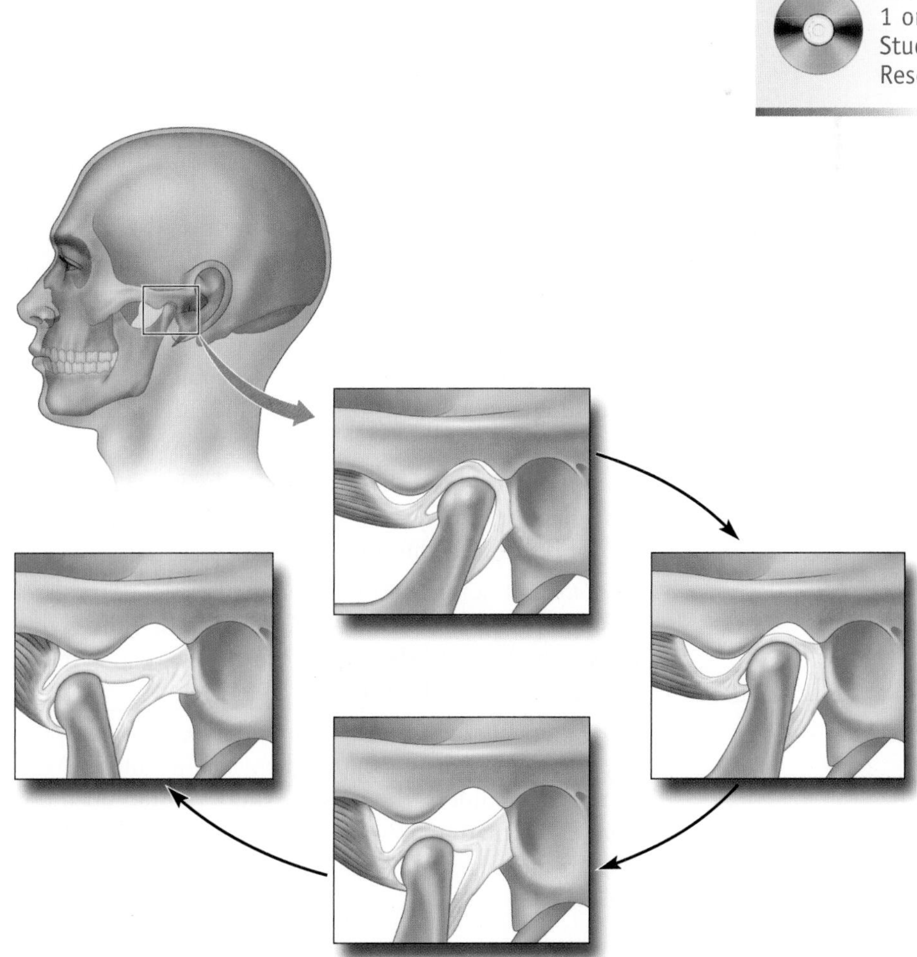

Figure 3.30. The temporomandibular joint allows great mobility as the jaw protracts.

Causes

TMJ disorders can be initiated by trauma, such as a fall or motor vehicle accident; in these cases the condition is sometimes called "jawlash." They can also arise spontaneously, often as a result of unusual emotional stress that is manifested as chronic jaw clenching.

TMJ problems are often circular. That is, the factors that cause TMJ disorders can also be the symptoms. In this way, tight muscles can lead to pain and tissue damage, which can lead to arthritis at the jaw, which reinforces muscle tightening. Rheumatoid arthritis occasionally strikes here, but osteoarthritis is a far more frequent contributor to TMJ problems. Other factors include misalignment of the bite and congenital malformations of the bones.

The fact that most of the people diagnosed with TMJ disorders are women of child-bearing years has led to the finding that women have estrogen receptors in the jaw and men do not. This may indicate that TMJ disorders are hormone-related problems. Alternatively, a high overlap between TMJD patients and people with hypermobile ligaments and mitral valve prolapse raises the question of a disorder of connective tissue quality.[39] Other conditions commonly seen with TMJD include FMS, chronic MPS, and irritable bowel syndrome.

Signs and Symptoms

The signs and symptoms of TMJ disorders are as follows:

- *Jaw, neck, and shoulder pain.* This can be from actual deterioration of bony structures inside the capsule (arthritis), or it can be local and referred pain generated by tight, trigger point–laden muscles.
- *Limited range of motion.* Deformation or displacement of the cartilage inside the joint can make it difficult or impossible to open the mouth all the way.
- *Popping in the jaw.* This is usually attributed to having the disc or bone out of alignment, which interferes in jaw opening. A similar clicking sensation is sometimes felt by people with knee problems involving the discs there.
- *Locking of the joint.* Again, this is a result of having the fibrocartilage disc interfere with normal joint movement.
- *Grinding teeth (bruxism).* Like many issues with this disorder, this symptom is also a possible cause of the problem. Chronically shortened jaw elevators contribute to clenching and grinding of teeth, especially during sleep, when the joint should be as relaxed as possible.
- *Ear pain.* Because of the location of the joint, pressure may be exerted directly on the eustachian tubes. Symptoms in this case include a feeling of stuffiness in the ears, and loss of hearing or tinnitus.
- *Headaches.* The pressure exerted at the second molar when the teeth are clenched is 2,000 lb per square inch. It is no surprise that the cranial bones are affected if this happens all night long. Headaches can also be related to trigger points of muscles in spasm and to cervical subluxation.
- *Chronic misalignment of cervical vertebrae.* This is probably a result of the muscular hypertonicity that is generated by this problem. As pain refers from the jaw to the neck and shoulders, the muscles there tighten up and pull asymmetrically on the neck bones. No matter how often the neck is adjusted or how brilliantly the neck muscles are massaged, this pain-spasm cycle will not abate until the jaw situation is addressed.

Diagnosis

Many conditions present signs and symptoms similar to TMJ disorder, but they don't respond at all to the most advanced kinds of interventions. Therefore, it is important to differentiate between true TMJ disorder, which involves bony or cartilaginous deformation inside the joint capsule, and the other diseases and conditions that can cause head, neck, and shoulder pain.

First among these diagnostic differentials is MPS. More than any other condition, this one is both a precursor and a complication of TMJ disorder. Jaw surgery won't resolve trigger points, but resolving trigger points could eliminate the need for future jaw surgery. However, true TMJ disorder can be (and usually is) present simultaneously with MPS. Other conditions that cause head, neck and shoulder pain include:

- *Sprain* of the ligament that attaches the stylomandibular joint to the base of the skull can cause pain in the jaw and head. This is also called *Ernest syndrome.*
- *Trigeminal neuralgia*, also called *tic douloureux*, is an extremely painful result of damage to the trigeminal nerve.
- *Occipital neuralgia* is damage to the greater or lesser occipital nerves.
- *Osteomyelitis* is a complication of dental surgery in which tissue death occurs at the site of extracted teeth, which causes pain in the face.

Some diagnostic tools that identify TMJ disorder include MRI, which can show whether or not the internal cartilage is chipped or subluxated; radiography of the jaw and head; and electromyography, which shows muscle function around the joint. A trained clinician can also feel a subluxation when fingers are inserted in the ear of the patient during chewing.

Treatment

Treatment for TMJ disorder is divided into surgical and nonsurgical options. In most cases nonsurgical options are tried first. These include applying heat or cold to painful areas, physical therapy, ultrasound and massage for jaw muscles, anti-inflammatories, and local anesthetics. Special splints that reduce bone-to-bone pressure may be prescribed, although some specialists feel that ill-fitting splints make matters worse rather than better. Proliferant injections to tighten the ligaments that surround the jaw may also be effective. If these noninvasive techniques are successful, the TMJ disorder may be averted before permanent bony distortion or cartilage damage inside the joint occurs.

In some situations the onset of symptoms may be very fast, for instance with a car wreck or a fall. If such a patient has been severely debilitated, or if noninvasive techniques have been unsuccessful and other problems have been ruled out, surgery may be considered. Several surgeries have been developed. These range from an outpatient procedure in which scar tissue and adhesions are dissolved with injections into the joint, to arthroscopic surgery to manipulate the cartilage, to full prosthetic joint replacement.

Massage?

Massage can be especially useful in the early teeth-clenching stages of TMJ problems, not only by addressing the muscles, but also by helping to increase the client's awareness of this habit. It's surprising how often people grit their teeth without realizing it; the proprioceptors can adapt to assume that this is normal, even if it's not optimal. And of course, in addition to helping reduce excessive muscle tone, massage can also deal with some of the referred pain patterns that can be such a problem with this condition.

Modality Recommendations for Temporomandibular Joint Dysfunction	
MODALITY	RECOMMENDATION
Deep tissue massage	Indicated to release jaw flexors, increase client awareness. Use active movement as release is performed.
Lymphatic drainage	Supportive after standard massage of face.
Polarity	S: Indicated. R/D: Indicated for gentle work when subacute.
PNF/MET/stretching	Indicated in all stages.
Reflexology	Indicated; work side of neck, jaw, ear, neck, throat, shoulder, lymph drain plug, upper glandular system, brain, top of head points.
Shiatsu	Indicated. Treat GB, TH, SI, ST, LI in head, face, neck.
Swedish massage	Avoid inflamed regions; work for proprioceptive release.
Trigger point therapy	Indicated while subacute.

See Chapter 1 for a brief description of each modality, including definitions of abbreviations.

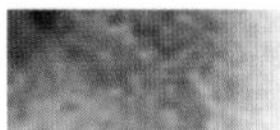

Genetic Musculoskeletal Disorders

Ehlers-Danlos Syndrome

Definition: What Is It?

Ehlers-Danlos syndrome (EDS) is a group of genetic disorders that lead to problems in the production of various types of connective tissue proteins. The first references to this disorder date to the fourth century B.C., but it wasn't fully explored and delineated until the early part of the twentieth century, when two doctors (Ehlers from Denmark and Danlos from France) combined their observations to outline the specifics of these disorders.

Demographics: Who Gets It?

EDS is relatively rare. It is estimated to affect 1 or 2 people in 10,000. About 50,000 Americans may have this disorder, but for many people it is mild and may not be easily recognized. EDS affects men and women equally and is distributed evenly throughout racial groups.[40]

Etiology: What Happens?

EDS is the result of genetic mutations that affect the production of collagen, elastin, and some other parts of the extracellular matrix that forms the bulk of connective tissues. The net result for most people with this disorder is hypermobility of the joints, along with chronic joint pain, delicate skin, and poor wound healing.

EDS is an inherited disorder, but that inheritance may be through autosomal dominant, autosomal recessive, or X-linked chromosomes. The most common forms of EDS are transmitted through autosomal dominant genes, which means that one parent must have the condition or be a carrier to have a 50% chance of passing the condition to a child. The rarer forms of the disease are autosomal recessive, which means both parents must carry the mutation and both must pass the gene on to the affected child. For more information on inherited disorders, see Sidebar 3.9.

Ehlers-Danlos Syndrome in Brief

Pronunciation: A-lurz don-LOS SIN-drome

What is it?

Ehlers-Danlos syndrome (EDS) is a collection of genetic disorders that lead to problems with connective tissues. It affects the musculoskeletal, cardiovascular, and integumentary systems.

How is it recognized?

Most people with EDS have hypermobile joints. They may also have delicate skin that is abnormally stretchy. They are prone to forming extensive scars wherever the skin has been injured. Some EDS patients also have delicate blood vessels and other tissues that are vulnerable to damage or rupture. Very rare forms of this disorder can also cause extreme postural deviations and eye problems.

Is massage indicated or contraindicated?

Massage is fine for people with EDS as long as the joints are not stretched beyond a normal range of motion and the cardiovascular system is healthy.

Signs and Symptoms

The signs and symptoms of EDS are mainly related to the type of genetic mutation that is present. Most symptoms are related to extremely delicate skin, hypermobile joints, and chronic joint pain. Common signs include easy bruising, poor wound healing, frequent joint dislocations, and eye problems, including myopia, detached retina, and damage to the connective tissue that maintains the globular shape of the eyeball. The risk of mitral valve prolapse is higher for EDS patients than for the rest of the population. Rarer signs of EDS include extreme postural deviations and slack, baggy skin.

Several types of EDS have been identified and classified according to different criteria, leading to a lot of confusion in how these conditions have been discussed. Recently the labeling of EDS types by number (I–XI) has been replaced by descriptive titles:

- *Classic EDS* involves stretchy, delicate skin that is fragile and prone to bruising. Wounds heal slowly and leave excessive scar tissue. Joints are loose and vulnerable to injury.
- *Hypermobility EDS* has hypermobility as its primary feature. Patients are prone to multiple dislocations, joint pain, and early-onset osteoarthritis.
- *Vascular EDS* has the most serious repercussions; it affects the connective tissues in the blood vessels and other tubes. People with vascular EDS have a life expectancy of 50 years, and their midsized blood vessels and gastrointestinal tract are vulnerable to damage or even rupture.
- *Kyphoscoliosis EDS* is extremely rare. It leads to very excessive scoliosis with hyperkyphosis, and it can affect the strength of the sclera of the eyes.
- *Arthrochalasia EDS* is a rare type involving joints (especially hips) that dislocate extremely easily.
- *Dermatosparaxis EDS* is a rare type involving loose, sagging skin (even in young children) and ligament laxity.

Diagnosis

EDS can be difficult to identify if symptoms are not extreme. Genetic testing is not conclusive for several varieties, so doctors rely on family history along with signs and symptoms to make a diagnosis.

Because EDS has varying genetic expression (in other words, it occurs in varying levels of severity), people with mild EDS may never be identified or diagnosed. This becomes a problem for their children, who may inherit this disorder and have it in a more extreme form. Genetic counseling is recommended when people are diagnosed with EDS so they can make informed decisions about childbearing.

Treatment

Because no treatment can reverse a genetic mutation, EDS is treated according to symptoms or related problems. People with hypermobile joints are taught how to preserve joint function and are discouraged from stretching joints beyond a healthy range of motion. Skin wounds are typically treated with bandages or wound glue rather than sutures because the skin is so delicate. Any surgery or dental work is conducted with extreme care because of poor wound healing and because people with a risk of mitral valve prolapse are also at risk for endocardial bacterial infections.

Pregnancies of women with EDS tend to be high risk because they are more than usually vulnerable to uterine tearing, prolapse, and early rupture of the membranes, leading to premature birth.

High doses of vitamin C, even in patients whose vitamin C levels are normal, may contribute to improved strength of connective tissues. This avenue is being pursued by some researchers, but no specific protocols have been developed.[40]

Massage?

Massage is appropriate for people with EDS as long as the cardiovascular system is healthy and hypermobility of the joints is respected. Massage therapists should be aware that these clients have extremely delicate skin and may be prone to bruising, so pressure must be adjusted accordingly.

Most people with EDS have normal life spans, and although they are counseled to avoid contact sports or activities that stretch their joints, other types of physical activity are safe. This indicates that most types of massage are likewise healthy and appropriate.

Modality Recommendations for Ehlers-Danlos Syndrome

MODALITY	RECOMMENDATION
Deep tissue massage	Contraindicated due to hypermobility in joints.
Lymphatic drainage	Indicated with gentle work to reduce joint swelling.
Polarity	S: Indicated. R/D: Supportive, depending on client's comfort and fragility.
PNF/MET/stretching	Contraindicated due to hypermobility in joints and general fragility.
Reflexology	Contraindicated because of general fragility.
Shiatsu	Supportive, especially with systemic treatment of LV, K. Avoid ROM.
Swedish massage	Supportive, within client's limits; avoid tapotement, friction, deep effleurage, pétrissage.
Trigger point therapy	Supportive, with caution for client fragility.

See Chapter 1 for a brief description of each modality, including definitions of abbreviations.

Marfan Syndrome

Definition: What Is It?

Marfan syndrome is the result of a genetic mutation that leads to the production of dysfunctional ***fibrillin***, a key connective tissue fiber. This is an autosomal defect, which means it is not gender specific, and each child of a parent with Marfan syndrome has a 50-50 chance of having it.

Demographics: Who Gets It?

Marfan syndrome affects about 1 in 5000 to 10,000 people. Some 200,000 people have Marfan syndrome of a related connective tissue disorder.[40] While it is usually passed from parent to child, about 25% of cases are spontaneous mutations.

Etiology: What Happens?

Marfan syndrome is a result of the production of faulty protein fibers with the consequence that certain connective tissues throughout the body may be weak or otherwise dysfunctional. The musculoskeletal system, the meninges, the heart and aorta, and the eyes are most at risk for problems related to Marfan syndrome.

Marfan Syndrome in Brief

What is it?
Marfan syndrome is a genetic defect leading to problems in the construction of fibrillin, a connective tissue fiber. Consequently all connective tissues are affected, with the most serious problems occurring in the skeleton, cardiovascular system, and eyes.

How is it recognized?
Marfan syndrome patients tend to be taller than average, with very long fingers. Joints tend to be hypermobile. Patients are prone to postural deviations and problems with the shape of the thorax. Their heart valves and aorta may be weak. Many Marfan syndrome patients are myopic, and up to half have a detached retina or dislocated lens in the eye.

Is massage indicated or contraindicated?
Marfan syndrome patients must adjust their daily activities to accommodate for fragility in their connective tissues. Massage must likewise be adjusted to meet the reduced capacity to adjust to changes in their environment.

Signs and Symptoms

Marfan syndrome is a multisystem disorder, but it manifests most often as problems with the musculoskeletal system, heart and aorta, eyes, and nervous system. Marfan symptoms appear on a continuum of severity; some people have it in a mild form, while others have a more severe form of the disease.

- *Musculoskeletal system anomalies.* People with Marfan syndrome frequently have unusually long fingers and toes (Figure 3.31) and disproportionately long arms and legs. One sign of this disorder is the wrist test: persons with Marfan syndrome can overlap the thumb and fifth digit (little finger) of one hand while encircling the opposite wrist. Ligament laxity and joint hypermobility are also common in this population. Other skeletal signs include chest deformities: a flat chest with a protruding sternum (*pectus carinatum*) or a sunken sternum (*pectus excavatum*) is common. This anomaly can contribute to serious lung problems and may have to be surgically corrected. Early onset and rapidly progressive postural deviations (especially scoliosis and hyperkyphosis) are other indicators of this disorder.
- *Cardiovascular system anomalies.* The aortic and mitral valves are particularly vulnerable to problems with connective tissue stability. Prolapsed valves lead to regurgitation of blood and an irregular heartbeat. Furthermore, people with Marfan syndrome develop an enlarged aorta, especially at the ascending section. A ruptured aneurysm or aortic dissection is a common cause of death for this population if the disorder is not treated.
- *Eye disorders.* ***Myopia*** (nearsightedness) is very common with Marfan syndrome. Up to 50% of

SIDEBAR 3.8: MARFAN SYNDROME: HISTORY OF A GENETIC DISORDER

Antoine Bernard Marfan was a pioneering specialist in pediatric medicine in Paris at the end of the nineteenth century. At a meeting in 1896 he presented a case of a 5-year-old girl who was abnormally tall and whose fingers, arms, and legs were disproportionately long. Later studies of this patient revealed other anomalies that were eventually classified and named after Marfan.

As the ability to recognize specific genetic defects developed, Marfan syndrome continued to generate a lot of interest. In 1991, the specific chromosome, gene, and component of connective tissue affected by this mutation were finally identified. Future studies of fibrillin and its role in the creation of healthy connective tissue may reveal new treatment options for people affected by Marfan syndrome.

SIDEBAR 3.9: WHAT'S IN YOUR GENES?

Genes are part of the building blocks of human cells. They are arranged along pairs of chromosomes, and each parent contributes one side of the pair. Some diseases are caused by anomalies in genetic structure. While these anomalies can be inherited from one or both parents, they can also occur with no family history as spontaneous mutations. Breakthroughs in the study of molecular genetics have revealed the specific anomalies responsible for various forms of muscular dystrophy, as well as other inherited disorders such as sickle cell disease, Marfan syndrome, hemophilia, and osteogenesis imperfecta.

Inherited diseases have three variations: they can be autosomal dominant, autosomal recessive, or X-linked disorders.

- **Autosomal dominant** inheritance means that one parent has a defective gene and the other does not. Each child has a 50% chance of inheriting the defective but dominant gene, which causes the disease. Males and females are at equal risk for autosomal dominant inheritance.
- **Autosomal recessive** inheritance means that each parent carries one defective gene, but it produces no symptoms. Each child has a 25% chance of inheriting both defective genes and developing the associated disease. Alternatively, each child has a 50% chance of inheriting only one gene and becoming a carrier for the next generation.
- **X-linked** inheritance means that a woman carries a defective gene on one X chromosome. Each of her sons has a 50% chance of inheriting the faulty gene from her. Each of her daughters has a 50% chance of carrying the faulty gene to her sons. It is rare for females to be severely affected by X-linked diseases. Women who carry these genetic defects are at increased risk for developing some but not all of the characteristics of the genetic disease. Men who have X-linked mutations may pass the genes onto their daughters, who may become carriers, but no sons are directly affected.

patients have a dislocated lens. A high risk of detached retina, a medical emergency that can lead to blindness, is also present.

- *Nervous system anomalies.* People with Marfan syndrome are vulnerable to ***dural ectasia,*** in which the dura mater stretches and weakens as a person ages. It can erode the vertebrae, especially in the lumbosacral area, leading to pain in the pelvis and down the legs.
- *Other symptoms.* People with Marfan syndrome tend to develop stretch marks on the skin with little or no provocation. Connective tissue weakness also puts them at risk for hernias, flat feet, ***spondylolisthesis,*** and hammertoes.

Diagnosis

At present no easily accessible blood or genetic test is available to identify Marfan syndrome, so it is usually diagnosed through clinical examination, family history, and careful observation.

Many of the indicators of Marfan syndrome don't become obvious until adulthood, so this condition is difficult to identify in children. When symptoms are present in children, they tend to be severe.

Treatment

Marfan syndrome can be treated only by symptoms because no therapy can reverse the action of mutated genes. Beta-blockers are frequently prescribed to reduce the load on the aorta. Other blood pressure medications show promise in preventing rather than slowing damage to the aorta; these may significantly extend life expectancy for people with Marfan syndrome. ***Prophylactic antibiotics*** are recommended when even distant procedures are performed, because heart valves are highly susceptible to infection.

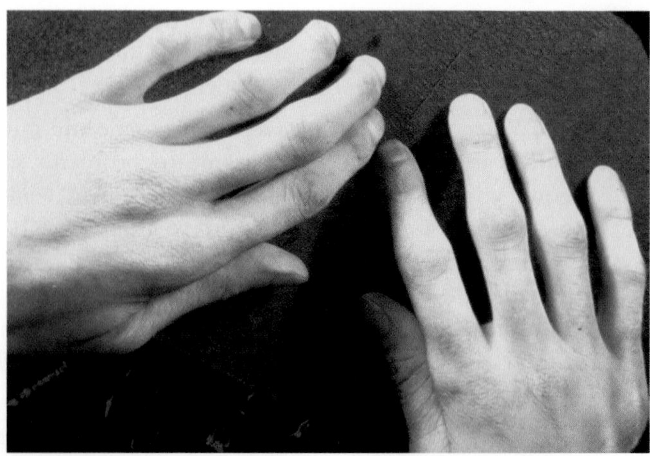

Figure 3.31. Marfan syndrome: abnormally long fingers.

Surgical interventions are not always necessary, but when the curve of scoliosis or the shape of the thorax interferes with normal breathing, this may be corrected. Similarly, if early-stage aneurysm or mitral valve prolapse is identified, these situations can be surgically addressed.

Massage?

Marfan syndrome weakens connective tissue and interferes with some activities of daily living. Patients are advised not to engage in contact sports or activities that put undue stress on the heart and aorta. With these cautions in mind, careful massage that respects the fragility of connective tissues and the cardiovascular system may be appropriate for clients with Marfan syndrome. This is a good situation in which to work as part of a well-informed health care team.

Modality Recommendations for Marfan Syndrome

MODALITY	RECOMMENDATION
Deep tissue massage	Contraindicated unless working with health care team.
Lymphatic drainage	Supportive.
Polarity	S: Indicated. R/D: Gentle work is supportive, depending on client comfort.
PNF/MET/stretching	Supportive.
Reflexology	Indicated.
Shiatsu	Supportive.
Swedish massage	Supportive, within client's limits; avoid tapotement, friction, deep effleurage, pétrissage.
Trigger point therapy	Supportive, within tolerance of the client.

See Chapter 1 for a brief description of each modality, including definitions of abbreviations.

Muscular Dystrophy

Definition: What Is It?

Muscular dystrophy is a group of several closely related diseases characterized by genetic anomalies. These mutated genes lead to the degeneration and wasting away of muscle tissue. It usually begins in skeletal muscles of the extremities but ultimately can affect the breathing muscles and the heart.

Demographics: Who Gets It?

The two most common varieties of muscular dystrophy are X-linked inherited diseases. This means the affected gene is carried by the mother but passed on only to her sons. About 400 to 600 boys are born with these types of muscular dystrophy each year.[41] Other types of muscular dystrophy are autosomal dominant or recessive; they may affect females as often as males.

Muscular Dystrophy in Brief

Pronunciation: MUS-kyu-lar DIS-tro-fe

What is it?

Muscular dystrophy is a group of related inherited disorders characterized by degeneration and wasting of muscle tissue.

How is it recognized?

Different varieties of muscular dystrophy destroy different areas of skeletal muscles. The age of onset, initial symptoms, and long-term prognosis depend on what kind of genetic problem is present.

Is massage indicated or contraindicated?

In early muscular dystrophy, some muscles waste away and their antagonists become tight. Physical therapy is often used to prevent or delay contractures as long as possible; massage can fit in this context as well, as long as the massage therapist is working as part of a health care team.

Etiology: What Happens?

Normal muscles convert fat or glycogen into fuel to do their work of pulling bony attachments together. They do this with the assistance of a special protein, **dystrophin**. Dystrophin is produced by specific genes close to the periphery of muscle cells, just under the sarcolemma. The most common versions of muscular dystrophy involve a genetic mutation that either prevents the production of dystrophin altogether or allows its production in only subnormal levels. Other forms of muscular dystrophy involve inadequate production of other vital proteins.

In the absence of dystrophin or other key chemicals to help create energy, muscle cells atrophy and die, to be replaced by fat and connective tissue. Antagonists to affected muscles have no resistance, and eventually their connective tissue shrinks, pulling bony attachments closer together in a permanent contracture.

Several varieties of muscular dystrophy have been identified, but two are more common than others, and one specifically affects adults; these are described in some detail. Other types of muscular dystrophy are much rarer, and are listed just for identification.

- *Duchenne muscular dystrophy* is the most common and most severe variety of the disease. It affects 1 in 3500 boy babies. The genetic anomaly with this condition prevents the production of any dystrophin at all.
- *Becker muscular dystrophy* is less common, affecting approximately 1 in 30,000 boys. It is also less severe, because while the production of dystrophin is lower than normal, some of this important protein is available to help muscles do their work.
- *Myotonic muscular dystrophy* is the most common form of adult-onset muscular dystrophy. Its primary symptom is ***myotonia:*** stiffness or spasm following muscular contraction. This is a progressive disorder that affects many systems. It can cause cataracts, gastrointestinal dysfunction, and heart problems.
- *Other varieties* of muscular dystrophy include the following: *Congenital muscular dystrophy* includes several rare varieties that are diagnosed at birth or in early infancy. *Facioscapulohumeral dystrophy* is a variety that primarily affects the muscles of the face, shoulder, and upper arm. *Limb girdle dystrophy* begins in the shoulders, upper arms, and pelvic area. *Emery-Dreifuss muscular dystrophy* shows contractures of the Achilles tendon, elbow, and spine. *Oculopharyngeal muscular dystrophy* affects the eyes and pharynx muscles first.

Signs and Symptoms

Signs and symptoms of muscular dystrophy vary according to type, but the two most common varieties, Duchenne and Becker, are very similar in presentation. A toddler might begin to have difficulty walking or climbing stairs. He may complain of leg pain. He develops a waddling gait with an accentuated lumbar curve to compensate for the weakness in his legs. Eventually he may not put his whole foot down at all but walk on tiptoes. His calves may seem to become disproportionately large in a condition called ***pseudohypertrophy;*** in actuality the muscle mass is being replaced with fat and connective tissue.

This condition can progress to affect the spine, joints, the heart and the lungs. Most muscular dystrophy patients die at a young age of cardiac or respiratory failure.

Duchenne muscular dystrophy is usually diagnosed between 3 and 5 years of age, and an affected child will probably be in a wheelchair by his twelfth birthday. Its progression is fairly dependable, and most patients don't live into their middle 20s.

Becker muscular dystrophy has a similar progression, but it is usually diagnosed later and has a less severe impact. The outlook may be a great deal brighter, depending on how much dystrophin individual patients may produce.

Muscular dystrophy is occasionally but not always accompanied by mental retardation. Other conditions that accompany these diseases include contractures and postural deviations that develop as the skeletal muscles tighten and pull on the spine and rib cage.

Diagnosis

The ability to identify various kinds of muscular dystrophy has taken some giant steps forward in the past two decades. It was just in 1987 that the protein dystrophin was isolated and named. Further discoveries in molecular genetics have made it possible to categorize the different types of muscular dystrophy much more accurately than ever before.

A child who shows signs of muscular problems will probably be given a blood test to look for signs of ***creatine kinase,*** an enzyme produced by damaged muscles. This may be followed by tests to rule out neurological problems. Finally a tissue biopsy may be taken to look for signs of decreased or missing dystrophin.

Treatment

If a diagnosis of some variety of muscular dystrophy is made, the family may be encouraged to meet with a genetic counselor to discuss the implications for future children. However, no treatment to reverse or cure muscular dystrophy exists. Some interventions have been developed to prolong the use of muscles and limbs. For instance, massage and physical therapy may be used to minimize the progression of contractures. Surgery is sometimes recommended to release tight tendons or to straighten a distorted spine. Prednisone is a steroidal anti-inflammatory that can preserve function temporarily, but the side effects of long-term use are very serious.

Outside of these interventions, a child with muscular dystrophy is aided to be as comfortable and as functional as possible. This usually means learning to use leg braces, a standing walker, and ultimately a wheelchair.

Massage?

This is a disorder of muscle function, but sensation is intact. This makes it a relatively safe condition for massage as long as the circulatory system is strong and healthy. Massage can be used along with physical therapy to stretch muscles and slow the progression of contractures, but it is recommended that massage therapists work as an integrated part of a health care team if they have an opportunity to work with a client who has muscular dystrophy.

Modality Recommendations for Muscular Dystrophy

Modality	Recommendation
Deep tissue massage	Contraindicated unless working with health care team.
Lymphatic drainage	Supportive.
Polarity	S: Indicated. R/D: Indicated, depending on client limitations and comfort.
PNF/MET/stretching	Indicated when symptoms are not acute.
Reflexology	Indicated.
Shiatsu	Supportive.
Swedish massage	Supportive; stay within client's activity limitations, pain tolerance.
Trigger point therapy	Indicated for trigger points that develop in unopposed muscles.

See Chapter 1 for a brief description of each modality, including definitions of abbreviations.

Osteogenesis Imperfecta in Brief

Pronunciation: os-te-o-GEN-eh-sis im-per-FEK-tah

What is it?

Osteogenesis imperfecta (OI) is a group of genetic disorders that affect the formation of type I collagen fibers. It results in bones that fracture easily, along with decreased muscle mass, ligament laxity, postural deviations, and several other problems.

How is it recognized?

The primary feature of OI is bones that fracture easily. In some types this can even happen prenatally. Other signs depend on what subtype of OI is present. Some common signs are a triangular face, a bluish tint in the sclera of the eyes, brittle teeth, and hearing loss.

Is massage indicated or contraindicated?

The treatment goals for people with OI include exercise and physical therapy to maintain muscle and bone mass. Stress reduction is another important coping mechanism for this potentially painful life-long disorder. Bodywork that respects the possible fragility of these clients' bones is appropriate and can be helpful.

Osteogenesis Imperfecta

Definition: What Is It?

Osteogenesis imperfecta (OI) is a group of genetic disorders that change the quality or the quantity of type I collagen fibers. Four main subtypes of OI have been identified, each with a different set of characteristics and prognosis. Further subtypes exist, but they are extremely rare.

Demographics: Who Gets It?

Type I osteogenesis imperfecta is the most common version, and it occurs in 1 in 30,000 live births. Type II occurs once in 60,000 live births. Type III occurs in 1 in 70,000 live births. Type IV and other variations are very rare.[42] It is estimated that between 20,000 and 50,000 people in the United States have OI; males and females are affected equally.[43]

Most versions of OI are autosomal dominant. This means that if one parent has the gene, he or she has a 50% chance of passing it to each child. About 25% of patients have no family history of this disorder; in these cases it is the result of a spontaneous mutation.

Etiology: What Happens?

OI is the result of a genetic mutation that alters the formation of type I collagen fibers. These fibers are formed of a triple helix of intertwining procollagen fibers. A problem in the coding for these chains leads to the production of faulty type I collagen or an inadequate number of fibers.

Type I OI is the most common and least severe form of this disorder. It involves an inadequate supply of type I collagen. People with this version have most of their fractures in early childhood and live normal lifespans with normal mobility, although they are prone to a number of secondary problems. Type II OI is the most severe form of this disorder; these babies are often born with broken bones, and many do not survive childbirth or early infancy. Other types of OI involve poorly formed collagen (rather than an insufficient amount) and range in severity between types I and II.

Signs and Symptoms

Signs and symptoms of OI vary with the type, but the primary feature is having bones that fracture extremely easily, especially in infancy and early childhood. Children with OI are sometimes mistaken for victims of child abuse because their radiographs show a history of multiple broken bones. Other signs and symptoms include brittle teeth, ligament laxity, easy bruising, short stature (for some types), postural deviations (especially hyperkyphosis with scoliosis), hearing loss, and low muscle mass.

Some particular physical characteristics are seen with many OI patients, including a triangular face and a blue or gray tint to the sclera of the eye. Often the chest is barrel shaped and the long bones are bowed.

Complications

People with OI are prone to several other disorders that can be associated with poorly formed or inadequate collagen. Besides the symptoms listed previously, many people with OI have an increased risk of heart valve problems, dilation of the aorta, gastroesophageal reflux disorder, vision loss related to distortions in the sclera, and muscle weakness. In addition, people with OI tend to have more pulmonary infections, kidney stones, and osteoporosis than the general population.

One particularly serious complication for types III and IV of OI is a condition called *basilar impression* or *basilar invagination.* In this situation ligament laxity allows the base of the skull to put pressure on the spinal column, leading to headaches and tingling or paresthesia in the extremities.

Diagnosis

OI is usually diagnosed in infancy or early childhood, when a child has obvious fractures with minimal stress. A biopsy of a collagen sample or a DNA test is the usual starting point. These are definitive for most cases, but some forms of OI require further testing.

Treatment

Because it is a genetic disorder, OI has no cure. Parents of OI patients are taught the safest ways to lift and hold their children to minimize the risk of fractures. The main goals of OI treatment are to maintain health and independence, to preserve bone density, and to minimize cardiovascular problems. Children and adults are encouraged to be physically active, but not with contact sports or activities that involve jumping or twisting; water sports seem to be the safest kind of exercise. A healthy diet is strongly promoted to control weight and assist with bone density.

A surgical procedure called "rodding" is sometimes performed to straighten and support bowed long bones. Any other assistive devices, from crutches to wheelchairs, may be used to improve mobility.

OI can be painful. Pain management for these patients can range from over-the-counter medications to TENS units or nerve blocks.

Massage?

Bodywork for a person with OI is determined mainly by how stable his bones are and what degree of mechanical stress he is able to take. For people with especially fragile bones, deep or percussive work is obviously contraindicated. Other health concerns should be explored as well, particularly for the risk of pulmonary or cardiovascular problems.

If major concerns are accommodated, OI patients can derive many benefits from massage, including pain reduction, stress relief, and support for a healthy active lifestyle.

Modality Recommendations for Osteogenesis Imperfecta

MODALITY	RECOMMENDATION
Deep tissue massage	Contraindicated unless working with health care team.
Lymphatic drainage	Supportive.
Polarity	S: Indicated. R/D: Gentle work supportive, depending on client limitations, comfort.
PNF/MET/stretching	Contraindicated unless working with health care team.
Reflexology	Locally contraindicated; work all gland points.
Shiatsu	Supportive, especially with K, BL, SP meridians and extensions.
Swedish massage	Supportive; stay within client's activity limitations and pain tolerance.
Trigger point therapy	Supportive, with caution for fragility of the bones.

See Chapter 1 for a brief description of each modality, including definitions of abbreviations.

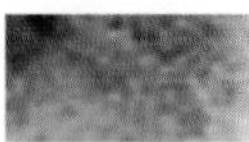

Other Connective Tissue Disorders

Baker Cysts

Definition: What Are They?

Baker cysts are synovial cysts found in the popliteal fossa, usually on the medial side. They are also called popliteal cysts.

> **Baker Cysts in Brief**
>
> **What are they?**
> Baker cysts are synovial cysts, usually found on the posterior aspect of the knee. They are often connected to the synovial capsule of the knee.
>
> **How are they recognized?**
> Baker cysts are sacs that are palpable deep to the superficial fascia in the popliteal fossa. They may cause pain on extension or a feeling of tightness in the knee in flexion.
>
> **Is massage indicated or contraindicated?**
> Massage is locally contraindicated in the popliteal fossa, especially if a Baker cyst is present. In addition, if any signs of circulatory disruption (coldness, clamminess, heat, edema) are present distal to the cyst, the client must be cleared of the possibility of thrombosis.

Etiology: What Happens?

Baker cysts form when the joint capsule at the knee develops a pouch at the posterior aspect. They usually protrude into a small gap between the medial head of the gastrocnemius and the tendon of the semimembranosus.

Baker cysts are relatively common in children, in whom they usually spontaneously resolve within a few months. When they occur in adults, they are almost always connected to general joint disruption: osteoarthritis, rheumatoid arthritis, cruciate ligament tears, or meniscus tears.

Complications

Baker cysts are not usually dangerous. The only risks they pose is that a cyst can become big enough impair blood flow through the lesser saphenous vein in the back of the leg. If that is the case, the patient is at risk for thrombophlebitis or deep vein thrombosis. Other complications include the risk of rupture, bleeding into the joint, infection, or posterior compartment syndrome (blockage of fluid flow from the posterior compartment of the lower leg).

Signs and Symptoms

Baker cysts themselves are generally asymptomatic, but the affected knee is often painful from the underlying cause of inflammation. The cysts usually extend into the medial side of the popliteal fossa and may protrude down the leg, deep to the gastrocnemius. Patients with Baker cysts often report a feeling of tightness or fullness when the knee is in flexion and mild pain on extension.

Treatment

Most Baker cysts are first treated with ice and nonsteroidal anti-inflammatories in the hopes that they will resolve spontaneously. If this is unsuccessful, they may be aspirated, followed by cortisone shots to resolve joint inflammation. This is often an impermanent solution, however, as they easily recur until the underlying joint disruption has been resolved.

Massage?

It is possible, though unlikely, that massage could rupture a Baker cyst, but a therapist would have to be working much deeper in the popliteal fossa than good sense allows. Baker cysts are considered local contraindications for massage, however, because of their proximity to the lesser saphenous vein. Therapists should watch for signs of fluid accumulation and poor blood return below the knee: heat, cold, clamminess, or edema that is more pronounced on the cysted side than the uncysted side (Figures 3.32 and 3.33). These are all signs that the cyst is big enough to cause a problem. If this is the case, the client should visit a doctor to rule out the possibility of thrombophlebitis or deep vein thrombosis.

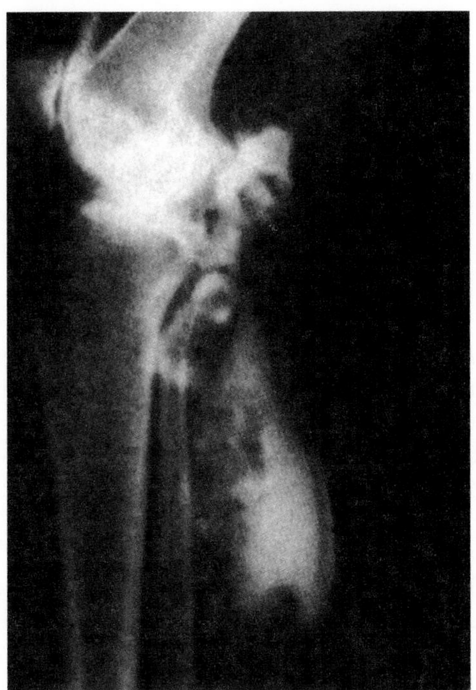

Figure 3.32. Baker cyst: the mass posterior to the femoral condyle is probably the original cyst; the mass in the gastrocnemius is leaked fluid.

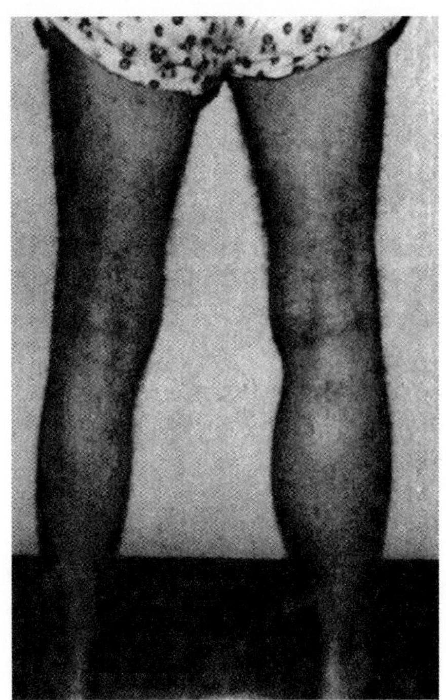

Figure 3.33. Disparity in size and color between two calves.

Modality Recommendations for Baker Cyst

MODALITY	RECOMMENDATION
Deep tissue massage	Locally contraindicated; otherwise supportive.
Lymphatic drainage	Indicated; may be effective locally to reduce swelling.
Polarity	S: Indicated. R/D: Locally contraindicated; otherwise supportive.
PNF/MET/stretching	Locally contraindicated; otherwise supportive
Reflexology	Indicated; work knee and lymphatic system points.
Shiatsu	Supportive.
Swedish massage	Locally contraindicated; otherwise supportive.
Trigger point therapy	Locally contraindicated; otherwise supportive.

See Chapter 1 for a brief description of each modality, including definitions of abbreviations.

Bunions

Definition: What Are They?

Bunions are also known as ***hallux valgus,*** which means laterally deviated big toe. The first phalanx of the great toe is distorted toward the lateral aspect of the foot. The joint capsule stretches, and callus grows over the protrusion. A smaller version of the same problem sometimes appears at the base of the little toe; this is called "tailor's bunion" or "bunionette".

Bunions in Brief

Pronunciation: BUN-yunz

What are they?
A bunion is a protrusion at the metatarsophalangeal joint of the great toe that occurs when the toe is laterally deviated.

How are they recognized?
Bunions are recognizable by the large bump on the medial aspect of the foot. When they are inflamed, they are red, hot, and painful.

Is massage indicated or contraindicated?
Massage is locally contraindicated at the point of a bunion, especially when or if it is inflamed. Massage elsewhere on the foot or body is very much indicated within pain tolerance to help with compensation patterns that occur when it is difficult to walk.

Demographics: Who Gets Them?

Bunions occur approximately 10 times more often in women than in men. The condition is linked to a habit of wearing high-heeled, narrow-toed shoes. A genetic weakness in the toe joints may predispose some people to bunions regardless of footwear, but most people can develop bunions if they wear the wrong kind of shoes.

Etiology: What Happens?

Several factors can contribute to the misalignment between the first metatarsal and the proximal phalanx of the great toe. Overarched feet (pes cavus) can force weight bearing to the medial aspect of the foot. Flat feet (pes planus) can contribute as well. An overly tight Achilles tendon can limit dorsiflexion; this puts stress on the affected joint. The shape of the head of the first metatarsal determines the stability of the metatarsophalangeal joint: the rounder the head, the less stable the joint and the more prone it is to valgus stress. Finally, four muscles cross this joint; if any of these is too tight or too loose, equilibrium can easily be lost.

Any of these issues, in combination with footwear that squeezes the toes or forces weight onto the medial aspect of the foot (i.e., high-heeled, narrow-toed shoes or cowboy boots), can open the door to the painful distortion that bunions involve.

The pressure at the metacarpophalangeal joint can cause erosion and irritation, but the acute pain of bunions is also often related to local bursitis. The bump formed by hallux valgus is a natural spot for protective bursae to develop. If that bursa should get irritated and inflamed, it becomes a case of friction bursitis, which can be extremely painful, even debilitating. Ultimately, if this badly misaligned weight-bearing joint is not corrected or supported in a way that limits erosion of the joint structures, the bunion patient can also develop bone spurs and/or arthritis, which can make it prohibitively painful to walk.

Signs and Symptoms

Bunions look like an enormous lump on the medial side of the metatarsophalangeal joint of the great toe. If the bunion is not irritated, a simple protrusion, often covered with a thick layer of callus, is obvious (Figure 3.34). If the bursa is inflamed, the area is red, hot, and extremely painful.

Treatment

The first steps in treating a bunion are to remove whatever irritants are causing the problem or making it worse. This usually means switching footgear or even cutting holes in shoes to make room for the protrusion. Other noninvasive techniques include the use of massage and exercise. Range-of-motion stretches, gentle traction, and friction around the affected area are recommended to limit pain and slow progression, but these interventions do not permanently realign the toe. Elevating the heel to an appropriate height can diminish pain, and a corticosteroid injection can reduce inflammation. But if damage has developed inside the joint and if the bunion is painful enough to limit the patient's activity, surgery may be recommended. A variety of surgeries have been developed to remove the bunion, reshape the foot bones, or fuse the joint. The success rates are determined by how badly the foot was distorted and whether joints other than the metatarsophalangeal joint were involved.

Massage?

Acutely inflamed bunions locally contraindicate massage; massage elsewhere on the body is perfectly safe. If no acute inflammation is present, massage is appropriate, although the bump

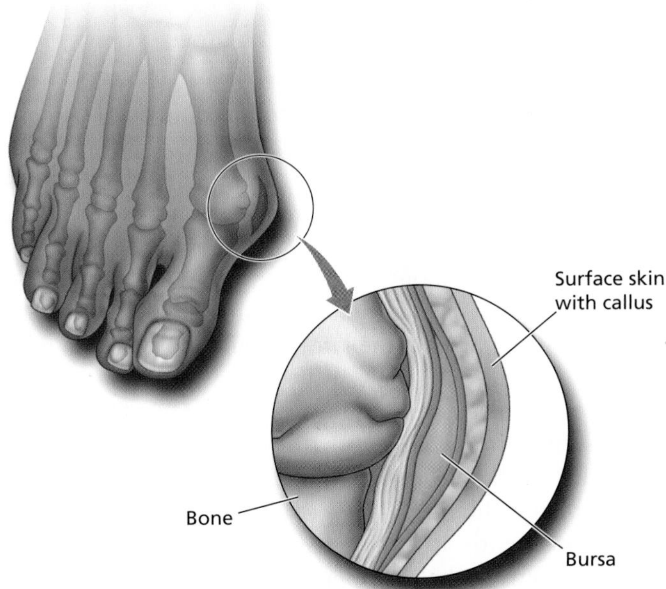

Figure 3.34. Bunion.

itself is still a local contraindication if pressure irritates the area. Massage does not make bunions go away. Therapists don't have access to genetic patterning or to the inner workings of the affected joint. The best massage can do is work with the compensation patterns that inevitably ripple through a body that is forced to move differently because of foot pain. This can mean concentrating on the intrinsic muscles of the affected foot, and it can mean working with the extrinsic muscles for postural distortion everywhere else.

Modality Recommendations for Bunions

MODALITY	RECOMMENDATION
Deep tissue massage	Contraindicated while acute; otherwise indicated. Work to release layers of plantar fascia and intrinsic foot muscles; address leg and hip compensation.
Lymphatic drainage	Supportive.
Polarity	S: Indicated. R/D: Locally contraindicated; otherwise supportive.
PNF/MET/stretching	Locally contraindicated while acute; otherwise supportive.
Reflexology	Locally contraindicated; work spine, hips, knees, leg points.
Shiatsu	Treat SP, GB meridians, especially in foot.
Swedish massage	Locally contraindicated while acute; otherwise supportive.
Trigger point therapy	Locally contraindicated; otherwise supportive.

See Chapter 1 for a brief description of each modality, including definitions of abbreviations.

Bursitis in Brief

Pronunciation: bur-SY-tis

What is it?

A bursa is a fluid-filled sac that acts as a protective cushion at points of recurring pressure, eases the movement of tendons and ligaments moving over bones, and cushions points of contact between bones. Bursitis is the inflammation of a bursa.

How is it recognized?

Acute bursitis is painful and is aggravated by both passive and active motion. Muscles surrounding the affected joint often severely limit range of motion. It may be hot or edematous if the bursa is superficial.

Is massage indicated or contraindicated?

Acute bursitis locally contraindicates massage, which can exacerbate inflammation. Massage elsewhere on the body during an acute phase and directly to the muscles of the affected joint (within pain limits) in a subacute phase is perfectly appropriate. Bursitis due to infection contraindicates massage until the infection has been eradicated.

Bursitis

Definition: What Is It?

Bursae are small closed sacs made of connective tissue. They are lined with synovial membrane and filled with synovial fluid. Bursitis is inflammation of the bursae. When these fluid-filled sacs are irritated, internal cells proliferate and generate excess fluid, which causes pain and limits mobility.

The human body has about 160 bursae, but new ones can be generated in areas that need protection. Most bursae are very small, but the ones that protect the knee, shoulder, and hip can be quite large.

Bursitis comes in all shapes and forms, some of which have descriptive names, like *housemaid's knee* and *student's elbow*, which occurs on the point of the olecranon. *Weaver's bottom* is bursitis on the ischial tuberosity. Bursitis at the greater trochanter is a common variety, as is bursitis at the insertion of the iliopsoas on the lesser trochanter and at the calcaneus (Figure 3.35). The most common type of bursitis, at the pad between the humerus and the acromion, is called subacromial bursitis but could be labeled *jack hammerer's shoulder*.

Etiology: What Happens?

Imagine stretching a rubber band over the sharp edge of a table. Now imagine moving it back and forth for several minutes. In a short time, the rubber band frays and then breaks. But if a tiny water balloon is placed between the rubber band and the edge of the table, the rubber band (i.e., tendon) has freedom to move without the friction from the table (i.e., bone). The water balloon (i.e., bursa) protects it from damage. Bursae are the water balloons; they serve to ease the movement of tendons over bony angles (Figure 3.36). They also cushion the bones where they would otherwise bang against each other. Bursae pad people's sharpest corners:

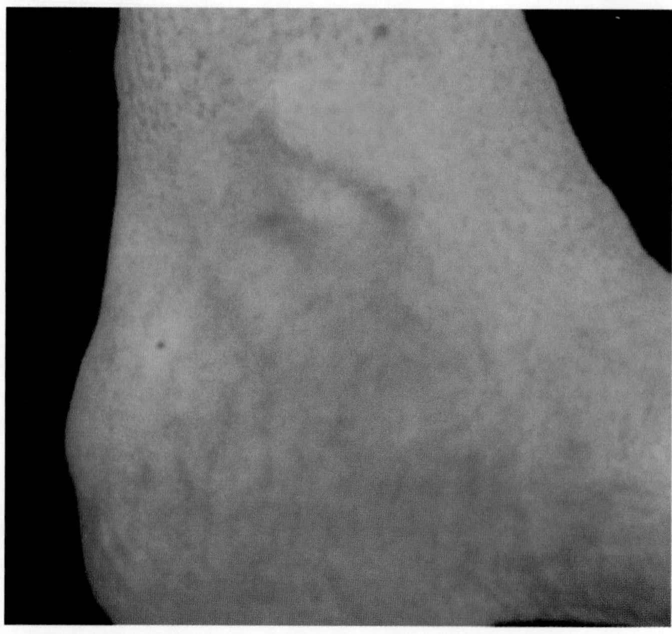

Figure 3.35. Calcaneal bursitis.

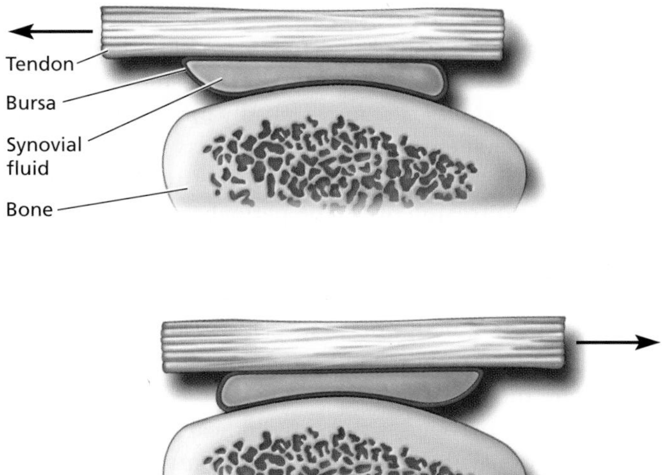

Figure 3.36. Bursae allow tendons to move freely over bony prominences.

they are on elbows, knees, heels, and ischial tuberosities and between layers of fascia. Bursae can grow anywhere around a joint that takes extra wear and tear.

Without bursae to protect them, several tendons would fray and rupture in short order. Some bones that are not meant to touch *would* touch, with great force. Sharp corners, such as elbows or bunions, would have no protection.

Repetitive stress is usually the culprit behind bursitis. Performing the same movement or rubbing the same spot over and over, day after day, sooner or later irritates that fluid-filled sac. Then the inflammatory process tries to pack a tangerine's worth of fluid into a sac the size of a grape, which *hurts*. In response to the pain, the muscles that surround the joint go into spasm, splinting the injury. This drastically limits the range of motion of the affected joint. Sometimes the muscles actually aggravate and prolong an attack of bursitis by compressing the joint and the bursa at the same time.

Bursitis often occurs in concert with other inflammatory conditions. It tends to accompany general area inflammation, so if a person has shoulder tendinitis, bursitis is often present as well. (Unfortunately, it's hard to treat the tendinitis if the bursitis is in the way.) It also attends gout, rheumatoid arthritis, and tuberculosis.

Bursae can be inflamed by infection in addition to overuse. This happens most often with superficial bursae, especially at the elbow and the knee.

Signs and Symptoms

The symptoms of bursitis include pain on any kind of movement, passive or active, along with extremely limited range of motion because of the muscular splinting reaction to pain. Superficial bursitis may also show palpable heat and swelling. If the affected bursae are deep, no heat or edema may be palpable, but pain and limitation of movement are still present.

Diagnosis

The diagnosis of bursitis is made mainly through the patient's history. It is important to consider other local injuries, which could include tendinitis, arthritis, ligament sprains, and any other problems specific to the joint or area being affected.

Treatment

Treatment strategies for bursitis range from anti-inflammatories to warm, moist applications (cold is too intense for this inflammation; the muscles seize up and make it worse), to aspiration of excess fluid, to corticosteroid injections. One or two injections generally clear away even chronic inflammation, and since the chemical is being injected into a closed cavity, one doesn't have to deal with the side affects that accompany a systemic dose of steroids.

As a last resort, some doctors suggest a ***bursectomy*** to remove a badly inflamed bursa. But the only way to be sure that the bursitis is permanently cured is to address the factors that caused it. No matter how often or how effectively bursitis is treated, if the stimulus that irritated the bursa to begin with is not removed, no treatment can be permanently successful.

Massage?

Bursitis is a local contraindication for most types of bodywork, especially in an acute phase. If local muscles can be released without irritating the area, some range of motion may be restored, but care must be taken not to irritate the bursa again.

When bursitis doesn't involve an infection, massage is certainly indicated for the rest of the body. If the bursitis is caused by an infectious agent, it systemically contraindicates massage until the infection has subsided.

In the subacute stage, a skilled massage therapist can address the muscles that cross over the affected joint and may well have some success at decompressing the bones that are irritating the affected bursa. And as with any condition that involves prolonged discomfort and immobility, it's a good idea to look for compensation patterns that may contribute to pain.

Modality Recommendations for Bursitis

MODALITY	RECOMMENDATION
Deep tissue massage	Supportive while subacute; work to decompress fascias that cross affected joints.
Lymphatic drainage	Indicated while subacute.
Polarity	S: Indicated. R/D: Locally contraindicated; otherwise supportive.
PNF/MET/stretching	Locally contraindicated while acute; otherwise supportive.
Reflexology	Locally contraindicated; work lymphatic system points.
Shiatsu	Indicated. Treat TH/SP/K to reduce swelling, inflammation. Use gentle pressure at local site when acute.
Swedish massage	Locally contraindicated while acute; otherwise supportive.
Trigger point therapy	Locally contraindicated; otherwise indicated to minimize excessive muscle tension in the region.

See Chapter 1 for a brief description of each modality, including definitions of abbreviations.

Dupuytren Contracture

Definition: What Is It?

This condition, also called *palmar fasciitis,* is an idiopathic thickening and shrinking of the palmar fascia that limits the movement of the fingers. Usually the ring and little fingers are most severely affected, although the index and middle fingers may also be bent (Figure 3.37).

Demographics: Who Gets It?

This condition strikes mostly middle-aged men of northern European descent. It is rarer among females. Some Dupuytren contracture patients have other family members with the same condition, so a genetic component is probably part of this process.

A statistical link between Dupuytren contracture and some other conditions has been observed. Smoking and alcohol use are recognized risk factors. Men with long-term seizure disorders are at increased risk as well, although researchers speculate that the connective tissue changes are related to anticonvulsant medications rather than to the seizures themselves. Men with type I and type II diabetes develop palmar fasciitis more often than others, but they are generally spared the contracture aspect of this disorder.[44]

Dupuytren Contracture in Brief

Pronunciation: du-pwe-TRON kon-TRAK-chur

What is it?

Dupuytren contracture is an idiopathic shrinking and thickening of the fascia on the palm of the hand.

How is it recognized?

This is a painless condition that usually affects the ring and little fingers, pulling them into permanent flexion.

Is massage indicated or contraindicated?

Massage is indicated for Dupuytren contracture as long as sensation is present, although it may do little to reverse the process if it has progressed too far.

Etiology: What Happens?

It is unclear exactly why the palmar fascia shrinks. The development of Dupuytren contracture resembles the growth of scar tissue in response to trauma, but to an excessive degree. Specialized fibroblasts and other cells contribute to proliferations of type III collagen fibers, both in the fascia on the palm and in the fingers. As the condition progresses, the collagen thickens and toughens, but the active cells recede, leaving tight, thick bands of connective tissue that interfere with the use of the hand.

Flexion of the fingers is normal for patients of Dupuytren contracture, but they cannot extend their fingers normally. When the extension is limited by 30 degrees or more, patients are considered to be candidates for corrective surgery.

In some cases the tendency for fascial sheaths to thicken and shrink extends beyond the palms. Three conditions are associated with the most severe presentations of Dupuytren contracture:

- *Plantar fibromatosis* (*Ledderhose disease*) is essentially the same as Dupuytren contracture, but it develops on the plantar aspect of the foot.
- *Peyronie disease* is a condition in which scar tissue develops under the skin of the shaft of the penis.
- ***Knuckle pads*** (*Garrod's nodes*) are deposits of tissue at the DIP joints of the hands.

Signs and Symptoms

The typical pattern of Dupuytren contracture is that a middle-aged man develops a mildly tender or painless bump just proximal to his ring finger on the palmar aspect of the hand.

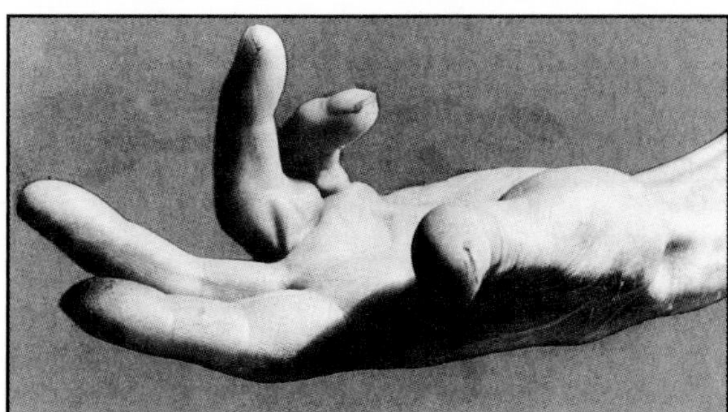

Figure 3.37. Dupuytren contracture.

Over months or years the nodule extends into a cord in his palm and out to the PIP joint. The little finger might develop a cord as well. Slowly the fingers are drawn toward the palm, and they can't be straightened out. Dupuytren contracture is bilateral in almost half of cases.

This condition may be mildly painful in early stages but then often becomes painless. It is usually slowly progressive, although some people (younger patients, as a rule) have a relatively fast onset. Some people have only the growth of tough, fibrous bumps on their hands, while others end up with severely bent, strangulated, unusable fingers. If the constriction to nerve and blood supply is very severe, the affected fingers may be amputated.

Treatment

If Dupuytren contracture is left untreated, the connective tissue may simply strangle the muscles and nerves until the affected fingers lose all function. If it is caught before too much atrophy occurs, corticosteroid injections can be an effective treatment. Injections of collagenase, an enzyme that dissolves collagen, is another treatment option in development, and release of the cord by way of tiny punctures ***(needle aponeurotomy)*** is a new procedure with little risk of complications.

Surgical intervention is generally not recommended until fingers become bent and too stiff to move. At that point, the surgery involves making several zig-zag cuts in the palm to release the fascia, followed by skin grafts, physical therapy, and massage to limit the growth of scar tissue. Even when surgery is successful, Dupuytren contracture recurs in about one-third of cases.

Massage?

Clients with Dupuytren contracture have sensation in the hand, at least before nerve damage develops, and for that reason massage is appropriate. But the connective tissue involved with this disorder is particularly tough and strong. While massage will certainly not make the condition any worse, it may not make it better either. Massage is a good preventive measure for contractures, and it is frequently used in postoperative rehabilitation, but if this condition is already present, massage may not reverse it.

Modality Recommendations for Dupuytren's Contracture

MODALITY	RECOMMENDATION
Deep tissue massage	Supportive; may help to reduce contracture. Work slowly with dense tissue.
Lymphatic drainage	Indicated; focused work at contracture may be very effective.
Polarity	S: Indicated. R/D: Supportive within client comfort.
PNF/MET/stretching	Indicated in all stages.
Reflexology	Locally contraindicated; work circulatory system points.
Shiatsu	Indicated. Hold fingers outstretched while applying point pressure to ligaments and tendons of hand.
Swedish massage	Indicated.
Trigger point therapy	Supportive.

See Chapter 1 for a brief description of each modality, including definitions of abbreviations.

Ganglion Cysts

Definition: What Are They?

Ganglion cysts are small connective tissue pouches filled with fluid. They grow on joint capsules or tendinous sheaths. They usually appear on the wrist, the hand, or the top of the foot.

> **Ganglion Cysts in Brief**
> Pronunciation: GANG-le-on sists
>
> **What are they?**
> Ganglion cysts are small fluid-filled synovial sacs that are attached to tendinous sheaths or joint capsules.
>
> **How are they recognized?**
> Ganglion cysts form small bumps that usually appear on the hand, wrist, or ankle. They are not usually painful unless they are in a place to be injured by normal wear and tear.
>
> **Is massage indicated or contraindicated?**
> Ganglion cysts locally contraindicate massage. Friction or direct pressure may irritate them by increasing local inflammation.

Etiology: What Happens?

While some ganglion cysts seem to grow in response to direct trauma or overuse, most simply appear without an identifiable reason. A ganglion cyst is essentially a synovial pouch that forms as an extension of a joint capsule or tenosynovial sheath. They are filled with a viscous fluid that contains ***hyaluronic acid, glucosamine,*** and other substances. They may have a single chamber, but some cysts have multiple lobes that are connected by tiny channels.

Ganglion cysts are not inherently dangerous, but they can grow in a place that allows them to put enough pressure on nearby structures to interfere with function. This can lead to pain, tingling, weakness, and loss of range of motion. They usually grow on the wrist, hand, or foot, but have been found in many other locations.

One type of ganglion cyst is also called a ***mucous cyst.*** This grows on the DIP joint, usually of older people with osteoarthritis at the same joints. Mucous cysts can damage the joint capsule or distort the growth of the fingernail.

Signs and Symptoms

Ganglion cysts may be too small to notice or they may grow nearly to the size of a tennis ball, obstructing joint function and interfering with normal range of motion. Most ganglion cysts are not painful except that they have a habit of growing in places where they can be easily irritated, such as on the fingers and around the wrists (Figure 3.38). This can put them in a state of chronic irritation, and it can be difficult for them to heal and subside. Sometimes ganglion cysts grow on the dorsal aspect of the wrist, where they may be too small to see or palpate but large enough to cause pain and limit range of motion. These occult cysts may only be detected with an MRI.

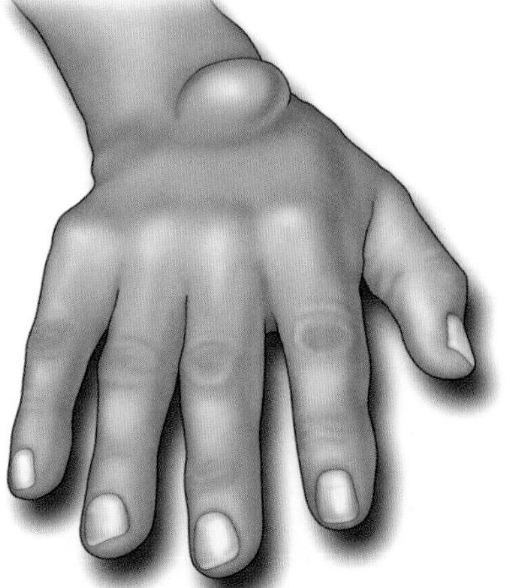

Figure 3.38. Ganglion cyst.

Treatment

Generally the treatment for ganglion cysts is to leave them alone. It may take a while, but they usually resolve without interference. They may be injected with cortisone or aspirated to relieve internal pressure, but they grow back about half the time. The traditional home remedy for ganglion cysts used to be to smash them with a Bible. Patients are not advised to use this option, however, as smashing a ganglion cyst with a book or any other heavy object can cause a lot of other soft tissue damage.

Cysts may be surgically excised if they are big enough to be a significant problem. If they grow back, they are usually not as large as the original cyst.

Massage?

Ganglion cysts are a local contraindication. Massage doesn't make ganglion cysts bigger, worse, or more painful *unless* they are overstimulated. Massage can't make them go away either, so massage therapists should leave them alone. If a client has a mysterious bump on her wrist, foot, or anywhere else, it is important to get a diagnosis before working anywhere in the area.

Modality Recommendations for Ganglion Cysts

MODALITY	RECOMMENDATION
Deep tissue massage	Locally contraindicated; otherwise supportive.
Lymphatic drainage	Supportive.
Polarity	S: Indicated. R/D: Locally contraindicated; otherwise supportive.
PNF/MET/stretching	Supportive.
Reflexology	Locally contraindicated; work circulatory system points.
Shiatsu	Supportive. Treat all meridians and extensions above and below cyst.
Swedish massage	Locally contraindicated; otherwise supportive.
Trigger point therapy	Locally contraindicated; otherwise supportive.

See Chapter 1 for a brief description of each modality, including definitions of abbreviations.

Hernia

Definition: What Is It?

Hernia means hole. Specifically in this case it means "hole through which contents that are supposed to be contained are protruding". Muscles may herniate through fascial walls; vertebral discs may herniate; the brain may even herniate through the cranium. Discussed here are the hernias that occur in various places around the abdomen.

Demographics: Who Gets Them?

Hernias are quite common; it is estimated that about 1 in 10 people in the United States will have some kind of hernia at some point. About 5 million hernias are diagnosed every year, leading to approximately 700,000 surgeries. Men with hernias of the abdominal wall outnumber women by a ratio of about 7 to 1.[45]

Etiology: What Happens?

Hernias can be caused by a number of factors, from congenital weakness of the muscular wall, to childbirth, to abnormal straining, which increases internal abdominal pressure. Inguinal hernias are the most common; they develop along the pathway where the testicles descend from the abdominal cavity during gestation. This is why men are so much more likely to develop hernias than women.

Most hernias are reducible, which means that the contents can be put back where they belong without surgery. Generally, though, hernias get worse, bulging more and more often, while a bigger hole develops. Therefore, once a hernia has been identified, surgery to tighten up or close the hole is recommended sooner rather than later. Where a hernia develops and what it feels like depend mainly on gender and what forces push the abdominal contents against their walls.

Hernia in Brief

Pronunciation: HUR-ne-a

What is it?

A hernia is a hole or rip through which the abdominal contents may protrude.

How is it recognized?

Abdominal hernias usually show some bulging and mild to severe pain, depending on whether a portion of the small intestine is trapped. Hiatal hernias usually involve heartburn or other signs of gastroesophageal reflux disorder.

Is massage indicated or contraindicated?

Untreated hernias locally contraindicate massage. If the hernia is accompanied by fever or other signs of infection, it systemically contraindicates massage, and the person should seek immediate medical attention. Recent hernia surgeries are vulnerable to infection, but old hernia surgeries with no complications are fine for massage.

Signs and Symptoms

The signs and symptoms of hernias depend on what part of the abdominal wall has been compromised.

- *Inguinal hernia* is the most common variety. Inguinal hernias are holes in the abdominal wall at the inguinal ring. This opening for the spermatic cord to enter the abdomen is a structurally weak spot. A sudden change in internal abdominal pressure, like coughing, sneezing, or heavy lifting (especially with simultaneous twisting) may force a section of small intestine right through this weak spot (Figure 3.39). Inguinal hernias are especially common in infant boys, whose peritoneum may not be fully formed.
- *Epigastric hernia* is a bulge superior to the umbilicus. In this condition the linea alba is split and a portion of the omentum pushes through. The symptoms, besides a visible lump above the navel, may include a feeling of tenderness or heaviness in the area but seldom extreme pain. This hernia happens with women and men, but it is more common in men.

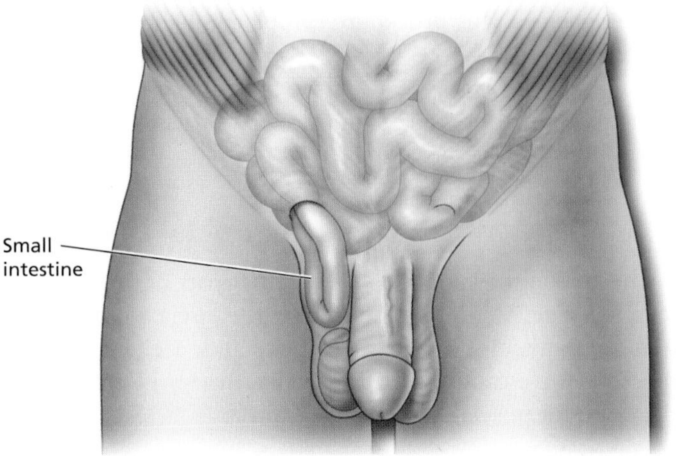

Small intestine

Figure 3.39. Inguinal hernia.

- *Paraumbilical hernia* is another split of the linea alba, this time right at the navel. It is sometimes a complication of childbirth. The symptoms are the same as for the epigastric type, but the bulge is lower. This type of hernia is almost always found in women.
- *Umbilical hernia* is a hernia directly at the umbilicus. It is a common condition in newborn babies, and it usually closes without intervention by age 2. In adults umbilical hernias may occur with obesity, ascites, or as a result of multiple pregnancies.
- *Femoral hernia* is the female equivalent to the inguinal hernia. In this case the abdominal contents protrude through the femoral ring just below the inguinal ligament. Femoral hernias usually affect women, and they can be hard to detect. They can be very dangerous, however, because the hole around the intestine is usually quite small, which increases the chance of strangulation or obstruction of the intestine.
- *Hiatal hernia* is an enlargement of the diaphragmatic hiatus, the opening in the dome of the diaphragm where the esophagus and other structures pass from the thorax to the abdomen. When this opening is enlarged, the stomach can protrude up into the thoracic cavity. Hiatal hernias are a major contributor to gastroesophageal reflux disorder.
- *Other hernias* are rare. *Incisional hernia* is a bulge at the site of an incisions. *Obturator hernia* is a bulge of pelvic contents into the obturator foramen. *Spigelian hernia* is a bulge at the lateral aspect of the rectus abdominus.

Complications

The seriousness of a hernia is determined by how big it is. Paradoxically, the bigger the hernia, the safer it is, at least for the short term. Small holes, as seen with femoral hernias, can be more dangerous: the small intestine becomes obstructed, in which case the patient has abdominal pain, nausea, and vomiting; or it becomes strangulated, cut off from its blood supply. In this case the area rapidly becomes red, enlarged, and extremely painful. Without medical intervention the strangulated loop of intestine may become infected and possibly gangrenous.

Treatment

Surgery is frequently recommended even for mild hernias because they tend to get worse and worse as time goes on. Sewing up a small stretch of abdominal fascia is easier than repairing a big rip. The standard surgical technique entails inserting a small piece of mesh at the site of the tear. This helps to distribute the force of abdominal pressure more evenly than stitches or staples alone, reducing the risk of a recurrence. This procedure can be conducted as open or laparoscopic surgery.

If a person doesn't need immediate surgery, a special corset or truss may be recommended to prevent sudden changes in abdominal pressure, but these days trusses are considered only temporary measures, not a solution to the problem.

Massage?

If a client has been diagnosed with a hernia but has not had surgery, that part of the body locally contraindicates any kind of deep massage. Vigorously stretching the fascia around an already weakened area could have disastrous results. If, on the other hand, a client has had surgery, follow the guidelines for postoperative cautions. If the hernia surgery is ancient history and no pain is present, massage does not pose a danger in any way.

Modality Recommendations for Hernia

MODALITY	RECOMMENDATION
Deep tissue massage	Contraindicated while acute. Work with postsurgery compensation patterns.
Lymphatic drainage	Supportive.
Polarity	S: Indicated. R/D: Locally contraindicated; otherwise supportive.
PNF/MET/stretching	Locally contraindicated; otherwise supportive.
Reflexology	Indicated; work points for solar plexus, spine, hip, lymphatic system, adrenal glands, organs of affected area.
Shiatsu	Indicated. Treat above and below hernia site.
Swedish massage	Locally contraindicated; otherwise supportive. Avoid compressing abdomen or stretching nearby fascia.
Trigger point therapy	Locally contraindicated; otherwise supportive.

See Chapter 1 for a brief description of each modality, including definitions of abbreviations.

Osgood-Schlatter Disease

Definition: What Is It?

Osgood-Schlatter disease (OSD) is irritation and inflammation at the site of the quadriceps insertion. It can also be called **tibial tuberosity apophysitis**. It occurs when the quadriceps muscles are vigorously used in combination with rapid growth of the leg bones.

Demographics: Who Gets It?

OSD is practically exclusive to adolescent athletes. It is especially common among people who participate in sports that involve running, jumping, and making fast, tight turns. Soccer, basketball, figure skating, and dancing are all sports with a high incidence of OSD.

OSD occurs in both boys and girls, although it is more common in boys. The average age of onset for boys is 13 to 14 years; for girls it occurs a little earlier, between 10 and 11 years of age. It can also affect older adolescents.[46]

Etiology: What Happens?

When children enter their teens, they begin a time of rapid bone growth, especially in their femurs and tibias, the bones that determine how tall they will be. Most of the time the muscles, fascia, and other connective tissues in the legs can easily keep up with the accelerated growth rate during this time, but when the quadriceps muscles are particularly taxed through demanding athletics, the combination of stresses can cause the insertion of this powerful muscle group to become irritated and inflamed.

Osgood-Schlatter Disease in Brief
Pronunciation: OZ-good SHLAH-ter dih-ZEZE

What is it?
Osgood-Schlatter disease (OSD) is the result of chronic or traumatic irritation at the insertion of the quadriceps tendon in combination with adolescent growth spurts.

How is it recognized?
When OSD is acute, the tibial tuberosity is hot, swollen, and painful. The bone may grow a large protuberance at the site of the tendinous insertion.

Is massage indicated or contraindicated?
An acute flare-up of OSD locally contraindicates circulatory massage, which could exacerbate inflammation. Techniques for reducing lymphatic retention and work elsewhere on the body are certainly appropriate. A client with a history of OSD but no current inflammation at the knee may benefit from the pain relief and balance in quadriceps muscle tone that massage can supply.

With acute inflammation of the quadriceps insertion the tendon can pull away from the bone, causing microscopic fractures and enlargement of the tibial tuberosity. In extreme cases the tibia can develop an ***avulsion***, a forceful separation of a part of the bone from chronic tendinous tension. It is common for OSD patients to develop a large, permanent bump at the tibial tuberosity; this is where the bone adapts to the constant pull of the quadriceps insertion (Figure 3.40) OSD is usually unilateral, but some athletes develop inflammation in both knees.

The severity of OSD varies greatly from one person to the next; one person may have to be careful about not overstressing her knee, while another athlete may have to quit the team altogether. It is generally a self-limiting condition, which means that when the connective tissue growth catches up with the bone growth, the pain and irritation subside. This can take anywhere from several months to 2 years.

Signs and Symptoms

OSD is easy to identify because the people susceptible to it are such a well-defined group: athletic teens. In acute stages of OSD the knee is hot, swollen, and painful just distal to the patella at the tibial tuberosity. Any activity that stresses or stretches the quadriceps aggravates symptoms.

When OSD is not acute, pain and inflammation are resolved, but the characteristic bump of the remodeled tibia may be permanent. A person who had OSD as a child may never be comfortable kneeling because of tibial distortion.

Treatment

Treatment for OSD focuses on reducing pain and limiting damage to the quadriceps attachment at the tibia. Mild cases can be managed by heating the knee with hot packs before athletic events and icing them afterward. Nonsteroidal anti-inflammatories may be suggested to help with pain and inflammation, and doctors or physical therapists may recommend that stretches designed to reduce tension in the quadriceps be performed several times a day.

Severe cases may require that the athlete suspend activity until the pain and inflammation have been gone for several weeks. In the meantime, the knee may be supported with a brace or cast. This period is followed by rehabilitative exercise to strengthen the muscles and reduce the chance of a recurrence when the athlete becomes active again.

In rare cases, the knee may need surgery to remove bits of the tibia that were pulled off and suspended in the tibial tendon. Studies of patients with OSD suggest that the long-term outcomes of surgery are essentially the same as for no surgery, so this is avoided whenever possible.

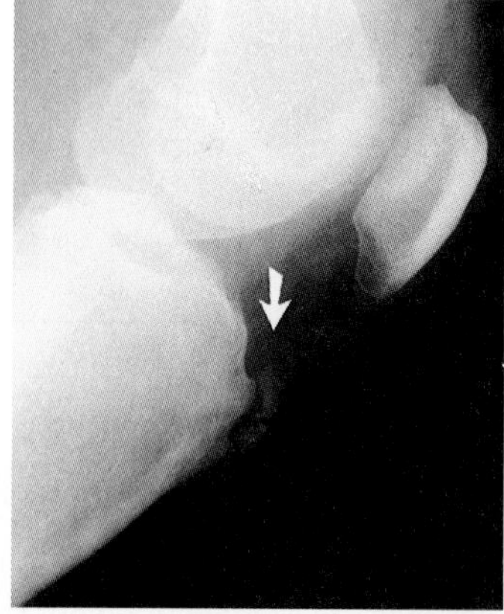

Figure 3.40. Osgood Schlatter disease: a protuberance at the tibial tuberosity is visible, and the blurry area (arrow) shows where inflammatory edema has accumulated.

Massage?

In its acute stages OSD locally contraindicates circulatory massage, which only exacerbates inflammation. Other techniques that may reduce edema can be appropriate, as is work anywhere other than the affected knee.

When the knee is not acutely painful, massage may be useful in reducing quadriceps tension that pulls on the tibial tendon. Massage is unlikely to resolve or reverse a case of OSD, but it may help to deal with the pain and speed up recovery so that a teen athlete may more quickly and safely resume activity.

Modality Recommendations for Osgood-Schlatter Disease

MODALITY	RECOMMENDATION
Deep tissue massage	Locally contraindicated while acute. Otherwise may support relief of pain from quadriceps. Work to reduce tension on quadriceps and anterior fascia latae.
Lymphatic drainage	Supportive.
Polarity	S: Indicated. R/D: Locally contraindicated while acute; otherwise indicated.
PNF/MET/stretching	Locally contraindicated while acute. Indicated when subacute; releasing quadriceps tension can help decrease pain and irritation.
Reflexology	Indicated; work hips, legs, knees, endocrine system points.
Shiatsu	Indicated. Treat ST, SP, K, GB meridians, TH extension in thigh and leg, especially at joints. Use light pressure at knee when inflamed or swollen.
Swedish massage	Indicated when subacute; releasing quadriceps tension can help decrease pain and irritation.
Trigger point therapy	Locally contraindicated while acute; indicated while subacute.

See Chapter 1 for a brief description of each modality, including definitions of abbreviations.

Pes Planus, Pes Cavus

Definition: What Are They?

Pes planus (flat feet) is the medical term for feet that lack the medial arch between the calcaneus and the great toe, the lateral arch between the calcaneus and the little toe, and the transverse arch that stretches across the ball of the foot.

Pes cavus (caved feet) is the term for feet with jammed arches, or a hyperaccentuated arch that does not flatten out with each step but instead stays high and immobile.

Etiology: What Happens?

The feet are architecturally complex. Each one has 26 bones, 33 joints, and more than 100 muscles, tendons, and ligaments to mediate our relation to gravity when we stand. Imbalance at the forefoot, midfoot, or hindfoot can lead to problems in how weight is distributed over the whole surface and how the stress of weight bearing is translated to the rest of the body.

> **Pes Planus, Pes Cavus in Brief**
> Pronunciation: pes PLANE-us, pes KAV-us
>
> **What are they?**
> These are the medical terms for flat feet or jammed arches.
>
> **How are they recognized?**
> In pes planus the feet lack arches. Eversion of the ankle may also be present. Persons with pes cavus have extremely high arches that don't flatten with weight bearing.
>
> **Is massage indicated or contraindicated?**
> Pes planus and pes cavus usually indicate massage. In some cases the health of intrinsic foot muscles and ligaments can be improved to the point where alignment in the foot is also improved. If the ligaments are lax through genetic or other problems, massage may not correct the situation, but neither will it make it worse.

Pes planus and pes cavus may develop because of a congenital problem in the shape of the foot bones or the strength of the foot ligaments. They may arise from the unending battle between the deep flexors and everters combined with footwear that offers little or no support to the intertarsal ligaments that are meant to hold up the arches (Figure 3.41).

Pes planus in particular has been studied in relation to a poorly functioning tibialis posterior tendon. This leads to hypertonicity and imbalanced pulling, especially at the peroneus muscles on the lateral aspect of the foot. Consequently, while the medial arch is flattened, the foot veers laterally, putting excessive pull on the medial deltoid ligament.

Pes cavus, when it is serious enough to interfere with function, is often examined as a complication of an underlying or preexisting disorder. Malunion fractures and shin splints are often considered. Neuromuscular disorders, such as Charcot-Marie-Tooth syndrome, muscular dystrophy, polio, or cerebral palsy, may contribute to jammed arches. When pes cavus has a sudden onset and is bilateral (i.e., not related to a specific trauma) a neurological cause is investigated: it could be related to a tumor or other problem in the central nervous system leading to spasticity in lower leg muscles.

Complications

Whichever direction the tarsal bones go—to the floor or to the roof—if they lack mobility, a critical function is lost: shock absorption. Each time the foot hits the ground, thousands of pounds of downward pressure should be softly distributed through the tarsal bones, which flatten out and then rebound in preparation for the next step. If the arches are somehow compromised and the bones lose their rebound capacity, all that force reverberates through the rest of the skeleton. This is how flat feet or jammed arches can lead to arthritis in the feet, heel spurs, plantar fasciitis, ***neuromas***, knee problems, hip problems, back problems, even headaches and TMJ disorders. Furthermore, foot problems can be especially dangerous for people with poor peripheral circulation because chronic friction and irritation at isolated spots can lead to sores on the feet.

All of these processes point back to the central idea that should echo throughout good anatomy training: *everything in the body is connected to everything else*. Pes planus and pes cavus are excellent examples of how an "insignificant" problem in one place can create very significant problems elsewhere. These problems can be difficult to track down and correct unless a therapist knows where to look.

Treatment

Unless they lead to serious arthritis or plantar fasciitis, flat feet or jammed arches often don't hurt in the feet as much as causing dysfunction in other places in the body. When this is the case, they may never be treated at all. A person who is aware that the alignment of the feet is a problem may be recommended to switch to highly supportive shoes, perhaps with orthotic inserts. Physical therapy to rebalance the peroneus longus and tibialis posterior muscles may be suggested. Rarely, surgery may be performed to repair injured tendons that can contribute to flat feet, to reshape foot bones, or to fuse foot joints for reduced pain and improved stability.

When pes cavus is related to an underlying condition and function could be restored by surgically releasing tight tissues, this may be considered a viable choice.

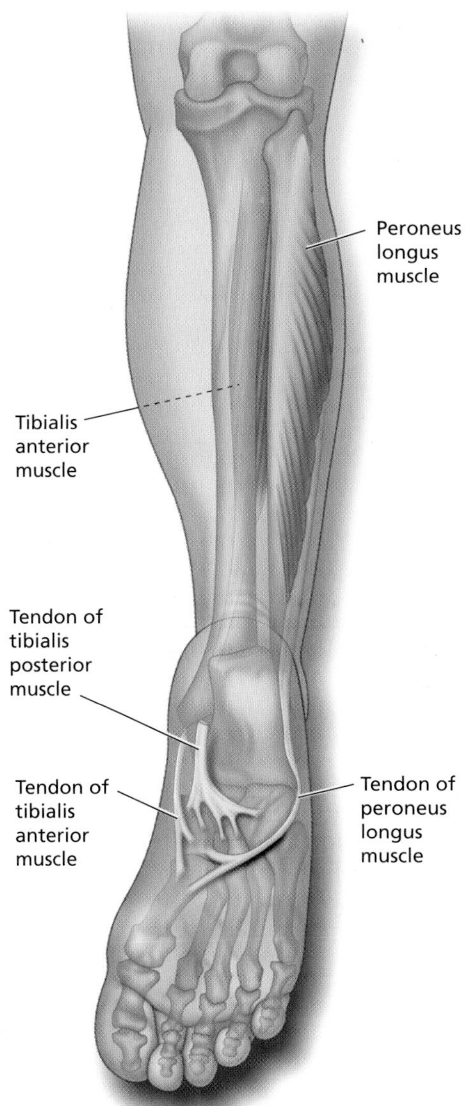

Figure 3.41. Pes planus: the stirrup of lower leg muscles that supports the medial arch of the foot.

Massage?

Pes planus and pes cavus indicate massage if they are unrelated to a contraindicating condition. If the problems are congenital, massage won't have much lasting effect, but even temporary relief from pain is better than nothing. Furthermore, massage can ameliorate some of the distant effects of foot problems, such as knee strain and hip rotation.

If flat feet or jammed arches are related to muscular or ligamentous stresses, massage may have some success at equalizing the tensions between antagonistic muscles and stimulating energy and circulation to the ligaments. Deep, specific massage tips the scales, drawing lots of fresh nutrition to ligaments that otherwise wouldn't get it.

Modality Recommendations for Pes Planus, Pes Cavus

MODALITY	RECOMMENDATION
Deep tissue massage	Indicated; work slowly and deeply with plantar and associated fascias, lower leg muscles and compartments.
Lymphatic drainage	Supportive.
Polarity	S/R/D: Indicated.
PNF/MET/stretching	Indicated in all stages.
Reflexology	Indicated if no foot inflammation is present.
Shiatsu	Indicated. Treat all meridians and extensions in feet. Use all stretches and joint movements in feet.
Swedish massage	Indicated.
Trigger point therapy	Indicated.

See Chapter 1 for a brief description of each modality, including definitions of abbreviations.

Plantar Fasciitis

Definition: What Is It?

Plantar fasciitis is a condition involving pain at the plantar fascia, which stretches from the calcaneus to the proximal phalanges on the plantar surface of the foot. While *-itis* implies that this is an inflammatory condition, it is probably related to the degeneration of collagen rather than to chronic inflammation.

Demographics: Who Gets It?

This is a common problem; most heel pain is diagnosed as plantar fasciitis. Up to 2 million cases are reported each year, and that includes only people who seek treatment.[47] It affects men and women equally, and though children can get it, adults are far more susceptible because their plantar fascia has generally lost some of its youthful elasticity.

Two populations seem to be at highest risk for developing plantar fasciitis: runners (some estimates are that up to 10% of runners have plantar fasciitis at some time) and nonathletes who may be overweight, especially if a sudden change in activity puts unusual stress on the foot.[48]

Plantar Fasciitis in Brief

Pronunciation: PLAN-tar fah-she-Y-tis

What is it?
Plantar fasciitis is a condition caused by repeated microscopic injury to the plantar fascia of the foot.

How is it recognized?
Plantar fasciitis is acutely painful after prolonged immobility. Then the pain recedes but comes back with extended use. It feels sharp and bruiselike, usually at the anterior calcaneus.

Is massage indicated or contraindicated?
Plantar fasciitis indicates massage. Bodywork can help release tension in deep calf muscles that put strain on the plantar fascia; it can also help to affect the quality of collagen at the site of the injury.

Etiology: What Happens?

The plantar fascia is a tough, thick band of connective tissue that supports the medial longitudinal arch of the foot. It is thickest in the middle of the band and thinner on the medial and lateral aspects. It is vulnerable to damage through anatomic and repetitive biomechanical forces.

Being overweight can predispose someone to plantar fasciitis, as can wearing shoes without good arch and lateral support. Unequal leg length and flat or pronated feet are associated with this problem, as are jammed arches. Very tight calf muscles are also contributing factors, especially for runners. And plantar fasciitis may occur as a secondary complication to an underlying disorder such as gout, rheumatoid arthritis, or diabetes.

When the plantar fascia is overused or stressed, its fibers tend to fray or become disorganized (Figure 3.42). Recent research indicates that plantar fasciitis is not usually an inflammatory condition but rather the degeneration of the collagen matrix of the plantar aponeurosis. This finding puts plantar fasciitis more in the category of tendinosis than tendinitis. The absence of acute inflammation has some implications for determining the best treatment options, so it is an important point to consider.

Radiographs of people with plantar fasciitis often show that a bone spur has developed at the attachment to the calcaneus. It was once assumed that these bone spurs caused the pain of plantar fasciitis. It is now clear that the chronic irritation of injured fascia stimulates the growth of bone spurs, not that bone spurs cause fascial irritation. Furthermore, up to 15% of the population with no heel pain shows bone spurs on the calcaneus, so the automatic assumption that these are always the source of heel pain has been dropped.

The pain that accompanies plantar fasciitis occurs when the foot has been immobile for several hours and then used. The fibers of the fascia begin to knit together during rest and are irritated again each time the foot goes into even gentle weight-bearing dorsiflexion.

Signs and Symptoms

Plantar fasciitis follows a distinctive pattern that makes it easy to identify. It is acutely painful for the first few steps every morning. Then the pain subsides or disappears altogether but becomes a problem again with prolonged standing, walking, or running. A sharp bruised feeling either just anterior to the calcaneus on the plantar surface or deep in the arch of the foot often marks this disorder.

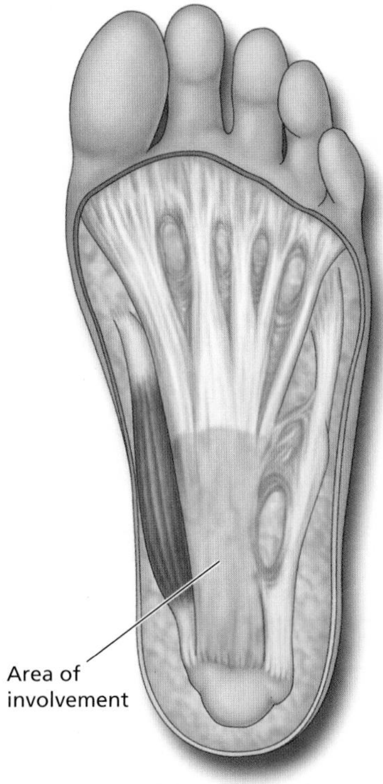

Figure 3.42. Plantar fasciitis.

Treatment

The most important thing to do for plantar fasciitis is to remove the tensions that cause the plantar fascia to be injured every morning when the foot first hits the floor. This can be accomplished in a number of ways. Warming and massaging the foot and lower leg before getting out of bed can make the tissue more flexible. Shoe inserts can keep the foot from going into deep dorsiflexion; these should be in all shoes, including bedroom slippers. Someone with plantar fasciitis should *never* go barefoot until the fascia can stretch without tearing. Another helpful device is a night splint that holds the foot in a slightly dorsiflexed position. This allows the plantar fascia fibers to knit in a way that won't be stressed and retorn so easily.

Nonsteroidal and topical anti-inflammatories, ice, stretching, and deep massage to the calf muscles and at the site of the irritation are frequently prescribed for plantar fasciitis. Corticosteroid injections are sometimes given if other interventions are unsuccessful, but steroids damage the fat pads on the heels and may weaken the collagen fibers and increase the risk of plantar fascia rupture, so they are used only sparingly. Shockwave ***lithotripsy***, similar to that used to break up kidney stones, is being used with some success for plantar fasciitis. As a last-ditch option surgery may be performed to divide the plantar fascia.

No single treatment is universally effective; each patient must experiment with the treatments that meet his or her own needs. Most people eventually find relief, but it may take 6 to 18 months before all symptoms are resolved.

Massage?

Plantar fasciitis responds well to bodywork. Massage is often suggested both to decrease tension in the deep calf muscles and to have an organizing influence on collagen fibers within the plantar fascia itself.

Modality Recommendations for Plantar Fasciitis

MODALITY	RECOMMENDATION
Deep tissue massage	Indicated when subacute; work with crural fascia and compartments, then muscles and tendons to foot. Use ROM at ankle and toes.
Lymphatic drainage	Supportive if used after standard massage treatment.
Polarity	S: Indicated. R/D: Work gently while acute; otherwise indicated.
PNF/MET/stretching	Indicated in all stages.
Reflexology	Locally contraindicated with severe pain; otherwise use light pressure with shorter and more frequent sessions.
Shiatsu	Indicated. Treat all meridians and extensions in feet. Use all stretches and joint movements in feet.
Swedish massage	Indicated.
Trigger point therapy	Locally contraindicated while acute; indicated while subacute.

See Chapter 1 for a brief description of each modality, including definitions of abbreviations.

Scleroderma

Definition: What Is It?

Scleroderma is a disease in which fibroblasts in the smallest blood vessels produce abnormal amounts of collagen. This frequently occurs in the skin, hence the name: *sclero* (Greek for *hard*) *–derma* (Greek for *skin*), but other tissues and organs may also be affected.

Demographics: Who Gets It?

Scleroderma is considered by most experts to be an autoimmune disease. Like many other autoimmune disorders, scleroderma affects women more often than men; in this case during the peak years for diagnosis (age 30 to 55) the ratio of women to men is 3 or 4 to 1. It is a relatively rare disease, affecting approximately 300,000 people in the United States.[49] Some forms of scleroderma are slightly more common in some groups, but overall its incidence is about the same across ethnic groups. It is rare in children and elderly people.

Scleroderma in Brief

What is it?
Scleroderma is a chronic autoimmune disorder involving damage to small blood vessels. It leads to abnormal accumulations of collagen in the skin and other tissues.

How is it recognized?
Scleroderma has varied symptoms, depending on which tissues are involved. The most common outward signs are edema followed by hardening and thickening of the skin, usually of the hands and face. Lesions may be oval or linear. Other symptoms are determined by what other organs are affected.

Is massage indicated or contraindicated?
Scleroderma may indicate massage if circulatory and kidney damage is not advanced. Clients who are not capable of keeping up with the changes circulatory massage brings about may benefit from bodywork with less mechanical impact.

Etiology: What Happens?

Scleroderma is the result of an immune system attack against the lining of small blood vessels, the arterioles, capillaries, and venules. Damage to these tiny blood vessels causes local edema and the stimulation of nearby fibroblasts to spin out huge amounts of type III collagen, the basis for scar tissue. Eventually the edema subsides, but the scar tissue deposits remain hard and unyielding for years at a time. Scleroderma takes two forms: local and systemic.

Local scleroderma When scleroderma is local, the areas of damage are limited to the skin. The initial edema may last for several weeks or months, the thickening of the skin may accumulate over a course of about 3 years, and then the symptoms gradually stabilize or even reverse. Local scleroderma is often discussed in two forms:

- *Morphea scleroderma* takes the shape of discrete oval patches that develop on the trunk, face, or extremities. The lesions first appear as areas where the skin seems dry and thick. Eventually they become pale in the center and purplish around the edges.
- *Linear scleroderma* appears as a discolored line or band on a leg or arm or over the forehead. In this location it may be called **coup de sabre** because it resembles a sword-fight scar.

Systemic scleroderma When scleroderma is a systemic problem, blood vessel damage occurs in the skin but also in other organs and systems. CREST syndrome (see Signs and Symptoms, discussed later) is usually a part of systemic scleroderma. Tissues most at risk are in the digestive tract, heart and circulatory system, kidneys, lungs, and various parts of the musculoskeletal system, especially synovial membranes in joints and around tendons. When systemic scleroderma affects the lungs, kidneys, or heart, the prognosis becomes much more serious. This disease may stabilize and even reverse itself, but it can also be fatal. Systemic scleroderma is also called "systemic sclerosis", and it is recognized in three forms.

- *Limited systemic scleroderma* has a slow onset and begins as CREST syndrome but may eventually infiltrate internal organs.
- *Diffuse scleroderma* has a more sudden onset and earlier involvement of internal organs.
- *Sine scleroderma* doesn't involve the skin at all; it only involves internal organs. (*Sine* means *without*.)

Causes

The cause of scleroderma is unknown, but several contributing factors have been identified. Abnormal immune responses and chronic inflammation stimulate the fibroblasts to produce excessive collagen. Some patients have accumulated *chimeric* cells that contain genes not only of the affected person but of someone else as well. Probably they are leftover fetal material from pregnancies that may date from many years previously.

Other factors associated with scleroderma include exposure to specific chemicals, including vinyl chloride, epoxy resins, uranium, and aromatic hydrocarbons. Organic solvents, silica, and viral infections (especially with cytomegalovirus or human herpesvirus 5) are also being examined as environmental triggers.

Signs and Symptoms

Scleroderma can produce a huge variety of symptoms, depending on which blood vessels are under attack. The term *CREST syndrome* has been coined as a mnemonic for the most common scleroderma symptoms:

- **C:** *Calcinosis* refers to accumulation of calcium deposits in the skin, especially in the fingers.
- **R:** *Raynaud phenomenon* is a result of impaired circulation and vascular spasm in the hands.
- **E:** *Esophageal dysmotility* refers to sluggishness of the digestive tract and chronic gastric reflux.
- **S:** *Sclerodactyly* is hardening of the fingers, a result of the accumulation of scar tissue in the hands (Figure 3.43).
- **T:** *Telangiectasia* is a discoloration of the skin caused by permanently stretched and damaged capillaries. It is also known as "spider veins".

Other symptoms of systemic scleroderma include skin ulcers in which circulation prevents normal nutrition for healthy cells, changes in pigmentation, and hair loss in the affected patches. Muscles may become weak, while tendons and tendinous sheaths become swollen. Lungs may accumulate edema or fibrosis where blood vessels are under attack. Heart pain, arrhythmia, and heart failure may develop as the heart tries to push blood through a system that cannot accommodate it. And kidneys, working under high blood pressure and with damaged arterioles, may fail. Trigeminal neuralgia and carpal tunnel syndrome may develop as a result of nerve entrapment. Finally, Sjögren syndrome (pathologically dry mucous membranes) may be a part of the picture.

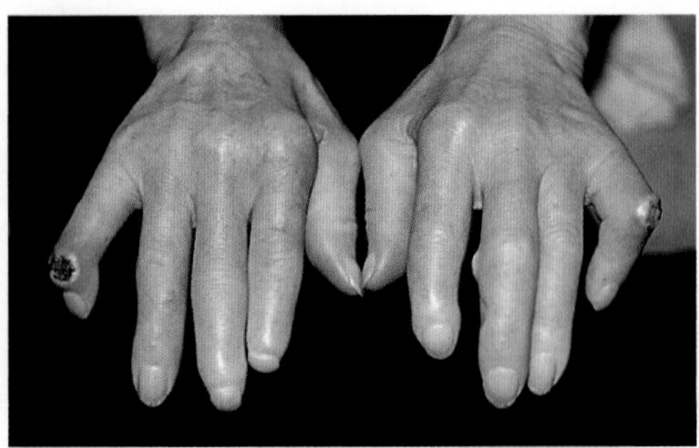

Figure 3.43. Scleroderma.

Treatment

Treatment for scleroderma is directed at managing the symptoms and complications of the disease. Calcium channel blockers may be recommended for Raynaud phenomenon; angiotensin-converting enzyme (ACE) inhibitors and diuretics for kidney function; antacids for gastric reflux; nonsteroidal anti-inflammatories for muscle and joint pain. Other drugs have been developed to prolong and improve lung function. DMARDs may be prescribed to suppress immune system overactivity. Physical or occupational therapies are employed to maintain flexibility in the hands. Patients are usually advised to avoid smoking, cold conditions, and spicy foods to minimize symptoms.

Massage?

Scleroderma presents very differently in each client. One person may have some stiffness and coldness in her hands, while another may be undergoing dialysis because her kidneys are failing. The decision about massage in the context of scleroderma must be based on the client's circulatory health and resiliency. It is inappropriate to try to mechanically push fluid through a system whose blood vessels are either inflamed or severely scarred. Bodywork that does not challenge fluid flow but works to restore immune system balance, however, can be beneficial.

MODALITY RECOMMENDATIONS FOR SCLERODERMA

MODALITY	RECOMMENDATION
Deep tissue massage	Contraindicated while acute; otherwise work with health care team. May help with contractures.
Lymphatic drainage	Supportive.
Polarity	S: Indicated. R/D: Supportive within client's limitations and comfort.
PNF/MET/stretching	Supportive.
Reflexology	Indicated; work all glands and solar plexus points.
Shiatsu	Indicated. Treat K/TH/SP for immune system.
Swedish massage	Supportive; stay within client's activity limitations and pain tolerance.
Trigger point therapy	Locally contraindicated; otherwise supportive,

Tendinopathies

Definition: What Are They?

Tendinopathies are injury and damage to tendons. The injury process has a lot in common with strains, sprains, and tenosynovitis. In fact, these conditions may sometimes be difficult to delineate from each other.

Etiology: What Happens?

Tendons are made primarily of type I collagen fibers suspended in liquid ground substance. A small number of elastin fibers are woven into the structure to lend some limited stretch and

> **Tendinopathies in Brief**
> Pronunciation: ten-dih-NOP-ath-ez
>
> **What are they?**
> Tendinopathies are injuries or damage to tendons. While it is possible for them to involve acute inflammation (as indicated in the traditional term *tendinitis*), most long-term tendon injuries are probably related to collagen degeneration rather than inflammation. The term for this condition is *tendinosis*.
>
> **How are they recognized?**
> Pain and loss of range of motion are often present with tendinopathies. Pain is exacerbated by resisted exercise of the damaged muscle-tendon unit.
>
> **Is massage indicated or contraindicated?**
> Tendinopathies indicate massage. If they are acute, lymph drainage techniques may help to limit and resolve inflammation. When inflammation is not present, massage may influence the production of useful scar tissue, reduce adhesions and edema, and reestablish range of motion.

rebound, but the bulk of tendons are dense, linearly arranged thick collagen fibers. Healthy tendons look hard, shiny and white.

When tendons are injured, a number of changes in the tissue occur. Acute injuries involve inflammatory cells (various types of white blood cells), edema, and pain; the correct term in this situation is *tendinitis*. But histological studies have revealed that most tendinopathies do not involve acute inflammation. Rather, they are conditions in which the collagen degenerates and the tendon loses its weight-bearing capacity. This situation is more correctly termed ***tendinosis***, or pathologic condition of the tendon.[50]

The causes for the chronic degenerative processes of tendinosis are probably a combination of intrinsic and extrinsic factors. Intrinsic factors can include direct or shearing forces transferred through the tendon, overuse without recovery time, poor flexibility, underlying disease, or a history of corticosteroid injection. Extrinsic factors can include training errors of athletes, problems with equipment, or a fall or blow that damages the tendon from the outside.

Tendinosis has a particular appearance, both to the naked eye and under the microscope. While healthy tendons are white and shiny, tendinosis looks dull, gray or brown, and soft. Microscopy shows more liquid ground substance in a structure with tendinosis than in a healthy tendon. The collagen fibers are clearly disrupted and discontinuous. Fibroblasts are active, and excessive blood vessels are present also, probably to provide the fibroblasts with fuel to produce more collagen and more ground substance. The collagens produced by fibroblasts in tendinosis tend to be type III fibers, which are thinner and weaker than the normal type I fibers of healthy tendons. The result is that the affected tendon becomes weaker and is increasingly vulnerable to damage and a repeating cycle of microtrauma and poor-quality collagen production.

Notably absent in this scenario are inflammatory white blood cells. This has some repercussions for massage therapists but even more significant ones for other medical professionals who deal with this type of soft tissue injury.

Tendon damage can occur anywhere in the tendon, but the tenoperiosteal junction and the musculotendinous junction are most vulnerable to mechanical stresses. The Achilles tendon, rotator cuff tendons, and tendons of the extensor compartment of the forearm (associated with tennis elbow) have been studied most closely in this research.

Signs and Symptoms

The symptoms of tendinopathies are very similar to those of muscle strains, though they may be more intense. The acute stage may show some heat and swelling, depending on which tendons are affected. Most tendon swelling is not visible or palpable with a few exceptions: the Achilles tendon and the posterior tibialis tendon at the medial ankle may swell significantly with injury. In all stages of tendinosis, stiffness and pain are present on resistive movements and in stretching.

Treatment

The quality of the healing of a damaged tendon depends largely on what happens with the production of new collagen. New understanding of the process of tendinosis has changed the expected outcome for these injuries. While athletes and others used to be told that their healing process would be completed within a few weeks, it is now clear that it may take significantly longer to return a degenerated tendon to its previous weight-bearing capacity.

Because inflammation turns out not to be a significant issue in most stubborn tendon injuries, the use of anti-inflammatories is being reconsidered. Corticosteroid injections into damaged tendons have been shown to offer short-term pain relief but no long-term benefits; indeed, they may in fact increase the risk of future injury by weakening existing collagen.[51]

Rest, ice, stretching, and carefully gauged exercise turns out to be the best treatment for these injuries. Emphasis on eccentric contractions is particularly useful to rebuild a damaged tendon and can often make planned surgery unnecessary.[52] Some orthopedists recommend that patients wear a splint or brace to help bear some of the force of a damaged tendon, but not all experts agree on this strategy.

Massage?

Tendinopathies definitely indicate massage. If the injury is acute, this phase must be respected to allow the body to begin the process of cleaning up debris and laying down new fibers in peace. Practitioners familiar with lymph drainage techniques may be able to limit the accumulation of edema and minimize scar tissue. In chronic tendinopathy, massage has been shown to be valuable for the mechanical action it can have on poorly formed collagen fibers and for its influence on local tissue nutrition.[53]

MODALITY RECOMMENDATIONS FOR TENDINOPATHIES

MODALITY	RECOMMENDATION
Deep tissue massage	Indicated while subacute. Work slowly around affected area to reduce tension in fascia.
Lymphatic drainage	Indicated while subacute.
Polarity	S: Indicated. R/D: Locally contraindicated while acute; otherwise supportive.
PNF/MET/stretching	Indicated in all stages.
Reflexology	Indicated.
Shiatsu	Indicated in all stages.
Swedish massage	Locally contraindicated while acute; proximal centripedal flushing can help decrease swelling. Supportive when subacute.
Trigger point therapy	Locally contraindicated; otherwise supportive.

See Chapter 1 for a brief description of each modality, including definitions of abbreviations.

Tenosynovitis

Definition: What Is It?

Tenosynovitis is irritation and inflammation of tendons that pass through a synovial sheath.

Etiology: What Happens?

Some tendons have to pass through very narrow, crowded passageways or around sharp corners to get to their bony attachments. Without any lubrication those tendons and their neighbors would soon be worn and frayed. But they do have lubrication, provided by special sheaths made of connective tissue and lined with synovial membrane: tenosynovial sheaths. The syn-

Tenosynovitis in Brief

Pronunciation: ten-o-sin-o-VY-tis

What is it?

Tenosynovitis is inflammation of a tendon and/or its surrounding tenosynovial sheath. It can develop wherever a tendon passes through a sheath but is especially common in the wrist and hand.

How is it recognized?

Pain, heat, and stiffness mark the acute stage of tenosynovitis. In the subacute stage only stiffness and pain may be present. The tendon may feel or sound gritty as it moves through the sheath. It is difficult to bend fingers with tenosynovitis but even harder to straighten them.

Is massage indicated or contraindicated?

Tenosynovitis contraindicates massage in the acute stage of inflammation and indicates massage when the swelling has subsided.

ovial sheath may also be called the *epitenon.* As the tendon or group of tendons pass through the epitenon, synovial fluid is secreted to provide lubrication and ease of movement (Figure 3.44).

Repetitive stress, percussive movement, or constant twisting can irritate the tendons inside tenosynovial sheaths. The sheath may become inflamed and then shrink around the tendons to inhibit freedom of movement. A cycle of stiffness followed by irritating movement, which creates more stiffness, pain, and inflammation, may develop.

Causes

Tenosynovitis is usually caused by trauma, repetitive movement, or infection, especially with gonorrhea. It can happen anywhere synovial sheaths protect tendons: the wrist, the ankle, the long head of the biceps, or near the thumb, where it has a special name: *de Quervain tenosynovitis.* Tenosynovitis also occurs as a complication of other diseases, such as rheumatoid arthritis, gout, or diabetes.

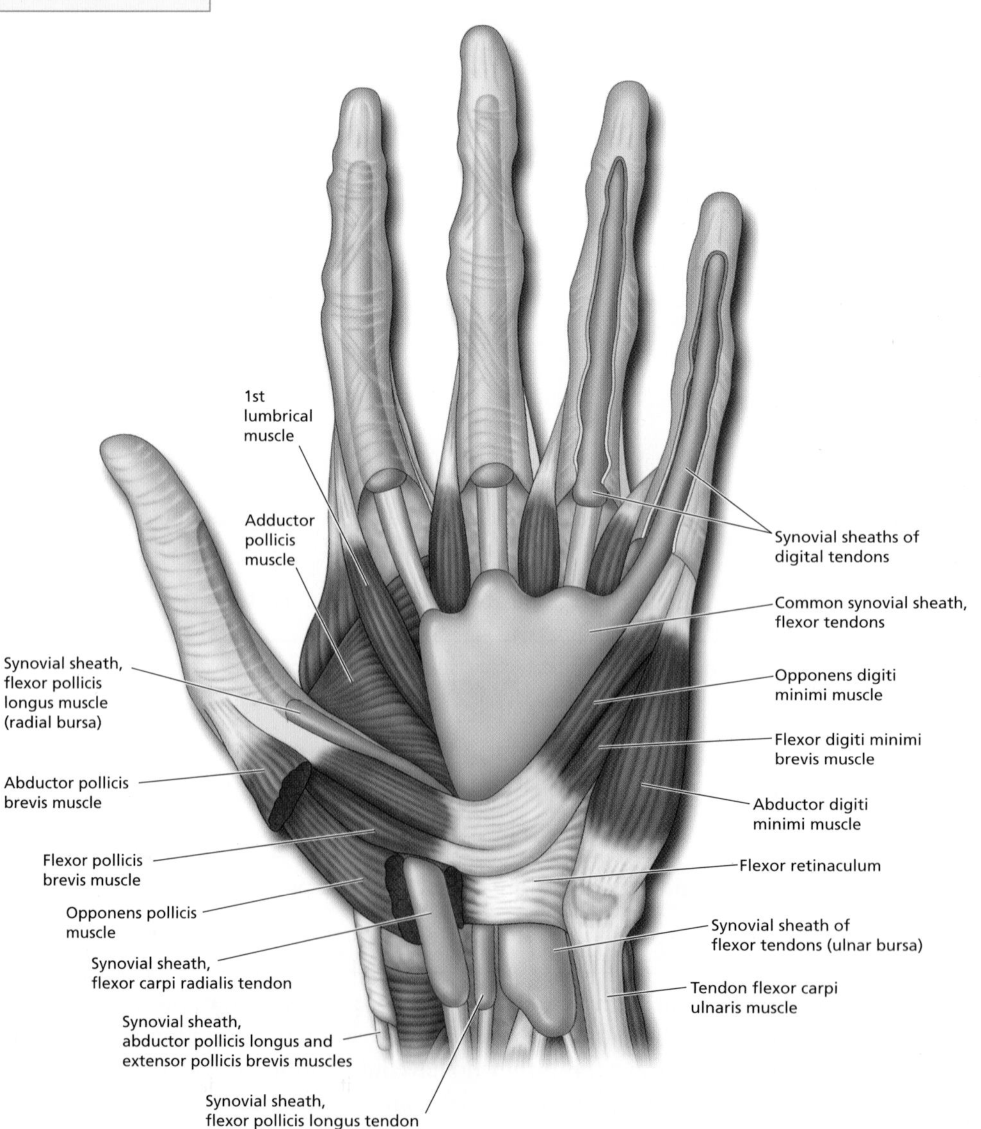

Figure 3.44. Synovial sheaths allow groups of tendons to slide easily over each other.

Signs and Symptoms

Symptoms of tenosynovitis are predictable: local pain, sometimes with swelling, heat, and a palpable nodule at the base of the fingers. When it occurs in the hands, the pain and limitation are often focused at the PIP. It maybe difficult flex the joint, but extending it is even harder; excessive force must be applied to slide the tendon through its sheath, and the joint usually straightens with a sudden pop. A grinding noise or gritty feeling called crepitus occurs when the affected joint is moved.

Movement of the tendon through the sheath tends to exacerbate the problem, but lack of movement decreases the production of synovial fluid. It can be a very frustrating condition because nothing seems to make it better.

Treatment

If the synovium is inflamed because of infection, the obvious course is to treat it with antibiotics. Noninfectious tenosynovitis is typically treated with anti-inflammatory drugs, then injected with steroids, and if that is unsuccessful, the synovium is surgically split.

Massage?

When tenosynovitis is acute, it is an inflammatory condition, and the inflammation is confined to a very small, crowded space. This makes bodywork counterproductive.

When inflammation is not acute, however, massage can help to support the production of synovial fluid, flush out toxins, and create very specific movements of structures against each other to prevent the accumulation of scar tissue and/or adhesions. Massage may or may not actually solve the problem of irritation inside the synovial sheath, but it can improve the nutrition and freedom of movement available to the affected structures.

Modality Recommendations for Tenosynovitis

MODALITY	RECOMMENDATION
Deep tissue massage	Indicated while subacute. Work slowly around affected area to reduce tension in fascia.
Lymphatic drainage	Indicated while subacute.
Polarity	S: Indicated. R/D: Locally contraindicated while acute; otherwise supportive.
PNF/MET/stretching	Indicated in all stages.
Reflexology	Indicated.
Shiatsu	Indicated. Treat SP,K,TH,PC meridians and extensions at local area with light pressure.
Swedish massage	Locally contraindicated while acute; proximal centripedal flushing can help decrease swelling. Supportive when subacute.
Trigger point therapy	Locally contraindicated; otherwise supportive.

See Chapter 1 for a brief description of each modality, including definitions of abbreviations.

Whiplash in Brief

What is it?
Whiplash is an umbrella term referring to a collection of soft tissue injuries that may occur with cervical acceleration and then deceleration. These injuries include sprained ligaments, strained muscles, damaged cartilage and joint capsules, and TMJ problems. Although whiplash technically refers to soft tissue injury, damage to other structures, including vertebrae, discs, and the central nervous system, frequently occurs at the same time.

How is it recognized?
Symptoms of whiplash vary according to the nature of the injuries. Pain at the neck and referring into the shoulders and arms, along with chronic headaches, is the primary indicator.

Is massage indicated or contraindicated?
An acute whiplash injury contraindicates circulatory or mechanical massage. In the subacute and maturation phases of scar tissue formation, however, massage along with chiropractic or manipulation can be important contributors to a positive resolution to the problem.

Whiplash

Definition: What Is It?

Whiplash, or CAD (cervical acceleration-deceleration) is a broad term used to refer to a mixture of injuries, including sprains, strains, and joint trauma. Bone fractures, herniated discs, and concussion are commonly seen along with these soft tissue injuries and so are often addressed simultaneously. Whiplash injuries are usually, but not always, associated with car accidents in which the head whips backward and then forward in rapid succession (Figure 3.45).

Demographics: Who Gets It?

Whiplash injuries are common in this country. It is estimated that 85% of neck pain derives from a neck injury. About 1 million cases of whiplash related to motor vehicle accidents are recorded each year. About 15.5 million people in the United States have had whiplash.[54]

Etiology: What Happens?

The nature of damage incurred by whiplash accidents depends on many variables, including the direction of impact, the speed with which the vehicles were moving, the relative weight of the vehicles involved, whether the individual was wearing a seatbelt, the position of the individual's head, and whether the person was aware of the impending impact and had time to brace. Analysis of rear-impact accidents shows that as the momentum of the car seat forces the thorax forward, the head initially stays stable. About 100 milliseconds later, the head is propelled into flexion. The momentum of this movement is magnified by the leverage of the neck. At an impact of 20 miles per hour the maximum acceleration of the head has been measured at 12*g*![54]

Accidents of this nature put the cervical muscles (especially the sternocleidomastoid, scalenes, and splenius cervicis) at risk for strains. Supraspinous and intertransverse spinal ligaments are frequently stretched. Two ligaments that massage can't touch, the anterior and posterior longitudinal ligaments, may also be traumatized.

Other structures that may be injured with CAD include the capsules of the facet joints; the esophagus and larynx; spinal discs, which may herniate or rupture; vertebrae, which may subluxate or fracture; the temporomandibular joint; the spinal cord, which may be compressed or stretched; and the brain, which can be bruised and damaged in concussion.

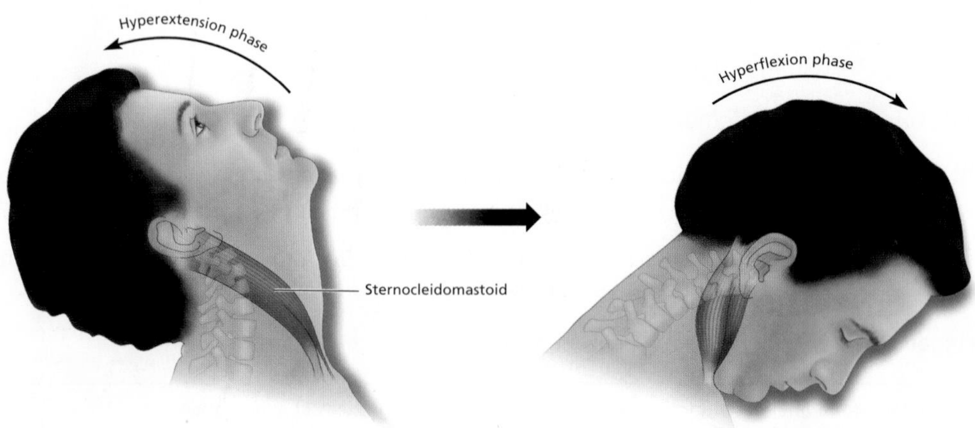

Figure 3.45. Cervical acceleration and deceleration: whiplash.

Signs and Symptoms

A lot of crossover exists between what may be considered a symptom of whiplash and what is a complication, or resulting disorder, so the following is a list of both. Basic signs and symptoms include head and neck pain, which may radiate into the trunk or arms; loss of range of motion; and paresthesia. One of the curious aspects of whiplash is that it is common for symptoms to be delayed for days, weeks, and occasionally months before coming to full intensity. This phenomenon is not well understood.

- *Ligament sprains.* The supraspinous and intertransverse ligaments, which connect the vertebrae to each other, are at risk for injury in a whiplash type of accident. These ligaments can refer pain up over the head, into the chest, and down the arms. It is important to know about these structures because referred pain from ligaments can easily be misdiagnosed as pain from nerve damage. Ligament sprains often take a long time to heal, and they tend to accumulate excess scar tissue. They may be the most common cause of lasting pain and dysfunction when a whiplash injury occurs.
- *Damaged facet joint capsules.* One area of study in whiplash research is the role of facet joint capsules. It has been found that these structures are often irritated in CAD events and that they, like spinous ligaments, can refer pain to the head. Furthermore, these joint capsules are well equipped with nociceptors that may intensify pain messages sent to the spinal cord. They also have proprioceptors that can send confusing messages to the brain, leading to dizziness or disorientation.
- *Misaligned cervical vertebrae.* This generally shows clearly on radiographs. Vertebrae may be displaced to the front, back, or side or rotated one way or another. In some very extreme cases fractures may occur. Left untreated or incompletely treated, misaligned vertebrae with lax ligaments and lack of structural support may develop spondylosis.
- *Damaged disc.* This is not inevitable, but it may happen that the neck ligaments are so stressed in a trauma of this force that the annulus cracks, allowing the nucleus pulposus to seep into spaces where it doesn't belong. Car wrecks and other major traumas of this type are the easiest way to cause a herniation in the cervical region.
- *Spasm.* When a neck injury is acute, the paraspinals and other neck muscles go into spasm to splint, or give extra support to, the stretched neck ligaments. But this reaction has a tendency to outlive its usefulness. Spasm of neck muscles also significantly limits range of motion and blood flow to nearby connective tissues.
- *Trigger points.* Traumatized muscles often develop trigger points: local tight areas that refer pain, often into the head, causing chronic headaches. This is one form of MPS.
- *Neurological symptoms.* These can include dizziness, blurred vision, abnormal smell or taste, tinnitus (ringing in the ears), or loss of hearing. These signs indicate cranial trauma: the brain has been bruised and may have some internal bleeding. This is usually the result of a specific blow, hitting the head on the steering wheel, for instance, but postconcussion syndrome can also happen without direct impact.
- *TMJ disorders.* Again, direct impact of the jaw on a steering wheel or dashboard can damage the TMJ, but some research suggests that the joint can be traumatized just by the rapid acceleration and deceleration that accompany whiplash injuries. This is sometimes called "jawlash."
- *Headaches.* These arise for a variety of reasons, including but not limited to referred pain and trigger points from spasms in the neck, sprained ligaments that refer pain up over the head, irritated facet joint capsules, cranial bones that may be out of alignment, stress and its autonomic action on blood flow, muscle tightness in the neck and head, TMJ problems, and concussion.

Diagnosis

Some assumptions can be made about which precise structures have been injured based on whether the car wreck was a direct head-on or a rear-end collision. But these assumptions will not hold true if the impact occurred at an angle or if the person's head was turned at the moment of contact.

The techniques to measure the extent of injury (MRI, radiography, CT, nerve conduction velocity tests) are extremely valuable for evaluating one particular type of whiplash damage: direct mechanical nerve pressure. Pressure on a nerve causes **radicular pain**, or pain that radiates directly along the distribution of the affected nerve. Care must be taken, however, to delineate between what these tests show and what patients report: very frequently MRIs or radiographs show anomalies that don't actually create symptoms for the patient.

Unfortunately, much of the pain associated with whiplash injuries is not radicular pain but referred pain brought about by trauma to connective tissue and muscle tissue that feed into the same nerve root as the associated spinal nerve. This type of damage is much harder to quantify. It is best evaluated with good palpation skills that reveal information about local tenderness, muscle spasm, and trigger point activity.

Treatment

Neck collars are used for acute whiplash patients to take the stress off their wrenched ligaments and to try to reduce muscle spasm. But the sooner the injured structures are put back to use, the less scar tissue accumulates. Therefore, collars are strictly for short-term use, as this kind of immobilization can create more long-term problems than benefits.

Medical intervention typically focuses on pain relievers, anti-inflammatories, and muscle relaxants. These substances can change the quality of the tissues, so massage therapists should be aware when clients use them. Physical therapy and massage to strengthen injured neck muscles, reduce spasm, and deal with trigger points are usually recommended later in the recovery process.

Other treatments for whiplash depend on the type and severity of specific injuries. Research shows that about 40% of patients still have symptoms 3 months after their accident, while about 18% report symptoms 2 years after their accident.[53] The goal with treatment is to prevent these symptoms from becoming chronic pain, which is of course much harder to treat successfully.

Massage?

The acute stage of this injury contraindicates mechanical massage. This is an important phase of healing that massage therapists must not disrupt. Gentle reflexive work with the intention of balancing the autonomic nervous system rather than making changes in the tissue may ameliorate the emotional trauma and shock such an injury often incurs. As long as it doesn't disrupt the cellular activity at the site of the injury, this type of work is a fine idea.

If it has been established that no other serious disorder is present, such as a herniated disc or spinal fracture, chiropractic or manipulation alone can be sufficient to undo the damage done to the cervical vertebrae in a whiplash injury. But if muscle spasm is not addressed, bony adjustments are difficult to perform and often don't hold for long because the muscles simply pull the bones out of alignment again. Furthermore, in the absence of the circulation that can be stimulated by massage, the injured ligaments have little access to nutrition. They tend to accumulate masses of scar tissue that bind to other ligaments and other muscles sheaths, thus turning a temporary loss of range of motion into a permanent one.

Chiropractic or manipulative therapy *with* massage can yield good results, blending the best of soft tissue work (to prevent or reduce muscle spasm, scar tissue accumulation, adhesions, fibrosis and ischemia) with the best of bony alignment. It is fairly common for someone to emerge from a whiplash recovery with this kind of care in better shape than before the injury.

CASE HISTORY 3.2

Whiplash

Client X: The sneezer

A massage therapist met with a first-time client approximately 1 year after the client was in a car accident. The client was still in considerable pain. He was diagnosed with whiplash and was seeking massage under prescription from his doctor.

The therapist worked slowly and carefully and was encouraged by the client to go deeper into his neck muscles, all the way down to the transverse processes of the neck vertebrae. He felt better after the massage; his muscles were looser, and he had an improved range of motion.

Several hours later, the client sneezed. The force of the motion wrenched his neck and reinjured the tissues so that he was in greater pain, more spasm, and had much less range of motion than he had before his massage. He returned for another session, but it was ineffective at reducing his pain and dysfunction. He never sought massage again.

What is the moral here? It is utterly unclear whether the first massage put the client at risk for reinjuring himself just by sneezing. The therapist followed all the rules of good sense, worked under medical supervision, and let the client guide her into how much pressure felt comfortable. Yet it is necessary to entertain the possibility that the massage somehow *did* put the client at risk, even though the therapist was well informed and made what seemed to be the right decisions. No two people go through the same kind of healing process, and no two people respond to massage the same way. Massage therapists must weigh the benefits and risks of their work on a case-by-case basis. It is impossible to rely only on books and rules to make decisions about whether to give massage.

Modality Recommendations for Whiplash

MODALITY	RECOMMENDATION
Deep tissue massage	Contraindicated while acute. During recovery consult with health care team for best outcome; focus on paravertebral muscles and fascias.
Lymphatic drainage	Supportive.
Polarity	S: Indicated. R/D: Locally contraindicated while acute; otherwise indicated.
PNF/MET/stretching	Locally contraindicated while acute. Indicated when subacute if bone or nerve injury ruled out.
Reflexology	Indicated; work head, neck, throat, upper vertebrae points.
Shiatsu	Indicated. Treat SI, TH, BL, GB, LI, K meridians and extensions in the neck, shoulders, upper back, clavicle.
Swedish massage	Locally contraindicated while acute; indicated while subacute.
Trigger point therapy	Locally contraindicated while acute; indicated while subacute.

See Chapter 1 for a brief description of each modality, including definitions of abbreviations.

Carpal Tunnel Syndrome in Brief

What is it?
Carpal tunnel syndrome (CTS) is irritation of the median nerve as it passes under the transverse carpal ligament into the wrist. It can have any of several causes.

How is it recognized?
CTS can cause pain, tingling, numbness, and weakness in the part of the hand supplied by the median nerve.

Is massage indicated or contraindicated?
Depending on the underlying factors, some CTS cases respond well to massage. Work on or around the wrist must stop immediately if any symptoms are elicited. It is necessary to get a medical diagnosis in order to know which type of CTS is present.

Neuromuscular Disorders

Carpal Tunnel Syndrome

Definition: What Is It?

Carpal tunnel syndrome (CTS) is a set of signs and symptoms brought about by entrapment of the median nerve between the carpal bones of the wrist and the transverse carpal ligament that holds down the flexor tendons (Figure 3.46). The median nerve supplies the thumb, forefinger, middle finger, and half of the ring finger (Figure 3.47). If it is caught or squeezed in any way, it creates symptoms in the part of the hand the nerve supplies.

Demographics: Who Gets It?

CTS is the most common peripheral nerve compression syndrome. It affects up to 10% of adults at some point.[55] CTS is an occupational hazard for massage practitioners and anyone else who performs repetitive movements for several hours every day, including people who work with keyboards, string musicians, bakers, assembly line workers, and checkout clerks.

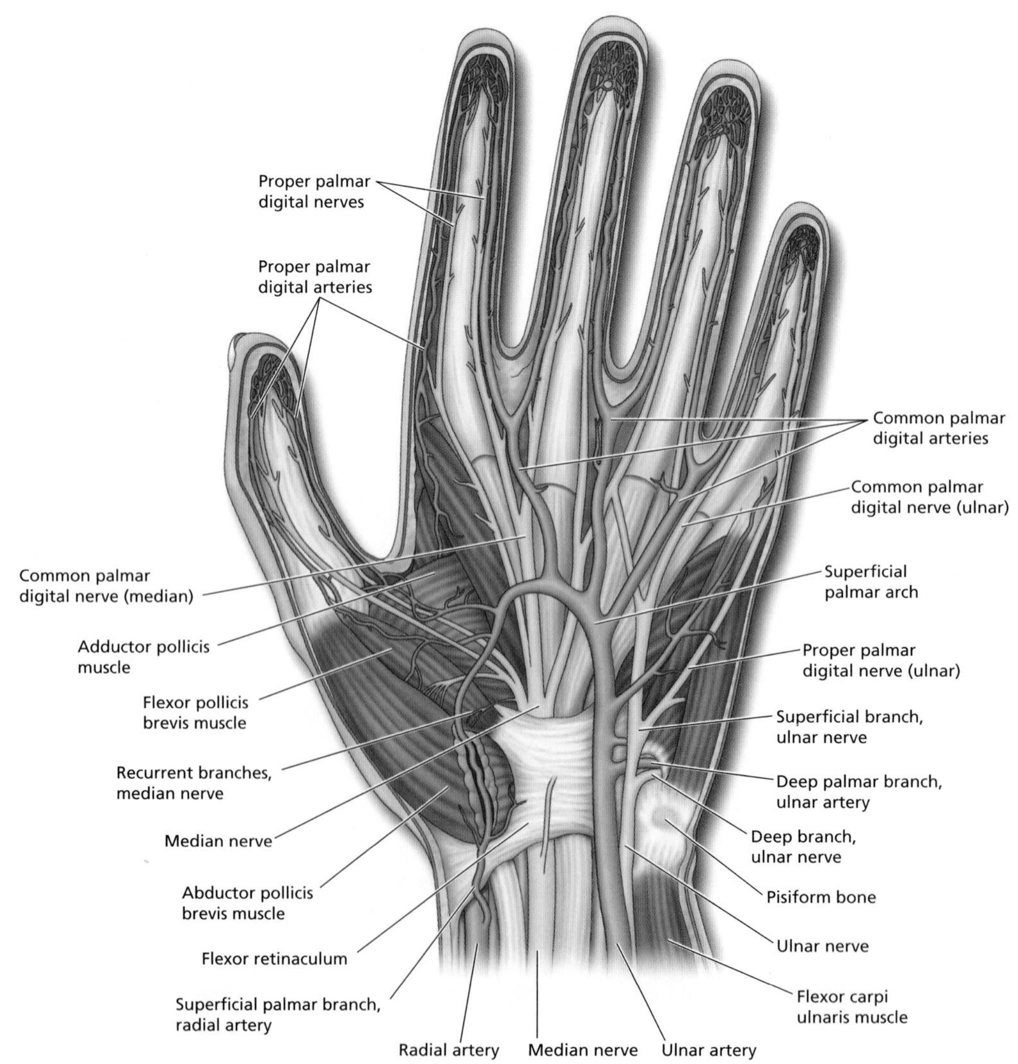

Figure 3.46. The carpal tunnel, formed by the transverse ligament (flexor retinaculum) and the carpal bones.

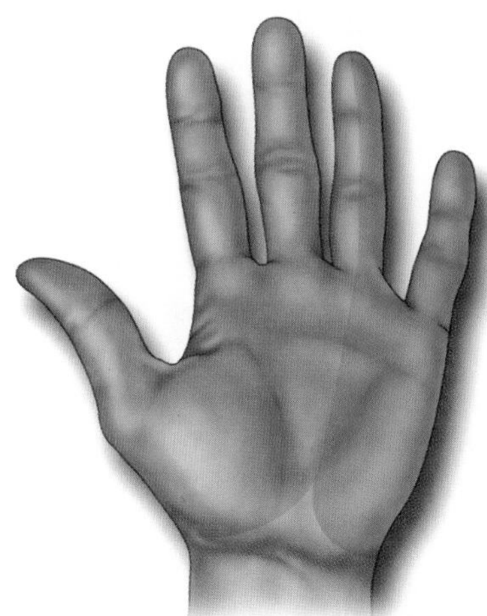

Figure 3.47. Carpal tunnel syndrome affects the thumb, index finger, middle finger, and half of the ring finger.

Women with CTS outnumber men by about 3 to 1; this may be because their carpal tunnels are smaller to begin with, and so less irritation may lead to symptoms.

Etiology: What Happens?

The source of the pain associated with carpal tunnel syndrome is debatable. While some experts claim that pressure directly on the nerve causes pain, others suggest that pressure impedes blood flow to the nerve, and that is the source of the problem.

Whether the damage is to the nerve itself or to its blood supply, pressure within the carpal tunnel may arise from several sources. To develop a treatment strategy (and to assess the appropriateness of massage), the aggravating factors must be determined.

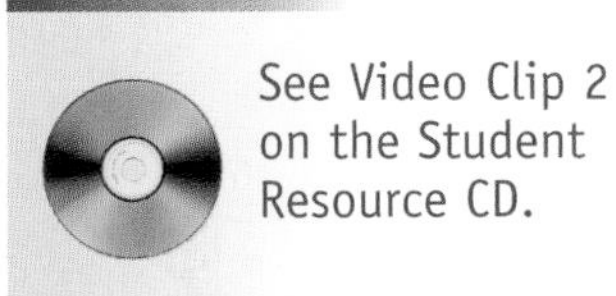

See Video Clip 2 on the Student Resource CD.

- *Edema.* Fluid retention, which is common for overweight people as well as menopausal and pregnant women, creates extra pressure in an area with no room to spare. The wrist is particularly susceptible because of its normal gravitational position; it's easy for fluid to pool here. CTS due to edema is usually bilateral and is quite common. It is most often treated with diuretics or other methods designed to help get rid of excess fluid.
- *Subluxation.* Sometimes the carpal bones, especially the capitate bone in the center of the distal row of carpal bones, subluxate toward the palmar side. This can put mechanical pressure on the median nerve that is not relieved by diuretics, anti-inflammatories, or any other drugs. This type of CTS is almost always unilateral. Manipulation is the treatment of choice, although the bones often move back into place back without intervention. Waiting for that to happen can be something of a gamble, though, because the longer the irritation goes on, the higher the chances of sustaining nerve damage and the less likely it is that the problem will resolve spontaneously.
- *Fibrotic buildup.* This is the most common variety of carpal tunnel syndrome. The human body simply wasn't designed to perform the same movements for 8 hours a day, 5 days a week. In an attempt to keep up with demands, the body tends to ***hypertrophy***, or grow bigger and thicker wherever we use it most. This is true of muscles and bones, and it also happens with the synovial sheaths at the wrist. When they thicken because of overuse, they press on anything else that has to travel through the tiny tunnel formed by the carpal bones and the transverse carpal ligament—namely, the median nerve. The ligament may also swell with chronic irritation, adding to the pressure on the median nerve.

CTS can also be a symptom or consequence of several other systemic diseases. Diabetes mellitus, hypothyroidism, lymphedema associated with cancer staging, acromegaly, rheumatoid arthritis, and gout can all involve pressure at the carpal tunnel.

Signs and Symptoms

Depending on the source and severity of the problem, CTS can manifest as tingling; pins and needles; burning, shooting pains; intermittent numbness; and weakness as innervation to the hand muscles is interrupted. The thenar pad may flatten out as the thumb muscles atrophy from lack of nerve stimulation. It is often worse at night, when people may sleep on their arm or turn their wrist into awkward positions. It can be painful enough to wake someone out of a deep sleep. If pressure is taken off the nerve promptly, symptoms tend to disappear. But the worst-case scenario is permanent damage to the median nerve resulting in some loss of muscle function and sensation in the hand.

The median nerve supplies the lateral aspect of the hand with sensation and motor function. About 90% of the fibers in the median nerve are sensory, and 10% are motor. This means that motor problems (weakness or atrophy) in the affected area may indicate more significant nerve damage than is seen with sensory problems alone.

Diagnosis

Carpal tunnel syndrome is generally diagnosed by the description of symptoms and two simple tests: *Tinel's test* involves tapping on the wrist while the hand is extended; ***Phalen's maneuver*** involves holding the wrist in flexion for 1 minute or more to see whether symptoms occur in this position. These are often followed by a nerve conduction test or electromyogram that measures nerve impulses passing through the wrist into the hand. Unfortunately, these tests are not conclusive.

One of the challenges with CTS is that many factors can contribute to pain or reduced sensation in the wrist and hand. All of them must be considered before reaching a conclusive diagnosis of carpal tunnel syndrome. The possibilities include but are not limited to the following:

- *Neck injury.* Herniated discs and irritated neck ligaments refer pain distally. The worse the irritation, the further the pain refers.
- *Thoracic outlet syndrome.* Nerve and vascular entrapment at the pectoralis minor and/or scalenes can create pain in the wrist.
- *Nerve entrapment elsewhere in the arm.* The pronator teres is especially likely to trap a piece of the median nerve between its attachments on the forearm. This can lead to symptoms in the wrist and hand, but it also tends to affect the forearm, whereas the symptoms of true CTS only radiate distally.
- *Nerve elongation elsewhere in the arm.* When nerves are inappropriately stretched along bones or around joints, they sustain damage and transmit pain signals.
- *Other wrist injuries.* These can include osteoarthritis, rheumatoid arthritis, tendinitis, and ligament sprains, all of which can cause pain in the wrist and hand and none of which will be affected by any of the standard treatments for CTS.
- *Double crush syndrome.* This is a situation in which the median nerve may be impeded at multiple sites. Research shows that compression at the neck or elbow can create enough irritation that only minimal compression at the wrist can cause significant symptoms.[56]

Treatment

Treatment for CTS often begins with a wrist splint. The goal is to keep the carpal tunnel in a neutral position (in which it is as open as possible) and to require less work from the supportive tissues. Steroidal or nonsteroidal anti-inflammatories may be prescribed. Corticosteroid injections into the wrist may also be recommended to reduce inflammation and melt excess connective tissue. Exercises to stretch and mobilize tight wrist tendons may be recommended. If the ligaments surrounding the wrist have become loose enough to allow nearby structures to become irritated, proliferant injections may be recommended to tighten them up.

If no other interventions are successful, CTS treatment culminates with surgery. The transverse carpal ligament is split, and some of the accumulated connective tissue is scraped away. Innovations in endoscopic surgery techniques allow surgeons to use tiny incisions and pencil-thin cameras to cut through the transverse ligament from the inside of the carpal tunnel without opening the rest of the tissues of the hand. This allows for a much shorter recovery time and a reduced risk of fresh scar tissue accumulation that would lead to a recurrence of symptoms.

Massage?

The appropriateness of massage depends on which kind of CTS the client has, and that determination is not a massage therapist's job. The most responsible choice then, is to work conservatively, check with the client's health care team, and monitor results. Edematous CTS responds well to massage that focuses on draining the forearm. Fibrotic CTS may or may not improve with massage, depending on how thick and where the fibrosis is. CTS due to a subluxation *may* respond to massage and traction, but wrist adjustments are *not* in the scope of practice of massage.

If work on or around the wrist creates symptoms, stop immediately! If, on the other hand, a client has some improvement, the therapist may be on the right track. Bodyworkers should proceed slowly, have a clear image of what should be accomplished, and work with a doctor for a definitive diagnosis.

Modality Recommendations for Carpal Tunnel Syndrome

MODALITY	RECOMMENDATION
Deep tissue massage	Contraindicated while acute; otherwise indicated. Work whole arm, shoulder girdle, neck. Use active movements of wrist and hand to assist release.
Lymphatic drainage	Supportive, especially after a focused standard massage treatment.
Polarity	S: Indicated. R/D: Indicated within client comfort.
PNF/MET/stretching	Indicated in all stages.
Reflexology	Locally contraindicated; work shoulder, chest, arm, sides of neck points.
Shiatsu	Indicated. Treat all meridians and extension in forearm, especially yin side. Hold carpal tunnel lightly; make sure carpals don't separate.
Swedish massage	Indicated if massage does not elicit symptoms; stay within pain tolerance.
Trigger point therapy	Locally contraindicated; otherwise supportive.

See Chapter 1 for a brief description of each modality, including definitions of abbreviations.

Disc Disease in Brief

What is it?
In disc disease the nucleus pulposus or the surrounding annulus fibrosus of an intervertebral disc protrudes in such a way that it puts pressure on nerve roots, the cauda equina, or the spinal cord.

How is it recognized?
The symptoms of nerve pressure include local back or neck pain, radiculopathy (pain along the dermatome), specific muscle weakness, paresthesia, and numbness.

Is massage indicated or contraindicated?
Back or neck pain that is not acutely inflamed or undiagnosed indicates massage with caution.

Disc Disease

Definition: What Is It?

Disc disease is an umbrella term referring to a collection of problems in which the nucleus pulposus and/or the annulus fibrosus extends beyond its normal borders. If the disc presses on the spinal cord or spinal nerve roots, pain will be present. If the bulge doesn't happen to interfere with nerve tissue, no symptoms may be present at all.

Etiology: What Happens?

A typical intervertebral disc is quite a complex package. It has an outer wrapping of three layers of very tough, hard material called the ***annulus fibrosus.*** This envelopes a soft, gelatinous center called the ***nucleus pulposus.*** Ideally, the nucleus should be roughly spherical, with the harder annulus layers forming flat surfaces above, below, and around the ball. This combination of textures gives the disc the advantages of strength and resiliency, which it needs to do its job of separating and cushioning the vertebrae (Figure 3.48). The spine is capable of bearing a great deal of weight, partly thanks to this arrangement of the discs.

The ring of annulus fibrosus is an arrangement of concentric circles of collagen fibers. These fibers are arranged in such a way that the tighter they're pulled, the stronger they become. On the other hand, the closer the vertebrae are, the looser (and weaker) the annulus is. This has great implications for the nucleus pulposus, which relies on a tight, solid exterior wall for support.

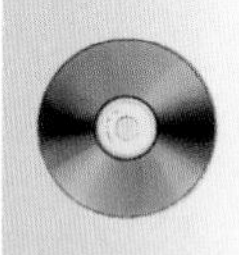

See Video Clip 3 on the Student Resource CD.

The annulus fibrosus is very strong, but studies show that it starts to degenerate sometime during the second or third decade of life. It can sustain multitudes of microtraumas, but they all contribute to setting the stage for future trouble. At the same time, the nucleus pulposus tends to shrink and dry with age. By the time most people are in their 50s, the nuclei of

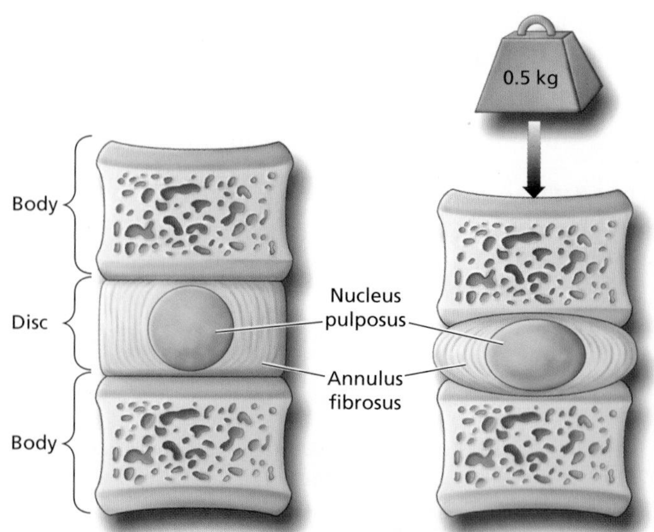

Figure 3.48. Intervertebral discs increase the weight-bearing capacity of the spine.

their discs are no longer soft and gelatinous; they have hardened and thinned. This process begins in the neck, where the discs are thinner but eventually also affects the more massive lumbar discs.

As the nucleus pulposus becomes thin and dry, more stress is placed on the annulus to bear weight and absorb shock. This puts the annulus at increased risk for tiny cracks or fissures. The whole degeneration of the disc then adds stress to the connecting vertebrae; osteophytes frequently develop on the lip of the vertebral bodies or around the facet joints. In this way disc disease is closely aligned to spondylosis, or osteoarthritis at the spine.

Compare and Contrast 3.4

Is It Really Disc Disease?

Disc injury is generally diagnosed through a combination of radiography, CT, myelography, and MRI. It is important to arrive at a clear diagnosis because similar symptoms may be exhibited by three other conditions that require vastly different treatment: spondylosis, ligament sprains, and, infrequently, bone tumors.

Spondylosis may lead to osteophytes that can put direct pressure on nerve tissue.

Irritated spinal ligaments running between spinous or transverse processes can refer pain along the same dermatomes as the nearby discs. Ligament sprains do *not* cause total numbness or specific muscle weakness, however, and they respond well to specific types of massage.

Bone tumors, by far the least common of these disorders, may involve growths in the spine that put mechanical pressure on nerve roots in much the same way that bulging discs may.

Individuals seeking a definitive diagnosis for their back, neck, arm, and/or leg pain may be frustrated by the fact that spondylosis, herniated discs, and irritated spinal ligaments may all exist simultaneously and in any combination. Here are some guidelines for sorting out the most common sources of pain.

FEATURES	DISC DISEASE	SPONDYLOSIS	LIGAMENT IRRITATION
Best diagnostic tool	MRI to see soft tissue distortion.	Radiography or CT scan for bony definition.	Skilled clinical exam to identify areas of injury.
On coughing, sneezing	Symptoms are elicited.	Symptoms don't change.	Symptoms don't change.
Things that make it worse	Sitting for long periods, flexion of the spine.	Extension of the spine.	Standing, twisting movements.
Pattern of weakness	Specific weakness in muscles supplied by affected nerve root.	Specific weakness in muscles supplied by affected nerve root.	General muscle weakness may appear gradually over time.
Pattern of pain	Shooting electrical pain along dermatome; numbness; reduced sensation; parasthesia. May be intermittent as disc changes shape and size.	Same symptoms as with disc disease dependably elicited when osteophytes press on nerve tissue.	Pain (usually not electrical) along dermatome; reduced sensation, paresthesia.

Types of Disc Problems

It is useful to be able to recognize the terminology for disc problems that may turn up in a diagnosis. Disc problems are generally discussed as three major issues:

Herniated nucleus pulposus In this case the nucleus pulposus extends beyond the posterior margin of the vertebral body. These injuries are most common in young adults. The nucleus may be damaged in these ways:

- *Bulge.* The entire disc protrudes symmetrically beyond the normal boundaries of the vertebral body.
- *Protrusion.* The nucleus pulposus extends out of the annulus at a specific location. If it protrudes posterolaterally (the most common version) it may press on nerve roots. If it protrudes straight back, it may press on the spinal cord or cauda equina.
- *Extrusion.* A small piece of the nucleus protrudes, with a narrow connection back to the body of the nucleus. In some cases the protrusion can separate from the nucleus altogether; this is called a *sequestration.*
- *Rupture.* The nucleus pulposus has burst and leaked its entire contents into the surrounding area.

Degenerative disc disease This refers to small, cumulative tears of the annulus, along with decreased disc height and dehydration of the nucleus. Eventually or in relation to a specific trauma, the annulus may press against a nerve root of the spinal cord. Degenerative disc disease is often considered a normal part of the aging process, although it is accelerated by smoking, obesity, and a sedentary lifestyle.

Internal disc disruption This condition is often related to trauma in addition to cumulative degenerative disc disease. In this case the nucleus protrudes through the annulus but stays within the boundaries of the whole disc.

Causes

Causes of disc injury may vary according to the general health of the connective tissues of the person involved. For some people a major trauma such as a car accident or a bad fall will damage the tissues enough to cause pain. People with weak, loose intervertebral ligaments have a higher risk of disc damage from ordinary everyday activity. The classic scenario for this kind of disc damage is an incident that involves simultaneous lifting and twisting.

Progression

When an intervertebral disc is injured and presses on nerve tissue, it's often because of a certain sequence of events on top of a lifetime of normal wear and tear. Here is a typical example of how a lumbar disc may herniate:

- A person bends over to pick up something heavy, a basket of laundry, for example. Going into trunk flexion flattens the anterior portion of the nucleus and opens up a posterior space while stretching the posterior fibers of the annulus.
- The person jerks into an erect posture, possibly twisting at the same time, while carrying a heavy load. Suddenly coming back into extension, especially while carrying something heavy, quickly redistributes the nucleus and shoots it into that posterior space with great force.
- The protruding section of nucleus presses against the weakest part of the posterior annulus and breaks through, which puts pressure on nerve roots. Or the force of the motion, combined with the brittleness of the annulus, causes the annulus to crack and put pressure on nerve tissue. The chemical substance of the nucleus pulposus creates a very extreme inflammatory response that can be a major contributor to the nerve pain that accompanies these injuries.

Many variations may develop on this theme. Discs that cause pain usually bulge posterolaterally because that is the path of least resistance in the tight space they inhabit, but they can also go to the left or the right side (Figure 3.49). Occasionally a disc bulges directly posteriorly, which puts pressure on the spinal cord or cauda equina rather than nerve roots. This is a very serious situation that can lead to permanent damage. But usually the protrusion is on nerve roots rather than the spinal cord, and the amount of herniated material is very small. It dries up and takes pressure off the nerve roots within a few days or weeks. This leaves the disc permanently thinned but doesn't necessarily lead to long-lasting problems.

L4 and L5 injuries are the most common with the kind of lifting or lifting and twisting injury described here. Cervical disc lesions are an occasional problem for car crash survivors; the action of a whiplash injury can be similar to the lifting and twisting injury. Thoracic injuries are possible but rarer, since the ribs make the thoracic spine much more stable than its cervical and lumbar counterparts.

Signs and Symptoms

Symptoms associated with disc disease arise from pressure on nerve tissue or from the exaggerated inflammatory response that occurs when the nucleus pulposus leaks. Nerve pressure can come and go as the patient's position and alignment shift, and so once the initial inflammation subsides, pain may be intermittent.

- *Local and radicular pain.* Pain is felt locally from inflammation and ligament irritation and along the dermatome for the affected nerve roots. A dermatome chart is a critical piece of equipment for a massage therapist working with this population.
- *Specific muscle weakness.* It is important to clarify the difference between general weakness, which occurs after a time of disuse or injury to whole muscle areas, and specific weakness, which develops fairly quickly and only in the muscles supplied by the affected nerve.
- *Paresthesia.* Pins-and-needles sensation is felt along the affected dermatomes.
- *Reduced sensation.* Poor sensation but not total numbness is a common symptom of ligament damage (which may frequently accompany disc damage).

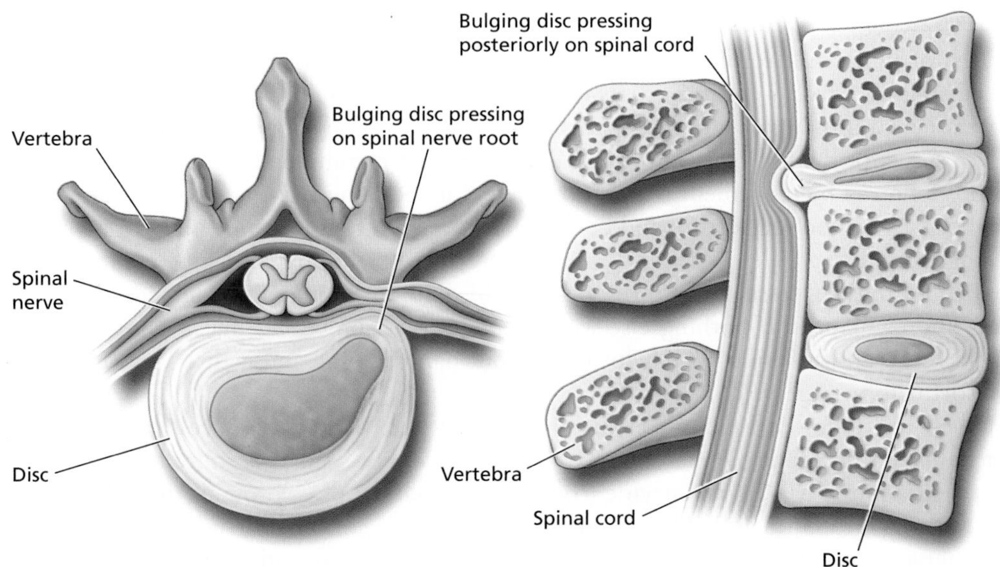

Figure 3.49. Herniated nucleus pulposus.

- *Numbness.* Total numbness is one distinguishing factor between disc problems and ligament injuries. A disc protrusion can completely cut off sensation to areas within a particular dermatome, but a ligament injury cannot. Numbness in a "saddle distribution," that is, in the low back, groin, and medial thigh, is an indication of pressure on the cauda equina, or cauda equina syndrome. This is a medical emergency that requires immediate attention.

Complications

The most serious complication of a disc injury is the threat of pressure exerted directly posteriorly. In the neck this means the spinal cord is compressed; in the lumbar spine it is called cauda equina syndrome because the disc material presses on the extensions of spinal nerves between T1 and S5 called the *cauda equina.* Direct spinal cord compression leads to some specific signs, including hyperactive reflexes; bilateral pain, paresthesia, or numbness; and the loss of bladder or bowel control. Any of these problems can become permanent, or paralysis can develop, if pressure is not removed quickly.

See Video Clip 4 on the Student Resource CD.

Diagnosis

It is important to get an accurate diagnosis for disc injuries, because many of the signs and symptoms may be caused by other disorders entirely. Doctors are especially vigilant to rule out the possibility of tumors or infection in the spine; these two conditions can create symptoms similar to those of disc disease but are much more serious.

Discs are generally examined through a combination of radiography, CT, and myelography, but MRI is the gold standard for identifying disc problems. However, many people show signs of disc injuries and are completely asymptomatic.[53] This raises the question whether a patient's significant back and radicular pain are brought about by disc disease or by some other soft tissue injury.

One situation that mimics a disc problem but is actually much less serious is a ligament sprain. Irritated spinal ligaments running between spinous or transverse processes can refer pain along the same dermatomes as the nearby discs. Ligament injuries do not cause total numbness or specific muscle weakness, however, and they respond well to specific types of massage. Further, one predictable feature with disc pain is that symptoms are reliably exacerbated by sitting, forward bending, and vibration. This is in contrast to ligament injuries, which tend to be irritated with side bending or twisting to the opposite side.

Treatment

The best of all possible resolutions for a damaged disc is for the bulging nucleus pulposus or cracked annulus fibrosus to return to its normal boundaries and remove pressure from nearby nerve tissue. Chiropractors and osteopaths work to correct bony alignment to create a maximum of space for the nucleus to retreat. Medical doctors recommend short-term bed rest or traction, followed by movement within tolerance, for the same reason. Physical therapy and special classes on correct posture and body mechanics are often recommended to people recovering from disc problems. Drugs that are prescribed for herniated discs are aimed at the tendency for muscles to seize up in response to this kind of trauma; these include muscle relaxants and painkillers. If nothing else works, cortisone is sometimes injected into the area. This powerful anti-inflammatory helps only about half the time and is often considered the last resort before surgery.

If bed rest followed by physical therapy doesn't help, it may be necessary to consider other kinds of intervention. One option is *chemonucleolysis.* This procedure involves injecting a preparation of papain, an enzyme from papayas that dissolves proteins (it is also used in meat tenderizer) into the disc. This material reduces the size of the protrusion, takes pressure off the nerve tissue, and so restores the patient to a pain-free state, all without major surgery. This procedure works best with young patients. *Transcutaneous discectomy*, the removal of disc material through a tiny incision, is sometimes also possible. Laser discectomy and microdiscectomy are newer procedures that are not yet widely available.

Massage?

Most people with disc problems have good days and bad days. Massage therapists should avoid intrusive techniques on the bad days. On the good days, they should work with the intention of creating space for the retreat of the bulging tissue. Referred pain and muscle spasms always accompany this condition. Compensation patterns that develop with chronic back pain also demand attention.

It is especially important not to work alone with a disc injury. Muscle spasm can serve an important protective function for newly damaged discs, and releasing it too soon may put a client in danger. Working with another professional who can handle the bony and/or medical end of the injury helps the client recover faster and more completely than with either professional alone.

MODALITY RECOMMENDATIONS FOR DISC DISEASE

MODALITY	RECOMMENDATION
Deep tissue massage	Supportive when not inflamed. Work paravertebral fascias from superficial to deep.
Lymphatic drainage	Supportive.
Polarity	S: Indicated. R/D: Indicated within client comfort.
PNF/MET/stretching	Supportive.
Reflexology	Indicated; work spine and endocrine system points.
Shiatsu	Indicated. Treat BL meridian and SI extension on the back, points in popliteal crease, K meridian in calf.
Swedish massage	Indicated when subacute; work to alleviate compensatory distortion when muscle splinting is no longer necessary.
Trigger point therapy	Indicated with careful pressure; use for associated muscle spasm.

See Chapter 1 for a brief description of each modality, including definitions of abbreviations.

Myasthenia Gravis

Definition: What Is It?

In 1890 a German doctor, Welhelm Erb, documented several patients with a "grave muscular weakness." This was the first written reference to what is now called *myasthenia gravis* (MG). MG is an autoimmune disease that involves degeneration or destruction of specific receptor sites at neuromuscular junctions. It is a progressive disease that involves but it is usually manageable with medical and surgical intervention.

Demographics: Who Gets It?

Although MG has been diagnosed in babies as young as 1 year and in adults as old as 80, it seen most often in women in their 20s and men in their 50s. It affects about 14 in 100,000 people, and about 36,000 Americans live with this condition.[57]

Myasthenia Gravis in Brief

Pronunciation: mi-as-THE-ne-a GRAV-is

What is it?

Myasthenia gravis (MG) is a neuromuscular disorder in which an autoimmune attack is launched against acetylcholine receptors at the neuromuscular junction. This makes it difficult to stimulate a muscle to contract, leading to fatigue and weakness.

What does it look like?

MG can develop at any age but is most common in women in their 20s and in men in their 50s. It often begins with weakness in facial muscles and in the muscles used in speech, eating, and swallowing. MG is a progressive disease, but it is usually treatable with medical intervention.

Is massage indicated or contraindicated?

Massage can be appropriate for persons with MG because this disease does not affect sensation. Massage may not affect ACh uptake in any positive way, but it won't make it worse either. Care must be taken to respect the side effects that accompany medications used to treat MG.

Etiology

MG is one of the best-understood autoimmune diseases. In learning about this condition, we have come to a much clearer understanding of the chemistry of muscular contractions. Before examining the disease process, however, it is worthwhile to review how nerves normally work with muscles.

Every motor neuron contacts its muscle cell at a specific area on the cell membrane called the motor end plate. At this junction, the chemical *acetycholine* (**ACh**) is released from bulbs in the motor axon. ACh moves across the synaptic cleft onto specialized receptor sites within the motor end plate. This stimulates the opening of channels into the membrane of the muscle cell. Sodium ions that have traveled the length of the motor neuron then flow through the channels, stimulating the release of positively charged calcium ions from the *sarcolemma*, or muscle cell membrane. The release of these calcium ions initiates muscular contraction. ACh, a neurotransmitter associated with increased excitability, is a key player in the lightning-fast cascade of events that translates electrical stimulation into chemical reactions.

In MG, the ACh receptor sites don't function correctly. While ACh may be released normally, the muscle loses the ability to respond and ultimately to contract. It is not clear exactly why autoantibodies attack the ACh receptor sites at the motor end plate, but it is clear that the thymus gland is involved. The thymus is abnormal in up to 90% of people with MG. Thymic abnormalities usually involve hypertrophic thymuses, or the growth of benign tumors (**thymomas**) that are easily removed.

Signs and Symptoms

Most people with MG report weakness and fatigability in affected muscles. The process begins most often around the eyes or lower face. Early signs include a flattened smile, droopy eyelids *(ptosis)*, and difficulty with eating, swallowing, and speech.

Symptoms tend to fluctuate during the day and are worst early in the morning and late at night. Repetitive activity, emotional stress, overexertion, exposure to heat, and some medications can make symptoms much worse.

The typical MG patient's muscle function degenerates for 2 or 3 years after diagnosis, and then symptoms tend to level off, sometimes even going into complete remission. However, MG is a progressive disease, and without intervention it can move from the muscles of the face and head to those of the arms and legs and ultimately to those that control respiration. This is the final stage of the disease, although it is rarely seen now that effective treatments have been developed.

Treatment

Before the 1970s the prognosis for MG was indeterminate at best. When the relation between ACh and muscle contractions was finally unraveled, it opened new possibilities for treating this disease.

Most treatment of MG has a double intention: to boost nerve transmission and to suppress immune system activity at neuromuscular junctions. Medications include drugs that limit the normal destruction of ACh by local enzymes (this allows the ACh more time and opportunities to bind with whatever receptor sites are functioning) and steroids that suppress immune system activity. Surgery is occasionally recommended to remove an abnormal thymus gland. In the event of a crisis (a sudden onset that threatens the patient's ability to breathe), *plasmapheresis* may be used to remove antibodies from the blood. This is an invasive procedure with only short-term benefits, so it is usually saved for extreme circumstances.

Massage?

MG is associated with motor loss but no sensory loss. It is exacerbated by stress, repetitive motion, and overexertion. Massage may be appropriate for MG patients, bearing in mind that excessive heat can also aggravate symptoms and that these clients may be taking immunosuppressive medications that put them at increased risk for picking up other people's infections.

MODALITY RECOMMENDATIONS FOR MYASTHENIA GRAVIS

MODALITY	RECOMMENDATION
Deep tissue massage	Contraindicated unless working with health care team.
Lymphatic drainage	Supportive.
Polarity	S: Indicated. R/D: Indicated, depending on client comfort.
PNF/MET/stretching	Indicated while subacute.
Reflexology	Indicated; work shoulder, chest, arm, side of neck, breast, chest, upper spine points.
Shiatsu	Indicated. Treat BL, K, LV, SP meridians and extensions.
Swedish massage	Indicated; supports homeostatic response.
Trigger point therapy	Supportive with gentle pressure on affected areas.

See Chapter 1 for a brief description of each modality, including definitions of abbreviations.

Thoracic Outlet Syndrome

Definition: What Is It?

Thoracic outlet syndrome (TOS) is a neurovascular entrapment. The nerves of the brachial plexus or the blood vessels running to or from the arm (or some combination thereof) are impinged or impaired at one or more of three places: between the anterior and medial scalenes; between the clavicle and the first rib, or under the coracoid process (Figure 3.50).

Etiology: What Happens?

The brachial plexus, the network of nerves that supplies the arm with sensation and motor control, consists of spinal nerves C5 to T1. These nerves interweave as they travel a complicated path to get to their final destinations in the arm: they go from intervertebral foramina through the anterior and medial scalenes, between the clavicle and the first rib, under the pectoralis minor, and around the humerus. If some part of the plexus is somehow compressed along

Thoracic Outlet Syndrome in Brief

Pronunciation: thor-AS-ik OUT-let SIN-drome

What is it?
Thoracic outlet syndrome (TOS) is a collection of signs and symptoms brought about by occlusion of nerve and blood supply to the arm.

How is it recognized?
Depending on what structures are compressed, TOS shows shooting pains, weakness, numbness, and paresthesia (pins and needles) along with a feeling of fullness and possible discoloration of the affected hand and arm from impaired circulation.

Is massage indicated or contraindicated?
If TOS is related to muscle imbalance, it indicates massage. TOS due to other problems, such as structural anomalies or neck trauma, may not respond as well to bodywork.

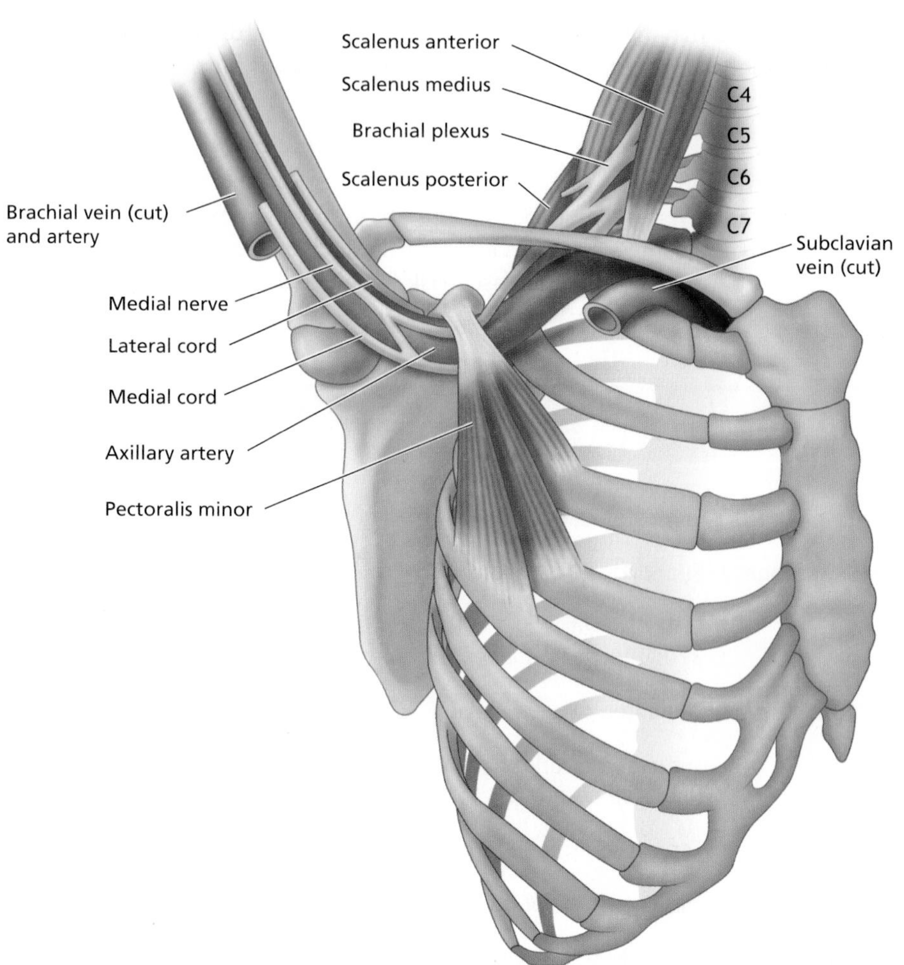

Figure 3.50. Thoracic outlet syndrome.

the way, a person feels it somewhere along the distance of that nerve. The nerve roots C8 and T1, both of which contribute to the ulnar and median nerves, are most at risk for compression with TOS.

Pinched nerves are only one part of TOS. This is a neurovascular entrapment, and the vessels at risk are the subclavian vein and the axillary artery, which is the distal portion of the subclavian artery. These vessels are also at risk for compression that can develop when muscles in small spaces get too tight.

TOS is discussed in many ways in medical literature: It is labeled as *neurological TOS* if it involves only nerve compression (the most common presentation). It is called *vascular TOS* if it involves only blood vessels. Often it is called *disputed TOS* because while the patient may have severe symptoms, the exact point of nerve or vascular impression may not be identified.

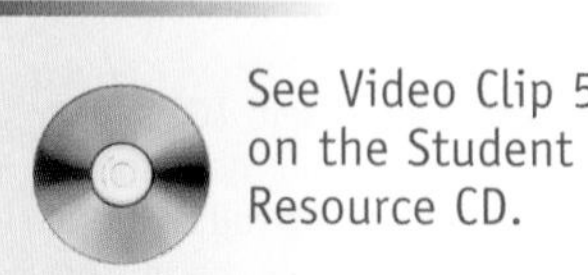

See Video Clip 5 on the Student Resource CD.

Contributing Factors

TOS can be caused by any factor that impinges brachial plexus nerves or blood vessels, anywhere from the anterior neck to the anterior chest. Although postural habits and bony growth patterns can make a person susceptible to TOS, it often seems to be precipitated by a specific traumatic event: a hyperextension injury or a repetitive stress situation similar to the factors seen with CTS.

The most common contributing factors to TOS include the following:

- *Cervical ribs.* In about 1% of the population, the transverse processes of the cervical vertebrae grow longer than normal, extending into territory where they don't belong. On radiography they actually look like little ribs sticking out into the soft tissues of the neck. They are usually unilateral, and C7 is the vertebra that grows them most frequently.

- *Muscle imbalance.* The anterior and medial scalenes and the pectoralis minor are the muscles most immediately involved with TOS. These tight muscles tend to become shrunken and fibrotic, while their antagonists (rhomboids, trapezius, neck extensors) become weak. This leads to a characteristic stooped or caved-in posture that significantly raises the risk of TOS.
- *Connective tissue bands.* Many people with TOS symptoms are found to have excessive connective tissue accumulation around the attachments of the scalenes. This material can put mechanical pressure on nerves and blood vessels. Whether the connective tissue bands are a congenital problem or a result of long-term postural habit is debatable.

Differential Diagnosis

Although TOS is diagnosed only when the impingement occurs at the scalenes, costoclavicular space, or under the coracoid, other factors can contribute to identical symptoms. To treat this condition successfully, it is important to find out exactly where that interference is happening. Some possibilities include the following:

- *Cervical misalignment.* This could be a subluxation but is more likely to be a rotation with subluxation of any combination of lower cervical vertebrae. Which nerves are affected (and therefore the location of the symptoms) depends on what level or levels of spinal nerves are being compressed.
- *Spondylosis.* If a bone spur intrudes at the nerve root at C6 (or any other cervical nerve root), symptoms are similar to those of true TOS.
- *Rib misalignment.* The joints that join the ribs to the spine are full synovial joints, called ***zygapophyseal*** joints. Like the intervertebral joints, the rib joints sometimes subluxate. When this happens to the first rib, either of two spots may cause problems: inferior to the anterior scalene and between the coracoid process and the ribs. In both of those locations the brachial plexus nerves can easily be caught between a bone (the first rib) and a hard place (a tight muscle or another bone).
- *Other injuries.* The list of other injuries that can create TOS-like symptoms is long. Possibilities include rotator cuff injuries, elbow and wrist injuries, CTS, nerve entrapment at the cubital fossa (cubital tunnel syndrome), disc disease, spondylosis, and injured cervical ligaments that refer pain into the shoulder and arm.
- *Nonorthopedic conditions.* More serious developments can put direct or indirect pressure on brachial plexus nerves or local blood vessels. Lung cancer with tumors in the apex of the lung, aneurysm or thrombus, or nerve damage to the spinal accessory nerve during a cervical lymph node biopsy can all lead to the collapse of the shoulder girdle and pressure on delicate structures.

Signs and Symptoms

Symptoms of TOS include all signs of nerve irritation: shooting pains, numbness and similar sensations, weakness, tingling, and pins and needles. Spinal nerves C8 and T1 are affected most often; these contribute to the ulnar nerve. Vascular symptoms include a feeling of fullness when blood return from a vein is blocked or cold and weakness when blood flow to the axillary artery is impaired. A difference in color or temperature of the affected arm may also be noticeable. Symptoms tend to be worst at night, when the patient lifts the affected arm over the head, or when the person is tired from other activities.

Diagnosis

Several tests for TOS have been developed. Unfortunately, none of them is always accurate for every patient, so a diagnosis is usually based on a physical examination combined with a description of symptoms from the patient. The challenge then is to locate exactly where the impingement is taking place.

One of the most dependable tests for TOS is the EAST (elevated arm stress test). The patient is seated, and his arms are abducted to 90 degrees. His elbows are flexed and his hands point toward the ceiling. He opens and closes his fists for 3 minutes. Most people with TOS are unable to complete this task before their symptoms interfere.

In the *Wright hyperabduction test,* the hand is placed over the head and the head is turned toward the affected side. If this exacerbates symptoms or reduces the strength of the pulse of the affected side, impingement to the axillary artery and lower brachial plexus nerves is suspected.

For *Adson's test* the head is extended and rotated toward the affected side. The client takes a deep breath, and the radial pulse on the affected side diminishes or even completely disappears. TOS that is due to muscle atrophy may show best when a client lies on his affected side and the pulse is diminished by axillary artery compression.

Nerve velocity conduction tests and electromyography (tests that measure electrical activity during muscle action) are sometimes used, but they are often inconclusive. Radiography, MRI, and other imaging techniques may be used to look for bone spurs, cervical ribs, or other mechanical obstructions, but they yield little information about chronic muscle tightness or atrophy.

Treatment

The treatment for TOS depends entirely on its causes, which is why it is important to get an accurate diagnosis. Some strategies are more appropriate for spondylosis than for tight scalenes, for instance. TOS due to muscle atrophy or tightness responds best to strengthening exercises and stretching. A small percentage of TOS patients are good candidates for surgery to release pressure on the affected nerves. This can mean the removal of a cervical rib or resection of the first rib or both.

Massage?

If the TOS is related to issues other than muscular imbalance, massage is unlikely to make much lasting difference. But if it is related to muscular problems, it can respond very well to bodywork. The client should also learn some specific stretches and strengthening exercises for pectoralis minor, its antagonists, and the scalenes.

Modality Recommendations for Thoracic Outlet Syndrome

MODALITY	RECOMMENDATION
Deep tissue massage	Indicated; work to decompress brachial plexus. Use active movement to assist release.
Lymphatic drainage	Supportive.
Polarity	S/R/D: Indicated.
PNF/MET/stretching	Indicated in all stages.
Reflexology	Indicated; work shoulder, chest, arm, side of neck, breast/chest, upper spine points.
Shiatsu	Indicated. Treat all meridians and extensions at neck, shoulder, upper back, rib cage. ROM for the shoulder joint within client limits.
Swedish massage	Indicated, especially when pain is muscular.
Trigger point therapy	Indicated for muscular component to decompress the brachial plexus; supportive for neurological problems.

See Chapter 1 for a brief description of each modality, including definitions of abbreviations.

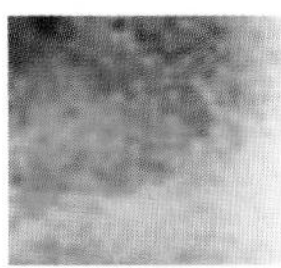

Chapter Review Questions: Musculoskeletal Conditions

1. What is the relationship between fibromyalgia and sleep disorders?
2. Why might fibromyalgia eventually be classified as a central nervous system disorder?
3. Name three injuries that might be present with shin splints.
4. What is the difference between a sprain and a strain?
5. What kind of muscle spasm serves an important function in healing?
6. What part of the bone is affected most severely by osteoporosis? What implications does this have for complications?
7. What does hernia mean? Name three kinds of abdominal hernias.
8. What condition is associated with the accumulation of trigger points?
9. Where do massage therapists often get osteoarthritis?
10. Describe how pes planus can lead to headaches.
11. Your client has excruciating pain at the base of the great toe on the left side. The skin is red, shiny, hot, and throbbing. What condition is probably present?
12. Your client has excruciating pain at the base of the great toe on the left side. The skin is thick and callused and a large bump protrudes medially. What condition is probably present?
13. Your client has electrical pain and weakness in the hand, especially at the thumb and first three fingers. What condition is probably present?
14. When a person has a herniated disc, what causes the pain?
15. What does RICE stand for?
16. What do ganglion cysts and tenosynovitis have in common?

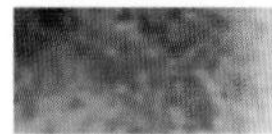

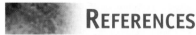

REFERENCES

1. Stedman's Medical Dictionary. 28th ed. Baltimore: Williams & Wilkins, 2000, p 1055.
2. Questions and Answers About Fibromyalgia. NIH Publication 04-5326. http://www.niams.nih.gov/hi/topics/fibromyalgia/fibrofs.htm. Accessed spring 2006.
3. Nye D. A Physician's Guide to Fibromyalgia Syndrome. Copyright © 1998, Missouri Arthritis Rehabilitation Research and Training Center. http://www.hsc.missouri.edu/~fibro/fm-md.html. Accessed spring 2006.
4. Chaitow L. Fibromyalgia An Evidence-Based Guide for Working with FMS Clients. © 2006 Massage Therapy Journal. Massage Therapy Journal spring 2006, pp 127–141.
5. Field T. Touch Therapy. London: Churchill Livingstone, 2000, p 73.
6. Fomby EW, Mellion MB. Identifying and Treating Myofascial Pain Syndrome. © 1998. The McGraw-Hill Companies. All Rights Reserved. The Physician and Sportsmedicine, Vol 25, No. 2, February 97.
7. Alvarez DJ, Rockwell PG. Trigger Points: Diagnosis and Management. © 2002. American Academy of Family Physicians. http://www.aafp.org/afp/20020215/653.html. Accessed spring 2006.
8. McPartland JM. Travell Trigger Points—Molecular and Osteopathic Perspectives. From Unitec Institute of Technology in Auckland, NZ. J Am Osteopath Assoc, Vol 104, No 6, June 2004, pp 244–249.
9. Travell J, Simons DG. Myofascial Pain and Dysfunction: The Trigger Point Manual. Baltimore: Williams & Wilkins; 1983.
10. Aiello MR. Avascular Necrosis. © 1996–2006 WebMD. http://www.emedicine.com/radio/topic70.htm. Accessed spring 2006.
11. Nochimson G. Legg-Calve-Perthes Disease. © 1996–2006 by WebMD. http://www.emedicine.com/emerg/topic294.htm. Accessed spring 2006.
12. Osteoporosis Overview. National Institutes of Health Osteoporosis and Related Bone Diseases National Resource Center. http://www.osteo.org/newfile.asp?doc=r106i&doctype=HTML+Fact+Sheet&doctitle=Osteoporosis+Overview+%2D+HTML+Version. Accessed summer 2006.
13. Beck BR, Shoemaker M. Rebecca. Osteoporosis: Understanding Key Risk Factors and Therapeutic Options. Physician and Sportsmedicine, Vol 28, No 2, February 2000. © 2000. The McGraw-Hill Companies. http://www.physsportsmed.com/issues/2000/02_00/beck.htm. Accessed summer 2006.
14. Fast Facts on Osteoporosis. National Institutes of Health Osteoporosis and Related Bone Diseases ~ National Resource Center. http://www.osteo.org/osteofastfact.html. Accessed summer 2006.
15. McCormick CC. Calcium & Osteoporosis - A Weak Link. © 1998–99 Cornell University. http://www.cce.cornell.edu/food/expfiles/topics/mccormick/mccormickoverview.html. Accessed summer 2006.
16. Barclay L. Calcium Plus Vitamin D May Not Reduce Hip Fracture or Colorectal Cancer Risk. Release Date: February 15, 2006 © 2006 Medscape. http://www.medscape.com/viewarticle/523698. Accessed summer 2006.
17. Depression, Bone Mass, and Osteoporosis. National Institute of Mental Health. http://www.nimh.nih.gov/events/prosteo.cfm. Accessed summer 2006.
18. Preventing and Reversing Osteoporosis. Physicians Committee for Responsible Medicine. http://www.pcrm.org/health/prevmed/osteoporosis.html. Accessed summer 2006.
19. Hobar C. Osteoporosis. © 1996–2006 by WebMD. http://www.emedicine.com/med/topic1693.htm. Accessed summer 2006.
20. Information for Patients About Paget's Disease of Bone. Osteoporosis and Related Bone Diseases ~ National Institutes of Health National Resource Center http://www.osteo.org/newfile.asp?doc=p110i&doctitle=Information+for+Patients+about+Paget%27s+Disease+of+Bone&doctype=HTML+Fact+Sheet. Accessed summer 2006.
21. Kurtzwei P. Help for People with Paget's Disease. FDA Consumer magazine (October 1996). http://www.fda.gov/fdac/features/896_pag.html. Accessed summer 2006.
22. Odom JA. Spinal Deformities: Benefits of Early Screening and Treatment. © June 1, 1995, Joel R. Cooper. http://medicalreporter.health.org/tmr0795/scoliosis0795.html. Accessed summer 2006.
23. Richardson M. Scoliosis. © 2000 University of Washington Department of Radiology. http://www.rad.washington.edu/mskbook/scoliosis.html. Accessed summer 2006.

24. Dalton E. Straight Talk: Symptomatic Scoliosis. Massage and Bodywork. ©2006 Associated Bodywork & Massage Professionals. April/May 2006, pp 62–70.
25. Mehlman C. Idiopathic Scoliosis. © 1996–2006 by WebMD. http://www.emedicine.com/orthoped/topic504.htm. Accessed summer 2006.
26. DiBacco TV. The pain of gout: Baffling condition left doctors guessing. Washington Post, October 11, 1994: p Z19.
27. Rothschild B. Gout. © 1996–2006 by WebMD. http://www.emedicine.com/orthoped/topic124.htm. Accessed spring 2006.
28. Gout. Copyright © 2006 University of Washington at Seattle. http://www.orthop.washington.edu/uw/tabID__3376/ItemID__34/mid__10313/Articles/Default.aspx. Accessed spring 2006.
29. Learn About Lyme Disease. Centers for Disease Control and Prevention. http://www.cdc.gov/ncidod/dvbid/lyme/index.htm. Accessed spring 2006.
30. Arthritis Related Statistics. Centers for Disease Control and Prevention. http://www.cdc.gov/arthritis/data_statistics/arthritis_related_statistics.htm. Accessed spring 2006.
31. Calculate Your Body Mass Index. National Institutes of Health. http://nhlbisupport.com/bmi/. Accessed spring 2006.
32. Hinton R, Moody RL, Davis AW, et al. Osteoarthritis: Diagnosis and Therapeutic Considerations. © 2002 by the American Academy of Family Physicians. http://www.aafp.org/afp/20020301/841.html. Accessed spring 2006.
33. Questions and Answers: NIH Glucosamine/Chondroitin Arthritis Intervention Trial (GAIT). NCCAM, National Institutes of Health. http://nccam.nih.gov/research/results/gait/qa.htm. Accessed spring 2006.
34. Osteoarthritis. © 1998–2006 Mayo Foundation for Medical Education and Research (MFMER). All rights reserved. http://www.mayoclinic.com/health/osteoarthritis/DS00019/DSECTION=2. Accessed spring 2006.
35. 1987 Criteria for the Classification of Acute Arthritis of Rheumatoid Arthritis. © 2005 American College of Rheumatology. http://www.rheumatology.org/publications/classification/ra/ra.asp. Accessed summer 2006.
36. Rheumatoid Arthritis and Complementary and Alternative Medicine. National Institutes of Health, National Center for Complementary and Alternative Medicine. NCCAM publication D282. http://nccam.nih.gov/health/RA/. Accessed summer 2006.
37. Rothschild BM. Lumbar Spondylosis. © 1996–2006 by WebMD. http://www.emedicine.com/med/topic2901.htm. Accessed summer 2006.
38. Trojian T. Ankle Sprains: Expedient Assessment and Management. © 1998 The McGraw-Hill Companies. Physician and Sportsmedicine, Vol 26, No 10, Oct 1998. http://www.physsportsmed.com/issues/1998/10Oct/mckeag.htm. Accessed summer 2006.
39. Basics – Overview. © 2002, 2003 TMJ Association, Ltd. http://www.tmj.org/basics.asp. Accessed summer 2006.
40. Shiel W. Ehlers-Danlos Syndrome. © 1996–2005 MedicineNet, Inc. http://www.medicinenet.com/ehlers-danlos_syndrome/article.htm. Accessed spring 2006.
41. Muscular Dystrophy: Hope Through Research. National Institute of Neurological Disorders and Stroke. http://www.ninds.nih.gov/disorders/md/detail_md_pr.htm. Accessed spring 2006.
42. Pattekar MA, Cacciarelli AA. Osteogenesis Imperfecta. © 1996–2006 by WebMD. http://www.emedicine.com/ped/topic1674.htm. Accessed spring 2006.
43. Osteogenesis Imperfecta: A Guide for Medical Professionals, Individuals, and Families Affected by OI. NIH Osteoporosis and Related Bone Diseases. http://www.osteo.org/newfile.asp?doc=i121i&doctitle=Osteogenesis+Imperfecta%3A+A+Guide+for+Medical+Professionals%2C+Individuals%2C+and+Families+Affected+by+OI&doctype=HTML+Fact+Sheet. Accessed spring 2006.
44. New Approach for Dupuytren's Contracture: A Newsmaker Interview With Charles Eaton, MD. © 2006 Medscape. http://www.medscape.com/viewarticle/531578. Accessed spring 2006.
45. Hernia. © Cleveland Clinic 2006. http://www.clevelandclinic.org/health/health-info/docs/3600/3619.asp?index=8823. Accessed spring 2006.
46. Chang AK. Osgood-Schlatter Disease. © 1996–2006 by WebMD. http://www.emedicine.com/emerg/topic347.htm. Accessed summer 2006.
47. Glazer JL. Plantar Fasciitis: Current Concepts to Expedite Healing. Physician and Sportsmedicine, Vol 32, No. 11, Nov 2004.
48. Singh D. Plantar fasciitis. © 1996–2006 by WebMD. http://www.emedicine.com/emerg/topic429.htm. Accessed summer 2006.

49. What Is Scleroderma? © 2004 Scleroderma Foundation. http://www.scleroderma.org/medical/overview.shtm. Accessed summer 2006.
50. Kahn K. Histopathology of Common Tendinopathies: Update and Implications for Clinical Management. © 2005 Clinical Sports Medicine. http://www.clinicalsportsmedicine.com/articles/common_tendinopathies.htm. Accessed summer 2006.
51. Standard of Care: Achilles Tendinopathy. © 2005 Brigham & Women's Hospital Department of Rehabilitation Services, Physical Therapy. http://www.brighamandwomens.org/RehabilitationServices/Physical%20Therapy%20Standards%20of%20Care%20and%20Protocols/Achilles%20Tendinopathy.pdf. Accessed summer 2006.
52. Hammer W.The Latest Scoop on Tendon Disorders and Treatment. All Rights Reserved, Dynamic Chiropractic, 2006. http://www.chiroweb.com/columnist/hammer/index.html. Accessed summer 2006.
53. Hunter OK. Cervical Sprain and Strain. © 1996–2006 by WebMD. http://www.emedicine.com/pmr/topic28.htm. Accessed summer 2006.
54. Mahar R. Musculotendinous Injuries of the Neck. St. Martha's Regional Hospital, Antigonish, Nova Scotia. http://www.theberries.ns.ca/Archives/Whiplash.html. Accessed summer 2006.
55. Norvell JG, Steele M. Carpal Tunnel Syndrome. © 1996–2006 by WebMD. http://www.emedicine.com/emerg/topic83.htm. Accessed spring 2006.
56. Osterman AL. The double crush syndrome. Orthop Clin North Am 1988 Jan;19:147–155. http://www.ncbi.nlm.nih.gov/entrez/query.fcgi?cmd=Retrieve&db=PubMed&list_uids=3275922&dopt=Abstract. Accessed spring 2006.
57. Howard JF. Myasthenia Gravis - A Summary. © 1997 by Myasthenia Gravis Foundation of America and James F. Howard, Jr, MD. All rights reserved. http://www.myasthenia.org/information/summary.htm. Accessed spring 2006.

4

Nervous System Conditions

Chapter Objectives

After reading this chapter, you should be able to . . .

- Name three diseases that could be confused with multiple sclerosis.
- Name two movement disorders in addition to tremor.
- Name the causative agent of herpes zoster.
- Name three types of depression.
- Name three types of anxiety disorders.
- Name the most subtle type of autism spectrum disorder.
- Name two types of stroke.
- Name the nerve involved in Bell palsy.
- Name three complications of spinal cord injury.
- Name two signs that a headache could be a medical emergency.
- Name the four classic symptoms of Ménière disease.
- Name three major cautions for massage in the context of nervous system disorders.

INTRODUCTION

By the time most massage therapists finish their training, they probably know more about the nervous system than they ever suspected existed, and they'll probably still feel like rank amateurs on the subject. That feeling is common to most people who study this topic. Fortunately, only a passing familiarity with the structure and function of this system is needed to make educated decisions about massage and many nervous system disorders. Most of the conditions considered here affect the peripheral nerves rather than the central nervous system (CNS), so this introductory discussion focuses mainly on the structure and function of the parts of the nervous system massage therapists can touch—which, not coincidentally, are also the parts of the system that are most vulnerable to injury.

Function and Structure

Nerves are bundles of individual neurons, fibrous cells capable of transmitting electrical impulses from one place to another. At their most basic level, the function of neurons is to transmit information from the body to the brain (sensation) and responses from the brain to the body (motor control). Interconnecting neurons in the brain also provide the potential for consciousness, learning, creativity, memory, and other fascinating abilities, but they are beyond the scope of this book.

Peripheral nerves are composed of bundles of long filaments (neurons) that run from the spinal cord to the area in the body for which they supply sensation or motor control. Each neuron is a single living cell. Some of them are tiny, but the neurons that signal when we stub our toe travel from the toe up the leg, through the buttock, into the spine, and up to the spinal cord, which terminates around T12 to L1. Each of these cells is several feet long.

Neurons have three parts: the ***dendrite*** (which carries impulses *toward* the cell body), the cell body with a nucleus, and the ***axon*** (which carries impulses *away* from the cell body). Sensory neurons therefore have exceptionally long dendrites to carry information from the periphery toward the cell body in the dorsal root ganglia; they have short little axons to continue carrying their impulses into the spinal cord. Motor neurons have tiny dendrites and cell bodies inside the spinal cord and very long axons to carry messages out to their terminating sites in the muscles and glands.

Motor and sensory neurons communicate via synapses, sometimes by way of some combinations of central, or association, neurons. At the same time that a response is generated at the spinal cord level, the information travels up the spine into the brain. This immediate reaction is called the reflex arc (Figure 4.1).

Most neurons in the peripheral and central nervous systems have a waxy insulating coating called myelin. This layer of material speeds conduction along the fiber and also prevents the electrical impulses from jumping from one fiber to another. In the peripheral nervous system, neurons have another protective feature in ***neurilemma***, an outside covering of special cells that can help to regenerate damaged tissue (Figure 4.2).

Peripheral nerves typically run close to the bone, where they are protected from most injuries. They are vulnerable in a few places, however. These spots are *endangerments* for massage therapists, who may cause injury to delicate tissues at these points; self-defense classes call them *targets*.

For specific information on nerve endangerment sites, refer to Appendix C on the Student Resource CD.

It is a convenient analogy to think about nerves as bun-

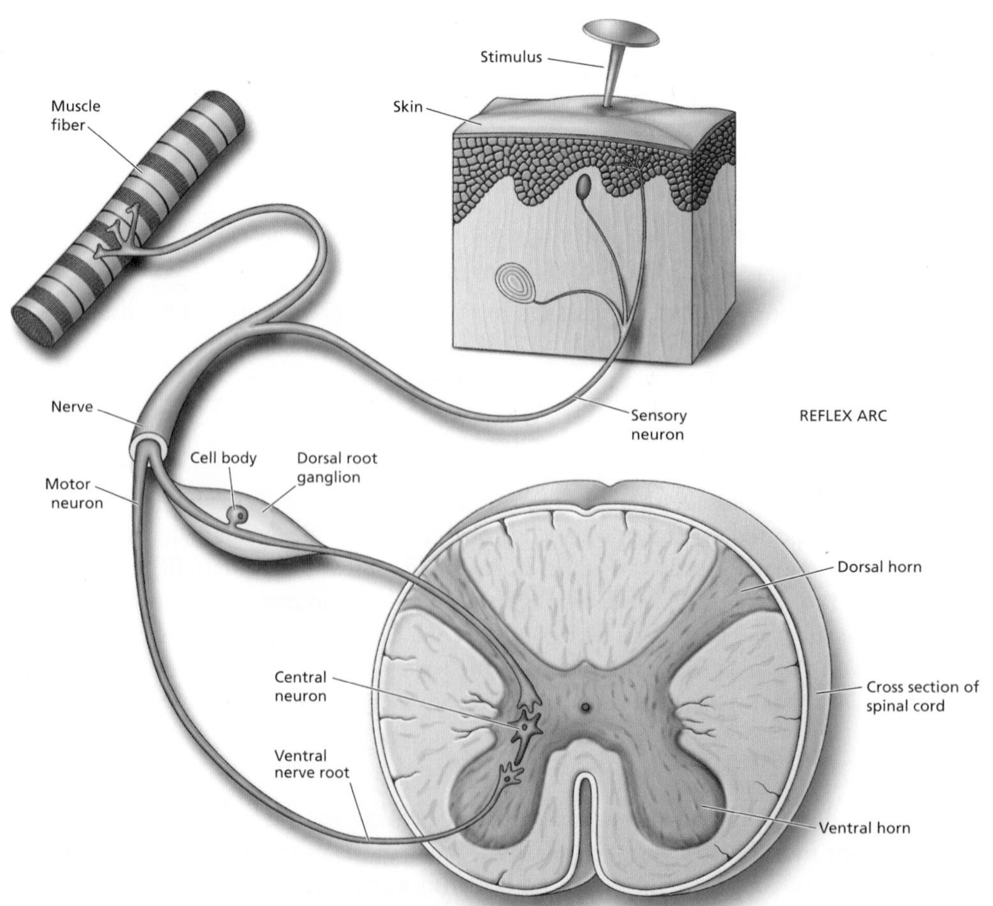

Figure 4.1. The reflex arc connecting sensation to motor response.

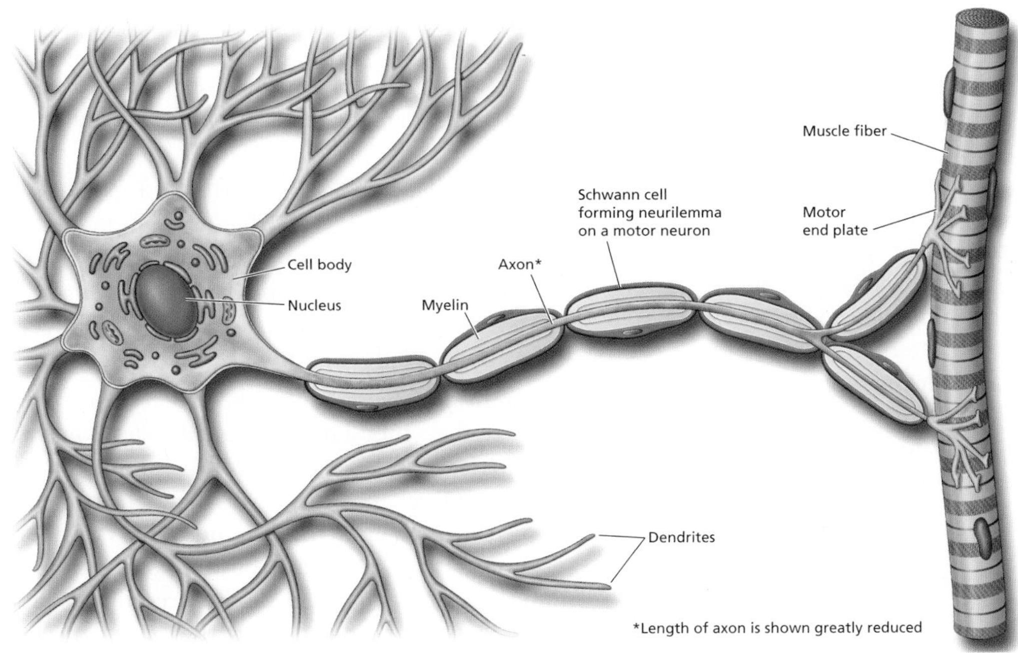

Figure 4.2. Neurons in the peripheral nervous system covered with Schwann cells, forming myelin and neurilemma.

dles of electrical wires. The similarities are obvious: here are thousands of filaments carrying electrical impulses, each one wrapped by an insulating layer of myelin, and they are bundled together for efficiency. The analogy stops, however, when one considers the effect of external pressure on nerve fiber transmission. In *Job's Body*, D. Juhan points out that a piece of electrical cable with a truck parked on it continues to carry its electrical messages, but a sciatic nerve squeezed by a tight piriformis has a drastically reduced flow of energy through it.[1] Nerves function with a combination of electrical and fluid flow; fluid flow may be severely limited by external pressure. Consider the implications of that pressure on a femoral nerve that is hugged by a psoas in spasm or the brachial plexus nerves running through a tangled maze of scalenes and pectoralis minor muscles.

General Neurological Problems

Most of the nervous system disorders that massage can mechanically affect involve some kind of pinching or distortion of peripheral nerves as they wend their way from the spinal cord to their destination in the body. Peripheral nerve damage has a generally good prognosis because of the regenerative properties provided by the neurilemma.

Other neurological problems involve the brain or spinal cord, which have very limited ability to regenerate and which massage obviously cannot directly access. But even when the spinal cord has been injured, overlapping patterns of innervation created by the twists and turns of the plexi often allow at least partial use of what would otherwise be a totally lost limb. This remarkable advantage begins to explain the benefits of the confusing routes that nerves take through the plexi. The best plan, when faced with a client who has sustained CNS damage, is to address the *symptoms* of these disorders as well as possible, looking for sensation where it is present, and to create as hospitable an internal environment as possible.

People with various kinds of CNS damage often progressively lose motor function. This has traditionally been viewed as an inevitable consequence, but this idea may prove to be a myth. It has been found in many cases that loss of motor function may be an issue of proprioceptive adaptation more than true nerve loss. In other words, a stroke or traumatic brain injury survivor may lose some strength in an arm or a leg, and the compensatory movement patterns allow for further degeneration of affected muscle fibers. Massage, stretching, and careful exercise may help make it possible to interrupt and even reverse this type of progressive loss.

Organic and mechanical problems with the central and peripheral nervous systems are one class of neurological problem massage therapists encounter. Psychiatric disorders, which can also be classified as neurological problems, are another matter altogether. Many people have a bewildering array of mental or psychological qualities that set them apart from the arbitrary standards called normal. Some of these people seek massage as a way to deal with some of the difficulties that their "abnormalities" create. This is often a good impulse; touch is an integral part of physical and psychological health. In fact, it could be said that touch is an important link between physical and psychological health (Sidebar 4.5).

Massage therapists can thus be put in the precarious position of deciding whether their work is an appropriate part of someone's healing (or even just coping) process. Sometimes the answer clearly is *no* (for instance with someone who obviously is in need of psychological counseling instead of or in addition to massage). At other times it may be less clear, and it is necessary to seek out the opinion of other professionals. Mental health patients who are on heavy, long-term doses of medication are in a particularly vulnerable position with regard to massage. Although bodywork is usually a good thing, it can change the internal chemistry of the body and brain significantly. When massage elicits a parasympathetic response, the types of neurotransmitters and hormones circulating in the body may shift radically away from fight-or-flight chemicals to substances that allow for relaxation and even sleepiness. If a client is taking medication to achieve equilibrium, it is inappropriate for a well-meaning but ignorant massage therapist to throw him off balance. It is important in these cases to consult with the client's medical and health care team before proceeding.

Major Cautions for Massage Therapists

In the context of nervous system problems and massage, a few cautions emerge as common themes:

- *Numbness.* When a client can't feel part of his or her body, it is inappropriate to try to change the quality of those tissues. It is fine to include the numb area with general, light pressure as a part of the incorporating aspect of massage, but extra care must be taken not to damage tissues where the client has no sensation.
- *Verbal communication.* Some types of nervous system problems make it difficult or impossible for clients to communicate verbally. While massage can still be safe and supportive, it is especially important for therapists to be sensitive to nonverbal cues about comfort and pain from these clients.
- *Medications.* Clients who take medication to help manage their mood or other mental states may find that massage is especially helpful—so much so that they want to change or stop taking their medication altogether. While this sounds like wonderful progress, it can be dangerous and should only be done with the guidance of the prescribing physician. Massage therapists must be careful never to step into that role.

Disorders of the nervous system can produce a bewildering variety of startling and sometimes intimidating symptoms. In working with these patients, as with all others, massage therapists must remember that their highest priority must always be to do no harm.

Nervous System Conditions

Chronic Degenerative Disorders

Alzheimer disease
Amyotrophic lateral sclerosis
Multiple sclerosis
Peripheral neuropathy

Movement Disorders

Dystonia
Parkinson disease
Tremor

Infectious Disorders

Encephalitis
Herpes zoster
Meningitis
Polio, postpolio syndrome

Psychiatric Disorders

Anxiety disorders
Attention deficit hyperactivity disorder
Autism spectrum disorders
Chemical dependency
Depression
Eating disorders

Nervous System Injuries

Bell palsy
Cerebral palsy
Complex regional pain syndrome
Spina bifida
Spinal cord injury
Stroke
Traumatic brain injury
Trigeminal neuralgia

Other Nervous System Conditions

Guillain-Barré syndrome
Headaches
Ménière disease
Seizure disorders
Sleep disorders
Vestibular balance disorders

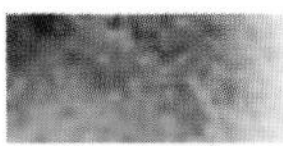

Chronic Degenerative Disorders

Alzheimer Disease

Definition: What Is It?

Alzheimer disease (AD) is a progressive degenerative disorder of the brain causing memory loss, personality changes, and eventually death. The precise causes are not fully understood, but it is now known that while most people can anticipate a certain degree of memory loss as they age, the severe dementia associated with AD is not normal and not an inevitable fate for every person.

> **Alzheimer Disease in Brief**
> Pronunciation: ALZ-hy-mur dih-ZEZE
>
> **What is it?**
> Alzheimer disease (AD) is a degenerative disorder of the brain involving shrinkage and death of neural tissue.
>
> **How is it recognized?**
> AD is difficult to definitively diagnose in a living person, but signs and symptoms include progressive memory loss, deterioration of language and cognitive skills, disorientation, and lack of ability to care for oneself.
>
> **Is massage indicated or contraindicated?**
> If an AD patient feels comfortable and nurtured while receiving touch, massage is very much indicated. But if the patient feels disoriented and threatened, the therapist must change tactics. Alzheimer patients may not be able to communicate verbally, so therapists must be sensitive to nonverbal cues.

Demographics: Who Gets It?

AD affects about 5% of the U.S. population, or about 4.5 million people. It affects about half of people living in nursing homes and costs some $100 billion per year in direct and indirect medical expenses.

The incidence of AD increases with age. About 10% of people over 65 are diagnosed with AD, and the prevalence doubles every 5 years after age 65. Close to half of those over 85 have AD. Because baby boomers are beginning to enter the at-risk age group, it is estimated that by 2050 this disease will disable some 16 million people.[2]

AD affects more women than men, but this may be related to the fact the women generally live longer than men rather than to a gender-based predisposition.

Etiology: What Happens?

AD is named for a German doctor, Alois Alzheimer, who in 1906 first documented the trademark lesions in the brain seen with this disorder. He performed an autopsy on a female patient who died in a mental institution in her mid-50s, and he noticed two specific changes in her brain tissue: plaques and tangles. These observations have become the primary postmortem diagnostic features of this disease, and they have become the focus of the leading edge of research today.

These are the features of AD:

- *Plaques.* Sticky deposits of a naturally occurring cellular protein called *beta amyloid* have been noted on neural cells of people with AD. Beta amyloid is produced by many cells throughout the body, and it occurs in various lengths and qualities, depending on where it is found. In the brain it seems to be particularly adhesive. When it accumulates in sufficient amounts, the deposits stimulate an inflammatory response in the brain that kills off not only the cells affected by the plaques but nearby unaffected cells as well.
- *Neurofibrillary tangles.* Another Alzheimer-related protein is called *tau*. This substance helps physically support long fibers in the CNS so they can connect at synapses. When tau proteins in AD patients degenerate, the long fibers collapse and become twisted and tangled together. Eventually the cells, which are incapable of transmitting messages to each other, shrink and die. The brain of a person with AD shows predictable patterns of atrophy, with deeper sulci (Figure 4.3), a smaller hippocampus, and larger ventricles.

The presence of beta amyloid plaques and tau-related tangles means that fewer brain cells function at normal levels. With the loss of neural tissue, levels of neurotransmitters in the

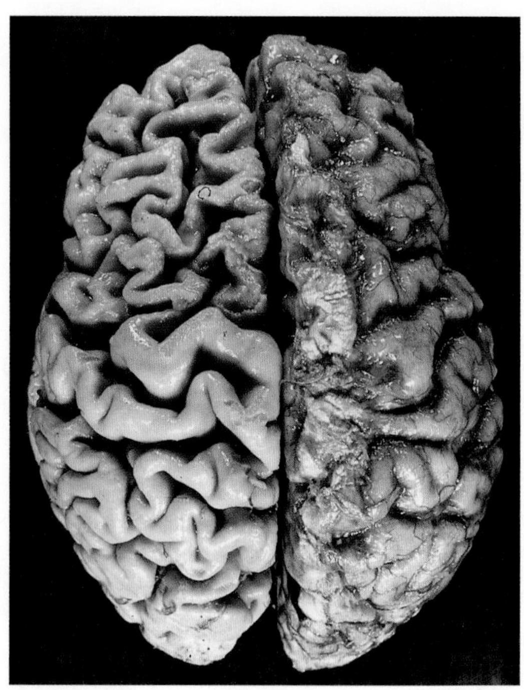

Figure 4.3. Visible atrophy associated with Alzheimer disease.

brains of AD patients become pathologically low. This makes it difficult for the functioning nerve cells that remain to communicate with each other. Further, the hippocampus (the part of the brain that processes and stores new information and knowledge) shrinks and loses function. Consequently, the AD patient loses access to memories and loses the ability to process new information.

Most of the information we have about how AD develops has been gathered in the past several years and is still in rapid development. Just recently it has been found that other issues, including genetics, chronic inflammation, a history of head injury, exposure to environmental toxins, high cholesterol levels, low estrogen levels (in women), and many other variables are contributing factors for many patients. These discoveries reveal many new possibilities for treatment and prevention of this disease.

Signs and Symptoms

The protocol for staging AD is somewhat variable. Some experts identify seven distinct phases ranging from no impairment to very severe dementia in which many mental and physical processes are lost, while others simply separate it into mild, moderate, and severe disease.

One recent development in the study of AD is that an early stage, called *mild cognitive impairment*, is the transition period between having no impairment and having advanced AD. Some medications appear to prolong this transitional period, which delays the onset of debilitating disease.

Most people with AD live about 8 years after their diagnosis, but this number can range from 3 to 20 years.

Diagnosis

Diagnosis of AD has always been problematic, because the presence of plaques and tangles can be confirmed only posthumously. This disease is diagnosed through a variety of tests to rule out other causes of dementia in combination with mental status examinations. It is important to try to come to an accurate diagnosis of AD for two reasons. First, the earlier treatment is introduced, the longer memory may be preserved. Second, dementia and loss of memory can sometimes be indicators of problems other than AD, some of which are reversible.

As the ability to gather information about living brains develops, it may become easier to diagnose AD. New technologies (positron emission tomography [PET] and single-photon emission computed tomography [SPECT]) allow doctors to observe interactions of brain chemicals at a molecular level in living, conscious patients. Nonetheless, a diagnosis of AD today is still based on physical and mental examinations and ruling out other dementing diseases.

Differential Diagnosis

AD is only one of several conditions that can cause dementia and memory loss. Some conditions involve permanent brain damage, whereas others may be only temporary problem, if they are treated appropriately. Causes of permanent memory loss other than AD include the following:

- *Vascular dementia* is caused by a narrowing of the arteries to the brain, usually associated with advanced cardiovascular disease.
- *Stroke and TIA* cause brain tissue to die because of an interruption in blood supply. These issues are more fully discussed later in this chapter.
- *Parkinson disease* nvolves the degeneration of certain motor centers in the brain, but it also often involves dementia. Parkinson disease is discussed later in this chapter.
- *Lewy body dementia* is the result of protein deposits (***Lewy bodies***) similar to the beta amyloid plaques that lead to dementia. This disease has features in common with both Alzheimer and Parkinson disease.
- *Huntington disease* is another progressive degenerative CNS disease. It is characterized by destruction of nerve cells and resulting changes in personality and intellect. Huntington disease is a genetic disorder.
- *Creutzfeld-Jakob disease* is a type of dementia that can affect young and middle-aged people as well as the elderly. It is the human variant of ***bovine spongiform encephalopathy*** (mad cow disease).

Other conditions can cause memory loss that is recoverable. Naturally, it is important to consider these possibilities before concluding that a patient has irreversible AD. Some examples of conditions that are important to rule out include high blood pressure, depression, diabetes, hypothyroidism, side effects of medication, and vitamin B_{12} deficiency.

Treatment

Treatment options address the deficit of neurotransmitters in the brain that make it difficult for nerves to communicate. ***Cholinesterase inhibitors*** are often prescribed to prevent reuptake of acetylcholine, an essential neurotransmitter that is often in short supply for AD patients. These drugs effectively improve memory, at least in the short term. Other medications may be prescribed to address some of the behavioral and mood distortions seen with this disease.

Other promising options include the use of some nonsteroidal anti-inflammatory drugs (NSAIDs) (specifically ibuprofen, naproxen sodium, and ***indomethacin***—*not* aspirin or acetaminophen) that seem to limit the inflammatory reaction to plaques that causes cell damage. Antioxidants (vitamin E, vitamin C, and others) are being studied, along with ginkgo biloba for their memory-saving effects. The role of estrogen in AD is not well understood; for some populations it seems to have a protective effect, but for others supplementing estrogen may increase the risk of dementia.

Massage?

AD patients, even in advanced stages of the disease when language is difficult or impossible, still respond positively to touch. Research done with AD patients shows that although bodywork doesn't slow or reverse the disease, it improves the quality of life for patients to the extent that they become measurably less disruptive, show better sense of orientation, and have more positive social interactions in nursing home settings.[3]

Two cautions must be kept in mind when working with AD patients. One is that most of these clients are elderly and consequently may have a number of other complicated disorders that may or may not contraindicate various kinds of bodywork. The other is that when a client cannot communicate clearly, it becomes the responsibility of the massage therapist to interpret nonverbal signals about how the bodywork is being accepted. Clients with AD generally respond well to massage, but if they become anxious and frightened for unknowable reasons, the therapist must be sensitive to the client's mental and emotional state.

Modality Recommendations for Alzheimer Disease

Modality	Recommendation
Deep Tissue Massage	Supportive: assist orientation through careful work on feet, legs, hips; also work with suboccipitals and erectors.
Lymphatic Drainage	Supportive.
PNF/MET/Stretching	Supportive.
Polarity	S: Indicated. R/D: Supportive, determined by client comfort.
Reflexology	Indicated; work brain, top of head, pineal, solar plexus points.
Shiatsu	Supportive. Work BL, K, H, SI meridians and extensions.
Swedish Massage	Indicated with caution for other conditions and as long as the client feels safe.
Trigger Point Therapy	Supportive with light work.

See Chapter 1 for a brief description of each modality, including definitions of abbreviations.

Amyotrophic Lateral Sclerosis

Definition: What Is It?

Also known as *Lou Gehrig disease* in the United States and *motor neurone disease* in Great Britain, ALS is a progressive condition that destroys motor neurons in the central and peripheral nervous systems, leading to the atrophy of voluntary muscles. The cells most at risk are the large motor neurons in the lateral aspects of the spinal cord. These are replaced by fibrous astrocytes, which make the spinal cord hard and scarlike: thus the name ***amyotrophic lateral sclerosis*** (ALS).

Amyotrophic Lateral Sclerosis in Brief

Pronunciation: am-e-o-TRO-fik LAT-er-al skler-O-sis

What is it?

Amyotrophic lateral sclerosis (ALS) is a progressive disease characterized by degeneration of upper and lower motor neurons and consequent atrophy of voluntary muscles.

How is it recognized?

Symptoms of ALS include weakness, fatigue, and muscle spasms. It appears most frequently in patients between 40 and 70 years old.

Is massage indicated or contraindicated?

ALS indicates massage, with caution, when the massage therapist works as part of the health care team.

Demographics: Who Gets It?

Three types of ALS have been identified: *sporadic*, which accounts for 90% to 95% of the cases in the United States; *familial*, which shows a genetic link for 5% to 10% of U.S. cases, and the *Mariana Island variety*, which is endemic to a specific population in the Western Pacific islands.

ALS usually affects people 40 to 70 years old; the average age at diagnosis is 55. Familial ALS tends to have a younger onset than the sporadic type. A little over 5,000 new cases of ALS are diagnosed in the United States every year (about 15 each day), and approximately 30,000 people in this country are living with this disease right now. Men get it slightly more often than women do.

Etiology: What Happens?

The cause or causes of ALS are unknown. When the disease develops, it leads to the degeneration of motor neurons in the spinal cord, which leads to the progressive and irreversible atrophy of voluntary muscle. About one-third of the motor neurons that supply a muscle must be destroyed before atrophy is apparent.

Several possible contributing factors have been identified, including some features that are strikingly similar to Alzheimer disease: tangled neural fibers and deposits of abnormal proteins on clumps of cells. This leads to degeneration of the neuron's cytoskeleton and strangulation of the presynaptic axons. ALS interrupts only motor function, however, and does not usually affect intellect or memory.

One well-established feature in ALS is the accumulation of the neurotransmitter ***glutamate*** in the synapses. This excitatory neurotransmitter is not neutralized or reabsorbed by the presynaptic neuron, and it eventually damages and even kills the motor neuron it is meant to stimulate.

Other contributors to ALS may include a genetic susceptibility to damage from free radicals (this has been reliably established in the case of familial ALS), autoimmune disease, mitochondrial dysfunction, and exposure to some environmental toxins. Another possible factor is absence of neurotrophic factors, or chemicals that support the health of nerve cells. Their absence may be a predictive factor for ALS.

Signs and Symptoms

Symptoms of ALS are sometimes classified by whether the disease affects spinal nerves or cranial nerves and whether the symptoms demonstrate damage to upper motor neurons or lower motor neurons. (Upper motor neurons are entirely within the CNS, and lower motor neurons begin in the ventral horn of the spinal cord and go to voluntary muscles throughout the body.)

About 75% of ALS cases are diagnosed as the spinal variation, with early symptoms in the arms or legs. Difficulty with fine motor skills in the hands (buttoning a shirt, turning a key) may be the first sign of a problem. When early symptoms occur in the legs, frequent tripping or stumbling may be the first indication of the disease. Both sides may be affected, but one side is typically worse than the other. Stiffness and weakness move proximally up the limb and eventually affect the voluntary trunk muscles that control breathing.

About 25% of ALS cases first present as difficulties with speech, swallowing, or motor control of the tongue. This is the *bulbar* form, and it is often more serious, with a faster progression, than the spinal form of the disease. Bulbar ALS is also associated with extreme and rapid mood swings, or "emotional incontinence".

Upper motor neuron problems manifest as progressive spasticity, exaggerated reflexes (including the gag reflex), and a positive ***Babinski sign*** (the great toe goes into extension rather than flexion when the plantar surface of the foot is stimulated). Lower motor neurons are involved when weakness, atrophy, muscle cramps, and ***fasciculations*** (uncontrolled twitching) are present. Both upper and lower motor neurons are damaged in ALS.

The nerve damage seen with this disease affects motor neurons only; sensory neurons are left intact. This can be a painful process, however, with muscle spasms, constipation, and the gradual collapse of the body as gravity puts stresses on muscles that have no power to respond.

ALS does not affect intellectual capacity at all.

CASE HISTORY 4.1

Amyotrophic Lateral Sclerosis

Eric: Without the weekly massage sessions, his medication level would be much higher, he would have more muscular spasms, and the pain in his shoulder would be unbearable.

Six months after he married the love of his life and built her a home, Eric was diagnosed with ALS. Rather than succumb to sadness, the couple decided to go to Paris for a vacation and try to conceive a child. Nine months later, a baby girl joined the household.

For the past 2 years I have treated Eric for 90 minutes in his home every week. Before he lost control of his facial muscles, I could understand his slurred speech; he sounded like a poststroke patient or a fellow hammered with too many whiskeys. Now all he can do is grunt and point, so he communicates with the aid of a small computer keyboard through which a stilted robotic male voice "speaks" as he types. He can no longer walk, and he moves about his huge home with a fancy battery-operated wheelchair.

In these 2 years he has changed from being a hearty, muscular chiseled strong man to a man who leans on one entire side of my body as he takes slow, uneven steps from his wheelchair to the massage table.

Eric says that without the weekly massage sessions, his medication level would be much higher, he would have more muscular spasms, and the pain in his shoulder would be unbearable.

Approaching a body with ALS is more than a little tricky. Spasms occur without warning; the beginning of slow, even, medium-pressure effleurage while applying lotion to a lower extremity can result in a board-hard leg that extends as if levitating off the table of its own accord. All I can do is place my hand on the leg and slowly coax it back down to the table. Arms that used to open wide to hug those around him would contract against his body were it not for the slow, sometimes painful range-of-motion exercises we perform on all arm joints each week. Every bit of therapy takes twice as long as working on a "normal" body: if he's not stretched, he contracts; if I go too fast, he spasms; communication is cumbersome; and causing pain, though unintended, is always a possibility.

The end of life for an ALS patient is often related to diaphragm function. It can slow down to the point that the decreased lung capacity invites pneumonia, which is the ultimate threat to any sedentary human. For this reason, aggressive (though careful) resisted breathing exercises are part of every session. This means I have to get up on the table and place my hands just at his tenth rib, trying not to dislodge his feeding tube or the dressing around his diaphragmatic monitor. Then I encourage him to push against me with his breath while I'm wobbling all over and trying hard not to fall off the table. This brings on a lot of laughter—therapeutic in itself for someone with limited lung capacity. I hover above him while he laughs and tries to take a deep breath. I watch as he deems himself victorious if he can take at least one deep inhale and exhale; it's enough to bring a strong woman to tears. The victory is minuscule to most of us, but this effort could help extend his life.

Presently, there is no cure for this frustrating and frightening disease. But massage therapy can make a profound difference in the patient's pain and in the progression of muscular contractions. Every case is different, but the intelligent and dedicated therapist can adapt her skills to these very special patients and help make the damnable progression of ALS more tolerable as it is accompanied by loving touch.

—*Charlotte Versag*

Diagnosis

No single test can identify ALS. It is typically diagnosed through history, physical examination, nerve conduction studies, and electromyographs. Tests are also conducted to differentiate ALS from other conditions that have some similar symptoms, such as muscular dystrophy, hyperthyroidism, multiple sclerosis (MS), postpolio syndrome, peripheral neuropathy, and pressure on the spinal cord from bone spurs, tumors, or other factors.

Treatment

Until very recently, treatment for ALS has been strictly palliative, that is, aimed at managing the severity of the symptoms only. Some of these options include moderate exercise and physical and occupational therapy to maintain muscle strength as long as possible. Heat and whirlpools are used to control muscle spasms, and speech therapy helps with difficulties in swallowing and speech. Assistive devices such as leg braces, arm braces, wheelchairs, voice aids, and computers can improve a patient's ability to function. In advanced cases swallowing may be so difficult that the insertion of a stomach tube (*gastrostomy*) may be recommended. Since this disease does not impede cognitive or emotional processes at all, psychological therapy for ALS patients and their families to deal with anxiety and depression is an important part of the treatment plan.

Drug treatment for ALS has traditionally been used only to help combat general fatigue, muscle spasms, or secondary infections, but new drugs limit the amount of glutamate in the CNS, so motor nerves live longer. These are not a cure for ALS, but they may significantly prolong the lives of people affected by this disease.

Treatment options that are still in development include the use of an antibiotic that stimulates a gene to produce extra glutamate transporters. This would help remove excess glutamate from synapses. Another option under development is introduction of drugs directly into the cerebrospinal fluid to bypass the blood-brain barrier for best effect.

Prognosis

Once diagnosed, this disease, which has no known cure, usually results in death within 2 to 10 years. Most ALS patients die of pneumonia or cachexia (extreme weight loss). Half of ALS patients succumb within 3 years of diagnosis, and 90% die within 6 years. Some ALS patients, however, have survived for decades, and it is unclear why.

Massage?

This disease is not blood-borne or lymph-borne, it doesn't involve sensory paralysis, and it's not contagious. It is treated with heat, exercise, and physical therapy. Furthermore, even with immobility and loss of muscle mass, most patients with ALS never develop decubitus ulcers. Therefore, in the absence of other contraindicated circumstances, massage may be appropriate and welcome. Massage therapists who get a chance to work with ALS patients should do so as part of a health care team, working primarily for comfort and pain relief.

Modality Recommendations for Amyotrophic Lateral Sclerosis

Modality	Recommendation
Deep Tissue Massage	Supportive, with health care team. Work within client comfort.
Lymphatic Drainage	Supportive.
Polarity	S: Indicated. R/D: Indicated, determined by comfort of client.
PNF/MET/Stretching	Indicated.
Reflexology	Indicated; work solar plexus and head points.
Shiatsu	Supportive. Treat LV, GB, ST, SP and BL meridians and extensions. Use passive stretches.
Swedish Massage	Indicated, with caution for other complications. Can help with pain relief.
Trigger Point Therapy	Supportive with light work.

See Chapter 1 for a brief description of each modality, including definitions of abbreviations.

Multiple Sclerosis

Multiple Sclerosis in Brief
Pronunciation: MUL-tih-pul skler-O-sis

What is it?
Multiple sclerosis (MS) is an idiopathic disease that involves the destruction of myelin sheaths around both motor and sensory neurons in the CNS.

How is it recognized?
MS has many symptoms, depending on the nature of the damage. These can include fatigue, eye pain, spasticity, tremors, and a progressive loss of vision, sensation, and motor control.

Is massage indicated or contraindicated?
Massage is indicated in subacute stages when the client is in remission, rather than during acute periods when symptoms flare.

Definition: What Is It?

Multiple sclerosis (MS) is a condition characterized by inflammation and then degeneration of myelin sheaths in the spinal cord and brain. It is thought to be an autoimmune disease, but the triggering pathogen or other stimulus has not yet been identified.

Demographics: Who Gets It?

MS affects whites about twice as often as any other ethnic group. Its highest incidence is among people who live in temperate climates (either north or south of the equator) or who did so before they were 15 years old. This group is five times more likely to develop MS than others. MS is rare in Native Americans and Asians.

Most MS patients are diagnosed when they are between 20 and 40 years old. Young women are diagnosed up to twice as often as young men, but among older patients, the gender distribution is about the same.

Between 300,000 and 350,000 Americans live with MS; about 25,000 new cases are diagnosed every year.[4]

Etiology: What Happens?

The word *sclerosis* means hardened scar or plaque. In MS myelin is attacked and destroyed. Research reveals that early in the process ***oligodendrocytes***, the myelin-producing cells in the CNS, multiply and attempt to repair the damage, but eventually they fail.

As attacks progress, normal myelin is replaced with scar tissue. Eventually the electrical impulses meant to tie the whole system together are either completely obstructed or significantly slowed. This results in motor and sensory paralysis instead of coordinated movement and feeling. The signs and symptoms of the disease, like so many disorders of the CNS, depend entirely on where and how much nerve tissue has been damaged.

MS, like many autoimmune diseases, often works in cycles of inflammatory flares followed by periods of remission. During flares the myelin is under attack and is replaced by scar tissue. During remission inflammation subsides and some myelin regenerates. In this way MS patients may lose some neurological function during flares but regain some or all of it during remission.

If flares are persistent and repetitive, the damage may affect the neuron itself. In this case, lost function is more likely to be permanent.

Causes

At present, the leading theories behind MS point to immune system attacks against some component of myelin sheaths in the CNS. This leads to an inflammatory response that destroys the protective myelin sheath and may eventually attack the nerve tissue itself. Many autoimmune diseases have a specific pathogenic trigger that begins the immune system mistake leading to tissue damage, but no specific trigger has yet been identified for MS. Pathogens under investigation include human herpesvirus type 6 (HHV-6) and *Chlamydia pneumoniae*.

It also seems clear that a genetic predisposition raises the risk of developing MS, but this seems to be a relatively small factor. The population-wide risk of developing MS is less than 1%. People with a first-degree relative who has the disease carry a risk of only 1% to 3%. If one identical twin has the disease, the other twin has only a 30% chance of developing MS.

This collection of information indicates that MS is probably an autoimmune disease to which some people are genetically predisposed but that requires some combination of environmental triggers to initiate the disease process. The fact that in a few isolated cases the incidence of MS among a local population (MS clusters) is much higher than the statistical norm supports the influence of environmental factors that are not yet understood.

Research into the development and progression of MS has revealed several issues in recent years. It is possible that a compromise in the blood-brain barrier allows into the CNS some immune system agents that would otherwise be blocked. A type of T cell that regulates autoimmune dysfunction in healthy people (T-reg cells) has been found to be underactive in mice with an MS-like disease; supplementing these T-reg cells improves function and decreases symptoms. Also, recent vaccination for tetanus has a statistical link with reduced incidence of MS.[5] Discoveries like these open new doors for treatment options and may one day lead to ways to prevent or cure this disease.

CASE HISTORY 4.2

Multiple Sclerosis

Tricia, Age 36: "It takes all the courage I can muster just to stand up in the morning."

Everyone has problems. Everyone gets in their own world so much. Now I look at someone with a disability and I wonder if they have it. You start to watch people walk and wonder if they've got it.

About a year and a half ago we had just moved into a new house and my youngest child had just started school. For the first time in 15 years I was looking forward to having some time, to getting on with my life.

Then there was a pain in my left heel that felt like a stone bruise. We were just back from a long vacation, so I thought it was from too much walking. Two weeks later there was a lack of sensation in my foot and it traveled up my leg to my knee. It began affecting my right leg too. Then there was numbness and tingling in my left hand. It felt like I had just had a shot of Novocain, it was that kind of tingling.

Try walking on the balls of your feet for a whole day. Then you'll get an idea of how hard it was. I couldn't put my heels down because there would be a sharp tingling funny bone feeling. My walking was so labored, I got to the point where I would rather shimmy on my chest like an army guy to get from room to room. I wasn't crying, I wasn't upset, it was just easier to crawl.

At the same time as feeling stressed about not knowing what was happening to me, I put off going to the doctor. I finally went to my obstetrician for my headaches. He gave me migraine medication, but it didn't work.

He sent me to a neurologist who checked me out and watched me walk. Then while I was sitting there he went out into the hall with another doctor and they started speaking in medical jargon that I couldn't understand; it made me really nervous. When he came back he asked me, "Will you come in for a spinal tap?"

"Why?"

"There are some things we want to check out."

"What do you think I have?"

"I think you have MS."

"Excuse me?"

I never *dreamed* it would be something like this.

They started me on intravenous steroids. The next morning I got up after a bad night, and for the first time in 2 months I could walk normally. I was so excited, I woke my family and called my mom on the phone. But by the end of that morning I was already beginning to feel tired. My condition deteriorated in spite of the steroids. By the end of the week I couldn't even get up off the couch to let the home care nurse in.

My neurologist finally sent me to the university hospital. There they did lots of other tests, more spinal taps and an MRI (magnetic resonance imaging). The MRI showed tiny spots in my brain but nothing like what they were expecting. The spinal taps all came back negative.

They had me talking to teams of doctors. I talked to neurologists, immune specialists, nutritionists, and psychiatrists. The head of the department was prepared to tell my family I had chronic progressive MS, which meant I could be dead in a matter of weeks. I finally decided that I needed to be home, I needed to be with my family, so I checked out even though they didn't want me to.

I continued physical therapy at a local clinic. At first they would have me sit in a warm pool with jets of water after I exercised, and I would go home feeling so drained and worn out, it was awful. Finally they adjusted that part of it and I did better.

Multiple Sclerosis *continued*

Today I still don't have much sensation below my knees. It takes all the courage I can muster just to stand up in the morning. I never know what kind of day I'll have, whether I'll be able to walk without a cane, whether I'll be tied to the house because my digestive system is unpredictable. I have terrible headaches that begin on the lower half of one side of my face and go up into my ear. I have days when I can't eat at all. I've had episodes of dizziness and double vision. I'm not on steroids now, but I take an antidepressant for the headaches. We're still struggling to find the right dose. My greatest fear, even more than being in a wheelchair, is that I will loose bladder or bowel control or go blind.

But my doctor says my scenario is good. It's been a year and a half without any exacerbations and he says I'm in remission. The only thing that's worse is my headaches, which are more painful and happen more often.

I think everything depends on your attitude. A major thing for me is to feel needed. If I have a purpose, I feel better. My aunt has MS, and she practically runs her family business. It's just amazing to see her get up and go. She says there are some days that if she didn't have that business to go to, she wouldn't be able to get out of bed. I have a chance now to see what other people have to deal with, and some of them are so much worse off than I am—because of physical problems but other kinds of problems too. I have five wonderful children and a husband who loves me. My doctor thought I was going to die, and here I am in remission. I just feel so lucky to be here.

Signs and Symptoms

This disease is sometimes called *the great imitator* because its initial symptoms can look like a variety of other diseases, depending on what area of nerve tissue has been affected. The order with which symptoms appear also varies greatly from one person to the next. Some of the most dependable signs and symptoms include these:

- *Weakness.* The onset of this problem may be gradual or sudden. It comes about because the loss of myelin makes nerve transmission slow.
- *Spasm.* This can take the form of chronic muscle stiffness or of active acute cramping.
- *Changes in sensation.* MS patients often report numbness or **paresthesia** (pins and needles) in various parts of the body. These sensations may last for hours or days at a time.
- *Optic neuritis.* Attacks on the myelin of the optic nerve result in extreme eye pain coupled with progressive loss of function. Vision may be minimally impaired (for instance, red-green color distortions) or it may be fully lost until the episode has passed. Most MS patients recover full or close to full vision when they go into remission.
- *Urologic dysfunction.* MS patients may find it difficult to urinate, or they may be incontinent.
- *Sexual dysfunction.* Difficulty maintaining an erection for men or having an orgasm in women are sometimes early signs of this disease.
- *Difficulty walking.* This problem can be a product of several factors, including muscle stiffness, numbness, and loss of coordination.
- *Loss of cognitive function.* A frequently overlooked issue for many MS patients is a change in mental ability. Short-term memory and the ability to learn and perform complex tasks are often challenged. Most MS patients have limited loss of cognitive function but can compensate. A smaller percentage undergo severe changes in cognitive skills.
- *Depression.* This is a complication of many chronic progressive diseases, especially in situations as unpredictable as those of MS. Up to 70% of MS patients live with depression, which can exacerbate symptoms.

- *Lhermitte sign.* In this neurological test electrical sensations run down the spine or into the extremities when the neck is in flexion.
- *Digestive disturbances.* Many MS patients have severe digestive disturbances (nausea, diarrhea, constipation) that vary greatly from day to day.
- *Fatigue.* Perhaps the most common symptom for MS patients is debilitating fatigue, which is particularly exacerbated by heat. The fatigue may be a result of slower or impaired nerve transmission (requiring fewer muscle fibers to work harder), muscle spasm, and other factors.

Progression

The progression of MS is highly unpredictable. It has a few characteristic patterns, but some patients move from one pattern to others within their disease process. Some of the basic patterns are these:

- *Benign MS.* The patient has only one flare in his or her lifetime, although CNS imaging may show progressive accumulation of plaques.
- *Relapse/remitting MS.* Definite periods of flare are followed by long periods of remission. It may be years between episodes. This is the most common presentation, but many patients eventually develop secondary progressive MS.
- *Secondary progressive MS.* Cycles of flare and remission occur, but recovery during remission is only partial.
- *Primary progressive MS.* Patients show a steady decline in function; episodes of flare are low grade but constant.
- *Malignant MS.* This is a rapidly progressive form of the disease, with little respite (if any) between flares. This is a rare form that may result in severe disability or death within a short time of onset.

Diagnosis

No single test can definitively diagnose MS. The medical convention is to describe a person's disease as *possible*, *probable*, or *definite* MS. It is identified through a description of symptoms, a family health history, a spinal tap to look for raised antibody levels and myelin fragments, and various types of MRI that can reveal CNS lesions and breaches of the blood-brain barrier. Nerve conduction tests to measure the speed of electrical impulses through nerves may also be conducted.

An official list of criteria has been developed to identify MS.[6] To achieve a positive diagnosis, a patient must have these findings:

- Objective evidence of at least two episodes. (This can be determined through MRI, examination of cerebrospinal fluid, or evoked potential tests that show the speed of nerve transmission in the brain.)
- Episodes of flare that are separated by at least a month and by location of affected function.
- No other explanation for symptoms that can be found.

Several conditions can produce MS-like symptoms. Part of a thorough diagnosis is ruling out the conditions listed in Table 4.1.

Treatment

Until recently, standard treatment options for MS included symptomatic treatment (e.g., for fatigue, muscle pain) with doses of steroidal anti-inflammatories to quell the severity of flares. Steroids can reduce symptoms in the short run but have not been shown to have long-lasting benefits, and their side effects can be severe. Therefore, they are usually used only as a temporary measure.

Drugs called *interferon betas* work specifically to limit immune system activity. These drugs can shorten the periods of flare and prolong periods between episodes. They are cumulatively toxic to the heart and liver, however, and must be used extremely carefully.

TABLE 4.1 Conditions that Can Produce Multiple Sclerosis–like Symptoms

Lyme disease	Herniated or ruptured disc
HIV/AIDS	Lupus
Scleroderma	CNS tumors
Vascular problems in the brain	Fibromyalgia
Complications of encephalitis	B_{12} or folic acid deficiency

Other possibilities include **plasmapheresis** to filter out overactive antibodies (this is recommended only for acute situations), and chemotherapeutic drugs to quell immune system activities. Many more treatments are in development, and new options may be available soon.

Non-pharmacological options for people living with MS include careful exercise and physical or occupational therapy designed to maintain strength and function as long as possible. Eating well and getting adequate amounts of high-quality sleep are important for maintaining health and prolonging remissions. Stress management techniques, including massage, are often recommended for the same reasons.

Massage?

MS usually has acute and subacute periods; massage is indicated in the subacute stages. Care must be taken not to overstimulate the client, which can result in painful and uncontrolled muscle spasms. Symptoms may also be exacerbated by heat, so therapists must avoid allowing their clients' core temperature to rise by working in an overly warm environment. Research on Swedish massage and reflexology has shown benefits for MS patients,[7] although the mechanism and duration of the benefits are not clear.

Every client with MS presents symptoms and problems differently. If sensation is present, massage can be useful as an agent against stress (which has been shown to exacerbate symptoms), depression, and spasticity, and it helps to maintain the health and mobility of the tissues. In areas where sensation is not present, nonmechanical types of work (i.e., very light effleurage and energy work) are more appropriate.

Modality Recommendations for Multiple Sclerosis

Deep Tissue Massage	Supportive when subacute and sensation is present to address spasticity. Avoid overstimulation of CNS.
Lymphatic Drainage	Systemically contraindicated while acute; otherwise supportive.
Polarity	S: Indicated. R/D: Indicated, adjusting for client comfort and sensitivity.
PNF/MET/Stretching	Indicated, with caution for sensory loss.
Reflexology	Indicated; work brain, spine, all glands, solar plexus, diaphragm points.
Shiatsu	Supportive. Treat BL, K, SP, ST, GB, LV meridians and extensions.
Swedish Massage	Supportive; be cautious about reduced sensation and staying within pain tolerance.
Trigger Point Therapy	Contraindicated while acute; indicated while subacute with caution for sensory loss.

See Chapter 1 for a brief description of each modality, including definitions of abbreviations.

Peripheral Neuropathy

Definition: What Is It?

Peripheral neuropathy (PN) is not a disease in itself but a symptom or a complication of other underlying conditions. Peripheral nerves, either singly or in groups, are damaged through lack of circulation, chemical imbalance, trauma, or other factors.

> **Peripheral Neuropathy in Brief**
> Pronunciation: per-IF-er-al nur-OP-ath-e
>
> **What is it?**
> Peripheral neuropathy (PN) is damage to peripheral nerves, often as a result of some other underlying condition or exposure to pathogens or toxic substances.
>
> **How is it recognized?**
> Symptoms include burning or tingling pain that begins distally and moves proximally, cramping or twitching, hyperesthesia, or autonomic dysfunction, such as problems with digestion, heart rate, breathing, or other issues.
>
> **Is massage indicated or contraindicated?**
> PN contraindicates massage when numbness interferes with the client's ability to give accurate feedback, or increased pain sensation makes massage impractical. In other cases, therapists must make case-by-case judgments about whether massage fits in the context of the underlying factors.

Etiology: What Happens?

PN can affect one nerve at a time (***mononeuropathy***) or multiple nerves (***polyneuropathy***). It is typically classified by whether it affects sensation, voluntary muscle control, or autonomic function.

PN is occasionally related to a genetic anomaly, but it is usually a consequence of some other injury, infection, or systemic disease; this is called acquired PN. Some common causes of acquired PN include the following:

- **Injury.** Carpal tunnel syndrome, thoracic outlet syndrome, Bell palsy, disc disease, and trigenurial neuralgia are all examples of PN related to acute or chronic injury.
- **Infection.** Herpes simplex, herpes zoster (shingles), HIV/AIDS, Lyme disease, hepatitis, syphilis, and Hansen disease (leprosy) can all cause damage and irritation to peripheral nerves.
- **Systemic disease.** Diabetes (type 1 or type 2), renal failure, vitamin B_{12} deficiency, cancer, and other tumors can all contribute to nerve damage, as can some autoimmune diseases, including lupus, Sjögren syndrome, sarcoidosis, and Guillain-Barré syndrome.
- **Toxic exposure.** Chronic alcoholism, sniffing glue, some medications, exposure to heavy metals (especially lead and mercury), solvents, and other environmental contaminants can damage peripheral nerves.

Signs and Symptoms

Most cases of PN begin subtly and slowly, and symptoms depend on what combinations of sensory, motor, and autonomic nerves are damaged. Injury to sensory neurons produces burning pain or tingling in the hands and feet, which gradually spreads proximally into the limbs and finally the trunk. Extreme sensitivity to touch (***hyperalgesia*** or ***allodynia***) can follow, but this may eventually be replaced by numbness. Numbness is problematic because a person who can't feel something—a toe, for instance—he or she can't tell if it's been injured or infected. Secondary ulcers and infections are common complications of numbness with any disease.

Damage to motor nerves can lead to twitching, cramps, and eventually to atrophy of the affected muscles.

Damage to autonomic nerves is often the most serious; this can interfere with digestion, maintaining heart and respiratory rates, sweating, blood pressure, and control of the bladder or bowel.

Treatment

Treatment for PN depends entirely on the underlying pathology that is causing the nerve damage. Chronic pain is often treated with tricyclic antidepressants or antiseizure medications. Topical ointments with lidocaine or pepper sometimes offer some relief. Other therapies include TENS units (transcutaneous electrical nerve stimulation that interrupts pain transmission), biofeedback, acupuncture, relaxation techniques, and massage to improve circulation in the affected extremities.

The good news is that if the disease is interrupted early, the peripheral nerves may be able to regenerate and the patient may regain full function. But if it is left untended, PN can progress to become a chronically painful long-term condition.

Massage?

If a client has undiagnosed tingling or numbness, he or she needs to see a doctor; it could be any number of things, PN included. Numbness and reduced sensation are contraindications too, since the client is unable to give informed feedback about comfort. Clients with nerve damage are likely to be hypersensitive; massage may exacerbate or soothe this symptom.

Massage therapists must make case-by-case decisions for clients with PN to balance the possible benefits (soothing irritable nerves, improving circulation) with the possible risks (further irritating irritable nerves, damaging numb tissue).

Modality Recommendations for Peripheral Neuropathy	
Deep Tissue Massage	Locally contraindicated in numb or painful areas; otherwise supportive. Decompress fascias proximal to affected areas.
Lymphatic Drainage	Indicated in all stages if used following a standard massage treatment.
Polarity	S: Indicated. R/D: Indicated within comfort of client. Extra light pressure in areas of atrophy or numbness.
PNF/MET/Stretching	Indicated in all stages. Be cautious about reduced sensation and staying within pain-free range.
Reflexology	Indicated; work all gland points.
Shiatsu	Indicated with respect for sensory deficit. Work K, LV, SP, GB constitutionally; use all possible joint movements between metatarsals and metacarpals.
Swedish Massage	Supportive; be cautious about reduced sensation and staying within pain tolerance.
Trigger Point Therapy	Contraindicated for numbness or atrophy; indicated for hypertonicity.

See Chapter 1 for a brief description of each modality, including definitions of abbreviations.

Movement Disorders

Dystonia

Definition: What Is It?

Dystonia is classified as a movement disorder. It involves repetitive, involuntary, sometimes sustained contractions of skeletal muscles. It often reaches a peak and then stabilizes or subsides in intensity, but it may recur. It can occur without an identifiable cause, due to a genetic anomaly, or as a secondary symptom of an underlying disorder or drug reaction.

Demographics: Who Gets It?

Dystonia is found among all ages and races. Most types of this disorder affect females more than males, by ratios of 2 or 3 to 1. Types of dystonia linked to genetic anomaly are most common among Ashkenazi Jews. Other types show no particular population spikes.

It is estimated that between 250,000 and 300,000 people in the United States have been diagnosed with dystonia. It is the third most common movement disorder, ranking just behind Parkinson disease and essential tremor.

Dystonia in Brief

Pronunciation: dis-TO-ne-ah

What is it?

Dystonia is a movement disorder resulting in repetitive, predictable, but involuntary muscle contractions.

What does it look like?

The primary symptom of dystonia is repetitive involuntary muscle contractions, especially during stress or in relation to specific tasks. It can involve only the head or face, the vocal cords, or one limb, but other forms are progressive or involve the whole body. The contractions themselves are not necessarily painful, but they can lead to painful tissue changes including arthritis, muscle strains, and contractures.

Is massage indicated or contraindicated?

Because this condition doesn't affect sensation, massage is safe and appropriate as long as the client is comfortable. Symptoms are often worse with stress or fatigue, so some dystonia patients may seek out massage as a coping mechanism. It is often treated with drugs that interfere with motor function, so the massage therapist should research the effect of bodywork in the context of these medications.

Etiology: What Happens?

Like other movement disorders, dystonia appears to be linked to problems with the basal ganglia. It involves an inability to process certain neurotransmitters, including dopamine, GABA (gamma-amino butyric acid, an inhibitory neurotransmitter), serotonin, and acetylcholine. The result is prolonged bursts of electrical activity in the affected muscles. This distinguishes it from other movement disorders such as Parkinson disease or tremor, which result in rhythmic, oscillating shaking on one plane of movement.

Dystonia can be classified by age of onset (childhood, adolescent, or adult) or by cause (primary, secondary, or dystonia-plus syndromes, which involve some rare neurochemical disorders). Most often, however, dystonia is described by what part or how much of the body is affected.

Focal dystonia affects only one area. Involuntary contractions are usually task specific, and they subside when that body part is not in use, but eventually contractions may happen at rest as well. Several subtypes of focal dystonia have been described:

- *Spasmodic torticollis* is the most common form of dystonia. It is sometimes mistaken for a simple stiff neck. It involves unilateral involuntary contractions of neck rotators, usually the sternocleidomastoid. For other types of torticollis, see Sidebar 4.1.
- *Vocal dysphonia* affects the vocal cords, leading to difficulty with speech.
- *Oromandibular dystonia* affects the face and lower jaw muscles. It can lead to problems with swallowing and eating.
- *Blepharospasm* leads to repetitive blinking and squinting of the eyes; it can be severe enough to cause functional blindness, even though the eyes themselves are not affected.
- *Writer's cramp* is a condition in which the dominant hand develops painful cramps during activity.
- *Other forms* of focal dystonia can affect other areas. It can make it difficult to lift the lower leg during walking, or cramps can occur in one foot. More rarely it affects the trunk or abdominal wall.

Segmental dystonia affects two adjacent or nearby areas of the body. One type of segmental dystonia is called *Meige syndrome*. This is a combination of *blepharospasm* and oromandibular dystonia.

- *Multifocal dystonia* affects disconnected parts of the body, the left leg and the face, for instance.
- *Hemidystonia* affects the left or right side of the body. It is an occasional repercussion of stroke.
- *Generalized dystonia* is the most severe form of this disorder. It usually starts in the leg and progresses to affect the whole body.

SIDEBAR 4.1: OTHER TYPES OF TORTICOLLIS

Spasmodic torticollis is classified as a type of dystonia, a movement disorder that starts in the CNS. Other forms of torticollis are related to musculoskeletal problems, which of course have very different implications for massage.

- **Congenital torticollis.** A genetic anomaly results in the development of only one sternocleidomastoid muscle. Because so many other muscles can rotate and flex the head, this problem may be dealt with through physical therapy.
- **Infant torticollis.** In the late stages of pregnancy the fetus may lie with the head twisted to one side. This can create a shortened or weakened sternocleidomastoid and cranial bone distortion. This condition is usually successfully treated with exercise and a special helmet designed to reshape the cranial bones.
- **Wryneck.** This is a simple stiff neck, often caused by irritation of the intertransverse ligament at C_7. A cervical misalignment may also create the problem, which will not be relieved until both the muscles and the bony alignment have been addressed. Trigger points and spasm in the splenius cervicis are another possible cause. Short-lived cases of wryneck may be brought about by sleeping in a bad position or some other event or trauma that might cause irritation in the neck muscles.
- **Other types.** Torticollis can, on rare occasions, be the earliest presenting sign of a more serious condition. In some documented cases it was the first symptom of bone cancer in the spine (the tumor may affect the motor and/or sensory neurons); bone infection; and even a bad infection of the adenoids. Adenoids or lymph nodes in the neck, can get so filled with pus that they irritate and cause spasm in the nearby muscles.

Signs and Symptoms

Signs and symptoms of dystonia are related to what type is present and at what age symptoms began. People who develop this disorder in childhood tend to have it in more severe forms than those who develop dystonia in maturity.

The primary symptom is involuntary contraction of an area. It tends to be exacerbated by stress or fatigue. Contractions are often related to specific tasks and disappear when other tasks that use the same muscles are substituted: walking backward instead of forward, for instance. Many dystonia patients develop a habit of repeatedly touching the affected area, which serves to reduce local contractions. This pattern is called ***geste antagoniste.***

The progression of dystonia varies greatly. Some people have a sudden onset, and then it quickly or eventually stabilizes or even subsides. When dystonia progresses, contractions may spill over to nearby muscles, or they may occur at rest as well as during activity. People diagnosed in childhood are most likely to have progressive loss of function as the muscle contractions spread to other areas in the body.

Dystonic contractions may not be painful, but they can lead to painful consequences. Headaches can result from spasmodic torticollis or facial contractions. Muscle irritation and arthritis may develop in areas where contractions are continually sustained. Eventually the muscle fibers may shrink and the connective tissue sheaths around them thicken into a permanent contracture. Another complication is the functional blindness that occurs when blepharospasm interferes with normal eyelid contractions.

Diagnosis

Dystonia is typically diagnosed through the patient's description of symptoms and by ruling out other possibilities, such as musculoskeletal problems with the neck, Parkinson disease, Tourette syndrome, and other movement disorders. Childhood-onset dystonia, which is often genetic, may be confirmed through testing for specific genetic anomalies.

Treatment

Treatment options for dystonia are attempts to modulate motor function in the affected muscles. This can be accomplished in several ways: Medications can affect neurotransmitter secretion or uptake. Injections of botulinum toxin (Botox) can block the acetylcholine receptors in the affected muscles. A device can be implanted in the brain to help regulate motor function (deep brain stimulation). Surgery can be conducted to disrupt dysfunctional portions of the basal ganglia or to interrupt nerve transmission to the muscle or in the spinal cord.

Massage?

Dystonia does not interfere with sensation, and it is exacerbated by stress or fatigue. These characteristics make massage safe and possibly helpful for a client with dystonia, although it is unlikely to create long-term changes. Massage therapists should be well informed about what medications or other treatments the client uses, however, since these may influence the safest forms of bodywork.

Modality Recommendations for Dystonia	
Deep Tissue Massage	Supportive with appropriate pacing. Monitor clients response.
Lymphatic Drainage	Supportive when used after standard massage treatment.
Polarity	S: Indicated. R/D: Supportive within client comfort.
PNF/MET/Stretching	Supportive.
Reflexology	Indicated; work brain, spine, all glands, solar plexus points.
Shiatsu	Supportive. Treat SP, ST, LV, GB, K, BL meridians and extensions.
Swedish Massage	Supportive; can help reinforce a parasympathetic state.
Trigger Point Therapy	Supportive: may help reduce trigger point formation due to repetitive muscle contraction.

See Chapter 1 for a brief description of each modality, including definitions of abbreviations.

Parkinson Disease

Definition: What Is It?

Parkinson disease (PD), first discussed by the British physician James Parkinson in 1817 as the "shaking palsy," is a movement disorder involving the progressive degeneration of nerve tissue and a reduction in neurotransmitter production in the CNS.

Parkinson Disease

James Parkinson (1755–1824) was a British physician who first documented this chronic degenerative movement disorder in 1817.

Demographics: Who Gets It?

PD affects 1 to 1.5 million people in the United States, with about 60,000 new diagnoses each year. It is rare in people under 40 but occurs in about 1% of people over 60. Men with PD outnumber women by about 3 to 2.

Etiology: What Happens?

PD is one of a variety of movement disorders. It involves changes in CNS structures that cause them to work inefficiently. To discuss this condition thoroughly it is necessary to review some of the inner workings of the brain.

Anatomy Review

The ***basal ganglia*** are structures in the brain that contribute to voluntary movement. They are little pockets of gray matter that work with several other structures to provide learned reflexes, motor control, and coordination. (*Coordination* here means the balance in action between prime movers and their antagonistic muscles.) The basal ganglia are found at the lower edges of the cerebrum.

Healthy basal ganglia cells are supplied with a vital neurotransmitter, ***dopamine***, by cells in a nearby structure, the ***substantia nigra*** (aka "black stuff"). In PD, the substantia nigra cells die off, depriving the basal ganglia of dopamine. Without dopamine, the basal ganglia cannot maintain the careful balance between agonists and antagonists in the body, and so coordination degenerates and controlled movement becomes very difficult.

Parkinson Disease in Brief

What is it?
Parkinson disease (PD) is a degenerative disease of the substantia nigra cells in the brain. These cells produce the neurotransmitter dopamine, which helps the basal ganglia to maintain balance, posture, and coordination.

How is it recognized?
Early symptoms of PD include general stiffness and fatigue; resting tremor of the hand, foot, or head; and slowed movement. Later symptoms include poor balance, a shuffling gait, a masklike appearance to the face, and a monotone voice.

Is massage indicated or contraindicated?
PD indicates massage with caution. Care must be taken for the physical safety of these clients, who cannot move freely or smoothly.

For PD symptoms to appear, 60% to 80% of the substantia nigra must be lost. This results in a significant loss of dopamine production in the area.

Causes

It is not clear why the substantia nigra degenerates in most PD cases. Environmental agents may be found to be one cause; risk factors for PD include exposure to some pesticides, fertilizers, and other industrial chemicals. The presence of Lewy bodies in the basal ganglia and other areas may predict PD, but these deposits are associated with other disorders as well. In some families a genetic connection is clear, and research has identified specific sites of genetic abnormality for those with familial PD.

The term *parkinsonism* refers to conditions that display Parkinson-like symptoms but differing etiologies. Some of these cases can be traced to specific issues, including certain drugs, repeated head trauma (pugilistic parkinsonism affects boxers), and neurovascular disease.

Signs and Symptoms

Symptoms of PD can be divided into primary and secondary problems. Primary symptoms arise from the disease itself, while secondary symptoms are results of primary symptoms.

Primary Symptoms

- *Nonspecific achiness, weakness, and fatigue.* PD has a slow onset and is most common in elderly people. Therefore, these early symptoms are often missed, either because they are too subtle to be seen or because of an assumption that a certain amount of fatigue and stiffness is a natural part of growing older.
- *Resting tremor.* This phenomenon is present in most PD patients and is often one of the first noticeable symptoms. A rhythmic shaking or pill-rolling action of the hand is often seen. Tremor may also affect the foot, head, and neck. This tremor is most noticeable when the patient is at rest but not sleeping. It often disappears entirely when the patient is engaged in some other activity.
- *Bradykinesia.* This is difficulty in initiating or sustaining movement. It can take a long time to begin a voluntary movement of the arm or leg, and the limb's movement may be halting and interrupted midstream. PD patients with **bradykinesia** sometimes report feeling rooted to the floor when they can visualize moving a leg but it doesn't happen without sustained effort.
- *Rigidity.* Gradually the muscles, particularly the flexor muscles, become permanently hypertonic. This can give rise to a characteristically stooped posture, as the trunk flexors contract more strongly than the paraspinals. This is particularly obvious when PD accompanies osteoporosis, as it often does in elderly patients. Rigidity also makes it difficult to bend or straighten arms and legs and can cause a particular masklike appearance as the facial muscles lose flexibility and ease of movement (Figure 4.4). This also accounts for a reduced rate of blinking, increased drooling, and difficulty with eating, swallowing, and digestion. The rigidity that accompanies PD is *not* the same thing as spasticity, which implies a different kind of nerve damage, discussed in the sections on spinal cord injury and traumatic brain injury. Rigidity indicates massage (with caution), while spasticity, which often accompanies numbness, must be approached more carefully.
- *Poor postural reflexes.* Disruption in the activity of basal ganglia cells results in uncoordinated movement and poor balance. PD patients are particularly susceptible to falling.

Secondary Symptoms

- *Shuffling gait.* Difficulty in bending arms and legs make walking a special challenge. Often the ability to swing the arm is noticeably diminished on one side. The patient

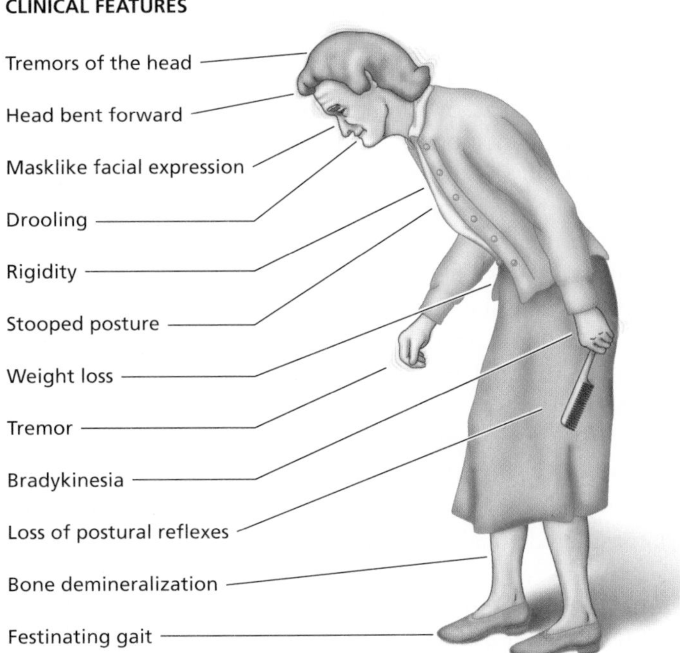

Figure 4.4. Clinical features of Parkinson disease.

takes small steps and may then have to stumble forward to avoid falling. This chasing after the center of gravity is called a *festinating gait*.

- *Changes in speech.* PD causes progressive rigidity of the muscles in the larynx that control vocalization. The speech gradually becomes monotone and expressionless and progresses toward whispering. Muscular changes in the mouth and throat also create problems with swallowing and drooling, particularly while lying down.
- *Changes in handwriting.* The loss of coordination in fine motor muscles changes the ability of a PD patient to write by hand. *Micrographia*, or progressively shrinking, cramped handwriting, is one of the later symptoms of this disease.
- *Sleep disorders.* PD patients are subject to a variety of sleep disorders, from a complete reversal of normal sleeping schedules to sleeplessness because it is difficult or impossible to move in bed.
- *Depression.* The progressive nature of PD makes anxiety and depression a very predictable part of the disease process. Depression can also be related to insomnia, or it can be a side effect of medication. Sometimes the symptoms of depression can outweigh the symptoms of the disease, and treatment for depression can lessen PD symptoms as well.
- *Mental degeneration.* This is a subject of some controversy. Some sources suggest that advanced PD patients have memory loss and deterioration of thought processes. Mental problems are often side effects of PD drugs, however, so it can be difficult to distinguish whether these symptoms are related to the disease itself or to treatments for it.

Treatment

In PD a dopamine deficiency develops in the basal ganglia of the brain. A manmade precursor of dopamine called *levodopa* (*L-dopa*) can cross the blood-brain barrier, especially with a companion drug called *carbidopa*, but it is usually a temporary solution. Patients often develop resistance to the drug, and it has a number of troubling side effects, including hallucinations and dementia. Some dopamine agonists can be substituted when it becomes necessary, or L-dopa can be prescribed with other drugs that serve to mediate side effects.

Other drug therapies include substances that slow the metabolism of dopamine so that whatever is available stays for a longer time, and substances that stimulate dopamine receptors in the basal ganglia so that uptake of the neurotransmitter happens more easily. ***Anticholinergic*** agents that work to limit muscle contraction, and antivirals are also employed. None of these is a permanent solution, however. Doctors working with PD patients must monitor their medications carefully and make frequent adjustments.

New discoveries about the pathology of neural tissue have yielded several other treatment options for PD patients who don't respond to medication. One of them is deep brain stimulation, in which an electrode is inserted in the thalamus. The patient can activate the thalamus by passing a magnet over a pacemaker-like device that is implanted in the chest. Stimulating the thalamus in this way causes an immediate cessation in tremors. Other surgical options include alterations to the thalamus and other midbrain structures to try to modulate motor dysfunction. As neurosurgery advances, these surgeries are becoming safer and more dependable, but they are still considered a viable option only when medications are no longer effective.

Physical, speech, and occupational therapies are often employed to maintain the health and general functioning levels of PD patients for as long as possible. Psychotherapy and support groups are recommended to cope with the effects of depression.

Massage?

PD patients have progressive stiffness and rigidity of voluntary muscles. Massage when the therapist is acting as part of a health care team can be a valuable tool not only to maintain flexibility and range of motion but also to reduce anxiety and depression. It is important to work in cooperation with a client's primary physician, because massage may affect the need for some kinds of medication. Be aware, however, that clients with PD do not have the freedom of movement that most other people do, and they may have great difficulty in getting on and off tables safely. Some massage therapists solve this by doing their work with these clients on mats on the floor.

Some PD patients receive tremendous benefits from various types of massage; frequent treatments with short duration seem to be the most effective.

Modality Recommendations for Parkinson Disease

Modality	Recommendation
Deep Tissue Massage	Supportive with adaptations for client comfort.
Lymphatic Drainage	Supportive.
Polarity	S/R/D: Indicated.
PNF/MET/Stretching	Supportive.
Reflexology	Indicated; work brain, spine, all glands, solar plexus points.
Shiatsu	Supportive. Treat BL, K, GB, SP, LV, SI meridians and extensions.
Swedish Massage	Indicated; can help with sleep and rigidity. Clients may need assistance getting on/off table.
Trigger Point Therapy	Indicated in all stages.

See Chapter 1 for a brief description of each modality, including definitions of abbreviations.

Tremor

Definition: What Is It?

Tremor is involuntary movements. It can be a freestanding disorder or a symptom of a number of different types of CNS problems. The key characteristics of tremor disorders are that the movements are rhythmic oscillations of antagonistic muscle groups and the movement occurs in a fixed plane. Tremor varies by velocity, body parts involved, and amplitude.

Chorea

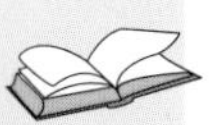

A synonym for tremor, *chorea* comes from the Greek *choreia*, a choral dance. It has the same root as the word *chorus*, which gives some insight into what those Greek choruses were doing during all those tragedies.

Etiology: What Happens?

Tremors can occur in a variety of ways. While the exact mechanisms in the brain are not well understood, new brain imaging techniques are beginning to yield more information about differences in CNS structure and metabolism in people who have various types of tremor. Most appear to be related to dysfunction in the links between the brainstem, the cerebellum, and the thalamus.

Tremor in Brief
Pronunciation: TREM-ur

What is it?
Tremor is rhythmic, involuntary muscle movement. It can be a primary disorder (unrelated to other problems), or it can be a symptom of other neurological diseases.

How is it recognized?
Tremor is identified through rhythmic, predictable, but uncontrolled fine or gross motor movements.

Is massage indicated or contraindicated?
Tremor may indicate massage as long as no contraindicating conditions are contributing factors.

Tremors are generally classified as *resting tremor*, *action tremor*, or *psychogenic tremor*. Resting tremor occurs when the person is at rest but not during sleep. This is the type of tremor seen with Parkinson disease. Action tremor is further classified as *postural tremor* (the ossillations occur when the patient attempts to hold a limb against gravity, i.e., holding an arm out in front); *isometric tremor* (shaking occurs with isometric contractions, i.e., squeezing the examiner's fingers); or *intention tremor* (this occurs when the patient attempts to use his or her hands for fine or complex tasks). Psychogenic tremor is present in everyone but is usually so subtle it is unnoticeable. When it becomes pronounced, it is often stress-related and disappears when the person is distracted.

Tremors may be further classified by whether they are *physiologic* (exacerbated by stress, fear, or underlying problems such as alcohol withdrawal, hypoglycemia, hyperthyroidism, or drug reactions) or *pathologic* (either idiopathic or caused by some other disease).

It is important to understand why a person may have tremors because treatment options for this disorder vary according to cause and classification. Some of the most common tremor types are listed here:

- *Essential tremor* is an idiopathic chronic tremor that is not secondary to any other pathology. Up to 10 million people in the United States have essential tremor. This condition is slowly progressive but not usually debilitating. Onset can occur as early as adolescence, but essential tremor most often shows up at about 45 years of age. It can be an inherited disorder. Neurological studies show that the cerebellum, thalamus, red nucleus, and ***globus pallidus*** are all more active than normal in persons with essential tremor.
- *Huntington disease* is a hereditary degeneration of nerve tissue in the cerebrum. Symptoms don't usually appear until adulthood, when tremors and progressive dementia become irreversible. The average age of onset is 35 to 50 years. It affects approximately 5 out of every 1 million people in the United States.
- *Multiple-system atrophy* can result in tremor, although it also involves stiffness, rigidity, loss of balance, poor coordination, orthostatic hypotension, fainting, blurred vision, and several other problems. Multiple-system atrophy is the term now given to what used to be three separate disorders: ***Shy-Drager syndrome***, ***striatonigral degeneration***, and ***olivopontocerebellar atrophy***.
- *PD* is another CNS disorder involving involuntary movement. It is discussed earlier in this chapter.
- *Other factors* that can cause tremor include alcohol withdrawal, PN, and damage to the cerebellum from stroke, MS, or tumors.

Treatment

Tremor is treated according to underlying causes. Dopamine precursors, beta blockers, tranquilizers, antiseizure medications, botulinum toxin (if it affects muscles of the voice or head), and small doses of alcohol may be suggested. Surgical intervention may be used if the tremor is debilitating and unresponsive to medication; options include surgical interruption at the thalamus or globus pallidus.

Massage?

If a client has episodes of uncontrolled muscular contraction and has not been diagnosed, it is important to get more information before performing massage. It may be that massage can help to reconnect these patients with their body in a way that is beneficial, but it is vital to work as part of a health care team.

Modality Recommendations for Tremor

Deep Tissue Massage	Supportive in conjunction with health care team. May improve client awareness with slow pressure.
Lymphatic drainage	Supportive.
Polarity	S/R/D: Indicated.
PNF/MET/Stretching	Supportive.
Reflexology	Indicated; work head, endocrine system, solar plexus points.
Shiatsu	Indicated. Treat BL, SI, LI, GB, LV meridians and extensions.
Swedish Massage	Supportive; can help reinforce a parasympathetic state.
Trigger Point Therapy	Indicated.

See Chapter 1 for a brief description of each modality, including definitions of abbreviations.

Encephalitis in Brief
Pronunciation: en-sef-uh-LY-tis

What is it?
Encephalitis is inflammation of the brain. It is usually brought about by a viral infection, but other agents can cause it as well.

How is it recognized?
Signs and symptoms of encephalitis include fever, headache, confusion, and personality and memory changes. In rare cases, encephalitis causes permanent neurological damage or even death.

Is massage indicated or contraindicated?
Acute encephalitis contraindicates massage, but if a client has had it in the past and has no signs of present infection or neurological damage, massage is perfectly safe.

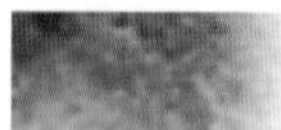

Infectious Disorders

Encephalitis

Definition: What Is It?

Encephalitis is an infection of the brain, usually caused by any of a variety of viruses. It frequently occurs along with inflammation of the spinal cord (myelitis) and/or inflammation of the meninges (meningitis).

Demographics: Who Gets It?

Until recently, some types of encephalitis were considered to be *endemic* to certain areas, that is, specifically limited to geographical regions. However, as the potential for international travel has essentially made the world smaller, strains of virus that used to be restricted to certain areas are being found all over the globe (Sidebar 4.2).

The most common varieties of encephalitis are not typically reported to public health organizations, so it is difficult to estimate how frequently they occur. It is a relatively rare problem, however, leading to fewer than 10,000 diagnoses per year overall.

The people at risk for the worst effects of encephalitis are infants and older people. Older children and young adults may be exposed to the infectious agents and never develop significant symptoms.

Etiology: What Happens?

Most cases of encephalitis are viral, although they can be related to bacterial infections (especially with Lyme disease) or fungi. Viral infections can be primary (a direct attack on the nervous system) or secondary (a complication of viral infection elsewhere in the body).

Primary viral encephalitis is often related to enteroviruses, which are spread directly from one person to another, or arboviruses, which are spread through an animal vector, usually mosquitoes. Another vector-borne form of encephalitis is spread through the bites of infected mammals: this is rabies, although it is rare in the United States today.

Secondary viral encephalitis is typically brought about as a complication of a viral infection that begins somewhere else. Causative agents include herpes simplex (this can cause a very dangerous form of encephalitis in newborns), mumps, measles, and herpes zoster (which is usually associated with chickenpox in childhood and shingles in maturity).

Encephalitis infections affect the *parenchyma* (working areas) of the brain and sometimes the meninges and spinal cord. Very often infections are mild and do not lead to long-lasting damage. Occasionally, and especially if the patient is very young or very old, encephalitis infections cause permanent neurological damage or even death.

SIDEBAR 4.2: WEST NILE ENCEPHALITIS: WATCHING A VIRUS TAKE HOLD

In August 1999, six residents of Queens, New York, checked into local hospitals with high fever in combination with debilitating headaches. Five of them also developed alarming neurological symptoms: weakness, paralysis, and even coma.

Initial tests suggested an outbreak of Saint Louis encephalitis, a mosquito-borne viral infection. But patients showed a different pattern from that usually seen with St. Louis encephalitis; several of them were much sicker than medical professionals expected to see. Within days several more people in the area were reporting similar symptoms.

At the same time, a few miles to the north of the epicenter, birds in the Bronx Zoo were dying at a startling rate. Crows all over the city were dying, too. Horses in nearby suburbs were falling to a mysterious brain fever.

It took some time, but epidemiologists finally put the phenomena together and realized that the viruses attacking humans were the same as those attacking the birds and horses. It was firmly established that the infectious agent was one never before seen in the United States: West Nile encephalitis virus was being transmitted from horses and birds to humans by common mosquitoes.

By the time the first frost killed the mosquito population, 56 confirmed cases were identified among humans, with 7 deaths. The people who died of encephalitis were all over 68 years of age.

It has never been firmly established exactly how the West Nile virus got to New York. One of the patients had been to Africa the previous June and might have been infected then, or it is possible that one of the birds in the Bronx Zoo carried the virus into the United States. Aggressive mosquito abatement programs limited the spread of the disease for that season, but studies of both mosquitoes and birds indicate that the virus has now expanded over much of the continent.

In 2005, 3,000 people in the United States were diagnosed with West Nile virus, and 119 of them died of it. The disease has been reported in every state in the contiguous United States.[8] The virus continues to be watched closely, but a general pattern has emerged: during the first summer that it appears in a new area diagnosis and mortality rates tend to be high. In subsequent summers they tend to fall. This indicates that a portion of the population may have low-grade exposure to the virus and develop protection from subsequent exposure. It is still important to be vigilant about this infection, which can be life threatening, but the initially aggressive phase may be over.

Signs and Symptoms

Symptoms of encephalitis can range from so mild they're never even identified to extremely severe. How the disease presents depends on the virus and the age and general health of the patient. Infants, the elderly, and immunosuppressed people are most vulnerable to the very extreme forms of the disease, while others only rarely have any lasting damage from the inflammation.

The mild end of the symptomatic scale includes a sudden onset of fever with headaches, drowsiness, irritability, and disordered thought processes. In severe cases drowsiness can progress to stupor and then coma. The patient may also have double vision, confused sensation, impaired speech or hearing, convulsions, and partial or full paralysis. Changes in personality, intellect, and memory may develop, depending on which parts of the brain are affected.

Diagnosis

The presenting symptoms for any CNS disturbance are so varied and individualized it is difficult to make a conclusive diagnosis without a full range of intrusive testing. For encephalitis this means a spinal tap to look for signs of inflammation in the cerebral spinal fluid, along with computed tomography (CT) or MRI to look for signs of inflammation. Blood tests can identify the presence of some viruses, and an electroencephalogram (EEG) can show signs of disrupted brain activity.

Treatment

Viruses don't respond to antibiotic therapy, which is designed to disable bacteria only. Encephalitis is treated with antiviral medications to slow viral activity, along with steroids to limit inflammation, sedatives to moderate convulsions, and "supportive therapy," which is to say, tender loving care.

Prognosis

The prognosis for encephalitis depends on the vulnerability of the patient, the virulence of the pathogen, and how early treatment is administered. Very often healthy people can emerge from a short-term infection with no lasting damage. But prolonged inflammation in the CNS may cause permanent damage to structures that have little or no capacity to heal. Thus permanent paralysis or cognitive changes may be the result of a serious bout with this disease.

Massage?

If a client exhibits the major signs of an encephalitis infection, especially headache, fever, and irritability, it systemically contraindicates massage. If, on the other hand, it shows up on the medical history as a long-ago infection and the client has no permanent damage, massage should be just fine.

Modality Recommendations for Encephalitis	
Deep Tissue Massage	Systemically contraindicated while acute.
Lymphatic Drainage	Systemically contraindicated while acute; otherwise supportive.
Polarity	S: Indicated for immune system support. R/D: Contraindicated while acute; otherwise supportive within client comfort.
PNF/MET/Stretching	Systemically contraindicated while acute; otherwise supportive.
Reflexology	Systemically contraindicated while acute; otherwise work endocrine system, lymphatic system, heart points.
Shiatsu	Systemically contraindicated while acute; indicated for immune system treatment via TH, SP.
Swedish Massage	Systemically contraindicated while acute; otherwise supportive.
Trigger Point Therapy	Systemically contraindicated while acute; otherwise supportive.

See Chapter 1 for a brief description of each modality, including definitions of abbreviations.

Herpes Zoster

Definition: What Is It?

Also known as *shingles*, herpes zoster is a viral infection of the nervous system. In this case the targeted tissues are the dendrites at the end of sensory neurons, which leads to painful, fluid-filled blisters on all of the nerve endings of a specific dermatome. Shingles affects about

500,000 people in the United States every year: about 2 in 10 people have this infection at some point. It seldom affects the same person twice unless that person is severely immunocompromised.

Etiology: What Happens?

The pathogen at fault here is the chickenpox virus, which can be called *varicella zoster virus.* When a person is exposed to chickenpox in childhood, the normal course of events is to have painful itchy blisters along with fever and malaise. The infection runs its course within a few days, and everything goes back to normal. The difference with varicella zoster virus is that although a full complement of chickenpox antibodies is present after the infection, the virus is never fully expelled from the body. Instead, it goes into a dormant state in the dorsal root ganglia (the meeting point for all the sensory neurons in each dermatome) or the ***geniculate ganglion*** of the trigeminal nerve. Then later in life, when circulating antibodies are low, the virus may reactivate, this time as shingles.

It is hard to predict what might trigger a reactivation of the herpes zoster virus. Contributing factors include stress, old age, and impaired immunity because of other diseases. Shingles is notorious for accompanying HIV, Hodgkin lymphoma, advanced tuberculosis, pneumonia, chemotherapy, or having had an initial infection before 18 months of age. Shingles occasionally occurs after severe trauma or as a drug reaction.

Although the fluid in zoster blisters is filled with virus, shingles isn't particularly contagious because most people have already been exposed to chickenpox and have protection. This does not hold true, however, for a person who comes in contact with shingles while his or her own immune system is depressed or who has never been exposed to the virus in the first place. In this case an adult is may get either shingles or chickenpox, but shingles is more likely.

Shingles 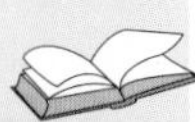

The name *shingles* derives not from the appearance of the infection, but from the Latin *cingulum*, which means girdle or belt. This describes the typical distribution of blisters around the chest or abdomen on a single dermatomal line.

Signs and Symptoms

Pain is the primary symptom of this disease. Pain is present for 1 to 3 days before the blisters break out. Pain is present for the 2 to 3 weeks in which blisters develop, erupt, and scab over. Pain is often present for months even after the lesions have healed and the skin is intact again.

The blisters may grow along the entire dermatome of the host dorsal root ganglion, but more often they appear along an isolated stretch. It is nearly always a unilateral attack (Figure 4.5). Sensory nerves that supply the trunk and buttocks are the most frequently affected, although the trigeminal nerve may also be attacked.

Occasionally a person can have a reactivation of varicella zoster virus with all of the pain sensation but with no visible lesions. This condition, called *zoster sine herpete* (*sine* means *without*, so this means *zoster without herpes lesions*) can be easily misdiagnosed as a herniated disc, a heart attack, or multiple other painful but invisible conditions.

Complications

The most common complication of herpes zoster is secondary bacterial infection of the blisters. Another common complication is a viral attack on the trigeminal nerve, which can lead to eye damage, hearing loss, and temporary or permanent facial paralysis resembling Bell palsy. This is sometimes referred to as ***Ramsay-Hunt syndrome type 1.***

Herpes Zoster in Brief

Pronunciation: HUR-peze ZOS-ter

What is it?

Herpes zoster, or shingles, is an infection of sensory neurons with the same virus that causes chickenpox.

How is it recognized?

Shingles produces a rash with extremely painful blisters unilaterally along the colonized dermatomes. The trigeminal nerve, trunk, low back, and buttocks are most often affected.

Is massage indicated or contraindicated?

This is an extraordinarily painful condition, and it contraindicates massage in the acute stage. After the blisters have healed and the pain has subsided, massage is appropriate.

SIDEBAR 4.3: CHICKENPOX VACCINE

A chickenpox vaccine for young children was licensed in the United States in 1995. Many schools now require that children entering kindergarten be vaccinated against this infection. While this protects children from an uncomfortable time (and a small but significant risk of dangerous complications), perhaps the greater incentive is for their parents, who would otherwise have to miss a week of work to stay home with a sick child.

But further research has revealed some unexpected consequences of this vaccination campaign. The chickenpox vaccine wears off within several years, leaving vaccinated children vulnerable to breakout infections with the virus, although these tend to be less severe than typical infections. But to retain full immunity, vaccinated people need to encounter this pathogen from time to time to boost their immune system responses. With the success of the chickenpox vaccination campaign, it is now rare to spend time with a child who has chickenpox.

A similar pattern has been seen with the incidence of shingles (herpes zoster) among older adults: those who are able to spend time with children who have chickenpox are much less likely to have shingles. It seems this exposure helps the immune system to remain armed against varicella zoster. This has led to research toward an adult booster shot for varicella zoster that will prevent the outbreak of shingles and its painful complication, postherpetic neuralgia.

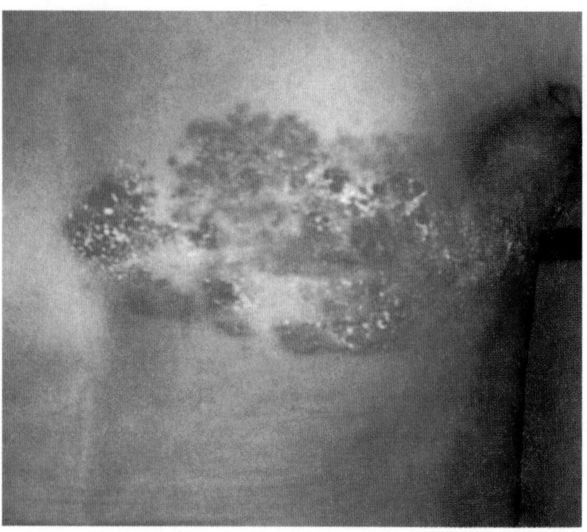

Figure 4.5. Herpes zoster, or shingles.

In rare situations a person with shingles develops lesions outside the affected dermatome. When 20 or more blisters are present beyond the initial area, a viral infection of the blood (***viremia***) may be present; this can be a life-threatening condition.

An additional complication of shingles is postherpetic neuralgia. In this situation the pain generated by the viral infection outlives the blisters by a minimum of 3 months and may persist for years. The risk of developing postherpetic neuralgia rises significantly with age: 60% of 60-year-old patients with herpes zoster develop it, and 75% of 70-year-old patients have this complication.

Treatment

Herpes zoster is treated mainly palliatively. Acyclovir, an antiviral medication, has some success with herpes zoster; it is believed to shorten any possible bouts with postherpetic neuralgia. Beyond that, soothing lotion, steroids for anti-inflammatory action, and painkillers are the interventions used most often. If postherpetic neuralgia develops, more aggressive pain interventions may be recommended, including antidepressants, antiseizure medications, topical lidocaine or capsaicin patches, and nerve blocks.

Massage?

Herpes zoster is the kind of disease that is very kind to massage practitioners: during an acute outbreak of this condition, the *last* thing a client wants for is someone to *touch* him or her. Occasionally very mild outbreaks occur, for which massage may be only locally contraindicated, according to the tolerance of the client. When the infection has passed and the lesions have completely healed, massage is perfectly appropriate.

For clients with postherpetic neuralgia, massage therapists must be guided by their comfort and feedback. Of course, any stimulus that exacerbates symptoms must be avoided, but if cooling energy can be shared in a way to alleviate symptoms, this can be a wonderful benefit.

Modality Recommendations for Herpes Zoster

Deep Tissue Massage	Systemically contraindicated while acute; otherwise supportive.
Lymphatic Drainage	Systemically contraindicated while acute; otherwise supportive.
Polarity	S: Indicated for immune system support. R/D: Contraindicated while acute; otherwise supportive within client comfort.
PNF/MET/Stretching	Systemically contraindicated while acute; otherwise supportive.
Reflexology	Indicated if not acute; work brain, spine, lymphatic system points.
Shiatsu	Systemically contraindicated while acute; then indicated for immune system treatment via TH, SP.
Swedish Massage	Systemically contraindicated while acute; otherwise supportive.
Trigger Point Therapy	Locally contraindicated while acute; otherwise supportive.

See Chapter 1 for a brief description of each modality, including definitions of abbreviations.

Meningitis

Definition: What Is It?

Meningitis is *meninges* + *-itis*: an inflammation of the meninges and the cerebrospinal fluid that surround the brain and spinal cord.

Demographics: Who Gets It?

About 5,000 cases of meningitis are diagnosed each year in this country. Most infections are in children under 5 years of age or elderly people, although in recent years other high-risk groups have been identified: first-year college students living in dormitories and military recruits also living in close quarters. Most dangerous cases of meningitis are among people whose resistance is low: the immunosuppressed, babies, and the elderly.

Etiology: What Happens?

Meningitis is usually caused by bacterial or viral infection. It is important to find the causative factor because the severity and treatment options vary according to the pathogen.

- *Bacterial meningitis.* This infection is usually due to an invasion of *Streptococcus pneumoniae* (also called *pneumococcus*) or *Neisseria meningitides* (also called *meningococcus*). Bacterial meningitis tends to be more severe than the viral infection, and the risk of long-term CNS damage, specifically hearing loss or loss of mental function, is much higher. It does respond to antibiotics if the correct ones are administered early in the disease process.
- *Viral meningitis.* The viruses that can cause meningitis are many and varied, including a number of enteroviruses (usually associated with intestinal infections), herpes, coxsackievirus, and others. Viral meningitis tends to be less severe than bacterial meningitis and seldom causes permanent damage.

Meningitis in Brief
Pronunciation: men-in-JY-tis

What is it?
Meningitis is an infection of the meninges, specifically the pia mater and the cerebrospinal fluid.

How is it recognized?
Symptoms of acute meningitis include very high fever, rash, photophobia, headache, and stiff neck. Symptoms are not always consistent, however; they may appear in different combinations for different people.

Is massage indicated or contraindicated?
Meningitis, a communicable inflammatory disease, strictly contraindicates massage in the acute phase. People who have recovered from meningitis with no lasting damage are perfectly fine to receive massage.

When a pathogen enters the CNS (usually in the bloodstream), it causes a number of changes that can be very dangerous. Bacteria in the CNS find a hospitable environment: cerebrospinal fluid is rich with nutrients but poor in white blood cells, antibodies, and complement factor that would otherwise work together to dismantle potential invaders elsewhere in the body.

Infection in the cerebrospinal fluid increases the permeability of the blood-brain barrier. This in turn leads to cerebral edema and adds toxins to cerebrospinal fluid. Intracranial pressure can damage cranial nerves (CN VIII is especially at risk, and damage here can lead to permanent hearing loss or deafness); obstructive ***hydrocephalus*** (which limits the normal circulation of cerebrospinal fluid within the brain and spinal cord); and inflammation of internal blood vessels with a high risk of blood clots and ischemic damage to brain cells.

Ultimately, without treatment the body's autoregulating centers are damaged, and the person dies of diffuse brain injury. Untreated meningitis, especially when it is bacterial, has a high mortality rate. Even when it is treated aggressively, 10 to 14% of cases are fatal, and 11 to 19% of patients have permanent damage.[9]

The bacteria that cause meningitis can infect other tissues as well. Most people with pneumococcal infections of the CNS concurrently have pneumonia, for instance. And bacterial infections of the blood can lead to the distinctive reddish-purple rash associated with meningitis, along with a risk of blood clotting in capillaries, which opens the door to gangrene in the extremities.

Signs and Symptoms

The symptoms of an acute meningitis infection include a rapid onset of very high fever and chills, a deep red or purple rash, extreme headache, irritability, aversion to bright light, and a stiff, rigid neck. The neck is held tightly because any movement or stretching of the swollen meninges is excruciatingly painful. Drowsiness and slurred speech may be present. More extreme infections cause nausea, vomiting, delirium, and possibly convulsions or coma.

Bacterial meningitis incubates for several hours to 10 days. It is imperative to treat bacterial meningitis quickly to avoid complications.

It takes up to 3 weeks for viral infections to develop. Symptoms generally peak and then recede over 2 to 3 weeks.

Diagnosis

Meningitis is diagnosed through a spinal tap to examine the cerebrospinal fluid for pus, fragments of pathogens, and reduced glucose levels. (The infectious agents consume the glucose that would normally be available to the CNS.)

Treatment

If the pathogen is identified as a bacterium, large doses of antibiotics are administered immediately to forestall the possibility of CNS damage. Steroids may also be prescribed to limit inflammation in the brain. Viral meningitis is generally treated with supportive therapy consisting of rest, fluids, and good nutrition while the patient's immune system fights back.

Most people emerge from meningitis with no lasting damage if the correct treatment is administered early in the infection.

Communicability

Meningitis can be contagious. Its mode of transmission is much like the common cold: an infected person sneezes or coughs and then touches some surface, such as a doorknob or light switch. An uninfected person touches the surface, then touches his or her eye or mouth.

Meningitis brought about by the intestinal enterovirus family can also be spread by oral-fecal contact, which is an issue when it occurs in young children or in day care settings.

Some parts of the world are subject to epidemics of meningitis. The meningeal belt of sub-Saharan Africa has seasonal outbreaks of the severe bacterial version of this disease.

Prevention

In the United States the *Haemophilus influenzae* type B (HiB) vaccine is probably the most effective prevention against childhood meningitis; before the vaccine was available, this was the most common causative agent of bacterial meningitis. Vaccines against two of the three types of meningococcus bacteria have been developed, but they are generally recommended only for people planning to travel to places where epidemics are in progress or college students who plan to live in a high-density dormitory.

Massage?

Meningitis contraindicates massage in the acute stage. These people don't just need bed rest; they may need hospital care. Clients who have recovered from meningitis with no lasting effects are perfectly appropriate candidates for massage.

Modality Recommendations for Meningitis	
Deep Tissue Massage	Systemically contraindicated while acute; work with affected areas during recovery.
Lymphatic Drainage	Systemically contraindicated while acute; otherwise supportive.
Polarity	S: Indicated following contagious stage. R/D: Systemically contraindicated while acute; otherwise supportive.
PNF/MET/Stretching	Systemically contraindicated while acute; otherwise supportive.
Reflexology	Systemically contraindicated while acute; otherwise work brain, lymphatic system points.
Shiatsu	Systemically contraindicated while acute; then indicated for immune system treatment via TH, SP. Add BL, GB to target brain.
Swedish Massage	Systemically contraindicated while acute; otherwise supportive.
Trigger Point Therapy	Systemically contraindicated while acute; otherwise supportive.

See Chapter 1 for a brief description of each modality, including definitions of abbreviations.

Polio and Postpolio Syndrome

Definition: What Is It?

Poliomyelitis, or *infantile paralysis*, as it used to be known, is a viral disease. The poliovirus targets intestinal mucosa first and anterior horn nerve cells later.

Postpolio syndrome (PPS) is a progressive muscular weakness that develops 10 to 40 years after an initial infection with the poliovirus.

Demographics: Who Gets It?

The last case of wild polio infection (that is, infection unrelated to weakened virus in vaccines) in the United States was in 1979, so the risk of encountering this disease in its acute state is low for people who live in this country (Sidebar 4.4).

Polio

Polio is from the Greek word for gray. Polio denotes damage to the gray matter of the CNS. Poliomyelitis indicates damage and inflammation in the gray matter, specifically in the spinal cord (**myelos** means marrow).

Polio and Postpolio Syndrome in Brief

What are they?
Polio is a viral infection, first of the intestines and then (for about 1% of exposed people) the anterior horn cells of the spinal cord. Postpolio syndrome (PPS) is a group of signs and symptoms common to polio survivors, particularly those who had significant loss of function in the acute stage of the disease.

How are they recognized?
The destruction of motor neurons leads to degeneration, atrophy, and finally paralysis of skeletal muscles in polio patients. Later in life they may develop a sudden onset of fatigue, achiness, and weakness. Breathing and sleeping difficulties may also occur.

Is massage indicated or contraindicated?
The poliovirus does not affect sensation or cognition. Therefore, massage is appropriate for polio survivors, as long as the acute phase of the infection has passed. PPS also indicates massage.

SIDEBAR 4.4: POLIO: IT'S ALMOST EXTINCT

The statistics on polio are extremely promising. In 1988 the Global Poliomyelitis Eradication Initiative combined efforts by the World Health Organization (WHO), UNICEF, Rotary International, and the Centers for Disease Control in the largest public health effort for the eradication of a disease. As a result of this effort, the last new case of wild poliovirus in the Western Hemisphere was diagnosed in Peru in August 1991. The western Pacific region was certified polio free in October 2000. The last reported case in Europe was in 1998.

As of 2003 wild poliovirus was endemic to only six countries (India, Pakistan, Nigeria, Niger, Afghanistan, and Egypt), and outbreaks occurred in tightly restricted areas. About 90% of the new cases of polio were in small areas of India, Pakistan, and Nigeria. Fewer than 800 new cases of polio paralysis were reported in all of 2003; this is in contrast to more than 1,000 cases per day reported in 1998.[10]

Countries with little or no incidence of polio infection are still vulnerable to invasion with the virus, especially along borders with countries where the virus is still active. Therefore, it is recommended that even "safe" countries maintain their vaccination schedules until the globe is free of the poliovirus.

PPS is a different matter, however. It is estimated that 440,000 people in the United States may be at risk for this condition.[11] It is difficult to gather statistics on what proportion of polio survivors eventually develop PPS; estimates range from 25% to 60%, but because it can be very mild, some people may never seek attention for this problem.

Etiology: What Happens?

The poliovirus is spread most efficiently through oral-fecal contamination. It usually enters the body through the mouth in contaminated water. It gets past the acidic environment of the stomach and sets up an infection in the intestine. New virus is concentrated and released in fecal matter, possibly to contaminate water elsewhere.

For over 99% of people exposed to the poliovirus, this is the end of the story. Symptoms resemble severe flu: headache, deep muscular ache, and high fever. These are followed by an intestinal infection, a bout with diarrhea, and then the infection is over. But in fewer than 1% of people who are exposed, the virus travels into the CNS, where it targets and destroys nerve cells in the anterior horn cells of the spinal cord. This impedes motor messages leaving the spinal cord, which in turn leads to rapid deterioration and atrophy of muscles and motor paralysis.

The paralysis caused by polio is motor only; sensation is still present. And because the motor nerves overlap muscle groups in the extremities, some muscle fibers may still function, even though a whole level of motor neurons may have been damaged. In other words, consider the dermatomes for the quadriceps. Even if all of the impulses to the motor neurons in L2 have been eliminated, L3 supplies other motor neurons to the same muscle group (Fig. 4.6). Furthermore, anterior horn cells that survive the initial attack can grow new terminal axons to enervate muscle cells that were otherwise cut off. This increases the size of each motor unit and puts excessive demand on the cell body of the enlarged motor neuron to supply the fiber with nutrition. In the long run, these motor neurons may wear out, leading to muscle weakness and possible atrophy: this is PPS.

Signs and Symptoms

Polio is little more than a memory for most people in this country, but some people who had polio as children, especially those who had significant loss of function with a good recovery in childhood, find as they reach middle age that they have a sudden and sometimes extreme onset of fatigue, achiness, and weakness: PPS. Breathing difficulties, sleep disturbances, and trouble swallowing may also develop. These symptoms usually begin 10 to 40 years after the original infection. They tend to run in cycles in which function is progressively lost, followed by periods of stability and then more loss of function.

Diagnosis

PPS is diagnosed by looking for a confirmed prior episode of paralytic polio along with other criteria that include a gradual onset of muscle weakness and loss of stamina persisting for at least a year as well as exclusion of other conditions that can cause similar symptoms.

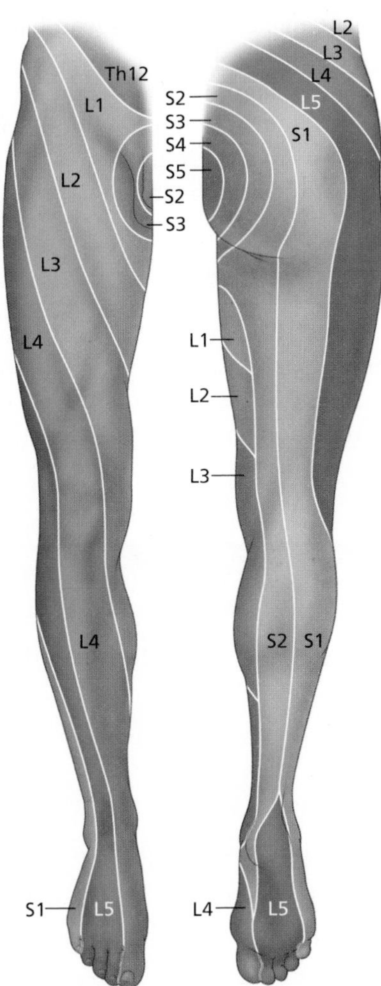

Figure 4.6. Dermatome patterns in the leg muscles allowing multiple nerves to supply muscle groups; if one nerve root is damaged, the muscle group is still usable.

Treatment

Moist heat applications, physical therapy, and massage have been used to treat polio survivors once the initial infection has subsided. Together, hydrotherapy and massage can help to keep functioning muscle fibers healthy and well nourished.

PPS is treated as a problem that may be addressed by reducing muscular and neurological stress: adjusted braces, a change in activity levels, and exercise programs that encourage the use of muscles *not* supplied by the damaged nerves. People with PPS should avoid excessive use of affected muscles, since exercise to these compromised tissues can cause permanent damage to the working fibers.

Prevention

Polio is not difficult to prevent. Two inexpensive, stable, easy-to-administer vaccines are effective against this disease.

The Sabin vaccine, an oral medication, introduces weakened viruses into the digestive system, where they attract antibodies exactly where the virus first tends to reside. The advantage of the Sabin vaccine is that because it is given orally rather than by injection, it can be administered by anyone. However, because it contains live virus, it carries a small risk that a person being vaccinated can become infected. Also, it is possible for the vaccinated person to transmit the disease to someone else. People who handle the diapers of infants who have received the oral vaccine need to be aware that live virus may be in the fecal matter. Immunosuppressed persons should avoid contact with infants who are undergoing this treatment.

The Salk vaccine is an injection of inactivated poliovirus into the bloodstream, causing the recipient to produce a set of antibodies against it. In the United States the injected form of vaccine is now the only one recommended; the oral version is still in use in worldwide vaccination programs.

Massage?

Massage therapists in the United States are *extremely* unlikely to encounter an acute case of polio in their practice. Polio survivors have only motor paralysis; sensation is still intact. Massage can be performed for these clients with good possibility of benefit and little risk of danger.

PPS indicates massage: it can improve local nutrition and generally decrease strain on the nervous system.

MODALITY RECOMMENDATIONS FOR POLIO, POSTPOLIO SYNDROME	
Deep Tissue Massage	Indicated for PPS within client tolerance to release fascia, restore mobility, relax CNS.
Lymphatic Drainage	Supportive.
Polarity	S: Indicated. R/D: Contraindicated while acute; otherwise indicated.
PNF/MET/Stretching	Systemically contraindicated while acute; otherwise supportive.
Reflexology	Indicated; work brain, spine, solar plexus, lymphatic system points.
Shiatsu	Indicated; treat BL, K, SI, L, GB, LV, SP, TH to target nerves, muscles, immune system.
Swedish Massage	Contraindicated while acute; otherwise indicated for improved muscle function.
Trigger Point Therapy	Contraindicated while acute; otherwise indicated for improved muscle function.

See Chapter 1 for a brief description of each modality, including definitions of abbreviations not spelled out here.

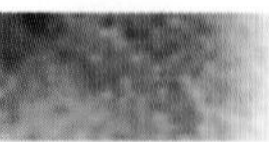

PSYCHIATRIC DISORDERS

Anxiety Disorders

Definition: What Are They?

Anxiety disorders are a collection of distinct psychiatric disorders that have to do with irrational fears and extensive efforts to avoid or control them. Anxiety disorders range in severity from mild to completely debilitating.

Demographics: Who Gets Them?

Statistics for specific types of anxiety disorders are discussed individually, but overall it is estimated that within a given year, up to 40 million people in the United States over age 18 have some type of anxiety disorder. Types of anxiety disorders have enormous overlap; most people with one meet the diagnostic criteria for one or more others.[12] Women outnumber men with anxiety disorders by a ratio of about 3 to 2, but it is unclear whether this is an issue of hormones, social conditioning, or other factors.

Anxiety disorders take a huge toll on a person's ability to complete school or hold a job. Consequently, a disproportionately high percentage of people with anxiety disorders never earn a high school diploma and are in the lowest end of socioeconomic ranking. Furthermore, people with anxiety disorders are far more likely than the general population to become substance abusers and to struggle with depression and suicidal tendencies.

Anxiety Disorders in Brief

What are they?
Anxiety disorders are a group of mental disorders that have to do with exaggerated, irrational fears and the attempts to control those fears. Some anxiety disorders come and go; some are chronic progressive problems; others reach a peak and then recede or remain stable. All anxiety disorders begin as emotional responses that create inappropriate sympathetic reactions.

How are they recognized?
While triggers for individual cases may vary, many anxiety disorders involve sympathetic reactions in the body, including fast heart rate, sweating, dizziness, faintness, nausea, and other signs and symptoms. In addition, some disorders bring about feelings of impending death, a sense of physical detachment, unwelcome or frightening thoughts, and other reactions.

Is massage indicated or contraindicated?
If the stimulus of bodywork is perceived as something safe and welcome, massage can have a useful place in dealing with a variety of anxiety disorders.

Etiology: What Happens?

"*Am I safe?*" At this moment every person who is alive and awake is asking this question at some level of consciousness. The answer for people with anxiety disorders is "*Probably not.*" This misinterpretation of environmental signals is reflected in emotional and physical experiences that can be completely debilitating. Contributing factors include a combination of genetic vulnerability, a history of traumatic events, and situations or circumstances that trigger an inappropriate stress response.

For investigation of these conditions, careful distinctions have been drawn between the key terms *arousal*, *fear*, and *anxiety*. *Arousal* is preparation for the possibility of a stressful event. It is directly linked to a perceived trigger or stressor (the deer that could dart across the darkened highway; the hurricane warnings on the radio). *Fear* occurs when the possibility of a stressful event is confirmed. The deer is in front of you; the wind is blowing shingles off the roof. *Anxiety*, by contrast, is a state of prolonged heightened arousal or fear with no discernible immediate or significant threat: no deer, no storm, but all the physical and emotional reactions that go with the feeling of impending disaster.

CNS studies have investigated two major issues with anxiety disorders: problems with the limbic system and the hypothalamic-pituitary-adrenal (HPA) axis, and neurotransmitter imbalances.

- *The limbic system and the HPA axis.* The limbic system is a part of the brain that is primarily responsible for determining a person's sense of safety in any given moment. It does this through two regulatory centers, the amygdala and the hippocampus. These structures govern memory storage and emotions, and they are directly linked to the hypothalamus, the mediator of sympathetic or parasympathetic response. The hippocampus has been found to be a center for verbal memory, while the amygdala catalogues a history of fear responses. When a person experiences a threatening stimulus, these structures work together to recognize the threat and translate this information to the hypothalamus, which uses the HPA axis to establish a stress response. The HPA axis produces electrical and chemical signals that allow a person to respond appropriately to a stressor. When the HPA axis is overactive, it can cause the release of excessive amounts of glucocorticoids (of which cortisol is the dominant hormone) from the adrenal glands. Research reveals that excessive levels of glucocorticoids in the blood can damage several processes. They can weaken connective tissue, suppress immune system responses, and—most pertinent to a discussion of psychiatric disorders—they can *shrink* the hippocampus.[13] One line of thought about anxiety disorders links the atrophy of the hippocampus (by up to 20% in some circumstances) to a problem in relating triggers to appropriate responses.

- *Neurotransmitters.* The neurotransmitters that are most frequently disturbed in anxiety disorders include ***norepinephrine*** (chemically related to adrenaline), ***gamma-aminobutyric acid*** (GABA), ***serotonin***, corticotrophin-releasing factor, and some others. These are so tightly interdependent that disruption in one of these chemicals tends to cause disruptions in all of them.

Types of Anxiety Disorders

Dozens of distinct anxiety disorders have been documented, each with specific criteria for diagnosis. This list includes of some of the most common versions, along with brief descriptions.

General anxiety disorder (GAD) This disorder affects some 6.8 million people in this country. Women with GAD outnumber men by about 2 to 1. GAD consists of chronic, exaggerated, consuming worry and the constant anticipation of disaster. It does not cause the person to avoid stressful situations, but he or she lives in a constant state of anxiety that makes it difficult to accomplish many tasks. It appears earlier and develops more slowly than other anxiety disorders.

GAD is diagnosed when at least three of the following symptoms persist for 6 months or longer: restlessness or a feeling of being on edge, easy fatigability, poor concentration, irritability, muscle tension, and sleeping problems.

Panic disorder Panic disorder is characterized by the sudden onset (often with no identifiable trigger) of very extreme sympathetic symptoms: a pounding heart, chest pain, sweatiness, dizziness, faintness, and alternating flushing and chilling. Hyperventilation causes numbness and tingling in the lips and extremities. A feeling of being smothered, of impending doom, and the nearness of death usually lasts for about 10 minutes but may persist for many hours.

A person can have a panic attack *without* having panic disorder; this happens to as much as 10% of the population each year. But when episodes repeat, especially if they are associated with a certain place or situation, panic disorder is diagnosed.

Panic disorder affects about 6 million American adults. It is complicated by worrying about having another attack: fear of fear. When it causes a person to avoid situations in which panic attacks have happened before or may happen in the future, it can cause another anxiety disorder, ***agoraphobia***, or fear of open places. Gradually a person's perceived safety zone shrinks to the point where he or she becomes reluctant to leave the immediate environment. About one-third of panic disorder patients develop agoraphobia.

Panic disorder is one of the most successfully treated of all anxiety disorders, but treatment is most successful if it is initiated before the onset of agoraphobia.

Acute traumatic and posttraumatic stress disorders Acute traumatic stress disorder is characterized by development of symptoms within 1 month of a triggering event; posttraumatic stress disorder (PTSD) is identified when symptoms have persisted for 3 months or more.

Traditionally associated with soldiers returning from the horrors of war, PTSD has also been known as "shell shock". PTSD affects about 7.7 million Americans.

Acute traumatic stress disorder and PTSD are characterized by persistent visceral memories of a specific ordeal, such as combat, physical or sexual abuse, rape, assault, torture, natural disaster, terrorist attack, or any other life-threatening event. Sometimes a patient was a witness to an attack or threat to someone else. Memories of the event are relived in nightmares and waking flashbacks. The patient often becomes withdrawn, irritable, and occasionally aggressive as these memories intrude more and more frequently into his life. Startle reflexes tend to be exaggerated. Dissociation, the detachment of the mind from physical or emotional experiences, is a hallmark of PTSD. Some patients find that their symptoms subside with time and eventually no longer affect them, but others find that without treatment this is a lifelong problem.

Symptoms of PTSD usually appear within 3 months of the triggering event, but some patients aren't affected until many months or years later; this is called delayed-onset PTSD.

People with PTSD tend to be hypervigilant, always on the lookout against the possibility of a repeated attack or trauma. Studies of the brain activity of PTSD patients show some differences depending on whether the trauma was impersonal, such as a hurricane or flood, or a personal attack, such as a rape or kidnapping. Generally, survivors of impersonal experiences have less extreme symptoms, although the severity of the stressor does not necessarily correspond to the severity of the symptoms.

Obsessive-compulsive disorder (OCD) OCD is a combination of intrusive, uncontrollable, unwelcome thoughts (*obsessions*) and highly developed rituals designed to try to quell or control those thoughts (*compulsions*). About 2.2 million Americans have it, and the gender ratio is about even. Unlike many other anxiety disorders, OCD can come and go throughout a lifetime and is not always progressive.

Some of the most common obsessions of OCD patients include fear of contamination by dirt, germs, or sexual activity; fear of violence or catastrophic accidents; fear of committing violent or sexual acts; and fears surrounding disorder or asymmetry. The rituals used to battle these fears include repeated hand washing (often to the point of damaging the skin); refusing to touch other people or contaminated surfaces; repeatedly checking locks, stoves, irons, or other appliances; counting telephone poles; carefully and symmetrically arranging clothes, food, or other items; and persistently repeating words, phrases, or prayers. While many people occasionally engage in some of these behaviors, OCD patients often devote hours every day to the rituals that are designed to keep them safe.

Phobias, Social and Specific

- *Social phobia.* Also called *social anxiety disorder*, social phobia is characterized by intense, irrational fears of being judged negatively by others or of being publicly embarrassed. It can involve specific situations, such as speaking or performing in public, or it can involve any social setting at all. Physical symptoms include blushing, sweating, trembling, and nausea, but many social phobia patients display no outward signs of their disorder. While many people feel shy or nervous among strangers, patients with social phobia are significantly distressed and even disabled by their fear, which can interfere with work, school, or relationships. Social phobia affects some 15 million adults in the United States.
- *Specific phobias.* A phobia is an intense, irrational fear of something that poses little or no real danger. Some common phobias include fear of animals (including larger animals such as dogs, cats, or birds but also insects and spiders); closed-in places (claustrophobia), heights (acrophobia), flying, elevators, and blood. Untreated phobias can severely restrict a person's ability to hold a certain kind of job, live in a certain kind of building, or perform mundane tasks, such as grocery shopping. About 19.2 million people have specific phobias. Persons with this disorder often respond better to controlled desensitization and relaxation techniques than they do to medication.

Signs and Symptoms

Signs and symptoms of anxiety disorders vary according to type. While they usually involve irrational fears and inappropriate sympathetic nervous system responses, they present differently by variety and patient. Brief descriptions of their signs and symptoms are included in the descriptions.

Treatment

Most anxiety disorders are treated with a combination of medication and psychotherapy. Some varieties respond better to psychotherapy and the development of coping skills alone, while others also require chemical intervention to reestablish neurotransmitter balance in the CNS. Most patients with anxiety disorders can find some combination of therapies that successfully treat their problem—if they seek treatment. Sadly, many patients are incorrectly diagnosed or never seek treatment at all.

Medications to treat anxiety disorders fall in three classes: antidepressants, antianxiety drugs, and beta blockers. Antidepressants include ***selective serotonin reuptake inhibitors*** (SSRIs), ***tricyclics***, and ***monoamine oxidase inhibitors*** (MAOIs). These drugs often take several weeks to become effective, and they cause unpleasant side effects in the initial stages. Antianxiety medications include ***benzodiazepines***: tranquilizers that influence levels of the neurotransmitter GABA. These can be effective drugs, especially since they can produce results in a short time. Unfortunately, they can also be highly addictive, and they react dangerously with alcohol. Therefore, they are not appropriate for long-term treatment or for anxiety patients who are also chemically dependent on alcohol or other drugs (which is a high percentage of this population). Beta blockers are usually prescribed for high blood pressure patients to decrease the force of heart contractions. They can also help to ameliorate some of the heart-pounding discomfort of panic attacks and social phobias, but they are strictly palliative; they do nothing to fix the problem, they simply quell some of the symptoms.

Psychotherapeutic techniques used for anxiety disorders vary from supported resistance to compulsive behaviors for OCD patients, to controlled exposure to frightening stimuli for people with specific phobias, to various forms of behavioral-cognitive therapies to help patients learn ways to address and often overcome the irrational fears that limit their lives.

Massage?

Relaxation techniques, breathing exercises, and biofeedback are often taught to anxiety disorder patients as coping mechanisms; it seems reasonable that massage and bodywork would fit under this heading as well. Indeed, several research projects under way have shown that touch in general and massage in particular are effective in reducing self-reported anxiety in various populations.[14] However, massage therapy is a fine choice for a person with anxiety disorders *only as long as the stimulus is perceived as safe and nurturing*. While a therapist's intent may be completely benign and supportive, the survivor of touch abuse or other types of trauma may not be able to interpret it as such.

Some people with issues and phobias about touch may specifically seek out massage as a way to experience positive touch in their life. It is a privilege to work with these clients, but massage therapists must be especially vigilant about maintaining clear and careful boundaries around these relationships, so that no one—neither the therapist nor the client—feels abused or taken advantage of.

Modality Recommendations for Anxiety Disorders

Modality	Recommendation
Deep Tissue Massage	Indicated within client tolerance. Invite client to participate with movement and breathing.
Lymphatic Drainage	Supportive.
Polarity	S: Indicated. R/D: Indicated within client comfort and perceived safety.
PNF/MET/Stretching	Supportive.
Reflexology	Indicated; work brain, solar plexus, heart, lymphatic system and endocrine system points.
Shiatsu	Indicated; treat SI, PC, BL, K, GB to calm the mind, nerves, tension.
Swedish Massage	Indicated; can help reinforce a parasympathetic state if client feels safe.
Trigger Point Therapy	Supportive with light work.

See Chapter 1 for a brief description of each modality, including definitions of abbreviations.

Attention Deficit Hyperactivity Disorder

Definition: What Is It?

Attention deficit hyperactivity disorder (ADHD) is a neurobiochemical disorder resulting in difficulties with attention, movement, and impulse control. Recognized in children since the early 1900s, it has had several names, including minimal brain dysfunction. It was not discussed in medical literature as an issue for adults until 1976.

An argument can be made that ADHD is a misnomer. This condition describes a person who pays attention to matters that are considered irrelevant to a central task: this is not attention *deficit*; it is rather *too much* attention to too many things.

Attention Deficit Hyperactivity Disorder in Brief

What is it?
Attention deficit hyperactivity disorder (ADHD) is a neurobiochemical imbalance in the brain resulting in problems with focus, impulse control, and motor activity. It occurs among children and adults.

How is it recognized?
ADHD is recognized by the behavior changes it brings about: inattention, inappropriate impulsivity, and when hyperactivity is present, difficulty with controlling movement. The diagnosis of ADHD depends on the observations of people close to the patient along with ruling out other possible sources for the problems.

Is massage indicated or contraindicated?
ADHD indicates massage, although the preference for the type of bodywork and the length of time it can be administered may vary greatly from one client to another.

Demographics: Who Gets It?

Most estimates suggest that about 4.3% of school-age children (about 4.4 million) have been diagnosed with ADHD. Some surveys, however, show that up to 18% of school-age children within certain areas are medicated for ADHD, and the numbers are disproportionately high among upper middle class white boys.[15] Many authorities recognize that nonwhite children and children with limited access to health care are probably an underserved population in regard to this disorder. This gives ADHD the distinction of being both overdiagnosed and underdiagnosed.

Boys with ADHD are diagnosed about 2.5 times more often than girls. This may be because the way boys often manifest this disorder is with hyperactivity and inappropriate attention-getting behaviors, while girls with the disorder are more often simply inattentive but not disruptive. The gender ratio is beginning to equalize as researchers recognize that many girls show ADHD differently than boys.

Studies suggest that about 30% to 75% of children who have ADHD continue to struggle with it as adults. Symptoms, especially the inability to control movement, are often less severe, but many complicating factors contribute to difficulties in the life of an adult with ADHD, including the high probability that he or she may be raising a child with ADHD.

Etiology: What Happens?

The etiology of this disorder remains a mystery, although new technologies that allow researchers to watch chemical pathways in conscious brains are beginning to offer some new ideas about how ADHD works.

ADHD is clearly a neurochemically mediated disorder. It has been traced to problems with dopamine production, transportation, and reabsorption and with ***noradrenaline*** disruption in the frontal cortex and basal ganglia: areas in the brain that have to do with decision making and movement.

Comparisons of the brains of children with and without ADHD yield some interesting differences. Overall, the brains of children with ADHD are 3% to 4% smaller than the brains of children without ADHD, although this is not reflected in comparative intelligence. Brains of children with ADHD who are medicated for their dysfunction show the same volume of white matter (myelinated fibers that connect various regulatory centers in the CNS) as children without ADHD. Brains of unmedicated children with ADHD show significantly less white matter than others.

While its causes are still unclear, some contributing factors have been identified. Genetics is certainly an issue, since many ADHD patients have a first-degree relative with the same disorder. Altered brain function is observable, as motor control and planning centers in the brain are affected by disturbed chemical levels. And maternal behaviors (smoking and alcohol consumption) and exposure to toxins (lead, dioxins, and PCBs) have been seen to increase the risk of ADHD in children.

Signs and Symptoms

Three specific patterns of behavior indicate ADHD: inattentiveness, hyperactivity, and impulsivity. A person with ADHD may only be inattentive or have a combination of these patterns, but they are consistent in multiple settings, that is, at school or work, at home, and in social situations.

Signs of inattention include becoming easily distracted by irrelevant sights and sounds; failing to pay attention to details and making careless mistakes; rarely following instructions carefully and completely; and losing or forgetting things such as toys, or pencils, books, and tools needed for a task.

Some signs of hyperactivity and impulsivity include feeling restless, fidgeting with hands or feet, or squirming; running, climbing, or leaving a seat when sitting or quiet behavior is expected; blurting out answers before hearing the whole question; and having difficulty waiting for others to complete a task.

Diagnosis

No conclusive test reliably and definitively identifies ADHD. In children it is usually diagnosed by ruling out other possibilities and then gathering observations from teachers, parents, coaches, and other adults in the child's life. In adults the same procedure includes feedback from family members and work associates. Perhaps the most important part of an ADHD diagnosis is ruling out other disorders that can lead to the same symptoms and recognizing how other psychiatric conditions often coexist and influence the behavior of a person with ADHD.

- *Differential diagnosis.* A number of things can cause children to become easily distractible and disruptive. It is important to rule these out before assuming that ADHD is the primary cause of their trouble. Depression, anxiety disorders, learning disabilities, sleep disorders (specifically sleep apnea or snoring), fetal alcohol syndrome, vision or hearing problems, Tourette syndrome, mood disturbances, and seizure disorders could all be considered.
- *Coexisting conditions.* Diagnosis of ADHD is complicated by several disorders that commonly occur concurrently with it. These include oppositional defiant disorder, depression, and anxiety disorders.

Complications

Untreated ADHD carries the risk of several serious consequences. Children with this disorder have difficulty with self-esteem, maintaining relationships, and performing well with schoolwork or other jobs. Later in life, untreated or unsuccessfully treated ADHD patients have a high rate of automobile accidents and an elevated risk of developing substance abuse or other addictive behaviors (i.e., gambling, shopping, engaging in sexual encounters) in attempts to self-medicate to manage their disease.

Studies show that teenagers who medicate for ADHD have a lower risk of engaging in substance abuse than teenagers who don't take medication.[16]

Treatment

At this moment the most successful treatment for ADHD is the use of psychostimulants, usually from classes of drugs called ***methylphenidates*** or ***dextroamphetamines***. These drugs work by stimulating areas in the brain where activity is diminished. Another option is a norepinephrine reuptake inhibitor; this is not a stimulant; it works to keep norepinephrine available in some synapses for a longer period.

Studies have been conducted to compare the success of children treated with medication alone; medication in addition to counseling and training in coping skills; and treatment with just counseling. Analysis shows that the best results occur with medication, but that when medication is coupled with family counseling or parental training, the average required dosage is smaller than for children who are treated with medication alone.[17]

Side effects of ADHD medications are a concern, especially if the patient is a young child. They can include appetite suppression, increased blood pressure and heart rate, sleep problems, and sometimes the development of facial or vocal tics. These signs indicate that a medication is poorly tolerated or the dosage needs to be adjusted. Some ADHD medications cannot be combined with some asthma medications.

Other approaches for ADHD include the use of nutritional supplements and adjusting the diet to avoid sugar, caffeine, and other stimulants. While these are recognized as good options, research indicates that they are not as successful at dealing with the symptoms of ADHD as pharmacological intervention.

Massage?

Massage holds no risks for children or adults with ADHD. Bodywork has been seen to improve classroom behavior and interpersonal relationships in children with this disorder.[15] It is important to have realistic expectations about what a child or adult with ADHD can tolerate in a bodywork session. While some love the stimulation of a rigorous, fast-paced sports massage type of modality, others prefer the chance to achieve the stillness found with subtler energy techniques. But regardless of preference, many ADHD patients cannot be expected to receive massage for a full hour or more.

MODALITY RECOMMENDATIONS FOR ATTENTION DEFICIT HYPERACTIVITY DISORDER	
Deep Tissue Massage	Indicated: can help with relaxation and client awareness. Use active movement and breathing to assist release.
Lymphatic Drainage	Supportive.
Polarity	S: Indicated with short, frequent sessions. R/D: Indicated within client comfort.
PNF/MET/Stretching	Supportive.
Reflexology	Indicated with short, frequent sessions; work brain, endocrine system, lymphatic system, liver, kidney points.
Shiatsu	Indicated, especially with passive meridian stretches.
Swedish Massage	Indicated; can help reinforce a parasympathetic state.
Trigger Point Therapy	Supportive with light work.

See Chapter 1 for a brief description of each modality, including definitions of abbreviations.

Autism Spectrum Disorders

Definition: What Are They?

Autism spectrum disorders (ASD) are a group of mental disorders characterized by problems connecting with other people, including parents and family members; communication difficulties; specific and predictable movement patterns; and sensory problems. ASD begins

Autism Spectrum Disorders in Brief

Pronunciation: AW-tizm SPEK-trum dis-OR-derz

What are they?

Autism spectrum disorders (ASD) are a group of CNS conditions that are usually recognized in infants and young children. They involve problems with communication, socialization, and movement behaviors.

How are they recognized?

ASD range from mild to severe. They can involve language development, difficulties in connecting to other people, hypersensitivity and hyposensitivity, repetitive and restrictive movement patterns, and several other issues, depending on the type and severity of the individual disorder.

Is massage indicated or contraindicated?

Massage can be beneficial if the person with autism welcomes it. Some patients may have a hard time accepting touch, and therapists may have to experiment to find approaches that are well tolerated.

in early childhood. It is usually diagnosable by age 3, although up to half of children with ASD aren't identified until they start kindergarten.

These problems have also been called *pervasive developmental disorders*, but ASD has become the standard term.

Demographics: Who Gets Them?

The incidence of ASD is about the same throughout ethnic and geographical groups. It is estimated that 3 or 4 in every 1,000 school-age children meet the diagnostic criteria for these disorders. That number has grown significantly since 1985. A change in the definition of the disorders accounts for part of that growth, but it is suggested that true rates of ASD are rising in addition to a broadening of the diagnostic criteria.[18]

Etiology: What Happens?

The difference in CNS function between people with ASD and people without it is the subject of intense study. It seems clear that abnormalities are present within various neural systems linking the brainstem, limbic system, basal ganglia, cerebellum, corpus callosum, and cerebral cortex, but no predictable pattern is present for all patients.

The most easily distinguishable factor behind some cases of ASD is a genetic anomaly. *Fragile X syndrome* is a condition in which a pinch appears in the X chromosome; this is the most common form of inherited mental retardation, and it affects 2% to 5% of ASD patients. *Tuberous sclerosis*, another genetic anomaly, involves the growth of benign tumors in the CNS and other vital organs. It affects 1% to 4% of children with ASD. The fact that siblings of children with ASD have a six times greater chance of having ASD than the general public (and the chances for identical twins is much higher still) clearly points to a genetic factor, although the specific mutations are not always identifiable.

Other theories for the development of ASD include mitochondrial dysfunction within neurons (a new field of study); early exposure to some virus that stimulates an autoimmune response; exposure to mercury, lead, or other heavy metals; and allergies, as indicated by the presence of high levels of eosinophils, basophils, and immunoglobulin-E. All are associated with allergic reactions.

Signs and Symptoms

Signs and symptoms of ASD vary according to what type is present. Three major issues are present for most types: deficits in verbal and nonverbal communication, problems with social interaction, and repetitive behaviors or movements. These occur in varying combinations and severity for each person. In addition, many ASD patients show unusual reactions to some sensory stimuli: they often seem to be impervious to cold or pain, while some sounds and textures, even soft ones, appear to be unbearable.

One common theme that many people with ASD share is the phenomenon of being locked within their own perspective. The recognition that other people also have consciousness is slow to come and difficult to integrate. People with ASD don't automatically register nonverbal signs such as facial expressions or body language, and it is difficult to interpret the emotional tone behind speech. "Come here" to a child with ASD means the same thing whether it's offered with a kiss and a cookie or with a frown and a punishment in store.

Consequently, the people in these children's lives, including parents and family members, can appear to be completely unpredictable and therefore to be avoided.

ASD frequently occurs with other conditions. About 25% of ASD patients also have seizures, and up to 75% have some level of cognitive disability. By contrast, of ASD patients with an IQ of 35 or above, 25% show signs of savant characteristics, that is, extremely highly developed skills with some narrow set of interests, such as numbers, music, reading, or other talents.

Signs and symptoms of ASD can usually be identified by age 3, but many children are not diagnosed until much later. This is unfortunate, because early intervention has been seen to improve the level of function and decrease self-destructive and inappropriate behaviors. Early indicators of ASD include the following: no babbling, pointing, or smiling at 12 months; no word use at 16 months; no word linkage at 24 months; no response to the child's name; and observable regression in language and social skills. Other signs include little or no eye contact, no imaginative play with toys, obsessive lining up of objects, extreme attachment to one object, and the appearance of a hearing deficiency. Many children show restricted, repetitive behaviors, such as hand wringing, rocking, or other movements, especially when they are tense or upset.

Diagnosis

Suspicion of ASD is usually aroused in the course of regular child developmental screenings and then further specified through evaluations by specialists. Some genetic anomalies can be confirmed through testing. Other disorders that could cause similar symptoms (hearing loss or lead poisoning, for instance) must be ruled out.

Each subtype of ASD has specific diagnostic criteria, which include age at onset along with particular signs and symptoms.

Types of Autism Spectrum Disorders

The spectrum of autistic disorders covers a broad range, but five major conditions are listed under this heading.

- *Autistic disorder* may also be called severe autism to distinguish it from the milder form. It is characterized by the three basic traits associated with ASD: impairment in communication skills; poor social interactions; and restricted, repetitive patterns of movement.
- *Asperger syndrome* is a mild form of ASD involving difficulties with socializing, but language skills and mental development are often normal or above normal. Some people classify Asperger syndrome as an entity distinct from mild autism, but not all experts agree on this. Many people with Asperger syndrome develop a consuming interest in some subject that completely engages them.
- *Pervasive developmental disorder, not otherwise specified* is a condition in which the child exhibits several ASD signs but doesn't meet the diagnostic criteria for any other label.
- *Rett syndrome* is a genetic disorder that typically results in severe symptoms. Almost all diagnoses are in girls, because affected boys are usually lost through spontaneous abortion or miscarriage. Where this was once considered a rare and extreme form of ASD, genetic testing is now able to identify milder cases of Rett syndrome.
- *Childhood disintegrative disorder*, a rare condition, occurs mostly in boys and has a later onset than other forms of ASD, around age 3 or 4. It is characterized by a dramatic loss of vocabulary, motor, and communication skills.

Other recognized conditions don't fit the descriptions of ASD but are clearly related to this spectrum of disorders:

- *Semantic pragmatic communication disorder* is delayed language development and problems with understanding words in context, but socialization skills are generally normal.
- *Nonverbal learning disabilities* produce an inability to understand nonverbal signs such as facial expression or body language; these children also tend to have problems with spatial perception and motor coordination.
- *High-functioning autism* could be synonymous with Asperger syndrome, but not all experts agree on this point. In any case, this condition shows some signs of ASD without cognitive impairment.
- *Hyperlexia* is an unusually early interest and skill with written language. Children with this condition typically teach themselves to read at an early age, although they may have little understanding of the words they are reading.

Treatment

ASD is treated according to type and the individual characteristics of the child. Most experts agree that children with ASD do best in highly structured, specialized programs that reinforce positive behaviors and work to reduce negative ones. Indeed, some ASD patients become extremely attached to the structure of their day and are severely disoriented by any interruptions to their routine.

Applied behavioral analysis is an intensive one-on-one intervention that occurs for many hours every week. Children who undergo this kind of therapy, especially in early years (preschool is preferable) often have significant improvement in function. Sensory integration therapy uses touch, pressure, vibration, massage, and lots of play equipment to help patients better organize their sense of touch.

Some parents find that dietary adjustments help their children. Avoiding gluten and casein (a protein found in dairy products) reduces symptoms for some, but not all, ASD patients. Supplementing vitamin B_6 with magnesium has similar results: some patients benefit, and others have no response.

In addition to these interventions, medication may be prescribed to help manage seizures, anxiety, and depression, but no medication addresses the issue of autism itself.

Massage?

Massage has been seen to have an extremely positive effect for ASD patients.[19] When compared with children who were read a story every day, children who received massage displayed fewer stereotypical behaviors, had better sleep, and more positive social interactions, and spent more time on task.

The major caution for children or adults with ASD is that the sensation of touch is not always positive. If a client with ASD doesn't perceive touch to feel safe or nurturing, the therapist must find ways to offer bodywork that is welcomed rather than avoided.

MODALITY RECOMMENDATIONS FOR AUTISM SPECTRUM DISORDERS	
Deep Tissue Massage	Indicated within client tolerance: build rapport with slow, firm touch.
Lymphatic Drainage	Supportive.
Polarity	S: Indicated with short, frequent sessions and client/practitioner rapport. R/D: supportive within client comfort and perceived safety.
PNF/MET/Stretching	Supportive.
Reflexology	Indicated with short, frequent sessions; work brain, endocrine system points.
Shiatsu	Supportive with short treatments if well tolerated. Brushing strokes from heel to toe on SP5 to SP1 may be helpful, as this area connects to embryological development.
Swedish Massage	Supportive, as long as the client feels safe and a trust bond has been established.
Trigger Point Therapy	Supportive with light work.

See Chapter 1 for a brief description of each modality, including definitions of abbreviations.

Chemical Dependency

Definition: What Is It?

Here is a controversial topic! While definitions of chemical use, abuse, and dependency are relatively clear, the whole issue is clouded by value judgments imposed by whether a substance is legal or not. A person may become addicted to nasal decongestants or to cocaine, but decongestants are not generally considered a substance abuse problem, while cocaine certainly is.

Alcoholism is form of chemical dependency that because of its prevalence in the culture and the profound effects it has on virtually every system of the body is discussed as a separate subset of chemical dependency in this article. The issue of chemical dependency falls into three categories: use, abuse, and dependency, or addiction.

- *Use. Use* is easy to identify: if a person ingests a substance specifically to change mood or physical experience, it is substance use.
- *Abuse.* One definition of abuse is simply "the use of a substance in a way that is potentially harmful to the user or to other people." Officially, abuse is identified when substance use leads to impairment or distress and when within a 12-month period at least one of the following facts is true: the user finds that he or she cannot fulfill obligations to work, family, or school; recurrent use puts the user in dangerous situations; the user has legal problems in relation to substance use; or the user has social or interpersonal problems in relation to substance use.[20]
- *Dependency.* The line between substance *abuse* and chemical *dependency* is sometimes blurry. The official identification of

Chemical Dependency in Brief

What is it?
Chemical dependency is the use of substances in methods or dosages that result in damage to the user and people close to the user. Chemical dependency can involve the use of both legal and illegal substances.

How is it recognized?
Specific symptoms of chemical dependency are determined by what substances are being consumed. Generally speaking, the symptoms of dependency include a craving for the substance in question, an inability to voluntarily limit use, unpleasant or dangerous withdrawal symptoms, and increasing tolerance of the substance's effects.

Is massage indicated or contraindicated?
People who are recovering from chemical dependency can benefit from massage, as long as no contraindicating conditions have developed as part of the abuse. Massage is contraindicated for people who are intoxicated at the time of their appointment.

dependency occurs when three or more of the following are true: the user develops increasing tolerance for the substance; the user has withdrawal symptoms when access to the substance is interrupted; increasing amounts of the substance are used; the user cannot voluntarily limit use; the user devotes significant time to using or recovering from use; the user replaces other activities with substance use; or the user continues to abuse the substance even when fully aware of the dangers involved.

Demographics: Who Becomes Chemically Dependent or Alcoholic?

Statistics on alcohol and chemical dependency are difficult to gather, especially since many people never get medical treatment, and they may move back and forth between using and being free from use.

The National Survey on Drug Use and Health Issues estimates that between 2002 and 2004, 22.5 million Americans over 12 years old were ongoing abusers of drugs or alcohol, but only about 3.8 million people got help for their problem.[21] Alcoholism is the third leading cause of death from a preventable cause (after smoking and obesity): each year this country sees average of 85,000 alcohol-related deaths and over $185 billion in health care costs.[22]

Etiology: What Happens with Chemical Dependency?

The process of developing dependency on a particular substance depends on the chemical makeup of that product and the susceptibility of the user. Some drugs work in the CNS by slowing the rate at which neurotransmitters are reabsorbed at key synapses. This can lead to changes in the numbers of neurotransmitter receptors, which can in turn be perceived as an increased need for the drug. Other disruptions in neural pathways and neurotransmitter relationships have been noted as well; positron emission tomography has revealed inherent characteristics that predispose some people to addiction, even before the addictive substance has been introduced.[23]

Etiology: What Happens with Alcoholism?

Alcohol and sedatives such as tranquilizers and barbiturates work by depressing CNS arousal, enhancing the activity of the inhibitory neurotransmitter GABA. Alcohol slows activity of the brain and nervous system. While it is technically a depressant, the loss of inhibitions felt by the drinker can give the impression that alcohol is a stimulant. Some people bear a genetic susceptibility to alcohol addiction, but many alcoholics develop the disease over many months or years of repeated use that finally and permanently changes the chemistry in the brain. Consequently, a physical addiction develops: the person is incapable of functioning normally without the substance. The effect of alcohol on specific organ systems is discussed in more detail in the section on *complications*.

Risk Factors

Several risk factors contribute to a person's susceptibility to chemical dependency.

- *Genetic predisposition.* The rate of drug abuse and alcoholism is demonstrably greater in the families of other addicts than in the general population. This is partly an environmental and availability issue, but studies have shown that even children who are not raised with their chemically dependent parents have a higher than normal incidence of addiction.
- *Other mental illness.* Depression and/or anxiety disorders raise the risk of a person becoming a substance abuser, as he or she may attempt to self-medicate to cope with problems.
- *Environmental factors.* These include availability of the substance in question, peer pressure, low self-esteem, a history of physical or sexual abuse, being a child in the household of a substance abuser, and other stressors that may make drug use look like a reasonable choice.

- *Type of drug being used.* Some drugs are simply more addictive than others, but most substances can cause dependency if they are used consistently enough.
- *Age.* The younger a person is at the beginning of use of an addictive substance, the more likely he or she is to develop a long-term dependency on it.
- *Medical reasons.* A patient's need for medication sometimes outlives the problem that required the initial prescription. Addictions to painkillers and sleeping pills are examples of this phenomenon.

Two issues are especially important in any discussion of chemical dependency. One is that even over-the-counter drugs can change body chemistry and make it very hard to cope without them. Nasal decongestants are an excellent example. Why should a person's own antihistamines do any work if some externally supplied nasal decongestant will do it for them? The difficulty lies in how long it takes to convince the body that no more decongestants will be consumed. The same kinds of dependency can develop with the use of sleeping pills, muscle relaxants, and some kinds of painkillers.

The other thing to remember is that the body builds up chemical tolerances to most kinds of drugs. That is, it takes more and more decongestant to clear up that stuffy nose, more sleeping pills, more painkillers, more caffeine, and so on. The higher the dose a person needs to feel satisfied, the harder it is to shake off the dependency.

Types of Addiction

Once a person becomes dependent on a substance, two things happen: it takes more and more of the substance to achieve the desired affects and to *stop* using the substance can create physical responses that are daunting to contemplate. Addiction is defined in two categories: psychological and physical. Most addicts deal with both problems, and treatment programs that don't address both of these issues tend not to be successful.

- *Psychological addiction* is dependency on the pleasurable or satisfying sensations that some substance provides—in other words, the addict *loves* the feeling the drug gives.
- *Physical addiction* is a dependency arising from the need to avoid withdrawal symptoms, which can include hallucinations, nausea, vomiting, seizures, and general physical pain.

Signs and Symptoms of Chemical Dependency and Alcoholism

Symptoms of chemical dependency vary according to the substance, but these main features are consistent:

- The person feels a persistent craving for the substance.
- The person goes to great lengths, including actions that are out of character (stealing, using violence) to ensure that the substance is always available.
- The person cannot voluntarily control use of the substance.
- The person develops an increasing tolerance to the effects of the substance and so must consume more to achieve the same results; the substance is necessary for the person to feel "normal".
- The person puts him or herself and others at risk for harm while under the influence.
- Cessation of use creates unpleasant, alarming, and even physically dangerous withdrawal symptoms.

In addition to these signs, the addict or alcoholic may devote a significant amount of time to using and then recovering from substance use. He or she may neglect responsibilities to family, job, friends, and other relationships while distracted by substance use. And finally, the addict often denies that substance use seriously impedes or endangers his or her life: "I'm not dead yet, so that proves I'm okay."

Complications of Chemical Dependency

Complications depend on the substance in question. They can range from paranoid delusions to coma or even death. Some of the worst effects of drug use are not limited to the users, however. People close to substance abusers also suffer tremendously. Drug-related violent crime, car accidents, industrial accidents, impaired judgment leading to the spread of HIV, and high rates of domestic violence and child abuse are other complications of chemical dependency that affect many people beyond the user.

Complications of Alcoholism

One drink is equal to 12 oz of beer *or* 4–5 oz of wine, *or* 1.5 oz of 80-proof liquor. Moderate consumption means one or two drinks per day. Heavy drinking is two to four drinks per day, and binge drinking means having more than four drinks in a row for a man or more than three drinks in a row for a woman.[24]

Alcohol use affects virtually every system of the body. Here is a brief synopsis:

The digestive system Alcohol irritates the stomach lining, and high levels of consumption are responsible for a specific type of gastritis. It is also very rapidly absorbed through the gastric mucosa into the portal system. The portal vein dumps the alcohol directly into the liver, where it enters the rest of the bloodstream. The effects of alcohol are felt until the liver has finished neutralizing it.

People who have preexisting gastrointestinal problems are especially vulnerable to the worst effects of alcohol. It is implicated in the development of cancer in the upper gastrointestinal tract, especially in the esophagus, pharynx, larynx, and mouth. Alcoholism can cause ulcers, internal hemorrhaging, and pancreatitis. About 20% of long-term drinkers develop cirrhosis.

The cardiovascular system Alcohol use decreases the force of cardiac contractions and can lead to irregular heartbeat, or arrhythmia. Alcohol is also toxic to myocardial tissue and can lead to alcoholic cardiomyopathy. Alcohol tends to agglutinate red blood cells, making them stick together. This leads to the possibility of thrombi, not only in the brain but in the coronary arteries as well. Alcohol use can also have the opposite effect: liver damage can lead to reduced clotting factors and poor vitamin K synthesis, which may result in uncontrollable bleeding.

Moderate alcohol consumption may actually help prevent cardiovascular disease by increasing high-density lipoprotein levels (the "good" cholesterol) in the blood.

The nervous system Memory loss frequently occurs for biochemical reasons as well as from agglutinated red blood cells getting stuck in the cerebral capillaries, causing brain cells to starve to death. Even some social drinkers sustain measurable brain damage from repeated agglutination. In the short term alcohol slows reflexes, slurs speech, impairs judgment, and compromises motor control. In the long term the same effects can happen on a permanent basis, often due to a thiamine deficiency. This is also known as **Wernicke-Korsakoff syndrome**. In advanced stages of cirrhosis the blood accumulates toxic levels of metabolic wastes that can cause brain damage.

The immune system Prolonged alcohol use severely impedes resistance, especially to respiratory infections. Alcoholics are especially vulnerable to pneumonia.

The reproductive system Alcoholism can cause reduced sex drive, erectile dysfunction, menstrual irregularities, and infertility. Babies of alcoholic women are susceptible to fetal alcohol syndrome, the most common type of environmentally caused mental retardation in the United States. Fetal alcohol syndrome affects about 2,000 babies every year.

Alcoholic families Children raised in homes with one or more alcoholic adults show a threefold increase in the risk of becoming substance abusers themselves. Their chances of developing depression, general anxiety disorders, and phobias are higher than in the general population. And their health costs are higher than those of other children. About 75% of children in foster care settings are from alcoholic homes.[25]

Other complications Alcohol is frequently a factor in traffic injuries, drownings, falls, burns, and unintentional shootings.

Treatment

The first and most important step in treating any kind of chemical dependency is recognizing that a problem exists. Once a person has reached that point, many treatment programs have good success rates, although the recurrence rate is high until a person reaches about 5 years of sobriety. Treatment goals for chemical dependency are threefold: abstinence, rehabilitation, and prevention of relapses.

Most programs begin with detoxification, during which the drugs are expelled from the body. This may be ameliorated with sedatives, tranquilizers, or even less potent versions of the drug in question until all chemical remnants have been processed out of the body. The time this takes varies according to the substance in question.

Detoxification is followed by rehabilitation, during which the patient is taught about the effects of chemical use and trained in avoidance behaviors to provide some ammunition against the temptation to fall back into old habits.

Aftercare has been shown to be the most important part of treatment for chemical dependency. This sets up the patient with a support system that will carry him or her throughout a lifetime choice of total drug abstinence.

Some medications can help to suppress the craving for alcohol or can cause violent physical illness when alcohol is consumed. The potential for relapse into substance abuse lasts indefinitely, so this is a condition that is treated most successfully with long-term coping skills rather than short-term patches. Total abstinence is essentially the only successful conclusion to treatment for most types of chemical dependency.

Massage?

Massage has a useful place in the treatment of chemical dependency. Some rehabilitation facilities employ massage therapists to help ameliorate withdrawal symptoms, speed detoxification, and reduce the need for tranquilizers and other drugs. Perhaps the most valuable thing massage has to offer an addict in recovery is a chance to reconnect with his or her body in a way that is pleasurable and healthy. But a client with a history of alcohol or drug abuse is at high risk for secondary health problems. For this reason, it is important to work as part of a health care team and to beware of complications associated with hard drug use: staphylococcal or streptococcal infections, cirrhosis, hepatitis B or C, HIV, and heart problems.

Clients who are in long-term recovery with no lasting contraindications are good candidates for massage.

Current alcohol or other drug use at the time of an appointment contraindicates massage, mainly because of the risk of overtaxing a liver that is already occupied. This guideline can be a judgment call, based on the level of intoxication (one glass of wine poses less stress on the liver than a fifth of vodka), the setting of the massage session, the behavior of the client, and the safety boundaries set by the therapist.

MODALITY RECOMMENDATIONS FOR CHEMICAL DEPENDENCY	
Deep Tissue Massage	Indicated when client is sober. Work for client awareness with slow pressure.
Lymphatic Drainage	Contraindicated while client is detoxifying; otherwise supportive.
Polarity	S: Indicated. R/D: Supportive within client comfort. Take extra care and caution for emotional releases.
PNF/MET/Stretching	Supportive.
Reflexology	Indicated; on ears work appetite suppression points. On feet and hands, work all glands, liver, solar plexus points.
Shiatsu	Supportive, especially in conjunction with acupuncture.
Swedish Massage	Supportive, with caution for drug or medication use that could require modality adjustments.
Trigger Point Therapy	Contraindicated while intoxicated; otherwise supportive.

See Chapter 1 for a brief description of each modality, including definitions of abbreviations.

Depression

Definition: What Is It?

Depression is a group of disorders that involve negative changes in emotional state. One of the best descriptions of this disease is "a genetic-neurochemical disorder requiring a strong environmental trigger whose characteristic manifestation is an inability to appreciate sunsets."[26]

In other words, depression is a CNS disorder involving a genetic predisposition, chemical changes, and often a triggering event that results in a person losing the ability to enjoy life. Depression is more than a temporary spell of the blues; it can be a long-lasting, self-propagating, and ultimately debilitating disease.

Depression in Brief

Pronunciation: de-PRESH-un

What is it?
Depression is an umbrella term covering a number of mood disorders that can result in persistent feelings of sadness, guilt, and/or hopelessness.

How is it recognized?
Symptoms vary according to the type of depression and the individual, but they usually include a sad mood and loss of enjoyment derived from usual hobbies and activities, along with some combination of disappointment with oneself, hopelessness, irritability, a change in sleeping habits, and thoughts of suicide.

Is massage indicated or contraindicated?
Most types of depression indicate massage, which can work in several ways to alleviate symptoms both temporarily and in the long run.

Demographics: Who Gets It?

Statistics on the incidence of depression in all its forms are hard to gather, because many affected people never seek help. Experts believe that up to 20% of women and 12% of men have some type of depression in their lifetime.[27] Within every 1-year period, 9.5% of the U.S. population, amounting to 20.9 million people, have a form of depression.[28]

Depression can affect people of any age. It has been observed in young children up through senior adults, in whom its symptoms can mimic or coexist with other specifically geriatric diseases.

Etiology: What Happens?

No one really knows how depression comes about. Several distinctive features have been noted in the brain and endocrine system of depressive individuals, but whether these features *cause* the problem or are *caused by* the problem is still a mystery. Nonetheless, as we learn more about the chemical changes associated with depression, we also learn new ways to attempt to treat it.

- *Neurotransmitter imbalance.* Three main neurotransmitters have been associated with depression: serotonin, norepinephrine, and dopamine. The assumption is that these neurotransmitters are in short supply, and if medical interventions make them more readily available, the patient will improve. Some research, however, points in a slightly different direction: that these neurotransmitters are actually present in *too much* concentration, and the brain builds up resistance to receiving them. Regardless, the drugs most often prescribed for depression change brain chemistry by increasing the accessibility of these important neurotransmitters.
- *Hormonal imbalance.* Neurotransmitter disruption leads to disruption in hormonal secretions, especially progesterone, estrogen, endorphins (which increase the sensation of pleasure), and cortisol, the hormone most closely related to long-term stress. It is also possible that this is a two-way street, in other words, that the hormonal shifts associated with long-term stress can disrupt neurotransmitter secretion.
- *Hypothalamus-pituitary-adrenal axis.* This is the tight connection between the CNS and the endocrine system. The pituitary gland, under the control of the hypothalamus, controls the adrenal glands (which secrete adrenaline and cortisol, among other things) by way of corticotrophin-releasing hormone. Depressive people tend to secrete excessive amounts of corticotrophin-releasing hormone, meaning that they create stress responses to minimal stimuli, and those responses tend to have a longer-lasting effect on the body (Sidebar 4.5).
- *Atrophy in the hippocampus.* The hippocampus is a structure deep in the brain that is involved with learning and memory. The hippocampus in persons with major depressive disorder is often smaller than normal, showing up to 20% atrophy. The causes of hippocampus atrophy vary, but the hypersecretion of cortisol is a factor; this is also seen with anxiety disorders.

Causes

Many factors contribute to a depressive episode. Some of them are controllable, but many are not. Whether or not someone becomes depressed depends on personal chemistry, genetics, and something much harder to quantify: the personality.

- *Genetics.* The rates of various kinds of depression show higher than normal incidence among family members, pointing to a distinct genetic predisposition to this disorder. Because this is such a common and widely distributed disease, many sites of genetic abnormality may be responsible.
- *Environmental triggers.* Most episodes of depression can be related to specific life events that initiate a slide into a depressed state. Sometimes the triggers are less clear, or they could be not recent. Triggers can range in severity from losing a loved one to losing a phone number. The more depressive episodes a person has had, the smaller the trigger may be.
- *Personality traits.* Some people, through their childhood experiences and family history, are simply

SIDEBAR 4.5: THE STRESS RESPONSE SYSTEM

The *stress response system* is the link between the CNS and the endocrine system that allows humans to respond to both short-term and long-term stressors. It is controlled by the HPA axis, the communication between the hypothalamus, the pituitary gland, and the adrenals. A healthy stress response system allows immediate reactions that are appropriately gauged to the circumstances: big reactions to big threats, small reactions to small threats. And when the stress response system works well, the chemical changes it brings about are transitory and quickly neutralized once the threat has passed.

Some people have a stress response system that doesn't work well. The chemical messages issued first from the hypothalamus, then by the pituitary gland, are slow to leave the brain and reach the adrenals. This takes longer to have an effect on the body, decreasing the ability to respond quickly to threat. But the stress reaction, once it takes hold, is tenacious. Its aftereffects linger much longer than for someone who has a healthy stress response system. Furthermore, people who have a sluggish stress response system also tend to have *more* stress responses *more* often to *less threatening* stimuli, and those responses have longer-lasting effects on the body than those with normal stress responses. This is a person who fumes in a long checkout line, who frets in heavy traffic, and who blows up when the kids leave their bikes in the driveway. This is someone who may have a sluggish but overactive stress response, and this person has a high propensity to develop, among other things, depression.

What determines the health of the stress response system? Studies with animals reveal one reliable predictor for a sluggish stress response: lack of tactile stimulation, or touch. Understimulated animals have consistently slower, longer-lasting, and more frequent stress responses than animals that were regularly petted and fondled. Consider what this means for the average undertouched person in our society: most us have low-functioning but longer-lasting stress reactions, and they occur with unnecessary and unhealthy frequency. The good news is that the health of the stress response system can be improved with an abundance of healthy, nurturing touch.

more prone to depression than others. Psychological testing can identify people with a pessimistic or passive "things in my life happen to me; I don't make things in my life happen" kind of attitude. These people carry an increased risk for developing depression.

- *Chronic illness.* People who live with chronic illness show a much higher rate of depression than the general population. This is easy to understand, as chronic pain or the prospect of sliding into inevitable disability naturally deprives a person of a sense of hopefulness or investment in life. Furthermore, the neurotransmitters associated with depression (serotonin, norepinephrine, and dopamine) are also strongly implicated in various chronic pain syndromes, including fibromyalgia, postherpetic neuralgia, and others. Research into chemical interactions in the brain may eventually yield some new and more effective interventions for both these problems. Often the symptoms of depression outweigh the symptoms of the chronic illness. If the depression can be resolved, coping skills for the illness may also improve.
- *Other problems.* Several other problems can contribute to depression, but these are often much more easily controlled than the ones so far discussed. Hypothyroidism, smoking, alcohol, drug use, or side effects of medication can all create depressive symptoms. Also, certain nutritional deficiencies, notably vitamin B_{12} and folate, can contribute to depressive symptoms.

Signs and Symptoms

The signs and symptoms of depression depend partly on what type is present. The two leading symptoms include a persistent sad or empty feeling and experiencing less enjoyment from usual activities (including sex) and hobbies. Other common symptoms include a deep sense of guilt or disappointment with oneself, a feeling of hopelessness—that things will never get better—irritability, and a change in sleeping habits: either the person sleeps very little or sleeps much more than usual.

Additional signs and symptoms can include a decreasing ability to concentrate, weight changes (the person either eats much more than usual or loses interest in food), a loss of energy, a feeling of helplessness, persistent physical pain that is unresponsive to treatment (especially headaches, backache, and digestive discomfort), and suicidal thoughts, plans, or attempts. A person is typically diagnosed with depression when five or more of these symptoms are present for in a new pattern for a minimum of 2 weeks.

Types of Depression

The Diagnostic and Statistical Manual of Mental Disorders (DSM-IV-TR) recognizes several etiologically distinct types of depression. Six of them are relatively common and are discussed here:

- *Major depressive disorder* is classic debilitating clinical depression. It is recognized by the major symptoms listed earlier in very severe form for periods longer than 2 weeks. Left untreated, episodes of major depression may last anywhere from 6 to 18 months and on average recur anywhere from four to six times over a lifetime. That means someone who doesn't seek treatment for a major depressive disorder can expect to spend up to 10 years feeling hopeless, helpless, and worthless.
- *Adjustment disorder* is related to a specific event that triggers an emotional response, but the symptoms significantly outlast what might be considered a normal recovery or grieving period.
- ***Dysthymia*** is a less extreme version of depression, with fewer symptoms in less extreme forms, but it can last for years. Someone who has dysthymia can function but won't ever feel normal or at his or her best.

- *Bipolar disease* is also called *manic depression*. It is marked by mood swings from major depression to mania. This is a state defined by heightened energy, elation, irritability, racing thoughts, increased sex drive, decreased inhibitions, and unrealistic or grandiose notions that lead to decisions made with extremely poor judgment. Someone in a manic state might spontaneously quit a job, buy a car, or make some other major life change without realizing the long-term implications—which will of course be waiting when the manic episode subsides.
- *Seasonal affective disorder* is depression related to the absence of sunlight. Its incidence in the general population goes up according to distance from the equator. It is thought to be related to low levels of melatonin, a neurotransmitter stimulated by exposure to sunlight. It is most prevalent during December, January, and February.
- *Postpartum depression*, the depression that affects new mothers, is different from other types. It is related to several factors, including sleep deprivation, vast hormonal shifts, and the challenge of matching expectations of parenthood with reality. A woman with postpartum depression has all of the symptoms of major depression along with the deep-rooted fear of having harm come to or of actually doing harm to her baby. In the most extreme version of postpartum depression a woman can become psychotic and have hallucinations that may put herself or her baby in danger. A woman with a history of postpartum depression with one infant is at increased risk for repeated episodes with other children.

Diagnosis

Depression is diagnosed with a combination of physical tests to rule out factors such as hypothyroidism, vitamin deficiencies, or underlying disease and psychological tests to identify exactly which type of depression might be present. Unfortunately, depression is often missed if the person never seeks treatment or if symptoms suggest other or underlying disorders. Also, if the depression occurs in an older person, the presenting symptoms are likely to be physical rather than emotional. Headaches, back pain, and digestive discomfort are the leading symptoms for elderly patients, and they are unlikely to be recognized as signals for major depressive disorder.

Complications

The most obvious and serious complication of depression is suicide. About 30,000 people successfully commit suicide each year in the United States, and up to 200,000 suicide attempts are recorded. It is estimated that half of those attempts are related to depressive episodes. About 15% of people with major depressive disorder kill themselves. Although men have depression about half as often as women, they are four times more likely to commit suicide. Suicide is the second leading cause of death among adolescents.[29]

In addition to suicide risk, a history of depression is now found to be a risk factor for several other conditions, notably stroke, heart attack, and other forms of cardiovascular disease. Further, the severity of the preexisting depression can be a predictor for how well a person recovers from a stroke or heart attack.[30] Although the cause-and-effect relationships between depression and cardiovascular disease have not been fully identified, an obvious connection can be made between depression and the physical manifestations of long-term stress.

Finally, depression frequently accompanies other long-term diseases. Unfortunately, the symptoms of depression can make the consequences of other conditions worse (e.g., pain sensation is amplified, sleep is disrupted), and people who are depressed are not likely to take good care of themselves by eating well, taking medication according to prescription, and staying in contact with family and other community support groups. The consequence is that when depression is treated successfully, other disorders that it accompanies are often also easier to treat.

Treatment

Most types of depression are treatable, although finding the right combination of therapies can be time-consuming, frustrating, and expensive. Several different classes of antidepressant medications have been developed, each with advantages and disadvantages, and new medications are in development all the time.

The success of a person's treatment for depression depends largely on patience, as many medications can take several weeks to achieve their full potential. New protocols for combining drugs or switching from one type to another (even when the underlying mechanism is virtually identical) are finding increasing success. It is important to try to treat depression fully, because when people find relief but have lingering symptoms, they are at high risk for recurrent episodes.

Antidepressant drugs Medications used for depression usually fall into one of four categories: SSRIs (selective serotonin reuptake inhibitors), SNRIs (serotonin norepinephrine reuptake inhibitors, including Effexor and Cymbalta), MAOIs, and tricyclic antidepressants (TCAs). All of these classes of medication aim to make neurotransmitters more easily accessible in the mood-determining areas of the brain.

SSRIs, which include Prozac and Zoloft, work by preventing the recycling of secreted serotonin into axon terminals. In this way, serotonin lingers in synapses for longer than it normally would. SNRIs work to retain higher levels of both serotonin and norepinephrine in the synapses. TCAs, including amitriptyline (Elavil), do essentially the same thing, although they don't focus specifically on serotonin or norepinephrine. TCAs have also been seen to ameliorate some chronic pain symptoms. MAOIs limit the action of an enzyme that would normally break down and clear away secretions of neurotransmitters. Nardil and Parate are examples of MAOIs. These are among the first antidepressants developed, but they are associated with a high risk of toxic interactions with other drugs or foods, so they are seldom used anymore.

Antidepressants are effective for most people, but they have two major disadvantages: they take several weeks to establish any noticeable mood changes, and they tend to produce unpleasant side effects during that initial adjustment period. Side effects usually include dry mouth, dizziness, constipation, skin rashes, sleepiness or sleeplessness, sexual dysfunction, and restlessness. Side effects generally subside within 4 to 6 weeks, which is about when the benefits of the medication begin to be felt.

Lithium is used specifically with bipolar depression. Rather than altering levels of neurotransmitter reuptake or recycling, lithium works simply to smooth out mood swings. It can be toxic and is associated with several complications, so several alternatives to lithium for bipolar disease have been developed.

Psychotherapy Psychologists and psychiatrists may also employ various types of talk therapy to help patients improve coping skills and reduce both the effects and the recurrence of depressive episodes. Three major approaches have been found to be most useful, depending on the personality and needs of the affected individual. *Cognitive-behavioral therapy* focuses on the patient's skills at managing life and making beneficial choices. *Interpersonal therapy* focuses on how relationships color a person's life for better or worse. And *psychodynamic* therapy looks at how unresolved inner conflicts can affect the way a person makes choices and lives with those choices.

Psychotherapy in addition to medication often works better than medication alone, because it can help the patient take some control of his or her life, a feeling many depressive people don't often have.

Other therapies

- *Light therapy.* Persons living with seasonal affective disorder may not need medication or talk therapy; they need sunlight. Exposure to broad-spectrum lights can help to reduce symptoms.

- *Electroconvulsive therapy.* Some major depressive disorder patients don't respond to medication, and they are at high risk for suicide. Electroconvulsive, or shock, therapy may be the best choice for these patients. While this may bring up disturbing memories of *One Flew Over A Cuckoo's Nest*, modern electroconvulsive therapy is conducted under light anesthesia and with muscle relaxants to limit uncontrolled contractions. It is not entirely clear why it works, but it can be a highly effective intervention for people who don't get relief from other options.
- *St. John's wort.* This herbal extract has received a lot of attention as a mood enhancer without the side effects that other antidepressants carry. While some studies indicate that it can be effective for mild dysthymia, it has been shown to be ineffective as a treatment for major depressive disorder. St. John's wort is not without its risks; if a person takes medication to control HIV or any cytotoxic drugs (to reduce the risk of organ rejection, for instance), St. John's wort has been seen to make these medications less effective.
- *Others.* A number of other interventions for depression continue to be explored. Transcranial magnet stimulation may have the same benefits as electroshock therapy without the risks. Vagus nerve stimulation is being explored as an option when other interventions are not successful. A dietary supplement called SAM-e (***S-adenosyl-methionine***), omega-3 fish oil, 5-hydroxytryptophan (a supplement that provides the building blocks for serotonin), and others are under investigation as possible alternatives to standard antidepressant medications.

CASE HISTORY 4.3

Depression

Dave, Age 50: "Everybody wants to see the evidence!"

I don't know for sure when I first started to notice any symptoms of depression. Maybe when I was around 45. I remember I spent about a year trying to figure out what was wrong. I thought I had an infection or something, maybe a sinus infection that was making me feel tired all the time.

One day I went to get a physical, and my doctor asked me a couple of questions about things, about my life. I didn't think anything of it; I thought he was just making conversation. Then he said, "You know, Dave, you have depression." I laughed at him because there wasn't anything to be depressed about. My life was wonderful, I had no real problems, everything was good.

When I was first diagnosed, my problem was nowhere near its peak. After that, though, it got really bad. I couldn't concentrate on anything, and I spent weeks in bed. I couldn't respond to any questions, I didn't even know what was going on. When I did tune in, I had this indescribable horrible feeling. The only way I made it through that time was by asking Jesus to hold me. I just pulled the covers up over my head and asked God to just hold me. That gets me through the bad times.

I took short-term disability, for 6 months, from my job as a safety engineer. When it was over I tried to go back to work, but it wasn't any good. I used up all my sick leave, and one day the personnel officer came and told me I was through. I haven't worked since then. I got 18 months of disability, and they shut the door. If I'd broken my back, they would have paid disability for the rest of my life. But this kind of illness gets no respect. With mental illness, people think you're either slothful or insane. Slothful people are expected to get up and pull their own weight. Insane people are just ignored.

My illness is not the result of any outside situation; it is a chemical thing, an imbalance. I tried antidepressant drugs. They're hard, though, because when you try one you have to give it a good 2 months before you know if it'll do any good. For about 90% of people with depression, those drugs help them out. I'm in the 10% they don't help.

Depression *continued*

I've taken lots of tests in the past 2 years. My latest diagnosis is that I have schizoid-affective disorder along with depression. It's hard to categorize. Now I'm taking antipsychotic drugs. I had a really bad episode about a month ago. I was in tears, tearing out my hair, just crawling out of my skin. I ended up in the hospital. I thought it was a reaction to the medication, but apparently the medication wasn't working yet. It was just my disease, hitting a big crest.

That's how it goes, in cycles, from day to day, hour to hour, week to week. It's impossible to predict, but it's always wavelike, never steady. Medications are a crap shoot. You take your meds and hope something happens. By now I've taken so many, and the combinations are so complicated, it's really hard to make any changes. I think I developed tolerance to all the antidepressants. The antipsychotics are new, and there are times when I feel pretty good.

The worst part of all this for me is that on my bad days I have no energy to do anything. I just lie there and sleep. I'm completely unreliable. I can't be sure I'll show up for church or for choir practice. It's a real bummer.

I get lots of support at home. My wife has an incredible burden, but she's been behind me 100% all the way. She knows that when I'm in bad shape there's nothing to do but wait until I'm feeling better. Then we just go on with life without dwelling on what we've missed—that's a good approach for me.

I know I'm in lots of people's prayers. I feel that's a powerful tool. I know the prayers being lifted up for me are helping, without a doubt. But when I'm feeling bad, you can't come over and cheer me up, because that's not what I need. When people come visit me in the middle of the day and I've been in bed, I'm not showered or shaved, then I get so embarrassed, almost paranoid. It's not an atmosphere I like to see people in.

I don't think I'm at risk for suicide, although since I've had this disease I know more about why people do it. You get to a point where you say, " This. Is. Intolerable. This. Cannot. Go on." But it does. For now I don't see suicide being a danger for me.

At this point the only people who really understand depression are people in the medical profession, people who *have* it, or people who have someone in their family who has it. No one else really gets it. They all want to see the proof: where's the blood test, where's the x-ray, where's the *evidence*? I see a lot of the attitude that if you don't have the evidence, you must be faking it. I would like for everyone to understand that mental illness can be as debilitating as any other disease, and it deserves the same respect and concern that any other kind of disease gets.

Massage?

The ways massage can help a depressed person are many and varied. Although some cautions must be borne in mind, most people with depression can reap several benefits from bodywork.

Touch improves the efficiency of the HPA axis. Receiving nonsexual, nurturing, nonthreatening touch is one of the most important ways humans and other mammals have of keeping a healthy stress response.

Massage moves people from a sympathetic into a parasympathetic state. This brings about several physiological and chemical changes in the body, including an increase in serotonin secretion and a decrease in cortisol.

Research about how massage affects mood indicates a shift in EEG activation from the right frontal lobe (usually associated with sad affect) to the left frontal lobe (usually associated with happy affect), or at least to a symmetrical reading.[31]

Receiving massage is one of the few distinctively pleasurable things people can do that is also really good for them. The act of scheduling and receiving this gift is a step toward self-determination that depressive people can take with little risk of having it backfire on them.

Some cautions about working with depression patients remain, however. Some clients who receive massage and enjoy its benefits may wish to stop taking their medication. Well-meaning massage therapists may view this as a successful outcome and encourage their clients to try it, but balancing medication for depressive people is a difficult business. The only ones who should get involved in changing doses are the depressed person and his or her doctor.

Depression often accompanies complex emotional issues that a client may have trouble sorting out without help. Client-therapist relationships run the risk, in some cases, of becoming distorted when boundaries are not carefully respected. If a massage therapist has a client who is depressive in connection with other problems (for instance, if that person is recovering from emotional or physical or sexual abuse), that relationship can be precarious, especially if the client is not getting adequate support outside the massage clinic. Therapists in cases like these have the obligation to refer clients for other kinds of help and to prevent the client-therapist relationship from becoming more central to the client's life than it should be.

Modality Recommendations for Depression	
Deep Tissue Massage	Indicated when client is stable. Enlist client in process with slow, deep pressure.
Lymphatic Drainage	Supportive.
Polarity	S: Indicated. R/D: Indicated within client comfort.
PNF/MET/Stretching	Supportive.
Reflexology	Indicated; work brain, head, all glands, solar plexus, liver points.
Shiatsu	Indicated. Treat nerves, hormones, state of mind, muscular tension via BL, K, PC, SI, H, TH, GB.
Swedish Massage	Indicated; can help restore a healthy stress response system.
Trigger Point Therapy	Supportive.

See Chapter 1 for a brief description of each modality, including definitions of abbreviations.

Eating Disorders

Definition: What Are They?

Eating disorders include a variety of unhealthy eating habits that may begin slowly but over time become difficult or even impossible to break. Eating disorders often arise in response to specific kinds of emotional or physical stressors, although these may be difficult to identify. They often begin as a coping mechanism but become a serious impairment to health.

- *Anorexia nervosa* is the use of fasting, severely restricted eating, and/or compensatory activities to drastically reduce the number of calories that enter the digestive system. It is essentially self-starvation.
- *Bulimia nervosa* is normal or higher than normal calorie consumption followed by compensatory activities to prevent the absorption of those calories.
- *Binge eating* is patterns of overeating that are not followed by compensatory behaviors. Although it is a common eating pattern, it has only recently been recognized as a specific disorder.

Demographics: Who Gets Them?

The typical anorexia or bulimia patient is a female 12 to 35 years of age. Some estimates predict that up to 1% of females in this age range may have anorexia, and 2% to 5% of girls may

Eating Disorders in Brief

What are they?
Eating disorders are a group of psychological problems consisting of compulsions about food and weight gain or loss. Anorexia, bulimia, and binge eating are distinct problems, although they frequently overlap.

How are they recognized?
Signs and symptoms of anorexia and bulimia may be hard to recognize in early stages, since these behaviors are often done in private. Long-term consequences include esophageal and colon damage, tooth damage, arrhythmia, low cardiac stroke volume, electrolyte imbalance, hormonal disturbance, osteoporosis, and many other problems. Binge eating is recognizable by eating habits in combination with significant weight gain, often in a short period of time.

Is massage indicated or contraindicated?
Massage may be very supportive and appropriate for all types of eating disorders, as long as the body's chemistry can keep up with the changes bodywork brings about. If a client is in an advanced stage of anorexia or bulimia, modalities may have to be adjusted to respect the delicacy of the client's system.

have bouts of bulimia. Although some men also have this problem, more than 90% of eating disorder patients are female.[32]

Statistics on binge eating are difficult to gather, but surveys suggest that 2% to 5% of the U.S. population engages in this behavior within a 6-month period and up to 10% of the population does it at least twice a week for long periods. This disorder is more common in males than other forms; up to 35% of binge eaters may be men.[33] Given the fact that 64% of the adults in the United States are overweight and 59 million adults are classified as obese (with a body mass index of 30 or above), it is reasonable to suggest that many people have a dysfunctional relationship with food.

Etiology: What Happens?

Anorexia and bulimia The personality profiles of anorexia and bulimia patients point toward people with high expectations of themselves. They are often eager-to-please overachievers who do well in school and may be involved in athletics that emphasize thinness: dancing or gymnastics, for instance. Anorexia and bulimia are often control issues for a population that feels powerless: adolescent girls in a culture that bombards them with impossible standards to live up to. A young woman may not be able to control how people treat her, but she can at least control what goes into her mouth. For many, that feels like a major victory, at least in the short run.

Most people in this society are exposed to essentially the same cultural pressures, but not all young women develop eating disorders. This has led some researchers to look for organic causes in the chemistry of the brain. Not surprisingly, serotonin levels are found to be generally lower in eating disorder patients than in the general population. Whether this is a cause or a result of anorexia and bulimia is debatable, but it does open the door to some extra treatment options.

When a person begins to change the way she eats, ultimately it doesn't matter whether it's because of a neurotransmitter imbalance or because she's desperate to get on the track team. The impact of her choices on her body eventually change the way it functions. If her problems go on long enough, she may even reach the point at which it's impossible for her digestive system to work properly; she can lose the ability to break down nutrients, absorb nutrition, or process waste. Anorexia and bulimia can be terminal illnesses.

Binge eating The etiology of overeating is a complex mixture of physical and psychological issues. It has significance for massage therapists for several reasons:

- *Touch.* The experience of touch is a basic human need. Touch deprivation in infancy has been shown to lead to sluggish stress response systems and all manner of severe psychological dysfunction. When adults are deprived of touch, they have weakened immune systems, a high incidence of chronic diseases, and shortened life spans. What does this mean for this undertouched society? It means that if a person doesn't get touch on the *outside*, she can at least get touch on the *inside*. Think of the digestive tract as a seamless continuation of the external skin. Eating to the point of satiation causes a specific snug, comforting feeling that may be in short supply for some people. Eating for comfort can become a vicious circle, as this culture places a high premium on physical attractiveness (i.e., being slender), which means that overweight people may have a harder time making and keeping supportive touch-rich relationships. This can drive them to the short-term comfort measure of overeating more frequently. Massage therapists are in a position to provide nurturing, restorative, educated, and *nonjudgmental* touch to a population of people who may have little or no other access to this important sensory nourishment.

- *Protection.* Weight gain creates a physical barrier between a person and the world. This protective device may be a person's conscious or subconscious attempt to protect and distance herself from experiences she wants to avoid. It is common to see overeating and weight gain, for instance, in people who are subject to physical, verbal, or sexual abuse. Survivors may use overeating as a strategy to discourage their abusers. If they can make themselves unattractive by gaining weight, they can hope to lose the sexual interest of the person who abuses them. Many survivors of touch abuse are binge eaters. Many survivors also eventually explore massage as a way to experience touch that is positive and nurturing. Massage therapists who work with this population must be very aware of how closely these clients' emotional state may be reflected in their physical state.

Signs and Symptoms

Anorexia As a person moves toward being anorexic, she may begin to avoid social eating situations, in which people may notice her new habits. Anorexics often don't see themselves accurately. Seeing herself as fat, a pathologically thin woman may dress herself in large, shapeless, baggy clothes. These serve to hide her weight loss as well as they would to hide her perceived weight gain.

Anorexia has been divided into two varieties: *restrictive*, in which a person simply doesn't take in enough calories to sustain her, and *purge type*, in which calorie intake may be adequate for sustenance, but it is negated by compensatory activities, including vomiting; use of laxatives, diuretics, and/or enemas; and excessive exercise.

Advanced anorexics, in addition to being extraordinarily thin, sometimes develop *lanugo*: fine, downy hair usually seen only in early infancy. This grows all over the body, possibly as an effort to compensate for the absence of any insulating fat in the superficial fascia.

Bulimia Bulimia patients may appear to eat normally in public but then binge in private. Bingeing episodes are often triggered by emotionally stressful experiences: a fight with a loved one, a failed test, or some other disappointment.

The bingeing food is usually chosen to be self-indulgent. Bulimics don't binge on celery; they binge on candy bars. These episodes of drastic overeating are then followed by some kind of compensatory activity. *Purge-type* bulimics will attempt to prevent calorie uptake by removing the food they've just eaten through vomiting, laxatives, diuretics, or enemas. In *non-purge type* bulimia, eating episodes are followed by excessive exercise or periods of fasting.

Bulimia patients don't lose weight as anorexics do; this can make it harder to recognize the disease in early stages. The complications they develop, however, can be more visible than those seen with anorexics.

Binge eating Binge eating may be done in public, in private, or both. The reasons behind it often have the same roots as the triggers for anorexia and bulimia: stress and a feeling that the person has little or no control over what happens to her. Because the overeating is not followed by excessive exercise, fasting, or purging, binge eaters tend to gain a lot of weight. If the behavior is related to a specific trauma or emotional problem, this can take place over a relatively short time. The good news is that the long-term physical damage and dangers to the body from compulsive overeating are much easier to undo than those associated with anorexia and bulimia.

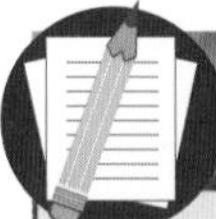

CASE HISTORY 4.4

Eating Disorders

Jessica, age 19: "Food was the one thing I thought I could control completely."

I think my eating problems began when I was around 12 years old. I was an only child and a gymnast, working hard in my program. All my coaches wanted muscle, muscle, muscle—no flab. At that time I got in the mindset that the more I worked out, the more muscle I'd have, so I started skipping meals to have more body-building time. Having muscles and doing my routines perfectly were the only things on my mind.

I went on a pretty much just rice diet. Rice doesn't have any fat but lots of carbs to burn for energy. I'd have a bowl of rice and some water, which would make me feel really full. I think because of that my stomach shrank; just eating regular foods became really hard. Since I was always by myself, my parents didn't realize my problem. I always wore baggy clothes because I was constantly cold, and if I wore something tighter, my mother would say I looked fat; but in truth I was barely 5 feet tall and about 70 or 75 pounds. When I was in seventh grade I got food poisoning from a school lunch. I ended up in the hospital. After that I couldn't eat lunch anymore until I was 18.

When I was 15 my grandfather, who had been the center of my life, died. I went into a deep depression. I had already lost gymnastics because of an injury. So I'd just go to school, go home, go to sleep, get up for a little bit to eat, and go back to sleep to do it all over again. When I slept, I had terrible dreams, and I heard voices when I was awake. I started to lose a lot of hair and have irregular menstrual cycles.

At this time and up until I turned 18, I felt like my parents controlled everything: what I wore, who I spent time with, where I was, every minute of the day. Food was one thing I thought I could control completely. Sometimes I'd get up in the middle of the night and eat and eat like I was about to die. I would feel awful later, but I would never make myself throw up. I saw a movie on bulimia once and saw how much damage it caused, so instead I would not eat for a day or two after I binged. I still do that sometimes, but not as severely as I used to.

I was always a straight-A student in school until my senior year in high school. That is when I learned of my eating problem. Several of my friends noticed how I never seemed to eat and started to help me break out of my cycle. The best thing I did was to go to Europe by myself. That gave me a chance to break out of my box, which opened a whole new world of options to me. I'd say that was when I began to heal from both my depression and my eating problems.

Now I'm in massage school. I eat about two and a half meals a day. I was kind of surprised that getting massage was so easy for me. I did have some fears about lying supine on the table, but I'm over it. I have chronic back pain, and I enjoy deep massage. I still have some fears about long-term problems from anorexia. My periods were irregular then, and they're painful now. I lose a lot of blood every month; I'm definitely anemic.

Still, I know I was lucky. I was able to control my eating before it got so bad that I needed to be admitted to the hospital. My whole sense of who I am and what makes me feel good is different now. I still really like getting compliments. If I hear, "You look great," or "That shirt looks good on you," then I feel like I can eat a chicken sandwich or a bowl of ice cream without feeling guilty later. But for the most part, for stuff like the grades I get in school or what courses I take, no one decides what I need now. I am my own person, and I am in control of my life once again. It feels really good.

Complications

The complications associated with eating disorders can be divided into mental/emotional issues and physical issues. Many eating disorder patients also struggle with depression, irritability, sleep disorders, and anxiety disorders, especially obsessive-compulsive disorder. Physical disorders vary according to eating behaviors.

Anorexia Physical problems related to self-starvation include a slow heart rate (bradycardia), low blood pressure, and arrhythmia. Severely reduced caloric intake interferes with hormone secretion, and amenorrhea (loss of the menstrual period) and osteopenia or osteoporosis can be consequences. Because this happens when bones would normally be *gaining* mass, the signs of reduced bone density can be observed relatively quickly: 6 months of anorexic behavior may lead to observable levels of bone loss in young women. Overuse of laxatives can cause colon dysfunction, and self-induced vomiting can lead to tooth damage, esophageal erosion, and dangerously imbalanced electrolytes. In addition, anorexia is a specific risk for girls with type 1 diabetes, an autoimmune dysfunction of the pancreas. Young women who have both type 1 diabetes and anorexia are at significantly increased risk for vascular and metabolic problems.

Bulimia The physical complications seen with bulimia are all related to repeated vomiting or the use of laxatives or enemas to empty the bowel. Advanced erosion of the enamel of molars is a hallmark of bulimia, along with characteristic calluses on the knuckles that indicate self-induced vomiting. The esophagus may develop ulcers or strictures (scar tissue that restricts movement), or it may rupture altogether. The colon may lose function as its work is replaced by laxative or enema use. And electrolyte imbalances brought about by vomiting and diarrhea may reach life-threatening levels. Eventually a bulimic person may find it difficult to keep food down even if she wants to.

Binge eating Binge eaters are at risk for cardiovascular disease, osteoarthritis, type 2 diabetes, and other physical problems associated with being overweight if their eating habits are never modified. However, these patients do not accrue the same life-threatening chemical imbalances that anorexic or bulimic patients do. If eating behaviors are changed, binge eaters may sustain few if any long-term problems.

Diagnosis

The DSM-IV-TR has identified four main criteria for the diagnosis of anorexia and five for the diagnosis of bulimia.[30]
The four criteria for a diagnosis of anorexia include the following:

- Refusal to maintain weight at or above a normal level; weight is below 85% of normal body mass index.
- Intense fear of gaining weight.
- Distorted self-perception; the patient sees herself as heavier than she is.
- Lack of menstrual periods (amenorrhea) for at least 3 months in a row.

The five criteria for bulimia include the following:

- Recurrent episodes of binge eating.
- A sense of lack of control; the patient couldn't stop eating even if she wanted to.
- Inappropriate compensatory behaviors, including self-induced vomiting, laxative or enema use, or excessive exercise (persisting in exercise when exhaustion or injury is present).
- A binge/compensation pattern that occurs at least twice a week for at least 3 months in a row.
- Behaviors influenced by body image.

Binge eating is still being researched as a specific disorder. The most common diagnostic features include that a person eat an excessive amount of food in a short period and that this occurs at least twice a week for 6 months or more. These eating habits are marked by a feeling of a lack of control along with significant distress about the habit.

Treatment

Treatment for eating disorders is most successful when the emphasis is *not* on gaining or losing weight but on resolving the issues that led to the behaviors in the first place. While it is important to stabilize weight and teach patients about good eating habits, these interventions are generally unsuccessful until the patient's psychological and emotional issues have been addressed.

New research revealing neurotransmitter imbalances in the brain of many eating disorder patients has opened the door to medications that may help. Addressing some of the emotional and psychological complications of eating disorders can also help to stabilize a patient's emotional state so that she can begin to understand more clearly the consequences of her actions.

Massage?

If a client with an eating disorder is stable and her circulatory system is not overtaxed (as might be seen with an advanced anorexic client, for instance), massage can be a wonderful experience for a person who has a generally negative perception of her body. Several studies have shown that anorexia or bulimia patients who received massage over time reported fewer symptoms than other patients who were treated only with traditional interventions.[34,35]

Overeaters, undereaters, and people who interfere with the absorption of food can all benefit from time spent focused on how *good* they can feel. The main cautions for bodywork concern the possibility of cardiovascular weakness, and these can be circumvented by choosing modalities that do not focus on challenging circulation.

Modality Recommendations for Eating Disorders

Deep Tissue Massage	May be indicated to increase relaxation and body awareness.
Lymphatic Drainage	Supportive.
Polarity	S: Indicated. R/D: Indicated within client comfort.
PNF/MET/Stretching	Supportive.
Reflexology	Indicated; work solar plexus, brain, stomach, all glands. For overeating, work appetite suppression points on ears.
Shiatsu	Supportive, especially with psychotherapy.
Swedish Massage	Indicated, with caution for complications that may require modality adjustments. Massage can help restore a realistic body image.
Trigger Point therapy	Contraindicated if very severe; otherwise supportive.

See Chapter 1 for a brief description of each modality, including definitions of abbreviations.

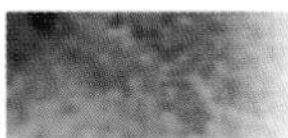

Nervous System Injuries

Bell Palsy

Definition: What Is It?

Bell palsy is the result of damage to or impairment of CN VII, the facial nerve. This nerve is composed almost entirely of motor neurons and is responsible for providing facial expression, blinking the eyes, and providing some taste sensation (Figure 4.7). It travels a complicated route from its origins to the face and exits the cranium through a small foramen just behind the earlobe.

Demographics: Who Gets It?

Bell palsy is a fairly common condition, affecting about 40,000 people per year in the United States. It is most common among young and middle-aged adults, although it has been seen in children. People most at risk for Bell palsy are pregnant women, people with diabetes, and people who are immunosuppressed.

Etiology: What Happens?

Bell palsy is a type of peripheral neuritis, that is, inflammation of a peripheral nerve. The facial nerve (CN VII) begins in the brain and passes through several narrow spaces before emerging to supply the tongue with some taste sensation and the muscles of the face with motor control. When the nerve is inflamed in a tight passageway, it sustains damage.

Several factors contributing to Bell palsy have been identified, but most cases are evidently linked to the herpes simplex virus, the same virus that causes cold sores. This pathogen,

Bell Palsy

Sir Charles Bell (1774–1842) was a Scottish surgeon, anatomist, and physiologist. He pioneered neurological research in several areas, including damage to the facial nerve and the structure of the spinal cord. (Bell's law states that the ventral horns of the spinal cord are for motor function, while the dorsal horns are for sensory function.)

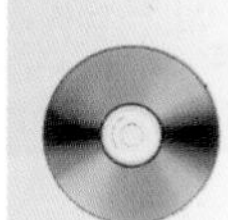

See Video Clip 6 on the Student Resource CD.

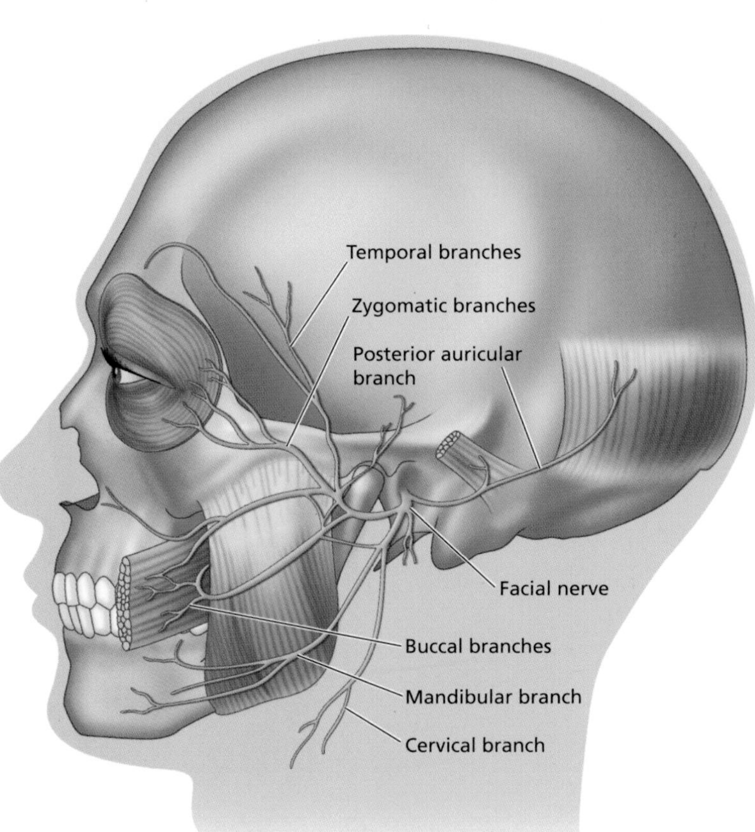

Figure 4.7. The facial nerve.

Bell Palsy in Brief

What is it?
Bell palsy is flaccid paralysis of one side of the face caused by inflammation or damage to CN VII, the facial nerve.

How is it recognized?
Symptoms of Bell palsy include a sudden onset of weakness in the muscles of the affected side of the face. Ear pain, headaches, hypersensitivity to sound, and drooling may also occur.

Is massage indicated or contraindicated?
Bell palsy indicates massage to maintain flexibility and good circulation in the affected muscles. It is important, however, to rule out causes of the nerve damage that may contraindicate massage.

which lies dormant in the nervous system until it reactivates, stimulates the production of antibodies and elicits an inflammatory response against the facial nerve. A mild case may cause damage only to the myelin sheath, but a more serious episode can damage the facial nerve itself. Since CN VII provides motor control for muscles of facial expression and the platysma, damage to this nerve results in weakness or total paralysis of the face on the affected side. The good news is that because the facial nerve is a peripheral nerve, it has the potential to regenerate, at a rate of about 2 millimeters per day.

Signs and Symptoms

Symptoms of Bell palsy are brought about by loss of enervation to the muscles on one side of the face. Classic signs include a sudden onset of flaccid paralysis of the muscles of the upper and lower face (Figure 4.8). It is difficult to eat, drink, and close the eye of the affected side. Production of saliva may be increased or decreased, and taste may be distorted. Sometimes the ear on the affected side becomes hypersensitive, because a muscle connected to the eardrum (the stapedius) is paralyzed; this is called ***hyperacusis***. The affected side may have pain, but it is more likely to be in the form of headaches or an ache behind the ear than electrical nerve pain. This is motor, not sensory, paralysis (except for some taste buds that may be affected), so sensation throughout the face stays intact.

Complications

Bell palsy is usually a short-lived disorder with few serious complications. About 85% of people who have it regain full or nearly full function within a few months.

One serious problem that can occur is damage to the eye. This can develop if the lubrication and cleaning of the eyeball provided by blinking is impaired. Another rarer complication occurs when the facial nerve forges some new and inappropriate connections as it heals. The result may be unpredictable muscle activity in the face (***synkinesis***), or secretion of excessive tears during salivation.

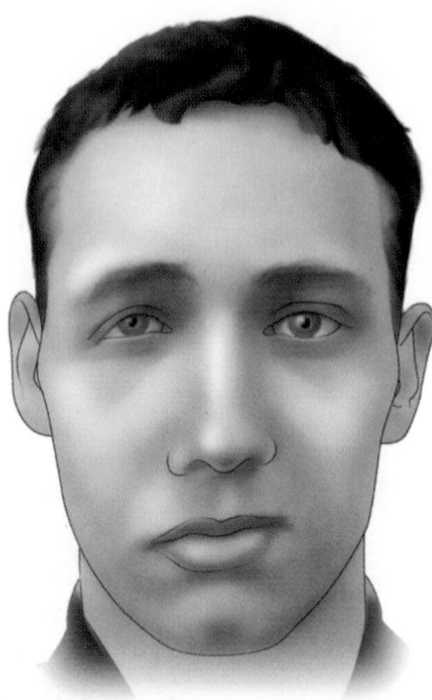

Figure 4.8. Bell palsy.

CASE HISTORY 4.5

Jim S: *"No dimple for a year!"*

When I think about what may have precipitated my bout with Bell palsy, I remember one of the most stressful years of my life. I had recently moved to the Pacific Northwest and had to go back to school to receive Washington State licensure as a massage practitioner. I was working three jobs and going to school. I had also spent some days plunging into the cold water of a tributary of the Breitenbush River. I was overcooked!

When the paralysis started, I thought it was a temporary effect of some bodywork I had received. I was told to take Advil and ice my neck. I was given massage to help with the pain. But nobody recognized the seriousness of the symptoms. Within a day I had full-on Bell palsy complete with hyperacusis (abnormal acuteness of hearing), full facial muscle paralysis, an eyelid that would not blink (with the inherent rolling of the eye up and out of danger when the lid would normally blink), and a distorted soapy beer taste on the affected side of my tongue.

It was clear in my subsequent research that these symptoms could not have been caused by a massage. With Bell, the location of impediment on the facial nerve is described by the symptoms. In other words, if I had only had facial paralysis, I would know that the nerve was impaired at a point above the jaw line. As you add symptoms (hyperacoustic sensitivity, taste impairment), you trace farther up proximal to the geniculate ganglion, inside the area near the ear.

Because I neglected to see a neurologist for over a week, my facial nerve degenerated, and it took almost a year for nearly full function to resume. I couldn't use my dimple for a year! I'm adamant about people seeing a neurologist immediately these days when I hear of a case of Bell palsy.

The whole experience was generally frustrating because there's a lot of poor information out there, but it was a great emotional process; when you've used your face for a calling card all your life and suddenly it's not available to you anymore, you have to really deal with what's underneath.

Diagnosis

Bell palsy is usually diagnosed through the client history. A sudden onset of motor paralysis to one side of the face is unique to this disorder. Herpes simplex has been identified as a causative factor in most cases of Bell palsy, but some other pathogens can cause the same kind of damage. *Borrelia burgdorferi* is the bacterium that causes Lyme disease, which can also damage the facial nerve. Other possibilities include cytomegalovirus and Epstein-Barr virus, both members of the herpes family.

Other problems can compress the facial nerve, however, and it is important to rule these out. While it is possible for Bell palsy to occur bilaterally, it is quite rare. Bilateral facial paralysis is more likely to be related to MS, Guillain-Barré syndrome, sarcoidosis, or tumors on or around CN VII or CN VIII. Ramsay-Hunt syndrome is a complication of herpes zoster (shingles) that can affect the facial nerve, but it tends to be much more painful and longer-lasting than Bell palsy.

Treatment

Treatment for Bell palsy is usually conservative because most cases are self-limiting, that is, they resolve without interference. A combination of steroidal anti-inflammatories and acyclovir to slow down herpes activity is effective for most Bell palsy patients. Patients are counseled to tape the affected eye closed at night and to protect it from drying and dust during the day. Massage is often recommended to stretch and mobilize facial muscles until the nerve is repaired.

Massage?

Bell palsy is a flaccid paralysis with sensation left intact. If the underlying cause of the neuritis has been diagnosed, then massage is a very appropriate treatment choice. Massage keeps the facial muscles elastic and the local circulation strong. This sets the stage for a more complete recovery when nerve supply is eventually restored.

Modality Recommendations for Bell Palsy	
Deep Tissue Massage	Indicated when subacute. Focus on suboccipitals, temporalis fascia, masseter, cervical paraspinal fascias.
Lymphatic Drainage	Supportive if used after a focused standard massage treatment.
Polarity	S/R/D: Indicated.
PNF/MET/Stretching	Supportive.
Reflexology	Indicated; work brain, head, face, neck, eyes, ear points.
Shiatsu	Indicated. Treat all meridians, extensions, points in face, neck, shoulders.
Swedish Massage	Indicated to help restore function to facial muscles.
Trigger Point Therapy	Indicated on facial muscles with caution for depth of pressure; supportive for rest of body.

See Chapter 1 for a brief description of each modality, including definitions of abbreviations.

Cerebral Palsy

Definition: What Is It?

Cerebral palsy (CP) is an umbrella term for many possible injuries to the brain during gestational development, birth, and early infancy. Several types of CP have been identified, each involving damage to different parts of the brain at different moments in development.

Demographics: Who Gets It?

The incidence of CP in the United States is 2 to 4 in every 1,000 live births. Between 500,000 and 1 million CP patients live in the United States today. About 8,000 babies and 1,500 preschoolers are diagnosed each year.[36] In spite of improved prenatal care, the rate of CP has remained unchanged and in some areas has even gone up. This may be related to the fact that more premature babies are surviving than ever before, and they are especially vulnerable to these problems. Other high-risk populations are hard to identify, but statistics are highest among children of mothers who smoke, who live in poverty, who don't receive prenatal care, and who have previously had preterm babies.

Cerebral Palsy in Brief

Pronunciation: ser-E-bral (or SER-eh-brul) PAWL-ze

What is it?

Cerebral palsy (CP) is an umbrella term used to refer to a variety of CNS injuries that may occur prenatally, at birth, or in early infancy. These injuries usually result in motor impairment, but they may also lead to sensory and cognitive problems as well.

How is it recognized?

CP is usually diagnosed early in infancy, when voluntary motor skills are expected to begin to develop. CP patients may have hypertonic or hypotonic muscles, suppressed or extreme reflexes, and poor coordination, and they may show random involuntary movement.

Is massage indicated or contraindicated?

As long as sensation is intact and the patient is able to communicate with the therapist in some way, massage is appropriate and potentially very useful for persons with CP, as they work to maintain muscular elasticity and improve motor skills.

Etiology: What Happens?

CP is the result of brain damage, usually to motor areas of the brain, specifically the basal ganglia and the cerebrum. Intracranial hemorrhage, damage to the white matter around the ventricles, and toxicity due to extreme jaundice are leading factors in CP. The causes of most cases are probably multifactorial events that often occur early in pregnancy. Causes of CP can fall into three groups, according to when they occur.

- *Prenatal causes.* Most cases of CP can be traced to problems during pregnancy, often due to maternal illness. Contributing factors include infection with rubella or toxoplasmosis, hyperthyroidism, diabetes, Rh sensitization (the mother essentially has an allergic reaction to the blood type of her unborn child), toxic exposure, or abdominal trauma. Pregnancy-induced hypertension and infection of the placental membrane can also increase the risk of CP.
- *Birth trauma.* CP can result if the child undergoes ***anoxia*** or ***asphyxia*** (lack of air from a mechanical blockage) during birth. Respiratory distress and head trauma (often from a difficult presentation or the use of forceps in delivery) may also increase the risk of brain damage. Anoxia and asphyxia account for less than 10% of cases of CP.
- *Acquired CP.* This is CP that is acquired in early infancy. Causes include very extreme jaundice that can lead to brain damage and deafness, head trauma (often from car accidents or child abuse, as in shaken baby syndrome), infection with meningitis or encephalitis, vascular problems (brain hemorrhages), or neoplasms in the brain that may lead to brain damage.

Regardless of the cause of the brain damage, the child with CP has some impairment of function. The problem could be so minor that only people who know what to look for may see it, or it may be completely debilitating both physically and mentally. It all depends on what part and how much of the brain has been affected.

Types of Cerebral Palsy

CP is classified into five types: spastic, athetoid, dystonic, ataxic, and mixed.

- *Spastic CP* is the most common form of the disorder, accounting for 50% to 80% of CP cases. In some areas of the body muscle tone is so high that the tight muscle's antagonists have completely let go. This is called the clasp-knife effect.
- ***Athetoid CP*** is less common than spastic CP, accounting for up to 30% of cases. It involves very weak muscles and frequent involuntary writhing movements of the extremities, face, and mouth.
- ***Ataxic CP***, a rare variety of the disorder, involves chronic shaking, intention tremors, and very poor balance.
- *Dystonic CP* involves slow, involuntary twisting movements of the trunk and extremities.
- *Mixed CP*, or a combination of the forms, affects many CP patients.

CP may also be classified by what part of the body is affected. These terms are consistent with those used for other CNS disorders: hemiplegic CP means the left or right side is affected; diplegic CP means either two arms or two legs are affected; and quadriplegic CP means all the extremities are affected to some extent.

CP is not a progressive disorder, but as a child matures, it may seem to present differently. In some children, mild forms of CP that are diagnosed in early childhood appear to resolve spontaneously by around age 7. The child's nervous system is able to adapt, and symptoms disappear.[37]

Complications

Damage to the motor systems of the body is only the beginning for many CP patients. Complications of this disorder include several other serious challenges. Many CP patients have changes in sensation, including partial or total hearing loss. Up to 75% have some amount of ***strabismus*** (eyes that don't focus on the same axis). This condition can be corrected to prevent further sight loss.

Digestive difficulties, including gastroesophageal reflux disease and poor gastrointestinal motility are common, as are low bone density and heart disease. CP is associated with excessive drooling and a high risk of cavities.

Although it doesn't always involved cognitive problems, many CP patients have some level of mental retardation, and fully cognizant patients may have challenges in communicating clearly. About 50% of CP patients have seizure disorders, which can require very powerful medication to control.

And finally, the muscles of CP patients can become so chronically tight that they are replaced with tight, restrictive connective tissue called contractures. Contractures can pull on the skeleton so constantly and so powerfully that the patient is at risk for developing hip dislocation or extreme scoliosis that can make it painful to sit or stand and difficult to breathe.

Perhaps the most pervasive and least studied complication of CP is the *pain* that these children and adults must deal with on a daily basis. The disorder itself can be painful as it twists the body into stressful postures and positions, but the treatments, from frequent injections, to surgeries, to aggressive rehabilitation exercises, can also be severely painful.

Signs and Symptoms

Signs and symptoms of CP vary according to the location and extent of brain injury. Some of the most common features of CP include hypotonicity, hypertonicity, poor coordination and voluntary muscle control, unusually weak muscles, random movements, and early hearing and/or vision problems.

Because infants don't develop voluntary motor skills until they are around 6 months old, CP may be difficult to diagnose earlier than this point. Children with this disorder often show a preference for using their left or right side before age 1, however, and this is a marker for CP.

Treatment

The CNS damage that occurs with CP is incurable and irreversible. CP is therefore managed, rather than treated, by providing skills and equipment to live as fully and functionally as possible. For some CP patients, this means braces for one foot that is slightly weaker than the other; for others it means intensive occupational, physical, and speech therapy for many years. Computers have become an important tool for many patients with CP; these appliances can improve communication and open many new opportunities for this population.

Interestingly, many CP patients who undergo extensive and aggressive physical therapy and massage have a surprising recovery or maintenance of function. This indicates that the proprioceptive response to the motor loss in the CNS reinforces and exacerbates the process in the musculature. Therapies to maintain peripheral function may be able to interrupt this self-fulfilling prophecy.

Medication for CP is prescribed to help manage seizures and to reduce muscle spasm. Botox injections can limit excessive salivation and involuntary muscle contractions for several months at a time. Some surgical interventions have been developed to correct hip dislocations, to lengthen contracted muscles, to realign vertebrae that have become distorted by scoliosis, to sever some motor neurons to the legs, and to alter nerve pathways in the brain to reduce the severity of tremors.

Adults with Cerebral Palsy

Coping mechanisms for CP have improved significantly in the past decade, and the life expectancy for people with mild versions of this disorder is close to that for people with no disability. But because these advances are so recent, adults with CP are essentially a new phenomenon, and they have some difficulties that have yet to be fully explored.

Adults with CP tend to age faster than others. They are far more likely than the general population to have vision problems. A person with CP who can walk is likely to have a longer, healthier life than someone who is confined to a wheelchair. Even so, it takes several times more energy and effort to walk for someone with CP than for someone without. Simple activities are more draining, and adult patients tend to be prone to fatigue, exhaustion, and overuse syndromes.

Massage?

Massage therapy can have a valuable role in improving the quality of life of a person with CP. As stated earlier, if physical therapy is used to stretch and strengthen skeletal muscles, massage is also a safe choice. The only caution is that people with very severe CP may not be able to communicate their wants or concerns clearly. If a massage therapist works with a client who cannot speak, other modes of communication, including nonverbal signals, become especially important. It is the responsibility of the massage therapist to make sure that his or her work is welcome and freely accepted at all times.

Modality Recommendations for Cerebral Palsy	
Deep Tissue Massage	Indicated when sensation is present and client can communicate; may help to release hypertonic tissues.
Lymphatic Drainage	Supportive.
Polarity	S: Indicated. R/D: Indicated with rapport and within client comfort.
PNF/MET/Stretching	Indicated for hypertonicity where sensation is intact.
Reflexology	Indicated; work brain points.
Shiatsu	Indicated. Treat BL, K, SP for brain development; LV, GB, SP, ST for muscle tone, tension.
Swedish Massage	Supportive, with caution for clear communication between client and therapist.
Trigger Point Therapy	Contraindicated for numbness or flaccidity; indicated for hypertonicity where sensation is intact.

See Chapter 1 for a brief description of each modality, including definitions of abbreviations.

Complex Regional Pain Syndrome

Definition: What Is It?

Complex regional pain syndrome (CRPS) is a collection of signs and symptoms including long-lasting pain and changes to the skin, muscles, joints, nerves, and blood vessels of the affected areas. CRPS 1 is the most current label for what used to be called *reflex sympathetic dystrophy syndrome* (RSDS); this is abnormal pain and other signs related to soft tissue or other injuries, usually to a distal portion of the arm or leg. CRPS 2 (formerly known as *causalgia*) is pain related to a specific nerve injury that again outlives a normal process and often exceeds the boundaries of the affected nerve (Sidebar 4.6).

Complex Regional Pain Syndrome in Brief

What is it?
Complex regional pain syndrome (CRPS) is a chronic condition in which an initial trauma (usually to the distal part of the arm or leg) causes pain that is more severe and longer lasting than is reasonable to expect. The pain can become a self-sustaining phenomenon that is a lifelong problem.

How is it recognized?
CRPS is identified primarily by pain that outlasts a normal healing period for a trauma or injury. Other signs include changes in the quality of the skin around the area, muscle weakness, joint stiffness, and eventual atrophy.

Is massage indicated or contraindicated?
Most CRPS patients have little or no tolerance for touch of any kind, at least in the area where the pain syndrome began. Physical therapy is often recommended to keep the affected joints movable and functioning; massage may help to relieve some of the pain associated with this therapy. Massage within tolerance in other parts of the body may be welcome and supportive.

Demographics: Who Gets It?

Statistics on CRPS have been difficult to gather, largely because not all specialists follow the same diagnostic criteria. Although it has been observed in all ages from babies to elderly adults, most CRPS patients are diagnosed when they are 40 to 60 years of age. Women are diagnosed about three times more often than men.

Etiology: What Happens?

When a person receives a stimulus, a sensory neuron carries that information to the spinal cord, where a reflex response begins. At the same time, that impulse travels up the spinal cord to the brain, where the stimulus is interpreted at a conscious or subconscious level. The response might be regulated by the parasympathetic nervous system, for instance, if the stimulus was a soothing, confident gliding massage stroke. But if the stimulus is threatening or painful, the sympathetic nervous system responds with the release of norepinephrine from motor nerve endings and the potential for pain activation.

In CRPS, an initial trauma (often to a hand or foot, but anywhere on the body can be affected) begins a pain sensation that is managed by the sympathetic nervous system. This disorder is often associated with high-velocity trauma such as bullet or shrapnel wounds, but it has also been seen with minor strains and sprains, as a postsurgical complication, with fractures, at injection sites, following strokes, as a consequence of disc disease, and sometimes with no identified causative trauma at all.

The pain, whatever its trigger, creates a sympathetic response, which reinforces the pain sensation. In addition, pain sensors in the affected area become increasingly sensitive to sympathetic chemicals such as norepinephrine. In other words, the pain becomes a self-fulfilling prophecy: a person hurts, which causes anxiety, which makes the hurt worse, and the normal healing processes that would interrupt this sequence are unable to overcome the power of the vicious circle.

Eventually the physiological changes that occur when a specific part of the body is stuck in a sympathetic loop cause their own kinds of damage, which may eventually be irreversible. This pain cycle also has the potential to spread proximally on the affected limb and even to the contralateral limb.

The pain generated with CRPS is sometimes discussed as two separate phenomena: *sympathetically maintained pain* and *sympathetically independent pain*. In sympathetically maintained pain, the source of the pain is sympathetic nervous system activity. Blocking the action of sympathetic nerves effectively relieves pain. In sympathetically independent pain, the pain becomes more resistant to treatment and sympathetic blockades are no longer effective. Sympathetically independent pain is recognized as an advanced or late-stage phenomenon of CRPS. It may come about because of less contribution from the sympathetic nervous system or because sympathetic nerve ganglions develop fibrosis at the sites where nerve-blocking drugs are injected.

SIDEBAR 4.6: PAIN BY ANY OTHER NAME...

In October 1864, a group of doctors compared their observations of Civil War soldiers recovering from gunshot wounds. Their comments were remarkably astute and constitute a vivid picture of the experience of the condition eventually termed *causalgia*, from the Greek *kausis* (burning) and *algia* (pain).

"In our early experience of nerve wounds, we met with a small number of men were suffering from a pain which they described as `burning' or as `mustard red-hot' or as `red-hot file rasping the skin' . . . Its intensity varies from the most trivial burning to a state of torture, which can hardly be credited, but which reacts on the whole economy, until the general health is seriously affected . . . "[38]

Over the years this condition, now called complex regional pain syndrome (CRPS) has been known by many names. Sympathetic maintained pain syndrome is another term, along with shoulder-hand syndrome and Sudeck atrophy. Causalgia itself is now considered to refer to pain related to peripheral nerve injury (CRPS 2), while reflex sympathetic dystrophy syndrome refers to pain that begins in the extremities (CRPS 1).

Signs and Symptoms

Signs and symptoms of CRPS vary widely, but three major issues are usually present: One is burning pain around the site of initial injury. Another is autonomic dysfunction that shows as changes in skin temperature and texture, edema, hair and nail growth, and changes in local blood supply that can lead to characteristic bone density loss. Third is motor dysfunction that begins as weakness in local muscles along with joint stiffness but may progress to contracture and atrophy of muscle, bone, and joint structures.

CRPS 1 has been broken into three loosely defined stages. Not all experts agree on the sequence of progression, as this disorder is experienced differently by every person who has it, but they can be a useful organizing principle to understand the process of the problem.

- *Stage I* signs and symptoms are prevalent during the first 1 to 3 months of pain. They include severe burning pain at the site of the injury; muscle spasm; reduced range of motion, excessive hair and nail growth if the injury is on a hand or foot; and shiny, hot, red, sweaty skin (Figure 4.9). Stage I is sometimes called the acute stage.
- *Stage II* is characterized by changes in the growth pattern of the affected tissues. The swelling spreads proximally from the initial site, the hair stops growing, and the nails become brittle and easily cracked. Skin that was red in stage I takes on a bluish cast in stage II. In this intensely painful stage the muscles begin to atrophy from underuse, and the nearby joints may thicken and become stiffer. Stage II usually lasts 3 to 6 months. It is also called the ***dystrophic*** stage.
- *Stage III* CRPS 1 shows signs of irreversible changes to the affected structures. The bones become thin and brittle, the joints become immobile, and the muscles tighten into permanent contracture. The condition may spread proximally up the limb, to the contralateral limb, or anywhere else in the body. At this point the pain sensation is a self-sustaining phenomenon in the brain. In other words, the neurotransmitter balance and pain sensation centers in the brain are essentially incapable of letting go of this sensation. This is known as the ***atrophic*** stage.

Diagnosis

CRPS is typically diagnosed through the client history, a physical examination to rule out other possible factors, and two tests: a triple-phase bone scan to find characteristic changes in bone density, and thermography to look for differences in skin temperature in the affected areas.

Recent meetings of pain specialists have led to the development of an agreed-upon set of diagnostic criteria for CRPS 1 and 2; the hope is that a more systematic collection of information will eventually lead to better treatment options for this very difficult disorder. The diagnostic criteria are as follows:[39]

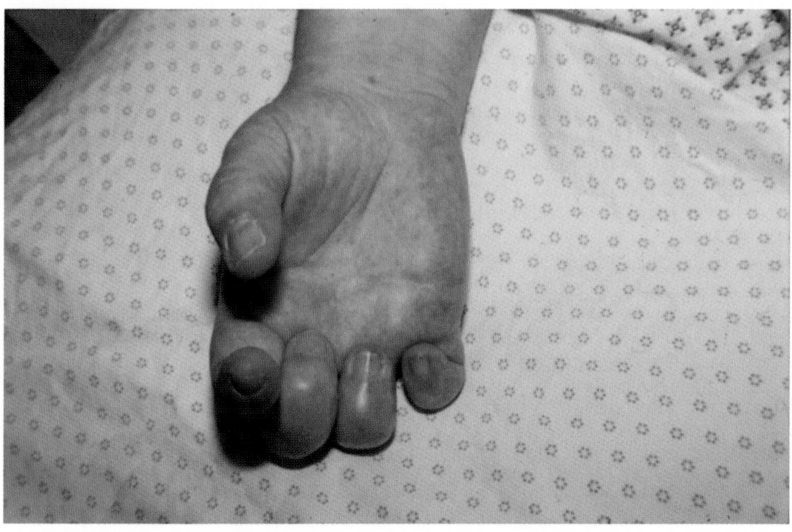

Figure 4.9. Complex regional pain syndrome.

- An initiating trigger or event (type 1) or a specific nerve injury (type 2).
- Persistent pain that outlasts a typical healing process; in type 2 the pain may exceed the boundaries of the affected nerve.
- Marked edema, sweating, hair or nail growth, shiny skin, discoloration, and temperature differences in the affected area; this also includes changes in bone density as regulated by local blood vessels.
- No other identifiable contributing factors; these would include nerve entrapment, arthritis, thrombophlebitis, or local infection.

Treatment

Treatment for CRPS is a long-term process. Aggressive physical and occupational therapy are recommended to preserve function and prevent or delay atrophy of the affected areas; this is problematic for many people who are in significant pain that is exacerbated by movement or exercise.

Psychotherapeutic intervention is suggested, as the pain and disability involved with this condition can lead to extreme forms of depression, anxiety, and sleep disorders. All of these can make CRPS symptoms worse.

Chemical nerve blocks are often used to block nerve transmission at the sympathetic ganglia near the spinal cord. These are often useful, but they are temporary and cannot be used indefinitely.

Intrathecal pumps that deliver painkilling medications directly into the spinal cord allow patients to manage their own pain. These bypass the blood-brain barrier to allow the same results with smaller doses of drugs.

Some patients undergo a full *sympathectomy*, that is, their sympathetic motor neurons are surgically severed. While it has been effective for some, others find that this extreme intervention is also temporary and has many serious side effects.

Massage?

CRPS locally contraindicates massage in acutely affected areas, where any stimulus is painful and unwelcome. When it is treated with physical therapy to limit bone and joint atrophy, massage that is well tolerated may be appropriate and important in this context as well. If massage is perceived as pleasant anywhere else on the body, it could certainly add to the quality of life of a person who has some extreme physical challenges.

Modality Recommendations for Complex Regional Pain Syndrome	
Deep Tissue Massage	Indicated within early stages. Desensitize with slow, gentle touch; then go deeper within client tolerance.
Lymphatic Drainage	Supportive.
Polarity	S: Indicated. R/D: Locally contraindicated depending on stage; otherwise indicated.
PNF/MET/Stretching	Indicated while subacute.
Reflexology	Indicated; work brain, spine, solar plexus, affected area points.
Shiatsu	Locally contraindicated in severe swelling or pain. Indicated elsewhere to resolve trauma; reduce pain, swelling; maintain muscle function, especially via SI meridian and extension.
Swedish Massage	Locally contraindicated; otherwise supportive.
Trigger Point Therapy	Locally contraindicated; otherwise supportive.

See Chapter 1 for a brief description of each modality, including definitions of abbreviations.

Spina Bifida

Definition: What Is It?

Spina bifida (literally, "cleft spine") is a neural tube defect in which the vertebral arch fails to close completely over the spinal cord. This defect can be so subtle it is found only through incidental radiography or MRI, or it can be so severe that it the spinal canal is open and the baby may not survive the birth.

Spina Bifida in Brief

Pronunciation: SPY-nah BIF-ih-dah

What is it?

Spina bifida is a neural tube defect resulting in an incompletely formed vertebral arch, damage to the meninges and/or spinal cord, and a high risk of distal paralysis and infection.

How is it recognized?

Spina bifida occulta can be completely silent and detected only through incidental tests. Cystic spina bifida can be detected through prenatal testing, but the most obvious sign is a protrusion, sometimes covered by skin, of a cyst containing the dural and arachnoid layers of the meninges, and usually the spinal cord as well.

Is massage indicated or contraindicated?

Infants with spina bifida surgery are given rigorous physical therapy to establish and maintain function, especially in the abdomen and legs. Massage is appropriate in this context as well. For adults with spina bifida, the judgment about massage depends on the extent of the damage, complicating factors, and the presence or absence of sensation.

Demographics: Who Gets It?

Spina bifida statistics in the United States have recently been declining, but it still occurs about once in every 1,000 live births, or 1,500 to 2,000 times per year. It clearly has a genetic component, because having this disorder in the family raises the risk of having a child with spina bifida, but about 95% of cases occur in families with no history of the disease.

Hispanics and European whites have a higher incidence of spina bifida than other races. Women who have spina bifida themselves or who have diabetes or seizure disorders have a higher than normal chance of having a child with this disorder.

Etiology: What Happens?

Several types of neural tube defects may occur between day 14 and day 28 after conception (Sidebar 4.7).

At this time the woman may not know she is pregnant, and the fetus is about the size of a grain of rice, but the cells that eventually differentiate into connective, muscle, and epithelial tissue at various levels of the spinal cord are in place. If something interrupts their development, spina bifida may occur.

The main risk factor for spina bifida is a deficiency of folic acid at conception and in the earliest weeks of fetal development. Because this condition may be determined before a woman knows she is pregnant, it is especially important for women who want to have children to be sure they are getting enough folic acid in their diet.

Spina bifida can be classified as occult (invisible without looking for it) or cystic.

- *Spina bifida occulta*. The vertebral arch, usually in a lumbar vertebra, does not completely fuse, but no signs or symptoms are obvious. Indeed, a person with spina bifida occulta may never be aware of the condition unless a low back radiograph is taken for another reason. It is difficult to estimate how common it is; some sources suggest that 5 to 10% of the population may be affected.[40] Some people with spina bifida occulta have a small dimple, birthmark, or tuft of hair on the spine at the location of the abnormality, but they have no dysfunction because of it. While spina bifida occulta is usually inconsequential, it can be serious. Two or more vertebrae may be affected, and the person may develop a tethered spinal cord. This

SIDEBAR 4.7: OTHER NEURAL TUBE DEFECTS

The neural tube is composed of specialized fetal cells that fold in on themselves during the earliest days of development. Under normal circumstances the tube is complete and closed by day 28, when the fetus is about the size of a grain of rice.

Sometimes those cells, which are the starting material of the vertebrae, skull, spinal cord, spinal nerves, and brain, deform. Spina bifida occulta, meningocele, and myelomeningocele describe problems with the spinal cord, but the brain can also be affected. Some neural tube defects that can occur apart from or along with spina bifida include the following:

- **Encephalocele.** In this condition the bones of the skull don't develop properly. A cyst protrudes from the head, containing cerebrospinal fluid and possibly brain tissue as well.
- **Anencephaly.** In this condition the brain forms incompletely or doesn't form at all. These babies tend to be stillborn or die soon after birth.
- **Arnold-Chiari malformation.** This is a rare disorder except in the presence of myelomeningocele, with which it is relatively common. In this situation the brainstem and some of the cerebellum protrude into the spinal canal in the neck. This leads to hydrocephalus, difficulties with swallowing and breathing, and impaired coordination of the arms.

can manifest as problems in the feet (especially pes cavus) and problems with bladder and bowel control. These often arise during puberty, when the child goes through a growth spurt that stretches the spinal cord.

- *Spina bifida meningocele.* This is the rarest type of cystic spina bifida. Only the dura mater and arachnoid layers of the meninges press through at the site of the vertebral cleft, forming a cyst that is visible at birth. It is easily reparable with surgery and generally has few or no long-term consequences for the baby.
- *Spina bifida myelomeningocele.* This is the most common and most severe version of cystic spina bifida, accounting for about 94% of cases. In this case the spinal cord or extensions of the cauda equina protrude along with the meninges through several incompletely formed vertebral arches. Occasionally the skin doesn't cover the protrusion, raising a serious risk of CNS infection if no immediate intervention takes place.

Signs and Symptoms

Spina bifida occulta is not obvious at birth, although it sometimes causes a birthmark, patch of hair, or a dimple at the site of the abnormality. Cystic spina bifida is obvious, because a sac containing meninges and/or spinal cord material protrudes on the back of the newborn infant. It usually occurs in the lumbar spine, and the sac is often red and raw looking (Figures 4.10–4.12).

The severity of cystic spina bifida is determined by the location and size of the cyst. The higher the defect, the more paralysis tends to be present. Fortunately, most cases present in the thoracic or lumbar spine.

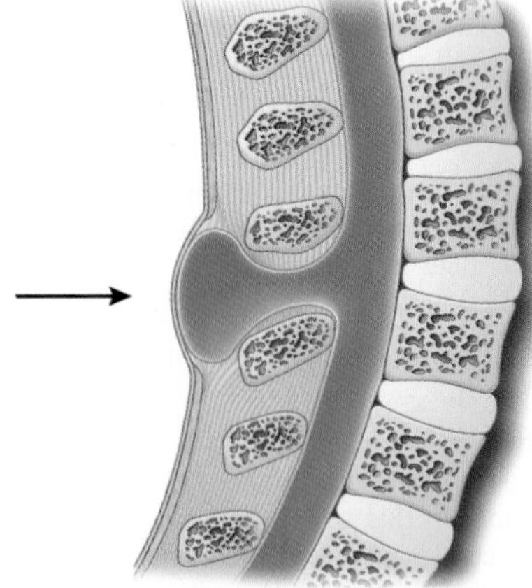

Figure 4.10. Spina bifida occulta. The vertebrae are incompletely fused; no external sac is present.

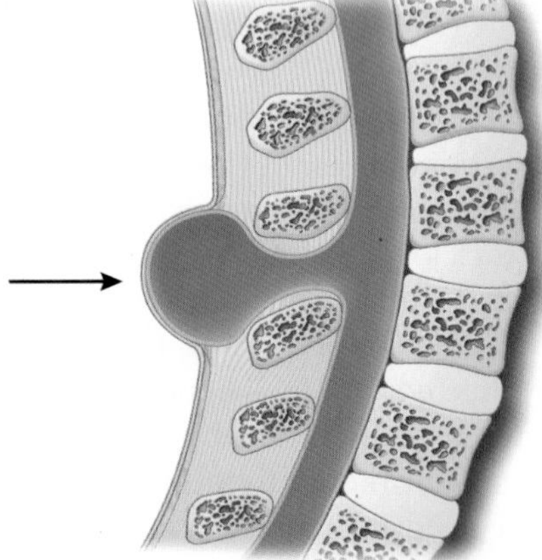

Figure 4.11. Spina bifida meningocele. An external sac contains the meninges and cerebrospinal fluid.

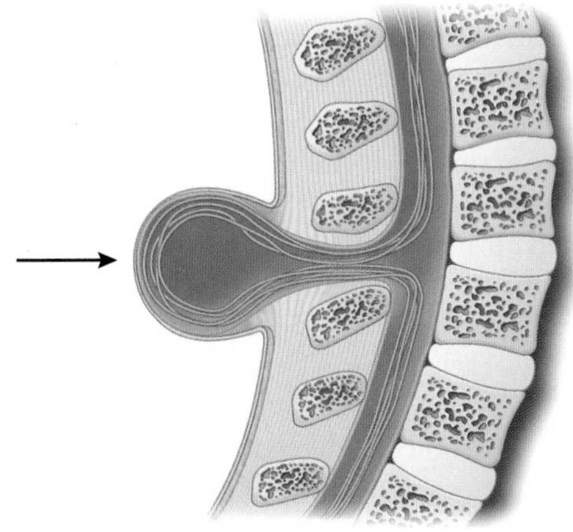

Figure 4.12. Spina bifida myelomeningocele. An external sac contains the meninges and cerebrospinal fluid, peripheral nerves, and spinal cord tissue.

CASE HISTORY 4.6

Spina Bifida

While the lower half of his body revealed a life of disease, death, and despair, his upper body reflected a life filled with drive, determination, ambition, and hope.

With an effortless motion, he pulled himself onto the table. He grasped his lifeless legs and twisted his whole body until he was lying prone. To gaze on his body was to grasp two opposing realities at once. His legs, clad in a loose-fitting pair of sweatpants, were shriveled and limp. Even his hips and buttocks were hollowed out and gaunt after years of frustrated growth and nearly useless service to the greater whole.

Yet beginning with his lower back and especially with the lower border of his rib cage, a transformation of epic proportions occurred. The sides of his torso tapered out dramatically to accommodate his thickly muscled back. Indeed, his entire upper body resembled that of a professional bodybuilder. Thus, while the lower half of his body revealed a life of disease, death, and despair, his upper body reflected a life filled with drive, determination, ambition, and hope.

At the end of the session, when my client had gotten off my table, dressed, and left the building, I reflected on the meaning of wholeness. It dawned on me that wholeness is not a disease-free condition, at least in this life, in this reality.

Instead, wholeness is a realized and used connection between the human will and a greater purpose, a greater goal. This athlete thrives because his sights are set on goals that diminish the significance of his lower body and magnify the significance of his upper body, including and especially his mind. Similarly, I thrive when my sights are set on goals that are adorned in truth and immersed in love—on my best days and even on my worst days.

—Jan Fields, observations on the 2002 Paralympic Games

Complications

Spina bifida is a complex disorder with several possible complications. ***Hydrocephalus***, or water on the brain, affects about 85% of children with cystic spina bifida. The insertion of a shunt that drains cerebrospinal fluid from the brain down the neck and into the abdominal cavity prevents hydrocephalus from damaging the brain.

While most children with spina bifida have normal intelligence, many have mild to severe learning disabilities that may make it difficult to function in a mainstream classroom. Many spina bifida patients develop very severe latex hypersensitivity, possibly from having multiple intrusive surgeries and other medical procedures early in life. This allergy may create a dangerous anaphylactic reaction later in life.

Other common complications include decubitus ulcers, digestive tract problems, urinary tract problems, obesity, and severe muscle imbalances that can lead to flaccidity on one side, contractures on the other, and severe scoliosis.

Diagnosis

Spina bifida is detectable prenatally. Testing begins with a blood sample; if that comes up positive for a substance called ***alfa-fetoprotein***, a follow-up ultrasound and/or ***amniocentesis*** may be scheduled. If a woman is found to be carrying a child with spina bifida, a number of options can be considered. Some research indicates that a cesarean section is safer than vaginal birth for a baby with spina bifida; this can be planned. Furthermore, a few facilities have begun to try in utero corrective surgery. This approach is very new, but early reports suggest a lower risk of hydrocephalus for these children. This procedure carries very high risks, however, to both the mother and the child.

Treatment

A baby born with cystic spina bifida needs surgery within a few days to reduce the cyst and preserve as much spinal cord function as possible. Afterward, even tiny babies are supported with rigorous physical therapy and exercises to maintain function in the leg muscles as much as possible. As children mature and their functional level becomes clear, they may be taught to use crutches, braces, wheelchairs, or other equipment as necessary.

Many spina bifida patients undergo multiple surgeries, not only to reduce the protruding cyst but also to correct a tethered cord, in which the spinal cord doesn't slide freely within the spinal canal; to deal with the complications of hydrocephalus as discussed earlier; and to address whatever complications may be brought about by severe scoliosis.

Massage?

The guidelines for massage and spina bifida are the same as for most CNS disorders. Judgments must be based on the presence of sensation, the level of function, and other contraindications that may accompany this complex and serious CNS dysfunction. Many patients engage in physical therapy and exercise to preserve function, and massage can certainly be appropriate in this context.

Modality Recommendations for Spina Bifida

Deep Tissue Massage	Indicated within limits of client activity and sensitivity. Work to reduce contractures.
Lymphatic Drainage	Supportive.
Polarity	S: Indicated. R/D: Locally contraindicated depending on stage; otherwise indicated.
PNF/MET/Stretching	Supportive with caution for complications, areas of reduced sensation.
Reflexology	Indicated; work brain, spine, lymphatic system, endocrine system points.
Shiatsu	Indicated to maintain function, tonus, activity. Treat BL, K, SI meridians.
Swedish Massage	Supportive, with caution for local contraindications and comfortable position on table.
Trigger Point Therapy	Locally contraindicated over affected spinal region and for numbness; otherwise supportive.

See Chapter 1 for a brief description of each modality, including definitions of abbreviations.

Spinal Cord Injury

Definition: What Is It?

The definition of spinal cord injury (SCI) is self-evident: damage to nerve tissue in the spinal canal. How that damage is reflected in the body depends on where and how much of the tissue has been affected.

Traumatic SCI falls into one of five categories: In *concussion* tissue is jarred and irritated but not structurally damaged. In *contusion* bleeding in the spinal cord damages tissue. In *compression* a damaged disc, a bone spur, or a tumor puts mechanical pressure on the cord. In *laceration* the spinal cord is partially cut, as with a gunshot wound. In *transection* the spinal cord is severed.

An injury that affects the lower abdomen and extremities but leaves the chest and arms intact is called paraplegia. An injury that affects the body from the neck down is called tetraplegia or quadriplegia. For more terminology in the context of CNS injuries, see Sidebar 4.8.

Demographics: Who Gets It?

Frequency of traumatic SCI in the United States is estimated at about 10,000 to 11,000 per year, excluding those who die at the scene of the accident. About 250,000 people in this country live with permanent SCI. Male patients outnumber females by more than 4 to 1.

Motor vehicle accidents cause about 50% of SCIs. Gunshot wounds and other acts of violence cause 11%; this figure has fallen

Spinal Cord Injury in Brief

What is it?
In spinal cord injury (SCI) some or all of the fibers in the spinal cord have been damaged, usually by trauma but occasionally by other problems such as tumors or bony growths in the spinal canal.

How is it recognized?
The signs and symptoms of SCI vary with the nature of the injury. Loss of motor function follows destruction of motor neurons, but that paralysis may be flaccid or spastic, depending on the injured area. Loss of sensation follows the destruction of sensory pathways. If the injury is not complete, some motor or sensory function may remain in the affected tissues.

Is massage indicated or contraindicated?
Vigorous massage is appropriate only where sensation is present and no underlying pathologies may be exacerbated by the work. Areas without sensation contraindicate massage that intends to manipulate and influence the elasticity of tissue.

SIDEBAR 4.8: NERVE DAMAGE TERMINOLOGY

Nerve damage can manifest in several ways. Familiarity with some of the vocabulary of nervous system damage can make it much easier to "talk shop" with clients and doctors dealing with these problems.

- **Paresthesia** is any abnormal sensation, particularly the tingling, burning, and prickling feelings associated with pins-and-needles sensation.
- **Hyperkinesia** is excessive muscular activity.
- **Hypokinesia** is diminished or slowed movement.
- **Hypertonia** is a general term for extreme tension, or tone, in the muscles.
- **Hypotonia** is an abnormally low level of muscle tone, as seen with flaccid paralysis.
- **Spasticity** is a type of hypertonia in which the stretch reflex is overactive. The flexors want to flex, but the extensors don't want to give way. Finally the extensors are stretched too far, and they release altogether. This phenomenon is called the clasp-knife effect.
- **Paralysis** is loss of any function controlled by the nervous system. The word comes from the Greek for *loosening*.
- **Paresis** is partial or incomplete paralysis.
- **Flaccid paralysis** is typically a sign of peripheral nerve damage. It accompanies conditions such as Bell palsy. Flaccid paralysis occurs with muscles in a state of hypotonicity.
- **Spastic paralysis** is the result of CNS damage. It combines aspects of hypertonia, hypokinesia and hyperreflexia. It is never resolved, which distinguishes it from mere spasm. These are types of spastic paralysis:
    - **Hemiplegia** means the left or right side (or hemisphere) of the body is affected. This is the variation that most often accompanies stroke.
    - **Paraplegia** means the bottom half of the body or some part of it has been affected. These patients still have at least partial use of their arms and hands.
    - **Diplegia** is symmetrical paralysis of upper or lower extremities resulting from injuries to the cerebrum.
    - **Tetraplegia**, or quadriplegia, means that the body has been affected from the neck down. Tetraplegics can eat, breathe, talk, and move their head because these functions are controlled by the cranial nerves, which are usually protected from injury.

significantly in the past few years. Falls are responsible for 24%, and sports injuries account for 9% of SCIs.

Statistics on other forms of SCI are not kept, but some estimates suggest that more people have been disabled by nontraumatic damage to the spinal cord (from arthritis, bone spurs, tumors, or other causes) than from accidents and injuries.[41]

Etiology: What Happens?

A primary injury to the spinal cord is usually a crushing blow (Figure 4.13), but the cord can also be injured through direct compression exerted by tumors, bone spurs, or cysts or by stretching the spinal column (this is most frequently seen in children). Gunshot wounds may lacerate the cord. Spinal cords are rarely completely transected; when they are, the mortality rate is very high.

A newly injured spinal cord goes through a period called spinal cord shock. During this time many body functions are severely impaired: blood pressure is dangerously low, the heart beats slowly, peripheral blood vessels dilate, and the patient is susceptible to ***hypothermia***.

During the acute phase of injury the affected muscles may be flaccid, or hypotonic. When the inflammatory process begins to subside, the muscles supplied by damaged axons begin to tighten, and their reflexes become hyperreactive. ***Spasticity*** along with ***hyperreflexia*** is a hallmark of SCI. If muscles stay flaccid and reflexes are dull or nonexistent, the damage is probably to the nerve roots rather than to

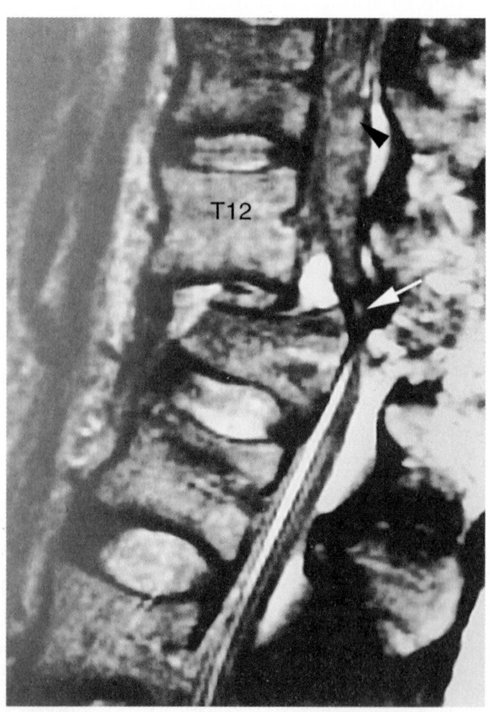

Figure 4.13. Spinal cord injury.

the spinal cord itself. Injuries to the low back often show this pattern, as the spinal canal is occupied by the cauda equina nerve extensions from T12 down to the sacrum. Depending on the nature of the accident, it is perfectly possible to sustain injury to both the spinal cord and the nerve roots.

As researchers learn more about SCI, some very exciting information has emerged: a large part of the damage to delicate CNS tissue is incurred not by the trauma itself but by posttraumatic reactions in the body. These secondary reactions can cause significantly more damage than the initial injury, but as we discover new secrets about the workings of the CNS, new ways to interfere with these secondary processes continue to improve the prognosis for SCI survivors.

Some of the most serious secondary injuries include these:

- *Excessive bleeding* into and inside the spinal cord; this can also contribute to circulatory shock and dangerously low blood pressure and slowed heart rate.
- *Local edema* of the spinal cord; both these issues can lead to the death of CNS neurons through hypoxia.
- *Free radical activity*: these specialized oxygen molecules can destroy cell membranes.
- *Excitotoxicity*: the secretion of excessive glutamate, an excitatory neurotransmitter in the spinal cord can damage motor neurons.
- *Immune system activity*: under normal circumstances specialized cells in the CNS provide immune system protection, and other white blood cells are blocked by the blood-brain-barrier. When the spinal cord has been injured, white blood cells flood the area. This turns out to be a two-edged sword: while they are effective at cleaning up debris and limiting infection, they secrete inflammatory cytokines that contribute to cell damage and the accumulation of scar tissue in the spinal cord.
- *Apoptosis*: It was originally thought that the cell damage with SCI was due to mechanical trauma, but tests now show that many neurons die in the days and weeks following an injury through "cellular suicide" or *apoptosis*. This process seems to affect the oligodendricytes in particular: these are glial cells that form myelin in the CNS. When they degenerate, CNS cells are stripped of the covering that would otherwise speed transmission and provide electrical insulation from other fibers.

Ultimately, secondary damage increases the extent of CNS injury, contributes to the formation of scar tissue and cysts in the spinal canal, and reduces post-injury function. Interventions to limit this process are being aggressively pursued.

Signs and Symptoms

The motor and sensory impairment caused by SCI is entirely determined by what parts of the cord are damaged and at what levels. Obviously, the higher the damage, the more of the body is affected. Injuries to the anterior cord affect motor function, while damage to the posterior aspect affects the senses of touch, proprioception, and vibration. Damage to the lateral parts of the cord interrupts sensations of pain and temperature.

Complications

Spinal cord injuries can lead to many serious long-term complications. An SCI patient must invest a lot of time and energy in working to prevent, manage, or recover from these secondary problems:

- *Respiratory infection.* SCI patients are at high risk for respiratory infection, especially if the damage is higher than T12. When the chest can't fully expand and contract and the cough reflex is limited, it is difficult to expel pathogens from the body. The leading cause of death among SCI patients is pneumonia.

- *Deep vein thrombosis, pulmonary embolism.* The formation of blood clots in the venous system is a high risk for new SCI patients, and the risk decreases only slightly with the passage of time. Blood that goes into the legs but that lacks the muscular support to get back up the leg veins can pool and thicken, causing deep vein thrombosis. If a fragment of a clot breaks loose, it will inevitably go to the lungs, causing a life-threatening pulmonary embolism; this is the second leading cause of death for SCI patients.
- *Urinary tract infection.* SCI patients who must use a catheter to urinate are at high risk for contamination and infection of the urinary tract. Left untended, the risk of these infections invading the kidneys is significant.
- *Decubitus ulcers.* Also known as bedsores or pressure sores, they can arise anywhere circulation is limited by mechanical compression of the skin. Because these wounds don't heal quickly or easily, they are highly susceptible to infection, which can easily complicate to septicemia or blood poisoning.
- *Heterotopic ossification.* This is the formation of calcium deposits in soft tissues. It is very similar to myositis ossificans, but this particular process is seen only in SCI patients. It typically occurs around the hips or knees, where it can be acutely painful. Heterotopic ossification can be corrected only with surgery.
- *Autonomic hyperreflexia.* Damage to the spinal cord above T6 raises the risk of developing ***autonomic hyperreflexia***, in which a minor stimulus (e.g., a full bladder or bowel, a ridge of cloth caught under the skin, menstrual cramps) creates an uncontrollable sympathetic reaction. It causes a pounding headache, increased heart rate, sweating, and other fight-or-flight symptoms, including dangerously high blood pressure. Autonomic hyperreflexia can be a medical emergency.
- *Cardiovascular disease.* Suddenly changing from an active life to confinement in a wheelchair means a significant reduction in physical activity for most SCI patients. The risk of developing hypertension, atherosclerosis, and other cardiovascular problems is high for this sedentary population.
- *Numbness.* Most SCI patients have some numbness or reduction in sensation, depending on which part of the spinal cord has been damaged. The absence of pain is a dangerous feature, because it allows damage to occur without warning. Small cuts or abrasions can become infected, and an SCI patient may never know.
- *Pain.* Many SCI patients have various kinds of pain along with numbness and lack of sensation. Some chronic pain is generated in the nerve tissue itself but refers to the damaged limbs. Nerve root pressure may refer pain along the associated dermatome. Pain may be generated by the development of calcium deposits. Also, pain may be related to musculoskeletal injury, as a person must learn to use the arms and shoulders in new ways to propel the wheelchair and get into and out of it.
- *Spasticity, contractures.* As the muscles supplied by damaged motor axons begin to tighten, an SCI patient loses range of motion. Some spasticity may become a permanent feature of the injury. Chronically tight muscle fibers eventually atrophy, to be replaced by thick, tough layers of connective tissue; this is called a contracture. If any sensory or motor function is left in the limb, temporary episodes of spasticity may also be a problem. These may be caused by any kind of stimulus; the reflexes of active muscle fibers in SCI patients are very extreme and sensitive.

Treatment

If something presses directly on the spinal cord or cauda equina, emergency surgery to remove it is indicated. The other very important early intervention with these traumas is to limit inflammation and other secondary body reactions that may damage uninjured tissue, so anti-inflammatories and other medications that limit this kind of activity are usually administered as quickly as possible.

Some later treatments for SCI include the implantation of electrodes in muscles that are controlled from an external computer. These neural prostheses can provide pinching and gripping capabilities for people who otherwise would not have the use of their hands.

Surgical transfer of healthy tendons can also be helpful. For some people the triceps muscle is paralyzed, but the deltoid is not. Surgically extending the posterior deltoid tendon and attaching it to the olecranon can provide these people with the power it takes to use a wheelchair.

Another new line of treatment focuses on spinal reflexes for walking and other movements. Even when the patient needs extensive help, going through the motions on a treadmill or stationary bike improves motor function, exercises functioning muscles, and benefits the cardiovascular system. Furthermore, these interventions appear to improve reflexes in general, which leads to a better overall prognosis.

Treatment for SCI survivors is targeted at providing them with the skills to live as fully as possible. Physical and occupational therapists specialize in helping these patients gain the skills they need to function; mental/emotional therapists are also essential, especially for those who are adapting to their paralysis as a new way of life. Ultimately, about 90% of SCI patients are able to live independently with these new skills.

The focus of research in SCI treatment is on influencing the growth of CNS neurons. It has been found that some proteins in cerebrospinal fluid inhibit neuronal growth, while others stimulate it. Further, it may be that different types of neurons require different chemical environments for repair. Eventually, through a combination of stem cell implantation, genetic manipulation, and the creation of highly conducive chemical environments, it may be possible for someone with extensive spinal cord damage to regenerate damaged tissue and emerge with full or nearly full function.

Massage?

Massage can be an important part of the life of people with SCI, as long as the complications are considered and respected.

One aspect of living with SCI that may be frequently missed is that in incomplete injuries where part of the spinal cord still functions, sensation and some motor control are still present. Some of the proprioceptors in these muscles still send messages about tightness and movement. If those messages are consistently relaying information about limitation, that can become a self-fulfilling prophecy: a muscle that is partially limited can become completely unusable. It is vital that the proprioceptors in affected muscles be stimulated to allow the *most* use possible, rather than the least. When physical therapy and massage for SCI survivors focus on this goal, the long-term prognosis for maintaining function is much improved.

SCI patients have very different physical and emotional stressors than the rest of the population, but they are prone to the same kinds of injuries as anyone else. Imagine being in a wheelchair and having a rotator cuff injury; wouldn't it be a relief to get rolling pain free again?

It takes a lot of courage to work with SCI survivors; massage therapists may have fears of accidentally hurting them, physically or emotionally, by saying or doing the wrong thing. But within this group is a population waiting eagerly for the chance to enjoy all the benefits bodywork.

Modality Recommendations for Spinal Cord Injury	
Deep Tissue Massage	Indicated within limits of client activity and sensitivity. Work to improve proprioception; encourage client movement with releases.
Lymphatic Drainage	Indicated, especially in early stages of recovery.
Polarity	S: Indicated. R/D: Indicated above/below injury within comfort of client.
PNF/MET/Stretching	Supportive with caution for complications, areas of reduced sensation.
Reflexology	Indicated; work brain, spine, lymphatic system points.
Shiatsu	Indicated to maintain function. Treat BL for nervous system, SI for trauma.
Swedish Massage	Supportive with caution for complications and areas of reduced sensation.
Trigger Point Therapy	Indicated proximal to injury; otherwise strongly cautioned.

See Chapter 1 for a brief description of each modality, including definitions of abbreviations.

Stroke

Definition: What Is It?

Stroke, also called brain attack or cerebrovascular accident (CVA), is damage to brain cells due to oxygen deprivation.

Stroke in Brief

What is it?
A stroke is damage to brain tissue caused either by a blockage in blood flow or by an internal hemorrhage.

How is it recognized?
The symptoms of stroke include paralysis, weakness, and/or numbness on one side; blurry or diminished vision on one side with asymmetrically dilated pupils; dizziness and confusion; difficulty in speaking or understanding simple sentences; sudden extreme headache; and possibly loss of consciousness.

Is massage indicated or contraindicated?
Most people who survive strokes are at high risk for other cardiovascular problems. Rigorous circulatory massage should probably be avoided with this group, although they may certainly benefit from other types of bodywork to augment their rehabilitative physical therapy. Massage around the neck should also be avoided for stroke survivors until the client has reached prestroke levels of activity.

Demographics: Who Gets It?

Stroke is the single most common type of CNS disorder. It is the third leading cause of death in the United States, coming in behind heart disease and cancer. It is the leading cause of adult disability.

About 700,000 people have a stroke each year in this country: that's one every 45 seconds. Of them, 500,000 will have their first attack, while 200,000 will have a repeat stroke. About 160,000 Americans die of stroke each year (one every 3.3 minutes). Of the survivors, 15 to 30% are permanently disabled, and 20% require institutionalized care. About 4.7 million stroke survivors are alive in this country today.[42]

Demographic statistics have revealed that stroke is by far most common in the southern United States; this is known as the "stroke belt". Further, especially high concentrations of stroke incidence have been found in the "stroke buckle" of the stroke belt: North Carolina, South Carolina, and Georgia have the highest rates of stroke in the country.

Etiology: What Happens?

Oxygen deprivation in the brain can be caused by ischemia or bleeding in the cranium. Ischemic strokes account for about 80% of CVAs. They typically occur in one of two forms:

- *Cerebral thrombosis.* In this condition a clot develops in and eventually blocks a cerebral artery, starving off nerve cells.
- *Embolism.* Emboli are fragments of blood clots or atherosclerotic plaque that travel to the brain from elsewhere in the body. Atherosclerosis in the carotid arteries can be one source; others come from ***atrial fibrillations***: incomplete and arrhythmic contractions that allow blood in the left atrium to thicken and form clots before being forced out into the bloodstream (Figure 4.14).

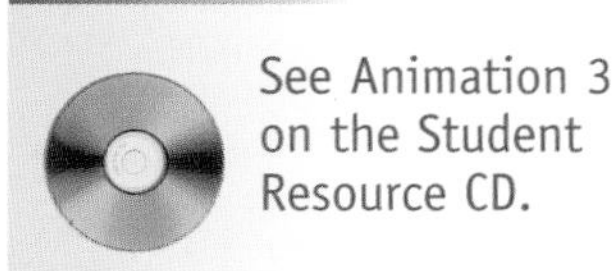

See Animation 3 on the Student Resource CD.

Ischemic strokes are distinct from but closely related to another phenomenon: *transient ischemic attacks*, or TIAs. In a TIA a very tiny blood clot creates a temporary blockage in the brain, but it disperses before any lasting damage can occur. Symptoms of TIA are very similar to those of stroke, except that they last only a few minutes or hours. They are, however, like the muffled rumblings of an incipient eruption; about one-third of all people who have a stroke had a TIA beforehand.

A CVA with no known cause is called a ***cryptogenic*** stroke. The causative factor in this case is often a ***patent foramen ovale***, an abnormal opening in the septum of the heart that allows blood from the pulmonary circuit to cross over into the systemic circuit. This is especially likely when a stroke occurs in a person younger than 55 years of age.

Another type of stroke has to do with bleeding inside the cranium (Figure 4.15). These are called hemorrhagic strokes, and they also occur in two forms, comprising about 20% of strokes:

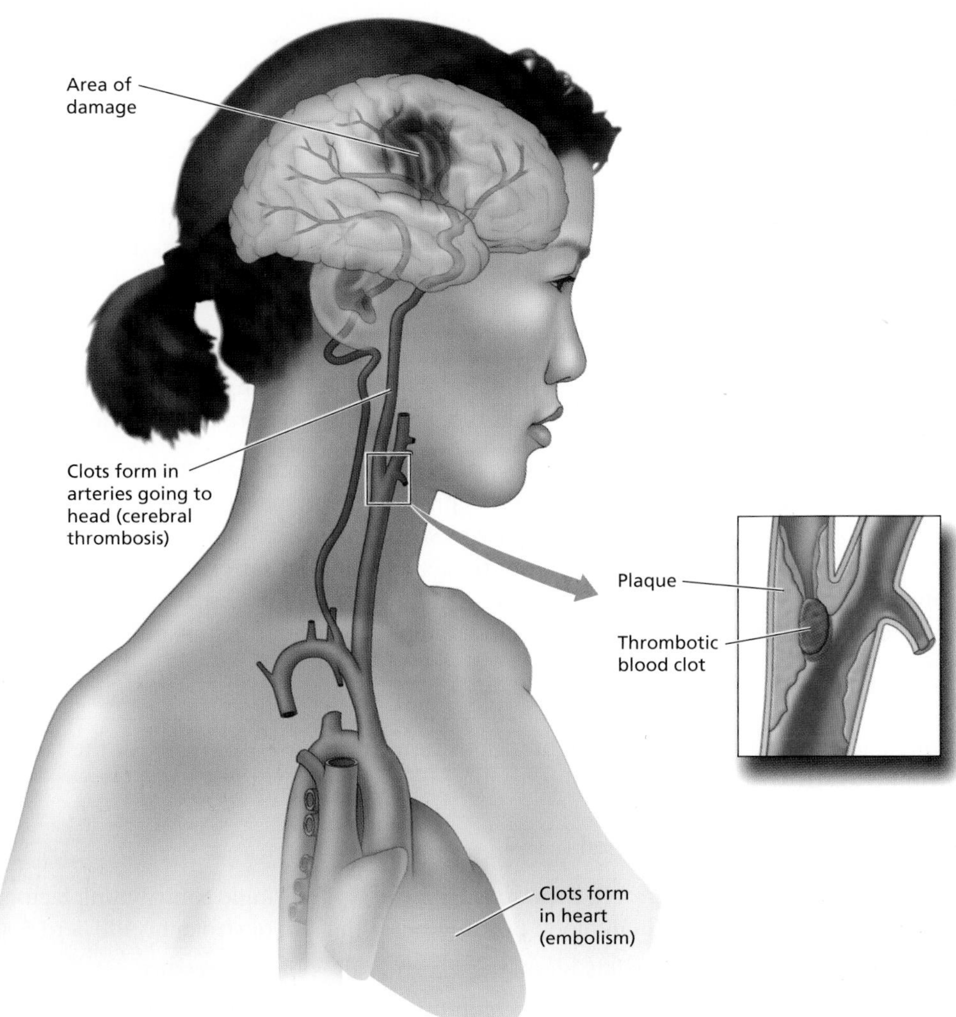

Figure 4.14. Ischemic stroke.

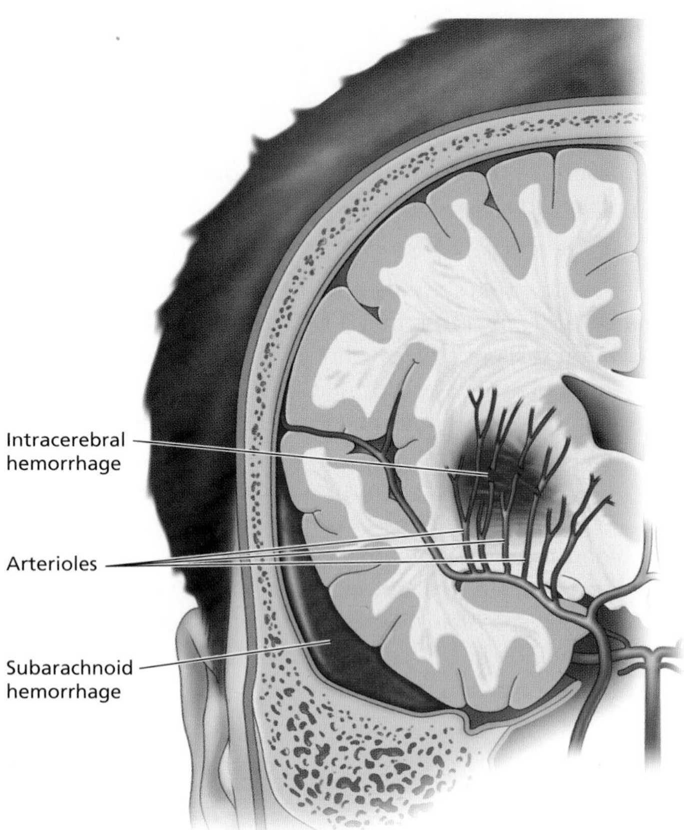

Figure 4.15. Hemorrhagic stroke.

- *Intracerebral hemorrhage.* This is the rupture of a blood vessel that can cause tissue death in the brain. Intracerebral hemorrhages are often associated with aneurysms, which may be a result of chronic hypertension, bleeding disorders, head trauma, or malformation of blood vessels.
- *Subarachnoid hemorrhage.* This is the rupture of a blood vessel on the surface of the brain rather than within the brain tissue itself. The leaking blood fills the space between the brain tissue and the arachnoid, eventually compressing the nerve cells.

The amount of damage a stroke causes is determined primarily by the location and number of neurons that are damaged by oxygen deprivation. Secondary responses to tissue damage have also been seen to contribute heavily to stroke damage. Inflammatory reactions, free radical activity, and other factors can cause tissue damage that far exceeds the oxygen deprivation brought about by the stroke itself. The good news in this discovery is that these secondary responses can be interrupted and moderated if treatment begins quickly enough.

Risk Factors

Although a person can have a genetic predisposition toward a CVA, many of the factors that contribute to stroke are well within the reach of personal control.

Risk Factors That Can Be Controlled

- *High blood pressure.* Untreated hypertension is the biggest single contributing factor to the risk of stroke. Chronic high blood pressure raises the risk of stroke by 400% to 600%.
- *Smoking.* Nicotine constricts blood vessels and raises blood pressure.
- *Atherosclerosis, high cholesterol.* These conditions also contribute to high blood pressure and raise the risk of emboli.

- *C-reactive protein.* This substance is present with long-term low-grade inflammation. A high C-reactive protein level is a dependable predictor for both ischemic stroke and atherosclerosis.
- *Atrial fibrillation.* Left untreated, this condition can help to form the emboli responsible for some ischemic embolic strokes.
- *High alcohol consumption.* This is generally considered to be more than 2 drinks per day.
- *Drug use.* Cocaine, crack, and marijuana have all been seen to increase stroke risk.
- *Obesity and sedentary lifestyle.*
- *Diabetes.* Untreated, this condition can contribute to high blood pressure and atherosclerosis. Poorly treated diabetes triples the risk of stroke.
- *High-estrogen birth control pills.* These pose a risk especially when taken by a person who smokes.
- *Hormone replacement therapy.* Some women who supplement estrogen and progesterone as a way to manage symptoms of menopause have a significantly increased risk of stroke.
- *Depression.* Depression has been seen to be a predictive factor for stroke: one-third of stroke patients are diagnosed for depression before their CVA.
- *Overall stress.*

Risk Factors That Cannot Be Controlled

- *Age.* Three-quarters of stroke patients are over 65 years of age. The risk of stroke doubles each decade after 55.
- *Gender.* About 25% more men than women have strokes, but strokes kill more women than men.
- *Race.* African Americans have a higher incidence of hypertension than whites. They are about twice as likely to have a stroke as whites, and they are almost twice as likely to die of it.
- *Family history.* Having a family history of stroke and cardiovascular disease can be a predisposing factor. Structurally weak blood vessels can be an inherited problem. However, in cases of ischemic strokes, this question should be asked: what is inherited, the status of the blood vessels or the diet and exercise habits?
- *Previous stroke.* Having one stroke usually predisposes a person to having another. Predisposition is not predestination, however; by taking control over whatever factors are within reach, a person can take big steps toward reducing the chances that he or she will have another stroke.

Signs and Symptoms

It is important to be able to recognize the signs of stroke; the sooner treatment is administered, the less damage will occur. Surprisingly, many Americans don't recognize the major symptoms of stroke, which are as follows:

- Sudden onset of unilateral weakness, numbness, or paralysis on the face, arm, leg, or any combination of the three.
- Suddenly blurred or decreased vision in one or both eyes; asymmetrical dilation of pupils.
- Difficulty in speaking or understanding simple sentences; confusion.
- Sudden onset of dizziness, clumsiness, vertigo.
- Sudden extreme headache.
- Possible loss of consciousness.

The symptoms of a TIA are very similar to those of a stroke. While TIA symptoms may subside after a few minutes or hours, it is *not* appropriate to take a wait-and-see approach to any stroke symptoms. The effectiveness of stroke treatments depends on how soon treatment begins, so any symptoms should be immediately investigated.

After a debilitating stroke the extent of the damage depends on what part and how much of the brain has been affected. Occasionally progressive degeneration may continue over 1 or 2 days, but usually a stroke is complete within a few hours.

SIDEBAR 4.9: DEPRESSION → STROKE → DEPRESSION . . .

The relation between stroke and depression is fascinating and complicated. It is well established that depression is an independent risk factor for stroke, but the mechanism is not well understood. One theory suggests that a low serotonin level changes the function of platelets (making them more sticky) and increases inflammation. This is also a big issue for heart attack and atherosclerosis. Interestingly, while cognitive-behavioral (talk) therapy is effective to relieve the symptoms of depression, it does *not* reduce the risk of other vascular problems—but antidepressants that improve the uptake of serotonin *have* been seen to reduce the risk of future vascular problems, especially heart attack.

Massage therapists should be interested in this phenomenon, since one of the most consistently measured effects of massage is a rise in serotonin.[43] Wouldn't it be interesting if massage and bodywork had an influence on the risk of depression-related stroke?

Many stroke survivors (up to 185,000 per year) develop depression *after* their incident; this is called poststroke depression. This number is not separated from the people who had depression *before* their stroke, however. Depression tends to make all stroke treatments less effective and significantly affects the prognosis for recovery. Issues that influence whether a person develops poststroke depression include the location of damaged neural tissue (areas where the serotonin or norepinephrine pathways are most active are sensitive to this); the severity of the stroke; gender (women are more susceptible than men); age; lack of a supporting community; and a history of depression before the stroke occurred.[44]

Complications

Motor damage from strokes can result in partial or full paralysis of one side of the body; this is called ***hemiparesis*** for weakness or ***hemiplegia*** for complete loss of function. ***Aphasia*** (loss of language), ***dysarthria*** (slurred speech), memory loss, and mild or severe personality changes may also occur. Sensory damage may result in permanent numbness and/or vision loss. Depression is another complication that is frequently seen after stroke; this condition has a complex intersection with stroke that is discussed in Sidebar 4.9.

Diagnosis

When a person may have had a stroke, the first priority is to determine whether it was an ischemic or hemorrhagic event, since these two phenomena require very different treatment. A diagnosis may be reached through a combination of a physical examination, CT, MRI, ultrasound, arteriography, and blood tests.

Treatment

Treatment for stroke is typically broken into three categories: prevention, acute care, and postacute, or chronic care.

Prevention includes identifying people at high risk for stroke and making preventive measures available. This may include exercise and diet changes, antiplatelet or anticoagulant drugs, or surgery on the carotid artery (Sidebar 4.10).

The treatment of choice for acute ischemic stroke is anticoagulant medication to minimize the risk of more clotting. One anticoagulant, called recombinant ***tissue plasminogen activator*** (r4-PA) has been found to be extremely effective for melting the blood clots associated with both stroke and heart attack if it is administered within the first 3 hours of onset. This can preserve a huge number of cells that would otherwise be lost to ischemia or edema, but only a minority of stroke patients makes it to a hospital within this narrow window of opportunity.

Another clot-melting drug has been derived from the natural anticoagulant found in a surprising source. This substance, called DSPA, for *Desmodus rotundus* (the Latin name for vampire bat) salivary plasminogen activator, is effective for up to 9 hours after a stroke. It is in final testing stages now.

These interventions, while extremely effective, are appropriate only for an ischemic stroke. If the CVA was from a hemorrhage, anticoagulant treatment could be dangerous or even deadly. A brain aneurysm caught before it ruptures may be treated with surgery to take the pressure off or strengthen the affected artery.

Once the dust has settled and it is clear how much function was lost during a stroke, postacute care begins. Therapy may begin to help a patient relearn how to do basic tasks such as walking, speaking, eating, and self-care. Because the brain has a vast resource of backup wiring, this is often a very successful part of recovery. It should be started as soon as possible after the CVA, though, to prevent the fibrosis and atrophy of muscle tissue that happen so quickly when nerve signals have been interrupted.

A new option in physical therapy is called *constraint-induced movement therapy*. This technique involves tying down the more functional arm for many hours each day to encourage the use of the affected arm. Patients who complete this course of therapy have better function of their affected side than patients who go through traditional physical therapy rehabilitation.[29] Occupational and speech therapists may be enlisted in this process as well; massage, with respect for the risk of cardiovascular disease, may have a role here too.

SIDEBAR 4.10: CAROTID ARTERY DISEASE: NOWHERE TO GO BUT UP

The discussion of atherosclerosis points out that because of chronically high blood pressure, both the aorta and coronary arteries are particularly prone to the development of atherosclerotic plaque. The carotid arteries, which emerge from the aortic arch, are similarly vulnerable. Although they are farther from the heart, blood pressure in the arteries that supply the head is ordinarily very high to ensure adequate blood flow to the brain. This puts the carotid arteries at risk for the same endothelial damage and plaque development seen with the aorta and the coronary arteries; this is called carotid artery disease.

The problem with carotid artery disease is that if any fragment of plaque or blood clot should break free, it has only one direction to go: straight up into the brain. When this happens in very tiny increments, it is called transient ischemic attack, or TIA. But the presence of carotid artery disease significantly raises the risk of a major stroke—so much so that identifying this disorder often leads to aggressive treatment, in the shape of carotid endarterectomy: the artery is surgically opened, cleaned out, and closed up again.

Massage therapists working with clients who know they have carotid artery disease must stay away from the neck, especially the anterior triangle, which is bordered by the sternocleidomastoid muscle, which runs superficially over the carotid arteries.

Massage?

Massage can play a role in the recovery of a stroke survivor, but some cautions must be considered. First and foremost is the client's general cardiovascular health. Most stroke patients have other circulatory problems, some of which can affect easily accessible blood vessels in the neck. Therefore, it's very important to work as part of a client's health care team. Second, hemiplegia is a type of spastic paralysis, which carries specific cautions and guidelines for massage.

Persons who are in physical and occupational therapy for stroke recovery may derive significant benefit from massage as well; remember that proprioceptors in affected limbs may misinterpret the amount of limitation that occurs, leading to an unnecessary degeneration of muscular function. Stretching, exercising, and improving circulation in areas that have good sensation can slow that process.

MODALITY RECOMMENDATIONS FOR STROKE

Modality	Recommendation
Deep Tissue Massage	Indicated within limits of client activity and sensitivity. Work to improve proprioception; encourage client movement with releases.
Lymphatic Drainage	Indicated after initial inflammation has subsided.
Polarity	S: Indicated. R/D: Supportive within client comfort.
PNF/MET/Stretching	Indicated after initial inflammation subsides, with caution for sensory deficit.
Reflexology	Indicated; work brain, spine, neck, adrenals, heart points.
Shiatsu	Indicated. Treat PC, H, SI meridians and extensions.
Swedish Massage	Supportive with caution for cardiovascular problems and areas of reduced sensation.
Trigger Point Therapy	Supportive with caution for sensory deficit.

See Chapter 1 for a brief description of each modality, including definitions of abbreviations.

Traumatic Brain Injury in Brief

What is it?
Traumatic brain injury (TBI) is damage to the brain brought about by trauma rather than congenital or chronic degenerative disease.

How is it recognized?
Symptoms of TBI vary according to the location and severity of the injury. Long-term effects range from mild cognitive impairment, learning problems, and motor control difficulties, to varying types of coma or persistent vegetative state.

Is massage indicated or contraindicated?
Many TBI patients undergo intensive physical, occupational, and speech therapy to preserve or recover motor function. Carefully administered massage is also appropriate, as long as it is incorporated into the patient's health care plan and doesn't pose any risk in the presence of spasticity, numbness, or psychiatric disturbance.

Traumatic Brain Injury

Definition: What Is It?

Traumatic brain injury (TBI) is an insult to the brain not brought about by congenital or degenerative conditions, that leads to altered states of consciousness, cognitive impairment, and disruption of physical, emotional, and behavioral function.

TBI is usually due to external force: a direct blow or a rapid acceleration/deceleration incident. Motor vehicle accidents, gunshot wounds, falls, sports injuries, and physical violence are leading causes.

Demographics: Who Gets It?

About 1.5 million TBIs are reported every year, with 1 million emergency department visits. Roughly 270,000 TBIs are classified as moderate to severe; the rest are considered to be mild (although even mild carry some significant risks). Approximately 80,000 people are disabled, 60,000 develop new seizure disorders, and 70,000 people die of head injuries every year.[45]

Between 2.5 and 6.5 million TBI survivors are living in the United States today. The direct and indirect costs of treating this injury are about $56 billion per year.[45]

Most TBI patients are 15 to 25 years of age or older than 75. The older patients are injured most often in falls; younger patients are injured in motor vehicle accidents, sports, and personal violence, including gunshot wounds, shaken baby syndrome, and other incidents. About half of TBI injuries are related to alcohol or drug use.[46]

Etiology: What Happens?

Several classifications for head injuries have been created to try to organize the vast number of ways the brain, although encased in a protective casing, can be injured.

- *Skull fracture* occurs when the bones around the skull are broken, usually by a direct blow. This can lead to a number of internal injuries, but interestingly, the prognosis for an open head injury is often better than for a closed head injury, because the risk of damage from too much pressure is somewhat less.
- *Penetrating injury* is usually due to a gunshot wound, but may also be from a knife or other object. Penetrating injuries are the leading cause of death among TBI patients.
- *Concussion* is any temporary loss of brain function. It can include loss of consciousness, often brought about by jarring of the cranium. Concussion is the most common type of TBI. When concussion occurs in an athlete (as it does about 300,000 times per year),[47] it is essential that the tissues heal completely before the athlete returns to play. If he has another head injury too soon, he can develop *second impact syndrome*, a much more serious condition than a simple concussion.
- *Contusion* is bruising inside the cranium. When a contusion happens at the point of impact and also where the brain hits the opposite wall, it is a ***coup-contrecoup***.
- *Diffuse axonal injury* is internal tearing of nerve tissue throughout the brain. It is often related to acceleration/deceleration accidents, as seen with whiplash or shaken baby syndrome.
- *Anoxic brain injury* is complete lack of oxygen in the brain. It can be brought about by airway obstruction or sudden apnea.

- *Hypoxic brain injury* is an inadequate supply of oxygen, often associated with ischemic stroke, edema, or toxic exposure, especially carbon monoxide poisoning.
- *Hemorrhage* is bleeding inside the brain, often associated with ruptured aneurysms.
- *Hematoma* is development of a large amount of coagulated blood, either pressing outside or within the brain.
- *Edema* is a secondary inflammatory response that can follow any or all of the causes of TBI. The swelling of brain tissue and action of free radicals against healthy tissue may ultimately be responsible for more damage than the original source of the trauma.

Signs and Symptoms

Signs and symptoms of a TBI vary according to what areas of the brain are affected and how severe the injury is. Trauma to the frontal lobes is most common and may result in language and motor dysfunction; trauma to structures close to the brainstem is more likely to lead to massive loss of autonomic function.

Symptoms of an acute TBI include leakage of cerebrospinal fluid from the ears or nose; dilated or asymmetrical pupils; visual disturbances; dizziness and confusion; apnea or slowed breathing; nausea and vomiting; slow pulse and low blood pressure; loss of bowel and bladder control; possible seizures, paralysis, numbness, lethargy, or loss of consciousness. In infants chronic crying, lethargy, or unusual sleep patterns are cause for concern. Symptoms may occur immediately or grow in severity over a course of days or even weeks.

Long-term consequences of TBI include mild to severe cognitive dysfunction, especially with memory and learning skills. Movement disorders may range from hypertonicity to spasticity. Seizures are a frequent complication. Permanent changes in behavioral and emotional function are also common; many TBI survivors are emotionally volatile and may develop new patterns of aggressiveness and hostility. More severe cases of TBI (usually ones that affect the brainstem) may lead to various levels of coma or a persistent vegetative state.

Treatment

TBI is treated with surgery to remove pressure on the brain if necessary, followed by intensive physical, recreational, occupational, and speech therapy to preserve or recover function. The prognosis with children is generally best, since their brains seem to be most capable of establishing new pathways to relearn skills. Nonetheless, brain plasticity, or the ability to tap into unused areas for motor and mental function, is a new field and further research continues to brighten the outlook even for mature TBI survivors.

Prevention

Preventive measures to guard against the risk of TBI are self-evident but worth repeating. Most TBIs happen as a transport injury, that is, in an event involving cars, motorcycles, bicycles, scooters, skates, or skateboards. Driving only while alert and sober, using a seat belt, and wearing a helmet can reduce the risk and severity of these accidents. Other preventive measures include making sure the home is safe for young children and elderly people to reduce the risk of falls, and ensuring the appropriate storage of firearms.

Massage?

Decisions about bodywork in the presence of a TBI must be based on the client's ability to adapt to the changes massage brings about. If sensation is present and the client is able to communicate clearly about comfort, massage is not only appropriate but could be an important part of the rehabilitation picture to assist in the maintenance of healthy muscles and connective tissues.

If a client is comatose, massage or other stroking techniques may be performed to help preserve the health of the tissues and prevent complications such as decubitus ulcers, but these must be performed with caution, since the client cannot give feedback to manage the risk of overtreatment.

In either case, TBI is a complicated, serious problem with many long-term problems that affect many aspects of health. Any TBI survivor who receives massage as part of a rehabilitative process should do so as part of integrated health care management, incorporating massage with other therapies for the best result.

Modality Recommendations for Traumatic Brain Injury	
Deep Tissue Massage	Indicated within limits of client activity and sensitivity. Work to improve proprioception; encourage client movement with releases.
Lymphatic Drainage	Indicated, especially in early stages of recovery.
Polarity	S: Indicated. R/D: Supportive with light pressure within client comfort; use caution.
PNF/MET/Stretching	Supportive with caution for sensory deficit.
Reflexology	Indicated; work brain and solar plexus points.
Shiatsu	Indicated. Pressure must be gentle, extremely sensitive to avoid overtreating. Hold points at occiput, temples, supraorbital ridge.
Swedish Massage	Supportive, with caution for clear communication between client and therapist.
Trigger Point Therapy	Supportive with caution for sensory deficit.

See Chapter 1 for a brief description of each modality, including definitions of abbreviations.

Trigeminal Neuralgia

Definition: What Is It?

Trigeminal neuralgia (TN) is *neuro-algia* ("nerve pain") along one or more of the three branches of Cranial Nerve V, the trigeminal nerve (Figure 4.16) It is also called ***tic douloureux***, which is French for *painful spasm* or *unhappy twitch*.

Demographics: Who Gets It?

TN is a relatively rare disorder; it affects about 40,000 people in the United States. Women have it more often than men, with a ratio of about 3 to 2. The average patient is 60 to 70 years old, although it has been documented among all ages. When it occurs in younger people, it is most likely to be a complication of an underlying problem such as MS or a tumor.

Etiology: What Happens?

TN is usually classified as primary or secondary. In either case, the trigeminal nerve is irritated, and the result is brief, repeating episodes of sharp, electrical, burning, or stabbing pain on one side of the face.

Trigeminal Neuralgia in Brief

Pronunciation: try-JEM-ih-nul nur-AL-je-ah

What is it?

Trigeminal neuralgia (TN) is a condition involving sharp electrical or stabbing pain along one or more branches of the trigeminal nerve (CN V), usually in the lower face and jaw.

How is it recognized?

The pain of TN is very sharp and severe. Patients report stabbing, electrical, or burning sensations that occur in brief episodes but that repeat with or without identifiable triggers. A muscle tic is often present as well.

Is massage indicated or contraindicated?

Trigeminal neuralgia is intensely painful, and even very light touch may trigger an attack. It therefore contraindicates massage on the face unless the client specifically guides the therapist into what feels safe and comfortable. Massage elsewhere on the body is appropriate, although clients with TN may prefer not to be face down.

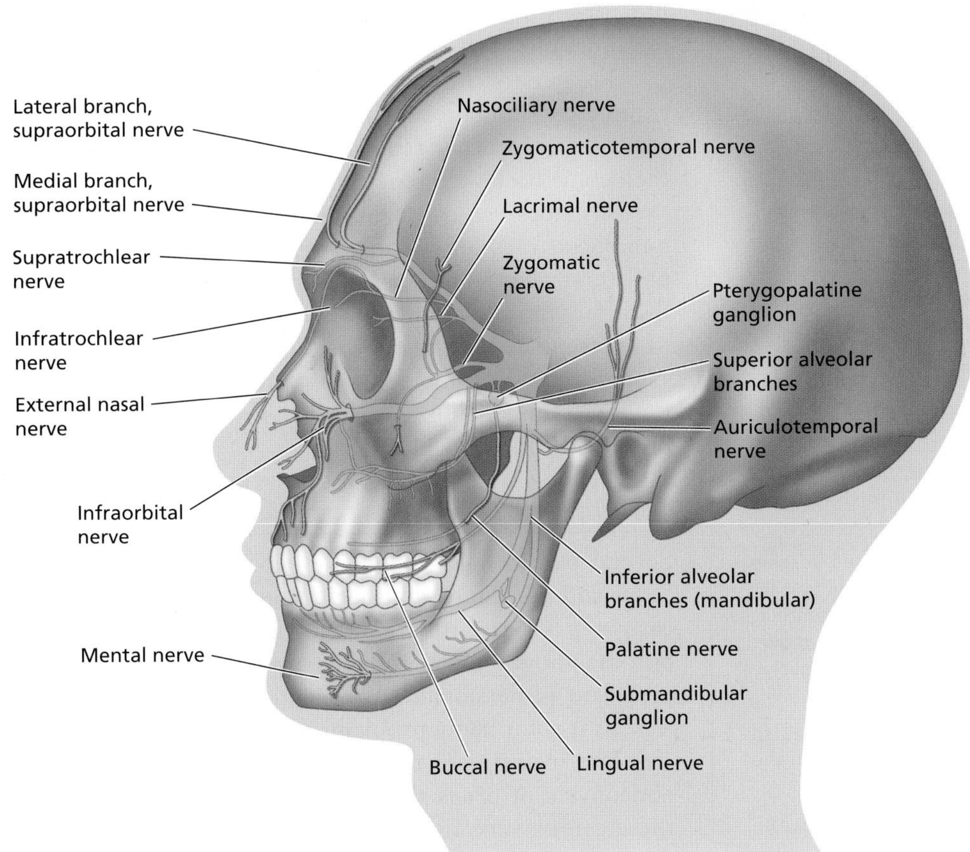

Figure 4.16. The trigeminal nerve.

The cause of primary TN is somewhat controversial. Most experts agree that the typical presentation is probably related to an artery or vein that wraps around or irritates the trigeminal nerve where it emerges from the pons at the base of the brain. This blood vessel may essentially wear away the myelin covering on some of the fibers, which allows the nerve to misfire. Autopsies of people with TN are not always consistent about this, however, and many people have this structural anomaly with no painful symptoms.[48] Ultimately the source of the pain may be a combination of peripheral and central nervous system factors.

Secondary TN is due to some other structural problem. Causative factors include tumors, bone spurs, recent infection, complications of dental surgery, and MS.

Some specialists divide TN into type 1 and type 2. Type 1 TN is the more common presentation. Most of the episodes take the form of sharp blasts of pain on one side of the face in response to some mild trigger. Type 2 TN is less typical. In this form the pain is long lasting and described as a constant ache or burning sensation that may be interrupted by bolts of electrical stabbing or burning pain.

Episodes of trigeminal nerve pain can be triggered by speaking, chewing, swallowing, sitting in a draft, a light touch to the wrong spot, and sometimes by no stimulus at all. Episodes may happen several times a day for days, weeks, or months and then suddenly disappear—only to begin again months or years later. TN can be a debilitating lifelong condition if it is not treated.

Signs and Symptoms

Some people call the pain of TN among the worst in the world. It's often described as a sharp, electrical, stabbing, or burning sensation. These episodes may last for 10 seconds to 2 min-

SIDEBAR 4.11: OTHER CRANIAL NERVE DISORDERS

Any damage or irritation to a cranial nerve may lead to symptoms in the face. TN and Bell palsy are two of the most common disorders that may cause facial symptoms. But a few other cranial nerve disorders deserve a passing glance as well:

- **Postherpetic neuralgia** is a complication of herpes zoster. It may occur wherever the shingles blisters appeared but can outlast the visible lesions by several weeks or months. When the herpes infection affects the optic nerve, postherpetic neuralgia can create extremely painful facial symptoms.
- **Glossopharyngeal neuralgia** is etiologically identical to vascular compression on the trigeminal nerve, but this condition affects CN IX, which supplies sensation to the back of the throat.
- **Atypical face pain** is a condition similar to TN and in some cases may be a predecessor to it. It is characterized by pain that is less severe than TN, but it tends to involve continuous rather than intermittent pain. The pain may go up over the back of the head and into the scalp, and it may involve the occipital as well as the trigeminal nerve.
- **Hemifacial spasm** creates a painless tic that is related to blood vessel compression of the facial nerve rather than the trigeminal nerve.

utes, or several jabs may occur in rapid succession. A muscle tic sometimes develops along with the nerve pain.

Triggers of TN attacks may vary, or episodes may be completely spontaneous. The incidence of attacks may also vary; they can occur regularly, then disappear for a while, then come back with renewed vigor.

TN does *not* give pain during sleep, nor does it cause numbness, muscle weakness, or hearing loss. It is usually unilateral. (For some reason the right side is affected about five times more often than the left.) All of these factors help to differentiate TN from other conditions that might cause similar symptoms, including migraine or cluster headaches, Ramsay-Hunt syndrome, stroke, or other cranial nerve problems (Sidebar 4.11).

Treatment

Several treatment strategies for TN have been developed. Sinus and tooth infections can sometimes mimic TN, so an early step is to rule those out. Cervical misalignment or temporomandibular joint problems can be sorted out by the appropriate professionals. Acupuncture can be effective for TN, as it is for many problems with nerve conduction.

The mainstream medical approach to TN starts with anticonvulsant drugs that inhibit nerve conduction. While these can be very effective in the short run, many patients don't tolerate them well, or they build up resistance and the drugs provide less and less relief. Muscle relaxants may be prescribed in addition to an anticonvulsant; the two drugs together seem to increase their effectiveness.

Several more invasive interventions have been developed to treat TN. These usually involve the controlled destruction of part of the nerve with lasers, radiation, a heated probe, or injected chemicals. These options often provide some relief, with the understanding that the patient may have permanent numbness and some facial muscle weakness as a result. Microvascular surgery to relieve pressure on the trigeminal nerve is the most invasive procedure. It entails unwrapping the strangulating blood vessel from around the trigeminal nerve. This process leaves sensation intact and is successful for many patients, but because it is surgery so close to the brain, it carries more risks of complication than other approaches.

Massage?

Clients who are having TN attacks may feel unsafe with any pressure or work on their face; massage therapists should respect this caution. Face cradles may also be uncomfortable; it may not be possible to work with TN clients in a prone position. Massage anywhere else on the body is certainly indicated.

Modality Recommendations for Trigeminal Neuralgia	
Deep Tissue Massage	Locally contraindicated; otherwise supportive to encourage parasympathetic response.
Lymphatic Drainage	Contraindicated while acute; otherwise indicated.
Polarity	S: Indicated. R/D: Locally contraindicated when acute; otherwise supportive.
PNF/MET/Stretching	Locally contraindicated; otherwise supportive.
Reflexology	Indicated; work brain, cervical spine, neck, face points.
Shiatsu	Indicated. Treat local area according to pain tolerance, along with meridians, extensions of head and neck.
Swedish Massage	Supportive, with caution for positioning client and comfort of face.
Trigger Point Therapy	Locally contraindicated; otherwise supportive.

See Chapter 1 for a brief description of each modality, including definitions of abbreviations.

Other Nervous System Disorders

Guillain-Barré Syndrome

Definition: What Is It?

Guillain-Barré syndrome (GBS) is a condition involving acute inflammation and destruction of the myelin layer of peripheral nerves. It usually starts in the extremities and moves toward the trunk, but some variants of this syndrome affect only cranial nerves or have other patterns.

Demographics: Who Gets It?

GBS can affect anyone at any time, but most affected people are 15 to 35 or 50 to 75 years old. Men with GBS slightly outnumber women. Although it is not a particularly common problem, affecting about 1 in every 100,000 people (about 3,000 people in the United States each year), it is the most frequently seen form of acute neuromuscular paralysis since the eradication of polio in the Western Hemisphere.

Etiology: What Happens?

GBS was first described in 1916, but our understanding of how this disease comes about has not progressed a great deal since then. Many patients have an infection of the respiratory or gastrointestinal tract several days before developing GBS symptoms. It is believed that this preceding infection stimulates an immune system attack mistakenly directed against the myelin sheaths of peripheral nerves. Research indicates that a common cause of food poisoning, the bacterium *Campylobacter jejuni*, may trigger many cases of GBS in the United States. Other pathogens that have been linked to GBS include *Haemophilus influenzae*, *Mycoplasma pneumoniae*, *Borrelia burgdorferi*, *cytomegalovirus*, *Epstein-Barr virus*, and HIV.

Guillain-Barré Syndrome in Brief

Pronunciation: ge-YAHN bar-RAY SIN-drome

What is it?

Guillain-Barré syndrome (GBS) is a demyelinating disorder of peripheral nerves. It usually begins in the feet and moves proximally. It appears to be an autoimmune condition, but consistent triggers have not been identified.

How is it recognized?

GBS is marked by its sudden onset (symptoms usually begin quickly and peak within 2–4 weeks) followed by gradual remission (most patients have nearly full recovery within 18 months). Furthermore, GBS affects limbs symmetrically and moves proximally toward the trunk, which distinguishes it from other peripheral nerve problems.

Is massage indicated or contraindicated?

When a person has begun to recover from a GBS attack, physical and occupational therapy are often employed to speed recovery and prevent muscle atrophy. Massage at this stage may be useful to limit pain, improve circulation, and reduce fatigue and anxiety.

Some GBS patients don't experience a preceding infection. This disorder has also been seen in conjunction with immune system changes brought about by pregnancy, surgery, and administration of certain vaccines, specifically the swine flu vaccine that was distributed in 1976.

Regardless of what initiates the disease process, the end result is that the myelin sheaths on peripheral nerves are attacked and destroyed by macrophages and lymphocytes. The damage progresses proximally and may also affect cranial nerves. This can be life threatening if the nerves that control breathing are damaged; many GBS patients spend time on a ventilator before they recover.

GBS is now recognized as several different subtypes of demyelinating diseases. The most common form in the United States is *acute inflammatory demyelinating polyneuropathy*; this accounts for 90% of GBS diagnoses. Other types include these:

- *Acute motor axonal neuropathy* affects motor neurons only. It is most common in children and has a good prognosis.
- *Acute motor-sensory axonal neuropathy* affects motor and sensory function. It is most common in adults and has a poorer recovery rate than other forms of GBS.
- *Miller-Fisher syndrome* is a rare variant of GBS that involves only the cranial nerves. It leads to poor control of the eyes and other facial muscles.

Signs and Symptoms

GBS is notorious for being unpredictable, but it has a few features that distinguish it from other peripheral nerve disorders. Onset is typically fast and severe; a patient may go from being fully functional to being hospitalized within a matter of hours or a couple of days. GBS is usually symmetrical, affecting both legs equally. Also, myelin damage progresses proximally, moving up toward the trunk rather than distally; this pattern is unique among peripheral nerve problems.

When GBS first appears, it often involves weakness or tingling in the affected limbs. Reflexes become dull or disappear altogether. Loss of sensation progresses proximally, although pain frequently develops in the hips and pelvis. If the GBS affects cranial nerves of the face, facial weakness, pain, and difficulty with speech and swallowing may develop. As the disease progresses, the nerves that supply respiratory muscles are affected, and problems with breathing develop.

GBS symptoms usually peak 2 or 3 weeks after onset, and they may linger for several weeks before they begin to subside. The amount of damage that accrues while the nerves are inflamed depends on what treatments were introduced when and on how soon the patient can begin to use the affected muscles after the paralysis resolves.

Diagnosis

The signs and symptoms of GBS are so distinctive that it is usually not difficult to diagnose. A lumbar puncture may be performed to look for elevated proteins in cerebrospinal fluid, and a nerve conduction test may be recommended to confirm that nerve transmission to the extremities is impaired.

Treatment

Because GBS is an idiopathic disease, no specific cure has been developed. Two treatment options have been successfully used to shorten recovery time: plasmapheresis (blood cleansing) and injections of high concentrations of immunoglobulin (donated antibodies).

Plasmapheresis is a process by which blood cells are removed from the patient's blood by centrifugation, placed in fresh donated plasma or a plasma substitute, and then replaced in the body. This removes autoimmune antibodies and reduces attacks against myelin. This procedure is most effective within 2 weeks of onset.

Immunoglobulin administered intravenously is believed to inhibit the patient's antibody and cytokine activity, thus limiting the autoimmune attack against myelin sheaths on peripheral nerves.

Clinical trials of both treatment options show them to be about equally effective. They can shorten the recovery process by up to 50%.

Other interventions for GBS patients are dictated by their individual needs. About one-third of patients require the use of a ventilator until the respiratory nerves regain full function. Anticoagulants may be used against the danger of blood clots in immobilized legs. Pain management is problematic because powerful pain medications can depress the nervous system; massage and other nondrug options are often recommended for this purpose. Once the acute inflammation has passed, occupational and physical therapy is used to help the patient regain as much muscle function as possible.

Prognosis

The good news is most people who develop GBS have a full or nearly full recovery, although the process may take 18 months or longer. Many people live with permanent loss of some neurological function (foot drop or numbness in an area, for instance), but these are not considered disabling problems. A small number of patients (5%–15%) have permanent serious disability as a result of the disease. About 10% of GBS patients have a relapse later in life. About 5% to 7% of GBS patients die, usually of respiratory failure, pulmonary embolism, or cardiac arrest.

Massage?

A person in the acute stage of GBS is unlikely to seek massage, and it would be wisest to avoid trying to stimulate the body mechanically while this immune system confusion is still raging.

Once the client is stable, physical and occupational therapy play a key role in the rehabilitation of a person recovering from GBS. As long as sensation is present and accurate (i.e., the client can give feedback about pressure and comfort), massage can be a very useful adjunct in this long and frustrating process.

Modality Recommendations for Guillain-Barré Syndrome

Deep Tissue Massage	Indicated while subacute. Work in areas with full sensation to improve proprioception. Encourage active movement with release work during a long recovery.
Lymphatic Drainage	Supportive.
Polarity	S: Indicated. R/D: Locally contraindicated while acute; otherwise indicated.
PNF/MET/Stretching	Supportive.
Reflexology	Indicated; all glands, brain, head, spine, solar plexus points.
Shiatsu	Indicated. Treat immune system via TH/SP/K; nervous system via BL, SI.
Swedish Massage	Contraindicated while acute; otherwise indicated to help restore function. Caution for areas of reduced sensation.
Trigger Point Therapy	Locally contraindicated while acute; indicated when subacute with caution for areas of reduced sensation.

See Chapter 1 for a brief description of each modality, including definitions of abbreviations.

Headaches in Brief

What are they?
Headaches are pain caused by any number of sources. Muscular tension, vascular spasm and dilation, and chemical imbalances can all contribute to headache. Headaches only rarely indicate a serious underlying disorder.

How are they recognized?
Tension headaches are usually bilateral and steadily painful. Vascular headaches are often unilateral and have a distinctive throbbing pain from blood flow into the head. Headaches brought about by CNS injury or disease are extreme, severe, and prolonged. They can have a sudden or gradual onset.

Is massage indicated or contraindicated?
Headaches due to infection or CNS injury contraindicate massage. Persons with vascular headaches generally avoid stimuli like massage, but massage is definitely indicated for tension headaches.

Headaches

Definition: What Are They?

Headaches are one of the most common physical problems in the range of human experience. Up to 90% of adults in the United States have a headache each year. Although they can herald some serious underlying problems, most headaches are self-contained temporary problems, only peripherally related to other conditions in the body.

Types of headaches New advances in headache research have uncovered similarities between headache types that were never before suspected. As we learn more about the physiological processes of these disorders, our methods for classifying them may change, but for the present, many experts discuss headaches as primary or secondary. Primary headaches are unrelated to serious underlying pathology, while secondary headaches are symptoms of other problems. In addition, most headaches can be described as belonging one of four categories. These problems don't necessarily outline well, however, and many headaches share qualities from more than one of these classifications.

- *Tension-type headaches.* By far the most common type of headache people experience (90%–92%), these are triggered by muscular tension, bony misalignment, postural patterns, eyestrain, temporomandibular joint disorders, myofascial pain syndrome, ligament irritation, or other musculoskeletal imbalances. Tension-type headaches may also be described as episodic (happening fewer than 15 times per month) or chronic (happening more than 15 times per month).
- *Vascular headaches.* These include classic and common migraines, cluster headaches, and possibly sinus headaches. They account for a total of about 6% to 8% of headaches. Many vascular headaches are triggered by stress, food sensitivities, alcohol use, or chemical shifts seen with the menstrual cycle.
- *Chemical headaches.* The triggers for these headaches can be any kind of chemical disturbance.
- *Traction-inflammatory headaches.* These are the rarest type of headache and the most dangerous. They indicate severe underlying pathology, such as tumor, aneurysm, hemorrhage, or infection in the CNS.

Etiology: What Happens?

The common denominator that has been observed in tension and vascular headaches (by far the two most common types) is the activity of serotonin, a neurotransmitter that has been implicated in a number of other CNS disorders. Both migraine and tension headache episodes show significant changes in serotonin levels. This may lead to the dilation of arteries in the periphery of the brain. This excessive vasodilation stretches blood vessels, causing pain. In addition, local prostaglandin release may initiate an inflammatory response, adding to the fluid in a closed cavity.

The primary difference between migraine headaches and tension headaches, therefore, may simply be the triggers and the presence or absence of a throbbing sensation. Migraines are generally associated with throbbing pain and chemical triggers such as food sensitivities or hormonal shifts, while tension headaches are more often associated with compressive head-in-a-vise pain and mechanical triggers such as tight muscles or misaligned vertebrae. But both types of triggers evidently may lead to serotonin shifts and intracranial vasodilation.

Tension Headaches

Definition: What Are They?

Tension headaches are headaches triggered by mechanical stresses that initiate the CNS changes in serotonin levels and blood vessel dilation discussed previously.

Etiology: What Happens?

The average head weighs about 18 to 20 pounds. The area of bone-to-bone contact between the occipital condyles and the facets of C1 is about the same as two pairs of fingertips touching. The whole mechanism is kept in balance by tension exerted by muscles and ligaments around the neck and head. The muscles primarily responsible for the posture of the head form two inverted triangles just below the occiput (Figure 4.17). It is not surprising, then, that when this delicate balance is a little off, the resulting pain reverberates throughout the whole structure.

Similarly, when postural or movement patterns elsewhere in the body exert force on the spine, the end result can be tension at the occipital connection. In this way, a foot that strikes the ground too hard on the lateral side may pull on the knee, which may then demand compensation in the hip. The sacrum moves to adjust to the tip in the os coxae. This creates a slight twist in the lumbar vertebrae, which reverberates all the way up the spine to the head. The result: headaches because the feet are not in alignment.

Triggers These are almost too numerous to list here, precisely because staying pain free involves such a precarious balance of muscle tension, bony alignment, and a myriad of other factors. Here are some of the major causes of tension headaches:

- *Muscular, tendinous, or ligamentous injury to the head or neck structures.* The ligaments in the neck may be most easily injured; they are vulnerable to fraying and irritation with uncontrolled movement, and they refer pain over the back of the head.
- *Simple muscle tension in the suboccipital triangle or the jaw flexors.* These muscles are especially vulnerable to the effects of emotional stress. When people are worried or angry, they tend to clench their jaws and tighten their necks.
- *Subluxation or fixation of cervical vertebrae.* Disorders of these vertebrae can irritate ligaments and/or cause muscle spasms, both of which lead to headaches.

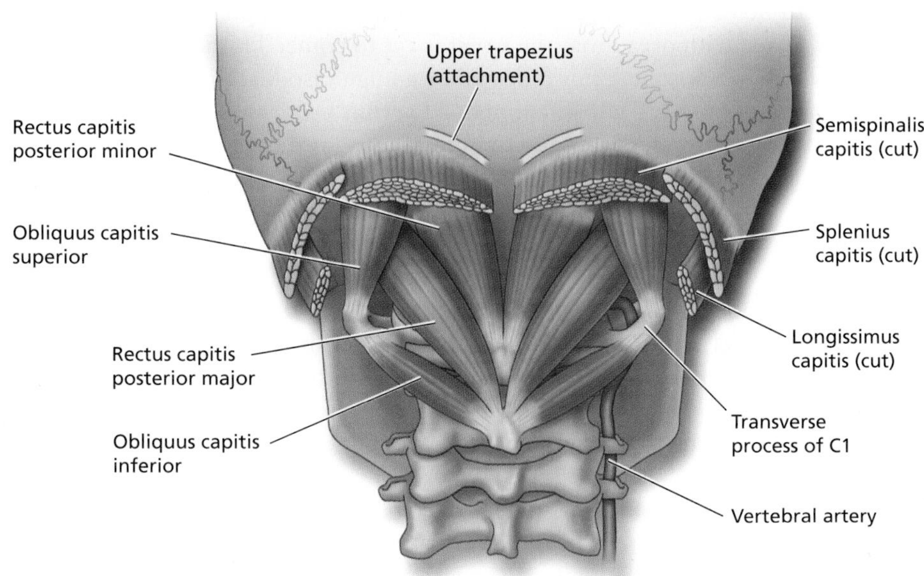

Figure 4.17. Muscular imbalance at the suboccipital triangle is a contributing factor in many headaches.

- *Structural problems.* Misalignment of the cranial bones (which are not completely immobile) or in the temporomandibular joint can cause headaches.
- *Trigger points in the muscles of the neck and head.* These can refer pain all around the head.
- *Eyestrain.* Chronic contraction of muscles in the eye to focus on reading material or other visual input may be relieved when corrective eyewear reduces eye muscle tension.
- *Any kind of ongoing mental or physical stress.* Stress can change postural and movement patterns, which will lead to muscle spasm, subluxation, fixation, and so on. Poor ergonomics, especially in repetitive work situations, are frequently the culprit behind chronic tension headaches.

Vascular Headaches

Definition: What Are They?

These headaches are often triggered by food sensitivities, hormonal shifts, alcohol use, stress, or other factors that are difficult to identify. The pain they cause comes from excessively dilated blood vessels in the meninges. They are characterized by pain that throbs with the patient's pulse.

Migraines

Demographics: Who Gets Them?

About 28 million people in the United States have diagnosed migraines. This malady is responsible for an overwhelming $50 billion in lost wages and medical expenses every year.

Women get migraines more than men do. It is estimated that up to 18% of women have a migraine at some time in their life; that number is closer to 6% for men. Many migraines are genetically linked; 70 to 80% of migraine patients have other family members with the same problem.

Etiology: What Happens?

Migraine headaches begin with extreme vasoconstriction in the affected hemisphere, which one would expect to be painful, but it's not. Instead, for some people, a sense of euphoria is felt, although it is mixed with dread that the worst is yet to come. This is the prodrome of the classic migraine. The vasoconstriction is followed by a huge vasodilation, a flood of blood into the affected part of the brain. It is all still contained within the vessels, of course, but the excessive pressure against the vessel walls and meninges causes excruciating pain.

Migraines are associated with increased risk of seizures and stroke.

Triggers No one has identified exactly what sets up the process for migraines to take place. Some triggers have been identified, such as the consumption of certain kinds of foods, including red wine, cheese, chocolate, coffee, tea, aspartame, monosodium glutamate, and any kind of alcohol. Abnormal levels of stress can bring them on, as can hormonal shifts such as menstruation, pregnancy, and menopause. (These hormonal shifts can also make preexisting migraines disappear.) The good news about migraines is that they usually subside by middle age. It is rare for mature people to have migraines.

Signs and Symptoms The word *migraine* comes from the French, *hemi-craine*, or *half-head*. This is because migraine headache has a characteristic unilateral presentation. In classic migraines the pain is preceded by the euphoric prodrome stage. Blurred vision, the perception of flashing lights or auras, and even auditory hallucinations may occur. Classic migraines constitute only about 15% to 20% of migraines. Then, as with the aura-free common migraines, (the other 80% to 85% of migraines) the patient has extreme throbbing pain on one side of the head, which may cause the ipsilateral eye and nostril to water. Hypersensitivity to light, nausea, and vomiting are all possible. Some patients have tingling or other sensation changes in their extremities. One rare version, called hemiplegia migraine, is accompanied by temporary paralysis on one side of the body; this version has a strong genetic link. Migraine can persist for several hours to several days and can leave the person exhausted.

Cluster Headaches

Definition: What Are They?

These are a fairly rare, not well understood variety of vascular headache. Cluster headaches affect men much more often than women, and they affect less than 1% of the United States population. Cluster headaches usually happen at night, with pain severe enough to wake a person out of a sound sleep. Like migraines, they cause the eye and nostril of the affected side to water. They may also cause facial swelling and unilateral sweating. Each headache lasts 30 minutes to 3 hours, and in an episode a person may have one to four headaches every day for 4 to 8 weeks.

Reliable triggers for cluster headaches, outside of alcohol, have not been identified. They may occur seasonally, once or twice in a year, or just once in a lifetime.

Sinus Headaches

Sinus headaches are worth a mention among the vascular headaches because they also have to do with too much fluid in the skull. The fluid is in the sinuses rather than the cranium itself. When a person has sinus allergies or sinusitis, the membranes can become irritated and inflamed. Sinusitis is discussed in more detail in Chapter 7.

Chemical Headaches

Definition: What Are They?

Chemical headaches are triggered by a variety of chemical imbalances in the body. They are often warning signs that the person has too much or too little of some substance vital to maintaining homeostasis. Causes of chemical headaches include the following:

- Very low blood sugar, indicating that the person needs to eat soon.
- Hormonal shifts like those seen with the menstrual cycle and childbirth.
- Extreme dehydration, either from physical exertion or from alcohol consumption. This is the typical "hangover" headache.
- Too much headache medication. These "rebound" headaches may last for 2 weeks or more, and the only way to treat them is to stop taking pain medication.

Traction-Inflammatory Headaches

Headaches are occasionally a sign of a serious CNS injury or infection. Headaches in combination with extreme fever often have a bacterial or viral precipitator. They are usually short-lived, subsiding when the fever passes the crisis point. The time to become concerned is when headaches are severe, repeating, and have a sudden onset ("thunderclap headache"), when they appear in a new pattern after age 50, or when they have a gradual onset but no remission. In these cases headache may be a symptom of some serious underlying condition. This is true particularly if the headache is accompanied by slurred speech, numbness anywhere in the body, and difficulties with motor control. The first things to investigate in cases like this are encephalitis, meningitis, stroke, tumor, and aneurysm.

Treatment

Avoiding or managing headache triggers is the most proactive and least invasive way to deal with this problem. People who have recurrent headaches of any type are usually encouraged to keep a headache journal to try to pin down their own specific triggers for headaches.

As understanding of the most common types of headaches changes, treatment options also shift. For the moment, medical headache treatment falls into two categories: prophylactic treatment, which works to prevent the headache from beginning, and abortive treatment, which works to end the headache once it has begun. Because migraines often are accompanied by nausea and vomiting, some medications are poorly tolerated when taken orally; nasal spray applications work well for some patients.

Cluster headaches respond well to pure oxygen inhalation if this can begin within the first few minutes of the first headache.

Tension-type headaches are still treated primarily with nonsteroidal anti-inflammatories when they require medical intervention at all.

Massage?

The appropriateness of massage depends on what kind of headache the client has. If it is related to a serious underlying pathology or to a bacterial or viral infection, any massage is obviously inappropriate.

Vascular headaches are usually so extreme and painful that clients prefer to wait until the acute stage has passed. Hydrotherapy to draw fluid out of the congested cranium may be successful if the client can tolerate it.

For the most common tension-type headaches, massage is resoundingly indicated. These episodes are an excellent opportunity to demonstrate how many seemingly disconnected postural and movement patterns can create pain in an entirely different area of the body.

Modality Recommendations for Headaches	
Deep Tissue Massage	Indicated for tension headaches. Work suboccipitals, cervical paravertebral fascias, jaw fascias.
Lymphatic Drainage	Supportive.
Polarity	S: Indicated. R/D: Indicated within client comfort.
PNF/MET/Stretching	Indicated in all stages.
Reflexology	Indicated; work head, neck, shoulder, eyes, spine, adrenals, pituitary, liver, solar plexus points.
Shiatsu	Indicated. Treat GB, TH for temporal, cluster, migraine headaches; ST, LI for sinus headaches; BL for frontal headaches. Treat all local points, meridians, extensions in head, face, neck for all headaches.
Swedish Massage	Indicated as long as headache is not a sign of a contraindicating underlying disorder.
Trigger Point Therapy	Indicated while subacute for TrPs related to tension and migraine headache pain; otherwise supportive.

See Chapter 1 for a brief description of each modality, including definitions of abbreviations.

Ménière Disease

Definition: What Is It?

Ménière disease is a group of signs and symptoms that center on inner ear dysfunction, leading to vertigo, tinnitus, and hearing loss. It was first described and documented by French physician Prosper Ménière in 1861.

Demographics: Who Gets It?

Most people diagnosed with Ménière disease are in their 20s to 50s, although it has been seen in children and older people. It is estimated that about 625,000 people in the United States have been diagnosed with Ménière disease, and about 45,000 new diagnoses are made each year. Men and women are affected about equally, and no specific racial or genetic predilection has been identified.

Ménière Disease in Brief

What is it?
Ménière disease is an idiopathic condition that affects the inner ear, leading to problems with vertigo, tinnitus, and hearing loss.

How is it recognized?
Signs and symptoms of Ménière disease include episodes of extreme vertigo, tinnitus, a sensation of pressure in the middle ear, and hearing impairment. Episodes last anywhere from 20 minutes to 24 hours.

Is massage indicated or contraindicated?
Ménière disease has no inherent contraindications for massage. If clients are comfortable on the table and techniques do not trigger symptoms, massage can be safe and supportive for a person with this condition.

Etiology: What Happens?

The inner ear is composed of several structures, including the bony labyrinth, which forms the semicircular ducts leading to the ampulla, the vestibule, and the snail-shaped cochlea. The bony labyrinth is filled with a sodium-rich fluid called ***perilymph***. Inside the bony labyrinth, the membranous labyrinth floats in the perilymph. The membranous labyrinth is filled with a potassium-rich fluid called ***endolymph*** (Figure 4.18). Together the endolymph and perilymph, separated by the membranous labyrinth, help to conduct sound vibrations. Furthermore, nerve endings from the vestibulocochlear nerve terminate in the ampulla, an enlarged space where the semicircular canals converge. These nerve projections are suspended in endolymph and move like seaweed in water whenever the head changes position. Signals from the vestibulocochlear nerve coordinate with the eyes and general proprioceptors throughout the body to help orient us in space.

The exact causes or sequence of events that lead to Ménière disease are not well understood. Several theories have been developed and are being intensively researched, but this dis-

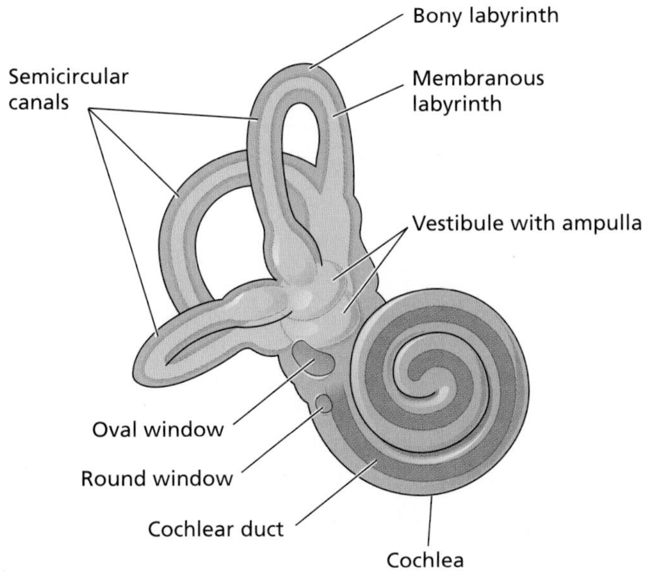

Figure 4.18. Semicircular canals. Perilymph fills the bony labyrinth, and endolymph fills the membranous labyrinth.

ease is still largely a mystery. Most researchers agree, however, that it has to do with the accumulation of excess fluid in the endolymph inside the membranous labyrinth. When no other cause can be found for this process, **idiopathic endolymphatic hydrops**, a synonym for Ménière disease, is identified. Possible causes for the accumulation of excess endolymph include rupture of the membranous labyrinth that allows the perilymph and endolymph to mix, autoimmune activity, viral infection, or pressure from a tiny blood vessel wrapping around the vestibulocochlear nerve.

Signs and Symptoms

Ménière disease has four classic symptoms, all of which appear intermittently and in any combination. It usually affects only one ear, but it can progress to affect the other ear as well. Onset of an episode is typically fast and unpredictable, and any given Ménière attack can last 20 minutes to 24 hours.

- *Hearing loss.* Hearing loss typically involves low-frequency sound. It is worst during flares but eventually becomes permanent. A person with a long history of this disorder may eventually become totally deaf.
- *Tinnitus.* This is an umbrella term for any unexplained ringing, whistling, or pounding noise in the ear. It can feel loud enough to interfere with the ability to sleep or concentrate. People describe tinnitus as sounding like a million crickets or like the whine of a jet engine.
- *A sense of fullness in the middle ear.* Many people with Ménière disease report that during flares they feel their ear is full, similar to the sensation of ascending or descending quickly, or coming in for a landing on an airplane. This is not relieved by yawning, as normal ear pressure is. Physical examinations of people with Ménière disease don't show a measurable increase in middle ear pressure, even during acute episodes.
- *Rotational vertigo.* This may be the most disabling symptom of Ménière disease. During an episode the person perceives that the world is spinning or the floor is sloping. *Nystagmus* (an abnormal rhythmic oscillation of the eyes) is observed as well. Nausea and vomiting are common results. Unlike the short-term vertigo that anyone gets when they spin or go on a Tilt-A-Whirl ride, this version lasts for several minutes or hours and is aggravated by any movement of the head.

Diagnosis

Ménière disease is diagnosed when no other cause for the dysfunction (e.g., MS, a neuroma on the acoustic nerve) can be found; when a person has at least two spontaneous episodes of vertigo and a feeling of fullness that last longer than 20 minutes; and when that person also has documented hearing loss.[49]

Treatment

Because Ménière disease is an idiopathic condition, treatment options focus on symptomatic control rather than trying to correct an identified problem. Some patients are able to identify triggers that increase their risk of having an episode. Many people are counseled to avoid foods and habits that raise blood pressure and increase fluid retention. A low-salt diet, avoiding monosodium glutamate, limiting caffeine and alcohol, and quitting smoking are usually recommended as early interventions. Medications to manage vertigo and nausea may be prescribed.

If diet and medications are unsuccessful, some patients explore chemical and surgical options to interfere with the sensation of vertigo. This can be accomplished by essentially disabling the vestibulocochlear nerve and relying on the unaffected side to compensate for the lost function. This is an option only when Ménière disease has not progressed to affect the contralateral side.

Massage?

Ménière disease has no direct contraindications for massage. If a person is not having an episode and feels comfortable on the table, any kind of bodywork is likely to be safe and appropriate. But if a client finds that certain positions or modalities trigger an episode, those should of course be carefully avoided.

Modality Recommendations for Ménière Disease	
Deep Tissue Massage	Supportive: work suboccipitals, cervical paravertebral fascias, jaw fascias for spacial orientation; work legs and hips to improve grounding.
Lymphatic Drainage	Supportive.
Polarity	S: Indicated. May have to prop client with pillows. R/D: Indicated within client comfort.
PNF/MET/Stretching	Supportive.
Reflexology	Indicated; work head, neck, face, ear points.
Shiatsu	Indicated. Treat all local points, meridians, extensions in neck, head, face.
Swedish Massage	Supportive; therapist may have to offer assistance with getting on/off table.
Trigger Point Therapy	Contraindicated when symptoms are acute; otherwise supportive.

See Chapter 1 for a brief description of each modality, including definitions of abbreviations.

Seizure Disorders

Definition: What Are They?

A seizure disorder is any kind of problem that can cause seizures. Epilepsy, one type of seizure disorder, is one of the oldest conditions recorded in medical history. It was first described about 2,000 years B.CE., but it was not studied as a specific problem other than "demonic possession" until the mid 19th century. Epilepsy is identified as a specific disorder when a person has two or more seizures that were not caused by some other medical problem.

Demographics: Who Gets Them?

Seizures are surprisingly common: about 10% of the U.S. population will have at least one seizure. About one-third of those have another seizure within an 8-year period, and most of those people have further repeated episodes.[50]

Approximately 2.7 million people in the United States have been diagnosed with epilepsy, and 200,000 new diagnoses are made every year, mostly among young children or elderly people. The incidence among children has been falling, but among elders it has been increasing to the point that 3% of people over age 75 have seizures.[51]

Seizure Disorders in Brief

Pronunciation: SE-zhur dis-OR-derz

What are they?

Seizure disorders are any condition that causes seizures. They are often related to some kind of neurological damage in the shape of tumors, head injuries, or infection, although it may be impossible to delineate exactly what that damage is. Epilepsy is a subtype of seizure disorder.

How are they recognized?

Seizures may take very different forms for different people. They can range from being barely noticeable to life threatening. Seizure disorders are diagnosed through physical examination, a description of symptoms, CT, MRI, and EEG.

Is massage indicated or contraindicated?

Seizure activity itself contraindicates massage, but bodywork is certainly appropriate for patients with most kinds of seizure disorders at any other time.

Etiology: What Happens?

When interconnecting neurons in the brain are stimulated in a certain kind of way, a tremendous burst of excess electricity may stimulate the neighboring neurons. The reaction is repeated, and soon millions of neurons in the brain are giving off electrical discharge. This is the CNS "lightning storm" of a seizure, and it affects the rest of the body in a number of ways.

For the most part, no one knows what starts the storm in the first place. Triggers vary from person to person. For some, sudden changes in light level from dark to light or vice versa trigger a seizure. For others, flashing or strobe lights or the strobe effect created by a ceiling fan or the sun shining through moving leaves is the trigger. Many children have their first seizure while watching television or playing video games. For others certain sounds or even particular notes of music trigger a seizure. High anxiety, sleep deprivation, hormonal changes around the menstrual cycle or pregnancy, and sicknesses such as fever, cold, or flu can also lead to seizures.

Whatever the trigger, the result is uncoordinated neuronal activity that allows electrical signals to get increasingly extreme, sometimes to the point of collapse and loss of consciousness. The ion pumps that regulate the potassium–sodium balance inside and outside neurons may malfunction. Some seizures are linked to underactive inhibitory neurotransmitters, overactive excitatory neurotransmitters, or both.

Causes

In some cases the cause of seizures can be definitively linked to a mechanical or chemical problem in the brain. Birth trauma, TBI, stroke, brain tumors, and penetrating wounds can all cause seizures, as can some types of metabolic disturbances, infections, exposure to some toxins (lead, carbon monoxide, and others), and extreme hypotension or hemorrhage. Alcoholism and drug abuse are risk factors. Alzheimer disease is a leading cause of seizures among the elderly. Some seizures can be traced to a hereditary issue. Even with all these possible factors, about half of seizures are idiopathic, untraceable to any identifiable problem.

Signs and Symptoms

Seizures take very different forms in each person they affect. From the original oversimplified categories of petit mal and grand mal seizures, more than 30 classes of seizures have been identified. Seizures are classified by the parts of the brain they affect when that information can be gathered. *Generalized* seizures affect the whole brain, while *partial* seizures involve abnormal activity in isolated areas. The most common types of seizures are described here.

Partial seizures These seizures involve abnormal activity only in isolated areas. The motor cortex and the temporal lobes are the sites most often affected. Partial seizures come in two subtypes:

- *Simple partial seizures.* In this type of seizure the patient doesn't lose consciousness. He or she may become weak or numb, may smell or taste things that aren't present, and may have some changes in vision or temporary vertigo along with some muscular tics or twitching.
- *Complex partial seizures.* This type of seizure is specifically associated with temporal lobe dysfunction. The patient may exhibit repetitive behaviors such as pacing in a circle, rocking, or smacking the lips. He or she may laugh uncontrollably or experience fear. Visual and olfactory hallucinations are other symptoms of complex partial seizures.

Generalized seizures These seizures involve electrical signals that occur all over the brain. They may be very subtle or dramatic. These are the major types:

- *Absence seizures.* These involve very short episodes of loss of consciousness. The patient doesn't fall to the floor but may simply "check out" for 5 to 10 seconds and have no memory of the lapse.
- *Tonic-clonic seizures.* These are what have traditionally been called grand mal seizures. They involve uncontrolled movement of the face, arms, and legs followed by loss of consciousness and a fall to the floor. They may last for 5 to 20 minutes, and the patient is usually tired and disoriented after an episode.
- *Myoclonic seizures.* These involve bilateral muscular jerking, which may be very pronounced or almost unnoticeable. They are usually seen among very young patients.
- *Status epilepticus.* These are a life-threatening variation of tonic-clonic seizures; they last for a long period and can put such a strain on the body that they can cause brain damage or death. Status epilepticus, or static seizures, are a medical emergency.

Diagnosis

Epilepsy is usually diagnosed by electroencephalogram (EEG), a test that measures electrical activity in the brain. Many people with epilepsy have a distinctive EEG even when they are not in the midst of a seizure. CT and/or MRI may be used to look for identifiable lesions. Tests are conducted in part to delineate seizures from other conditions that produce similar symptoms: migraine headaches, stroke, fainting spells, heart arrhythmia, narcolepsy, hypoglycemia, some anxiety disorders, withdrawal symptoms, and reactions to some medications.

Treatment

Seizures are generally treated with anticonvulsant medication, which acts to make neurons in the brain harder to stimulate. It can be difficult to find the right dosage of these powerful medications, and while most patients can find an anticonvulsant that works for them, some patients don't tolerate them well.

Some epilepsy patients find that their seizures are less frequent and less extreme when they follow a strict high-fat, low-fiber ketogenic diet.

Surgical intervention for seizure disorders is reserved for when an isolated and expendable mass (i.e., a tumor or clump of scar tissue) can be determined to be the cause of the seizures. Some patients with tonic-clonic seizures can control them when their corpus callosum is severed.

One device that is successful for some patients for whom medications don't work is a vagus nerve stimulator. This mechanism is implanted in the vagus nerves in the neck and sends pulses of electrical stimulation to the vagus nerve. It is believed that stimulating the vagus nerve in this way helps to activate some of the inhibitory neurotransmitters that seizure disorder patients lack.

Massage?

It is inappropriate to try to massage someone who is in the midst of a seizure of any kind. In the event of a tonic-clonic seizure, the practitioner's job is to make sure the client is safe and then wait until the seizure has subsided. Obviously, emergency services should be called if a client is injured during the seizure or has trouble breathing at any time.

It is perfectly fine to work with a client who has a history of seizures at any other time, although if the seizures tend to come on fast with no warning, the therapist should be alert to the possibility of its happening during an appointment. How the client would like to be treated in the event of a seizure can be discussed beforehand.

Someone recovering from a severe seizure often is sore and tender, as if he had been doing a lot of unaccustomed exercise, which in fact he has. It is also possible to sustain serious injury when these seizures happen in unprotected surroundings. Sprains, bruises, bloody noses, and even broken bones can happen during tonic-clonic seizures.

Modality Recommendations for Seizure Disorders	
Deep Tissue Massage	Indicated during recovery. Work slowly to increase relaxation, decrease contracture, soothe CNS.
Lymphatic Drainage	Supportive.
Polarity	S: Indicated when no signs of seizure present. R/D: Supportive when subacute.
PNF/MET/Stretching	Supportive.
Reflexology	Indicated with short, frequent sessions. Work brain, head, endocrine system, solar plexus, lymphatic system points.
Shiatsu	Indicated with caution when no signs of seizure are present. Treat water and fire element meridians and extensions.
Swedish Massage	Supportive, as long as no signs of seizure are present.
Trigger Point Therapy	Contraindicated during episode; otherwise supportive subacute.

See Chapter 1 for a brief description of each modality, including definitions of abbreviations.

Sleep Disorders

Definition: What Are They?

Sleep disorders are any disorders that interfere with the ability to fall asleep, to stay asleep long enough, or to wake up feeling refreshed. More than 70 sleep disorders have been defined. This section covers the most common varieties: insomnia, sleep apnea, restless leg syndrome, *narcolepsy*, and *circadian rhythm* disruption.

Sleep Disorders in Brief

What are they?
Sleep disorders are a collection of problems including insomnia, sleep apnea, restless leg syndrome, narcolepsy, circadian rhythm disruption, and others that make it difficult to get enough sleep or to wake up feeling rested and refreshed.

How are they recognized?
The primary symptom of sleep disorders is excessive daytime sleepiness. If this continues for a long period, a weakened immune system, memory and concentration loss, an increased risk of automotive or on-the-job accidents, and other complications may occur.

Is massage indicated or contraindicated?
Sleep disorders indicate massage. Bodywork may not correct a mechanical or psychological dysfunction that leads to sleep deprivation, but it can improve the quality of sleep and can reduce the mental and physical stresses that may interfere with sleep.

Demographics: Who Gets Them?

Approximately 40 million Americans report chronic, ongoing problems with sleep every year. While some disorders are specific to childhood, the incidence of sleep disorders increases with age; elderly people are less likely to feel refreshed by sleep than are younger people.

Etiology: What Happens?

To understand what happens when sleep is interrupted, it is useful to take a brief look at the phenomenon of sleep itself. Until recently, sleep was considered to be a strictly passive, uneventful activity. As researchers examined it more closely, however they have found that sleep occurs in cycling stages, and each of those stages performs specific functions in keeping the body healthy.

While human beings can adapt to live in colder or warmer temperatures, to living at high or low altitudes, or to living with more food or less, humans simply *cannot* adapt to sleep deprivation. Studies show that a healthy adult sleeps about 8 to 8.5 hours per night if not interrupted by an alarm clock or other disruption. Surveys show, however, that the average American adult gets only 6.9 to 7 hours of sleep on an average night.[52] The results of this chronic sleep deprivation show up in a multitude of short-term and long-term problems, including slowed reflexes and lower cognitive skills, poor immune system efficiency, fibromyalgia syndrome, chronic pain, depression, hallucinations, and psychosis. Poor sleep is now also being linked to weight gain, high blood sugar, and an elevated risk of developing type 2 diabetes.[52]

The circular relationship between poor health and poor sleep is another complicating factor. A person who doesn't feel well and consequently doesn't sleep well will probably continue *not* to feel well *because* of not sleeping well.

The need for sleep is determined partly by the accumulation of metabolic byproducts in the blood and by the hormone melatonin, a secretion of the pineal gland, deep within the brain. This hormone is secreted in the absence of full-spectrum sunlight. Melatonin contributes to a feeling of drowsiness. A standard rotation of wakefulness and sleepiness usually runs on a 24- to 25-hour cycle called the circadian rhythm.

Stages of Sleep

Sleep occurs in five distinct phases or stages:

- *Stage I.* In this light sleep a person is easily wakened. Eye movement is slow. A phenomenon called ***hypnic myoclonia***, the feeling that a person is suddenly starting to fall, occurs in this stage.
- *Stage II.* The eyes stop moving. Brain waves slow down but still show occasional bursts of activity called sleep spindles.
- *Stage III.* Brain waves are much slower. A particular deep-sleep pattern called delta waves are intermixed with slightly faster brain waves during this stage.
- *Stage IV.* Only delta waves are emitted from the brain. Stage IV sleep is when the body secretes the hormones that enable new growth for children and adolescents and repair and regeneration for adults.
- *REM sleep.* In REM (rapid eye movement) sleep breathing is rapid, shallow, and irregular. Eyes move quickly, but muscular activity in the limbs is usually absent. Heart rate and blood pressure approach waking levels. REM sleep is the stage in which dreams occur.

A person cycles through each of the five stages and then starts over again at stage I. It takes about 90 to 100 minutes to complete a sleep cycle, although the amount of time spent in each stage varies according to the time of night. In other words, a person spends more time in stages 3 and 4 at the beginning of the night and most time in stage 1 and REM sleep toward the morning. Overall a healthy balance of sleep stages allows an adult to spend 20% to 25% of the time in REM sleep, 50% of the time in stage II, and 30% of the time in the other stages.

Types of Sleep Disorders

Sleep disorders are loosely classified as *parasomnias* (disruptions of the sleep state) and *dyssomnias* (problems with initiating and maintaining sleep). Parasomnias include conditions such as night terrors, sleep talking, sleepwalking, and REM sleep behaviors: the person essentially acts out dreams. The most common dyssomnias among adults are the following:

Insomnia Literally, this means lack of sleep. Insomnia can involve difficulty falling asleep, difficulty staying asleep, or difficulty sleeping long enough for the body to get the rest it needs. Insomnia can be described as *transient*, in which case it occurs for less than 4 weeks at a time, or *chronic*, in which a person can't sleep most nights for more than a month at a time.

Transient insomnia is usually attributable to habits or environmental issues that are controllable. Caffeine taken too close to bedtime can ruin some people's sleep. (For many people, "too close to bedtime" means any time at all.) Alcohol, while being a depressant, reduces the quality of sleep. Some medications, including diet pills, antihistamines, and antidepressants, can interfere with sleep or reduce the time spent in REM stage. Cigarette smoking can cause a person to wake up too early from nicotine withdrawal.

Environmental conditions can also contribute to insomnia. Having a room that is too cold, too hot, too loud, or too light can make it hard to get to sleep or to stay asleep. Having a bed partner who snores or moves around a lot in the night can interrupt sleep. Exercising too late in the day or not exercising at all can also make it hard to fall asleep.

Emotional stress is of course a major contributor to sleep loss. Ironically, the longer a person lies in bed feeling the need to sleep, the less likely he or she is to drop off: the stress of waiting for sleep ensures that it never comes.

Chronic insomnia is usually examined as a sign of some deeper medical or psychological problem. Hyperthyroidism, fibromyalgia, depression, kidney failure, heart problems, and chronic fatigue syndrome are all possible factors when a person doesn't sleep well or long enough.

Obstructive sleep apnea *Apnea* means absence of breath. Sleep apnea is a disorder in which the air passage of a sleeping person temporarily shuts down, depriving him or her of oxygen for up to 60 seconds at a time. Repeated episodes may occur dozens or even hundreds of time each night, reducing the quality of sleep but more importantly, putting the person at risk for serious damage from oxygen deprivation.

Statistics on sleep apnea vary widely, with some estimates suggesting it affects up to 18 million Americans.

Obstructive sleep apnea is a mechanical problem in which the air passage collapses when muscles relax during sleep so that oxygen cannot enter during inhalation. When oxygen levels fall sufficiently, muscles tighten slightly, and air reenters the passageway with a loud snort or gasp; loud snoring is one sign of possible sleep apnea. Other signs are excessive daytime sleepiness and morning headache from oxygen deprivation.

Central sleep apnea Central sleep apnea is a neurological problem involving decreased respiratory drive. A rise in carbon dioxide in the blood is the signal to waken and breathe again. In some extreme cases central sleep apnea has caused brain damage or even death from respiratory arrest during sleep.

Frequent waking from central or obstructive sleep apnea leads to sleep deprivation and an increased risk of motor vehicle accident or on-the-job injury. Patients with either kind of sleep apnea also have an increased risk of stroke, heart attack, and hypertension.

Restless leg syndrome This disorder often runs in families, although it can also be associated with several other conditions, including pregnancy, diabetes, anemia, fibromyalgia, and ADHD. It involves a constant crawling, prickling, tingling sensation in the extremities, especially the legs, that is relieved only by rubbing and movement. It is closely related to another disorder called ***periodic limb movement disorder***, in which a person experiences repeated involuntary jerking movements of the legs every 20 to 40 seconds.

Although restless leg syndrome is present at all times, its symptoms are most pronounced when a person lies still in an effort to sleep. It is relieved by movement, massaging the affected areas, or warm baths. Symptoms tend to subside in the morning.

Some estimates suggest that restless leg syndrome affects up to 12 million Americans, most of them elderly.[53] It responds well to the dopamine-related drugs used to treat Parkinson disease, which reveals some clues about its etiology as a movement disorder.

Narcolepsy This chronic neurological dysfunction gets its name from the Greek *narco* for *stupor* and *lepsis* for *seizure*. It involves unpredictable "sleep attacks" at inappropriate times, often in response to intense emotional reactions such as laughing or anger.

Narcolepsy is generally diagnosed in adolescence; this is one sleep disorder that does not increase in incidence with age. Researchers suggest that it affects some 350,000 people in this country but has been diagnosed in only 50,000.[53]

Narcolepsy has three basic symptoms, which can appear in any combination for a positive diagnosis. *Cataplexy* refers to a sudden loss of muscle tone, even during waking hours. These events can last anywhere from several seconds to 30 minutes. *Sleep paralysis* is a phenomenon in which a person temporarily cannot speak or move while dozing. *Hypnagogic hallucinations* occur while drifting off to sleep. Narcolepsy patients often have poor nighttime sleep, which adds to a general problem with drowsiness during the day.

Circadian rhythm disruption The circadian rhythm is the normal cycle of drowsiness and wakefulness that all humans experience. It is regulated by exposure to ambient light and the secretion of melatonin. Most people run through this cycle every 24 to 25 hours. They feel drowsy as the sun goes down and wider awake as it rises. When people are forced to be physically or mentally active in a different cycle, their circadian rhythms are disrupted and the quality of their sleep, as well as the quality of their waking hours, is compromised.

Circadian rhythm disruption can occur in response to variable shift work, having to be awake all night for a graveyard shift, losing a night's sleep, or changing time zones through travel. Short-term difficulties associated with this problem are excessive sleepiness along with the degenerating reflexes and mental functioning that accompany exhaustion. Longer-term problems can include depression and other physical and psychological disorders brought about by sleep deprivation.

Some 25 million Americans don't work a standard daytime shift and are forced to adjust their sleep to accommodate a different schedule. While numbers on how many of those people are subject to dysfunction are difficult to gather, it has been found that these workers carry a higher than normal risk for motor vehicle accidents and on-the-job injuries. They also have more colds, flu, hypertension, weight gain, irregular menstrual cycles, and digestive discomfort than the rest of the population.[53]

Signs and Symptoms

The primary sign of a sleep disorder is excessive daytime sleepiness. Chronic sleep deprivation can also cause irritability, decreased ability to focus or concentrate, mood changes, and poor short-term memory. Other symptoms are associated with specific disorders, as described previously.

Complications

The National Sleep Foundation estimates that about 100,000 motor vehicle accidents each year have excessive fatigue as a primary cause. In addition to car crashes, fatigue and sleep deprivation contribute dangerously to on-the-job injuries that affect not only the sleep-deprived person but many others as well.

Deprivation of specific stages of sleep has also been associated with specific disorders. Lack of REM sleep over a long time can lead to hallucinations and psychosis. Fibromyalgia syndrome patients don't get adequate stage IV sleep, which means they don't secrete the hormones that stimulate healing and repair in adults. Other long-term consequences of sleep deprivation have already been discussed.

Diagnosis

If a person is so drowsy that it is difficult to accomplish basic tasks, it is worth pursuing with a medical professional on the chance that sleep apnea is interfering with the nighttime oxygen supply. Patients are often encouraged to keep a sleep diary in which they record activities in relation to how well they sleep. This is a useful tool to look for behavioral patterns that may interfere with a good night's rest. A physical examination is usually conducted to rule out other causes of insomnia, such as hyperthyroidism. A polysomnograph is a sleep study conducted in a laboratory, where a person's heart rate, respiratory rate, blood pressure, and other vital signs are measured during sleep. How much time a person spends in each stage may also be measured.

These tests can yield useful information about the nature of an individual's sleeping problem along with possibilities for treatment.

Treatment

Cases of transient insomnia are treated with lifestyle changes that better support healthy sleep. This can mean changes in diet and exercise habits, quitting smoking, adjusting temperature or sound levels in the bedroom, or other simple interventions. By the time insomnia has become a chronic problem, it can be difficult to recondition the body to sleeping well, so the earlier intervention can be taken, the better.

Over-the-counter sleep aids are generally discouraged, as they tend to create an imbalance in the time spent in each stage of sleep. Prescription sleep aids can be helpful for short periods, but several of them are habit forming, so long-term use is not a viable solution.

Sleep apnea can be treated in a variety of ways. Surgery to keep airways open may be conducted, or a nose mask to provide continuous positive airway pressure may be used. Apnea patients should not sleep on their back, and if they are overweight they should work to lose weight and reduce their risk of apnea complications. It is especially important that sleep apnea patients not drink alcohol or use sleep aids at night; these substances may interfere with their already challenged breathing mechanisms.

Restless leg syndrome is believed to be associated with dopamine deficiencies in certain brain areas. It is managed with dopamine agents, tranquilizers, and for very extreme cases, opioids and anticonvulsants. Less severe cases of restless leg syndrome can be managed with mild exercise, warm baths, and massage.

Narcolepsy is treatable with some medications and increasing exercise, which has been seen to reduce the number of sleep attacks.

Massage?

Most types of sleep disorders certainly indicate massage. Anyone who has restless nights and persistent daytime sleepiness appreciates the opportunity to tune out while receiving bodywork. Some studies indicate that massage increases the time spent in stage III or IV restorative sleep,[44] which decreases pain sensation and speeds healing. Massage can improve the quality of sleep for insomniac clients, and while it doesn't reverse sleep apnea, a massage therapist may be the first person to bring the habit of not breathing and then gasping during sleep to a client's attention.

Modality Recommendations for Sleep Disorders	
Deep Tissue Massage	Indicated for improved relaxation response.
Lymphatic Drainage	Supportive.
Polarity	S/R/D: Indicated within comfort of client.
PNF/MET/Stretching	Supportive.
Reflexology	Indicated; work solar plexus, diaphragm, brain, head, face, neck, spine, endocrine system points; focus on adrenal and pituitary glands.
Shiatsu	Indicated. Treat water and fire element meridians and extensions, esp. back, chest, abdomen.
Swedish Massage	Indicated; can improve quality of sleep.
Trigger Point Therapy	Supportive.

See Chapter 1 for a brief description of each modality, including definitions of abbreviations.

Vestibular Balance Disorders

Definition: What Are They?

Vestibular balance disorders are a group of conditions that can cause the vestibular branch of Cranial Nerve VIII to dysfunction, leading to debilitating vertigo that may last anywhere from a few seconds to many hours.

Vestibular Balance Disorders in Brief

Pronunciation: ves-TIB-yu-lar BAL-ens dis-OR-derz

What are they?
Vestibular balance disorders are problems with the vestibulocochlear nerve. They can be related to infection, inflammation, tiny calcium deposits, or other causes.

How are they recognized?
Vertigo, a sensation that the world is spinning, is the leading symptom of vestibular balance disorders. This may be accompanied by nausea, vomiting, and nystagmus.

Is massage indicated or contraindicated?
As long as a client is comfortable lying down, turning over, and getting up off a massage table, massage is fine for people with vestibular balance disorders.

Demographics: who gets them?

Vertigo can be reported by anyone, but it is most common in elderly people. About 30% of people over 65 years old, and over 50% of people 70 years and older have reported "dizzy spells." Many elderly people report that their vertigo significantly impacts their quality of life, and one-half of all accidental deaths among seniors are the result of balance-related falls.[54] Two million doctor visits are made each year to treat vertigo.[55]

Etiology: What Happens?

The vestibulocochlear nerve (CN VIII) terminates in the inner ear in two segments. The cochlear branch goes to the cochlea, where sound vibrations are transmitted to the brain for interpretation. The vestibular branch goes to the vestibule, an area of the inner ear where the semicircular canals converge. Vestibular nerve endings are suspended in fluid, and they sway like seaweed whenever the head moves or tilts in any direction. This information, when correlated with sensation from the eyes and general proprioceptors all over the body, provides our sense of position in relation to gravity.

Changes in the environment in the vestibule or other problems with the vestibular branch of CN VIII can lead to the sensation of vertigo. Some of the most common versions of vestibular balance disorders are these:

- *Benign paroxysmal positional vertigo*. In this common condition, small bits of calcium debris that are normally held within the vestibule are displaced into the semicircular canals. This is a common cause of a sudden onset of extreme vertigo that may last a few seconds to a few minutes. Special maneuvers of the head allow these tiny ***otoliths*** ("ear stones") to move back into the vestibule.
- *Labyrinthitis*. This is inflammation within the bony or membranous labyrinth. It is usually related to a self-limiting viral infection, but the pathogen is not always identified. This condition tends to last a few days or weeks and then gradually subsides.
- *Acute vestibular neuronitis*. This is inflammation of the vestibular portion of CN VIII. If the cochlear branch is affected, hearing loss may develop along with vertigo. Like labyrinthitis, this condition tends to be self-limiting and is usually resolved within a few days or weeks.
- *Ménière disease*. This idiopathic condition involves episodes of vertigo along with tinnitus, hearing loss, and a feeling of fullness in the middle ear. It is discussed elsewhere in this chapter.
- *Head injury*. Blows to the head, violent sneezing, or whiplash-type accidents can cause inner ear fluid to leak into the middle ear in a condition called perilymph fistula. This can also occur with a scuba diving accident, when it is called **barotrauma**.

Other less common causes of vestibular balance disorders include CNS problems such as stroke, tumors, MS, or migraine headaches. Allergies that block the eustachian tubes can interfere with fluid in the inner ear. Some psychological disorders (specifically anxiety and depression) can cause vertigo, as can medications used to treat them. Additional drugs, including alcohol, barbiturates, antihypertensives, diuretics, and cocaine, can also cause vertigo.

Signs and Symptoms

By definition, vertigo means a perception that the world is spinning or tilting. This delineates vertigo from other types of dizziness, which can include lightheadedness, disequilibrium, or feeling faint.

When a person has an episode of vertigo, associated symptoms also arise; nausea and vomiting are common. Nystagmus (abnormal rhythmic oscillations of the eyes) is frequent as well. The direction of the oscillations can sometimes yield clues about the source of the problem (peripheral nerve problems cause rotational and mixed nystagmus, while CNS trauma causes oscillations on only one axis).

Diagnosis

Diagnosis for vertigo can be a difficult process, because it has so many possible causes. Furthermore, the average patient is elderly and may have a combination of contributing factors. Clues can be derived from information about the speed of onset and the duration of symptoms. Brain imaging with MRI or CT is usually recommended to rule out CNS problems. Other evaluations include hearing tests, blood tests, ***electronystagmogram*** (to measure how well the eyes and vestibular mechanism work together), and ***posturography***, in which the patient stands on a tilting surface and the ability to adapt to changing positions is evaluated.

Treatment

Treatment for vestibular balance disorders depends on what the contributing factors are determined to be. Benign paroxysmal positional vertigo is treated with appropriate head maneuvers; medication is not necessary. Labyrinthitis and acute vestibular neuronitis are treated with drugs to control nausea and vomiting and exercises to help the CNS adapt to changes in sensation. These exercises have been found to be extremely helpful in managing vertigo and have the added benefit of giving elderly patients more confidence to avoid falls.[56] Other forms of vertigo are treated according to underlying causes.

Massage?

Massage is appropriate for clients who have vertigo as long as the bodywork or the actions of getting on, off, or turning over on the table don't aggravate symptoms.

Specialized maneuvers to help with benign paroxysmal positional vertigo may be learned to help affected clients. Trigger points in neck muscles may create some similar symptoms; resolving these may also offer some relief.

Modality Recommendations for Vestibular Balance Disorder	
Deep Tissue Massage	Indicated to improve proprioception. Work face, head, neck muscles and fascias; work legs and hips to improve grounding.
Lymphatic Drainage	Supportive.
Polarity	S: Indicated; may have to prop client with pillows. R/D: Supportive within client comfort.
PNF/MET/Stretching	Supportive.
Reflexology	Indicated; work brain, face, neck, ear points.
Shiatsu	Indicated. Treat H, SI, PC, TH, K systemically; all points, meridians, extensions in head and neck.
Swedish Massage	Supportive; therapist may have to offer assistance with getting on/off table.
Trigger Point Therapy	Supportive.

See Chapter 1 for a brief description of each modality, including definitions of abbreviations.

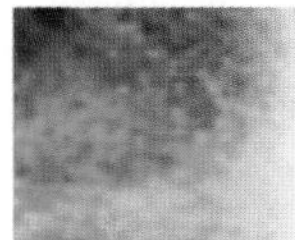

Chapter Review Questions: Nervous System Conditions

1. What is the difference between spastic and flaccid paralysis? Where in the nervous system does each indicate damage?
2. How can a person who has spinal cord damage at C6 still have control of his or her head and neck?
3. Why is massage indicated for Bell palsy when it is contraindicated for most other types of paralysis?
4. Is postpolio syndrome contagious? Why or why not?
5. Describe the safest course of action for a client who has an epileptic seizure during a massage.
6. A client who has MS comes for massage. The therapist performs a rigorous sports massage treatment and then recommends a soak in a hot tub. Is this a good idea? Why or why not?
7. Can a person who has had chickenpox catch herpes zoster from another person? Why or why not?
8. A person with CRPS may have poor circulation and bluish skin in the affected area. Is it appropriate to massage him or her here? Why or why not?
9. List five types of depression.
10. A client is recovering from a major stroke. What are some of the key criteria on which to base a judgment about the appropriateness of Swedish massage?

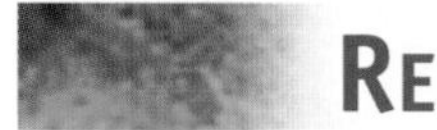

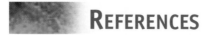

REFERENCES

1. Juhan D. Job's Body: A Handbook for Bodywork. Barrytown, NY: Station Hill, 1987, p 158.
2. Alzheimer's disease statistics. © Alzheimer's Association. http://www.alz.org/Resources/FactSheets/FSAlzheimerstats.pdf. Accessed summer 2006.
3. Therapeutic Touch Eases Agitation in People with Alzheimer's. © 2005 Digital Output Inc. DBA Massage Magazine, Inc. http://www.massagemag.com/Magazine/2004/issue107/research107.2.php. Accessed summer 2006.
4. Lazoff M. Multiple Sclerosis. © 1996–2006 by WebMD. http://www.emedicine.com/emerg/topic321.htm. Accessed summer 2006.
5. Tetanus vaccination lowers multiple sclerosis risk. Neurology 2006;67:212–215. © 2006 Reuters Ltd. http://www.medscape.com/viewarticle/542163. Accessed summer 2006.
6. Fox RJ. Multiple Sclerosis. © The Cleveland Clinic 2006. http://www.clevelandclinicmeded.com/diseasemanagement/neurology/multsclerosis/multsclerosis.htm. Accessed summer 2006.
7. Multiple Sclerosis Research, Alternative & Complementary Therapies. © Internet Health Library 1999–2001. http://www.internethealthlibrary.com/Health-problems/Multiple%20Sclerosis20-%20researchAltTherapies(incomp).htm. Accessed summer 2006.
8. 2005 West Nile Virus Activity in the United States. Centers for Disease Control. http://www.cdc.gov/ncidod/dvbid/westnile/surv&controlCaseCount05_detailed.htm. Accessed summer 2006.
9. Prevention and control of meningococcal disease. Morbidity & Mortality Weekly. Centers for Disease Control. Recommendations and Reports May 27, 2005. Vol. 54. No. RR-7. http://www.musa.org/pdfs/mmwr.pdf. Accessed summer 2006.
10. History. The Global Polio Eradication Initiative. http://www.polioeradication.org/history.asp. Accessed summer 2006.
11. Post-Polio Syndrome Fact Sheet. National Institute of Neurological Disorders and Stroke. http://www.ninds.nih.gov/disorders/post_polio/detail_post_polio_pr.htm. Accessed summer 2006.
12. The Numbers Count: Mental Disorders in America. National Institute of Mental Health. NIH publication 06-458. http://www.nimh.nih.gov/publicat/numbers.cfm. Accessed summer 2006.
13. Mental Health: A report of the surgeon general. http://www.surgeongeneral.gov/library/mentalhealth/chapter4/sec2.html. Accessed summer 2006.
14. Werner R. Jangled adults: Touch and the stress response system. Massage and Bodywork, Feb/March 2006, p 122.
15. Mental Health in the United States: Prevalence of Diagnosis and Medication Treatment for Attention-Deficit/Hyperactivity Disorder—United States, 2003. Centers for Disease Control Morbidity and Mortality Weekly Report. http://www.cdc.gov/mmwr/preview/mmwrhtml/mm5434a2.htm#top. Accessed summer 2006.
16. Attention Deficit Hyperactivity Disorder. NIH Publication 3572. National Institute of Mental Health. http://www.nimh.nih.gov/publicat/adhd.cfm1. Accessed summer 2006.
17. Dadson M. Nonpharmacologic approaches to treating ADHD. Medscape Psychiatry & Mental Health 2006;11(2) © 2006 Medscape. http://www.medscape.com/viewarticle/541193?src=mp. Accessed summer 2006.
18. Cullen-Powell LA. Exploring a massage intervention for parents and their children with autism: The implications for bonding and attachment. J Child Health Care 2005;9(4):245–255. http://chc.sagepub.com/cgi/reprint/9/4/245. Accessed summer 2006.
19. Autism Spectrum Disorders, or Pervasive Developmental Disorders. © 2002, 2003, 2004 The Children's Clinic. http://www.thechildrensclinic.ie/autism.html#cranialtherapy. Accessed summer 2006.
20. DSM-IV Substance Abuse Criteria. Diagnostic and statistical manual of mental disorders: DSM-IV. 4th ed. American Psychiatric Association, 1994:181. © 1994. http://www.dawnfarm.org/pdf/DSM_Abuse_and_dependence_criteria.pdf. Accessed summer 2006.
21. NIDA InfoFacts: Treatment Approaches for Drug Addiction. NIDA. http://www.nida.nih.gov/infofacts/treatmeth.html. Accessed summer 2006.
22. Thompson W. Alcoholism. © 1996–2006 by WebMD. http://www.emedicine.com/med/topic98.htm. Accessed summer 2006.
23. Jones EM. Common Problems in Patients Recovering from Chemical Dependency. © 2003 by the American Academy of Family Physicians. http://www.aafp.org/afp/20031115/1971.html. Accessed summer 2006.

24. Quick Stats: General Information on Alcohol Use and Health. Centers for Disease Control and Prevention. http://www.cdc.gov/alcohol/quickstats/general_info.htm. Accessed summer 2006.
25. Thompson W. Alcoholism. © 1996-2006 by WebMD. http://www.emedicine.com/med/topic98.htm. Accessed summer 2006.
26. Sapolsky RM. Why Zebras Don't Get Ulcers. 3rd ed. © 2004 by Robert M. Sapolsky. p 272.
27. Aronson S. Depression. © 1996–2006 by WebMD. http://www.emedicine.com/med/topic532.htm. Accessed summer 2006.
28. Depression. NIH Publication 00-3561: National Institutes of Mental Health. http://www.nimh.nih.gov/publicat/depression.cfm. Accessed summer 2006.
29. Rakesh J. Addressing Both the Emotional and Physical Symptoms in Depression. © 2003 Medscape. http://www.medscape.com/viewprogram/2240. Accessed summer 2006.
30. Williams L. Depression and stroke: Cause or consequence? Semin Neurol 2005;25(4):396–409. © 2005 Thieme Medical Publishers. Posted 02/15/2006.
31. Field T. Touch Therapy. London: Churchill Livingstone; 2000, p 165.
32. Pritts S. Diagnosis of Eating Disorders in Primary Care. © 2003 by the American Academy of Family Physicians. http://www.aafp.org/afp/20030115/297.html. Accessed summer 2006.
33. Eating Disorders: Facts About Eating Disorders and the Search for Solutions. National Institute of Mental Health publication 01-4901. http://www.nimh.nih.gov/Publicat/eatingdisorders.cfm. Accessed summer 2006.
34. Ives J. Massage in the Treatment of Eating Disorders. August 2006, Vol. 7, No. 8. © 2006 American Massage Therapy Association. http://www.amtamassage.org/etouch/etouch0806m.html#1. Accessed summer 2006.
35. Anorexia Symptoms are Reduced by Massage Therapy. © Touchpoints. Touchpoints Vol. 13, No. 1, Winter 2006.
36. Krigger K. Cerebral Palsy: An Overview. © 2006 by the American Academy of Family Physicians. http://www.aafp.org/afp/20060101/91.html. Accessed summer 2006.
37. Ratanawongsa B. Cerebral Palsy. © 1996–2006 by WebMD. http://www.emedicine.com/neuro/topic533.htm. Accessed summer.<<Au: What year?>>
38. Reflex Sympathetic Dystrophy Syndrome. © 1997–2006 American RSDHope. http://www.rsdhope.org/Showpage.asp?PAGE_ID=3&PGCT_ID=546. Accessed summer 2006.
39. Harmon R, ed. Complex Regional Pain Syndrome Treatment Guidelines. © 2006 RSDSA. http://www.rsds.org/3/pdf/Txguide_chap1.pdf. Accessed summer 2006.
40. Shutack J. Introduction to Spina Bifida. © 1999–2006 SpineUniverse.com http://www.spineuniverse.com/displayarticle.php/article234.html. Accessed summer 2006.
41. Spina bifida. © 1998–2006 Mayo Foundation for Medical Education and Research. http://www.mayoclinic.com/health/spina-bifida/DS00417. Accessed summer 2006.
42. Stroke. Centers for Disease Control and Prevention. http://www.cdc.gov/stroke/index.htm. Accessed summer 2006.
43. Barclay L. Constraint-Induced Movement Therapy May Be Helpful for Chronic Stroke. © 1994–2006 by Medscape. http://www.medscape.com/viewarticle/525520. Accessed summer 2006.
44. Massage Therapy Studies. Touch Research Institute. Copyright 1997–2006, University of Miami. http://www6.miami.edu/touch-research/touchpoints.htm. Accessed summer 2006.
45. Traumatic Brain Injury. © 2003 NeurosurgeryToday.org. All rights reserved. http://www.neurosurgerytoday.org/what/patient_e/head.asp. Accessed summer 2006.
46. Traumatic Brain Injury: Hope Through Research. National Institute of Neurological Disorders and Stroke NIH publication 02-2478. http://www.ninds.nih.gov/disorders/tbi/detail_tbi.htm. Accessed summer 2006.
47. Concussion. © 2003 NeurosurgeryToday.org. All rights reserved. http://www.neurosurgerytoday.org/what/patient_e/concussion.asp. Accessed summer 2006.
48. Trigeminal Neuralgia Discussion. Medscape Neurology & Neurosurgery 3(2), 2001. © 2001 Medscape Portals, Inc. http://www.medscape.com/viewarticle/430125_4. Accessed summer 2006.
49. Ménière's disease. © 1998–2006 Mayo Foundation for Medical Education and Research. http://www.mayoclinic.com/health/Menière s-disease/DS00535. Accessed summer 2006.
50. Seizures and Epilepsy: Hope Through Research. National Institute of Neurological Disorders and Stroke. NIH publication 04-156. http://www.ninds.nih.gov/disorders/epilepsy/detail_epilepsy.htm. Accessed summer 2006.
51. Epilepsy and Seizure Statistics. © 2001–2005. Epilepsy Foundation. http://www.epilepsyfoundation.org/answerplace/statistics.cfm. Accessed summer 2006.

52. Cauter E, Knutson K, Leproult R, et al. The Impact of Sleep Deprivation on Hormones and Metabolism. Copyright © 1994–2005 by Medscape. http://www.medscape.com/viewarticle/502825. Accessed summer 2006.
53. Your Guide to Healthy Sleep. National Heart, Lung and Blood Institute. NIH publication 06-5271. http://www.nhlbi.nih.gov/health/public/sleep/healthy_sleep.pdf. Accessed summer 2006.
54. Statistics: How many people have vestibular disorders? © 2005 VEDA. http://www.vestibular.org/vestibular-disorders/statistics.php. Accessed summer 2006.
55. Bredenkamp JK. Vestibular Balance Disorders: Vertigo, Motion Sickness, and Dizziness. © 1996–2005 MedicineNet, Inc. http://www.medicinenet.com/vestibular_balance_disorders/article.htm. Accessed summer 2006.
56. Sadovsky R. Exercise-Based Treatment for Chronic Dizziness. © 2005 by the American Academy of Family Physicians. http://www.aafp.org/afp/20050715/tips/4.html. Accessed summer 2006.

5

Circulatory System Conditions

Chapter Objectives

After reading this chapter, you should be able to . . .

- Name two deficiencies that may cause nutritional anemia.
- Define hemophilia.
- Name the most likely destination for loose blood clots on the venous side of the systemic circuit.
- Name three possible destinations for loose blood clots or other debris on the arterial side of the systemic circuit.
- Name two signs or symptoms of deep vein thrombosis.
- Name the tissue that is damaged first in chronic hypertension.
- Name three controllable risk factors for the development of atherosclerosis.
- Name the difference between primary and secondary Raynaud syndrome.
- Name two factors that determine the severity of a heart attack.
- Describe how right-sided heart failure can develop as a result of left-sided heart failure.

Introduction

The body's cells are highly specialized and complex. Most of them are fixed: unable to move toward nutrition or away from toxic wastes. They depend on the circulatory system for constant delivery of food and fuel and constant carrying away of garbage. Suppose a person needed someone to run to the grocery store and to flush the toilets and take out the trash. How long would the person last if this service were interrupted? Massage can promote circulatory health, but it can also interrupt or interfere with this service. For a massage therapist to make informed choices about to whom and when to give massage, he or she must have a strong understanding of the interaction between bodywork and the circulatory system.

General Function: The Circulatory System

The body depends on *diffusion*, the random distribution of particles throughout an environment, for the exchange of nutrients and wastes. For diffusion to happen, a medium must allow substances to move freely within small areas. What could be better than the combination of blood and lymph? People contain about 23 liter of liquid. In every milliliter of it particles are flowing this way and that, chemicals are reacting, and *life* is happening.

The circulatory system, through the medium of the blood, works to maintain homeostasis, which is the tendency to maintain a stable internal environment. It does this in a number of different ways:

- *Delivery of nutrients and oxygen.* The blood carries nutrients and oxygen to every cell in the body. If for some reason the blood can't reach a specific area, cells in that area starve and die. This is the situation with many disorders, including stroke, heart attack, pulmonary embolism, renal infarction, and decubitus ulcers.
- *Removal of waste products.* While dropping off nutrients, the blood, along with lymph, picks up the waste products generated by metabolism. These include carbon dioxide and more noxious compounds that can cause problems if left to stew in the tissues. Again, if blood and lymph supply to an area is limited, the affected cells can drown in their own waste products and be damaged or even die.
- *Temperature.* Superficial blood vessels dilate when it's hot, and they constrict when it's cold. Furthermore, blood prevents the hot places (the heart, the liver, working muscles) from getting too hot by flushing through and distributing the heated blood throughout the body. By helping us to keep a steady temperature, the circulatory system helps to maintain a stable internal environment.
- *Clotting.* This is an often overlooked but truly miraculous function of the circulatory system without which people would quickly die. Every time a rough place develops in the endothelium of a blood vessel, a whole chain of chemical reactions results in the spinning of tiny fibers that catch cells to plug any possible gaps. Unfortunately, in certain circumstances, this reaction is sometimes more of a curse than a blessing.
- *Protection from pathogens.* Without white blood cells we would have no defense against the hordes of microorganisms that try to gain access to the body's precious (and precarious) internal environment. For a closer look at what actually happens to those would-be invaders, see the introduction to Chapter 6.
- *Chemical balance.* The body has a very narrow margin of tolerance for variances in internal chemistry. A person can actually die if his or her blood gets even 15% too alkaline or too acidic. Happily, blood components, including red blood cells, are supplied with enzymes and other buffers specifically designed to keep pH balance within the safety zone.

Structure and Function: The Blood

Red Blood Cells (Erythrocytes)

Almost all of the blood cells, red and white alike, are made in the red bone marrow. Red blood cells are created at the command of a hormone secreted by the kidneys called ***erythropoietin***. Red blood cells are constantly being produced and dying, at about 2 million per second. They comprise 98% of blood cells. Their life span is about 4 months, and during that time they do a single job: they deliver oxygen to the cells and carbon dioxide to the lungs. They are so devoted to this task that they have given up their nuclei to make more room to carry their cargo.

Red blood cells are tiny; 1 mL of blood holds about 5 million of them. They are built around an iron-based molecule called ***hemoglobin***. This molecule (there are 250 million of them in each red blood cell) is extremely efficient at carrying oxygen and slightly less so at carrying carbon dioxide; most of that is dissolved in plasma. Another key quality to healthy red blood cells is their shape: they are discs that are thinner in the middle than around the edges. They are very smooth and should be flexible enough to bend and distort themselves to get through the tiniest capillaries. If for some reason they are not round, smooth, and flexible, big problems ensue.

White Blood Cells (Leukocytes)

Leukocytes aren't really white; they're more or less clear. Unlike red blood cells, which are all identical, different classes of white blood cells fight off different types of invaders in different stages of infection. Types of white blood cells include neutrophils, basophils, eosinophils, monocytes, and lymphocytes (Figure 5.1).

Platelets (Thrombocytes)

Thrombocytes are not whole cells at all but fragments of huge cells that are born in the red bone marrow. They are usually smooth, but when they are stimulated, they quickly become spiky and sticky. Thrombocytes travel the system looking for leaks or rough places in the blood vessels. If they find one, a series of chemical reactions causes tiny

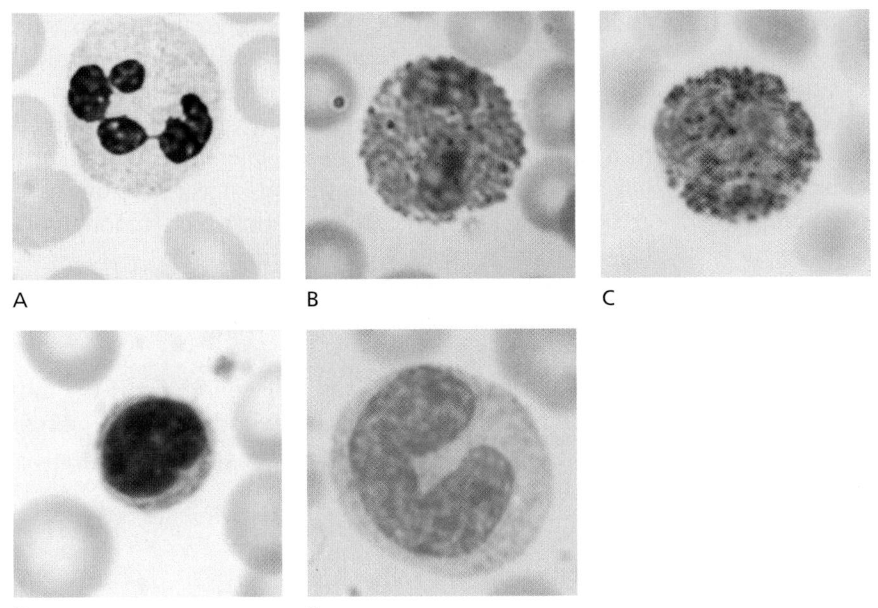

Figure 5.1. Varieties of white blood cells. A. Neutrophil. B. Eosinophil. C. Basophil. D. Lymphocyte. E. Monocyte.

threads of fibrin, a protein, to be woven from plasma proteins in the injured area. These fibers act as a net to catch not only passing thrombocytes but passing red blood cells as well, forming a *crust* on the skin or a *clot* (*thrombus*) internally. This is a good thing; it's very important, and it's usually not a problem because other chemicals whose job is to *melt* clots circulate in the blood. Under certain circumstances the clotting mechanisms work harder than the clot-destroying mechanisms. This ultimately can become life threatening.

Structure and Function: The Heart

The heart is divided by the septum into left and right halves. The right half pumps blood to the lungs (the pulmonary circuit), and the left half pumps to the rest of the body (the systemic circuit). Each half of the heart is further divided into top and bottom. The small top chambers, where blood returning from the lungs and body enters, are called the atria (the singular form is *atrium* from the Latin for *entrance hall*), and the larger bottom chambers are the ventricles (from the Latin for *belly*). The two-part "lub-dup" of the heartbeat is the closing of the valves that separate the chambers from each other and the ventricles from the arteries leaving the heart.

The cardiac muscle of the atria is much thinner and weaker than that of the ventricles. This is because the atrial contraction has to push blood only a few centimeters downhill into the ventricles. The cardiac muscle of the ventricles is thicker and stronger than that found in the atria because the ventricular contraction pushes blood into the circulatory system—through the pulmonary circuit to the lungs from the right ventricle, and through the systemic circuit to the rest of the body from the left ventricle. The differences in the workload of various parts of the heart have great implications for the seriousness of myocardial infarctions (heart attacks); the location of the damaged tissue determines how well the heart will function without it.

Structure and Function: Blood Vessels

The vessels *leaving* the heart are called *arteries* and *arterioles*; the vessels *going toward* the heart are called *venules* and *veins*; the vessels that connect them are called *capillaries*. Ideally this should be a closed system. That is, although white blood cells are free to come and go through capillary walls, the red blood cells should never be able to leave the 60,000 miles of continuous tubing that constitutes the circulatory system. If they *do* leak out, it's because the system has an injury, and a blood clot should be forming.

Arteries and veins share the basic properties of most of the tubes in the body. They have an internal layer of epithelium (it's called *endo*thelium here because it's on the inside); this layer is called the tunica intima, or inside coat. The middle layer (tunica media) is made of smooth muscle; and the external layer of tough, protective connective tissue is called the tunica externa, or the adventitia. This combination of tissues makes these tubes strong, pliable, and stretchy.

Capillaries are delicate variations of basic tube construction. As the arteries divide into smaller arterioles, their outer layers get thinner and thinner. Finally all that is left is one layer of simple squamous epithelium wrapped with smooth muscle cells: the capillaries. This construction is ideal for the passage of substances back and forth, because most diffusion happens readily through single-cell layers. But because capillaries lack the tougher muscle and connective tissue layers of the larger tubes, they are much more vulnerable to injury.

Blood cells leave the heart through the thick-walled arteries, crowd into arterioles, and line up one by one to squeeze through the capillaries. Once they've dumped their cargo of oxygen and picked up the carbon dioxide, they have more breathing room; now they're in the venules. Again the three-ply construction design is present, but with a difference. Much of the venous system operates against gravity. Blood flows upward in the legs, the arms, and the trunk, partly by indirect pressure exerted by the heart on the arterial system but also with the help of hydrostatic pressure and muscular contraction. To help the blood move along without backing up in the system, small epithelial flaps or *valves* line the veins. The smooth muscle layer here is thinner and weaker than in the arteries, which have to cope with much higher pressure coming directly from the heart. Veins get wider, bigger, and stronger as they approach the heart, but they are never as strong as arteries. Fortunately, the force with which blood moves through them is never as strong either.

When blood returns from the body to the heart (the systemic circuit), it goes to the lungs to be oxygenated (Figure 5.2).

The chapter on cardiovascular conditions is the most self-referential portion of this book. Most of the conditions discussed here are caused by or are complications of (or both) other conditions in this chapter.

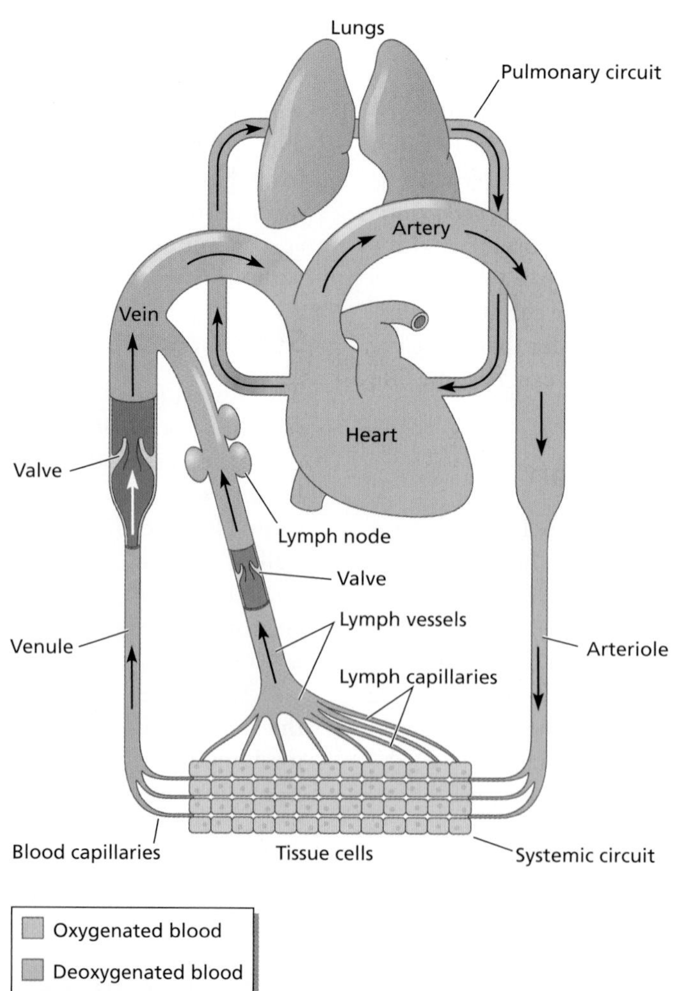

Figure 5.2. The right side of the heart pumps blood to the lungs in the pulmonary circuit; the left side of the heart pumps blood through the rest of the body in the systemic circuit.

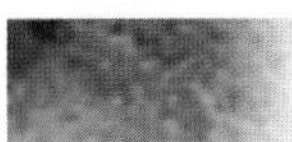

Circulatory System Conditions

Blood Disorders

Anemia
Embolism, thrombus
Hematoma
Hemophilia
Leukemia
Malaria
Myeloma
Sickle cell disease
Thrombophlebitis, deep vein thrombosis

Vascular Disorders

Aneurysm
Atherosclerosis
Hypertension
Raynaud syndrome
Varicose veins

Heart Conditions

Heart attack
Heart failure

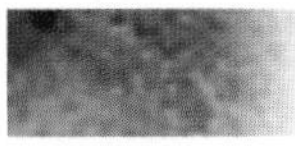

Blood Disorders

Anemia

Definition: What Is It?

Anemia is the condition of having either an insufficient supply of red blood cells, an insufficient or somehow functionally impaired supply of hemoglobin, or both. In any case, anemia by itself is not a diagnosis; it's a description. The diagnosis comes when one determines *why* a shortage of red blood cells or hemoglobin has developed.

Demographics: Who Gets It?

Anemia is a common problem, affecting about 3.4 million people in the United States.[1] Most anemia patients are women or people with a chronic disease, such as cancer, infection, or bone marrow suppression.

Etiology: What Happens?

Several kinds of anemia are possible, each with different guidelines for treatment and the appropriateness of massage. Some of the most common varieties are discussed here, with descriptions of the process and how massage might positively or negatively affect them.

Idiopathic anemias These conditions, which have no well-understood cause, may be due to poor nutritional uptake because of how stress affects gastric juices, or to other more mysterious factors. But once other pathologies are ruled out, these anemias (which are usually comparatively mild) may respond well to massage.

Nutritional anemias These anemias occur because the body is missing something vital in its diet and no amount of massage, no matter how brilliantly administered, can replace it. However, most of these conditions are not negatively affected by massage. The only exception to this rule is advanced pernicious anemia.

- *Iron deficiency anemia.* Iron is at the center of the hemoglobin molecule. An insufficiency of iron in the diet leads to insufficiency of hemoglobin, and then to pathologically small or

> **Anemia in Brief**
> Pronunciation: ah-NE-me-ah
>
> **What is it?**
> Anemia is a symptom rather than a disease in itself. It indicates a shortage of red blood cells, hemoglobin, or both.
>
> **How is it recognized?**
> Symptoms of anemia include pallor, shortness of breath, fatigue, and poor resistance to cold. Other symptoms may accompany specific varieties of anemia.
>
> **Is massage indicated or contraindicated?**
> Anemia that is idiopathic or due to nutritional deficiency may indicate massage, as long as no neurological damage has occurred. Anemia related to bone marrow suppression, chronic disease, inflammation, or premature destruction of red blood cells may contraindicate rigorous bodywork, although some types of energy work may be appropriate.

thin red blood cells and "iron-poor blood." Iron deficiency anemia is the most common variety of anemia around the world and in the United States. It can come about from a diet that is poor in iron, an inability to absorb iron from digestion, chronic bleeding, or lead poisoning. Women are at increased risk for iron deficiency anemia because they need about twice as much iron as men but consume fewer calories. Pregnant women have a radically increased need for iron, and about half of them in this country are anemic.

- *Folic acid deficiency anemia.* Folic acid is a nutrient found in green leafy vegetables that is critical for the formation of red blood cells. If a person doesn't get enough, it's impossible to produce the 2 million red blood cells per second that it takes to keep up with the cells that are dying off. Folic acid is water soluble. That means it can't be stored for later use; a steady fresh supply is necessary. Folic acid anemia is usually related to dietary insufficiency or malabsorption, often due to alcoholism or celiac disease.
- *Pernicious anemia.* Of all of the nutritional anemias, this is the most serious because it can lead to irreversible damage to the central nervous system. Vitamin B_{12} is necessary for the formation of red blood cells. Vitamin B_{12} is available only from animal food sources, including eggs and dairy products. Very few people in the United States have a B_{12} deficiency, yet pernicious anemia is relatively common. This is because a chemical in gastric secretions, ***intrinsic factor***, is necessary for absorption of vitamin B_{12}. Without it a person may take in all the B_{12} he or she requires, but the body has no access to it and cannot produce enough erythrocytes to keep up with its needs. Age, genetic predisposition, stomach surgery, autoimmune disease, alcoholism, tapeworms, celiac disease, and Crohn disease may all interfere with intrinsic factor activity. The only treatment for pernicious anemia is to supplement vitamin B_{12} in some form that the body can absorb it (this may involve injections). This pales in comparison to the alternative, however. B_{12} is also critical to the maintenance of the central nervous system. Without it, a person experiences the slow onset of paralysis, loss of proprioception, and brain damage.
- *Other nutritional deficiencies.* Anemia can be the result of shortages of several other substances, notably copper and protein. Massage does not improve this condition, and if it is very advanced (with extreme shortness of breath, fatigue, and low stamina), massage could possibly tax the already overworking heart in a dangerous way. Anemia this advanced is relatively rare, however.

Hemorrhagic anemias Hemorrhagic anemias are those brought about by blood loss. Usually it's from a slow leak, but occasionally it's from some trauma; this would be acute hemorrhagic anemia. The most common causes of hemorrhagic anemia are gastric or duodenal ulcers, chronic kidney problems leading to the loss of blood in the urine, heavy menstruation, and large wounds. Obviously, bleeding ulcers and large wounds contraindicate rigorous circulatory massage. Heavy menstruation isn't negatively affected unless the therapist works deeply in the abdomen during flow, but it is a sign that something may be wrong, and the client should consult with her health care team to rule out some other disorder, such as endometriosis or fibroid tumors. Blood in the urine contraindicates circulatory massage until the causes can be identified and addressed.

Hemolytic anemias These anemias are characterized by the premature destruction of healthy red blood cells. In addition to the basic symptoms of anemia, ***splenomegaly*** (enlarged spleen) and jaundice may be present. Another sign of hemolytic anemia is the presence of higher than normal numbers of ***reticulocytes*** in the blood. These are immature red blood cells that cannot carry as much oxygen as fully developed red blood cells. High numbers of reticulocytes are released from the bone marrow when the supply of erythrocytes is getting dangerously low.

Causes of hemolytic anemia include genetic predisposition, allergic reactions to certain drugs, and infection. Two types of hemolytic anemia, sickle cell disease and malaria, are discussed later in this chapter.

Aplastic anemia In aplastic anemia bone marrow activity is sluggish or even nonexistent. The production of every kind of blood cell is slowed or suspended. When this moment's 2 million cells report to the spleen for destruction, insufficient new red blood cell replacements are available. Likewise, no new white blood cells are manufactured, so resistance to infection is impaired. And finally the stream of thrombocytes has dried up too, making persons with aplastic anemia prone to uncontrolled bleeding. This sometimes shows as frequent bloody noses or bleeding from the gums.

Aplastic anemia can be caused by autoimmune attack against bone marrow, renal failure, folate deficiency, certain viral infections, exposure to some types of radiation, and some environmental toxins, namely benzene and some insecticides.

Myelodysplastic anemia is a closely related problem, but in this case the bone marrow makes multitudes of abnormal cells rather than being suppressed altogether. This can be a precancerous condition that indicates a risk of leukemia or myeloma.

Secondary anemias Anemia is a frequent complication of other disorders. Sometimes a direct cause-and-effect relationship is obvious, and sometimes the association is a less clear but still present. A partial list of the conditions that anemia frequently accompanies includes the following:

- *Ulcers.* Gastric, duodenal, and colonic ulcers can all bleed internally. This may not be very obvious, but it results in a steady draining of red blood cells, which can impair general oxygen uptake and energy levels. This is a type of *hemorrhagic anemia*, discussed earlier.
- *Kidney disease.* The capillaries inside the kidneys have a tremendous workload. Not only do they filter toxins and maintain water balance, but they do it under tremendous mechanical pressure from the renal arteries. Sometimes the kidney capillaries are damaged and leak red blood cells into the urine. Again, it's a leak rather than a gusher, but just as that dripping faucet drives up the water bill, a leaking kidney slowly but surely drains away viable red blood cells. Furthermore, the kidneys secrete the hormone that stimulates bone marrow to produce red blood cells (***erythropoietin***). When the kidneys are not functioning well, erythropoietin levels drop and red blood cell production goes down.
- *Hepatitis.* The liver contributes vital proteins to the blood, and it is responsible, with the spleen, for breaking down and recycling the iron from dead erythrocytes. If liver function is disrupted for any reason, the quality and amount of hemoglobin available to new red blood cells may decline.
- *Acute infectious disease.* Anemia is sometimes an indicator that the body is under attack. It is a frequent follower of pneumonia, tuberculosis, or other infection. Infectious disorders often cause iron to be used elsewhere in the body, reducing the amount of hemoglobin available to new red blood cells. Anemia in these cases usually clears up spontaneously once the primary condition has been resolved.
- *Leukemia, myeloma, lymphoma.* In these conditions masses of nonfunctional white blood cells are produced in bone marrow or in lymphatic tissues. These white blood cells essentially crowd out functional red blood cells.

Signs and Symptoms

No matter what the cause of anemia is, some signs and symptoms are consistent. These include the following:

- *Pallor.* Pallor is present because of a reduced number of red blood cells, or a reduced amount of hemoglobin to carry the oxygen that gives the red blood cells their color. Pallor is visible in the skin and in mucous membranes, gums, and nail beds. In dark-skinned people, pallor shows as an ashy-gray appearance to the skin.
- *Dyspnea.* This is shortness of breath. ***Dyspnea*** is a symptom of anemia because with less oxygen-carrying capacity, a person has to breathe harder and more often just to keep up. Another sign of anemia is a higher than normal respiratory rate.
- *Fatigue.* Often this is the first noticeable symptom of anemia. Less oxygen is available to go around, so muscles wear out sooner and stamina is nonexistent. Unfortunately, a host of other conditions may make a person feel worn out, so this is rarely enough to go on for a diagnosis.
- *Rapid heartbeat.* Another term for this is ***tachycardia***. It allows oxygen-poor blood to travel faster through the body.
- *Intolerance to cold.* Oxygen is needed for muscle contraction and for heat production (shivering). Someone who is in short supply of oxygen runs out of steam in a hurry.

Massage?

The appropriateness of massage for clients with anemia varies according to the cause. Massage has been seen to increase red blood cell count at least temporarily, but this is probably due to the action of pushing sluggish red blood cells back into circulation; these effects don't tend to last very long. Massage certainly doesn't provide missing nutrients, but the resulting parasympathetic response may improve uptake in the digestive system.

Anemia contraindicates massage when it accompanies other disorders that may be negatively affected. Specifically, if pernicious anemia has resulted in a decrease in sensation or if the anemia is due to acute infection, circulatory massage is inappropriate.

Very advanced anemia of any kind is fairly rare. However, if the blood is especially low in hemoglobin or oxygen, the heart has to work extremely hard to pump the diminished supply through the body. For this reason, very advanced anemia of any kind contraindicates vigorous circulatory massage.

Modality Recommendations for Anemia

Deep Tissue Massage	Contraindicated when severe; otherwise supportive.
Lymphatic Drainage	Supportive.
Polarity	S: Indicated. R/D: Supportive.
PNF/MET/Stretching	Supportive.
Reflexology	Indicated; work liver, spleen, thyroid, lymphatic points.
Shiatsu	Indicated, especially in conjunction with Chinese herbs. Treat LV, SP, BL, K meridians and extensions systemically.
Swedish Massage	Indicated with caution for underlying conditions; can help reinforce parasympathetic state.
Trigger Point Therapy	Supportive.

See Chapter 1 for a brief description of each modality, including definitions of abbreviations.

Embolism, Thrombus

Definition: What Are They?

An ***embolism*** is a traveling clot or collection of debris, and ***thrombus*** is a lodged clot (Figure 5.3). Thrombi that form on the venous side of the systemic circuit are discussed in the section of this chapter on thrombophlebitis and deep vein thrombosis. Emboli and thrombi that form on the arterial side of the systemic circuit are part and parcel of the whole interrelated cardiovascular disease picture. Having them can cause heart trouble, and heart trouble can cause them.

Embolism, Thrombus in Brief

Pronunciation: EM-bo-lizm, THROM-bus

What are they?

Thrombi are stationary clots; emboli are clots that travel through the circulatory system. Emboli are usually composed of blood but may also be fragments of plaque, fat globules, air bubbles, tumors, or bone chips.

How are they recognized?

If venous thrombi break loose, or *embolize*, they can only land in the lungs, causing pulmonary embolism. Symptoms include shortness of breath, chest pain, and hemoptysis, or coughing up sputum that is streaked with blood. Many venous thrombi and pulmonary emboli are silent: they create no symptoms until the damage has been done.

Clots that form on the arterial side of the system can lodge anywhere their artery carries them. Some of the most common (and dangerous) locations for arterial clots to land are in the coronary arteries (heart attack), the brain (transient ischemic attack or stroke), and the kidneys (renal infarction).

Is massage indicated or contraindicated?

Any disorder associated with the potential for lodged or traveling clots contraindicates circulatory massage.

Etiology: What Happens?

Blood leaves the left ventricle of the heart via the aorta and goes to its destination through smaller and smaller vessels: arteries, arterioles, and finally capillaries. Nutrient–waste exchange happens at the capillary level, and then the vessels get bigger and bigger as they lead toward the right atrium: from venules to veins to the vena cava. The same telescoping action happens in the pulmonary circuit: blood leaves the right ventricle through the huge pulmonary artery, and vessels going into the lungs get smaller and smaller. Oxygen and carbon dioxide are exchanged in capillaries in the lungs, and the freshly oxygenated blood goes back toward the heart through venules, veins, and finally the large pulmonary vein.

Platelets constantly flow through the circulatory system looking for rough spots, which indicate injury. If they find any disruption in the walls of the blood vessels, they quickly develop spikes and stick to that spot. Then they release the chemicals that cause blood proteins to weave fibers, making a net to catch other blood cells, and a clot is formed. Clots can also form in places where blood doesn't flow quickly; clotting factors accumulate enough to thicken the fluid even without an injury to initiate the action. This kind of stasis thrombosis happens frequently enough that it now has a name: "coach class syndrome".

The construction of the circulatory system is such that clots cannot pass through capillaries; they form and remain either on the arterial side of the systemic circuit or on the venous side. The damage that ensues depends on the origin of the clot, its size, and where it finally gets stuck.

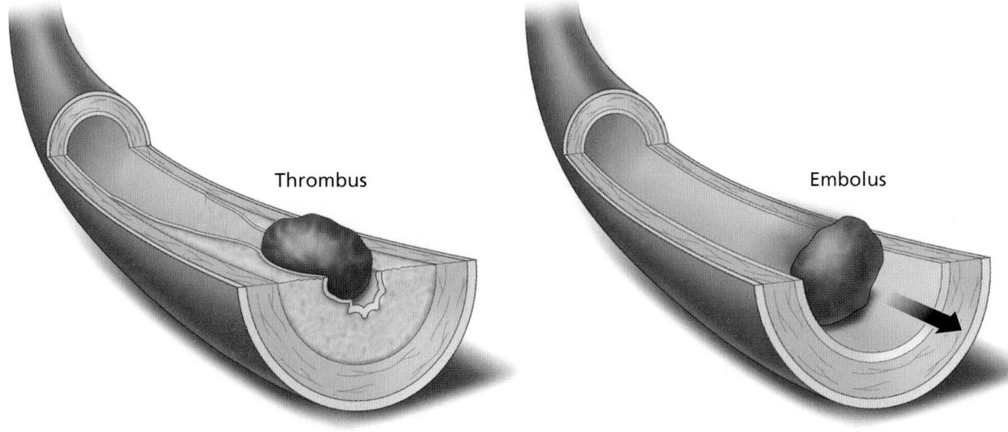

Figure 5.3. A. thrombus is a lodged clot; an embolus is a moving clot.

Pulmonary Embolism

The lungs are the one and only destination for clots or debris anywhere on the venous side of the systemic circuit, unless the heart has a structural defect called a patent foramen ovale, which allows communication between the left and right sides. When something, often a sudden movement after prolonged immobility, knocks any debris in any vein loose, it jets toward the heart in increasingly big tubes. It goes through the right atrium and ventricle, enters the pulmonary artery, and ends up in the lungs (Figure 5.4). Most pulmonary emboli are fragments that lodge in multiple places in both lungs simultaneously. The extent of damage can vary from a temporary loss of a tiny bit of lung function to total circulatory collapse when suddenly little or no blood returns to the heart from the lungs.

Every year about 650,000 people in the United States have a pulmonary embolism.[2] Many of them resolve spontaneously, but about 200,000 people die of pulmonary embolism every year.[3] This condition is usually related to thrombophlebitis or deep vein thrombosis as a complication of immobility, surgery, or trauma.

Risk factors for pulmonary embolism Risk factors for pulmonary embolism include other types of cardiovascular disease, recent trauma, extended bed rest, and any kind of surgery, although surgeries for femur and hip fractures or any gynecological problem have a particularly high embolism rate. Pulmonary embolism is the third leading cause of death in hospitals.[2]

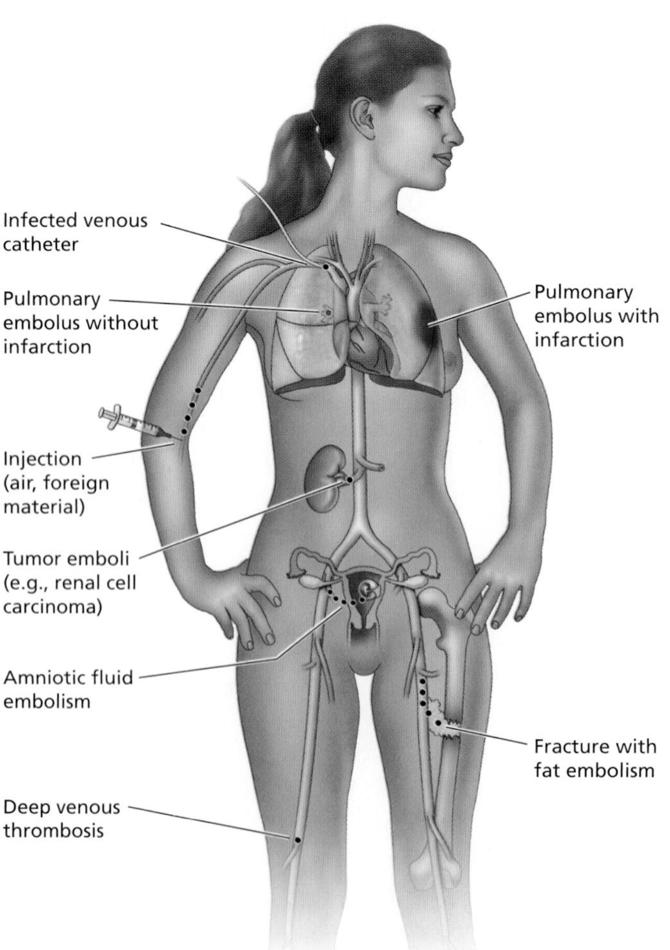

Figure 5.4. Sources of pulmonary embolism.

Women who are pregnant or who have recently given birth are at high risk for pulmonary embolism, as the weight of the uterus on the femoral vessels can cause blood to pool and thicken in the legs, and hormonal changes associated with pregnancy and childbirth can also thicken the blood.

Other risk factors include being overweight, smoking, and taking hormones for birth control or as hormone replacement therapy.

Signs and symptoms of pulmonary embolism Some studies estimate that up to 80% of pulmonary embolism cases show no discernible signs or symptoms until after lung damage has occurred. Classic symptoms of pulmonary embolism include difficulty breathing, chest pains, and **hemoptysis** (coughing with bloody sputum), but many people don't show this pattern. Other symptoms that may or may not be present are shortness of breath, lightheadedness, fainting, dizziness, rapid heartbeat, and sweating. Chest pain and chest wall tenderness along with back, shoulder or abdominal pain are also possible.

Complications of pulmonary embolism A person with a history of pulmonary embolism is at increased risk for having another episode. Further, if a significant amount of lung function is lost, pulmonary hypertension and right-sided heart failure may develop as the heart tries to push blood through the damaged, restricted pulmonary circuit.

Treatment of pulmonary embolism Treatment of non–life-threatening pulmonary embolism is usually an aggressive course of thrombolytics and anticoagulants and attention to the cause of the deep vein thrombosis. If it is a major embolism, surgery may be required to remove it from the lung.

Prevention of pulmonary embolism Pulmonary embolism is the leading cause of death from surgical complication. Because this condition is very difficult to diagnose early, emphasis has shifted from treatment to prophylaxis, or prevention. Preventive measures include identifying patients who are at particularly high risk for developing clots, administering low-dose anticoagulants starting shortly before surgery, elevation of the legs, external compression on the legs, and early walking following surgery.

Arterial Embolism

This is one of the many complications of atherosclerosis. Emboli in the arteries can also be a complication of bacterial infection, ***atrial fibrillation*** (uncoordinated flutter of the atrium instead of a rhythmic, strong contraction), or rheumatic heart disease, which can produce clots inside the heart. Emboli can be made of some foreign object in the bloodstream such as a bit of plaque, a bone chip, an air bubble, or a knot of cancer cells.

The main difference between arterial and venous emboli is the final resting place. If the clot is on the arterial side of the systemic system, it could wind up virtually anywhere *except* the lungs. Therefore, the damage it causes is very different. The brain, the heart, the kidneys, and the legs are statistically the most common sites for arterial emboli to lodge.

Signs and symptoms of arterial embolism Symptoms of emboli in organs may be nonexistent until the affected tissue has significant loss of function. This is particularly dangerous in the kidneys, where many tiny clots can come to rest somewhere in the renal arteries, leading to progressive renal failure. If clots lodge in the legs, however, symptoms are sharp, tingling pain followed by numbness, weakness, coldness, and blueness. Left untreated, this tissue may become necrotic in a matter of hours; immediate medical attention is necessary.

If the embolus lodges in the brain and the symptoms are short-lived, it is called a transient ischemic attack. A more serious brain embolism can cause an ischemic stroke. And finally, if it lodges in a coronary artery, it's called a heart attack.

Treatment

If a person has a tendency to form clots easily, anticoagulant medications may be prescribed to circumvent the complications of heart attack or stroke.

Massage?

The tendency to form thrombi or emboli systemically contraindicates rigorous circulatory massage. Lodged thrombi are a medical emergency. If a person knows an embolism is present in either the venous or arterial side of the system, he or she should be under treatment. Clients who take anticoagulant medications require extra care from massage therapists. These clients have two significant issues: they have a history of excessive clotting, and they are taking medication that limits their ability to clot, which means they bruise and bleed easily. Both of these contraindicate the use of techniques that push a lot of fluid or challenge the tissue to the point that bruising might occur.

Modality Recommendations for Embolism, Thrombus	
Deep Tissue Massage	Systemically contraindicated.
Lymphatic Drainage	Systemically contraindicated.
Polarity	S: Indicated; can help reinforce a parasympathetic state. R/D: Systemically contraindicated.
PNF/MET/Stretching	Supportive.
Reflexology	Systemically contraindicated.
Shiatsu	Systemically contraindicated.
Swedish Massage	Systemically contraindicated; later, be aware that anticoagulant use requires gentle touch.
Trigger Point Therapy	Systemically contraindicated.

See Chapter 1 for a brief description of each modality, including definitions of abbreviations.

Hematoma

Definition: What Is It?

The term ***hematoma*** refers to extensive bleeding and pooling of blood in hollow areas. This can happen in several locations. The leakage of blood from damaged superficial capillaries is called a bruise, or ***ecchymosis***. The familiar injury that happens when a person hammers his thumb or catches her finger in the door is called a subungual hematoma. Inside the cranium hematoma can be a result of traumatic brain injury or a ruptured aneurysm. Blood can also accumulate between muscle sheaths as a result of trauma or a complication of hemophilia.

Signs and Symptoms

Bruises are reddish or purplish (or black and blue) in the acute stage. They fade to yellowish green in the subacute stage, when the macrophages have migrated in to clean up the debris. The processes for cleaning up capillary leaks deeper than the skin, for instance in a gastrocnemius that has been kicked, are invisible but otherwise identical.

Larger bleeds can involve extensive inflammation along with discoloration. They can occur when an arteriole inside a muscle or between deep muscle layers is injured. It pours blood into an area until local pressure closes it off. A large acute hematoma feels like hot half-congealed gelatin under the muscle layers, and it is quite painful to the touch. They happen most often in large fleshy areas such as the calf, thigh, or buttocks.

Treatment

Small bruises require no medical intervention, although they respond well to alternating hot and cold applications, which stimulate macrophages to come into the area and flush away wastes from the tissue damage.

Bruises under fingernails or toenails require no attention if they discolor less than 25% of the nail area. Larger subungual hematomas are recommended for medical attention to drain the bleeding and to check for damage to the nail bed that may cause permanent disfiguration to the nail.

Large intermuscular bleeds can be complicated. If they're caught relatively early, they can be aspirated or drained, but if they're left too long, they are likely to congeal from the concentration of clotting factors in the blood. At that point only time, hydrotherapy, and gentle movement will help to break up the pooled blood into a form that the body can reabsorb.

Hematomas can complicate into more serious problems. A bleed on the anterior lower leg can cause *acute compartment syndrome*, which can lead to nerve damage and other problems. Another complication of hematoma occurs when the leaked blood calcifies into a mass that looks like a bone chip embedded in soft tissue; this is myositis ossificans.

Hematoma in Brief

Pronunciation: he-mah-TOE-mah

What is it?
A hematoma is a deep bruise (leakage of blood) between muscle sheaths or in other soft tissues.

How is it recognized?
Superficial hematomas are simple bruises. Deep bleeds may not be visible, but they are painful, and if extensive bleeding has occurred, a characteristic gel-like feel develops in the affected tissue.

Is massage indicated or contraindicated?
Massage is at least locally contraindicated for acute hematomas because of the possibility of blood clots and pain. In the subacute stage (at least 2 days later), when the surrounding blood vessels have been sealed shut and the body is breaking down and reabsorbing the debris, gentle massage around the perimeter of the area and hydrotherapy can be helpful.

Massage?

Hematomas and bruises contraindicate local massage in the acute stage because of pain and the possibility of disturbing blood clots. In the subacute stages (at least 2 days after the injury occurs) the local blood vessels are generally sealed off. Gentle massage may be appropriate around the edges of the lesions, always within the tolerance of the client. This can be coupled with alternating hot and cold applications to speed the turnover of circulation and the reabsorption of leaked blood.

Modality Recommendations for Hematoma

Modality	Recommendation
Deep Tissue Massage	Locally contraindicated; otherwise supportive.
Lymphatic Drainage	Indicated in subacute stage.
Polarity	S: Indicated. R/D: Locally contraindicated; light work above/below site to client comfort when subacute.
PNF/MET/Stretching	Locally contraindicated; otherwise supportive.
Reflexology	Locally contraindicated; work heart, solar plexus, and endocrine points.
Shiatsu	Locally contraindicated; indicated elsewhere. Treat LV and SP systemically. Avoid pressure at the local site.
Swedish Massage	Locally contraindicated; in subacute stage use local caution and stay within pain tolerance.
Trigger Point Therapy	Locally contraindicated; otherwise supportive.

See Chapter 1 for a brief description of each modality, including definitions of abbreviations.

Hemophilia

Definition: What Is It?

Hemophilia is a genetic disorder characterized by the absence of some plasma proteins that are crucial in the clot-forming process. It is actually a collection of genetic disorders, each one of them affecting a different clotting factor in the blood. Their presentations are all much the same, however, so the only people who need to know which type of hemophilia is present are the patients themselves and the people who care for them.

Demographics: Who Gets It?

In this country hemophilia affects about 18,000 men. The incidence of the most common variety is about 1 in 5,000 males, and the disease appears equally among races and socioeconomic status. It is identified in about 400 boys every year. The disease is carried on the X chromosome, so males with hemophilia pass the chromosome along to their daughters, who become carriers. These female carriers pass the mutation on to about half of their sons. About one-third of hemophilia cases occur as a spontaneous mutation, with no family history of the disorder.

It is possible for a girl to have hemophilia, but she would need positive X chromosomes from both her father and mother, and this is very rare.

Etiology: What Happens?

Thrombocytes constantly cruise around the circulatory system looking for signs of damage. When they encounter any kind of rough spot inside a blood vessel, they stick to that spot and secrete a series of chemicals that cause plasma proteins to weave nets of fibers called *fibrinogen*. These nets catch passing platelets and red blood cells, forming a plug to limit loss of blood through the damaged vessel. The plasma proteins that weave the fibrinogen have been identified as 12 distinct factors. Hemophilia occurs when a genetic mutation causes a deficiency in one or more of these clotting factors.

The most common variety of hemophilia is hemophilia A, which accounts for about 80% of all cases. It is characterized by a deficiency in clotting factor VIII. Hemophilia B, also called Christmas disease, is characterized by insufficient levels of factor IX. Hemophilia B accounts for about 15% of hemophilia cases. Other clotting factor deficiencies are possible, but they are much rarer than hemophilia A or B.

A person who is deficient in clotting factor VIII or IX has difficulty in forming a solid, long-lasting clot. Hemophiliacs don't bleed *faster* than average, but they do bleed *longer*. Hemophilia is rated as mild, moderate, or severe, depending on what percentage of normal levels of clotting factors the patient has. Severe hemophiliacs, who account for 60% of hemophilia patients, have lower than 1% of normal levels of clotting factors.

Hemophilia in Brief

Pronunciation: he-mo-FELE-e-ah

What is it?
Hemophilia is a genetic disorder in which certain clotting factors in the blood are either insufficient or missing altogether.

How is it recognized?
Hemophilia can cause superficial bleeding that persists for longer than normal, or internal bleeding into joint cavities or between muscle sheaths with little or no provocation.

Is massage indicated or contraindicated?
Severe cases of hemophilia contraindicate bodywork that can mechanically stretch, manipulate, or accidentally injure delicate tissues. Energetic work can be powerful and effective for pain management. Milder cases of hemophilia may be safer for circulatory massage.

Signs and Symptoms

Hemophilia first appears at birth, when the umbilical cord bleeds excessively, or in early childhood, as babies begin to engage in physical activities that involve minor bangs and bumps. These toddlers are subject to excessive bruising and bleeding with very mild irritation, and small scrapes and lesions tend to bleed for a long time.

As the person matures, he finds that he is prone to subcutaneous bleeding (bruising), intramuscular hemorrhaging (hematomas), nosebleeds (*epistaxis*), blood in the urine (*hematuria*), and severe joint pain brought about by bleeding in joint cavities. Bleeding episodes may follow minor trauma, or they may occur spontaneously.

Complications

The leading cause of death for children with hemophilia is intracranial bleeding: even minor head trauma can cause major bleeding episodes in and around the brain.

Bleeding into joint cavities is a significant problem for people with hemophilia. Unless clotting factors are administered very soon after an episode, the blood inside the joint may collect and lead to an inflammatory response that damages cartilage and articulating bones. This condition is called ***hemophilic arthritis***, and it occurs most often at the ankles, knees, and elbows.

Bleeding into muscles can cause pain and numbness as nerve endings are compressed. If the pressure is not quickly resolved, the muscle may develop a contracture, with a permanent loss of range of motion. The muscles most at risk for hematomas are in the calf, thigh, upper arm, and forearm. The psoas is also at risk for deep bleeds and stiffness.

Infected blood products used to be another major worry for people with hemophilia. Before screening methods were used consistently, contracting HIV or hepatitis was a significant risk for hemophiliacs. Blood and plasma screening now filters out most viruses, but some pathogens can still get through. It is recommended that hemophiliacs and other people who regularly use blood products be vaccinated for hepatitis A and B.

The development of genetically engineered clotting factor has improved the quality of life for many people with hemophilia, but a small number of patients develop resistance to this product. They may have to use other blood products until the hypersensitivity reaction subsides.

SIDEBAR 5.1: VON WILLEBRAND DISEASE: AN EQUAL OPPORTUNITY MUTATION

The kinds of hemophilia that most of us are familiar with involve X-linked genes that affect clotting factors VII or XI. But these types of hemophilia affect a relatively small proportion of the population. It turns out that another type of genetic mutation causes different clotting factor deficiency, and it is *not* on the X chromosome, which means men and women equally can be affected.

The condition is called von Willebrand disease, and it is a deficiency or poor quality of von Willebrand factor, one of the last clotting factors to participate in the cascade of chemical reactions that cause the spinning of fibrinogen to make blood clots. Von Willebrand disease is the most common genetically linked bleeding disorder in the world.

Von Willebrand disease is usually very mild. Signs and symptoms include frequent bloody noses, bleeding from the gums, and in women, heavy menstrual flow. A person may never be diagnosed until he or she has a tooth pulled or goes through childbirth or undergoes some other experience that can lead to prolonged bleeding.

If a client knows he or she has von Willebrand disease, no special precautions need to be taken for massage other than to avoid bruises and other lesions, but these are precautions for all clients.

Treatment

Treatment protocols for people with hemophilia have taken gigantic leaps forward in the past 30 years. Before 1965 the only treatment available was transfusion of whole blood, a time-consuming and inefficient means of replacing clotting factors for someone with an internal hemorrhage. Consequently, most hemophiliacs were in wheelchairs by their teens, and their life expectancy was much shorter than the norm. In 1965 techniques were developed to isolate the specific missing clotting factors, allowing a much more efficient treatment.

More recently, clotting factors have been manufactured in a form that can be stored at home and self-administered. These recombinant factors radically increase a hemophiliac's independence and ability to work and travel.

Synthetic or blood-based clotting factors can be administered after an injury takes place to limit bleeding into a joint or between muscles. They can also be taken prophylactically, before a surgical or dental procedure, for instance, to limit anticipated bleeding.

People with mild hemophilia A can also treat themselves with an injected or inhaled form of the hormone *desmopressin*, which stimulates production of extra clotting factor in response to an injury.

In addition to managing bleeding, people with hemophilia are counseled to exercise (although they must obviously avoid contact sports) and to keep their weight under control; both of these can limit the risk of arthritis and muscle contracture. Physical therapy may be suggested to help rehabilitate injured joints or muscles.

Massage?

Severe hemophilia contraindicates rigorous mechanical circulatory massage. Clients and therapists should consult with the client's medical team about receiving bodywork, and the therapist should use pressure that the client experiences as part of everyday activity.

Energetic and noncirculatory techniques are appropriate and welcome and often have powerful effect on stress and pain sensation.

Modality Recommendations for Hemophilia

Deep Tissue Massage	Contraindicated for deep work.
Lymphatic Drainage	Supportive.
Polarity	S: Indicated. R: Supportive with light touch. D: Systemically contraindicated.
PNF/MET/Stretching	Supportive.
Reflexology	Indicated for extremely light work: focus on heart, solar plexus, endocrine points.
Shiatsu	Supportive.
Swedish Massage	Supportive with gentle techniques; no tapotement or deep pressure.
Trigger Point Therapy	Systemically contraindicated for deep work.

See Chapter 1 for a brief description of each modality, including definitions of abbreviations.

Leukemia

Leukemia in Brief
Pronunciation: lu-KE-me-ah

What is it?
Leukemia is a collection of blood disorders characterized by production of nonfunctioning white blood cells in bone marrow.

How is it recognized?
Different types of leukemia have slightly different profiles, but all varieties include signs brought about by interference with the production of normal blood cells: anemia, bruising, bleeding, and low resistance to infection.

Is massage indicated or contraindicated?
Both leukemia and treatments for it wreak havoc with the immune system. While some types of bodywork may be supportive during this time, care must be taken to protect the client from any threat of infection.

Definition: What Is It?

Leukemia, or *white blood*, is a cancer of white blood cells produced in bone marrow. Some overlap has been established between types of leukemia that affect lymphoid cells and lymphoma: cancer associated with lymph nodes. Lymphoma is discussed in Chapter 6.

Dozens of types of leukemia have been identified, but this article focuses on the four most common classifications. These types of leukemia have much in common, but each has some unique features that are examined under individual headings.

Demographics: Who Gets It?

Leukemia in various forms is diagnosed in about 35,000 Americans every year, and it causes about 22,000 deaths. Although this disease is the leading cause of death from cancer in children, it is much more common in adults. About 208,000 leukemia patients are living in the United States today.[4]

The overall survival rate has tripled in the past four decades to about 48%. Children with this disease often have a better prognosis than mature adults. For more details about leukemia statistics, see Sidebar 5.2.

SIDEBAR 5.2: TYPES OF LEUKEMIA: INDIVIDUAL DISCUSSIONS

The four major classes of leukemia have some characteristics and statistical information[4] that distinguish them from each other. Massage therapists working with clients who have leukemia should become familiar with some of the basic features of their client's condition.

Acute Myelogenous Leukemia

Basic Information

Acute myelogenous leukemia (AML) is a rapidly progressive cancer of the myeloid group of white blood cells. The immature cancer cells are called blast cells, leading to the synonym *acute myeloblastic leukemia*. (Other synonyms are *acute myelocytic leukemia* and *acute granulocytic leukemia*.) The genetic damage that causes AML has been associated with certain specific environmental factors. High doses of radiation, chemotherapy for other types of cancer, and exposure to benzene all increase the risk of contracting AML in later years.

Because this variety of leukemia is aggressive and rapidly progressive, it is important to start treatment as soon as possible. The steps in administering chemotherapy are outlined in the general treatment section.

Statistics for AML

About 12,000 new cases of AML are diagnosed every year in the United States, and about 26,000 people are living with this disease. Although it can occur in young adults, this variety of leukemia is associated with age. Most cases occur in people over 50 years old; the average age at diagnosis is 65.

Chronic Myelogenous Leukemia

Basic Information

Chronic myelogenous leukemia (CML) is a slow-growing cancer of myelogenous cells in the bone marrow. It is also called *chronic granulocytic leukemia* and *chronic myeloid leukemia*. It involves the myeloid cells: granulocytes (which include neutrophils, eosinophils, and basophils) and monocytes.

CML is characterized by production of nonfunctioning white blood cells, but these are produced relatively slowly and they are released into the bloodstream when they are fully mature. These faulty cells can interfere with and slow down normal immune system activity, but they do not usually bring it to a halt.

CML patients often have an enlarged spleen and pain, as the cancerous cells congregate in this organ. Night sweats, unexpected weight loss, and a decreasing tolerance for warm temperatures are other signs and symptoms common to CML patients.

CML occasionally changes its pattern and becomes more aggressive. This is called an *accelerated phase* of the disease, and it is treated as if it were AML.

Statistics for CML

About 5,000 new cases of CML are diagnosed in the United States every year. Most patients are adults, but a small number of children contract CML.[5] The survival rate for untreated CML is poor: about 15 to 25% of patients survive for 5 years. When the cancer is treated with chemotherapy and/or bone marrow stem cell transplants, the survival rate is much better.

Acute Lymphocytic Leukemia

Basic Information

Acute lymphocytic leukemia (ALL) is a rapidly progressive, aggressive form of leukemia characterized by DNA mutations in stem cells that produce bone marrow lymphocytes. Synonyms for ALL include *acute lymphoid leukemia* and *acute lymphoblastic leukemia*.

ALL is an aggressive cancer of bone marrow lymphocytes. The proliferation of cancerous cells is so overwhelming that all other bone marrow activity is suppressed and immune system function is crippled. Cancerous lymphocytes are released into the blood before they are fully mature. These lymphocytes may gather in lymph nodes, or they may gain access to the central nervous system, where they accumulate and can cause severe headaches, vomiting, and seizures.

Causative agents and risk factors for ALL are not clear, but this disease has been associated with high doses of radiation and exposure to toxic substances during gestation or in early childhood.

Statistics for ALL

ALL affects young children more often than adults—until adults become mature. The incidence of this disease peaks among 4-year-olds and then subsides among older children and young adults. It becomes more common among people over 50.

ALL is most common in developed countries and among higher socioeconomic groups. About 4,000 new cases of ALL are diagnosed in the United States each year; about half of them are in children. The remission rate in children is 80%. Among adults the 5-year survival rate is 25% to 35%.

Chronic Lymphocytic Leukemia

Basic Information

Chronic lymphocytic leukemia (CLL) is a slow-growing version of lymphocytic leukemia. Although it can involve T cells or natural killer cells, most cases involve B-cell malignancies.

Sometimes CLL is so stable and so nonthreatening that no treatment is recommended. If numbers of functioning blood cells drop to dangerous levels, chemotherapy may be recommended, along with radiation to shrink enlarged lymph nodes or other tissues.

Statistics for CLL

CLL is found primarily in elderly people. Up to 95% of cases are among patients over 50, and the incidence rises sharply with age. About 10,000 cases of CLL are diagnosed every year.

CLL has the best prognosis of all the types of leukemia: 71% of patients make it to 5 years of remission.

Etiology: What Happens?

Healthy leukocytes come in several shapes and sizes, each with a specific role to play in the effort to keep us free from potential invaders.

Most white blood cells are produced in bone marrow. They develop from nonspecific blood stem cells into whatever type of cell is needed at the moment. Two types of stem cells, myeloid and lymphoid, manufacture white blood cells in bone marrow. Leukocytes are classified as myeloid or lymphocytic, depending on their origin. Leukemia occurs when a mutation in the DNA of one or more stem cells in the bone marrow causes the production of multitudes of nonfunctioning leukocytes. These cells can crowd out the functioning cells in the bone marrow and in the blood. Leukemia can be aggressive and quickly progressive, releasing immature cells into the circulatory system (acute), or it can be slowly progressive, leading to the release of mature but nonfunctioning cells (chronic). In either case, the mutated cells cannot function as part of the immune system, and they live far longer than normal cells, leading to dangerous accumulations of nonfunctioning cells. The four most common varieties of leukemia are as follows:

- *Acute myelogenous leukemia* (AML) is aggressive cancer of the myeloid cells.
- *Chronic myelogenous leukemia* (CML) is slowly progressive cancer of the myeloid cells.
- *Acute lymphocytic leukemia* (ALL) is aggressive cancer of the lymphocytes.
- *Chronic lymphocytic leukemia* (CLL) is slowly progressive cancer of the lymphocytes.

Each of these is discussed in more detail in Sidebar 5.2.

Unlike many types of cancer, leukemia spreads through the blood rather than the lymph. It can cause tumors in the lymph nodes (although not as readily as lymphoma), and it also affects the liver, spleen, testes, skin, and central nervous system.

The genetic mutations seen with leukemia are usually acquired rather than inherited. Exposure to environmental toxins and radiation are cited most often as contributing factors. Electromagnetic fields are being studied as possible risk factors for leukemia, but results so far are inconclusive. Some forms of leukemia are linked to a congenital problem: Down syndrome and some other genetic anomalies can increase the risk for these diseases.

Untreated leukemia results in death from excessive bleeding or infection.

Signs and Symptoms

Signs and symptoms of all types of leukemia point to bone marrow dysfunction. When the marrow is sabotaged by a genetic mutation that causes overproduction of nonfunctioning cells, functioning cells are produced in smaller numbers if at all. A leading sign of leukemia is fatigue and low stamina due to anemia: low numbers of red blood cells are available to deliver oxygen to working tissues. A person with leukemia bruises easily or may bruise with no particular trauma. Small cuts and abrasions may bleed for long periods. Unusual bleeding or bruising comes about because platelet production is suppressed (***thrombocytopenia***) and the person has limited ability to make blood clots. Finally, a person with leukemia is susceptible to chronic infections—these can be skin infections such as hangnails or pimples, or they can be respiratory infections such as colds and flu. They can even be chronic urinary tract infections. Whatever the infectious agent is, the person with leukemia has very limited resources to fight it off, because functioning white blood cells are in short supply.

Diagnosis

All types of leukemia are diagnosed by a combination of blood tests, bone marrow biopsies, and examination of cerebrospinal fluid for signs of metastasis. It is important to find out exactly which kinds of cells have been affected and whether the cancer is an acute or chronic variety. Furthermore, each type of leukemia has subtypes that respond differently to various treatment options.

Recent breakthroughs in the study of cell form and lineage have revealed that the lymphocytic leukemias that affect T cells, B cells, and natural killer cells are essentially the same as associated forms of lymphoma; the only difference is in whether the targeted cells are stationary or circulating. This has allowed for more accurate diagnoses and more effective treatments of these blood cancers.

Treatment

Leukemia treatment depends to a certain extent on what types of cells have been affected, how aggressive the disease is, and what kinds of treatments the patient has already had. Treatment usually begins with chemotherapy: administration of chemicals that are highly toxic to any cells that reproduce rapidly. Exactly which chemotherapy drugs are used depends on the type of cancer that is present. A course of chemotherapy for leukemia usually takes place in four stages:

- *Induction.* Chemotherapeutic drugs are introduced into the system, usually intravenously. The goal is to suppress cancer cells and to begin a period of remission.
- *Consolidation.* Once the process has begun, chemotherapy continues in high doses for several weeks or months in an effort to establish and maintain remission.
- *Central nervous system prophylaxis.* Some types of leukemia attack the central nervous system, but normal chemotherapeutic agents are blocked from these areas by the blood-brain barrier. To overcome this, chemotherapeutic drugs may be introduced directly into the central nervous system. Radiation therapy may be employed for this as well.
- *Maintenance therapy.* Continuing repeated tests and treatments as necessary are applied to keep the cancer in remission.

If a person doesn't respond well to chemotherapy or if the cancer keeps recurring (refractory leukemia), it is necessary to explore other treatment options. This can include adding radiation therapy or surgery, especially if cancerous cells have aggressively invaded any particular organ or location.

The treatment options for leukemia (and other types of cancer) are broadening every day. The use of bone marrow transplants with preserved marrow of the patient (*autogenic transplants*) or closely matched donors (*allogenic transplants*) is useful for some leukemia cases, but the incidence of complications is high. It is also possible to harvest stem cells from the bloodstream, bone marrow, or umbilical cords of healthy people and to transplant these "cellular blanks" into leukemia patients so that they can make healthy, functioning blood cells.

New treatments for leukemia also include the use of interferon or other medication to slow the production of cancerous cells and the use of manufactured antibodies that are designed to identify and destroy cancer cells. One new drug has been used successfully to suppress cellular replication for a previously untreatable form of leukemia; more drugs in this category are in development.

The treatment for leukemia, especially the acute varieties, can seem to take as hard a toll on the body as the disease itself. Chemotherapy introduces substances whose function is to kill off any rapidly reproducing cell. Unfortunately, this doesn't just mean cancer cells; it also means epithelial cells in the skin and the digestive tract and, ironically, healthy blood cells. The side effects of chemotherapy on epithelial tissues include development of ulcers in the mouth, nausea and diarrhea from gastrointestinal irritation, and hair loss as the epithelial cells in follicles are killed. One of the difficulties with digestive system disturbances is that if the patient can't eat well, the whole system becomes weaker and less able to cope with the stresses of both the disease and its treatment.

Chemotherapy also exacerbates symptoms of leukemia, as red and white blood cells and platelets are suppressed. Consequently, chemotherapy patients often have anemia, clotting problems, and low resistance to infection—all signs of leukemia itself.

Massage?

Leukemia is a type of cancer that can spread through the circulatory system. It involves seriously impaired immunity and a tendency to bleed easily. Some types of bodywork, especially those that enlist the healing energies of the client rather than trying to impose outside forces on blood flow or tissue manipulation, are helpful and supportive for a person going through a difficult, stressful, and often painful process. It is important in this situation to work as part of a well-informed health care team, so that the possibility of secondary infection or other complications can be carefully avoided.

The benefits massage can bring to cancer patients (reinforcing a parasympathetic state, improving immune system function, reducing pain perception) can be enjoyed with a minimum of risk if simple precautions are taken. For more guidelines about massage in the context of cancer and cancer treatments, see Chapter 12.

Modality Recommendations for Leukemia	
Deep Tissue Massage	Supportive as part of a health care team. Respect stage of recovery and treatment challenges.
Lymphatic Drainage	Supportive, especially during chemotherapy.
Polarity	S: Indicated. R/D: Supportive with light work.
PNF/MET/Stretching	Supportive.
Reflexology	Indicated; work lymphatic and pituitary points.
Shiatsu	Indicated to strengthen immune system. Treat K, TH, SP. Add fire meridians for blood and water meridians for bone/marrow/brain.
Swedish Massage	Supportive; stay within client's activity limitations.
Trigger Point Therapy	Supportive with light work.

See Chapter 1 for a brief description of each modality, including definitions of abbreviations.

Malaria

Definition: What Is It?

Malaria is a vector-borne infection of blood cells. The causative agent is one of four single-celled parasites from the *Plasmodium* genus of protozoa, and the vector is the bite of an infected female mosquito from the *Anopheles* species. This species is common all over the world, including in the United States, where it is also the vector for West Nile encephalitis.

Demographics: Who Gets It?

Globally, as many as 500 million people are infected with malaria each year. It causes 1.5 to 3 million deaths each year; the average age at death is 4 years. Most malaria cases (up to 90%)

are in sub-Saharan Africa, but it is also common in India, the Middle East, Southeast Asia, Oceania, and Central and South America.[5]

Malaria used to be common in the United States until massive eradication efforts essentially eliminated it by the early 1950s.[6] Nonetheless, between 1,000 and 2,000 cases of malaria are diagnosed here each year. Most of them are in recent travelers to areas where the infection is endemic, but some cases are native to this continent.

Malaria in Brief
Pronunciation: mah-LARE-e-ah

What is it?
Malaria is an infection of the blood with one of four parasites that invade erythrocytes. It is spread through the bite of *Anopheles* mosquitoes.

How is it recognized?
Malaria protozoa typically gestate for 1 to 3 weeks before causing symptoms, although it can take longer. When they appear, symptoms include extreme fluctuations of fever and chills along with nausea, vomiting, and diarrhea. Anemia and jaundice develop when red blood cells are destroyed. The most serious form of malaria can invade the brain and cause liver and kidney failure, coma, and death.

Is massage indicated or contraindicated?
Anyone displaying symptoms of malaria, especially someone who is a recent traveler from areas where this disease is endemic, needs to see a doctor, not a massage therapist. When the disease has been treated and all risk of liver or kidney damage has been addressed, massage can be safe and appropriate.

Etiology: What Happens?

The protozoa that cause malaria have a complex life cycle, requiring time to mature in both a mosquito and a human host. Four types of *Plasmodium* protozoa have been identified in this disease process: *P. ovale*, *P. vivax*, *P. malariae*, and *P. falciparum*.

When a human is bitten by an infected mosquito (only females take blood meals), an immature form of the parasite is introduced into the bloodstream. It travels to the liver, where it grows for 6 to 9 days. At that time it reenters the bloodstream, where it begins to invade healthy red blood cells.

The protozoa feed on hemoglobin and replicate inside the red blood cells. Finally the infected cells rupture, releasing toxic wastes and more protozoa. Newly released protozoa invade more erythrocytes. When an uninfected mosquito bites this person, immature protozoa enter the insect to begin the cycle again.

The less virulent forms of malaria protozoa are not life threatening, but *P. falciparum* can invade and damage tissues in the central nervous system, liver, and kidneys, leading to potentially fatal complications through liver failure, renal failure, and coma.

While malaria is usually spread through the bite of infected mosquitoes, it can also be transmitted through the placenta from mother to child or through blood transfusions or the use of shared needles.

Signs and Symptoms

The signs and symptoms of malaria include extreme fluctuations between fever and chills (these reflect whether red blood cells are being invaded or rupturing), in cycles that may recur over several days.

When enough red blood cells have been invaded, anemia develops. Malaria is a type of ***hemolytic*** anemia, in which red blood cells are destroyed faster than they can be replaced (Sidebar 5.3). Jaundice is another complication. It is related to the rapid destruction of erythrocytes that allows bilirubin to accumulate in the skin and mucous membranes.

A typical infection with the less virulent parasites lasts about 2 weeks and then subsides, but some parasites may remain in the liver to launch a new episode months or years later.

SIDEBAR 5.3: MALARIA AND SICKLE CELL DISEASE: A CLOSE CONNECTION

A person has sickle cell disease if he or she inherits a gene for it from *both* parents. If only one gene is present, a person has the sickle cell *trait* but not the disease. This is a crucial distinction because the sickle cell trait usually doesn't damage the body, although some people have mild anemia. But the presence of this single gene *does* limit the rupturing of erythrocytes during an attack of malaria. Sickle cell genes are mostly found in populations (and descendants of populations) from the Mediterranean, subtropical Africa, and Asia, otherwise called the *malarial belt*. Isn't it an amazing world?

Diagnosis

In areas where malaria is endemic, diagnosis is based on the presence of alternating fever and chills. In the United States many diagnoses are missed because the disease is so uncommon that practitioners often don't think to look for it; this leads to unnecessary illness and death each year.

The parasites can be identified in blood smears if technicians are skilled and know what to look for. Other tests to identify malaria-related antigens in the blood are in development. Some are available, particularly for use in developing countries where this disease is rampant, but they vary in accuracy and practicality because of costs.

Treatment

The treatment options for malaria are limited, and some parasites are developing an alarming resistance to chloroquine, the most common and cost-effective treatment option. This tendency, along with reports of increasing numbers of *P. falciparum* infections, is making the control of malaria an international health priority.

Most malaria patients can be treated successfully if they have full access to all the drugs necessary and if they take the drugs according to prescription. In developing countries, where malaria is most dangerous in young children, it costs about $19 to treat each case, and each household earns approximately $68 dollars per year.[7]

Prevention

Travelers to areas where malaria is common can take prophylactic medication that can help to prevent new malaria infections. Basic defense against mosquitoes is also recommended. This includes wearing long sleeves and pants; possibly using clothing treated with permethrin, which repels mosquitoes; and using treated netting over bedding.

A vaccine for malaria is in development but not yet available. Genome studies of both the parasites and the mosquitoes that carry them have revealed many potential ways to interrupt protozoan reproduction.

Massage?

A client who is having alternating bouts of high fever and bone-shaking chills is not a good candidate for massage. This person obviously needs to consult a doctor, especially after recent travel to an area where malaria is common. For people whose infection has been treated and who are not at risk for permanent kidney damage, bodywork is a safe and appropriate choice.

Modality Recommendations for Malaria	
Deep Tissue Massage	Contraindicated while acute; otherwise supportive.
Lymphatic Drainage	Contraindicated while acute; otherwise supportive.
Polarity	S/R/D: Contraindicated while acute; otherwise supportive.
PNF/MET/Sretching	Contraindicated while acute; otherwise supportive.
Reflexology	Indicated in remission; work lymphatic and pituitary points.
Shiatsu	Contraindicated when acute. Indicated, especially with Chinese herbs, in remission to strengthen the immune system and blood.
Swedish Massage	Contraindicated while acute, otherwise supportive when all signs and symptoms have resolved.
Trigger Point Therapy	Contraindicated while acute; otherwise supportive.

See Chapter 1 for a brief description of each modality, including definitions of abbreviations.

Myeloma

Definition: What Is It?

Myeloma (literally, "marrow tumor") is a blood cancer involving maturing B cells that are found in bone marrow.

Myeloma in Brief

Pronunciation: my-eh-LOE-mah

What is it?

Myeloma is a type of blood cancer that specifically affects B cells in bone marrow.

What does it look like?

The earliest sign of myeloma is usually bone pain associated with damage from growing tumors. Other signs can include low red blood cell count, low numbers of functioning white cells, kidney damage, and the presence of indicator proteins in the urine.

Is massage indicated or contraindicated?

As with all cancers, massage is indicated for support for a person going through an extremely difficult and challenging time. Myeloma patients require special care because of bone fragility, although they may also derive great benefit from the pain relief that careful massage can offer.

Demographics: Who Gets It?

Myeloma is diagnosed about 16,700 times each year in this country. About 58,300 people are living with this disease. Men slightly outnumber women. It is especially prevalent among African Americans, particularly older black men. It is usually diagnosed around age 70; it is rare in people under 45. Myeloma causes about 11,000 deaths per year.[4]

Etiology: What Happens?

The B cells that eventually produce antibodies to help fight off pathogenic invaders spend some time maturing in bone marrow. During this phase it is possible for some cells to undergo a mutation that causes them to do several things: they proliferate into tumors; they secrete cytokines that stimulate osteoclast activity; and they produce faulty antibodies.

Under normal circumstances the bone marrow holds only a few maturing B cells. When the cells are ready, they migrate to lymph tissue, where they operate as normal plasma cells, producing functioning antibodies. But when immature B cells become cancerous in the bone marrow, they rapidly proliferate into tumors. These usually grow in bone tissue (typically the spine, pelvis, ribs, or skull), but occasionally tumors form elsewhere: these are called ***plastocytomas***. Tumors inside bone marrow can interfere with normal blood cell production, leading to the signs and symptoms of other blood cancers: anemia, poor clotting, and reduced resistance to infection. But myeloma cells secrete cytokines that signal osteoclasts to dismantle bone tissue. This makes more room for the growing tumor, and it leads to pathologic thinning or even holes in bone tissue.

Healthy B cells produce many types of functioning antibodies (also called immunoglobulins) that work in different ways to neutralize pathogens. Myeloma cells, on the other hand, produce massive amounts of nonfunctioning antibody molecules, called ***monoclonal immunoglobulins:*** monoclonal because they are all alike, and immunoglobulins because they are technically antibodies even though they don't offer any protective properties. Another name for monoclonal immunoglobulins is M-proteins.

Normal antibodies are Y-shaped proteins, and they are too big to pass through the kidneys into the urinary system. M-proteins have branches that sometimes break off during formation. These fragments, called ***Bence Jones proteins***, are small enough to pass through the filters in the kidney to be excreted in the urine. The good news about this is that myeloma can be detected and to a certain extent tracked through urinalysis. The bad news is that if the disease is rapidly progressive, the kidneys can sustain extensive damage and even fail altogether. Three types of myeloma have been identified:

- *Multiple myeloma* produces tumors at several sites. It is the most common form, accounting for 90% of myeloma diagnoses.
- *Solitary myeloma* is development of a single myeloma tumor in the bone marrow.
- ***Extramedullary plastocytoma*** is growth of myeloma tumors outside of bone tissue. These growths can develop in the skin, muscle, lungs, or other areas.

Signs and Symptoms

Myeloma can be silent in early stages; it is sometimes found during a routine medical examination. The earliest symptom for most people is pain or even fractures that occur as tumors corrode bone tissue. Other signs include anemia, frequent and persistent infections, kidney problems related to the excretion of Bence Jones proteins, calcium in the blood, and the risk of **amyloidosis**: the accumulation of inflammatory proteins on organs such as the heart or lungs, where they can do significant damage.

Compare and Contrast 5.1
Blood Cancers

Blood cancers are a confusing collection of conditions because they seem to overlap each other. Indeed, it has been found that some forms of leukemia are essentially the same as some forms of lymphoma, because they affect the same cells. The only difference is that when the cells circulate, it is called leukemia, and when cells are fixed inside lymph nodes, the disease is called lymphoma.

Overall, about 785,000 people in the United States are living with some kind of blood cancer. About 118,000 new diagnoses are made each year (about one every 5 minutes); and about 54,000 deaths from blood cancers occur each year in this country (about one every 10 minutes). The death rates for all types of blood cancers are decreasing, although as always, children have a better survival rates than older adults.[4]

FEATURES	LEUKEMIA	MYELOMA	LYMPHOMA
Cells affected	Any white blood cell: myeloid (monocytes, neutrophils, basophils, eosinophils) or lymphoid (T cells, B cells, natural killer cells)	Nearly mature B cells in bone marrow only	B cells, T cells, natural killer cells in lymph nodes or spleen
Earliest signs and symptoms	Anemia, thrombocytopenia, poor immune function	Bone pain from corroding tumors in marrow	Painless enlargement of lymph nodes, especially at jaw, axilla, groin

Diagnosis and Staging

Several tests can give accurate information about myeloma and the extent of its progression. Urinalysis can show the presence of Bence Jones proteins; a blood test may show M-proteins circulating in the blood; and a bone marrow aspiration or biopsy can show the presence of abnormal cells and tumors. Bone imaging tests (radiography and magnetic resonance imaging) can reveal how much bone has been damaged and where tumors are growing.

Myeloma is rated as stages I to III depending on the extent of myeloma cells and how much bone and/or kidney damage has accrued.

Treatment

Myeloma is often not responsive to treatment. If it is slow-growing, and especially if the patient is elderly and in poor health, a period of watchful waiting is recommended to delay difficult procedures as long as possible. A combination of chemotherapy and bone marrow stem cell transplantation is usually suggested, but even with these intrusive interventions the 5-year survival rate is only 33%.

Massage?

The guidelines for massage and myeloma are like those for any other blood cancer. The client is facing difficult challenges, and bodywork should support rather than test stability. That said, gentle massage may be recommended to ease the bone pain that affects many of these patients; this must be done with great care to avoid the risk of fractures.

MODALITY RECOMMENDATIONS FOR MYELOMA

Modality	Recommendation
Deep Tissue Massage	Supportive for pain management; focus on low back and hips.
Lymphatic Drainage	Supportive, especially during chemotherapy.
Polarity	S: Indicated, can support immune system. R/D: Supportive with light touch within client comfort.
PNF/MET/Stretching	Supportive.
Reflexology	Indicated; work lymphatic and pituitary points.
Shiatsu	Indicated to strengthen the immune system. Treat K, TH, SP. Add fire meridians for blood and water meridians for bone/marrow/brain.
Swedish Massage	Supportive; stay within clientís activity limitations; be cautious of bone weakness.
Trigger Point Therapy	Supportive, with caution for bone fragility.

See Chapter 1 for a brief description of each modality, including definitions of abbreviations.

Sickle Cell Disease

Definition: What Is It?

Sickle cell disease is an autosomal recessive genetic condition that results in production of abnormal hemoglobin, the protein that carries oxygen in red blood cells.

Demographics: Who Gets It?

The sickle cell gene is most common in specific populations. Blacks, Hispanics, and people from Italy, Greece, Turkey, and the Middle East are most likely to be carriers. Roughly 2 million people in the United States have the sickle cell trait, and about 72,000 people have sickle cell disease. About 8,000 people are born with sickle cell disease each year, and about 500 people die of complications related to this condition.[8]

Etiology: What Happens?

The gene for sickle cell disease is recessive; this means if a person has only one copy of the gene, he or she has the sickle cell *trait* but not sickle cell disease. If two people who have the sickle cell trait have children together, each child has a 25% chance of inheriting a copy of the gene from each parent. This is the only way sickle cell disease is spread.

Being positive for the sickle cell trait carries no health consequences for the carrier and in fact may be beneficial if that person

Sickle Cell Disease in Brief

What is it?
Sickle cell disease is a disorder in which the gene that controls hemoglobin production is faulty. The result is short-lived, misshapen red blood cells that cannot pass through tiny blood vessels.

What does it look like?
The primary sign of sickle cell disease is the pain that occurs when abnormal erythrocytes block blood vessels. This can lead to organ damage, bone pain, kidney infarction, stroke, lung problems, and blindness. Other signs include a high risk of infection because the spleen is typically disabled and anemia with jaundice because the abnormal red blood cells die off faster than they can be replaced.

Is massage indicated or contraindicated?
Sickle cell disease patients often live in chronic pain, even when they are not in a sickle cell crisis. Gentle massage that works for stress relief and circulatory improvement and that is within the activities of daily living of the client is appropriate and helpful when the client is stable, but any rigorous circulatory modalities should be avoided during a sickle cell crisis.

lives in an area where malaria is endemic—interestingly, those areas also happen to be the places where sickle cell genes are most common (Sidebar 5.3). But having two copies of the sickle cell gene means that hemoglobin production is abnormal and red blood cells adopt a characteristic sickle shape (Figure 5.5). This prevents erythrocytes from squeezing through the smallest blood vessels and shortens their lifespan from about 4 months to about 10 days.

The most common form of sickle cell disease comes from inheriting two copies of the sickle gene: this is called the SS form. Other forms come from different genetic anomalies: the inheritance of one S gene and one C gene (for another abnormal form of hemoglobin) leads to SC sickle cell disease. A final form is called S-beta **thalassemia** sickle cell disease, referring to yet another type of genetic fault.

Signs and Symptoms

Having dysfunctional hemoglobin and brittle, fragile red blood cells produces many consequences in the body. The direct symptoms of sickle cell disease include fatigue, shortness of breath, and pallor related to inadequate oxygen-carrying capacity. Jaundice may develop as red blood cells die and bilirubin accumulates in the liver and backs up into the bloodstream.

Complications

Sickle cell disease can lead to many serious and potentially life-shortening complications:

- *Sickle cell crises.* An **infarction** is an area of tissue that dies because it is deprived of oxygen. A sickle cell crisis occurs when an infarction damages tissue. One example is *hand-foot syndrome.* This is often the first indicator of sickle cell disease in a young child. The hands and feet are vulnerable to sickle cell crises, and they swell and become extremely painful.
- *Organ damage.* The spleen, as a collection site for dead and damaged red blood cells, is often lost early in the disease process. This leaves the patient vulnerable to serious infections, as the spleen is also a key player in immune system function. Other organs that are frequently damaged include the liver, kidneys, and brain: even young children are vulnerable to ischemic strokes, which can lead to serious learning problems in a growing child.
- *Infection.* As mentioned earlier, the loss of spleen function makes a sickle cell disease patient vulnerable to serious and even life-threatening infections. Pneumonia is the leading cause of death among children with sickle cell disease.
- *Gallstones.* Accumulated bilirubin in the liver can concentrate into crystals that build up in the gallbladder.

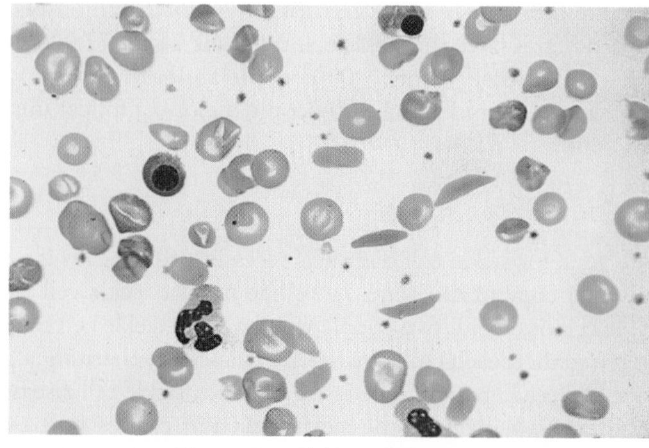

Figure 5.5. Sickle cell disease.

- *Vision loss.* The accumulation of fragile red blood cells in the arterioles that supply the retina can lead to blurred vision, hemorrhage, and even blindness.
- *Acute chest syndrome.* Damaged cells accumulate in the lungs, leading to inflammation and pneumonia-like symptoms. This puts excessive strain on the right side of the heart and can lead to pulmonary hypertension and right-sided heart failure.
- *Others.* Other complications of sickle cell disease include delayed growth in children; chronic ulcerations of the skin, usually at the lower legs; and *priapism*, a painful and long-lasting erection of the penis that occurs because the vessels that would allow blood to flow out are blocked with damaged red blood cells.

Treatment

Sickle cell disease is treated by trying to limit the severity and frequency of sickle cell crises. Mild episodes can be treated at home with over-the-counter pain medications and hot packs, but more severe attacks are often treated in the hospital with intravenous opioid drugs. One cancer drug, hydroxyurea, has been found to limit the frequency and severity of sickle cell crises in adults, but it carries many serious side effects and is not approved for use in children.

The leading cause of death in children with sickle cell disease is pneumonia. This risk is managed with doses of prophylactic antibiotics until age 5, along with careful immunizations for flu and other possible infections.

The life expectancy of a person with sickle cell disease has increased with better treatment options; today a person with this condition can expect to live well into his or her 40s or later.

No cure exists for sickle cell disease, which is an inherited genetic anomaly. However, new discoveries in gene therapy, stem cell transplants, and bone marrow transplants hold some promise for the future of this disease.

Massage?

Sickle cell disease is a painful, difficult problem. It involves poor circulation and the risk of organ damage. Clients who have this condition are counseled not to exercise vigorously and to avoid any activities that may trigger a sickle cell crisis.

For these reasons, vigorous circulatory massage is not appropriate for sickle cell disease patients. Energetic and reflexive work, however, may be extremely supportive and helpful. Research into gentle massage as a pain management technique is ongoing,[9] and many specialists recommend warm packs and gentle stroking for people undergoing a difficult time.

Modality Recommendations for Sickle Cell Disease	
Deep Tissue Massage	Systemically contraindicated.
Lymphatic Drainage	Supportive.
Polarity	S: Indicated; can support immune system. R/D: Supportive with light work within client comfort.
PNF/MET/Stretching	Supportive.
Reflexology	Indicated; work endocrine, heart, lung points.
Shiatsu	Supportive, especially with K, SP, H, TH meridians and extensions.
Swedish Massage	Contraindicated when symptoms are present; otherwise stay within activity limitations.
Trigger Point Therapy	Systemically contraindicated; *very* light work may be possible.

See Chapter 1 for a brief description of each modality, including definitions of abbreviations.

Thrombophlebitis, Deep Vein Thrombosis in Brief
Pronunciation: throm-bo-fleh-BI-tis

What is it?
Thrombophlebitis and *deep vein thrombosis* describe veins obstructed by blood clots.

How is it recognized?
Signs and symptoms of thrombophlebitis may or may not include pain, heat, redness, swelling, local itchiness, and a hard cordlike feeling at the affected vein. Signs and symptoms of deep vein thrombosis may be nonexistent or more extreme: possibly pitting edema distal to the site with discoloration and intermittent or continuous pain that is exacerbated by activity or standing still for a long time.

Is massage indicated or contraindicated?
Thrombophlebitis and deep vein thrombosis contraindicate any kind of bodywork that may disrupt clots, which could lead to a pulmonary embolism.

Thrombophlebitis, Deep Vein Thrombosis

Definition: What Is It?

Thrombophlebitis and *deep vein thrombosis* refer to veins that have become obstructed with blood clots. These clots can form anywhere in the venous system, but they develop most often in the calves, thighs, and pelvis. Thrombophlebitis is clots in superficial leg veins (lesser and greater saphenous), while deep vein thrombosis is much the same problem in deeper leg veins, specifically the popliteal, femoral, and iliac veins.

Demographics: Who Gets It?

The statistics on thrombophlebitis and deep vein thrombosis are difficult to gather because these conditions frequently go unrecognized and untreated. It is safe to say, however, that deep vein thrombosis is a leading cause of mortality in this country. It may happen up to 2 million times per year and is diagnosed in about 600,000 people, leading to about 200,000 deaths.[3,10] It is estimated that up to 5% of the population will have deep vein thrombosis at some point, although not all cases will be recognized.[3]

Etiology: What Happens?

These conditions are major concerns for well-trained massage practitioners. They involve thrombi, stationary clots in the venous system, where, if they break loose, nothing stops them from traveling up the vena cava, through the right atrium and ventricle, and into the pulmonary artery, causing pulmonary embolism.

The clotting mechanism is a normal part of homeostasis. We form blood clots in specific circumstances, but we also melt them with our own endogenous anticoagulants. Sometimes we form clots faster than we can melt them, and this is where we can run into trouble. In the mid 1800s a pioneer in pathology, Rudolf Virchow, first outlined three key factors in clot formation. The *Virchow triad*—injury to endothelium, hypercoagulability, and venous stasis, or slowed blood flow—is used today to describe the formation of blood clots in veins.

The triggers for thrombophlebitis and deep vein thrombosis can be many and varied. Any circumstance that involves part of the Virchow triad increases the chances of developing this problem. Here are a few of the most common precipitators of thrombophlebitis or deep vein thrombosis:

- *Physical trauma* is a predisposing factor; being kicked or hit in the leg can damage the delicate venous tissue, which is then prone to clot formation. Any fracture of bones in the leg can also increase risk (Case History 5.1).
- *Varicose veins* are another risk factor, since they too involve damaged tissue and the risk of clot formation. Fortunately, the clots that form in superficial veins tend to embolize, or break loose, much less frequently than those in deeper veins. However, many people with varicose veins also have deep vein thrombosis.
- *Local infection* can cause an inflammatory reaction leading to clot formation. These infections are often related to surgical procedures involving catheters.
- *Reduced circulation* from physical restriction, such as too-tight socks or leg braces, can cause the clotting factors in the blood to accumulate in amounts that cause coagulation without damage to a vessel wall.

- *Immobility*, often linked to sitting for long periods, can contribute to deep vein thrombosis. This phenomenon has given rise to a layman's term for this condition: "coach class syndrome". Some experts suggest that up to 50% of cases of deep vein thrombosis are related to recent air travel.[3]
- *Pregnancy* and *childbirth* can increase the risk of blood clotting. The weight of the fetus on femoral vessels slows blood return, and hormonal changes can cause the blood to thicken and become more viscous.
- *Certain types of cancer* can lead to thrombophlebitis or deep vein thrombosis, either because of changes in the blood or because of irritation at the site of a catheter.
- *Surgery* is another major risk for deep vein thrombosis. In fact, thrombosis and subsequent pulmonary embolism are the leading cause of death following orthopedic surgery, especially for knee and hip replacements. Heart and any kind of pelvic surgery also hold high risks of thrombosis.
- *High-estrogen birth control pills* or *hormone replacement therapy* can increase the risk of developing blood clots.
- *Other factors* that increase the risk for deep vein thrombosis include cigarette smoking, hypertension and other cardiovascular diseases, paralysis, and some genetic conditions that lead to excessive coagulation in the blood.

Most blood clots causing deep vein thrombosis or thrombophlebitis form in the lower legs, but they can develop elsewhere with surgery or other trauma. Sudden movement or change in position is often the factor that causes part of a clot to detach and travel to the lungs. Another alarming fact is that a patient who is immobile because of some leg injury is almost as likely to throw a clot from the *uninjured* leg as from the injured side. This is because lack of walking can thicken the blood systemically even where no damage to blood vessels has occurred.

One further twist on where clots travel occurs when a person has a defect in the cardiac septum. Some sources suggest that up to 25% of the adult population has a small hole in the wall between the left and right sides of the heart, usually at the atrium. This condition is called patent foramen ovale.[3] If clots from damaged veins that travel to the right side of the heart cross into the left side, they can go on through arteries to the brain as a stroke, to the cardiac muscle as a heart attack, or anywhere else as an arterial embolism.

Signs and Symptoms

Thrombophlebitis can show the major signs of inflammation: pain, heat, redness, and swelling. Sometimes itchiness, a hard cord where the vein is affected, and edema with discoloration distal to the area are present (Figure 5.6). Thrombophlebitis that has become a chronic problem may result in poor blood flow to the skin, leading to flaking, discoloration, and skin ulcers. If it is caused by a local infection, fever and general illness may also be present.

Deep vein thrombosis is considered the more dangerous of these two conditions because the clots in deeper veins can be big enough to do serious damage in the lungs and because clots in superficial veins usually melt under the influence of the body's own anticoagulants before they have a chance to break off and do any damage.

If deep vein thrombosis shows any signs (and it often doesn't), it may show more swelling and edema than thrombophlebitis, because the clot inhibits more blood flow back to the heart. The backup forces extra fluid out of the capillaries and into the interstitial spaces, thus adding general edema to any swelling of the vein. The capillary exchange may become so sluggish that the edema pits, or leaves a dimple wherever it's touched. Pitting edema is a red flag for massage therapists. It is an indication that this person's circulation is absolutely not capable of dealing with the internal changes brought about by massage.

It is important to point out that while the risks of pulmonary embolism from a clot in a superficial vein are minimal, many patients start with a superficial clot and have it intrude into deeper vessels with little or no sign of deep vein thrombosis.[10]

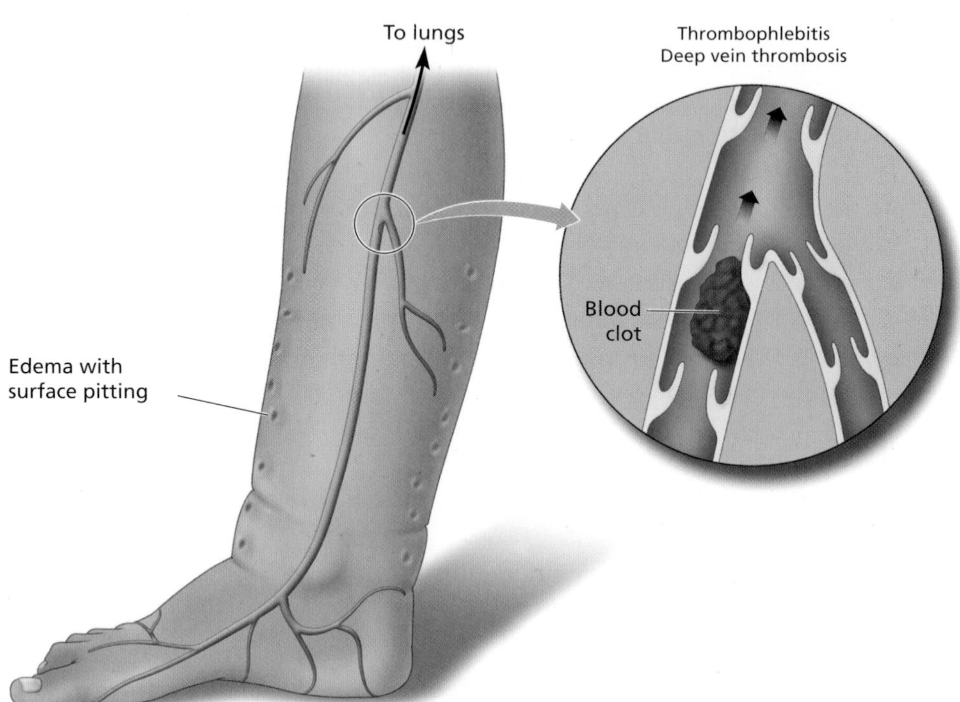

Figure 5.6. A. blood clot lodged in a vein can cause distal edema.

Diagnosis

Thrombophlebitis and deep vein thrombosis can be diagnosed in various ways, each with inherent benefits and disadvantages. Ultrasound is a fast and noninvasive technique, but it tends to yield a lot of false positives, leading to unnecessary prescriptions of anticoagulants, which can lead to risks of uncontrolled bleeding. ***Venography***—injecting the blood vessel with dye and watching how it moves through the system—can be more accurate, but it is slow and the injection itself can damage delicate tissue. MRI is fast, noninvasive, and accurate, but it is also expensive and not available at all medical facilities.

Treatment

The treatment for both thrombophlebitis and deep vein thrombosis is anticoagulants. These drugs can make a person prone to heavy bleeding, however.

A bedridden patient may be given pneumatic compression to reduce the risk of thrombophlebitis or deep vein thrombosis. A machine mimics the pumping action of exercise by inflating and deflating a tubular balloon around the affected leg. Support hose to prevent the accumulation of postoperative edema are also recommended.

People with thrombophlebitis in superficial veins are at much less risk for embolism than those with deep vein thrombosis. Self-care measures such as hot packs, analgesics, and gentle exercise may be recommended to resolve episodes of vein inflammation.

High-risk patients may have a filter implanted in the vena cava to prevent clots from reaching the lungs.

Thrombophlebitis and deep vein thrombosis may do permanent damage to leg veins, including destruction of valves that assist with blood return to the heart. These patients are at risk for ***chronic venous insufficiency***, which can include permanent edema, skin discoloration or ulcers, and very slow healing in the affected area.

CASE HISTORY 5.1

Deep Vein Thrombosis

Anne, aged 67: "It was just a broken knee!"

Anne is a retired schoolteacher who spends her winters in Arizona and summers in the mountains of Colorado. In May, a week after she moved to her summer home, she took a bad fall over a curb and sustained a lateral plateau fracture to the tibia of her left leg, with which she had a history of varicose veins and phlebitis.

Because her health maintenance organization was out of state (in Arizona), it was reluctant to cover any treatment for conditions not considered life threatening. For that reason Anne, a mildly overweight moderate smoker, spent 3 days sitting in a chair all day at 10,000 feet of altitude (which thickens the blood, because less oxygen is in the air). She was unable to move except with the use of a walker. Her broken knee was never set or seen by an orthopedist.

Eventually the swelling in the leg became so severely painful that she sought out a general practitioner in the Colorado town. He sent her to a local hospital for an ultrasound, which revealed a blood clot from her ankle to her groin. She immediately checked into the hospital and began receiving anticoagulant medication.

Then, 4 days later, she was sent home. Still basically immobile but taking anticoagulants, she returned to sitting in her chair with her leg elevated for 12 to 14 hours a day. On her second night home she woke in the night with severe chest pains and shortness of breath. The emergency medical team took her back to the hospital, where it was revealed that she had thrown a pulmonary embolism, a large clot to the lung. At this point her condition was too severe to be treated at a small rural hospital. After 2 days in the intensive care unit, she was transferred to a larger facility about 100 miles away, where a filter was inserted into her vena cava to prevent any further clots from reaching her lungs.

When she checked out of the second hospital, she was prescribed supplemental oxygen to compensate for the loss of lung function and the high altitude. She used an oxygen tank for several weeks and had to quit smoking in the process. Several months later Anne has no severe pain in her knee but does have constant achiness. She limps when she gets tired, which happens easily; her energy level never quite returned to what it used to be.

Massage?

A client who is at high risk for throwing a blood clot and developing pulmonary embolism is obviously not a candidate for circulatory or vigorous massage. The trick is that although thrombophlebitis *may* show obvious signs, it may *not*, or the signs may be indistinct. A client may come complaining of an ache deep in her calf that she really wants worked out. This is a reasonable request—except that the massage therapist may be working out a blood clot that will land the client in the hospital with the other 600,000 pulmonary embolism cases this year. This is one of the rare situations in which it is wisest to avoid the area and to refer the client emphatically and immediately to a primary health care provider.

MODALITY RECOMMENDATIONS FOR THROMBOPHLEBITIS, DEEP VEIN THROMBOSIS	
Deep Tissue Massage	Systemically contraindicated.
Lymphatic Drainage	Systemically contraindicated.
Polarity	S: Indicated. R/D: Locally contraindicated.
PNF/MET/Stretching	Locally contraindicated; otherwise supportive.
Reflexology	Locally contraindicated; work as part of health care team on lymphatic and endocrine points.
Shiatsu	Locally contraindicated.
Swedish Massage	Contraindicated when symptoms are present; **strongly** urge or require client to seek medical attention.
Trigger Point Therapy	Locally contraindicated.

See Chapter 1 for a brief description of each modality, including definitions of abbreviations.

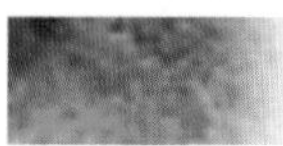

VASCULAR DISORDERS

Aortic Aneurysm

Definition: What Is It?

An aneurysm is a permanent bulge in the wall of a blood vessel or the heart. They happen most often at the aorta (aortic aneurysm) and in the brain (cerebral aneurysm). Cerebral aneurysms are discussed in the section on stroke in Chapter 4.

The damage may be brought about by any combination of injury, genetically weak smooth muscle tissue, high blood pressure, atherosclerosis, and compromised connective tissue. If an aortic aneurysm ruptures, the person can bleed to death in a very short time.

> **Aneurysm in Brief**
> Pronunciation: AN-yur-izm
>
> **What is it?**
> An aneurysm is a bulge or outpouching in a vein, an artery, or the heart. They usually occur in the thoracic or abdominal aorta or in the arteries at the base of the brain.
>
> **How is it recognized?**
> Symptoms of aneurysms are determined by their location. Thoracic aneurysms may cause chronic hoarseness; abdominal aneurysms may cause local discomfort, reduced urine output, or severe backache. Cerebral aneurysms may be silent or may cause extreme headache when they are at very high risk for rupture.
>
> **Is massage indicated or contraindicated?**
> If a client has been diagnosed with an aneurysm, circulatory massage must be conducted with great caution, and work in the abdomen should be avoided. Massage is also strongly cautioned for clients who fit the profile for aneurysms but have not been diagnosed.

Demographics: Who Gets It?

Most aortic aneurysm patients are men over 60 years old. By some estimates, about 5% of men over 60 will have an aortic aneurysm at some time.[11] About 15,000 aneurysm patients die every year.[12]

Etiology: What Happens?

The three-ply construction of the arteries includes the endothelial inside layer, the smooth muscle middle layer, and the tough connective tissue outer layer. Blood pressure in the aorta, the largest artery, is very high. If the walls of the aorta lose their elasticity, they can bulge wide with blood. This bulge is an aneurysm. As the aneurysm grows, the walls stretch and weaken, increasing the risk of rupture and death.

Aneurysms happen most often in the thoracic or abdominal aorta and at the base of the brain. Aneurysms sometimes develop in more distal vessels, but those cases are generally much less serious because the blood pressure drops with distance from the heart.

An occasional complication of a major heart attack is an aneurysm in the left ventricle of the heart itself. The damage to myocardium reduces elasticity to the point that chronic pressure causes the whole wall of the ventricle to bulge. This is discussed further in the article on heart failure.

Several factors can contribute to the chances of developing an aneurysm:

- *Compromised smooth muscle.* Atherosclerotic plaques invade and weaken aortal muscle. Aortic aneurysms are a serious and common complication of atherosclerosis and high blood pressure.
- *Smoking.* The damage incurred to endothelium by carbon monoxide from cigarette smoke and a rise in blood pressure from nicotine makes smoking a leading risk factor for aortic aneurysm.
- *Congenitally weak arterial wall muscle.* Sometimes the tissue simply isn't strong enough to put up with normal blood pressure, and with no warning an aneurysm can rupture. Inherited connective tissue diseases such as Marfan syndrome and Ehlers-Danlos syndrome can contribute to this kind of event.
- *Inflammation.* A few diseases, such as polyarteritis nodosa and bacterial endocarditis, can cause inflammation and weakening of the arterial tissue.
- *Untreated syphilis.* This can lead to damage in the aorta, sometimes decades after the initial infection.
- *Trauma.* Mechanical trauma, such as a car accident in which a person is injured by a steering wheel, may sometimes damage the outer layers of the aorta while leaving the inner one intact. This results in the characteristic bulging and stretching of the most delicate arterial tissue.

Types of aneurysm Aneurysms come in a variety of shapes and sizes, some of which are particular to where the lesion occurs (Figure 5.7).

- *Saccular aneurysm.* These usually occur with thoracic or abdominal aortic aneurysms. The aortal wall bulges like a rounded sack, which throbs and pushes against neighboring organs and other structures.
- *Fusiform aneurysm.* This is a common type of aortic aneurysm; in this case the bulge is less round and more tubular, as if the aorta were widened like a sausage for a few inches.
- *Berry aneurysm.* These small aneurysms are usually in the brain (Figure 5.8).
- *Dissecting aneurysm.* Also called false aneurysm, this is the least common and most painful type of aortic damage. The blood pressure actually *splits* the layers of the aorta

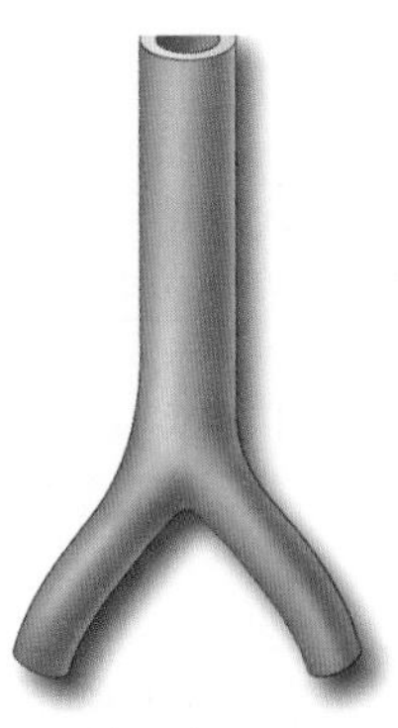
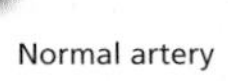

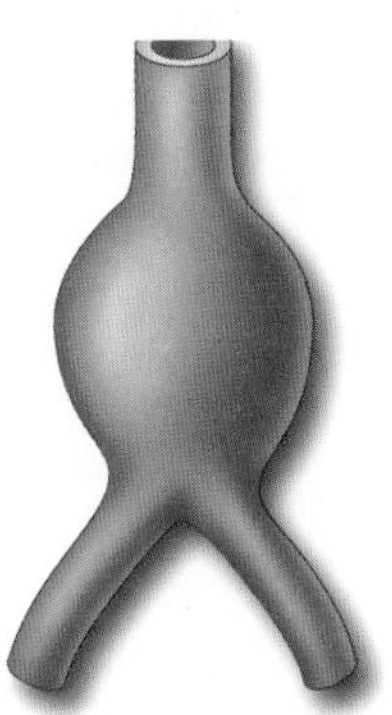

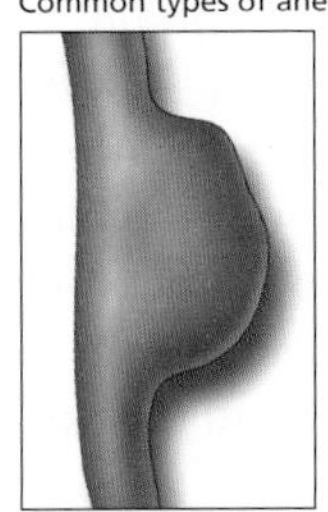

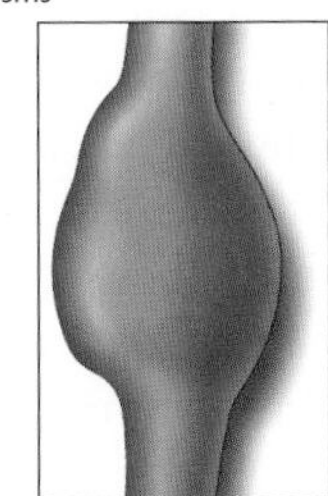

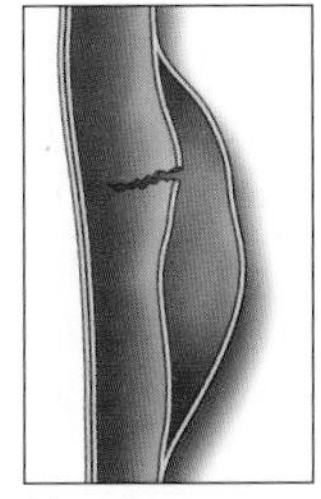

Figure 5.7. Aneurysms.

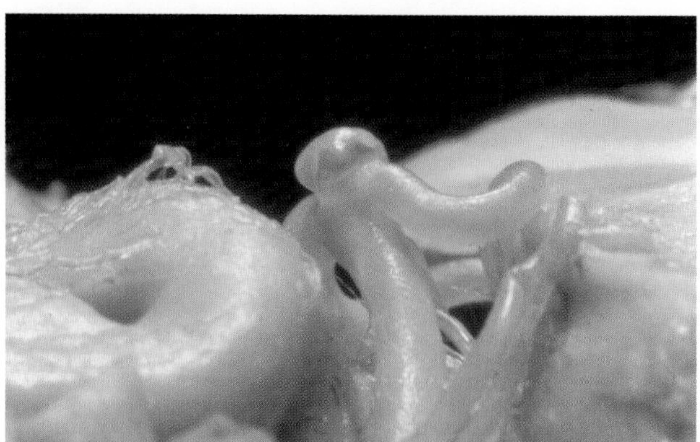

Figure 5.8. A berry aneurysm in a cerebral artery.

between the ***tunica intima*** (innermost layer) and the ***tunica media*** (muscular layer). In some cases this type of bulge can seal itself off when the blood trapped inside the split coagulates and solidifies. It is possible to have a dissecting aorta *without* an aneurysm.

Signs and Symptoms

Aneurysms can be difficult to identify by symptoms because they often aren't painful until they become a medical emergency. With aortic aneurysms the swelling might create some warning signals; this usually happens when the bulge is pressing on something else or interfering with another organ's functioning. Thoracic aneurysms sometimes cause difficulty with swallowing (***dysphagia***), chest pain, hoarseness, and coughing that is not relieved with medication, because the protrusion presses on and irritates the larynx. Abdominal aneurysms sometimes show as a throbbing lump near the umbilicus, loss of appetite, weight loss, reduced urine output, and if it's pushing against the spine, severe backache.

Diagnosis

Physical examinations often show signs of aneurysm; the turbulent movement of blood through the wide area of the aorta makes a specific sound called a ***bruit*** in stethoscopes. Large aneurysms in thin people can be palpated as a pulsating mass. Otherwise aneurysms are diagnosed by ultrasound, computed tomography (CT), and MRI; about three-quarters of the time, this happens when a patient undergoes tests for some other disorder and the aneurysm is found by accident.

Complications

For the rare aneurysms that are *not* in the aorta or the brain, no serious complications may develop unless the aneurysm gets large enough to impede blood flow, which can lead to gangrene. But the more typical aneurysm at the very least presses against its neighbors, which can be uncomfortable and can even interfere with function. If blood pools in an aneurysm for any length of time, clots may form and enter the bloodstream again. And of course, a rupture leads to hemorrhaging in the best case and shock followed by collapse of the circulatory system in the worst case. A ruptured cerebral aneurysm is fatal about 50% of the time; ruptured aortic aneurysms are fatal much more often than that.

Treatment

Aneurysms *don't* spontaneously retreat, because the pressure that causes them never lets up. They must be repaired, either with open surgery or with endovascular surgery. Open surgery involves clamping off the artery above and below the lesion and attaching either a replacement graft or a Dacron substitute to the two ends. This is usually successful, but it has to be done *before* a rupture.

Endovascular surgery involves inserting a catheter through the femoral artery and threading it up to the aorta to insert a patch or stent at the aneurysm site. This is a much less invasive procedure with a lower risk of surgical complications.

Some aneurysms don't require immediate intervention. Normal aortic size is about 2 cm; a dangerously distended aneurysm is about 5 to 6 cm. Many doctors recommend checking the growth of small aneurysms by ultrasound every 6 months until the benefits of intervention outweigh the risks.

Massage?

Any condition involving damaged blood vessels requires extreme caution for circulatory massage. *Massage changes the internal environment.* It dilates some blood vessels and constricts others. It reroutes circulation, mechanically through compression and friction on the skin, via the parasympathetic nervous system, and by changing hormonal balance (reducing adrenaline), which shifts blood from the skeletal muscles (a sympathetic state) to the internal organs (a parasympathetic state). A client who can't tolerate having the internal environment shifted in terms of blood vessel dilation, chemical distribution, and autonomic state isn't a good candidate for circulatory massage.

If a client has been diagnosed with a stable aortic aneurysm and wants to receive massage, the therapist should choose modalities that aim to lower blood pressure and support that parasympathetic state without putting undue mechanical force on the circulatory system.

Modality Recommendations for Aneurysm	
Deep Tissue Massage	Contraindicated, especially for deep work in abdomen.
Lymphatic Drainage	Supportive.
Polarity	S: Indicated.
	R/D: Supportive with light work within client comfort.
PNF/MET/Stretching	Supportive.
Reflexology	Contraindicated unless working as part of health care team.
Shiatsu	Supportive.
Swedish Massage	Contraindicated unless stable or repaired; then use caution and stay within activity limitations. Avoid deep centripetal work.
Trigger Point Therapy	Supportive with light work only.

See Chapter 1 for a brief description of each modality, including definitions of abbreviations.

Atherosclerosis

Definition: What Is It?

Arteriosclerosis is hardening of the arteries from any cause. Atherosclerosis is a subtype of arteriosclerosis. It is a condition in which deposits of cholesterol and other substances infiltrate and weaken layers of large and medium-sized blood vessels, particularly the aorta and coronary arteries. It is compounded by the facts that damage to these blood vessels can cause them to spasm and that blood clots form at the site of these deposits. These features contribute to

Atherosclerosis in Brief

Pronunciation: ath-er-o-skler-O-sis

What is it?
Atherosclerosis is a condition in which the arteries become inelastic and brittle as a result of the development of plaques.

How is it recognized?
Atherosclerosis has no symptoms until it is far advanced. However, it is connected to several other types of circulatory problems, including hypertension, arrhythmia, aneurysm, coronary artery disease, cerebrovascular disease, and peripheral vascular disease.

Is massage indicated or contraindicated?
Advanced atherosclerosis systemically contraindicates rigorous circulatory massage, but other modalities may offer many benefits with a minimum of risks.

occlusion of the diameter, or lumen, of the arteries Figure 5.9) and to the risk of forming and releasing blood clots on the arterial side of the systemic circuit.

Coronary artery disease is atherosclerosis specifically in the coronary arteries that supply the heart muscle (Figure 5.10).

Demographics: Who Gets It?

Random samplings of arteries taken from autopsies of people who died of something other than heart disease reveal that the incidence of atherosclerosis is very high in the United States, although it doesn't always become symptomatic. In some cultures, generally where dietary diseases are related to famine rather than to excess, atherosclerosis is all but unknown.

Certain populations carry a particularly high possibility of developing atherosclerosis. This is discussed in detail in the discussion of risk factors later in this article. For more information on the statistics on heart disease, see Sidebar 5.4.

Etiology: What Happens?

Development of atherosclerosis is a complex process that is not yet completely understood. It is clear that this multifactorial process varies slightly according to gender, age, race, diet, and other factors. At this point the most widely accepted idea of how atherosclerosis develops includes the following steps, although they may vary from one person to another:

1. *Endothelial damage.* The inside layer of arteries, also called the tunica intima, is made of delicate epithelial tissue and subject to a lot of abuse. A variety of things may hurl the first insult at the tunica intima: constant hypertension in the aorta and arteries surrounding the heart; carbon monoxide from cigarette smoke; high levels of oxidized low-density lipoproteins (LDL) and triglycerides; even a high level of iron in the blood may produce oxygen free radicals that begin endothelial erosion. This occurs most readily at branches or sharp curves in the arteries, where blood flow suddenly changes direction of force.

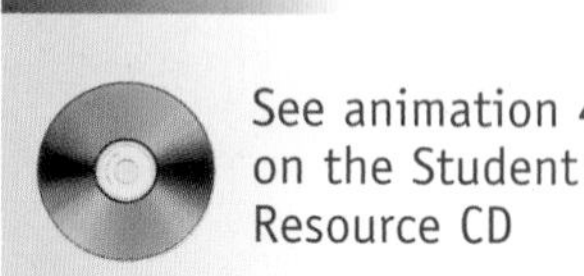

See animation 4 on the Student Resource CD

2. *Monocytes arrive.* These small white blood cells are attracted to any site of damage in the body. The monocytes infiltrate the epithelial layer and turn into macrophages, or big eaters.
3. *Macrophages take up LDL.* The reasons for this are unclear. For a quick overview, LDLs are the "bad guys" of the cholesterol world. Actually, they have an important job, which is to escort usable cholesterol to the cells in the body. But when those cells don't need any more cholesterol, they stop accepting it. This leaves those LDLs with nowhere to go. They are taken up by the white blood cells in the tunica intima, which are then called foam cells. This is the beginning of the development of fatty streaks that characterize atherosclerosis.

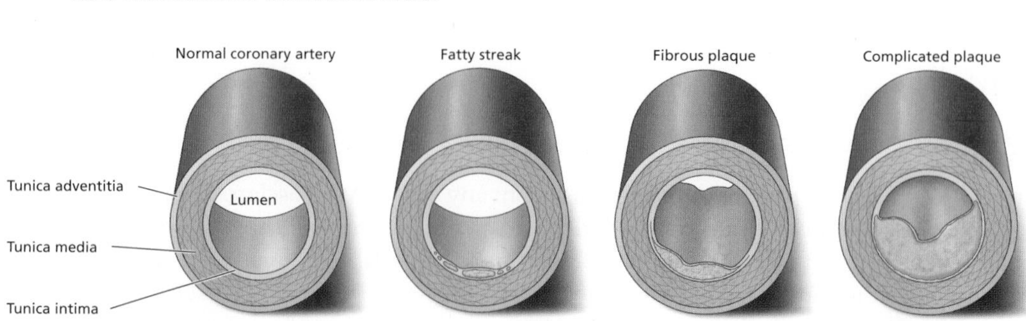

Figure 5.9. Atherosclerosis.

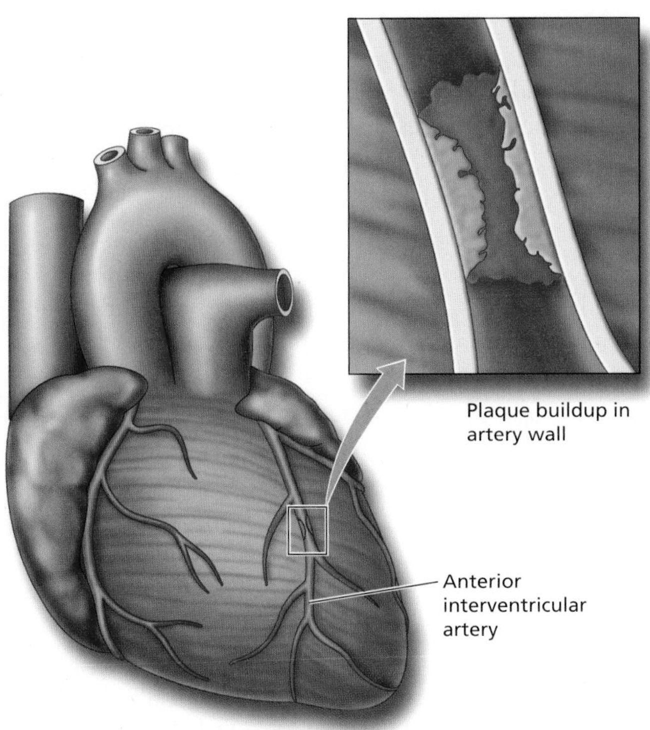

Figure 5.10. Coronary artery disease.

4. *Foam cells infiltrate and damage smooth muscle tissue.* Foam cells secrete growth factors; this causes the smooth muscle cells in the arterial wall to proliferate all around them. The grayish-white lumps of plaque that are inside dissected arteries are made of these extra muscle cells and cholesterol-filled macrophages. Furthermore, these foam cells can release enzymes that damage arterial walls and cause bleeding and clot formation.
5. *Platelets arrive.* Attracted by the changing texture of the arterial wall, platelets come and release their chemicals, which do three counterproductive things:
   a. *Growth factors are secreted,* and they reinforce the proliferation of new smooth muscle cells.
   b. *Clots form,* and they can further restrict the lumen of the artery.
   c. *Vascular spasm* occurs because the chemical that inhibits it can't get through all the plaque. This leads to a temporary lack of oxygen in the myocardium and the gripping chest pain called *angina pectoris.*

When vascular spasm and clots combine, partial or total occlusion of the artery can occur. Symptoms of this depend on the location of the blockage and the amount of tissue that is affected.

Risk Factors

Risk factors for atherosclerosis can be divided into modifiable and non-modifiable types.

Non-modifiable risk factors

- *Heredity, genetics.* Higher-than-average incidence of heart disease within families is clearly demonstrable, but a family history is not a death sentence; controlling modifiable factors significantly reduces the chance of developing problems.

SIDEBAR 5.4: HEART DISEASE IN THE UNITED STATES: SOBERING STATISTICS

The statistics for all varieties of cardiovascular disease are not generally separated from each other, since most of these conditions have a circular relationship. A person is unlikely to have atherosclerosis without high blood pressure, for instance, and a person is unlikely to have a heart attack without the predisposing factor of atherosclerosis, even if it never produces any symptoms.

Statistics for cardiovascular disease (this includes stroke, hypertension, heart failure, heart attack, angina, and congenital defects) are sobering. These conditions collectively account for about 2,500 deaths every day, or a death every 35 seconds. This group of diseases is the leading killer in the United States today, accounting for 37.3% of deaths, or 1 death in 2.7.

Here is a breakdown of reported heart disease statistics.[13] Understand that these conditions overlap each other significantly, so one person may have any combination of the following:

Condition	Incidence (millions)
High blood pressure	65.0
Myocardial infarct survivor	7.2
Angina pectoris	6.5
Stroke survivor	5.5
Heart failure	5.0

All combined, about 71.3 million Americans have some kind of cardiovascular disease. By contrast, behaviors that *limit* the risk of heart disease are now beginning to be studied. The four leading modifiable behaviors include not smoking, maintaining healthy weight, eating at least five servings of fruit and vegetables each day, and exercising for at least 30 minutes most days of the week. The breakdown of American adherence to these measures is as follows:

Healthy Behaviors	People who do them (%)
Not smoking	76
Maintain healthy weight	40
Eat five daily servings of fruits or vegetables	23
Get 30 minutes of exercise several days each week	22
Engage in all four risk-lowering behaviors	3

- *Gender.* While both men and women are affected by atherosclerosis, the average onset for men is typically around age 45, and for women it is around age 55. This reflects the shift in hormones that occurs after menopause.
- *Age.* The incidence of heart disease rises with age, but it is not a disease exclusively of the elderly.
- *Kidney disorders.* Atherosclerosis can sometimes lead to kidney problems. But if the kidney problems predate the circulatory ones, high blood pressure brought about by kidney failure can be a precipitator for atherosclerosis.

Modifiable risk factors

- *Smoking.* Carbon monoxide from cigarette smoke is extremely corrosive to endothelium. Furthermore, nicotine causes the release of epinephrine and norepinephrine, leading to vasoconstriction and high blood pressure. Studies show that cigarette smokers run a significantly higher risk of dying by heart disease than the general public.[14]
- *High cholesterol levels.* A predictable statistical link has been established between high cholesterol levels and the development of pathological atherosclerosis. Almost 100 million Americans have cholesterol readings above the recommended maximum of 200 mg/dL, and 34.5 million have readings over 240 mg/dL.[15] For more details on cholesterol, see Sidebar 5.5.
- *High blood pressure.* Chronic uncontrolled high blood pressure contributes to endothelial damage, which opens the door to the formation of plaques.
- *Sedentary lifestyle.* Regular moderate cardiovascular exercise, perhaps more than any other factor, can reduce the risk of atherosclerosis. It keeps arteries elastic and pliable; it reduces weight; it raises high-density lipoprotein levels for the reduction of plaques; it reduces the risk of diabetes; and it lowers blood pressure.
- *Diabetes.* People with uncontrolled diabetes are especially susceptible to atherosclerosis because of the way their body metabolizes food. However, if the diabetes is controlled, the risk of atherosclerosis is much lower.

Other risk factors

Continued study into who develops atherosclerosis and what makes them different from the rest of the population has yielded some additional risk factors. It is unclear whether these are modifiable or not, and the exact relationship between these issues and heart disease is not thoroughly understood. However, identifying these issues early and controlling them may improve the outcome for many people.

- *C-reactive protein* is a liver enzyme secreted in the presence of a systemic inflammatory response. It turns out to be a dependable predictor for heart attack, stroke, and other conditions related to atherosclerosis, although the mechanism is not clearly understood. The link between *C-reactive protein* and a high risk of atherosclerosis opens the door to questions about whether cardiovascular disease might be linked to chronic infection. Clear connections between gingivitis and other long-term, low-grade infections and a high risk of heart disease support this hypothesis.[17]

- *Homocysteine* is an amino acid in the blood. A small part of the population tends to have very high levels of *homocysteine*, which can contribute to endothelial damage. The exact relationship between homocysteine and atherosclerosis is not yet understood, but people with high levels are usually counseled to try to control this imbalance with folic acid and vitamins B_6 and B_{12}.
- *Other risk factors* that continue to be studied include body mass index, levels of fibrinogen, and subtypes of lipoproteins, some of which may be more involved with plaque formation than others. The goal of finding new predictors for heart disease is to be able to identify who is at risk as early as possible and to control those risk factors as carefully as possible.

Other contributors to atherosclerosis are somewhat harder to quantify. The way a person responds to stress, for instance, has a lot to do with his or her health profile. If stress makes him eat poorly, smoke more, and raises his blood pressure, his or her risk of developing atherosclerosis is higher than that of someone who deals with stress in different ways.

SIDEBAR 5.5: A BRIEF DIGRESSION ON CHOLESTEROL

Cholesterol is a fatty substance produced in the liver and available in any animal product. Saturated fats are particularly rich in easily absorbable cholesterol.

Cholesterol by itself has no access to the body's cells. Just as glucose must be escorted into cells by insulin, cholesterol must be escorted by *lipoproteins*, other chemicals also produced by the liver. When a cholesterol measurement is taken, it is actually the lipoproteins that are being counted.

Three varieties of lipoproteins are involved with the movement of cholesterol: low-density lipoprotein (LDL), high-density lipoprotein (HDL), and triglyceride. The LDLs ("bad cholesterol") deliver cholesterol to the body's cells. They are bad only when the body's cells have no more need for their cargo. At that point the LDLs deposit the cholesterol in artery walls. The HDLs ("good cholesterol") are involved in reverse cholesterol transport. In this process cholesterol is moved out of the arteries and back to the liver for metabolic processing. The third variety, triglycerides, are chemicals that help to convert fats and carbohydrates into energy for muscles. Studies have shown that elevated triglyceride levels contribute to plaque formation, so it is desirable to keep their numbers down.

When a person gets a cholesterol reading, it's useful to know not just what the overall levels are but in what ratios the fat types occur. An ideal reading would find total levels below 200 mg/dL, with a relatively high proportion of HDLs (over 35 mg/dL) and lower numbers of LDLs and triglycerides (less than 130 mg/dL combined).

Unfortunately, in the United States fewer than half the adult population can make this claim. About 100 million people have cholesterol readings over 200 mg/dL, and about 38% of those people have levels over 240 mg/dL.[16]

Signs and Symptoms

What are the symptoms of atherosclerosis? Until the damage has progressed to dangerous levels, *there are none*! An artery has to be 50% or more occluded before any tissue dysfunction occurs. This is largely because the body doesn't depend on any single artery to do a job. Most parts of the body have two or three alternative vessels, or the body can generate new vessels that can be pressed into service if one of them gets clogged up.

Once signs of atherosclerosis begin to develop, they arise from poor delivery of oxygen to the tissues. If the starved cells are in the heart, low stamina and shortness of breath are the earliest signs. More complications develop as other tissues are deprived of oxygen.

Complications

The complications of atherosclerosis are sometimes the first symptoms of the disease. They include but are not limited to these issues:

- *High blood pressure*. Hypertension is both a cause and a result of this disease; it contributes to the original damage to the tunica intima, and it is made worse when the arterial walls are too brittle to adjust to the constant changes in blood volume flowing through them.
- *Aneurysm*. When the wall of an artery is rendered inelastic and defective, it can bulge and become thin, weak, and susceptible to rupture.

- *Arrhythmia.* Advanced atherosclerosis can contribute to the development of irregular or uncoordinated beating of the cardiac muscle as blood supply through the coronary arteries is periodically interrupted. Arrhythmia can cause clots to form in the atria when the chamber doesn't empty completely. These clots can travel anywhere the aorta takes them.
- *Thrombus or embolism, peripheral circulatory damage.* A thrombus is a stationary clot; an embolism is a traveling clot. Thrombi are the link between atherosclerosis and stroke or transient ischemic attack when they travel to the brain, and between atherosclerosis and heart attack when they lodge in the coronary arteries. If a clot lodges in the renal artery, kidney damage occurs. Clots on the arterial side of the system may also end up in peripheral blood vessels, usually in the legs, where they can cause temporary pain and cramping (called ***intermittent claudication***), stasis dermatitis, gangrene, and skin ulcers,. This condition is called ***peripheral vascular disease*** (Figure 5.11).
- *Angina pectoris.* The process of developing atherosclerotic plaques also creates a higher risk of short-term vascular spasm, which leads to heart and chest pain.
  - *Stable angina pectoris* means that chest pain is predictable with exercise or exertion and subsides during rest.
  - *Unstable angina pectoris* means that chest pain varies in intensity, is not associated with exercise, and is unpredictable. Unstable angina is associated with a high risk of heart attack.
- *Heart attack.* When rough plaques form on smooth artery walls, they attract thrombocytes. If a clot or fragment of plaque breaks off in the coronary artery, it travels until its blood vessel becomes too small to let it pass. All of the myocardium that should have been supplied by that artery then dies. This is a myocardial infarction, or heart attack.

Diagnosis

The traditional way to check for ***stenosis***, or narrowing of arteries, is to inject them with dye and take a series of radiographs to watch to movement of fluid through the tubes in a procedure called an ***angiogram***. Other tests for atherosclerosis include CT, blood tests to look for targeted chemicals, echocardiography, ultrasound, and a test of the ***ankle-brachial index***, a comparison of blood pressure and the arm and lower leg to look for evidence of peripheral vascular disease.

Treatment

Treatment for atherosclerosis starts simply. If the situation is caught before it gets out of hand, it can often be managed or even reversed by changing eating and exercise habits.

More advanced cases of atherosclerosis often require drugs and/or surgery. The drugs are generally designed to influence blood pressure, cholesterol levels, and platelet activity.

Surgical intervention for atherosclerosis can include ***angioplasty, endarterectomy***, or bypass surgery. Angioplasty is a procedure in which the artery may first be treated with a laser, which vaporizes plaques (laser angioplasty), and then a small balloon is inflated to widen the artery (balloon angioplasty). Unfortunately, the scarring that occurs when the balloon is removed (***restenosis***) can be a difficult, even dangerous complication of this procedure; new cells rapidly proliferate where the endothelium was scraped. In an endarterectomy, a tiny rotating drill is inserted into clogged arteries to shave off plaque, and the shavings are trapped and removed. This is sometimes used for carotid arteries when the risk of stroke is high. In bypass surgery, surgeons remove the damaged piece of coronary artery and replace it, often with a

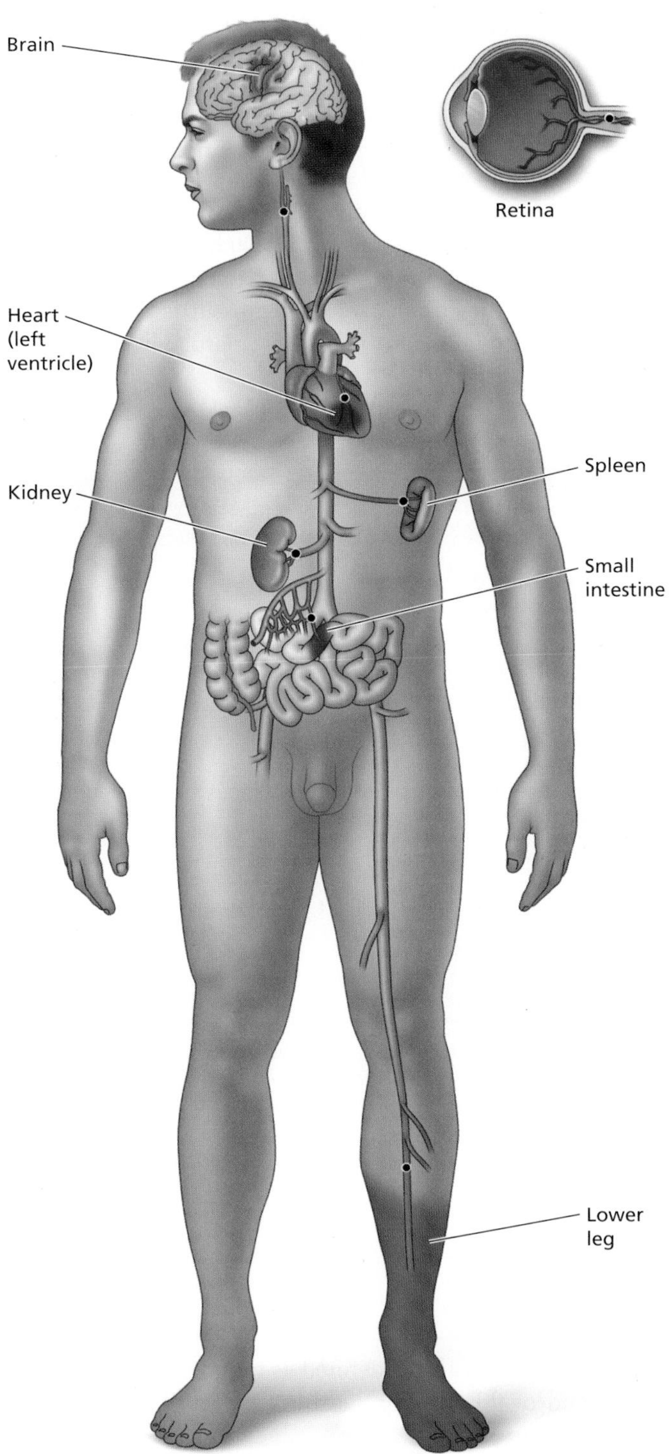

Figure 5.11. Arterial infarction sites.

graft from the internal mammary artery or a piece of femoral vein. A single, double, triple, or however-many bypass refers to the number of sections of artery being replaced.

With the exception of bypass surgery, these procedures can be done by inserting special tubes into arteries in the arms or legs and guiding the equipment to the target region. Obviously, the amount of shock to the system is less and the recovery process is much easier than it used to be. But new emphasis is being put on *maintaining* the structural changes brought about by intervention; if the patient reverts to former eating and exercise habits, his or her arteries can reach the same sorry state in just a few years.

Massage?

It is impossible to tell if a client has a subclinical buildup of plaque. The deciding factor is whether the client can adjust to the changes in internal environment that massage brings about. In other words, a person whose ability to maintain homeostasis is overly challenged by rigorous movement of fluid through the system is not a good candidate for circulatory massage.

If a client is taking *any* kind of medication for circulatory problems, it is important to clearly understand why and to adjust massage modalities to fit the circulatory limitations of the client.

Modality Recommendations for Atherosclerosis	
Deep Tissue Massage	Contraindicated in advanced stages.
Lymphatic Drainage	Supportive.
Polarity	S: Indicated. R/D: Indicated within client comfort.
PNF/MET/Stretching	Supportive.
Reflexology	Indicated with short sessions and light work; focus on solar plexus and endocrine and lymphatic system points.
Shiatsu	Supportive.
Swedish Massage	Indicated for parasympathetic effect; stay within activity limitations and adjust for medications.
Trigger Point Therapy	Supportive.

See Chapter 1 for a brief description of each modality, including definitions of abbreviations.

Hypertension

Definition: What Is It?

Hypertension is a technical term for *high blood pressure*. It is defined as blood pressure persistently elevated above 140 mm Hg systolic and/or 90 mm Hg diastolic.

Demographics: Who Gets It?

About 65 million people in the United States have high blood pressure: that's 1 in 3 adults.[18] It is seen in men more often than women until women reach age 65. Then it evens out and affects both genders equally. African Americans have higher hypertension rates than other races. Age is a predisposing factor; about half of those over 60 years of age have high blood pressure.

Other predisposing factors include obesity, smoking, high cholesterol levels, atherosclerosis, and water retention. A genetic predisposition may raise the risk of high blood pressure, but sometimes it's hard to know what's been inherited: high blood pressure genes, or high blood pressure habits.

Etiology: What Happens?

In hypertension, internal and/or external forces put pressure on the blood vessels. To understand how these forces can cause damage it is necessary to take a brief look at exactly what blood pressure is.

A *sphygmomanometer* is an instrument that measures the pressure blood exerts against arterial walls at two moments: ventricular contraction (*systole*) and ventricular relaxation (*diastole*). The blood pressure cuff converts the pressure in the arteries to millimeters of mercury.

Several variables influence blood pressure. Pressure from *inside* the vessel (which is increased with any buildup of material inside); pressure from *outside* the vessel (which is increased by having excess fluid pressing all around), blood volume, and blood vessel diameter are key factors. If any of these is out of balance, total body blood pressure may increase, which in turn influences the health and longevity of blood vessels.

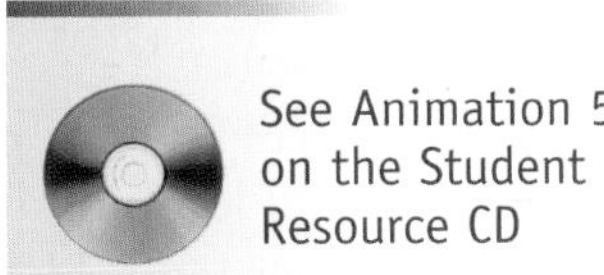
See Animation 5 on the Student Resource CD

Hypertension in Brief
Pronunciation: hy-per-TEN-shun

What is it?
Hypertension is the technical term for high blood pressure.

How is it recognized?
High blood pressure has no dependable symptoms. The only way to identify it is by taking several blood pressure measurements over time.

Is massage indicated or contraindicated?
For borderline or mild high blood pressure massage may be useful as a tool to control stress and increase general health, but other pathologies having to do with kidney or cardiovascular disease must be ruled out. High blood pressure that accompanies other cardiovascular disease may be inappropriate for circulatory massage but may respond well to other modalities.

Types of High Blood Pressure

Two types of high blood pressure have been identified: *essential*, or not due to some other pathology; and *secondary*, or a temporary complication of some other condition, such as pregnancy, kidney problem, adrenal tumor, or hormonal disorder. Secondary high blood pressure clears up when the precipitating cause is addressed. About 95% of hypertension is essential. In both essential and secondary high blood pressure another condition, ***malignant hypertension***, is possible. In this condition the diastolic pressure rises very quickly, over a matter of weeks or months. It is extremely damaging to the circulatory system, a high risk for ischemic or hemorrhagic stroke, and left untreated is often fatal. Malignant high blood pressure is a medical emergency.

The standard scale for hypertension in adults is based on how measurements correspond to the risk of developing cardiovascular disease, stroke, kidney disease, or heart failure. While a reading of 120/80 has traditionally been considered normal, research reveals that the risk of secondary disease increases significantly when the systolic reading is over 115 or when the diastolic reading is over 75. A person's blood pressure is based on the averages of two or more readings taken at each of two or more doctor visits.[19] Blood pressure ratings are shown in Table 5.1.

TABLE 5.1 Blood Pressure Ratings

Category	Systolic BP (mm Hg)	Diastolic BP (mm Hg)
Optimal	<120	<80
Prehypertension	120–139	80–89
Hypertension		
Stage 1 (mild)	140–159	90–99
Stage 2 (moderate)	160+	100+

Massage therapists are not generally required to take blood pressure measurements; these numbers are just an indicator of possible trouble. Be aware also that blood pressure can change significantly from hour to hour. It's fairly common to see it shoot up from anxiety while a person is in a doctor's office; this is known as "white coat hypertension".

Signs and Symptoms

Hypertension, which is often called the silent killer, has few recognizable symptoms. A few subtle signs are occasionally observed, however, so they are included here: shortness of breath after mild exercise; headaches or dizziness; swelling of the ankles, especially during the day-time; excessive sweating, or anxiety. Any combination of these symptoms is an indicator that a visit to the doctor would be a good idea.

Complications

This is a very important list. Having high blood pressure can shorten a person's life span. Here's how:

- *Edema.* High blood pressure forces fluid out of the capillaries at the nutrient–waste exchange sites. This adds to overall levels of interstitial fluid, causing edema. In a typically vicious circle, edema further raises blood pressure by putting external force on blood vessels.
- *Atherosclerosis.* Having blood pushing against arteries in an unceasing torrent simply wears out the walls, especially when the arteries have naturally lost some of their resiliency from age. As damage develops, the atherosclerotic process begins. This reinforces high blood pressure by narrowing arterial diameters.
- *Stroke.* Someone with hypertension is more likely to have a stroke than someone who does not have hypertension. The stroke may be from an embolism, or it may be from ruptured arteries in the brain.
- *Enlarged heart, heart failure.* Pushing against narrowed arteries causes the left ventricle to grow considerably, but the coronary arteries do not grow with it to handle the extra load. The muscle fibers also lose elasticity. Therefore, the contractions are actually weaker, because the muscle is not well supplied with blood and it can't contract fully. This can also cause angina, or heart pain. When the ventricles of the heart are so overtaxed that they simply cannot keep up with the workload, the patient risks heart failure.
- *Aneurysm.* This is the result of high blood pressure causing a bulge in the arteries.
- *Kidney disease.* This complication of high blood pressure demonstrates the circular relationship between hypertension and kidney dysfunction. If problems start with the circulatory system, hypertension causes atherosclerotic plaques to form in the renal arteries, which are subject to *huge* blood pressure. This causes changes in blood flow to the kidney, which impairs kidney function, leading to kidney damage, systemic edema, and yet more pressure exerted against vessel walls from that edema. If the problem starts in the kidneys, decreased kidney function causes fluid retention. This is often accompanied by extra release of ***renin***, the kidney-based hormone that regulates some electrolyte balance. Excess renin results in vasoconstriction, water and salt retention, increased edema, increased blood volume, and high blood pressure.
- *Vision problems.* Chronic high blood pressure can damage the blood vessels that supply the eyes, causing them to thicken and lose elasticity. Reduction of blood flow to eyes results in permanent visual distortion.

Treatment

Hypertension is a highly treatable disease, but because it has virtually no symptoms until it has progressed to very dangerous levels, it is frequently untreated or incompletely treated (e.g., someone not taking his medication because he feels fine). It is estimated that of the 65 million people who have high blood pressure in this country, 63.4% are aware of their problem; 45.3% are under treatment, and only 29.3% of all high blood pressure patients successfully control their disease. In other words, more than 70% of the people who have high blood pressure don't control it well enough to prevent other cardiovascular problems.[18]

Diet is the first way to manage this condition. The National Heart Lung and Blood Institute (NHLBI) has created the DASH (Dietary Approaches to Stop Hypertension) diet: a combination of high-fiber, low-fat foods that provide higher than average levels of calcium, magnesium, and potassium while cutting sodium by about 20%. Following the DASH diet (which is useful for anyone, not just hypertension patients) has been found to be as effective as treatment with one type of blood pressure medication, without side effects or long-term health risks.[19]

Exercise is also crucial for the development of healthy new blood vessels and for weight control. Losing even a small percentage of body weight for obese or overweight patients can have a profound effect on blood pressure and cardiovascular health.

Medication, if it's called for, includes diuretics, vasodilators, and beta blockers, which decrease the force of ventricular contraction. Controlling the systolic pressure turns out to be challenging but extremely important, especially in patients over 50 years old.

Medicating high blood pressure is a bit problematic. Because the disease itself has no strong symptoms and because the medicines often have unpleasant side effects (including dizziness, insomnia, impotence, and others), it can be difficult for hypertension patients to be consistent with their medications.

Massage?

If a client knows that he or she has high blood pressure but is *not* required to take medication for it, circulatory massage is probably fine, especially if the client is physically active or encouraged to become physically active. Massage can help to lower general blood pressure and the stress that contributes to it.[20] It is important, however, to rule out kidney disease and other advanced cardiovascular problems. Watch especially for signs that massage is overchallenging the body: clamminess, bogginess, and possible edema in the days after the treatment.

If a client *does* take medication for high blood pressure, circulatory modalities are strongly cautioned. Techniques that don't strongly influence fluid flow may be appropriate, but rigorous, fast-paced work may be too much of a challenge for an impaired ability to maintain homeostasis. As always, judgments about massage must be made by comparing the challenges of bodywork with activities of daily living.

Regardless of whether the client is on blood pressure medication, *high blood pressure contraindicates deep abdominal massage*. This is because it is possible to accidentally trip the vasovagal reaction. Unintentionally overstimulating the vagus nerve can result in amplified parasympathetic reactions. This leads to systemic vasodilation and faintness from lack of blood to the brain. Another possibility is a sympathetic rebound effect. Ordinarily a vasovagal reaction is unpleasant but not dangerous—*unless* the blood vessels are not equipped to handle a rapid demand to dilate and constrict. Once again, a client's health is determined by the ability to maintain a stable internal environment during massage.

Modality Recommendations for Hypertension

Deep Tissue Massage	May work slowly to assist relaxation if client manages condition with diet and exercise. Deep abdominal work is contraindicated.
Lymphatic Drainage	Supportive.
Polarity	S/R/D: Indicated.
PNF/MET/Stretching	Supportive.
Reflexology	Indicated; work head, neck, heart, kidneys, liver, solar plexus/diaphragm, endocrine points.
Shiatsu	Indicated. Treat all meridians and extensions of back, hips, and legs. Generally treat abdomen, rib cage, neck.
Swedish Massage	Indicated for parasympathetic effect; stay within activity limitations and adjust for medications.
Trigger Point Therapy	Supportive.

See Chapter 1 for a brief description of each modality, including definitions of abbreviations.

Raynaud Syndrome

Definition: What Is It?

Raynaud syndrome is a condition involving the status of the arterioles in the hands and feet, although it can also affect the nose, ears, and lips. Primary Raynaud disease is a vasoconstriction disorder, while secondary Raynaud phenomenon is a complication of an underlying problem.

Demographics: Who Gets It?

Raynaud disease, or primary Raynaud syndrome, is unrelated to underlying conditions. It usually affects women between 15 and 40 years of age; this population group makes up about three-quarters of all primary Raynaud syndrome patients. Secondary Raynaud syndrome, also called Raynaud phenomenon, is a symptom or complication of other disorders. Estimates vary, but it is suggested that some variety of Raynaud syndrome affects up to 5% to 10% of the general population.

Raynaud Syndrome

What is it?
Raynaud syndrome is defined by episodes of vasospasm of the arterioles, usually in fingers and toes and occasionally in the nose, ears, and lips.

How is it recognized?
Affected areas go through marked color changes of white, or ashy gray for dark-skinned people, to blue to red. Attacks can last for less than a minute or several hours. Numbness and/or tingling may follow during recovery.

Is massage indicated or contraindicated?
Raynaud syndrome that is *not* associated with underlying pathology indicates massage, even in the midst of an acute episode. For secondary cases, follow the guidelines for the precipitating condition.

Etiology: What Happens?

In both primary and secondary Raynaud syndrome the arterioles in the extremities develop vasospasm, or contraction of smooth muscle tissue. It occurs in temporary episodes at first, but especially if it is a secondary complication, the vasoconstriction can become permanent.

The chemical changes that occur with a Raynaud syndrome episode are the subject of intense study. The tunica intima is capable of secreting local chemicals that affect the constriction of arterioles and possibly even the viscosity of the blood. A high overlap between people with Raynaud syndrome and people with other vasoconstrictive disorders may eventually point to this condition as a chemical manifestation of hyperreactivity to cold or stress.

Primary causes *Raynaud disease* is a primary problem, that is, unconnected to underlying pathology. It may be due to emotional stress (the autonomic nervous system routes blood away from the skin during emergencies), cold, or a mechanical irritation, such as operating machinery that influences blood vessel dilation. Pianists and typists are particularly vulnerable. Raynaud disease generally has a very slow onset, and the attacks are less severe than when the symptoms occur as a secondary problem. If a person is prone to Raynaud disease, both the feet and hands tend to be affected.

Secondary causes Occasionally extreme vasoconstriction is a complication of some other disorder. In this case the condition is called *Raynaud phenomenon*. It generally has a much faster onset than Raynaud disease, the age at onset is typically older, and the risk of serious complications is much higher. Some conditions associated with Raynaud phenomenon include the following:

- Arterial diseases that involve occlusions, such as diabetes, atherosclerosis, and *Buerger disease* (a rare disease marked by inflammation and blood clots in the arteries)
- Autoimmune connective tissue diseases, such as scleroderma, lupus, and rheumatoid arthritis
- Sensitivity to some drugs, including beta blockers and ergot compounds
- Neurovascular compression, as seen with carpal tunnel syndrome, thoracic outlet syndrome, or crutch use

Signs and Symptoms

Raynaud syndrome is usually bilateral. During an attack the skin goes through a characteristic cycle of colors: white as the blood is shunted away from the area (on dark-skinned people the skin looks ashy gray); blue as the cells are starved for oxygen; and red as the attack subsides, the arterioles reopen, and the blood returns to the affected area (Figure 5.12). Some people only shift between blue and red; others show only pallor or blueness (cyanosis) during an episode. It usually affects distal fingers and toes, not the thumb or the rest of the hand. Sometimes only one or two digits are affected, and these may change from one episode to another.

Attacks of Raynaud phenomenon can last anywhere from less than a minute to several hours. Secondary Raynaud can be so extreme and long-lasting that atrophy and ulcerations on the starved skin may develop. Arterioles in the nailbeds can become thickened and distorted; this is identified in a test called a *nail fold capillaroscopy*. The fingers may taper, and the skin can become thin, smooth, and shiny. Gangrene is a rare but possible complication for these extreme cases.

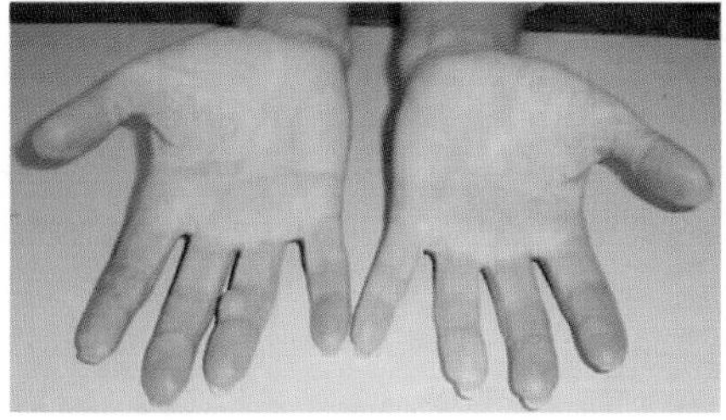

Figure 5.12. Raynaud syndrome.

Treatment

Treatment depends on whether the patient has primary or secondary Raynaud syndrome. Generally a noninvasive approach is taken first, at least for primary Raynaud disease. Quitting smoking, avoiding vasoconstrictors such as nicotine and caffeine, soaking in warm water, dressing appropriately for the weather, protecting the hands when working with cold or frozen foods, making sure that shoes aren't too tight, even moving to a warmer climate are all suggested before more intrusive intervention is suggested.

Because primary Raynaud disease can be exacerbated by emotional upset, patients are often encouraged to find productive ways to manage stress. This can range from learning biofeedback techniques, to exercising regularly, to receiving massage.

If results are unsatisfactory or if tissue damage from chronically impaired blood flow is a risk, the next step is medication to dilate the blood vessels. Other drugs work to counteract norepinephrine, the stress hormone that initiates vasoconstriction. Unfortunately, medical intervention is often unsuccessful for secondary Raynaud phenomenon. Surgery to interfere with sympathetic motor neuron stimulation of local capillaries may be conducted; this procedure, called a *sympathectomy*, is used only when no other options work, and it tends to be a temporary measure.

Massage?

The good news about Raynaud syndrome is that though the primary version of the syndrome is fairly common, the secondary version is rather rare. If Raynaud phenomenon is a part of lupus, scleroderma, or another vascular problem, the guidelines for massage must follow the cautions for the precipitating causes.

If any dangerous underlying causes of the vasoconstriction have been ruled out, primary Raynaud syndrome indicates massage, even during an episode. Massage can work mechanically with local blood vessels and reflexively with the parasympathetic nervous system to stimulate vasodilation.

Modality Recommendations for Raynaud Syndrome

Modality	Recommendation
Deep Tissue Massage	Contraindicated when associated with other conditions. Indicated if primary. Work to decrease fascial tension proximal to feet and hands.
Lymphatic Drainage	Supportive.
Polarity	S: Indicated. R/D: Supportive within client comfort.
PNF/MET/Stretching	Supportive.
Reflexology	Indicated; work endocrine, lymphatic, solar plexus points.
Shiatsu	Indicated. Treat the TH, PC, SP meridians and extensions in legs and arms. Add lots of ROM to joints of limbs.
Swedish Massage	Supportive if no contraindicated conditions are present.
Trigger Point Therapy	Locally contraindicated while acute; otherwise supportive.

See Chapter 1 for a brief description of each modality, including definitions of abbreviations.

Varicose Veins

Definition: What Are They?

Varicose veins are distended, often twisted or ropy superficial veins (*varix* means twisted). They occur when the valves that support blood flow against gravity are damaged. As blood collects in the system, the affected vein is stretched, distorted, and generally weakened (Figure 5.13). Varicose veins can develop at the anus (hemorrhoids), at the esophagus (esophageal varices) or at the scrotum (varicoles). But most often they are in the legs (Figure 5.14), which is the focus of the rest of this discussion.

Demographics: Who Gets Them?

Women get varicose veins more often than men; this is largely due to progesterone, which can weaken venous walls, and to a history of pregnancy. Increased blood volume, shifting hormones, and the weight of the fetus on the femoral vein all work together to set the stage for later problems. Varicose veins are very common; about half of people over 50 years old have them.[21]

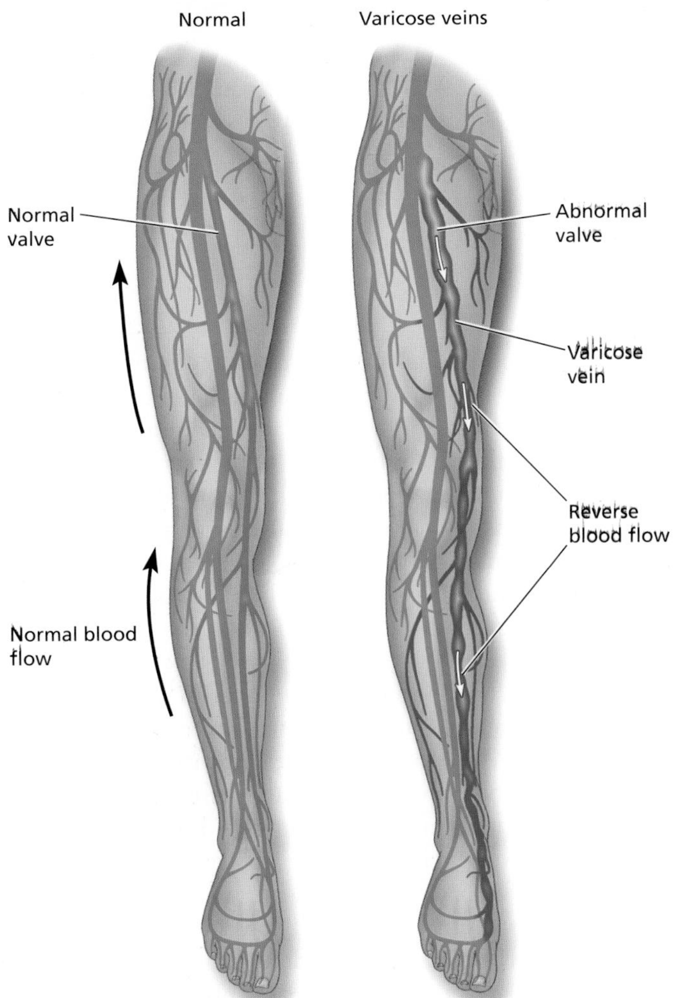

Figure 5.13. Varicose veins.

Varicose Veins in Brief

Pronunciation: VARE-ih-kose vanez

What are they?

Varicose veins are distended veins, usually in the legs, caused by venous insufficiency and retrograde flow of blood that should be moving against gravity.

How are they recognized?

Varicose veins are ropy, slightly bluish, elevated veins that twist and turn out of their usual course. They are most common in branches of the great saphenous veins on the medial side of the calf, although they are also found on the posterior aspects of the calf and thigh.

Is massage indicated or contraindicated?

Massage is locally contraindicated for extreme varicose veins and anywhere distal to them. Mild varicose veins contraindicate deep specific work but are otherwise safe for massage.

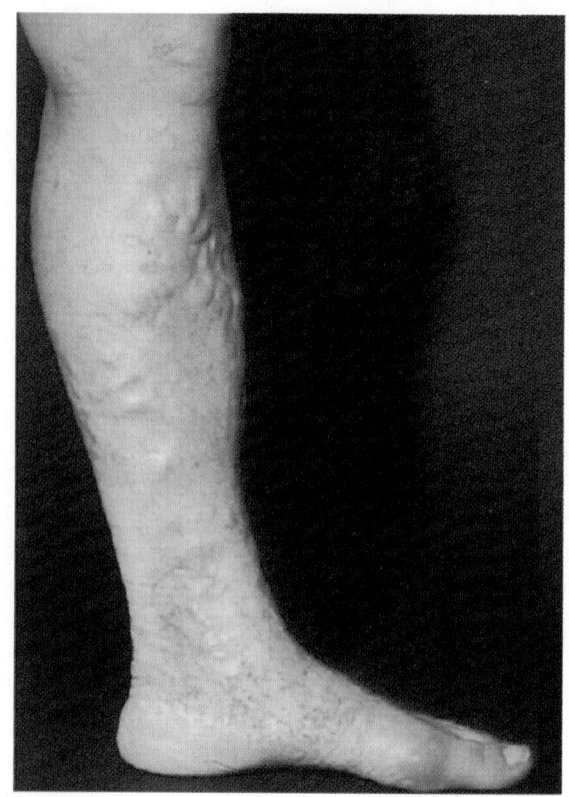

Figure 5.14. Varicose veins changing the contours of the skin.

Etiology: What Happens?

The veins in the legs have a fascinating construction that works to move blood from the toes all the way back to the heart. Small veins pick up the blood from the internal muscle capillaries. These veins tend to run on the superficial aspect of muscles. They feed into larger veins that perforate the muscle bellies and then into the really big deep veins that run under the muscles, close to the bones. When the leg muscles contract, the perforating veins are squeezed, sending their contents to the deep veins. When the leg muscles relax, the perforating veins draw in new blood from the smaller veins. The contraction and relaxation of the leg muscles (especially the soleus—"sump pump of the leg") is crucial to blood return. The valves inside the perforating veins and the deep veins ensure that blood does not collect in the smaller, weaker superficial veins.

What can damage the valves in the veins? It could be simple wear and tear: being on one's feet for many hours a day, especially if the leg muscles are not allowed to fully contract and relax during that time, weakens the veins. It could also be a mechanical obstruction to returning blood: knee socks that are too tight, a knee brace, or a fetus that presses on the femoral vein. Systemic problems from kidney or liver congestion have been seen to cause problems too. And finally, it could be simply congenitally weak veins or a structural anomaly at the junction between the great saphenous vein and the femoral vein.

Once a valve sustains damage, blood puts pressure on the next valve down. Vascular incompetence ultimately causes the weakest superficial veins to become distorted, dilated, and twisted off their regular pathway. Deeper veins are protected from this process because they have the external support of muscle tissue.

Signs and Symptoms

Varicose veins look like lumpy bluish wandering lines on the surface of the skin. They are often visible on the back of the calf, where they affect the lesser saphenous vein, but more often they affect the great saphenous vein, where they show up anywhere from the ankle to the groin on the medial side. They may be visible only when the patient is standing.

Varicose veins may itch or cause throbbing pain, especially at the end of the day, when legs feel tired and heavy. They can contribute to edema around the ankles as fluid backs up in the lower leg.

Complications

Although varicosities are seldom more than annoying, they can create some unpleasant or even dangerous complications. Chronically impaired circulation may result in varicose ulcers, which don't heal until circulation is restored. Skin irritation from poor circulation occasionally leads to a type of dermatitis that isn't resolved until the varicosity is relieved. Interruptions in blood flow increase the likelihood of annoying night cramps. And stagnant blood in a distended vein may coagulate, raising the possibility of clotting. Most clots that form in varicose veins are superficial and melt easily, however, so they are usually a lesser threat than clots that form in deeper leg veins. Be aware, however, that the presence of grossly distended varicose veins may indicate an increased risk of deep vein thrombosis. This is true especially when the varicosities have a sudden onset or change in size and quality very rapidly.[22]

Treatment

Mild varicose veins are usually treated with good sense. Using support hose or elastic bandages can give extra help to damaged veins, and avoiding long periods of standing up without full contraction and relaxation of the muscles is often recommended. Clothes that constrict at the leg, the groin, or the waist should be avoided. Reclining with the feet slightly elevated also reduces symptoms.

Whether or not the veins can actually *heal* is somewhat controversial. If the damage has not progressed too far, relieving the mechanical stresses while strengthening the smooth muscle tissue (with hydrotherapy, for instance) can yield good results.

Surgery for mild varicose veins is not generally recommended as a purely cosmetic intervention. However, varicose veins are a progressive condition; they don't usually spontaneously reverse, and if they are left untreated, their complications can be serious. Therefore, a certain number of patients eventually seek treatment for health rather than cosmetic concerns.

Several strategies for reducing varicose veins have been developed. These are appropriate when it is clear that the varicosity has *not* developed as a complication of a hidden obstruction or deep vein thrombosis. The traditional approach is surgery to tie off the proximal and distal sections of the great saphenous and remove the vein: this is called vein stripping. Ambulatory phlebectomy (ministripping) is a similar treatment that removes only small sections of the affected veins. Sclerosing involves injections of chemicals that cause the vein to close down completely; it eventually turns to scar tissue and fades. Applying laser energy or radiofrequency through a catheter to large veins is usually successful. In all of these treatments, the body's remarkable ability to generate new blood vessels quickly accommodates the closure or removal of the affected vein.

Massage?

Deep, intrusive massage is a local contraindication for varicose veins that are elevated from the skin and that are visibly distorted from their original pathway. Not only is the tissue injured and delicate, but it is inappropriate to push a lot of blood through vessels that may not be able to accommodate it. Heavy massage distal to these veins is cautioned also.

Clients with extreme varicosities who have a high risk of complications should be under a doctor's care and be checked regularly for signs of deep vein thrombosis.

If the vein is only slightly darkened and not raised or causing any pain, it is still wise to avoid local specific pressure, but otherwise massage is safe. Tiny reddened "spider veins" (*telangiectasias*) are slightly dilated venules and are safe for massage.

Modality Recommendations for Varicose Veins	
Deep Tissue Massage	Locally contraindicated.
Lymphatic Drainage	Supportive.
Polarity	S: Indicated. R: Supportive with light pressure. D: Locally contraindicated.
PNF/MET/Stretching	Supportive.
Reflexology	Contraindicated in extreme cases. Otherwise work liver, adrenals, hip, sacrum, legs, knee points; add lymphatic points if edema present
Shiatsu	Locally contraindicated. Otherwise treat PC, LV meridians and extensions.
Swedish Massage	Locally contraindicated for deep pressure; avoid inferior deep centripetal work.
Trigger Point Therapy	Locally contraindicated.

See Chapter 1 for a brief description of each modality, including definitions of abbreviations.

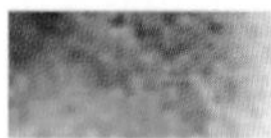

Heart Conditions

Heart Attack

Definition: What Is It?

A heart attack is damage to some portion of the cardiac muscle as a result of ischemia, which starves and kills some of the muscle cells. The ischemia is usually caused by coronary artery disease, or atherosclerosis of the coronary arteries, which supply the cardiac muscle with oxygen and nutrition. If these arteries are completely occluded by plaque, thrombi, or any combination of the two, some piece of the muscle dies (Figure 5.15). The muscle tissue does not grow back; it is replaced by inelastic, noncontractile scar tissue. The damaged area is referred to as an *infarct*. Another term for heart attack is *myocardial infarction*.

Demographics: Who Gets Them?

Coronary artery disease and heart attack is the leading cause of death in the United States, claiming over half a million lives every year, or 1 in 5 deaths. Over a million heart attacks occur every year, and about 40% of them result in death within the year. Over 13 million heart attack or angina survivors are alive in the United States today.[13]

Most people are familiar with the high-risk profile for heart attack victims: being sedentary, having hypertension, having high cholesterol levels, smoking, and being overweight. Being a man over 45 or a woman over 55, having a family history of cardiovascular disease, or being a woman over 35 who takes birth control pills also increases the chances of a heart attack.

That said, 50% of women and 64% of men who die of heart attack had no previous symptoms or warning signs on record.

Heart Attack in Brief

What is it?
A heart attack, or myocardial infarction, is damage to the myocardium caused by a sudden obstruction in blood flow through the coronary arteries, which results in permanent myocardial damage.

How is it recognized?
Symptoms of most heart attacks include a sensation of pressure on the chest, spreading pain, lightheadedness, dizziness, and nausea. Sometimes symptoms vary, and occasionally a heart attack may occur with no symptoms at all.

Is massage indicated or contraindicated?
Patients recovering from recent heart attacks are not candidates for circulatory massage, although techniques that do not challenge fluid flow may be appropriate. When they have completely recovered, they may be able to receive massage, depending on the rest of their cardiovascular health.

Etiology: What Happens?

A heart attack occurs when a portion of the cardiac muscle is killed off from lack of oxygen: an ischemic attack. Usually it comes from a blockage in the coronary artery that obstructs blood flow. It could also be from a loosened blood clot or a broken or torn piece of atherosclerotic plaque that blocks the coronary artery. Rarely, a heart attack may occur when a coronary artery goes into prolonged spasm; this is seen most often in cocaine or other drug overdose.

Examinations of exactly which plaques pose the greatest risk of heart attack have revealed that the size of the plaque evidently has little to do with its chances of breaking off or causing a heart attack. The more pertinent factor is how stable the plaque is. Older, harder plaques are relatively stable, but newer, softer plaques have a higher risk of breaking open and letting go of clots or atherosclerotic fragments that then block the coronary artery.

When a portion of the cardiac muscle is killed off by ischemic attack, the ability to contract with coordination and efficiency is badly damaged. If a heart attack is severe enough to trigger ventricular **fibrillations**, the risk of sudden death is very high.

The seriousness of a heart attack is determined by the size and location of the blockage. If it is relatively small and blood flow to an area that doesn't have to work especially hard is impaired, the heart attack is not a serious one. But if the infarct, or area of damaged tissue, is large enough to weaken the heart's ability to contract, or if the damaged tissue contains the electrical conduction system for the heart, major intervention is necessary to aid in recovery.

Signs and Symptoms

Heart attacks have a variety of signs and symptoms, some of which are extremely subtle and some of which are very severe. Some of the most common and dependable signs are these:

- *Pressure, pain in the chest.*
- *Spreading pain.* Pain may spread to the shoulder, arm, neck, and jaw of the left side of the body. This is the referred pain pattern for the dermatome shared by the heart.
- *Lightheadedness, nausea, sweating.* These usually occur along with chest pain. When they occur *without* chest pain they may still indicate a heart attack, but it is a less common presentation.

Other symptoms include shortness of breath with or without chest pain; unexplained nausea, anxiety, or weakness; fainting; palpitations; and cold sweat. Even stomach and abdominal pain may sometimes be signs of a heart attack.

- *Angina pectoris* (literally, chest pain). This is one of the few early warning signs for the risk of heart attack. Not all people have this symptom, but those who do should pay close attention.
- *Stable angina.* This is the simplest and most common form of angina. It affects about 6.5 million people and is diagnosed about 400,000 times a year. In this form of angina the heart can get enough oxygen to perform regular tasks, but any extra effort, such as carrying something heavy or running up a flight of stairs, demands too much of the

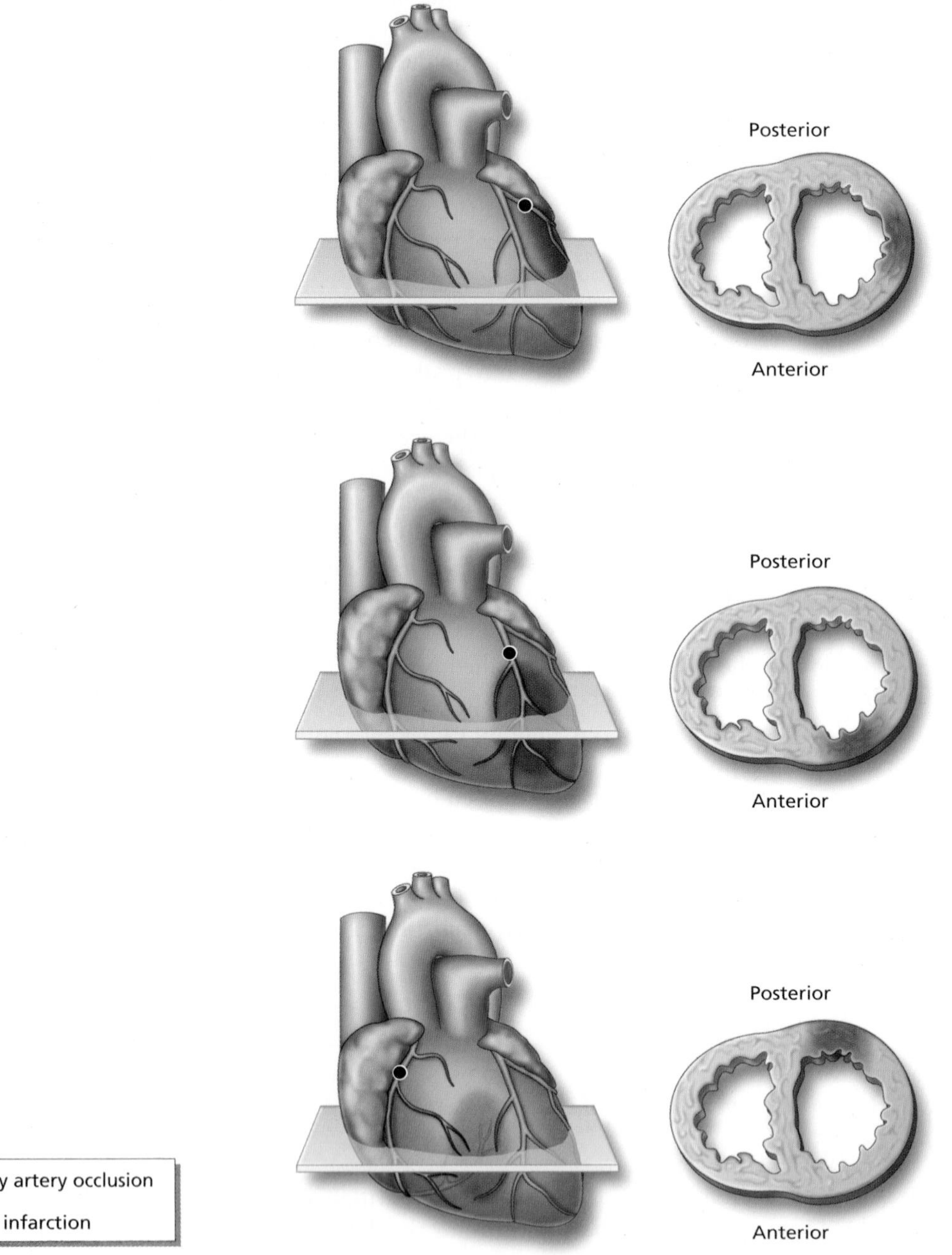

Figure 5.15. Heart attacks affecting the left ventricle.

clogged coronary arteries. The result is moderate to severe chest pain that is relieved with rest and/or angina medication, drugs that help blood vessels to expand.

- *Unstable angina.* This type of angina can occur *without* unusual physical activity. It often appears in the night, with very extreme but short-lived chest pain. It is caused by vascular spasm at or near the site of atherosclerotic plaques. This variety of angina is a reliable predictor of incipient heart attack.

A heart attack is a dynamic process. The critical blockage of the coronary artery may take place over several hours. This is good news because early intervention can preserve much of the myocardium: survival rates for heart attacks are better than ever. But this is also bad news, because many people tend to ignore early warning signs and don't seek attention until symptoms have been present for many hours or even days.

Complications

Several complicating conditions are discussed elsewhere in this chapter; diseases of the cardiovascular system are highly interrelated. Furthermore, with heart disease it's hard to say what comes first, the infarct or the thrombus. In other words, the chronology of these problems is often circular rather than linear.

- *Embolism.* A heart attack can cause blood clots to form in the heart itself. These clots exit through the aorta and travel to wherever the bloodstream takes them; these are arterial emboli, and they can land in the brain, causing a stroke, or the renal arteries, where they can contribute to renal failure. Prolonged bed rest can also promote deep vein thrombosis, which carries a risk of pulmonary embolism. Pulmonary embolism may also occur if clots form on the right side of the heart and are carried out by the pulmonary artery.
- *Atrial and ventricular fibrillations.* These are rapid, incomplete, weak attempts at contraction of the chambers. They occur most often if any part of the sinoatrial node, the heart's electrical pacemaker, has been damaged. These inefficient contractions allow blood to pool and thicken in the chambers of the heart and may contribute to the risk of stroke from the left side or pulmonary embolism from the right side. Ventricular fibrillations, because they interfere with blood flow to the entire body, may result in death if they are not treated quickly.
- *Aneurysm.* Weakened cardiac tissue can create a bulge in the heart muscle itself similar to aortic aneurysms.
- *Heart failure.* In heart failure the muscle is no longer strong enough to do its work, and the body pays the price. This condition is discussed further elsewhere in this chapter.
- *Shock.* In shock the circulatory system swings reactively from a sympathetic to a parasympathetic state, opening the arteries to a maximum diameter in the process. The main danger with shock is loss of oxygen to the brain from radically decreased blood pressure.

Diagnosis

Even with the new technologies that have been developed to deal with cardiovascular disease, the ability to identify and treat heart attacks *before* damage occurs is extraordinarily limited. Most of the time the best that can be done is to try to limit the damage as quickly as possible.

Screening for high-risk patients is usually conducted by angiogram: a flexible catheter is inserted into the femoral artery and snaked up to the coronary arteries. A contrast dye is injected, and pictures are taken to see how blood flows through occluded arteries. Unfortunately, this is an invasive procedure whose accuracy is somewhat limited. Although it can give useful information about arterial diameter, it doesn't measure risk of heart attack.

Much emphasis is being put on imaging techniques that may help to identify who is at most risk for having a heart attack and where that risk will come from *before* the heart is irrevocably damaged. Among the options that are becoming available are high-speed CT of the coronary arteries, contrast echocardiography, blood tests for C-reactive protein (an enzyme associated with inflammation), and MRI that can examine not only where plaques have developed, but also how dense they are and how deeply they penetrate into arterial walls.

Sidebar 5.6: Other Heart Conditions

Heart Murmurs

The heart can make several types of noise during its contractions. These are called murmurs. They often, but not always, point to some type of valvular dysfunction in the heart. A client with a persistent heart murmur may have an inefficient pump and may not be able to keep up with rigorous circulatory massage.

Hypertrophy of the Heart

This condition, which is seen most dramatically in the left ventricle, is brought about by chronically high systemic pressure in the blood vessels. If the heart has to fight against constricted arteries to push blood through the body, it can grow larger. It may also increase in strength for a while, but as the need for oxygen outgrows the supply from the coronary arteries, the tissue eventually undergoes ischemia, possible myocardial infarction, and eventually congestive heart failure.

Congenital Heart Problems

Any of 15 structural problems may affect the heart at birth. Approximately 36,000 babies with these are identified each year, but many more people are identified with minor problems in adulthood. About 1 million people in the United States have been identified as having a congenital heart problem. Defects often involve valve function or a hole in the septum that allows blood to cross from the right to the left side of the heart or vice versa.

Rheumatic Fever

Rheumatic fever is an autoimmune complication of exposure to streptococcus in which antibodies attack the heart valves, especially the mitral valve. It affects about 1.3 million Americans and is responsible for close to 6,000 deaths per year. Mitral valve damage affects the way the heart can pump blood through the body. It can lead to arterial emboli or congestive heart failure.

Infectious Diseases of the Heart

Different varieties of streptococcus may prey on endocardium. If they find a way in (which can happen from something as innocuous as an abscessed tooth but is more often a complication of open heart surgery), they cause clots that are released into the arterial system.

Massage?

Most of these conditions systemically contraindicate circulatory massage. Work that mechanically pushes fluid through the system will hinder rather than help these damaged structures.

Treatment

The first priority with heart attack patients is to determine where the blockage is and to get rid of it as quickly as possible. This is done with clot-dissolving drugs, which can take effect in 90 minutes or less, and with immediate balloon angioplasty, which can open up most clogged arteries in about an hour. The technical term for this procedure is ***percutaneous transluminal coronary angioplasty*** (PTCA). Other immediate-care options include the administration of oxygen and pain management with nitroglycerin and/or morphine.

Later care usually includes more clot dissolvers and nitroglycerin, which works to relax the smooth muscle tissue in the arteries. After the emergency has passed, the main treatment for heart attacks is observation. A barrage of tests is conducted to determine the location and extent of damage to the cardiac muscle. These tests indicate one of three future courses of action: that the infarct was minor and requires no further medical intervention; that prescription anticoagulants are indicated; or that a serious and permanent narrowing of a coronary artery requires surgery to open and repair it. This surgery may be a more complete version of the angioplasty or it may be coronary bypass surgery, in which damaged sections of the coronary artery are replaced with grafts of healthy vessels from elsewhere in the body.

Treatment in heart attack and heart surgery recovery must also embrace the lifestyle changes that will support a healthier future: eating sensibly, exercising regularly, controlling high blood pressure, and quitting smoking are the most important factors.

Compare and Contrast 5.2
Chest Pain, Chest Pain, Chest Pain

Not all chest pain means heart attack, although in a culture in which almost 40% of deaths are related to cardiovascular disease, it seems logical to jump to that conclusion. What follows is a comparison of types of chest pain with some indications of what might be heart attack and what probably is not. However, heart attack symptoms are notoriously variable, and it is *always* a good idea to consult a health care professional when the source of chest pain is not clear.

FEATURES	ANGINA	HEART ATTACK	PULMONARY EMBOLISM	OTHER
Duration	Chest pain lasts several minutes, subsides.	Chest pain progressively worsens.	Chest pain progressively worsens.	Chest pain subsides in <1 min.
Trigger	Usually triggered by activity.	May or may not be immediately triggered by activity.	May or may not be immediately triggered by activity.	May or may not be immediately triggered by activity.
Activity	Stops when activity stops.	Doesn't stop when activity stops; continues to worsen.	Doesn't stop when activity stops; continues to worsen.	Stops when person drinks water, changes position, or takes a deep breath.
Causes	Caused by transient ischemia; heart muscle temporarily doesn't get enough oxygen to function.	Caused by permanent ischemia; blockage deprives cells of oxygen, and heart is irrevocably damaged.	Caused by blood clot in lung. Small clot may have little impact. Large clot may lead to pulmonary and circulatory collapse.	Caused by any number of factors, e.g., musculoskeletal injury, gastroesophageal reflux.

Some studies have indicated that taking aspirin regularly can decrease the chance of a repeat heart attack for people with a history of heart disease. Specially coated tablets have been designed to minimize gastrointestinal problems, but this intervention carries a possibility of an increased chance of subdural hemorrhage, so patients must consider carefully all the implications of taking aspirin on a daily basis.

Massage?

The appropriateness of massage for heart attack survivors absolutely depends on the individual, the extent of the damage, and how long ago it occurred. Some survivors of mild heart attacks may make themselves healthier than they ever were before, while others will accumulate high levels of plaque on their arteries within just a few years of surgery. The safety of massage depends on how easily the client can withstand the changes in internal environment that this work will bring about. This means that modalities that support rather than challenge homeostasis are generally the safest choices.

CASE HISTORY 5.2

HEART ATTACK

Bob, Age 49: The wake-up call.

About 15 years ago my mom, who was 60 years old, had bypass surgery. I knew that having a female relative diagnosed with cardiovascular disease at 60 years old put me in a high-risk category for heart problems, especially since I've had type 2 diabetes for about 10 years. I know I didn't eat the healthiest diet in the world. At that time my regular lunch was a quarter-pounder and a bag of fries.

Last summer my mother went through a series of angina attacks followed by an angioplasty and having a stent inserted. After watching her, I began to seriously think about my own condition. I talked to my doctor, and he set me up with a low-cost on-site stress test that just used an exercise bike. He said if I could pass that I'd be okay. I took it, and in the words of the technician, "My heart was not happy with what I was doing to it." So my doctor scheduled me with a cardiologist for a full treadmill test.

After that first test I went out for what I knew would be my last double quarter-pounder with cheese.

I didn't last long on the treadmill. When it was over, my blood pressure dropped and I had some really unpleasant symptoms, like dizziness, nausea, and a general feeling of crappiness. My doctor called my wife in from the waiting room, and with both of us together he said, "My recommendation is to put you in the hospital now. We'll do an angiogram along with anything else that needs to be done."

"Well," I said, "I have a couple of things I need to finish up. Can I take care of them and come right back?"

"I'd rather you didn't."

I checked right in.

I went into the hospital the Tuesday after Labor Day. On Wednesday I had the angiogram followed by an angioplasty. They found that the main section of the left coronary artery was 100% blocked. They had trouble pushing a wire through it, but when they got that done, they put in the balloon and then a titanium stent. (They said it wouldn't set anything off, but I can't get into Target anymore without having all the alarms go off.)

They told me that they found evidence of a recent heart attack—one that was a fraction of an inch away from what they call a widow maker. This was amazing to me, because I have no memory of any chest pains. The only thing I can remember was when I went on a trip with my family at the beginning of the summer. I'd hiked around a little that day. That night in the motel I had a migraine headache. I felt sick and threw up. I took some ibuprofen and went to bed. That's the only time I can think of that I had any symptoms at all.

Three days after the angioplasty I went home. They started my cardiac rehab right away. I go to the hospital to exercise under supervision. I am next door to an emergency room, and medical staff is in the room with me, so if anything happens, the response time will be really quick. When I first started, I was hooked up to a heart monitor with four patches to measure my blood pressure before, during, and after my exercise. The first time I tried to exercise, they made me quit because I was about to go into ventricular fibrillation. Now I go exercise three times a week. I use the treadmill, the bike, weight machines, and free weights. I walk a lot at work, but I can't walk at home; it's too steep around my house. My doctors tell me I can't ever let my heart rate get over 120 beats per minute. If it gets any higher than that, I run the risk of forming clots around the stent.

I'm on several medications now. Some control my diabetes (I don't take insulin), and I'm also taking anticoagulants for 3 months, along with beta blockers and calcium channel blockers. And of course I've changed my diet. I eat so much chicken I feel like I'm growing feathers. It's all baked or grilled, and I take off the skin. We have little or no fried food, so no more french fries. Since I've made these changes, my blood glucose has been much more under control—I average about 115 now, and normal is anywhere from 80 to 120.

This episode was a real wake-up call for me. I'm the youngest man at my job and the last one they expected to have heart trouble. My identical twin went in for his own stress test and came back fine, but he was a couple of years later than me in developing his diabetes too, so he'll still have to keep an eye on it. I did some research about my situation, and I found that what I had—silent ischemia—is especially common in diabetic men over 40. I hope any man with type 2 diabetes over 40 or 45 will be sure to get his heart checked. You never know what you might find.

Modality Recommendations for Heart Attack	
Deep Tissue Massage	Contraindicated until the client is cleared for rigorous exercise.
Lymphatic Drainage	Systemically contraindicated.
Polarity	S: Indicated as part of health care team. R/D: Supportive when subacute.
PNF/MET/Stretching	Supportive.
Reflexology	As part of a health care team, work endocrine, heart, chest, solar plexus points.
Shiatsu	Indicated for prevention and recovery.
Swedish Massage	Contraindicated while symptoms are present; otherwise stay within activity limitations and adjust for medications.
Trigger Point Therapy	Contraindicated during acute stage; otherwise supportive.

See Chapter 1 for a brief description of each modality, including definitions of abbreviations.

Heart Failure

Definition: What Is It?

Heart failure is a term for the progressive loss of cardiac function that accompanies age and a history of cardiovascular disease. It does *not* mean that the heart has stopped working altogether (that would be cardiac arrest); it simply means that the heart cannot keep up with the needs of the body.

Demographics: Who Gets It?

The statistics on the incidence of heart failure in the United States are alarming but understandable, considering the changes in the health profile of the population. Heart failure is on a dramatic rise in this country; it affects about 3 million people, and the incidence is expected to rise in coming years. About 400,000 new cases are diagnosed every year.[23] Most of those cases are among people who have survived other cardiovascular crises: heart attacks, coronary artery disease, aneurysm, and others. Where many years ago these problems would have killed these patients, they now survive and their hearts simply wear out from progressive damage to the cardiovascular system.

More men than women have heart failure until age 75, when numbers are about even between genders. It affects African Americans about twice as often as whites. The incidence of heart failure rises dramatically with age: it affects about 1% of the population at age 50 and up to 10% of the population age 75 and older. Acute decompensated heart failure accounts for about 1 million hospitalizations per year.[23]

Etiology: What Happens?

When the heart is asked to pump 2,000 gal of blood each day through vessels that are progressively narrowed and resistant, it goes through a series of changes that ultimately limit its ability to function. Unfortunately, the heart can enter early stages of heart failure with no signs or symptoms.

Heart Failure in Brief

What is it?
Heart failure is a condition in which the heart no longer can function well enough to keep up with the needs of the body. It is usually slowly progressive, developing over a number of years before any changes in function may be noticeable.

How is it recognized?
The symptoms depend on which side of the heart is working inefficiently. Left-sided heart failure results in fluid congestion in the lungs with general weakness and shortness of breath. Right-sided heart failure results in fluid backups throughout the system, which shows as edema, especially in the ankles and legs. Both varieties of heart failure lead to chest pain; cold, sweaty skin; a fast, irregular pulse; coughing, especially when the person is lying down; and very poor stamina.

Is massage indicated or contraindicated?
Heart failure contraindicates circulatory massage, as it has the goal of pushing fluid through a system that is incapable of adjusting to those changes. Energetic work may be more appropriate to help clients lower stress and cope with the challenges of severely restricted circulation.

As resistance in the cardiovascular system increases (usually from atherosclerosis, hypertension, and other manifestations of cardiovascular disease), the heart compensates in various ways. Any of these mechanisms is appropriate for short-term challenges, but over the long term they add to the problem rather than helping to solve it.

The heart muscle cells respond to chronic stress by growing. The ventricles appear to become larger and thicker, allowing the heart to push harder against resistance in the pulmonary or systemic circuits. Ultimately, however, this cardiac hypertrophy causes the ventricles to become stiff so they don't fill or contract normally.

Some chemicals that influence heart function can also help to compensate for short-term problems but add to long-term ones. Resistance in the system or injury to the heart causes the release of stress hormones, especially epinephrine and norepinephrine. These make the heart beat harder, which is appropriate for short-term situations but damaging for chronic ones. Shifts in hormones also cause the body to retain salt and water. Both of these features end up increasing blood pressure and adding to the workload of the overburdened heart.

Finally, the muscle simply wears out and functions so inefficiently that blood flow to the rest of the body is insufficient for the most basic kinds of activities: climbing a set of stairs, walking across a room, even getting out of bed. Left untreated, the heart muscle goes into fibrillations and the circulatory system collapses.

Most cases of heart failure are related to underlying cardiovascular disease. A history of atherosclerosis or heart attack with resulting scar tissue in the heart muscle increases the risk of developing heart failure. High blood pressure, untreated diabetes, smoking, and alcohol and drug abuse can all be contributing factors as well. An especially potent setup for heart failure is any combination of these risk factors: uncontrolled high blood pressure along with smoking, for instance.

A smaller number of heart failure patients do not have a history of cardiovascular disease but have sustained damage to the heart muscle for other reasons. Cardiomyopathy, valve diseases, infections of the valves or heart muscle, and congenital problems may all be factors in these cases.

Types of heart failure: systolic versus diastolic Heart failure is sometimes classified by which cardiac function is most impaired.

- *Systolic heart failure.* The left ventricle has become enlarged and cannot contract efficiently. Consequently, it can't push blood out into the aorta and the systemic circuit well enough to keep up with a person's needs.
- *Diastolic heart failure.* The ventricles have become enlarged but stiff. They don't relax and expand well to allow the inflow of blood from the atria. This also leads to inadequate pumping of blood through the pulmonary and systemic circuits.

Types of heart failure: left side versus right side Heart failure is also classified according to which side of the heart is weaker.

- *Left-sided heart failure.* The left ventricle is impaired. A backup in the pulmonary circuit allows seepage of fluid back into the alveoli; this is pulmonary edema (Figure 5.16). Symptoms of left-sided heart failure include severe shortness of breath and stubborn coughing, perhaps with bloody sputum. Symptoms are worst when a person is active or lying down. One serious complication of this condition is the risk of pneumonia in the functionally impaired lungs.
- *Right-sided heart failure.* Also called ***cor pulmonale***, it commonly results from pulmonary disease and high vascular resistance in the lungs—often as a complication of the pulmonary edema that accumulates with left-sided heart failure. Consequently, it becomes difficult to pump blood through the pulmonary circuit, and the backup is felt through the rest of the body. Symptoms include severe edema, especially in the legs

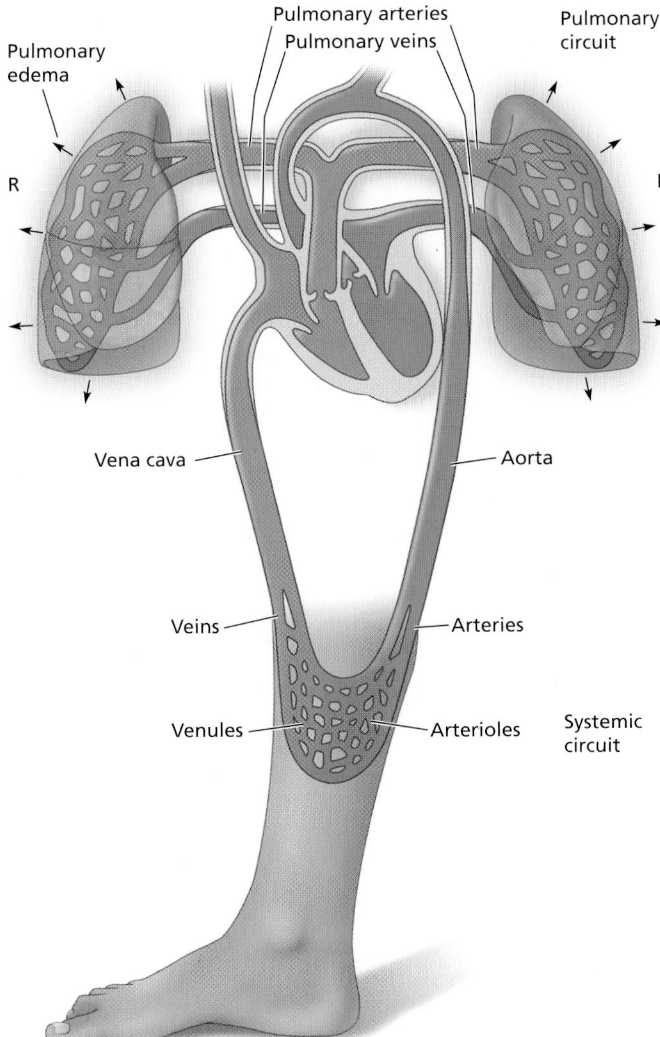

Figure 5.16. Left-sided heart failure leads to pulmonary edema.

(Figure 5.17). Someone with this type of heart failure has ankles that look like they're spilling over the sides of the shoes. If the patient is bedridden, the edema may occur in the abdomen (ascites) or in the pelvis—wherever gravity is pulling most. Right-sided heart failure is also closely linked to enlarged liver (hepatomegaly) and renal failure. As blood flow to the kidneys is reduced, the kidneys begin to retain water, which systemically increases blood pressure and makes the heart work even harder to push blood through narrow tubes.

- *Biventricular heart failure.* This is left- and ride-sided failure simultaneously. It is the end stage of the disease, and if the patient doesn't respond to medications, he or she may be a candidate for a heart transplant or other surgery.

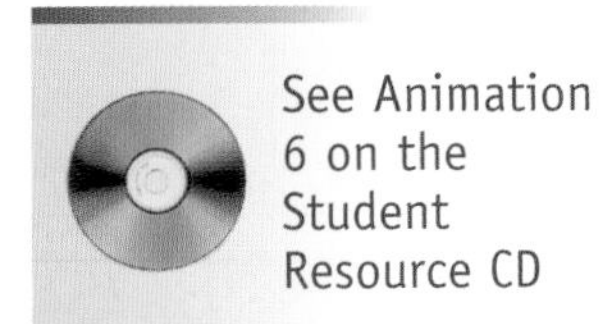

See Animation 6 on the Student Resource CD

Signs and Symptoms

Signs of heart failure depend on which side of the heart is dysfunctional, as already described. Along with shortness of breath (often exacerbated by lying down), low stamina, and edema, heart failure patients may also have chronic chest pain; indigestion; arrhythmia; visibly distended veins in the neck; cold, sweaty skin; and restlessness.

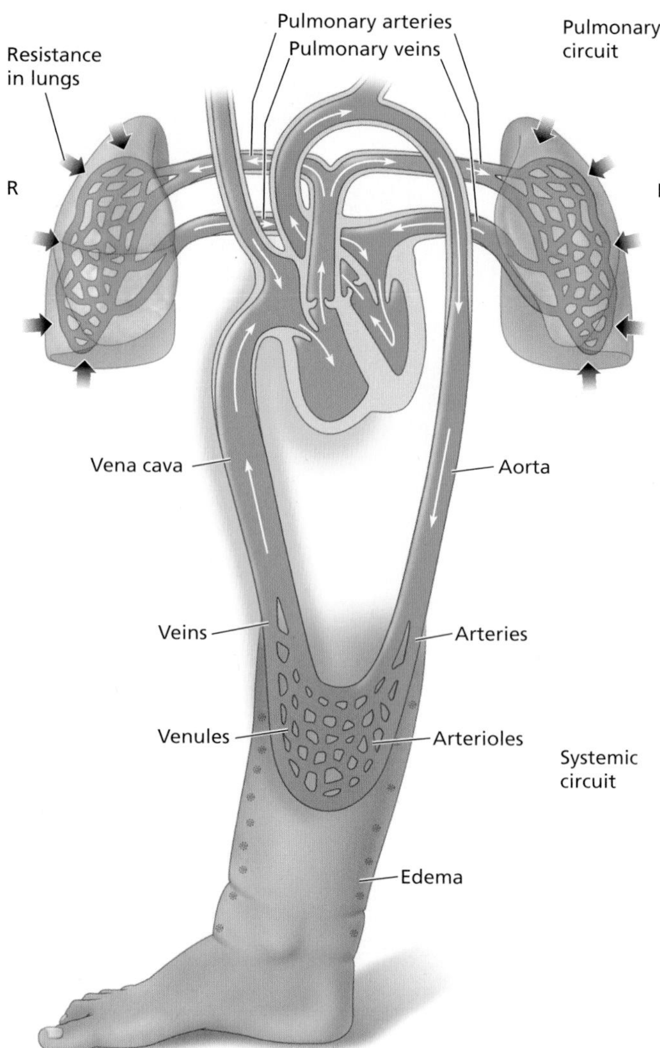

Figure 5.17. Right-sided heart failure leads to systemic edema.

Symptoms typically develop over a long period. If they have a sudden onset, they present a medical emergency.

Diagnosis

Heart failure isn't difficult to diagnose. It is often done through observation of systemic edema and *auscultation*, or listening to heart sounds and to the lungs for indications of fluid retention. Radiography may be indicated to look for cardiac enlargement, and an electrocardiogram may be conducted to analyze the efficiency of the heartbeat. An echocardiogram can show valve function if damage to these structures is suspected.

Heart failure may be rated on a scale of I to IV or from A to D. In either case, the mild end of the scale involves many risk factors but only minor symptoms or loss of function, while the extreme end of the scale indicates a life-threatening situation.

Treatment

The treatment options for heart failure depend on how severe it is and which side of the heart has been affected. Early interventions include rest, changes in diet, and modifications in physical activity so that the heart can be exercised without becoming overly stressed. Drugs for heart failure may include beta blockers, digitalis, diuretics, and vasodilators.

If a patient doesn't respond well to these noninvasive treatment options, surgery may be considered. Surgery can range anywhere from repair to damaged valves, to wrapping a strong mesh bag around the heart, to a complete heart or heart and lung transplant.

Massage?

Heart failure means that the heart can't function in a way that provides for essential needs. Most heart failure patients have other cardiovascular problems that contribute to their disease. Circulatory massage, which works with the intention of mechanically increasing blood flow through a basically healthy system, is inappropriate for clients whose blood vessels and heart cannot accommodate these changes in internal environment.

Energetic work that invites (rather than forces) the body to positive change may help to reduce blood pressure and perceived stress and so may be useful for heart failure patients, although it is not realistic to claim that massage can reverse the extensive damage seen with these clients.

MODALITY RECOMMENDATIONS FOR HEART FAILURE	
Deep Tissue Massage	Systemically contraindicated.
Lymphatic Drainage	Systemically contraindicated.
Polarity	S: Indicated when working as part of health care team. R/D: Supportive within client comfort.
PNF/MET/Stretching	Supportive.
Reflexology	As part of health care team, work endocrine, heart, chest, lymphatic, solar plexus points.
Shiatsu	Indicated. Treat H, K meridians and extensions systemically.
Swedish Massage	Supportive with light work; stay within activity limitations and adjust for medications.
Trigger Point Therapy	Supportive with light work.

See Chapter 1 for a brief description of each modality, including definitions of abbreviations.

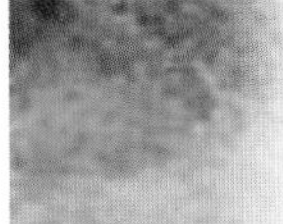

CHAPTER REVIEW QUESTIONS: CIRCULATORY SYSTEM CONDITIONS

1. What is the causative agent for malaria?
2. Why are fatigue and low stamina symptoms of anemia?
3. Name two types of blood cancer.
4. How does sickle cell disease lead to severely reduced immunity?
5. Where are the blockages that lead to heart attacks?
6. What is a term for uncoordinated contractions of heart chambers?
7. Why is hypertension called the "silent killer"?
8. Describe the circular relationship between high blood pressure and kidney dysfunction.

9. Describe how a person may have any three of the following conditions at the same time: high blood pressure, chronic renal failure, edema, atherosclerosis, diabetes, aortic aneurysm, stroke.
10. A client has a deep ache in the lower leg. Distal to the knee the tissue is clammy and edematous. Pressing at the ankle leaves a dimple, which takes several minutes to disappear. What cautions must be exercised with this client? Why?

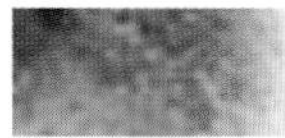

REFERENCES

1. Anemia. © 1998–2006 Mayo Foundation for Medical Education and Research. http://www.mayoclinic.com/health/anemia/DS00321. Accessed summer 2006.
2. Feied C, Handler J. Pulmonary Embolism. © 1996–2006 by WebMD. http://www.emedicine.com/emerg/topic490.htm. Accessed summer 2006.
3. Incidence. © Airhealth.org. http://www.airhealth.org/incidence.html. Accessed summer 2006.
4. Facts 2006–2007. Leukemia, Lymphoma, Myeloma. © The Leukemia & Lymphoma Society Inc. http://www.leukemia-lymphoma.org/all_mat_toc.adp?item_id=87311. Accessed summer 2006.
5. Malaria. Directors of Health Promotion and Education. http://www.dhpe.org/infect/Malaria.html. Accessed summer 2006.
6. Malaria. Centers for Disease Control and Prevention. http://www.cdc.gov/Malaria/features/surveillance_04.htm. Accessed summer 2006.
7. Malaria Fact Sheet. © 2006, Johns Hopkins University. http://www.jhsph.edu/Research Centers/malaria_facts.html. Accessed summer 2006.
8. Prognosis of Sickle Cell Anemia. Copyright © 2000–2006 Adviware Pty Ltd. http://www.wrong diagnosis.com/s/sickle_cell_anemia/prognosis.htm. Accessed summer 2006.
9. UF Pilot Study Shows Massage, Relaxation Reduce Sickle Cell Anemia Pain. © University of Florida. http://news.ufl.edu/2000/09/25/massage/. Accessed summer 2006.
10. Schrieber D. Deep Venous Thrombosis and Thrombophlebitis. © 1996–2006 by WebMD. http://www.emedicine.com/emerg/topic122.htm. Accessed Summer 2006.
11. Lee D. Abdominal Aortic Aneurysm. © 1996–2005 MedicineNet, Inc. All rights reserved. http://www.medicinenet.com/abdominal_aortic_aneurysm/article.htm. Accessed summer 2006.
12. Aortic aneurysm. © 1998–2006 Mayo Foundation for Medical Education and Research. All rights reserved. http://www.mayoclinic.com/health/aortic-aneurysm/DS00017. Accessed summer 2006.
13. Heart Disease and Stroke Statistics—2006 Update. © 2006 American Heart Association. http://www.americanheart.org/downloadable/heart/1140534985281Statsupdate06book.pdf. Accessed summer 2006.
14. Cigarette Smoking and Cardiovascular Diseases. © 2006 American Heart Association, Inc. http://www.americanheart.org/presenter.jhtml?identifier=4545..Accessed summer 2006.
15. Cholesterol Statistics. © 2006 American Heart Association. http://www.americanheart.org/presenter.jhtml?identifier=4506. Accessed summer 2006.
16. Health, United States, 2005. With Chartbook on Trends in the Health of Americans. National Center for Health Statistics. http://www.cdc.gov/nchs/data/hus/hus05. pdf#069. Accessed summer 2006.
17. Gingivitis. © 1995–2006 Life Extension Foundation. http://www.lef.org/protocols/dental/gin givitis_01.htm. Accessed summer 2006.
18. High Blood Pressure Statistics. © 2006 American Heart Association, Inc. http://www.american heart.org/presenter.jhtml?identifier=4621. Accessed summer 2006.
19. The Seventh Report of the Joint National Committee on Prevention, Detection, Evaluation, and Treatment of High Blood Pressure. National High Blood Pressure Education Program. NIH Publication 04-5230. http://www.nhlbi.nih.gov/guidelines/hypertension/jnc7full.pdf. Accessed summer 2006.
20. Research: Swedish Massage Massage Lowers Blood Pressure. Massage Magazine, April/May 2006. http://www.massagetherapyfoundation.org/pdf/MMagAprilMay2.pdf. Accessed summer 2006.

21. Varicose Veins and Spider Veins. National Women's Health Information Center. http://www.4woman.gov/faq/varicose.htm. Accessed summer 2006.
22. Feied C. Varicose Veins. © 1996–2006 by WebMD. http://www.emedicine.com/med/topic2788.htm. Accessed summer 2006.
23. Heart attack. © 1998–2006 Mayo Foundation for Medical Education and Research. All rights reserved. http://www.mayoclinic.com/health/heart-attack/DS00094. Accessed summer 2006.

6

Lymph and Immune System Conditions

Chapter Objectives

After reading this chapter you should be able to . . .

- Describe the difference between an allergy and an autoimmune disease.
- Identify one type of edema that indicates circulatory massage.
- Identify three types of edema that contraindicate circulatory massage.
- List two types of lymphoma.
- Explain why lymphoma causes anemia.
- Describe one risk of working with clients who have mononucleosis.
- Describe two central nervous system components seen with most chronic fatigue syndrome patients.
- Explain three benefits of not interfering with fever.
- Describe the four phases of HIV infection.
- State the most common symptom or complication of lupus.

Introduction

It is critically important for massage practitioners to understand the lymphatic system. It's a bit peculiar among systems: its components are not even vaguely symmetrical, and it functions as a sort of subsystem to both the circulatory and immune systems. The conditions listed under this heading may be influenced by either of the other two systems. Here is a brief overview of how the lymphatic system works.

Lymph System Structure

As blood travels away from the heart, it goes through progressively smaller tubes—the aorta branches into the arteries, which branch into arterioles, which finally divide into the very tiny and delicate capillaries. The pressure and speed with which blood travels decrease as blood gets farther from the heart. Still, everything keeps moving at a good pace; a blood cell can complete its circuit through the systemic circuit about every 60 seconds.

The walls of the capillaries are made of one-cell-thick squamous epithelium, designed for maximum efficiency of diffusion. Capillaries are so tiny that the red blood cells must line up one by one to pass through. This is the moment for the transfer of nutrients and wastes in the tissue cells. This is also where, having dropped off oxygen and picked up carbon dioxide, the blood vessels turn from arterial capillaries into venous capillaries. And finally, this is the moment when plasma from the arterial blood is squeezed out of the capillaries. In other words, *this* is the origin of interstitial fluid (Figure 6.1).

Interstitial fluid is absolutely vital. It is the medium in which all of the body's nutrients and wastes travel. But it must keep moving; if it stagnates, toxins or pathogens can accumulate and cause problems. Interstitial fluid keeps moving through the system by flowing into a different type of capillary, a lymphatic capillary. Lymphatic capillaries are similar to circulatory capillaries in construction, with one major difference: they are part of an *open* system. That is, interstitial fluid and even small particles can flow into lymphatic capillaries at almost any point along the length of that capillary. By contrast, circulatory capillaries are *closed* to the extent that red blood cells are *not* able to come and go unless the vessel has been damaged.

When interstitial fluid is drawn into a lymphatic capillary, it is called *lymph*. Lymph is composed mainly of plasma that has been pressed out of the bloodstream, loads of metabolic wastes that have been exuded by hardworking cells, and some chunks of particulate waste as well.

The new lymph is routed to a series of cleaning stations called nodes, where the wastes are neutralized and any small particles are filtered out. The nodes are also home to most of the body's specific immune-response cells, so if any pathogens have been picked up and marked by macrophages in the lymph, this is where the specific immune response gets started. The cleaned-up fluid is put back into the circulatory system just above the right atrium of the heart, where the right and left thoracic ducts empty into the right and left subclavian veins, respectively.

Lymph System Function

Lymph flows through the lymphatic capillaries into bigger and bigger vessels, usually against the pull of gravity and without the aid of the heart's direct pumping action. What moves it along? Several things:

- *Gravity* helps to move lymph if the limb is elevated.
- *Muscle contraction* pushes fluid through lymphatic vessels just as a hand squeezes around a tube of toothpaste. The larger lymphatic vessels also have smooth muscle tissue that contracts rhythmically.
- *Alternating hot and cold* hydrotherapy applications can increase contractions in the smooth muscle tissue of lymphatic vessels to move fluid along.
- *Deep breathing* draws lymph up the thoracic duct like an expanding bellows during inhalation and squeezes it out during exhalation.
- *Massage* with big mechanical manipulative strokes such as pétrissage and deep effleurage can increase lymph flow, but small, extremely superficial reflexive strokes can also cause fluid to be drawn into lymphatic capillaries. This is the mechanism employed with lymph drainage modalities.

If everything works well, fluid levels in the tissues are constant but not stagnant. The amount of fluid squeezed *out* of circulatory capillaries should be almost equal to the amount being drawn *into* lymphatic capillaries, with about 10% left over to become interstitial fluid; this is called the ***Starling equilibrium***. But a backup anywhere in the system can result in major changes in fluid balance. If veins,

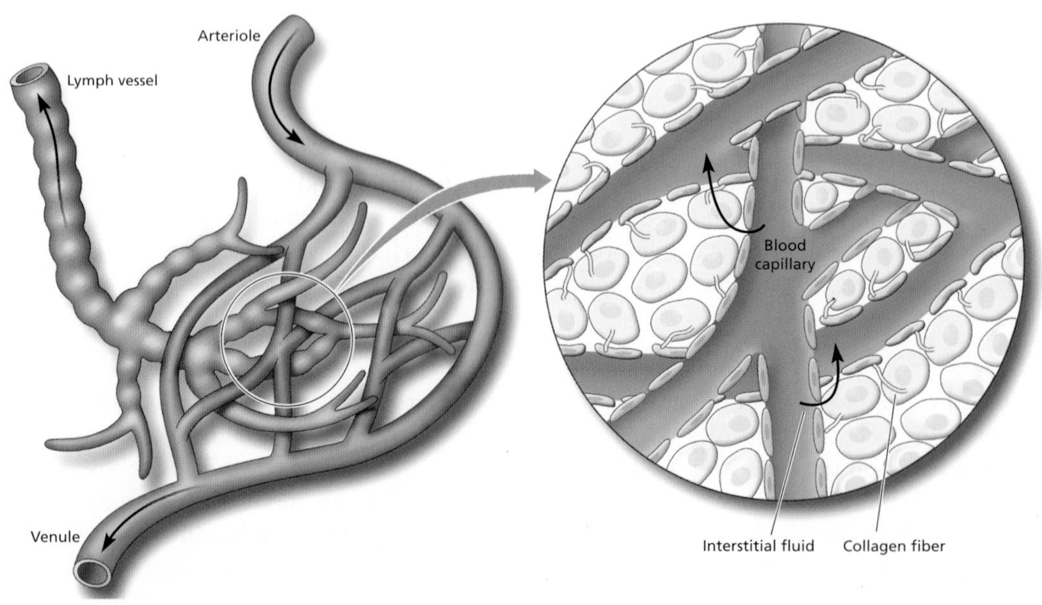

Figure 6.1. The origin of lymph.

lymph vessels, or nodes are blocked, fluid accumulates between tissue cells. The stagnant fluid quickly becomes a hindrance to diffusion and other chemical reactions rather than the transfer medium it is designed to be. This is the problem with many of the diseases of the lymph system, and it is a serious concern for massage practitioners, who generally should *not* be trying to push fluid through a system that is already overtaxed.

Immune System Function

The immune system is unique in that it is not composed of a collection of organs performing a task for a coordinated total effort, like other systems in the body. Instead, it is a nebulous, incredibly complex collection of cells and chemicals whose coordinated function is to keep the whole organism safe.

The primary function of the immune system is to distinguish what is *self* from what is *non self* and to eradicate anything that is *non self* as quickly as possible. Immune system devices range from very general to highly specific in identifying exactly which antigens they attack (Sidebar 6.1). Some white cells attack anything; others simply ignore a pathogen if it's not their particular target. Most of the nonspecific immune devices, such as intact skin and the acidity of the gastric juices, are not discussed here. However, it is worthwhile to look at some of the *specific* immune machinery, because when it's working well it's positively miraculous, and when it's *not* working well or when it makes mistakes, things can go terribly wrong.

T-Cells and B-Cells

The two interlocking branches of the specific immune responses are cellular immunity (T-cells) and humoral immunity (B-cells). Neither of these extremely complicated systems can work at all unless their target pathogen is displayed by a nonspecific white blood cell. So *that* is the first step in fighting off an infection: a white blood cell must find, destroy, and display a piece of the microorganism in question. Fortunately, white blood cells are distributed

SIDEBAR 6.1: DIFFERENT WHITE BLOOD CELLS FOR DIFFERENT FUNCTIONS

White blood cells come in various sizes, classes, and strengths. Each type of leukocyte has a specific role in the immune system and inflammatory response. As researchers learn more about how these cells work and communicate with each other, we gain ability to influence their activities.

Neutrophils

Neutrophils are the smallest, fastest, and most common of the white blood cells. They are produced in bone marrow, and chemicals that leak from damaged cells stimulate their production in even greater numbers. Neutrophils have a short life; they sacrifice themselves to disable potential invaders.

Monocytes

Monocytes begin as small white blood cells, but they have the power to change. When they are released into the bloodstream from the bone marrow, they circulate until they reach a target tissue. Then they leave the circulatory system to infiltrate that tissue and grow into *macrophages*, big eaters that can devour pathogens and display bits of cell membrane that begin the specific immune response.

Monocytes and macrophages move slowly; they are usually involved in the subacute or chronic phases of inflammatory response.

Eosinophils and Basophils

These inflammatory agents are not well understood. They have been observed most often in the context of allergic reactions and responses against invading parasites.

Lymphocytes

Lymphocytes include B cells, T cells, and natural killer cells. These are manufactured in both bone marrow and lymphoid tissue and are most often engaged in specific immune system responses to pathogens. These are the agents that allow us to develop immunity to infections.

That's a very brief summary of specific immunity, and it's a lot more than was known just 30 years ago. One of the most exciting discoveries about immune system function is that immune system cells actually *talk* to each other, discussing in a language of chemicals called cytokines their strategies in fighting off infection. These chemical messages are being deciphered, and some of them have been found to say things like *act like me, come over here*, and *eat this*. The ability to read these chemical codes and manufacture medicines that can influence immune system behavior by mimicking specific cytokines is opening whole new treatment options.

Furthermore, it turns out that immune system cells don't just talk to each other. Some of the chemical messages they send out are picked up and acted on by other systems in the body, especially the nervous and endocrine systems. White blood cells have receptors for central nervous system chemicals, for instance. In other words, the nervous system can talk directly to the immune system. Some of the lymphokines secreted by white blood cells are similar, even identical, to the neurotransmitters previously assumed to exist only in the central nervous system. Other lymphokines, specifically interleukin-1, are secreted by macrophages but relay information to the hypothalamus. This reveals some major implications about how health and resistance to disease are related to mental and emotional state. Intuitively this makes a lot of sense, and for the first time there is a way to back up these theories with empirical evidence. A branch of science called ***psychoneuroimmunology*** has been developed specifically to explore these relationships. Bit by bit, the imaginary division between mind and body is disappearing.

generously all through the blood and interstitial fluid, and they are concentrated in places such as the superficial fascia, lymph nodes, lungs, and liver, where the chance of meeting pathogens is especially high.

Consider what happens when someone touches a contaminated doorknob and then wipes his or her eye: rhinovirus 14 has just been introduced into the body. A passing macrophage eats the pathogen, and it is drawn through lymphatic capillaries into a nearby lymph node. A T-cell is waiting there. It just happens to be specially designed to recognize the flag of rhinovirus 14. The T-cell gets very busy, replicating itself into several forms that go out into the bloodstream in search of more viruses to attack. In the process, the original T-cell stimulates its B-cell partner. This B-cell clones, and the new cells start producing out rhinovirus 14–specific antibodies at a mind-boggling pace: 2,000 antibodies per second. Antibodies are *not* alive. They are Y-shaped chemicals forged especially to lock onto their target pathogen and retire it. This can happen in any of several ways, depending on the pathogen and the antibodies involved.

Back when the T-cells and B-cells were first becoming active, they each made a few copies of themselves that would outlive the infection and circulate through the body on the lookout for future attempts by the same pathogen to invade. These are *memory cells*, and thanks to them, people very seldom get sick with the same pathogen twice. If rhinovirus 14 gains access to the body again, an immune attack can mobilize against it so quickly that a person might never know he was even exposed.

Immune System Mistakes

The immune system is miraculous in how the T- and B-cells can somehow recognize their own special pathogen and launch just the right attack against it. It has even been shown that B cells produce antibodies that can disable synthetic pathogens that don't occur in nature. *That's* being prepared! But the immune system occasionally makes mistakes. Sometimes it launches a full-scale attack, with an inflammatory response, antibody production, and collateral damage to nearby cells, against an antigen that's not dangerous: cat dander, oak pollen, or peanuts, for instance: this is called an allergic reaction. Allergies range in severity from mildly annoying to life threatening.

The other slip the immune system can make is to mistake a part of the body for a dangerous pathogen. That is, it fails to distinguish *self* from *non-self*. Conditions involving this type of mistake are called autoimmune disorders. This group of diseases includes multiple sclerosis, lupus, scleroderma, rheumatoid arthritis, myasthenia gravis, and many other chronic, incurable problems. Both allergies and autoimmune dysfunction are sometimes discussed as *hypersensitivity reactions* (Sidebar 6.2).

SIDEBAR 6.2: HYPERSENSITIVITY REACTIONS AND MASSAGE OIL

Type I hypersensitivity reactions typically occur within several seconds to a few minutes of exposure to an irritating substance. However, a late-phase type I reaction can sustain allergic symptoms long after the irritation has been removed. *Arachidonic acid* is a substance associated with late-phase type I reactions, especially in the form of bronchial asthma. The significance of this for massage therapists is that some types of massage oils can break down into arachidonic acid on the skin. A client who is sensitive to this type of reaction may have no immediate skin symptoms but may wonder several hours later why he is coughing, wheezing, and feeling short of breath.

Oils that are particularly prone to breaking down into arachidonic acid are composed mostly of omega-6–sized molecules. These include safflower, soy, almond, sunflower, and corn oils. Although they can be pleasant and convenient to use for massage, they are the most likely to cause skin irritation and allergic reactions. Therefore, when it is important to avoid potentially irritating oils for certain conditions, these are the ones to eliminate first.

Four types of hypersensitivity reactions have been classified. Because two of them can involve the skin and the other two can involve systemic disorders, it's useful for massage therapists to be familiar with them.

- *Type I* hypersensitivity reactions are an immediate reaction to an antigen, or particle of nonself. In this situation immunoglobulin-E (IgE), a specific class of antibody, quickly sensitizes nearby mast cells to the presence of an "enemy," which may be a fragment of pollen, the proteins from peanuts or shellfish, or a droplet of bee venom. The alerted mast cells then release ***histamine*** and other chemicals that create dramatic changes in vascular permeability and that attract other white blood cells to the area. This inflammatory response produces the symptoms that are associated with typical allergic reactions: redness, swelling, itching, weepy eyes, and runny nose with hay fever; or nausea, vomiting, and diarrhea with certain food allergies.
- *Type II* hypersensitivity reactions are far less common than type I. They involve inflammatory cytotoxic (cell killing) reactions against a specific substance that may or may not belong to the body. Examples of type II reactions include hemolytic anemia, penicillin allergies, and reactions to the transfusion of mismatched blood.
- *Type III* reactions are those in which antibodies bind with antigens but the particles they form are

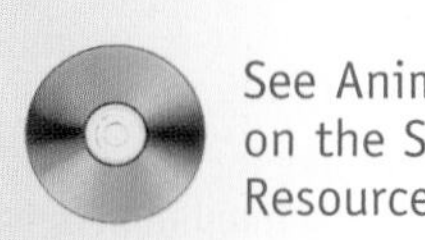
See Animation 7 on the Student Resource CD.

too small to be phagocytized. These tiny conglomerates, called *granulomas*, are eventually caught in the body's most delicate fluid filters: in the kidneys, the eyes, the brain, and the serous membranes surrounding the heart, lungs, and abdominal cavity. There they stimulate immune system activity, which results in inflammation and damage to these very delicate structures. Examples of type III reactions include systemic lupus erythematosus, a specific type of kidney damage called glomerulonephritis, and possibly rheumatoid arthritis.

- *Type IV*, or delayed, reactions are cell mediated; they rely on T cells to stimulate an immune response to an irritant. Contact dermatitis is an example of a type IV hypersensitivity reaction. In this case an inflammatory reaction appears on the skin after exposure to an irritating substance such as plant toxins, certain dyes, soaps, metals, or latex. This usually delayed reaction may occur 24 to 48 hours after exposure

Lymph and Immune System Conditions

Lymph System Conditions

Edema
Lymphangitis
Lymphoma
Mononucleosis

Immune System Conditions

Allergic reactions
Chronic fatigue syndrome
Fever
HIV/AIDS
Lupus

Lymph System Conditions

Edema

Definition: What Is It?

Edema is accumulation of fluid between cells. It may be local or systemic, and it is usually associated with inflammation or poor circulation. In any case the stagnant fluid must be pulled from the interstitial spaces into lymphatic capillaries to be processed by the lymph system.

Etiology: What Happens?

The Starling equilibrium states that the forces that cause fluid to leave blood capillaries should *almost* equal the forces that cause fluid to be reabsorbed by blood capillaries and that anything left over (which should be about 10%) should be taken in and processed by the lymph system. Lymph capillaries are perfectly designed to pick up excess interstitial fluid: each squamous cell is anchored to surrounding tissue by a collagen filament. When excess fluid accumulates in any area, these anchoring filaments pull back on the squamous cells, increasing the lymph capillary's ability to take in fluid. Sometimes, however, more fluid builds up in the tissues than the circulatory and lymph systems combined can take in, and this is called edema. Edema isn't generally noticeable until interstitial fluid volume is about 30% above normal.

Edema in Brief

Pronunciation: eh-DEE-mah

What is it?
Edema is retention of interstitial fluid because of electrolyte or protein imbalances, or because of mechanical obstruction in the circulatory or lymphatic systems.

How is it recognized?
Edematous tissue is puffy or boggy in early stages. It may become hard (indurated) if it is not resolved quickly. The area may be hot if associated with local infection, or quite cool if it is cut off from local circulation.

Is massage indicated or contraindicated?
Most edemas contraindicate circulatory massage. This is true especially of pitting edema, where tissue does not immediately spring back from a touch. Edemas that indicate massage include those due to subacute soft tissue injury or short-term immobilization caused by some factor that does *not* contraindicate massage.

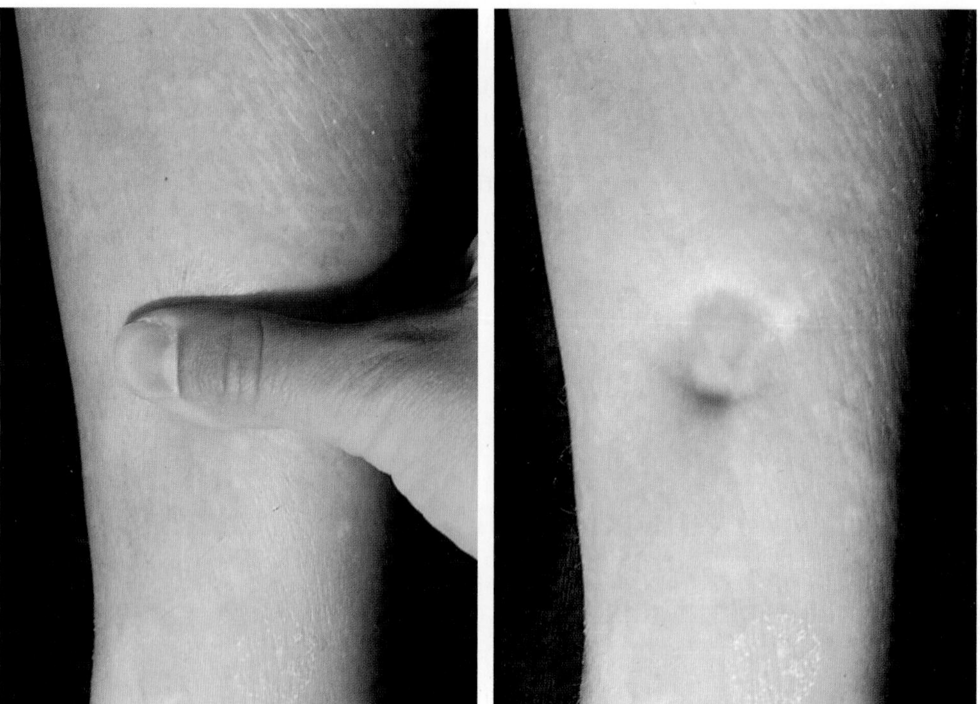

Figure 6.2. Pitting edema. **Left.** Before thumb pressure. **Right.** After thumb pressure.

Edema can have any of several causes; most of them are a combination of chemical and mechanical factors. Mechanical factors may involve a weakened heart or an obstruction to venous or lymphatic return. Chemical causes of edema usually have to do with accumulation of salts or proteins in the interstitial fluid, which causes the area to retain water.

Lymphedema is different from simple edema; this is the result of damage to lymphatic structures and accumulation of proteins in the interstitial fluid. It is discussed in Chapter 12.

Signs and Symptoms

Edema varies in presentation according to the source, the duration, and the area that is affected. Tissue is often soft, puffy, or boggy. The area may be hot if the edema is related to a recent injury or infection, or cool if the edema is long-standing and related to poor circulation.

When blood or lymphatic movement is chronically impaired, pitting edema may develop: a pit or dimple remains in the tissue for several minutes after it is gently compressed (Figure 6.2). Tissue that is edematous because of chronic problems such as heart failure or lymph node loss may become indurated, or hardened.

Massage?

Most types of systemic edema and *every* instance of pitting edema contraindicate circulatory massage because of the impact this kind of bodywork has on fluid flow.

Bodywork that is specifically designed to work with lymphatic flow can sometimes be used as long as the therapist is fully trained and knows how to avoid risks of infection or overtreatment.

Edemas that contraindicate circulatory massage Practitioners must be extremely careful to rule out these causes of edema before working with a client.

- *Heart problems.* If the heart is overtaxed, as seen with heart failure, and is not pumping the volumes it should be, fluid accumulates in the tissues. Massage does not improve this situation and could quite possibly make it worse by putting an even greater load on the system.

- *Kidney problems.* If the kidneys are not filtering blood fast enough or completely enough because of chemical imbalance or mechanical obstruction, massage could make the resulting systemic edema much worse.
- *Liver problems.* If the liver is congested, the puffiness and bogginess of typical edema may be less visibly apparent, but the same rules apply: pushing blood through a system that is chemically or mechanically impaired is likely to do damage.
- *Local infection.* If edema accumulates because of local infection, massage is contraindicated because of the risk of pushing pathogens into the lymphatic and circulatory systems before the body has had a chance to marshal appropriate defenses.
- *Blockage.* If a mechanical blockage develops anywhere in the circulatory system, massage is contraindicated because it can damage delicate structures, or worse, it could break loose a blood clot or other debris. Some examples of mechanical blockages include edema associated with pregnancy, thrombus, embolism, deep vein thrombosis, or lymph node damage that leads to lymphedema.

Edemas that indicate massage This is not to say that every kind of edema absolutely contraindicates every kind of massage under every circumstance. Edema is a red flag for massage therapists, and it calls for caution before proceeding. But if a client has fluid retention related to a subacute musculoskeletal injury, skilled massage is *very* appropriate, and in fact could contribute to the healing process. Likewise, if a client is confined to bed or is even partially immobilized for some reason that does *not* contraindicate massage, bodywork can be valuable to the health of his or her injured tissues as long as the risk of blood clotting has been ruled out. Bodywork modalities with minimal impact on fluid flow are more appropriate for edema than Swedish or other types of massage, but even practitioners of energy work need to know *why* their clients are retaining water to make the best possible choices for their care.

Modality Recommendations for Edema

Deep Tissue Massage	Locally or systemically contraindicated while acute, depending on cause.
Lymphatic Drainage	Indicated when infection is not present.
Polarity	S: Indicated. R/D: Supportive within client comfort; contraindicated for contraindicated edemas.
PNF/MET/Stretching	Supportive when no infection is present.
Reflexology	Indicated: work lymphatic system, kidneys, adrenals, heart points.
Shiatsu	Indicated. Treat K, SP meridians and extensions systemically and at site. Exercise caution if edema is pitting. Add movement and ROM to distal joint according to client comfort.
Swedish Massage	Locally contraindicated with trauma. Locally or systemically contraindicated with infection, heart or kidney failure, pitting. Can be beneficial if no other pathologies are present.
Trigger Point Therapy	Indicated while subacute for musculoskeletal problems; otherwise supportive.

See Chapter 1 for a brief description of each modality, including definitions of abbreviations.

Lymphangitis in Brief

Pronunciation: lim-fan-JY-tis

What is it?

Lymphangitis is an infection of lymph capillaries. If the infection invades the nodes, it is called *lymphadenitis*. If it gets past the lymphatic system and enters the bloodstream, it is called blood poisoning (*septicemia*), and it can be life threatening.

How is it recognized?

Lymphangitis has all of the signs of local infection: pain, heat, redness, swelling. It may also show red streaks from the site of infection running toward the nearest lymph nodes. Fever and malaise are often present as well.

Is massage indicated or contraindicated?

Lymphangitis contraindicates bodywork until the infection has been eradicated.

Lymphangitis

Definition: What Is It?

Lymphangitis is an infection with inflammation in the *lymphangions*, or lymphatic capillaries.

Demographics: Who Gets It?

People with depressed immunity and/or poor circulation are especially susceptible to lymphangitis because their white blood cell activity is sluggish, affording any available bacteria the opportunity to establish a stronghold in the lymphatic system.

Massage practitioners have a greater chance of developing lymphangitis than most clients do. This condition is an occupational hazard for bodywork professional because repeated immersions of the hands in soapy water may lead to hangnail formation and drying and cracking of nail beds. When these microscopic injuries are exposed to the pathogens that inhabit even healthy clients' skin, the risk of infection is significant.

Etiology: What Happens?

In lymphangitis the lymph capillaries become infected, usually with *Streptococcus pyogenes*, although other pathogens, including *Staphylococcus*, can also be the cause. This condition usually arises from a small injury on the skin. It can be a complication of cellulitis or of a viral or fungal infection such as herpes simplex or athlete's foot.

When the pathogens gain entry, they set up an infection in the lymph vessel before macrophages or other white blood cells can stop them. Infections that invade the lymph nodes are called *lymphadenitis*.

Signs and Symptoms

Lymphangitis starts with signs of local infection: pain, heat, redness, and swelling. The infected lymph vessel often shows a visible scarlet track running proximally from the portal of entry, which is usually some lesion in the skin such as a hangnail, a knife cut, or an insect bite (Figure 6.3).

If the infection is unchecked by white blood cells, it quickly moves farther into the lymph system, leading to swollen nodes, fever, and a general feeling of misery. Blisters may develop along the line of infection. Depending on the virulence of the bacteria, extensive tissue damage may also occur. This can happen surprisingly quickly; lymphangitis can become a systemic infection in a matter of hours.

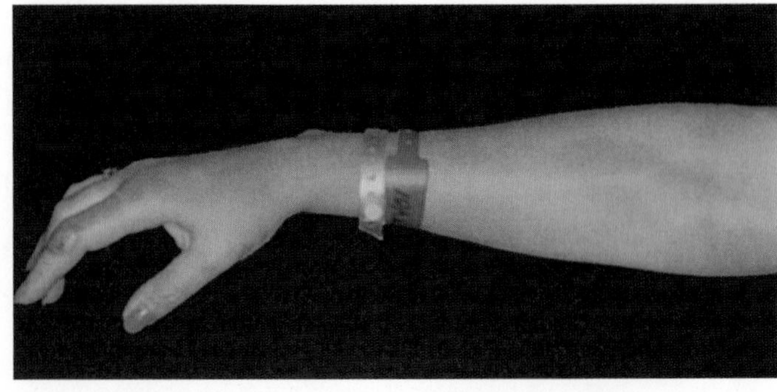

Figure 6.3. Lymphangitis: an infection of lymph capillaries.

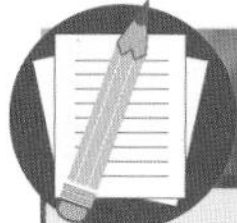

CASE HISTORY 6.1

Lymphangitis

Ruth, aged 24: "It was the most miserable night of my life."

One winter I was working four jobs at once. I was a tutoring for a massage school, I was setting up a small practice of my own, I was a nanny during the afternoons, and I was also working in a theater company, doing anything that needed doing, which was usually a lot. I enjoyed all of it, but I let myself get pretty run down.

I remember it was the week before Christmas, which was a really busy time for the theater company; we went on tour doing shows for young children. I had also done several massage treatments that week, which was unusual for me. I was working in the light booth at the theater one morning when I noticed that a hangnail on my right index finger suddenly seemed swollen, hot, and tender. There wasn't anything I could do about it. I remember sitting there for about an hour watching it get bigger, redder, and more painful.

That afternoon I had to leave town to be with my family over the holidays. The airport had been socked in with fog for 3 days, which delayed all the flights, so I missed my connection and had to spend the night on the floor of O'Hare Airport in Chicago. It was one of the most miserable times I can remember. I was feverish and shaking, and my hand hurt like hell.

By the time I finally reached Washington, DC, all I wanted to do was go to bed. I spent practically the entire holiday flat on my back. The swelling at my finger finally subsided, but not before I broke out in intensely painful blisters all over my mouth. My doctor back home told me they were probably just an opportunistic outbreak while my defenses were low. All I know is they made it impossible to eat and I missed all my favorite foods.

I found out much later that I had probably had lymphangitis and that I was very lucky it didn't develop into blood poisoning, especially since I didn't see a doctor until the whole thing was over. If I had it to do over again, I'd make sure I *never* let myself get so run down, and I'd be sure to cover any noticeable hangnails before doing massage. I wouldn't wish an experience like that on my worst enemy.

Complications

Lymphangitis is an infection of the lymph system, not the circulatory system. However, if even a few bacteria get past the filtering action of the lymph nodes, the infection *can* enter the bloodstream at the right or left subclavian vein. Then the situation is much more serious: the person has ***septicemia***, or blood poisoning, which is life threatening. This is why, if lymphangitis is a possibility, medical intervention is advisable at the earliest possible opportunity

Treatment

Lymphangitis is usually treated successfully with antibiotic therapy. Treatment must begin soon after the infection is identified, however, or the infection may complicate into blood poisoning.

Massage?

Lymphangitis patients feel so sick so fast that an infected client is highly unlikely to try to keep an appointment. While a client who has lymphangitis is contraindicated to *receive* massage, a practitioner who has it is likewise contraindicated to *give* massage. Therefore, massage therapists must keep their hands clean and own a good pair of cuticle scissors. They must *not* allow hangnails and other lesions to go uncovered or untrimmed, and perhaps most important, they must *not* allow their health to degenerate to the point that they are vulnerable to this kind of infection (Case History 6.1).

If a massage therapist has an open hangnail or other wound, the threat of lymphangitis is an excellent reason to cover it with a liquid bandage, finger cot, or other device during appointments.

Modality Recommendations for Lymphangitis

Deep Tissue Massage	Systemically contraindicated while acute.
Lymphatic Drainage	Systemically contraindicated while acute.
Polarity	S: Indicated for immune system support. R/D: Contraindicated while acute.
PNF/MET/Stretching	Systemically contraindicated while acute; otherwise supportive.
Reflexology	Systemically contraindicated while acute; otherwise supportive.
Shiatsu	Indicated for strengthening immune system via TH, SP.
Swedish Massage	Systemically contraindicated.
Trigger Point Therapy	Systemically contraindicated.

See Chapter 1 for a brief description of each modality, including definitions of abbreviations.

Hodgkin Disease

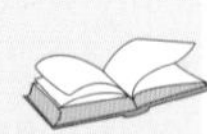

Thomas Hodgkin (1798–1866) was a British physician who documented this disorder.

Lymphoma

Definition: What Is It?

Lymphoma is any type of cancer of the lymph nodes. Like leukemia and myeloma, lymphoma involves a mutation of the DNA in specific white blood cells. These cancers usually start in the lymph tissues (including nodes and the spleen), but they can involve bone marrow cells as well. Some types of lymphoma are now understood to be lymphocytic types of leukemia, so the delineations between these labels are becoming hazy.

Demographics: Who Gets It?

About 67,000 people in the United States are diagnosed with lymphoma every year: 8,000 with Hodgkin lymphoma, and 59,000 with non-Hodgkin lymphoma. About 519,000 people in the United States are living with some form of lymphoma.[1] The rates of lymphoma diagnosis are climbing: its incidence is up 80% since 1973.[2] The reasons for this are not fully understood. Some factors include better screening and more accurate early diagnosis; an aging population; more survivors of immunosuppressant conditions, such as HIV/AIDS and organ transplants; and increased exposure to Epstein-Barr virus.

Although lymphoma does occur in children, most patients are adults. Hodgkin lymphoma most commonly affects people 15 to 34 years old or those over 55. Non-Hodgkin lymphoma is most common among people 60 to 70 years old.

Lymphoma causes about 20,500 deaths per year: 19,000 from non-Hodgkin lymphoma and 1,500 from Hodgkin lymphoma. Overall, death rates from lymphoma are declining for all populations.[1]

Lymphoma in Brief
Pronunciation: lim-FOE-mah

What is it?
Lymphoma is any variety of cancer that grows in lymph tissues. Many types have been identified; some are aggressive and very threatening, and others progress more slowly.

How is it recognized?
Painless swelling of lymph nodes is the cardinal sign of lymphoma, along with the possibility of anemia, fatigue, low-grade fever, night sweats, itchiness, rash, abdominal pain, and loss of appetite.

Is massage indicated or contraindicated?
Rigorous circulatory massage is generally not recommended for a person who is fighting lymphoma, although this may be a case-by-case decision. Any bodywork treatments must be incorporated into the rest of the client's treatment plan.

Etiology: What Causes It?

Lymphoma is cancer that originates in lymph tissues. Like leukemia, this disease begins with a mutation of the DNA of the affected cells, which in this case is usually some type of B-cell (these account for about 80% of cases) or of T-cells or natural killer cells. The mutated cell begins to replicate, producing massive numbers of nonfunctioning lymphocytes. This causes the lymph tissues to enlarge, and it initiates the other symptoms associated with lymphoma, namely, anemia, night sweats, itchy skin, and fatigue, among others.

The seriousness of lymphoma depends on what type of cell has mutated and how quickly it replicates. Over 30 different types of lymphoma have been identified, and they are categorized mainly by the appearance of the mutated cells.

Types of lymphoma Lymphoma is typically described as Hodgkin lymphoma or non-Hodgkin lymphoma. Hodgkin lymphoma involves the mutation of B cells into large, malignant, multinucleate cells called ***Reed Sternberg cells***. It is seen most often in the submandibular nodes but can also occur at the axillary and inguinal nodes. Eventually the growths metastasize to organ tissues, particularly the liver or bone marrow. The metastasis tends to be predictable and well organized, which distinguishes Hodgkin from non-Hodgkin lymphoma.

Recently the World Health Organization (WHO) worked with researchers to create the WHO-REAL (Revised European American Lymphoma) system to base classification of all types of lymphoma on cell morphology and lineage. This outline incorporates new understanding of the overlap between B-cell lymphocytic leukemia and lymphoma and helps to determine the best possible treatment options for various forms of lymphoma. A simplified version of the WHO-REAL classification follows:

- *Precursor and peripheral B-cell neoplasms* include many subtypes of B-cell lymphomas. Among them are B-cell acute and chronic lymphocytic leukemia, follicular lymphoma, hairy cell leukemia, Burkitt lymphoma, and several others.
- *T-cell and natural killer cell neoplasms* include T-cell chronic lymphocytic leukemia, aggressive natural killer cell leukemia, T-cell granular lymphocytic leukemia, and several others.
- *Hodgkin lymphoma* includes both nodular and classic Hodgkin lymphoma, with several subtypes.

Risk Factors

The increasing incidence of lymphoma in the past 30 years has raised the distinct possibility that this cancer can be linked to environmental exposure. Some research finds statistical relations between lymphoma and exposure to insecticides, herbicides, fertilizers, and even hair dye, but the direct cause-and-effect relationships have not yet been established.

Other environmental factors that increase the risk of developing certain types of lymphoma involve infection with specific pathogens. The incidence of lymphoma is 50 to 100 times higher among HIV-positive patients than it is among the general population. Epstein-Barr virus, which is associated with mononucleosis, has been linked to Burkitt lymphoma. Human T-cell lymphotropic virus is associated with T-cell lymphoma. And having the ***Helicobacter pylori*** bacterium raises the risk of developing lymphoma that originates in the stomach wall.

Signs and Symptoms

The primary sign of any kind of lymphoma is painless, nontender swelling of lymph nodes, especially in the neck, axilla, and inguinal area (Figure 6.4). Other signs and symptoms include anemia, fatigue, weight loss, night sweats, itchy skin, and loss of appetite. These typically have a relatively fast onset and persist for 2 weeks or more. Indolent varieties of lymphoma may have symptoms that come and go; this is problematic because it may cause a person to delay getting an important diagnosis.

In later stages lymphoma may show easy bruising and skin discoloration as platelet numbers drop, along with decreased resistance to cold, flu, and other infections.

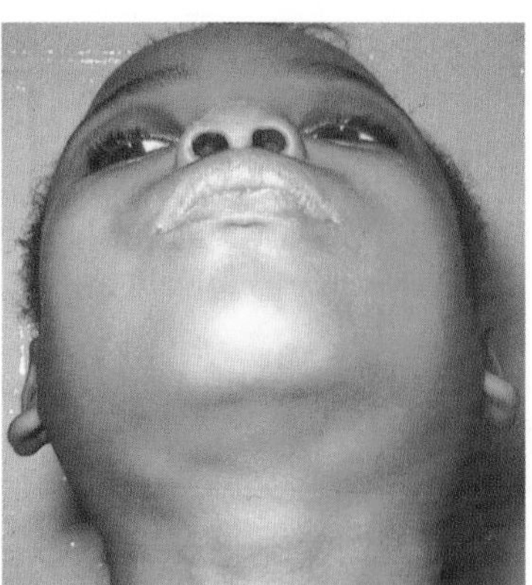

Figure 6.4. Hodgkin lymphoma: cervical and submandibular lymph nodes are visibly enlarged.

Diagnosis

The diagnosis of lymphoma begins with manual palpation of enlarged lymph nodes. If symptoms persist for 2 weeks or more, tests may be run to evaluate the node or nodes, and computed tomography (CT) or magnetic resonance imaging (MRI) may be used to look for signs of growth in the bones and other tissues so the cancer can be accurately staged.

Treatment

Treatment choices for lymphoma depend on several factors, including exactly which type of cells are affected, the progression of the disease, and whether it's a type A or type B presentation.

Chemotherapy and radiation are the usual choices, but some other options are providing success in dealing with lymphoma. These include allogenic and autologous bone marrow transplants, stem cell transplants, and various types of biologic therapy involving radioactive antibodies, cancer vaccinations, and other strategies.

SIDEBAR 6.3: STAGING LYMPHOMA

Lymphoma is staged by its degree of progression. In addition to a numerical stage, lymphoma is classified by whether symptoms other than enlarged glands accompany it. In other words, stage I-A means that the cancer is localized and not accompanied by fever, night sweats, or weight loss. Stage II-B means that the cancer has spread to nearby lymph nodes and the patient has fever and night sweats and has lost at least 10% of body weight within the previous 6 months.

- **Stage I.** The cancer is found in only one nodal region, or it has invaded only one nearby organ.
- **Stage II.** Two or more nodal regions are affected, and they are on the same side of the diaphragm; *or* multiple nodal regions along with one organ all on the same side of the diaphragm are affected.
- **Stage III.** Nodes on both sides of the diaphragm are invaded, along with organ involvement; the spleen may or may not be affected.
- **Stage IV.** The cancer is disseminated throughout the body, affecting nodes, organs, bone marrow, and/or the central nervous system.
- **Recurrent.** Recurrent lymphoma is cancer that reappears after a full course of treatment.

Prognosis

The prognosis for lymphoma depends on the type of cancer, the stage at which it is diagnosed, the age of the patient, and several other factors.

The 5-year survival rate for Hodgkin lymphoma is over 86%, and children fare even better, with a survival rate that tops 95%. The survival rates for other types of lymphoma vary, but collectively they have significantly improved to 62.9% for all patients and almost 82% for people diagnosed younger than age 20.

About 519,000 lymphoma survivors are living in the United States.[1]

Massage?

Rigorous circulatory massage is inappropriate for clients whose lymph tissue may be malfunctioning, regardless of whether it is possible for massage to speed up metastasis.

Noncirculatory work may be more appropriate, since the client may reap many supportive benefits without the risks of pushing a lot of fluid through a system that doesn't work smoothly. Massage is used increasingly to ameliorate the side effects of chemotherapy and radiation. Nonetheless, it's always a good idea to work as part of a fully informed health care team when a client is going through long-term, complicated, and life-threatening challenges to health.

Modality Recommendations for Lymphoma	
Deep Tissue Massage	Supportive as part of a health care team. Respect stage of recovery and treatment challenges.
Lymphatic Drainage	Supportive, especially during chemotherapy.
Polarity	S: Indicated. R/D: Supportive with pressure appropriate for stage.
PNF/MET/Stretching	Supportive.
Reflexology	Indicated when in remission: work lymphatic system and pituitary points.
Shiatsu	Indicated for strengthening the immune system via TH, SP.
Swedish Massage	Supportive as part of health care team and matched to client's activity levels and resilience.
Trigger Point Therapy	Supportive.

See Chapter 1 for a brief description of each modality, including definitions of abbreviations.

Mononucleosis

Definition: What Is It?

Mononucleosis is a viral infection of the salivary glands and throat that moves into the lymphatic system. The causative agent in about 90% of all cases is the Epstein-Barr virus, a member of the herpes family. Other pathogens that can cause mononucleosis include other members of Herpesviridae, specifically cytomegalovirus and human herpesvirus 6, along with adenovirus, *Toxoplasma gondii*, and others.

Demographics: Who Gets It?

Epstein-Barr virus is everywhere. Random blood studies show that the rate of infection in the United States and elsewhere is 90% to 95% by the time people reach 40 years of age. Not everyone who has been exposed develops the symptoms associated with mononucleosis, or mono, however. When young children are infected, their symptoms tend to be mild and are often missed entirely. When a first exposure to Epstein-Barr virus happens in adolescence or young adulthood, mononucleosis symptoms develop 35 to 50% of the time.[3]

Mono is diagnosed in the United States in about 45 of every 100,000 people. Most cases are found in people between 15 and 25 years old. Mononucleosis is diagnosed in as many as 3% of college-aged people every year.[3]

Mononucleosis In Brief

Pronunciation: mon-o-nu-kle-O-sis

What is it?

Mononucleosis is an infection, usually with the Epstein-Barr virus but occasionally with cytomegalovirus or other agents. The virus first attacks the epithelial tissue in the salivary glands and throat and then invades B-cells in lymph nodes, the spleen, and elsewhere.

How is it recognized?

The three leading signs and symptoms of mononucleosis are fever, swollen lymph nodes, and sore throat. Others may include profound fatigue, low stamina, enlarged spleen, and enlarged liver.

Is massage indicated or contraindicated?

Mononucleosis contraindicates circulatory massage in the acute stage, when the body is fighting hard to beat back this viral attack. In later stages, as long as circulation is healthy and the spleen and liver are not compromised, circulatory massage may improve recovery time. Noncirculatory types of bodywork may be appropriate as long as the possibility of lymphatic congestion is considered.

Etiology: What Happens?

Mononucleosis from Epstein-Barr virus spreads most efficiently through direct contact. This virus is fragile outside of a human host, and while it may remain viable for a short time on a dish or suspended in a droplet of mucus in the air, the most dependable way to catch it is through intimate saliva-to-saliva contact; it's not called the kissing disease for nothing.

Like many viral infections, mononucleosis moves through the body in two stages. In the first stage, the virus invades cells in the epithelial tissue of the throat and salivary glands. It can take a long time for the infection to get established; incubation can take up to 60 days, during which time the patient is infectious but not strongly symptomatic. Once established well in the epithelial tissue of the throat, however, the virus moves on to infect B-lymphocytes, which carry it to the lymph nodes, liver, and spleen.

The effect of the virus on its target B-cells is to make them immortal: that is, instead of dying at the end of a normal life span, the infected cells live on to replicate and produce a variety of antibodies, including antibodies to the virus itself but also nonfunctioning antibodies called ***heterophiles***. Changes to the infected B-cells cause them to resemble monocytes, an entirely different type of white blood cell. It is their resemblance to monocytes that led to the name *mononucleosis*.

As infected B-cells proliferate, the body responds by producing high numbers of cytotoxic (killer) T-cells. These T-cells eventually establish control over the rogue B-cells, and ultimately the virus becomes dormant in epithelial cells of the throat.

Once a person is infected with Epstein-Barr virus, the virus is present forever, although usually dormant. It may intermittently reactivate, however. During these episodes it is likely to be contagious but asymptomatic. This makes the spread of mononucleosis virtually impossible to control.

A history of exposure to Epstein-Barr virus is regarded as a risk factor for some types of cancer, specifically Burkitt lymphoma and nasopharyngeal carcinoma. These cancers are rare in the United States, but Epstein-Barr virus is not. The generally accepted conclusion is that the virus probably plays a role in the development of these cancers but is not the primary cause.

Signs and Symptoms

Mononucleosis is notorious for presenting different symptoms in different patients. The younger a person is at exposure to Epstein-Barr virus, the subtler the symptoms tend to be. Young children often go through exposure, infection, and recovery with no discernible symptoms at all.

In older patients, particularly adolescents and young adults, the signs and symptoms are more dependable. The prodromic stage, as the infection is becoming established but creates no strong symptoms, may be marked by general fatigue and *malaise*; the patient often does not feel well but may not feel sick, either. This may last anywhere from a few days to several weeks. Then as the infection becomes more aggressive, the leading triad of symptoms appears: fever of 102°F to 104°F (38.9°– 40°C), an extremely sore throat from the initial viral infection, and lymph nodes that are swollen from the production of massive numbers of B-cells and T-cells. The cervical lymph nodes are usually affected most, but submandibular, axillary, and inguinal lymph nodes may also be palpably swollen and tender.

Puffy, swollen eyelids are a common complaint among mononucleosis patients. *Splenomegaly* (enlargement of the spleen) occurs in about half of patients. Many also have inflammation of the liver. Some mononucleosis patients develop a splotchy, measly rash, especially if they are taking amoxicillin or ampicillin, two penicillin-family antibiotics that are prescribed for strep throat. Most mononucleosis patients taking these medications develop painful, alarming rashes.

Signs and symptoms of acute mononucleosis tend to last approximately 2 weeks before subsiding, but the whole infection is so wearing on the body that it can take several weeks or even months before a patient feels fully functional again.

Diagnosis

Recognizing exposure to Epstein-Barr virus is not difficult; the problem is in establishing the stage of the infection. Several features of this virus make it problematic to label: mononucleosis presents differently in different patients, the incidence of Epstein-Barr virus is nearly universal, and the virus can be present and active for many weeks or months after an infection. Furthermore, a person can have lifelong episodes of reactivation of the virus without symptoms. All of these issues can make it difficult to state definitively that a person's symptoms are due only or even primarily to this particular pathogen.

The starting place for a diagnosis of mononucleosis is a "monospot" test: this looks for signs of heterophile antibodies. Complete blood counts also reveal abnormally high lymphocyte counts: both atypical B-cells and extra T-cells to fight them.

Ultimately, since no medical intervention alters the course of mononucleosis, it isn't important to know the exact phase of the infection. It is important, however, to rule out some conditions that mimic this infection but that are either more serious or more treatable. Some of these possibilities include *rubella*, HIV/AIDS, *diphtheria*, measles, and strep throat—which is also a possible complication of the disease.

Complications

For most people mononucleosis is an unpleasant but basically benign, self-limiting infection. It can significantly disrupt a person's life because it has such a powerful effect on stamina, resiliency, and general strength, but it is seldom life threatening. A very small number of patients, however, do develop serious complications. These include infection of the central nervous system leading to Bell palsy, seizures, or meningitis; enlargement of the heart; and breathing problems when lymph nodes and tonsils get so inflamed that they block air passageways.

One fairly common complication of mononucleosis is a streptococcal infection of the throat. It is important to be clear about what infection is causing which symptoms in this case, since while strep throat is easily treatable with antibiotics, mononucleosis is not.

Perhaps the greatest danger for most mononucleosis patients is the potential for damage to the spleen. This gland, which is sometimes described as the body's largest lymph node, can become dangerously enlarged with lymphocytic activity. Since the spleen also breaks down and recycles dead red blood cells, it has a generous blood supply. If the enlarged organ should be injured by a fall or other trauma, it could rupture, which could lead to internal hemorrhage and rapid circulatory collapse. Persons recovering from mononucleosis are counseled to avoid contact sports for several weeks to reduce their risk of this kind of injury.

Treatment

Mononucleosis does not respond to antiviral medications. The typical approach is to treat the symptoms (*acetaminophen* to reduce fever and pain; rest; good nutrition; and generous hydration) and wait for it to be over. At one time mononucleosis patients were confined to bed for several weeks. More recently it has been concluded that they simply need to curtail activities that exhaust them and to avoid situations that could put them at risk for damaging the spleen.

Massage?

A person in an acute stage of mononucleosis has a fever and inflamed lymph nodes and feels generally sick and awful; all of these features contraindicate circulatory massage. When a person is in recovery from this infection, lymphatic congestion may linger, especially at the spleen; this is also a caution for circulatory massage and lymph drainage techniques. Energetic work that supports healing properties without taxing the lymph or immune systems may be a valuable addition to the lengthy healing process for mononucleosis.

A person with a history of mononucleosis but no symptoms is a perfectly fine candidate for massage.

MODALITY RECOMMENDATIONS FOR MONONUCLEOSIS	
Deep Tissue Massage	Systemically contraindicated while acute.
Lymphatic Drainage	Systemically contraindicated while acute.
Polarity	S: Indicated. R/D: Indicated with light pressure.
PNF/MET/Stretching	Contraindicated while acute; otherwise supportive.
Reflexology	Indicated when subacute: work lymphatic system, head, neck points.
Shiatsu	Indicated for strengthening immune system via TH, SP. Contraindicated when acute.
Swedish Massage	Contraindicated while acute; supportive while subacute if matched to client's activity level.
Trigger Point Therapy	Supportive with light work.

See Chapter 1 for a brief description of each modality, including definitions of abbreviations.

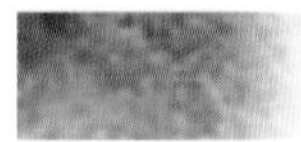

IMMUNE SYSTEM CONDITIONS

Allergic Reactions

> **Allergic Reactions in Brief**
>
> **What are they?**
> Allergic reactions are immune system mistakes in which an inflammatory response becomes irritating or dangerous as it reacts inappropriately to a variety of triggers.
>
> **How are they recognized?**
> The most dangerous acute sign of an allergic reaction is swelling around the face and throat that may obstruct airflow. This may be accompanied by decreased blood pressure and bronchospasm. Other signs include hives and other rashes, gastrointestinal discomfort with food allergies, and in the case of multiple chemical sensitivity, headache, disorientation, cognitive difficulties, joint pain, and other symptoms.
>
> **Is massage indicated or contraindicated?**
> Most hypersensitivity reactions contraindicate massage in the acute stage, since increasing blood flow to areas that are already congested is counterproductive. Between episodes, persons with allergies need to be careful about massage lubricants, essential oils, perfumes, candles, and other equipment that therapists often use but that may trigger a reaction.

Definition: What Are They?

Allergies are immune system reactions against stimuli that are not inherently hazardous. The immune system behaves as though an allergen, which could be oak pollen, cat dander, or another benign substance, were a potentially dangerous threat.

Demographics: Who Gets Them?

Allergies affect some 50 million Americans every year, and numbers appear to be increasing.[4]

Different types of allergies affect different parts of the population, depending on what substances people are exposed to and how often. The "hygiene hypothesis" suggests that rates of allergic rhinitis ("hay fever"), asthma, eczema, and some other allergies are on the rise in the United States because children are overprotected from allergens in early childhood, and this interferes with proper immune system development. Children raised in homes with pets and who spend time in day care with other children in their first year of life have lower rates of allergies than others.

Alternatively, repeated exposure to some substances, especially latex, can lead to dangerous allergic reactions later in life. This is a particular problem for people with spina bifida or another medical problems that require frequent surgeries, and for health care professionals who use latex gloves or latex-based equipment (e.g., catheters, syringes) on a regular basis. Allergies to latex are triggered by natural latex made from derivatives of rubber trees; synthetic latex does not appear to be a potent allergen.

Multiple chemical sensitivity syndrome (MCS) develops most often in people who undergo exposure to toxic substances and who consequently develop progressively more extreme reactions to other substances as well. MCS is discussed in Sidebar 6.4.

SIDEBAR 6.4: MULTIPLE CHEMICAL SENSITIVITY SYNDROME

Multiple chemical sensitivity syndrome (MCS) is also called *idiopathic environmental intolerance*. It is a condition in which a history of exposure to a trigger (usually an environmental toxin) results in a variety of possible reactions that become increasingly severe with repeated exposures. It is seen most often in people who have been exposed to chemical spills or other toxic exposures, who work in poorly ventilated buildings, or who have had other long-term toxic exposures. Military personnel have MCS more commonly than the rest of the population, and people who served in the first Gulf War have a higher incidence still.

The accepted description of MCS is as follows:

- A set of objectively observable signs and symptoms is acquired after documentable exposure to a triggering substance.
- Multiple body systems are affected.
- Severity of symptoms is in relation to measurable (but not usually toxic) levels of chemical triggers.
- Chemically unrelated substances can trigger a reaction.
- Episodes leave no objective evidence of permanent organ damage.

A few of the most common triggers of MCS include cigar and cigarette smoke; colognes, perfumes, and deodorants; diesel and gasoline exhaust; household and laundry detergents and cleaners; varnish, shellac, and lacquer; and tar fumes from roof or roadwork.

MCS symptoms vary widely, including chronic headaches, joint pain, cognitive difficulties, weakness, dizziness, and heat intolerance. Exposure to one trigger may permanently exacerbate responses to future exposures, even to different chemical triggers.

A massage therapist whose client has MCS must ensure that the work space is a safe and comfortable place. Detergents or bleach used to launder massage linens may be a trigger, as may be any candles, scents, incense, or the perfume worn by the client who just left. Any lubricant must be evaluated carefully not only for allergenic ingredients but for the risk of contamination from pesticides or the plastic bottle in which it is stored. If these hurdles can be overcome or if the client with MCS can tolerate whatever levels are present in a massage room, bodywork is be a supportive, strengthening, and preciously rare time for a person to feel that his or her body is a good place in which to live.

Etiology: What Happens?

Antibodies are the Y-shaped proteins manufactured by activated B cells against specific pathogens. Some classes of antibodies and some types of T cells are particularly reactive to noninfectious antigens, causing acute or chronic allergic symptoms. These hypersensitivity reactions have been classified as having four distinct types. For details on types of hypersensitivity, see the introduction to this chapter.

Several conditions involving allergic reactions are discussed elsewhere in this book, in the chapter dedicated to the system that is most significantly affected. Eczema, dermatitis and hives affect the skin; asthma and allergic sinusitis affect the respiratory system; and allergic gastroenteritis affects the digestive system. This article addresses two more general examples of hypersensitivity reactions: anaphylaxis and angioedema.

- *Anaphylaxis* is an acute, severe systemic allergic reaction leading to the release of massive amounts of histamine from previously sensitized mast cells. The result is a sudden drop in blood pressure (hypotension) and accumulation of fluid in the tissues (edema). If the reaction centers in the respiratory tract, it can dangerously interfere with breathing. Some of the most common triggers include antibiotics; blood products; the contrast medium used in diagnostic imaging; latex; stings of wasps, ants, and honeybees; and some foods, including peanuts and other nuts, soybeans, cow's milk, eggs, fish, and shellfish. The first exposure to a trigger may not cause a significant allergic reaction, but repeated exposures lead to increased antibody activity, complement activation, and mast cell activity, which causes and reinforces inflammation. Anaphylaxis is distinguished from angioedema because it occurs both at the site of exposure and systemically through the body. It is a medical emergency that results in about 500 deaths per year.[5]
- *Angioedema* is the rapid onset of localized swelling. The swelling can occur in the skin, genitals, extremities, or gastrointestinal tract. If it occurs in the tongue, larynx, or pharynx, angioedema can interrupt airflow, which is life threatening. Allergens commonly associated with angioedema include peanuts or tree nuts, chocolate, fish, tomatoes, eggs, fresh berries, milk, and food preservatives. Medicines associated with this condition include aspirin, angiotensin-converting enzyme (ACE) inhibitors, and some other hypertension medications. Exposure to poison ivy, poison oak, or poison sumac can also create this kind of reaction (Sidebar 6.5).

SIDEBAR 6.5: POISON IVY, POISON OAK, POISON SUMAC

Poison ivy, poison oak, and poison sumac all have a chemical in their sap called *urushiol*. Urushiol is a highly allergenic substance in leaves, stems, and roots that causes a type IV delayed reaction on the skin involving inflammation, itchiness, and blisters. Up to 85% of the population has an allergic reaction to urushiol.

Poison ivy, poison oak, and poison sumac reactions occur in three ways: through direct contact with the sap, indirect contact with equipment or a pet that has been running through the woods, or through the air when plants are burned.

Many people are familiar with the signs of poison ivy: the rash is red, hot, and very itchy. Blisters may form and crust over. The rash can take up to 10 days to heal fully. Poison sumac and poison oak produce the same symptoms because the allergen is the same chemical.

Occasionally a rash leads to a very extreme allergic reaction in the shape of angioedema or anaphylaxis; this is a risk especially when swelling takes place around the face or neck, where it can obstruct the airway.

Poison ivy and its relatives are of particular interest to massage therapists because they usually cause a delayed reaction: an exposed person may have no symptoms for 24 hours or more after contacting the plants, although the toxin is present on the skin. This means a massage therapist working with a client who had a pleasant walk in the woods that morning may spread the urushiol further or even pick up some of the toxin: not the way most people would prefer to spend time in the country!

Signs and Symptoms

Anaphylaxis in the skin creates hives, itchiness, and flushing. Excessive edema can cause respiratory symptoms, including shortness of breath, coughing, and wheezing. A person may have so much swelling around the throat that swallowing becomes difficult; this is *dysphagia*. Gastrointestinal symptoms include nausea, vomiting, cramps, bloating, and diarrhea. In extreme circumstances a person may have a slowed heart rate, hypotension, fainting, and shock.

Signs of angioedema depend on where the inflammation takes place. The skin may be puffy and hot, although if it appears without hives, it may not be itchy. It is often asymmetrical, affecting only one part of the lip, for instance, or one side of the face. It has a rapid onset but usually resolves within 72 hours (Figure 6.5).

Diagnosis

Diagnosis of angioedema and anaphylaxis is straightforward: visible swelling of various tissues (most often around the face and throat) along with shortness of breath or gastrointestinal symptoms indicate exposure to a triggering allergen.

Anaphylaxis may take several hours to develop, and symptoms can appear to subside before returning in a more extreme form. A person who is at risk for this type of reaction must be observed for a prolonged period to make sure he or she is stable.

Treatment

Antihistamines are usually recommended to treat mild allergies. These interrupt the inflammatory process that causes many allergy signs: itchy skin, runny nose, and irritated eyes.

Angioedema and anaphylaxis are more serious, and they are typically treated in the short term with epinephrine and oxygen if breathing is impaired and steroidal anti-inflammatories after the crisis has passed. People at risk for anaphylactic reactions are taught how to avoid triggers and trained to keep medication, usually injectable epinephrine (an EpiPen), close at hand in case of emergency. However, epinephrine doesn't work well for people who use smooth muscle relaxants to control their high blood pressure: the two medications work at cross-purposes, so an alternative to epinephrine must be used instead.

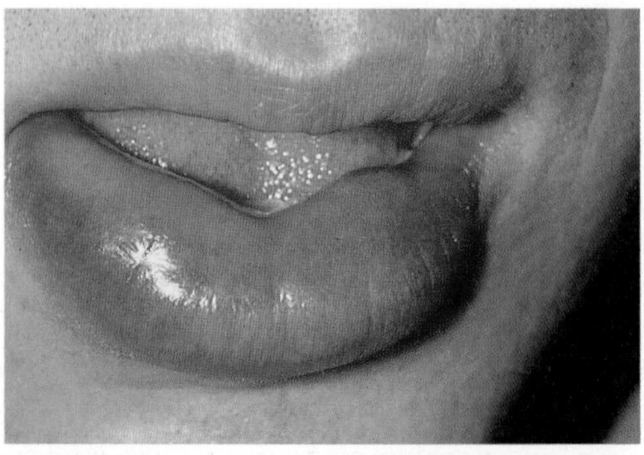

Figure 6.5. Angioedema.

When a person has dangerous allergic reactions to insect stings, a long-term course of desensitization may be recommended; this process can radically reduce the risk of dangerous anaphylactic reactions.

Massage?

Obviously, a person in the midst of an angioedema or anaphylaxis episode is not a good candidate for Swedish massage; this person needs to seek medical intervention if breathing becomes impaired and may consider massage only after the crisis has passed. At that point, the massage therapist should be aware of the person's history and choose a hypoallergenic lubricant without the use of essential oils, incense, or perfumes to reduce the risk of triggering another attack.

Modality Recommendations for Allergic Reactions	
Deep Tissue Massage	Systemically contraindicated while acute; otherwise supportive.
Lymphatic Drainage	Systemically contraindicated while acute; otherwise supportive.
Polarity	S: Indicated with medical attention for angioedema or anaphylaxis. R/D: Contraindicated while acute, otherwise supportive.
PNF/MET/Stretching	Systemically contraindicated while acute; otherwise supportive.
Reflexology	Indicated; work lymphatic system and affected areas.
Shiatsu	Indicated for strengthening the immune system via TH, SP, L, K.
Swedish Massage	Contraindicated during acute stages of types I–III reactions; may be locally contraindicated for type IV reactions. Use hypoallergenic lubricant.
Trigger Point Therapy	Systemically contraindicated while acute; otherwise supportive.

See Chapter 1 for a brief description of each modality, including definitions of abbreviations.

Chronic Fatigue Syndrome

Definition: What Is It?

Chronic fatigue syndrome (CFS) is a collection of signs and symptoms that affect multiple systems in the body. It varies in severity from mildly limiting to completely debilitating.

CFS was named in 1988 by scientists at the Centers for Disease Control, and its definition continues to evolve. The name is vague on purpose because this disease affects different people in very different ways; being any more specific about causes or symptoms, they feared, would exclude some people who are badly affected by this condition. Nonetheless, some people feel this title trivializes their condition, and CFS is therefore also called *chronic fatigue immune dysfunction syndrome* (CFIDS). In Europe and Canada a condition called ***myalgic encephalomyelitis*** is sometimes referred to as a synonym for CFS, but whether it is actually the same disease is not certain: the current description for CFS is so wide that it can encompass aspects of myalgic encephalomyelitis while not being the same entity.

CFS has probably been documented since at least the nineteenth century. Florence Nightingale had debilitating fatigue for

Chronic Fatigue Syndrome in Brief

What is it?
Chronic fatigue syndrome (CFS) is a collection of signs and symptoms that affect many systems in the body and result in potentially debilitating fatigue.

How is it recognized?
The central symptom to CFS is fatigue that is not restored by rest. It may be accompanied by swollen nodes, slight fever, muscular and joint aches, headaches, and excessive pain after mild exercise.

Is massage indicated or contraindicated?
CFS indicates massage, which can be a very helpful part of a treatment plan.

decades; it is suspected that she had CFS. This may also be the condition behind other vague diagnostic labels, such as "neurasthenia" and more recently, "yuppie flu".

Demographics: Who Gets It?

Statistics on the incidence of CFS are difficult to gather for several reasons. First, it is probably significantly underreported, since not all people who are affected attempt to be treated. The Centers for Disease Control suggest that only 20% of people who have CFS are diagnosed.[6]

CFS looks like several other disorders, any of which may affect a person simultaneously (this is called ***comorbidity***), so a definitive diagnosis is sometimes difficult. Further, statistics gathered from various cities show some vast differences in race, gender, and age distribution of the disorder. This means that while diagnostic criteria have recently been redefined for clarity, much disparity still exists in when and where it is identified.

When all of this disparate information is processed, estimates suggest that this disorder (or other CFS-like disorders) probably affects many thousands of Americans. It is diagnosed most often in women, but that may be a reflection of who seeks help rather than of who is most affected.

Etiology: What Happens?

The etiology of CFS is not well understood. It seems clear that it arises from a combination of factors that may or may not involve infectious agents, mentally or emotionally stressful events, endocrine and neurological dysfunction, and other factors.

For many years the leading theory was that a person was infected with a common virus (probably Epstein-Barr, the herpesvirus that causes most cases of mononucleosis) and then the body simply continued to behave as though the infection were acute long after the danger had passed. Although blood studies of patients with CFS often show some immune system abnormalities (levels of the inflammatory cytokine interleukin-1 are very high, while natural killer cell levels tend to be unusually low), it now seems clear that not all CFS cases begin with a viral infection.

Other pathogenic exposures have been implicated in CFS, specifically candida, mycoplasma (a bacterialike pathogen), some enteroviruses, *Chlamydia pneumoniae*, and other infectious agents. No single pathogen has been found to be present in most CFS patients, however, and most people who have been exposed to these agents do *not* develop CFS symptoms.

Three central nervous system components seem to be consistent problems for most CFS patients:

- *Hypothalamus-pituitary-adrenal (HPA) axis dysfunction.* This can lead to a sluggish but tenacious stress response and eventually to adrenal dysfunction. Interestingly, the HPA axis appears to be a factor in depression as well, and depression is recognized as a common complication of CFS. The differences lie in cortisol secretion. A problem with the HPA axis typically leads to excessive cortisol secretion: this is demonstrable with depression. But people with CFS usually have *lower*-than-normal levels of circulating cortisol. Whether this is because of adrenal depletion or simply poor adrenal regulation is still an unanswered question.
- *Neurally mediated hypotension.* Impulses from the brain to the circulatory system do not keep the blood vessels contracted enough to maintain a normal blood pressure. This condition is connected to an inappropriate response to adrenaline.
- *Neurotransmitter imbalance.* Recent research reveals that the cerebrospinal fluid of people with the symptoms of CFS has several proteins that are distinctive to the disease. This is one of the first consistent biological markers of the disease that has been discovered.

Signs and Symptoms

Fatigue is the central symptom of CFS. The fatigue is unending and not restored by sleep or rest. Most experts agree that unrelenting fatigue must persist for a minimum of 6 months to achieve a diagnosis of CFS. Additionally, at least four of the symptoms listed in Table 6.1 must be present.[6]

Of these, poor memory and concentration, along with significant postexertional pain, are the most consistent CFS symptoms. Patients may also report abdominal bloating, nausea, diarrhea, cramping, chest pain, irregular heartbeat, coughing, dizziness, dry eyes and mouth, weight loss, jaw pain, morning stiffness, night sweats, and psychological problems related to living with chronic illness, especially depression and/or anxiety.

This list of symptoms points to an important feature of CFS. It closely resembles two other chronic stress-related conditions: fibromyalgia syndrome and irritable bowel syndrome, and it frequently occurs along with them. In fact, so much overlap exists between these conditions that many people with aspects of all three disorders are simply diagnosed with whatever syndrome's primary features appear first: irritable bowel syndrome for gastrointestinal discomfort, fibromyalgia syndrome for predominant muscle and joint pain, or CFS if the leading symptom is unrelenting fatigue.

Diagnosis

No particular marker in the blood identifies CFS. It is diagnosed by ruling out other diseases with a similar profile. This is challenging, because many other disorders can cause long-term unexplained fatigue. It is important to clarify which condition or conditions are present, since some may be more serious than CFS and some can be successfully treated and resolved.

Some of the disorders that are ruled out when looking for a solid diagnosis include conditions listed in Table 6.2.

Treatment

The primary treatment for CFS is making lifestyle choices that support the body as fully as possible. This means avoiding stress (any stimulus, emotional or physical, that requires the body to adapt to a change) as much as possible. It also means avoiding stimulants (caffeine, sugar) and depressants (alcohol) as much as possible and exercising consistently and gently, within tolerance so as not to exacerbate symptoms.

An important part of treatment for CFS patients is education; the more they learn about their condition, the better equipped they are to handle its challenges.

TABLE 6.1 Symptoms of Chronic Fatigue Syndrome
Poor short-term memory
Sore throat
Muscle and/or joint pain
Poor-quality sleep
Poor concentration
Enlarged lymph nodes
Headache in a new pattern
Postexertional pain

At least four of these must be present for a diagnosis of CFS.

TABLE 6.2 Disorders to Rule out for a Diagnosis of Chronic Fatigue Syndrome

Hypothyroidism	Hepatitis B or C	Lupus
Postpolio syndrome	Lyme disease	Sleep apnea or narcolepsy
Cancer	Diabetes	Eating disorders
Bipolar disease	Alcohol or substance abuse	Severe obesity
Reactions to medication	General autoimmune dysfunction	Dementia
Chronic, subacute infection	Schizophrenia	

Medical intervention can be helpful, but it can be difficult to find exactly the right combination of drugs. Many CFS patients are hypersensitive to chemicals, and they often find that one-quarter of the regular dosage is adequate. A powerful combination for many people is immunosuppressant drugs combined with low-dose tricyclic antidepressants.

Massage?

Massage stimulates the parasympathetic response, cleanses tissues, and stimulates circulation when exercise may be too much to handle; it can relieve muscle and joint pain, and it can improve sleep. Studies show that people diagnosed with CFS report lower levels of anxiety and better quality sleep after receiving massage.[7]

Because CFS doesn't appear to be contagious or a condition that spreads through the circulatory system, gentle massage is a safe and appropriate choice for these clients.

MODALITY RECOMMENDATIONS FOR CHRONIC FATIGUE SYNDROME

Deep Tissue Massage	Indicated with caution; work slowly for parasympathetic response.
Lymphatic Drainage	Supportive.
Polarity	S/R/D: Indicated.
PNF/MET/Stretching	Supportive.
Reflexology	Indicated: work endocrine system, lymphatic system, solar plexus, liver points.
Shiatsu	Indicated for strengthening immune system via TH, SP.
Swedish Massage	Indicated to facilitate homeostasis.
Trigger Point Therapy	Indicated for muscular sequelae.

See Chapter 1 for a brief description of each modality, including definitions of abbreviations.

Fever

Definition: What Is It?

Fever can be recognized at a glance (or touch). Massage therapists are not required to keep thermometers or take clients' temperatures, but they do need to be familiar with the basic mechanisms of this important immune system activity.

Fever is an abnormally high body temperature, usually brought about by bacterial or viral infection but sometimes stimulated by other types of tissue damage. Exactly when fever is identified is a bit of a moving target: most people vary in internal temperature by a degree Fahrenheit or more throughout the day. Generally, fever is identified when an under-tongue thermometer registers 101°F (38.3°C) or more. Fever is a *controlled* change in temperature, which distinguishes it from other types of hyperthermia (Sidebar 6.6).

Fever in Brief

What is it?
Fever is a controlled increase in core temperature, usually brought about by immune system reactions, often in response to pathogenic invasion.

How is it recognized?
Fever is identifiable by readings on a thermometer.

Is massage indicated or contraindicated?
Most fever contraindicates massage, as it is an indication that the body is fighting an infection and should be allowed to do its work undisturbed.

Etiology: What Happens?

Several steps are involved in the development of an infection-based fever:

1. A person is infected with some microorganism, such as bacteria.
2. White blood cells find and eat those invaders.
3. Some pieces of the bacterial cell membranes are displayed by the macrophages. They stimulate other white blood cells to secrete a ***lymphokine*** called *interleukin-1.* Other lymphokines and substances that are secreted include interleukin-6 and tumor necrosis factor (TMF).

SIDEBAR 6.6: TYPES OF HYPERTHERMIA

Fever is a systemic rise in body temperature that is carefully controlled by the hypothalamus. It has the advantages of speeding up immune system activity while slowing and starving infectious agents. Fever is an extraordinarily efficient mechanism to fight infection.

Sometimes, however, a person's core temperature rises without hypothalamic control. This generally occurs when a person generates more heat than he or she can release. In this case the body temperature continues to rise until external factors work to cool off the person. If environmental factors don't allow this to happen, the person is at risk for brain damage or death.

The three levels of hyperthermia are heat cramps, heat exhaustion, and heat stroke. They are most commonly seen in people who are physically very active in warm, humid environments. Massage therapists who work at summertime sporting events can expect to see any of these manifestations of hyperthermia.

Heat Cramps

Muscle cramping is a frequent result of the dehydration that accompanies excessive heat production. The body sweats in an attempt to lower its temperature, and the result is a deficit in interstitial fluid. This makes it more difficult for the calcium ions that stimulate muscle contractions to be reabsorbed into their storage containers. Consequently, muscle contractions are sustained and uncontrolled. Fortunately, massage along with rehydration is an excellent way to move fluid back into the muscle bellies and stimulate the chemical and neurological reactions that reduce the spasm.

Heat Exhaustion

Heat exhaustion occurs when muscular activity generates more heat than a person can release. It is marked by excessive sweating, headache, vasodilation, and dehydration. Excessive sweating may lead to low blood pressure, lightheadedness, and fainting.

Heat Stroke

Heat stroke is the final stage of hyperthermia. In this condition body temperature rises to dangerous levels (approximately 104°F, or 40°C, for adults). Prolonged dehydration may lead to *lack* of sweating and circulatory shock from loss of water and electrolytes. The person may become confused or delirious. Heat stroke can be fatal if the core temperature is not quickly but carefully reduced to safe levels.

Malignant Hyperthermia

This is not a sports-related problem but rather a genetic anomaly that allows the body temperature to rise to dangerous, even fatal, levels with a minimum of muscular work. It is sometimes seen as part of an allergic reaction to anesthesia. Many people don't know they are at risk for this disorder until they have a dangerous episode.

4. Interleukin-1 circulates through the system, including the brain. It causes a series of chemical reactions involving prostaglandins that tell the hypothalamus to reset the body's thermostat to a higher level. In this situation interleukin-1 is acting as a ***pyrogen***, a fever starter.
5. Orders from the hypothalamus ripple through the body, setting up the muscular and glandular reflexes that raise the core temperature. These reflexes include shivering, constriction of superficial capillaries, and increased metabolism.

The characteristic shivering and chills that go along with a rising fever are part of the mechanism to increase the core temperature. Once that goal has been met, the shivering stops, but the body processes keep working to maintain the increased temperature until the stimulating chemicals have been removed. This peak is called the crisis of the fever. When the crisis has passed, the body's cooling mechanisms, sweating and capillary dilation, take over. That is the sign that the worst is over and the fever is broken.

Viral or bacterial infection is the causative factor of most but not all fevers. Severe injury can upset the hypothalamic thermostat, as can certain cancers and some autoimmune diseases. If fever, even low-grade fever, persists for more than a few days, it is important to find out the source of the problem.

This culture has a strange and troubling discomfort with discomfort. Often people would rather *hide* a symptom than *feel* it and figure out what it's trying to tell them. This is true particularly with fever, which can be disagreeable and inconvenient. In rare cases it can get high enough to do some serious damage. But most of the time fever is a sign that the body is working in the most efficient possible way to get rid of invading pathogens. Some of those mechanisms include the following:

- Interleukin-1 and other cytokines not only help to reset the body's thermostat, they also stimulate T-cell production. Increased T-cell production stimulates B cells and the production of antibodies.
- In the presence of fever interferon, a powerful antiviral agent, is much more active.
- Increased temperature limits iron secretion from the liver and spleen, starving off and slowing bacterial and viral activity.
- Increased temperature raises the heart rate (10 beats per minute per degree), which in turn increases the distribution of white blood cells throughout the body.
- Increased temperature increases cell wall permeability and speeds chemical reactions. This promotes faster recovery for damaged tissues.

Complications

Fever occasionally presents a danger, particularly when the temperature rises over 104°F (40°C). The most common complications are dehydration (from prolonged sweating), acidosis (the blood gets too acidic), and once in a great while brain damage. Death from fever occurs somewhere around 112°F to 114°F (44.4°C–44.5°C) for adults. If a fever comes down too fast, it can quickly dilate blood vessels. This can lead to shock, which can be dangerous, especially to older patients.

Treatment

Experts don't agree about the best time to treat simple fevers in adults. Suppressing symptoms may prolong an infection, and allowing a person to go back to work or school puts them in contact with other people who may become infected. On the other hand, fevers are uncomfortable and inconvenient, and it is natural to try to interrupt their course. Aspirin, ibuprofen, and acetaminophen all work to inhibit fever by interrupting the action of prostaglandins on the hypothalamus so the internal thermostat can be reset.

Massage?

Fever systemically contraindicates massage. Energetic techniques that don't affect blood flow may be helpful for someone having a hard time getting past the crisis point, as long as the therapist is safe from the threat of a contagious condition.

Modality Recommendations for Fever	
Deep Tissue Massage	Systemically contraindicated while acute.
Lymphatic Drainage	Systemically contraindicated while acute.
Polarity	S: Indicated. R/D: Contraindicated while acute, then supportive within client comfort.
PNF/MET/Stretching	Systemically contraindicated while acute; otherwise supportive.
Reflexology	Systemically contraindicated while acute.
Shiatsu	Systemically contraindicated while acute.
Swedish Massage	Systemically contraindicated while acute.
Trigger Point Therapy	Systemically contraindicated while acute.

See Chapter 1 for a brief description of each modality, including definitions of abbreviations.

HIV/AIDS

Definition: What Is It?

AIDS (acquired immune deficiency syndrome) was first recognized as a specific disease in the United States in 1983, but research since then indicates that it has been here since long before that. The causative virus, HIV (human immunodeficiency virus), attacks various agents of the immune system with disastrous results.

Demographics: Who Gets It?

Worldwide Current estimates suggest that about 40.3 million people are HIV positive. Most are adults, but 2.3 million are children under 15 years old. Slightly more men than women are infected except in developing countries, where women can make up three-quarters of the infected population. About 5 million new HIV infections occur every year: that's 14,000 per day. And each year about 3.1 million people die of complications of AIDS.[8] Worldwide, 90% of HIV infections are the result of heterosexual activity.[9]

United States In the United States it is estimated that about 950,000 people are infected with HIV, although about 240,000 don't know. About 40,000 new infections begin every year in this country, 70% among men and 30% among women. It is the cause of about 20,000 deaths each year. HIV is spreading fastest among minority populations. It is found seven times more often in African Americans than in whites, and three times more often in Hispanics than in

HIV/AIDS in Brief

What is it?
Acquired immune deficiency syndrome (AIDS) is a disease caused by human immunodeficiency virus (HIV), which attacks and disables the immune system. This leaves a person vulnerable to a host of diseases that are usually not a threat to people without HIV.

How is it recognized?
Most people with HIV have a week or two of flulike symptoms within several weeks of being infected, followed by an interval with no symptoms. When the virus has successfully inactivated the immune system, infection by opportunistic pathogens such as herpes simplex and zoster, cytomegalovirus, or *Pneumocystis carinii* occurs.

Is massage indicated or contraindicated?
All stages of HIV infection indicate massage as long as the practitioner is healthy and doesn't pose any risk to the client, and the client is able to keep up with the changes that massage brings about in the body.

whites. AIDS is the leading cause of death among African American men between 25 and 44 years old.

In the United States about 40% of new infections arise from sexual activity between men; 30% of new infections are the result of heterosexual activity; and 26% of new infections are related to shared needle use. Other infections are related to combinations of risk factors.[10]

Etiology: What Happens?

HIV enters the body by way of body fluids: blood (including contaminated transfusions and shared needles), semen, vaginal secretions, and breast milk.

HIV can attach to cells in mucosal epithelium to gain entry to the body. Any other sexually transmitted infection, such as syphilis, genital herpes, chlamydia, or gonorrhea, can significantly increase the risk of transmitting the virus. Once in the tissue, the virus invades a target cell through a molecular portal of entry on the membrane called CD4, along with coreceptor sites, which vary. Monocytes, macrophages, and T-cells have this molecular doorway and so are called CD4+ cells. HIV invades circulating monocytes and macrophages or directly invades helper T-cells. It uses its first hosts as transport to concentrations of T-cells in the bone marrow, lymph nodes, spleen, tonsils, and adenoids.

These targets are significant for a couple of reasons. First, when the virus pools in macrophages before moving up in the immune system hierarchy, its presence does not immediately trigger the production of antibodies, which makes it difficult to identify in a blood test. Second, consider the consequences of a virus that targets, as its ultimate goal, the helper T-cells. Helper T-cells are the vital link between humoral and cell-mediated immunity. They tell the B cells when to produce plasma cells and antibodies; they govern the activities of macrophages and monocytes through the secretion of lymphokines; they also stimulate killer T-cells and natural killer cells. Without helper T-cells, the entire immune system collapses and leaves the body vulnerable to a wide array of opportunistic diseases.

Most viruses invade active cells and enlist all that activity to produce new viruses (Sidebar 6.7). One of the more mysterious aspects of AIDS is that HIV works at an unusual pace. In addition to invading active cells, it invades *inactive* T-cells and lies in wait, its protein strands floating in the cytoplasm, until the day when the T-cell is activated by the presence of its target pathogen. Then the virus wakes up and disables the T-cell.

Blood-borne HIV can move from one CD4+ cell to another, and it can pool in the core of lymph nodes, where it eventually causes the cells to break down and the lymph node to lose all function. HIV has also been found in astrocytes and microglial cells in the central nervous system. This breaks down the blood-brain barrier, so toxic accumulations can lead to neurological symptoms.

HIV is composed of RNA rather than DNA, which holds the blueprints for our own cells. Once inside a target cell, this retrovirus uses the enzyme ***transcriptase*** to convert its RNA to DNA during replication. In the process, the virus is often minutely altered—just enough to make it resistant to identification or treatment. It is possible for new viral particles to escape the host cell without killing it, but ultimately CD4+ cells die in the disease process, through

SIDEBAR 6.7: A VIRUS PRIMER

Viruses consist of a protein coat of variable complexity wrapped around a core of DNA or RNA. Outside a host cell, viruses have no metabolic functions and cannot replicate. Inside a host cell, the virus reprograms the functions of that cell to replicate more viruses. In other words, the host cell becomes a virus factory. When the factory is full of inventory, it literally bursts at the seams, releasing hordes of new viruses in search of other hosts. Enormous amounts of damage occurs with any viral infection, not just to the cells attacked by the virus but to the cells the body sacrifices to fight back.

Most viruses cause short-term acute infections that spread easily. The coughing and sneezing seen with respiratory tract infections such as cold and flu are remarkably efficient distributors of virus. Likewise, the diarrhea that occurs with intestinal infections is an effective way to spread virus through fecal contamination. The immune system response to these viruses is severe and usually successful; most infections are curtailed, and the viruses are expelled in short order.

A few viruses, however, cause long-term chronic infections instead of short-term acute illness. Hepatitis B and C, herpesviruses, and HIV are notorious among these. For a virus to live in a body for a long time, it must be able to hide from immune system cells to escape attack and destruction. It is precisely the ability of HIV to hide from typical immune system activity that makes it so difficult to fight. In addition to being good hiders, chronic infectious viruses have been seen to produce decoy particles that draw antibody attack away from themselves and to secrete fake cytokines, chemical messengers that confuse and slow down immune system response.

As we learn more about how chronic infectious viruses pool in hidden reservoirs in the body, our ability to fight back will improve. We may someday be able to eradicate these hidden invaders permanently.

membrane rupture, apoptosis (where the cell essentially self-destructs), or ***anergy***, whereby the influence of the virus on the cell's DNA simply tells the cell to shut down and stop working.

Progression

Each stage of HIV/AIDS is associated with decreasing numbers of active helper T-cells and increased viral ***titers*** (counts of virus). The typical pattern looks like this:

- *Phase 1.* A person is infected with HIV. The virus is in the body but may be pooling in white blood cells rather than eliciting an immune response. Consequently, tests are negative, and no symptoms are present, but the person can transmit the disease because the viral load, that is, levels of virus in the blood, is very high. This incubation phase can last a year or more, although the average is 3 weeks to 6 months in sexually transmitted cases.
- *Phase 2.* In the acute primary phase HIV infection antibodies become detectable in blood tests. About 70% of people have fatigue, swollen glands, fever, weight loss, headaches, drowsiness, and confusion within several weeks of exposure. These signs and symptoms usually last about 2 weeks and are often mistaken for flu or mononucleosis.
- *Phase 3.* No signs, symptoms, or opportunistic diseases are obvious. Although the virus is continuing to replicate while decimating immune system cells, the body is able to keep up with the process. It is during this phase that medical intervention inhibits viral replication and prolongs life expectancy. The length of the asymptomatic phase varies widely, depending on the initial health of the person, what kind of treatment is given, and several other factors. It can last anywhere from 1 to 20 years or more, with a median of 10 years.
- *Phase 4.* Signs and symptoms of opportunistic diseases or AIDS-related cancers become apparent and eventually debilitating. A normal T-cell count is 800 to 1,000 cells per milliliter of blood. AIDS is diagnosed when these levels drop to 200 cells per milliliter or below and indicator diseases begin to develop.

HIV Resistance

Recent research has focused on the variables that determine how long a person who is HIV positive can keep the virus under control. Some people who are infected with HIV never develop symptoms, or develop them much more slowly than most people. These "long-term nonprogressors" can provide important clues to ways the virus may be fought once infection has been established. Three main factors have been identified:

- *Host resistance.* Some HIV patients have a genetic mutation in their immune system that produces few receptor sites on their macrophages and T-cells for the virus to latch on to. It takes more exposure over a longer time to establish an infection in these people, because the chance for a successful invasion is much lower.
- *Immune system response.* When most cells are invaded by a virus, they display a fragment of that virus on their membrane. This serves as a signal to immune system agents that the cell is compromised and should be destroyed. HIV is capable of slowing down this display reaction or of hiding from it altogether by mimicking normal cell membranes. If the efficiency of the display mechanism is improved, immune system response is more aggressive.
- *Virulence of the virus.* Sometimes HIV is partially weakened by medication or an immune system response but remains transmittable to another person. Infection with a weakened virus generally means the new host is better able to control it. Relative virulence of individual viruses is difficult to measure, however.

It seems clear that most long-term nonprogressors or very slow progressors have a combination of these factors working in their favor. It is estimated that approximately 5% of people who are HIV positive never develop symptoms or low CD4+ counts, even many years after their infection.[11]

Signs and Symptoms

Signs and symptoms of HIV depend on the stage of infection; these are described earlier in this section.

Communicability

HIV is spread from one person to another through the exchange of intimate fluids. These include blood (as from contaminated blood products, shared needles, or maternal-fetal circulation), semen, vaginal secretions, and breast milk. HIV does not accumulate in concentrations high enough to cause infection in other body fluids, such as sweat, saliva, or tears. The virus is unstable outside a human host, so it is not considered to be transmissible through contaminated surfaces or insect vectors such as mosquitoes, ticks, or bedbugs.

Complications

When HIV has virtually disabled normal immune function, the body is incapable of fending off attacks from pathogens that are not threatening to healthy people. A group of formerly obscure diseases are now so closely associated with AIDS they are called indicator diseases. Here are some of the most common and serious ones:

- ***Pneumocystis carinii*** **pneumonia.** This is a fungal infection of the lungs. It is now also called ***Pneumocystis jiroveci.***
- ***Cytomegalovirus.*** This member of the herpes family can cause retinitis and blindness, colitis, pneumonia, and infection of the adrenal glands.
- ***Kaposi sarcoma.*** This is a type of skin cancer (Figure 6.6) related to infection with human herpesvirus 8. Kaposi sarcoma is much more common in men with AIDS than in women.
- ***Non-Hodgkin lymphomas.*** HIV has been found to specifically initiate cancer cell replication with a variety of lymphomas. They tend to be aggressive, they frequently metastasize to the central nervous system, and they are highly resistant to treatment.

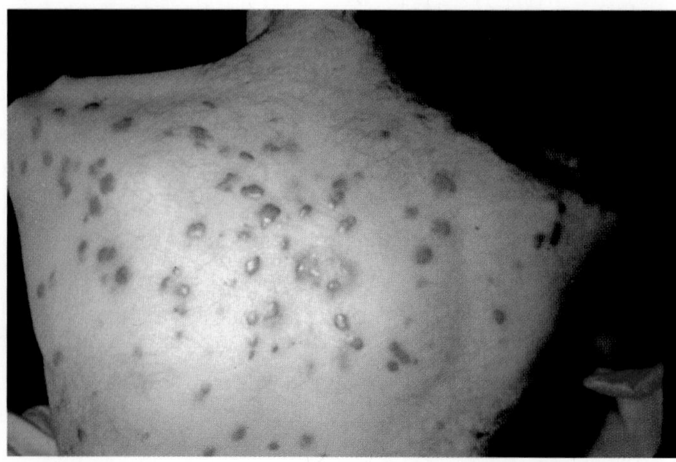

Figure 6.6. Kaposi sarcoma.

Other opportunistic indicator diseases include toxoplasmosis, a protozoan that can cause encephalitis or pneumonia; candidiasis, a yeast infection that can cause thrush or esophagitis; and *Cryptococcus neoformans*, a fungal infection that can cause meningitis and pneumonia.

In addition to these indicator diseases, people with AIDS are highly susceptible to gastrointestinal disturbances, herpes simplex, meningitis, shingles, cervical cancer, hepatitis C, and many other conditions. When tuberculosis occurs simultaneously with HIV, the risk of having tuberculosis become an active, contagious condition rises exponentially with each year of coinfection.

It is important to point out that while it is difficult to catch HIV from an infected person without some kind of intimate contact, it is *not* difficult to catch some of the contagious complications of AIDS. Tuberculosis, herpes, and other infections don't discriminate between HIV-positive and other persons.

Diagnosis

Infection with HIV is determined by the presence of antibodies in the blood. This is a bit problematic, since the peculiar nature of this pathogen prevents the body from tagging it and initiating antibody production until the virus is widespread. To get a truly dependable diagnosis, HIV tests must be conducted up to 6 months after the last incidence of high-risk behavior: sharing intravenous drug needles, unprotected sex with a possibly infected partner, or the use of blood or blood products.

Typically the first blood test given is ***ELISA*** (enzyme-linked immunosorbent assay). Because this extremely sensitive test sometimes yields false positives, a positive reading is followed by a second ELISA and/or a Western blot test. If both tests are negative and the person is clearly in a high-risk population and showing signs of being sick, tests may be conducted to look for signs of the virus itself in the blood rather than antibodies to the virus.

Recently the Centers for Disease Control issued a recommendation that all teenagers and adults be routinely screened for HIV in the same way that they are screened for other health issues such as cholesterol or high blood pressure. It is estimated that worldwide only about 10% of the people infected with HIV are aware of their status, so a public health effort like this could have significant ramifications for future infection rates.[8]

Treatment

One of the things that makes finding a cure for AIDS so difficult is that in the process of converting its core from RNA to DNA, the virus can minutely change, just enough to make it resistant to drugs as well as to immune system activation. The answer to that problem has been to combine various drugs to anticipate the mutations of the virus. This has been highly successful in laboratory settings, but these drug combinations are often prohibitively toxic to the actual patients.

The most successful AIDS treatments so far have involved using multiple strategies to interrupt viral replication. The use of *highly active antiretroviral therapy* (***HAART***) has been seen to slow progression in many patients, but it can't get at the virus when it hides in long-lived cells such as memory T-cells, which have a life expectancy of 60 years or more. Although the goal of eradicating the virus from an infected person is still a long way off, studies of patients who manage to control their infection efficiently continue to point the way to better treatment options, and the life expectancy for a person with HIV today (who can afford to treat it) is better than it's ever been.

The biggest controversy in HIV treatment today is in deciding when it is best to initiate antiviral therapy. It is clear that drugs prolong the lives of AIDS patients, but they are also highly toxic and have many serious side effects, including low blood cell count, peripheral neuropathy, pancreatitis, chronic diarrhea, liver inflammation, kidney stones, and many others. One of the most visible side effects of HIV medication is *lipodystrophy*. Fat in the cheeks and the buttocks degenerates, but fat in the upper back, breasts, and around the belly accumulates.

Furthermore, many AIDS patients live in isolation, and they are more likely than most to be depressed and/or substance abusers, which increases the risk of their not taking their medication according to prescription: this gives rise to ever more resistant strains of the virus.

Treatment recommendations vary. If HIV is identified during the primary phase of flu-like symptoms, some research suggests the best prognosis if therapy is started right away. Health care workers who get needle sticks with a risk of contamination are treated immediately to reduce the risk that the virus can take hold. But if the virus isn't identified until the person is asymptomatic, many experts recommend holding off on aggressive treatment until CD4+ levels drop to below 350/μL of blood.[12]

Research for more and better HIV/AIDS treatments continues. In the near future we may see more ways to interrupt the viral bonding with target cells, a topical antimicrobial cream that will prevent the virus from crossing through the mucous membrane, mechanisms to root out latent virus hiding in immune system tissues, and possibly even a vaccine that will prevent the infection altogether.

Massage?

HIV is spread through the exchange of intimate bodily fluids: semen, breast milk, blood, and vaginal secretions. No research has ever shown that it can be transmitted through sweat or casual contact. Obviously, the person most at risk for getting sick when an AIDS patient receives massage is not the therapist; it's the client. Therefore, care must be taken that the practitioner does not carry active pathogens that may put a client with AIDS at risk.

Massage for HIV-positive clients who are asymptomatic is certainly indicated. One study that compared massage with a friendly visit among children with no access to antiviral therapy found that the massaged group had consistently higher CD4+ counts at the end of the project.[13]

Although in advanced stages of AIDS opportunistic diseases can make rigorous massage problematic, other types of work may reduce stress, which in turn strengthens the immune system. Bodywork can be a wonderful treatment option and an important source of support and comfort for people who are often rejected, ignored, or actively persecuted by society.

Modality Recommendations for HIV/AIDS

Modality	Recommendation
Deep Tissue Massage	Indicated while asymptomatic; work for parasympathetic response.
Lymphatic Drainage	Supportive.
Polarity	S/R/D: Indicated within client comfort for immune system support.
PNF/MET/Stretching	Supportive.
Reflexology	Indicated within client tolerance: work endocrine and lymphatic systems, solar plexus points.
Shiatsu	Indicated for strengthening immune system via TH, SP, K, L systemically.
Swedish Massage	Indicated while asymptomatic; in AIDS depends on resilience of the client.
Trigger Point Therapy	Supportive.

See Chapter 1 for a brief description of each modality, including definitions of abbreviations.

Lupus

Definition: What Is It?

Lupus is an autoimmune disease in which various types of tissues are attacked by the body's own antibodies. Lupus can be mild, but has the potential to be life threatening. In extreme cases this disorder can attack the heart, the lungs, the kidneys, and the brain, with devastating results.

Lupus

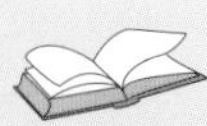

From the Latin word for wolf, this name could have come about for a couple of reasons. It could refer to the characteristic butterfly mask on the face that looks like the facial markings of a wolf, or it could refer to the circular lesions that may appear on the face or elsewhere on the body that were thought to resemble wolf bites.

Demographics: Who Gets It?

Statistics on this disease vary greatly because it is difficult to diagnose early in the process. Population surveys estimate that roughly 1.5 million people in the United States have some form of lupus. African Americans, Hispanics, Native Americans, and Asians have higher rates than whites.[14]

Lupus can affect people at any age, but it is most common in women of childbearing age. It affects women far more than men, by 9 to 1.

Etiology: What Happens?

Four varieties of lupus have been identified: drug-induced lupus erythematosus, neonatal lupus, discoid lupus erythematosus, and systemic lupus erythematosus.

- *Drug-induced lupus* is brought on by some prescribed medications for high blood pressure, heart arrhythmia, psychosis, and epilepsy. These symptoms resolve when the medications are discontinued.
- *Neonatal lupus* occurs when a mother's antibodies are transferred to a newborn baby and the baby sustains a skin rash, liver problems, or a low blood count for a few weeks or months until the antibodies are no longer active. At that time the symptoms disappear, usually with no long-term consequences.
- *Discoid lupus erythematosus* (DLE) is a chronic skin disease. It can involve small scaly red patches with sharp margins that don't itch, or the characteristic butterfly rash of redness over the nose and cheeks (Figures 6.7 and 6.8). The skin can become very thin and delicate, or lesions may become permanently discolored and thickened. DLE is sometimes described as a subset of skin disorders called *subacute cutaneous*

Lupus in Brief

Pronunciation: LU-pus

What is it?

Lupus is an autoimmune disease in which antibodies attack various types of tissue throughout the body. Four distinct types of lupus exist, but systemic lupus erythematosus is both the most common and the most serious.

How is it recognized?

A constellation of 11 specific signs and symptoms have been determined for a diagnosis of lupus; a patient must have at least four of them. They include, among other things, arthritis in two or more joints, pleurisy, pericarditis, kidney disease, and nervous system dysfunction.

Is massage indicated or contraindicated?

When lupus is in a state of acute flare, circulatory massage may exacerbate symptoms, while energetic or reflexive techniques may be supportive. When the condition is in remission, bodywork of any kind can help to reduce pain and anxiety and to help maintain flexibility.

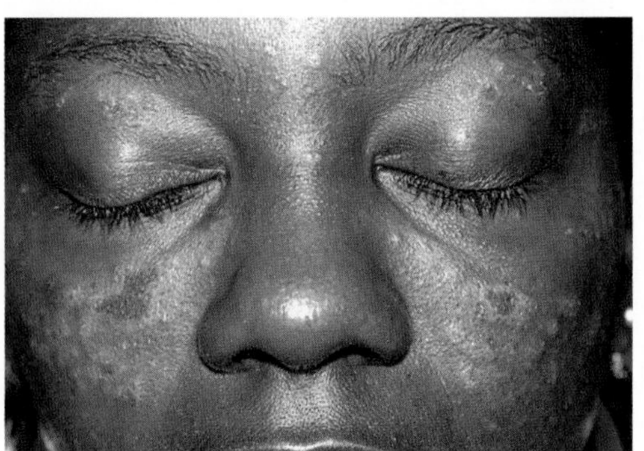

Figure 6.7. Discoid lupus.

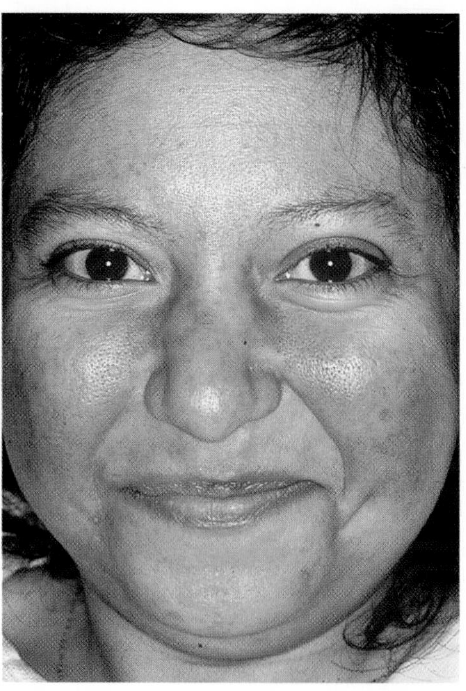

Figure 6.8. Malar rash.

lupus. A small number of people with DLE go on to develop systemic lupus erythematosus.

- ***Systemic lupus erythematosus*** (SLE) is caused by antibody attacks against a variety of tissues throughout the body. This can result in arthritis, renal failure, thrombosis, psychosis, seizures, coronary artery disease, inflammation of the heart, and ***pleurisy***. SLE can be very serious. It can usually be controlled, but at this time it cannot be cured. SLE sometimes begins as DLE, but not always. The rest of this discussion focuses on SLE, which has the farthest-reaching and longest-lasting signs and symptoms of the four varieties of lupus.

The precise cause or causes of lupus are unknown; most authorities suggest that it is the result of a combination of genetic predisposition, hormones, and environmental exposures. A genetic link is clearly a factor, but a child of a parent with lupus has only a 5% chance of developing the disease. Further, when one identical twin develops SLE, the other twin may not. This indicates that although a genetic susceptibility may be inherited, other factors must also contribute to the development of the disease. Another indicator that genetics is not the primary issue is that while lupus in the United States has the highest incidence among African American women, lupus is practically unheard of among women in Western or Central Africa.[15] This points to environmental influences along with genetic predisposition.

Environmental factors may include exposure to certain viruses, ultraviolet light, certain medications, and high levels of estrogen. Women with lupus often report a change in symptoms with their menstrual cycle, and research shows that estrogen replacement therapy that is employed to reduce the risk of osteoporosis can increase the risk of lupus for some women.[15]

Several theories are in development about the etiology of lupus; these change frequently as research reveals more and more details about the process of this disease. It seems clear that accelerated apoptosis (programmed cell death) is an issue for lupus patients, along with a hyperreactive immune response to material that is considered antigenic, or non-self. Abnormalities in blood clotting and some differences in inflammatory chemicals have been observed; these findings continue to open doors to new and more effective treatment options.

Signs and Symptoms

Lupus can affect virtually every system in the body (Figure 6.9). Usually the mechanism is damage to small blood vessels, which can lead to clotting, atherosclerosis, and prolonged and damaging inflammatory activity. Sometimes the problems associated with lupus are not serious or even detectable. At other times they can be life threatening. Because some of the features of this disease make profound changes in health, it is worth looking at how SLE affects several systems.

- *Integumentary system.* The characteristic butterfly or discoid rash that is seen with lupus has already been described. These rashes, which can appear anywhere on the body, may be exacerbated by sunlight in a condition called ***photosensitivity***. Lupus can also cause ulcers in the mucous membranes, particularly in the nose, throat and mouth. Lupus rashes may be acute or subacute; subacute rashes tend to be photosensitive but do not leave permanent scars. Photosensitive rashes can be prevented or reduced with the use of sunscreen and avoiding sun exposure during peak hours. When SLE causes superficial blood vessels to become inflamed, symptoms may appear on the skin in the shape of welts, red lines, and painful bumps.
- *Musculoskeletal system.* Some 80% to 90% of people with lupus eventually develop arthritis. Joint pain usually occurs at the hands and feet, seldom in the spine. Interestingly, even someone with longstanding lupus does *not* usually show signs of internal joint damage. Nonspecific muscle pain is another common symptom, and many lupus patients also meet the diagnostic criteria for fibromyalgia.
- *Nervous system.* Many people with lupus have some nervous system dysfunction. This can range from extreme headaches to psychosis (including paranoia and hallucinations) to high fever or seizures, depending on which part of the brain is adversely affected by

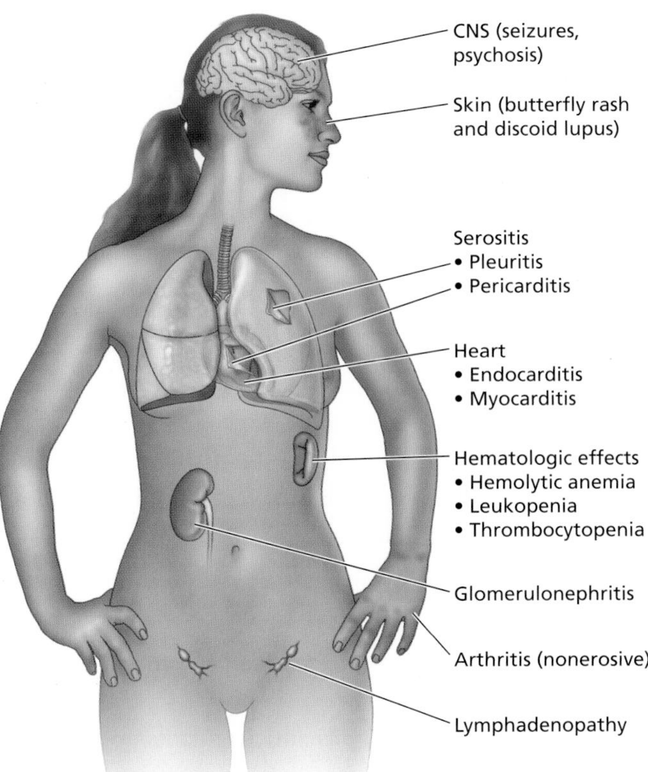

Figure 6.9. Sites affected by systemic lupus erythematosus.

blood vessel inflammation. When the clotting disorders that may accompany this disorder occur in the brain, the result is a transient ischemic attack or stroke.

- *Cardiovascular system.* Lupus is can lead to inflammation and damage of major blood vessels, opening the door to rapidly progressive atherosclerosis, even in young people. Women with lupus have a 50-fold greater risk of having a heart attack than women without lupus.[16] Lupus is also associated with slow clot formation and slow clot dissolving. This problem can lead to thrombophlebitis or pulmonary embolism. In addition to blood vessel damage, lupus may affect the serous membranes of the heart. This results in inflammation, arrhythmia, and severe chest pain. Anemia is a frequent complication of long-term inflammation and bone marrow suppression. Thrombocy-topenia, or a shortage of platelets, may occur when lupus antibodies have attacked thrombocytes. Raynaud phenomenon is a sign of vasculitis, or inflammation of the blood vessels.
- *Respiratory system.* A common complication of lupus is pleurisy, or inflammation and fluid accumulation in the serous membranes that line the lungs. This causes pain on inhalation and restricted movement of the lungs. Pleural effusion is the accumulation of fluid between the layers of the pleurae. If enough resistance in the lungs develops, a lupus patient may be at risk for pulmonary hypertension and right-sided heart failure.
- *Urinary system.* Tissue damage in the kidneys leads to a specific type of ***glomerulonephritis***. Kidney damage can accumulate without symptoms until the kidneys are on the brink of renal failure.
- *Reproductive system.* The clotting disorder associated with lupus can make it difficult to carry a child to term. Repeated spontaneous miscarriages are sometimes the first sign of the disease that will lead to a diagnosis. Pregnant women with lupus face special challenges, as some of the medications that control symptoms are not safe for the baby.

Diagnosis

It is clear from this long and varied list of symptoms that lupus can look like a lot of different diseases. Fortunately, it leaves some specific clues in the blood that can help to identify it. Unfortunately, those clues are sometimes present in people *without* lupus, so they can't be used as a definitive diagnosis.

A collection of 11 signs and symptoms has been developed as a diagnostic criterion for SLE. If any four of these criteria are present at any time, a positive diagnosis of lupus can be made. The four signs do *not* have to be present simultaneously.[16]

- Malar (butterfly) rash
- Discoid skin rash (can cause permanent scarring)
- Photosensitivity
- Mucous membrane ulcers, particularly in the mouth, nose, or throat
- Arthritis in more than two joints, specifically in the hands or feet (*not* in the spine)
- Pleurisy and/or pericarditis
- Kidney problems: blood or protein in the urine
- Brain irritation: headaches, seizures, or psychosis
- Blood count abnormalities: low red blood cell count, white blood cell count, or platelet count
- Immunologic disorders: special antibodies and/or lupus anticoagulants are present in the blood
- ***Antinuclear antibodies*** in the blood

Lupus, like other autoimmune conditions, is exacerbated by certain kinds of stimuli. Excessive exposure to ultraviolet light, emotional stress, injury, infection, or trauma can be triggers. Pregnancy is a trigger for some women, while for others it may suppress flares. Someone who has lupus must identify the stimuli that are particularly potent for her and avoid them carefully.

One of the challenges in the diagnosis of lupus is that symptoms fluctuate and may change entirely over time. In addition, other connective tissue diseases may occur simultaneously with lupus to further cloud the issue (Sidebar 6.8).

SIDEBAR 6.8: MIXED CONNECTIVE TISSUE DISEASE

About 10% of people diagnosed with lupus have it simultaneously with other autoimmune diseases. This combination of conditions is sometimes called *mixed connective tissue disease.*

The autoimmune diseases that are most often a part of mixed connective tissue disease include scleroderma, rheumatoid arthritis, lupus, polymyositis, and dermatomyositis. Rheumatoid arthritis and lupus occur together so often that a new name has been coined for this condition: rhupus.

In many cases a person presents over a long period with a range of fluctuating symptoms that are not specific to any particular autoimmune disease. These usually include fatigue, muscle weakness, joint pain and swelling, swollen fingers, mild fever, and bouts with Raynaud phenomenon. Much later, the symptoms often narrow down to point to just one condition, which is usually scleroderma.

The role of massage for a client with mixed connective tissue disease is to work conservatively, being supportive but not challenging during flares, and working to improve function during remission. Communication with a client's health care team is important to maximize benefits (e.g., reducing stress, improving attitude, easing pain) while minimizing risks (exacerbating inflammation, irritating damaged tissues).

Treatment

The treatment strategy for lupus is to minimize the negative impact of inflammation during flares. Lupus patients have essentially four levels of medical recourse in the effort to manage this condition. Each intervention has inherent risks, however, which must be weighed against the benefits.

If the case is not very severe, it may be managed with nonsteroidal anti-inflammatories. These drugs are inexpensive and easily accessible, and they are often effective against inflammation. Unfortunately, they are also associated with chronic stomach irritation, and long-term use can irritate and damage the kidneys. This a matter of concern for lupus patients, many of whom develop kidney damage from the disease process and don't want to speed that progression with medication.

Steroidal anti-inflammatories (especially prednisone) are sometimes prescribed for short-term use, especially during flares. These are very powerful anti-inflammatories, but they are also associated with many dangerous side effects, including mood changes, weight gain, liver damage, bone thinning, and ***osteonecrosis***, or death of bone and joint tissue, especially in the hips and shoulders.

Antimalarial drugs have found success in treating some of the symptoms of lupus, especially skin rashes and ulcers of mucous membranes. Some antimalarial drugs cause changes in eye function, so an ophthalmologist must closely monitor their use.

In very severe cases of lupus, ***cytotoxic*** drugs that entirely disable the immune system may be recommended. This of course leaves the patient vulnerable to secondary infections because the immune system has been suppressed to keep it from attacking.

Other treatment options for lupus depend on the presenting symptoms. Acute rashes may be treated with topical steroid creams or ointments. If a patient has blood clotting problems, anticoagulants may be administered. It is a high priority to treat lupus symptoms quickly as they arise; early intervention can reduce the amount of damage that accrues during flares and keep the body functioning at normal levels during periods of remission.

The treatment options for lupus sound alarming, but in truth it is usually manageable. When it was first recognized, most patients died within 5 years of diagnosis. Now, thanks to these medical interventions, 80% to 90% of lupus patients can expect a normal life span.[14]

Massage?

Active flares of lupus mark periods of inflammation that can damage the heart, lungs, and kidneys and cause painful swelling at joints. Circulatory massage during these acute episodes may exacerbate symptoms and put unhealthy stress on an inflamed cardiovascular system. Energy work during these episodes, however, may be supportive and helpful.

Circulatory massage is more appropriate during remission, especially as a treatment strategy against the stress that can trigger attacks, but care must be taken to ensure that the circulatory and urinary systems are capable of handling the changes in internal environment that massage brings about.

Modality Recommendations for Lupus	
Deep Tissue Massage	Supportive within client tolerance while subacute or in remission.
Lymphatic Drainage	Supportive.
Polarity	S: Indicated. R/D: Systemically contraindicated while acute, otherwise supportive.
PNF/MET/Stretching	Systemically contraindicated while acute; supportive between flares.
Reflexology	Indicated in remission; work lymphatic system and affected areas.
Shiatsu	Indicated for strengthening the immune system via TH, SP, L. Add H, SI to calm mind for restorative sleep.
Swedish Massage	Contraindicated while acute; indicated to facilitate homeostasis between flares.
Trigger Point Therapy	Systemically contraindicated while acute; supportive between flares.

See Chapter 1 for a brief description of each modality, including definitions of abbreviations.

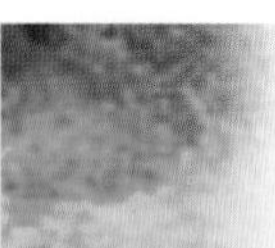

Chapter Review Questions: Lymph and Immune System Conditions

1. What is the main function of the immune system?
2. Why are massage therapists particularly at risk for lymphangitis?
3. What are lymphokines, and what do they do?
4. What is the most dependable early sign for any kind of lymphoma?
5. What is the causative agent for most cases of mononucleosis?
6. How is HIV communicable?
7. What type of cell is the *first* target for HIV?
8. Who is most at risk for getting sick when a massage therapist works with an AIDS patient? Why?
9. What is the difference between anaphylaxis and angioedema?
10. Your client has been diagnosed with systemic lupus. She takes anti-inflammatories and immune-suppressant drugs to control her symptoms. What are some cautions or concerns about massage in this situation?

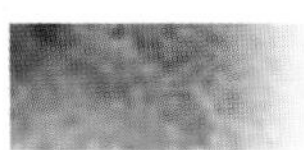

REFERENCES

1. Facts 2006–2007. Leukemia, Lymphoma, Myeloma. © The Leukemia & Lymphoma Society Inc. http://www.leukemia-lymphoma.org/all_mat_toc.adp?item_id=87311. Accessed summer 2006.
2. Gajra A, Vajpayee N, Grethlein S. Lymphoma, B-Cell. © 1996–2006 by WebMD. http://www.emedicine.com/med/topic1358.htm. Accessed summer 2006.
3. Epstein-Barr Virus and Infectious Mononucleosis. National Center for Infectious Diseases. http://www.cdc.gov/ncidod/diseases/ebv.htm. Accessed summer 2006.
4. Media Resources: Media Kit. © 1996–2006. All Rights Reserved. American Academy of Allergy Asthma & Immunology. http://www.aaaai.org/media/resources/media_kit/allergy_statistics.stm. Accessed summer 2006.
5. Anand MK. Hypersensitivity Reactions, Immediate. © 1996–2006 by WebMD. http://www.emedicine.com/med/topic1101.htm. Accessed summer 2006.
6. CFS: Basic Facts. Centers for Disease Control and Prevention. http://www.cdc.gov/cfs/. Accessed summer 2006.
7. Field T. Touch Therapy. Churchill Livingstone. © Tiffany Field, 2000, p 165.
8. HIV/AIDS. © 2000–2006 Global Health Council. http://globalhealth.org/view_top.php3?id=227. Accessed fall 2006.
9. HIV Infection in Women. National Institute of Allergy and Infectious Diseases. http://www.niaid.nih.gov/factsheets/womenhiv.htm. Accessed summer 2006.
10. Epidemiology of HIV/AIDS in the United States. © 2006, Regents of the University of California. http://hivinsite.ucsf.edu/InSite?page=kb-01&doc=kb-01-03. Accessed summer 2006.
11. How HIV Causes AIDS. National Institute of Allergy and Infectious Diseases. http://www.niaid.nih.gov/factsheets/howhiv.htm. Accessed fall 2006.
12. Human Immunodeficiency Virus. © 1996–2005 MedicineNet, Inc. http://www.medicinenet.com/human_immunodeficiency_virus_hiv_aids/article.htm. Accessed summer 2006.
13. Massage for HIV-Positive Children. Massage Therapy Foundation. http://www.massagetherapyfoundation.org/or_article_massagemag115B.html Accessed fall 2006.
14. Statistics about Lupus. © 2001 Lupus Foundation of America, Inc. http://www.lupus.org/education/stats.html. Accessed summer 2006.
15. Bartles C, Hildebrand J. Systemic Lupus Erythematosus. © 1996–2006 by WebMD. http://www.emedicine.com/med/topic2228.htm. Accessed summer 2006.
16. Lupus. © 1998–2006 Mayo Foundation for Medical Education and Research. All rights reserved. http://www.mayoclinic.com/health/lupus/DS00115. Accessed summer 2006.

7

Respiratory System Conditions

Chapter Objectives

After reading this chapter, you should be able to . . .

- Name what percentage of calories a healthy person invests in the act of respiration while at rest.
- Identify the oxygen saturation of an average inhaled breath compared with the oxygen saturation of an exhaled breath.
- Identify underlying triggers of acute bronchitis.
- Explain why no vaccine can permanently protect against colds or flu.
- Identify a synonym for the common cold.
- Name three causative agents for pneumonia.
- Identify which form of sinusitis is most appropriate for massage.
- Describe the difference between primary-phase and secondary-phase tuberculosis.
- Name the group of conditions to which chronic bronchitis and emphysema belong.
- Explain why persons with asthma, chronic bronchitis, or emphysema are often encouraged to be vaccinated against the flu.
- Name what kinds of glands are affected by cystic fibrosis.

Respiratory System Introduction

Structure

The easiest way to discuss the structure of the respiratory system is to follow a particle of air through it (Figure 7.1). Take a deep breath. Air drawn in through the nose encounters mucous membranes. Mucous membranes line any cavity in the body that communicates with the outside world: the respiratory, digestive, reproductive, and urinary systems. In the respiratory system the mucous membranes start inside the nose and mouth, and they line the sinuses and throat all the way down into the smaller tubes in the lungs. The wet, sticky mucous membranes in the respiratory system are responsible for warming, moistening, and filtering the air that passes by.

Once past the nose and mouth, air enters first the pharynx, then the larynx, the trachea, and the bronchi. The bronchi are asymmetrical. The right bronchus is bigger, wider, and straighter, leading into the three lobes of the right lung. The left bronchus is smaller in diameter, and it curves off to the side to reach the two lobes of the left lung. This

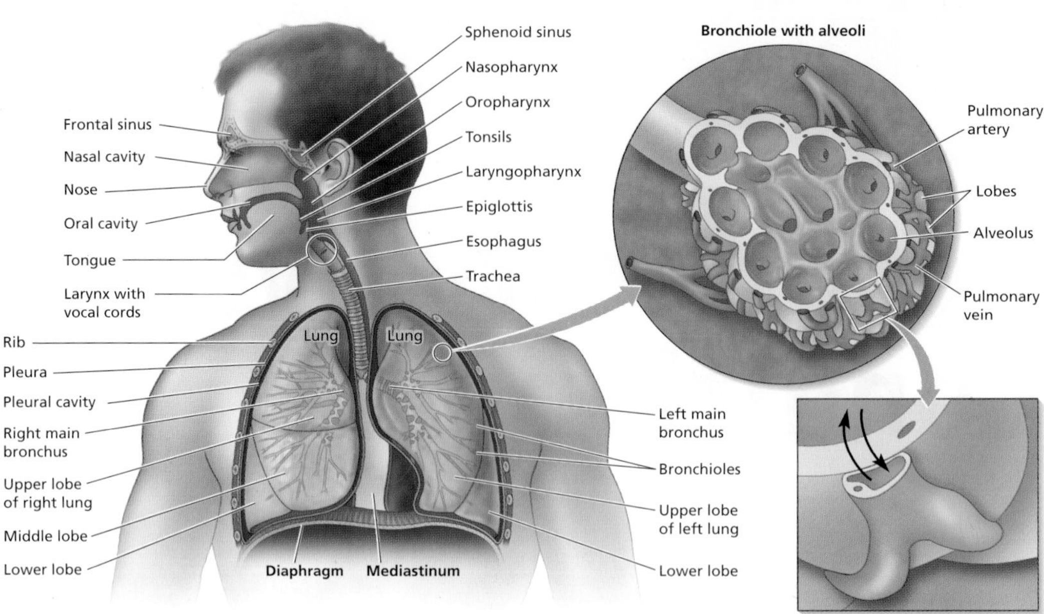

Figure 7.1. Overview of the respiratory system.

is significant if a foreign object is inhaled into the lungs; it almost always follows the path of least resistance to the right side.

The next section of tubing is the bronchioles, which subdivide 23 times until they end in microscopic ***alveoli***. These grape-shaped clusters of epithelial bubbles are like tiny balloons surrounded by blood capillaries. Gaseous exchange occurs through the permeable surfaces between the alveoli and the capillaries. If for any reason the alveoli are impaired or not functioning correctly, the body cannot make an efficient trade of carbon dioxide for oxygen.

The structure of the lungs themselves is well suited for fighting off infection. Each lung has two or three separate lobes, and each of those lobes has smaller separate segments called lobules. This isolation of areas makes it difficult for pathogens to infect the whole structure. All of the tubes are lined with mucous membrane, which traps pathogens and other particles. Then the cilia in the tract help move the mucus blanket toward the mouth and nose for expulsion. Smooth muscle tissue lines all of the tubes down to the smallest bronchi; when an irritant is trapped in these tubes, a healthy cough reflex quickly moves it out of the body.

Function

Air cycles through the lungs 12 to 20 times per minute. The lungs themselves do not have any muscle tissue to make them fill up or empty; they are simply limp-walled sacs that inflate or deflate according to the air pressure inside and outside of them. A change in air pressure is brought about by a change in the shape of the thoracic cavity. If the cavity is made larger, the air pressure inside is low until air rushes in to equalize it. In other words, the act of inhaling is simply filling a vacuum. When the pressure inside and outside the lungs has been equalized, air eases out again: exhalation. Exhalation is usually a passive process; it doesn't involve muscular activity unless a person specifically tries to remove air from the lungs.

The efficiency of this mechanism is astonishing. Even though oxygen–carbon dioxide exchange is only partial with each breath (a typical inhalation contains roughly 21% oxygen, while a typical exhalation still contains about 16% oxygen), the respiratory system supplies the entire body with enough oxygen to function with minimal effort. In fact, a healthy person invests only 5% of resting calories in the act of breathing.

The conditions examined in this chapter mostly have to do with the vulnerability of the respiratory system to infection. Fortunately, thanks to the sticky mucous membranes and lungs with isolated segments, those infections seldom get a strong enough grip to do lasting damage.

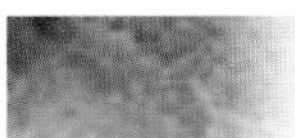

Respiratory System Conditions

Infectious Respiratory Disorders

Acute bronchitis
Common cold
Influenza
Pneumonia
Sinusitis
Tuberculosis

Chronic Obstructive Pulmonary Diseases

Asthma
Chronic bronchitis
Emphysema

Other Respiratory Disorders

Cystic fibrosis
Lung cancer

Infectious Respiratory Disorders

Acute Bronchitis

Definition: What Is It?

Acute bronchitis is a self-limiting inflammation of the respiratory tract, specifically of the bronchial tree. It is usually a complication of the common cold or flu. Acute bronchitis is usually resolved within 10 days to several weeks of onset. This helps to distinguish it from chronic bronchitis, which is an irreversible condition.

Demographics: Who Gets It?

It is estimated that about 12 million cases of acute bronchitis occur every year in the United States,[1] leading to about 3 million doctor visits.[2] Most cases are in young children, but adults are certainly susceptible. Adults who smoke or work in an environment with dust, fumes, or other pollutants are at higher risk for developing acute bronchitis than others. Other risk factors for acute bronchitis include being elderly, having heart problems, and being otherwise immunosuppressed.

Etiology: What Happens?

When the bronchi are irritated or infected by any kind of pathogen, an inflammatory response ensues. The tubes swell, the cilia are damaged, excessive mucus is produced, and the result is coughing and wheezing as air moves through obstructed passageways. Most cases of acute bronchitis are complications of a cold or flu in which the viruses simply move from the upper respiratory system to the bronchial tubes. Other causative agents include a variety of bacteria, fungi, and noninfectious irritants, such as fumes, air pollutants, and other contaminants. Chronic reflux from the esophagus can also irritate the bronchi.

An important feature of acute bronchitis is that it is self-limiting and results in no permanent changes to the bronchi, cilia, or mucous membranes. This distinguishes acute bronchitis from chronic bronchitis, which is typically irreversible.

> **Acute Bronchitis in Brief**
> Pronunciation: ah-KYUTE brong-KY-tis
>
> **What is it?**
> Acute bronchitis is inflammation of the bronchial tree anywhere between the trachea and the bronchioles. If inflammation extends into the bronchioles and alveoli, it is called bronchopneumonia.
>
> **How is it recognized?**
> The hallmark of acute bronchitis is a persistent cough along with sore throat, nasal congestion, fatigue, and fever. Although other symptoms generally subside within 10 days, the cough may last for several weeks while the bronchi heal.
>
> **Is massage indicated or contraindicated?**
> Acute bronchitis, like all acute infections, contraindicates circulatory massage. If the infection has passed and the cough is the only lingering symptom, massage may be appropriate as long as the client is comfortable on the table.

Signs and Symptoms

The primary sign of acute bronchitis is a persistent cough. It often starts as a dry cough but within a few days becomes productive. Sputum may be clear or opaque. Wheezing, nasal congestion, headache, low fever, muscle aches, chest pain, and fatigue may also be present. Most of the symptoms of acute bronchitis subside within about 10 days of onset, but the cough may persist for several weeks while the delicate lining of the bronchial tubes heals.

If fever persists or exceeds 101°F (38.3°C) or if the sputum becomes greenish, yellow, or blood-streaked, the possibility of pneumonia must be considered. This is a more serious condition that usually needs medical intervention.

Diagnosis

Acute bronchitis is usually diagnosed simply by its distinctive symptoms. However, several other respiratory disorders can create a similar picture. Bacterial sinusitis, mild pneumonia, and asthma can all involve wheezing and productive coughs. These disorders should be ruled out to be sure that treatment options are as effective as possible.

Treatment

The best treatment options for most cases of acute bronchitis are the same as those for cold or flu: plenty of rest, lots of fluids, and warm, humid air to liquefy mucus and aid in its expulsion. Antibiotics are not effective in most cases of acute bronchitis, but they are appropriate when the causative agent has been identified as bacterial.

Bronchodilators and cough suppressants can help to ameliorate some of the symptoms of acute bronchitis, but they do not eradicate the infection or speed recovery.

Massage?

Circulatory massage is inappropriate for someone in the acute stage of a bronchial infection. When the infection has passed, however, and the person is left with a persistent cough while the bronchial tubes heal, massage may be appropriate as long as the client is comfortable on the table.

MODALITY RECOMMENDATIONS FOR ACUTE BRONCHITIS	
Deep tissue massage	Systemically contraindicated while acute; otherwise supportive. Work respiratory muscles and fascias.
Lymphatic drainage	Systemically contraindicated while acute; otherwise supportive.
Polarity	S: Indicated. R/D: avoid while acute; otherwise supportive; determined by patient's comfort.
PNF/MET/stretching	Systemically contraindicated while acute; otherwise supportive.
Reflexology	Indicated: work lungs, chest, adrenal points.
Shiatsu	Contraindicated while acute; then systemically: L, LI. Locally: K, ST, SP in chest; BL in back.
Swedish massage	Systemically contraindicated while acute; otherwise supportive.
Trigger point therapy	Systemically contraindicated while acute; otherwise supportive.

See Chapter 1 for a brief description of each modality, including definitions of abbreviations.

Common Cold

Definition: What Is It?

The common cold is brought about by any of about 200 viruses. Over the course of a lifetime people are exposed to multitudes of cold viruses. They get sick, they establish immunity to that particular pathogen, and they move on to the next infection. Much of this happens in childhood; by adulthood people have encountered most of what they're likely to see, and the frequency of infections generally subsides. But no single infectious agent causes the so-called common cold, and the viruses themselves keep mutating and changing. This is why there may never be an effective vaccine for the cold.

> **Common Cold in Brief**
>
> **What is it?**
> The common cold is a viral infection from any of about 200 types of viruses.
>
> **How is it recognized?**
> The symptoms of colds are nasal discharge, sore throat, mild fever, dry coughing, and headache. Symptoms last anywhere from 2 days to 2 weeks.
>
> **Is massage indicated or contraindicated?**
> Colds indicate circulatory massage only when the acute stage has passed, and even then massage may exacerbate symptoms, as the healing process may be accelerated. Energetic types of bodywork may be supportive and helpful if a person has a hard time getting past the peak of a cold.

Demographics: Who Gets It?

It is difficult to project just how common the common cold really is. One estimate suggests that about 1 billion infections with common cold virus occur in the United States in an average year.[3] Children are most at risk for these infections until their immune system has built up a collection of protective antibodies. Children have an average of 6 to 10 colds per year, and adults generally have 2 to 4 per year. People over 60 years old may have fewer than 2 colds per year.

Colds cause about 26 million lost school days and 23 million lost work days each year, and they cost untold millions of dollars in health care and lost productivity.[4]

Etiology: What Happens?

The common cold, also known as an upper respiratory tract infection (URTI) or viral rhinitis, is caused by any of more than 200 different viruses. Rhinoviruses cause approximately half of colds; this group has about 110 subtypes and is most active in autumn and spring. Other pathogens include coronaviruses (these are the group that also cause severe acute respiratory syndrome, or SARS), adenoviruses, and respiratory syncytial virus. Most of these viral infections are low grade and not dangerous, but some can cause very severe infections, especially in infants and young children.

The viruses that cause the common cold enter the nose, where the temperature is about 91°F (32.8°C), a perfect growth environment. The cilia in the mucous membrane carry the viruses to the back of the throat, where they have access to their target cells in the lymphoid tissue of the adenoids. When a virus gains access to its target, it infiltrates that cell and takes over its processes until the cell literally bursts with new viruses. Cold viruses act fast: the incubation period between being exposed and developing symptoms can be as short as 12 hours.

While the damage that cold viruses cause is substantial, it pales in comparison with the damage caused by the immune system when it is fighting off a cold virus. Special signals released by infected cells attract immune system agents, which cause the area to be flooded with inflammatory chemicals and aggressive immune systems cells. It is the immune system response to a viral threat that causes most of the discomfort associated with common cold symptoms.

Research about whether *being* cold *causes* cold is inconclusive. Some studies do indicate that a drop in body temperature increases the risk of developing symptoms,[5] while others dispute this. Theories on why colds happen most in winter include the possibility that cold temperatures cause vasoconstriction in the nose, reducing immune system protection there; air tends to be drier in winter, which provides a better chance for the viruses to adhere to the lining of the sinuses; and cold outdoor temperatures makes people share indoor spaces more closely, increasing the likelihood of spreading infection.

Other factors that increase the risk of catching cold include psychological stress and allergies.[3]

Signs and Symptoms

The symptoms of a cold are probably familiar to everyone: runny nose, sneezing, sore throat, dry coughing, headache, and perhaps a mild fever. Colds are typically limited to the upper respiratory tract. Symptoms generally last less than 2 weeks, although the cough may linger for 3 weeks or more.

Complications

Colds are seldom dangerous except when they complicate into another disorder. The compromised integrity of the membranes and the accumulations of mucus, a perfect growth medium, leaves the body vulnerable to a bacterial onslaught that can include ear infection, laryngitis, acute bronchitis, sinusitis, and pneumonia. People with asthma also frequently find that colds exacerbate their respiratory symptoms.

Prevention

Cold viruses can stay viable for up to 3 hours outside the body. The viruses are airborne after an infected person coughs or sneezes, but they are much more readily spread when someone gets a virus on the hand or face, and it finds access to the body through a portal of entry: the mouth, the eyes, or the nose. Picking up a virus on the hands or from a light switch, a doorknob, a keyboard, or a piece of money and then rubbing the nose is a very efficient way to spread the disease.

The best way to prevent the spread of colds and other infectious diseases is by frequently washing the hands, focusing on the cuticles and nails, using soap or detergent and scrubbing for 30 seconds or more before rinsing. Using paper tissues and disposing of them carefully, avoiding contact with people who are sick, and using other good judgment about sleep, diet, and exercise can also help to prevent the spread of colds.

Treatment

Because they are viral infections, antibiotics are useless for treating colds. Getting extra rest, drinking lots of fluids, and isolating oneself from family, classmates, and coworkers who could get infected are all high priorities. Using a humidifier may relieve some of the irritation to mucous membranes, although some types of humidifiers can be breeding grounds for fungi or bacteria, so it's important to keep them scrupulously clean.

Over-the-counter drugs can relieve the symptoms of a cold, but they do *not* reduce recovery time. In fact, by inhibiting the ways a body fights off infection (reducing fever, drying up the sinuses), over-the-counter drugs may actually increase the amount of time the infection is present in the body. Some research shows that aspirin can also increase the concentration of virus shed in nasal secretions, increasing the possibility of spreading the disease.[3]

Alternative health care strategies for dealing with colds include plenty of vitamin C, echinacea, lysine (an amino acid with antiviral properties), zinc lozenges (also antiviral), and licorice root as an expectorant. Some of these interventions have been shown to reduce recovery time, but their efficacy as preventatives has yet to be proved. Hydrotherapy options include artificial fever to boost immune function and cold double compresses or packs.

Massage?

Circulatory bodywork is appropriate for colds only after the fever has peaked. If someone receives massage in the acute stage of a cold, it can spread it through the body *much* more effectively than would happen naturally, and that's *not* a benefit. On the other hand, if someone is on the postacute side of an infection, massage may help to speed recovery time. It's important to ask permission though, because it sometimes makes the person feel worse. It is, after all, squeezing 3 days of recovery into one day of feeling crummy again.

Modality Recommendations for Common Cold

Deep tissue massage	Systemically contraindicated while acute; otherwise supportive. Work respiratory muscles and fascias.
Lymphatic drainage	Systemically contraindicated while acute; supportive if treated early in onset.
Polarity	S: Indicated. R: Supportive. D: Avoid while acute.
PNF/MET/stretching	Systemically contraindicated while acute; otherwise supportive.
Reflexology	Work in subacute stage: adrenals, lymphatic and circulatory system, sinuses, ears, eyes, kidney points.
Shiatsu	Contraindicated while acute; then systemically: L, LI. Locally: K, ST, SP in chest; BL in back.
Swedish massage	Avoid while acute; work during recovery may temporarily increase symptoms.
Trigger point therapy	Systemically contraindicated while acute; otherwise supportive.

See Chapter 1 for a brief description of each modality, including definitions of abbreviations.

Influenza

Definition: What Is It?

Influenza, or flu, is a viral infection of the respiratory tract. Most of the time it is a relatively benign, self-limiting infection, but it can become life threatening if an aggressive virus invades a vulnerable patient.

Influenza 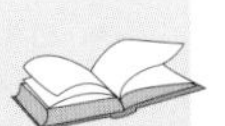

A synonym for flu is *grippe*, from the French *gripper*, to seize.

Demographics: Who Gets It?

Everyone can get the flu and probably does at least a few times over a lifetime. It is estimated that anywhere from 5% to 20% of the population has at least one bout of flu each year.[6] Children are two to three times more likely to contract flu than adults.

For most people flu is a significant inconvenience but not a serious problem. But for the very young, the very old, those with chronic heart or lung disease, the immunosuppressed, and those who spend a lot of time in hospitals or long-term care facilities, an outbreak of flu can be deadly. Flu and its complications hospitalize 200,000 people and kill 36,000 Americans each year.[6]

Influenza in Brief

Pronunciation: in-flu-EN-zah

What is it?
Influenza (flu) is a viral infection of the respiratory tract.

How is it recognized?
The symptoms of flu include high fever and muscle and joint achiness that may last for up to a week, followed by a runny nose, coughing, sneezing, and general malaise.

Is massage indicated or contraindicated?
Flu indicates circulatory massage only after the acute infection has subsided. Nonmechanical forms of massage may be appropriate to support a person who is fighting an infection, with respect for the fact that this condition is highly contagious and contact may put the therapist at risk.

Etiology: What Happens?

Flu viruses work in the usual way of infectious agents. They gain access to the body, usually by inhalation or touch on a contaminated surface. Then they invade and attack their target cells, in this case, mucus-producing cells that line the respiratory tract. Once the infection is established, the immune system response causes most of the extreme symptoms. White blood cells attack infected mucous cells, causing sore throat and coughing. They also release the chemicals that stimulate fever. It can take 2 or 3 days for symptoms to appear, but the person is shedding virus in oral and mucous secretions all the time. The peak of communicability is usually around day 4 of the infection. The person continues to shed virus throughout the acute and subacute stages.

Three classes of flu virus have been identified. The type A viruses are the most virulent, responsible for the major epidemics that claimed millions of lives in the early twentieth century (Sidebar 7.1). Type A viruses mutate quickly and so can cause repeated infections in the same person. Type B flu viruses can also spread, but they are not as aggressive or widely spread as type A viruses. Type C flu viruses are not associated with epidemics, and they are relatively stable. They create much less severe symptoms than the other types.

Type A flu viruses are remarkably adaptable. They can infect several species besides humans, including birds, pigs, seals, whales, and horses. It appears that when flu passes from one species to another, it undergoes some minor changes to its enzymes that allow it to invade its new host. In some cases it may move directly from animals to humans without mutation. So far, only type A viruses are capable of this process.

Flu viruses also have the ability to mutate as they develop resistance to attack. This makes it impossible for the body to establish permanent immunity, because each time it is exposed, the pathogen is different.

SIDEBAR 7.1: WE ARE ALL UNDER THE INFLUENCE: THE HISTORY OF FLU

Symptoms of the infectious disease now called flu have been documented since the fifth century B.C.E. It was observed in those early days of medicine that this disorder could spread throughout a population, but symptoms sometimes wouldn't appear for a few days after exposure, and it continued to spread for several days after all symptoms were gone among the original patients. Because its course seemed so mysterious, it was assumed to be controlled by the influence of the planets and stars. In the early 1500s, the Italian term for influence (*influenza*) became the common name for this disorder.

The first recorded pandemic of flu virus is known from records from Europe from 1580. The twentieth century saw three pandemics of flu infections and a strong threat of a fourth.

- 1918. The Spanish Lady was a flu virus that swept across the globe. In the course of 3 years it killed half a million people in the United States and more than 20 million people worldwide.
- 1957. Asian flu.
- 1968. Hong Kong Flu.
- 1977. Russian flu. These flu viruses killed a total of 1.5 million people worldwide.
- 1997. In Hong Kong another new flu virus was identified. This one had a previously unknown feature: it seemed to be directly communicable from birds to people. It infected 18 people and killed 6, but if it had escaped Hong Kong, it could have killed millions more. It was controlled by an aggressive public health effort that ended in the slaughter of all of Hong Kong's domestic poultry to limit the spread of the virus. The flu that appeared in 1997 is the same virus (H5N1) that we now call "bird flu".

Signs and Symptoms

Flu symptoms can range from subtle to fatal within hours or days. For most common infections the symptoms look like a bad cold: respiratory irritation with runny nose and dry cough, sore throat, headache, chills, and a long-lasting high fever. It's not unusual for flu-related fever to go over 102°F (38.9°C) in adults, and it may last for 3 days or more. Most flu infections cause symptoms that affect more than the upper respiratory tract, however. Many patients have aching muscles and joints and debilitating fatigue. (One area that flu viruses generally *don't* attack is the gastrointestinal tract. What is commonly referred to as stomach flu is far more likely to be infection with Norovirus or a case of food poisoning.) For more information on how flu differs from the common cold, see Compare and Contrast 7.1.

Flu symptoms usually appear about 3 days after exposure to the virus, and they may persist for up to 2 weeks. If they persist longer than that or if the coughing begins to produce a lot of phlegm, it may be that the original viral infection has complicated to a secondary infection of the lungs.

Complications

The greatest danger with flu is the possibility of an opportunistic viral or bacterial infection in the shape of pneumonia or acute bronchitis. This is a particular danger for high-risk populations: the very young; the very old; heavy smokers; diabetics; and people who are immunosuppressed, living in long-term care facilities, or affected by chronic lung or heart problems.

Treatment

As a viral infection, flu is unaffected by antibiotics. Good-sense measures include rest, liquids, alternative regimens, and lots of chicken soup. Over-the-counter drugs may abate the symptoms but do not speed healing. They can be useful, however, if the symptoms are preventing a person from getting the sleep necessary to heal.

Compare and Contrast 7.1: Is it a Cold? Is it the Flu? Does It Matter?

Colds and flu are both caused by viral attacks on cells in the respiratory tract. They have similar symptoms, and they carry similar cautions about working with clients who have these infections. Still, flu can be much worse than a cold. Flu is more contagious, and it can linger in the body much longer. Therefore, it's useful to have a clear idea of which pathogen a client is battling.

Presentation	Common Cold	Influenza
Duration	Usually less than a week.	Could be 10 days or more.
Fever	Usually low (under 102°F, 38.9°C) and short-term (resolves within 48 hours).	Usually high (over 102°F, 38.9°C) and long-term (may persist for 3 days or more).
Location	Symptoms strictly in upper respiratory tract.	Possible systemic muscle and joint pain, inflamed lymph nodes, debilitating fatigue.
Complications	Complications usually involve sinus or ear infection.	Complications affect the lower respiratory tract as bronchitis or pneumonia.
Communicability	Usually spread by hands touching contaminated surfaces. Contagious, but not usually epidemic.	Usually spread by inhalation of airborne virus. Often highly virulent; may infect high proportion of population.
Resolution	Quickly eliminated; when symptoms are over, no longer contagious.	May linger several days after symptoms abate, still communicable.

Some antiviral medications are finding use among flu patients. *Amantadine* can reduce the duration of symptoms of flu caused by a type A virus, but it is associated with central nervous system side effects, including sleeplessness, restlessness, and confusion, especially among elderly patients. A closely related medication, rimantadine, usually has fewer side effects. Neither amantadine nor rimantadine is effective against type B or C virus, and both medications have been seen to allow the mutation of flu virus into more dangerous drug-resistant strains. Further, they must be administered within 2 days of exposure to have any efficacy.

Another class of drugs, called *neuraminidase* inhibitors, includes the name brands Tamiflu and Relenza. These drugs have some advantages in that they tend to cause fewer side effects than amantadine and rimantadine. However, they are expensive and not suitable for use in children. Tamiflu in particular is associated with resistance in avian flu virus.[7,8]

Every year the Food and Drug Administration distributes a vaccine to fight a combination of type A and type B viruses. These vaccines are formulated about 9 months ahead of flu season (November through March). Consequently, the vaccine may or may not be fully effective against the viruses that are circulating when it's administered. Furthermore, because viruses mutate quickly, flu vaccines must be updated every year. Nonetheless, flu vaccines are recommended for high-risk populations to avoid complications and to avoid a new risk: the possible reassortment of avian flu virus with human flu virus (Sidebar 7.2).

Massage?

A person with flu who receives circulatory bodywork in the early stages of infection may have a much more serious infection than otherwise. A person who receives massage after the infection has peaked and is on the mend may recover more quickly. Two cautions must be kept in mind, however. One is that squeezing several days of recovery into 1 or 2 days may make the client feel sick again; he or she should know that this is a possibility. The other is that a person who is recovering from the flu may still be shedding virus. This puts the massage therapist at risk for getting sick.

SIDEBAR 7.2: AVIAN FLU

Avian, or bird, flu refers to a specific group of type A viruses. These viruses are labeled according to the presence of certain proteins, called **hemagglutinin** and **neuraminidase**, on their outer coat. Researchers have identified 15 subtypes of hemagglutinin and 9 subtypes of neuraminidase, and individual strains of virus are named for the subtypes they carry. For instance, the most common forms of human flu are H1N1, H2N2, and H3N1.

The most virulent variety of bird flu virus is called H5N1. Its distinguishing feature is the ability to jump from one species to another, specifically from birds to humans. The first recorded event like this took place in Hong Kong in 1997 (Sidebar 7.1).

The basic mechanism of the virus works like this: It is commonly carried in the digestive tract and mucous membranes of wild birds, especially water birds such as ducks, geese, or swans. In these hosts the virus may cause sickness but not death. When domestic poultry are exposed, however, the mortality rate approaches 100%. In other words, if domestic chickens or turkeys encounter fecal matter or respiratory secretions of wild infected birds, that flock is likely to be dead in a matter of days.

People who live or work closely with domestic poultry are exposed to the virus in secretions, fecal matter, and contaminated surfaces. In a few cases the virus has made the jump from a bird host to a human host, where it has a mortality rate near 60%. At this writing, human cases of bird flu have been recorded in nine countries in Asia and the Middle East. The latest numbers available indicate that 243 human cases have been confirmed, with 144 deaths.[9] Birds infected with H5N1 have been found all over Asia and the Middle East. Cases have been recorded in Western Europe and Northern Africa as well.[10]

Symptoms of bird flu in humans are similar to those in other types of flu, with the added complication of conjunctivitis and a very high risk of pneumonia and acute respiratory distress.

At this point, H5N1 spreads easily between birds and occasionally from birds to people, but it doesn't seem to move easily from one person to another (although in some isolated cases that may already have happened). If the virus mutates to be able to do that (an **antigenic shift**), we may be threatened with a pandemic to rival the outbreak of the Spanish flu in the early part of the twentieth century. That epidemic killed tens of millions of people in a 3-year period. The virus could make this shift in two ways: it could infect a person who already has human flu, or it could infect a pig that also harbors human flu. In either of these hosts the viruses could reassort to adopt the worst qualities of each: the high communicability of human flu and the high mortality rate of bird flu.

To prepare for this possibility, research into an H5N1 vaccine is in human trials.[9] Also, antiviral medication, specifically Relenza, is being stockpiled against the possibility of a widespread outbreak.

Modality Recommendations for Influenza

Deep tissue massage	Systemically contraindicated while acute; work during recovery may temporarily increase symptoms.
Lymphatic drainage	Systemically contraindicated while acute; supportive in early stages of recovery; can do harm in later stages.
Polarity	S: Indicated. R: Supportive; determined by patient's comfort. D: Avoid while acute.
PNF/MET/stretching	Systemically contraindicated while acute; otherwise supportive.
Reflexology	Indicated: work adrenals, lungs, chest, lymphatic system points.
Shiatsu	Contraindicated while acute; then systemically: L, LI. Locally: K, ST, SP in chest; BL in back.
Swedish massage	Systemically contraindicated while acute; work during recovery may temporarily increase symptoms.
Trigger point therapy	Systemically contraindicated while acute; otherwise supportive.

See Chapter 1 for a brief description of each modality, including definitions of abbreviations.

Pneumonia

Pneumonia 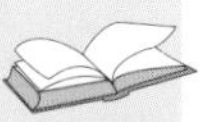

The Greek root is *pneumon*, or *lung*. The suffix *-ia* indicates *condition*.

Definition: What Is It?

Pneumonia is a general term for inflammation of the lungs, usually due to an infectious agent.

Demographics: Who Gets It?

Pneumonia can affect the entire age range of the population, from infants to senior adults. Because it is an opportunistic infection that takes advantage of weak immune systems, it combines with flu to be the seventh leading cause of death in the United States.[11] Every year between 3 and 5 million people in the United States get pneumonia; half a million of them receive hospital care, and about 60,000 die.[12] The severity of infection ranges from not much worse than a bad cold to a cause of death within 24 hours.

Pneumonia in Brief

Pronunciation: nu-MO-ne-ah

What is it?

Pneumonia is an infection in the lungs brought about by bacteria, viruses, or fungi.

How is it recognized?

The symptoms of pneumonia include coughing that may be dry or productive, high fever, pain on breathing, and shortness of breath. Extreme cases may show cyanosis, or a bluish cast to the skin and nails.

Is massage indicated or contraindicated?

Depending on the causative factor and the general resiliency of the person, pneumonia may indicate massage in the subacute stage.

Etiology: What Happens?

The alveoli are the most vulnerable structures in the lungs. They are the tiny air balloons with walls made of squamous epithelium. They are surrounded by the capillaries of the pulmonary circuit for the exchange of oxygen and carbon dioxide in the bloodstream. When an infectious agent is aspirated into the lungs, these tiny air balloons fill up with dead white blood cells, mucus, and fluid seeping back from the capillaries. Eventually diffusion of gases is impossible. Abscesses may form, and capillary damage may occur, allowing bleeding into the alveoli and eventually into the sputum.

In extreme cases the pleurae may be affected. Scar tissue can develop between layers, leading to pain and limited movement with each breath; this is called ***pleurisy***. Alternatively, the pleural fluid itself can host infection in a condition called ***empyema***.

Several infectious agents can cause pneumonia. Each of them has its own symptomatic profile, including what kind of sputum they produce and how they alter diagnostic tests. It is also possible for more than one type of pathogen to be present at a time, a fact that sometimes makes diagnosis and treatment of this condition a challenge.

- *Viruses.* Viral infections account for about half of pneumonia cases. Influenza and ***syncytial*** virus are the most common culprits. Other viruses include cytomegalovirus, *herpes simplex*, and adenovirus. The incubation period of viral pneumonia is 1 to 3 days. Viral pneumonia tends to be short-lived and not serious. It appears most frequently in children.
- *Bacteria.* Varieties of staphylococci and streptococci often live harmlessly in the nose and throat, but when resistance is low, they may invade the lower respiratory tract to set up an infection in the lungs. The toxins released by the bacteria initiate an inflammatory response, leading to edema in the alveoli and a reduced ability to draw oxygen into the system. This kind of infection usually responds well to antibiotics. *Streptococcus pneumoniae*, also called pneumococcus, is the most common form of bacterial pneumonia. Another bacterial pneumonia is caused by *Legionella pneumoniae*, named for the Legionnaires' convention where it was first identified in 1977. Chlamydia (a different pathogen from the chlamydia that causes sexually transmitted infections) and tuberculosis bacilli can also cause bacterial pneumonia.
- ***Mycoplasma.*** Often described as tiny bacteria, mycoplasma are the smallest free-living infectious agents ever found. The incubation period for mycoplasma pneumonia is quite long, 1 to 4 weeks, and because it tends not to be as severe as bacterial or viral types of infection, it is sometimes called "walking pneumonia" or "atypical pneumonia". Fortunately, like bacterial pneumonia, mycoplasma pneumonia responds well to antibiotics.

- *Fungi.* Some fungi that are endemic to certain areas of the United States are associated with pneumonia. The pathogen *Coccidiodes immitis* is indigenous to the desert Southwest; it causes a type of pneumonia called ***coccidioidomycosis***, also known as San Joaquin Fever or Valley Fever. The Ohio and Mississippi river valleys also host fungi which can cause lung infections called ***histoplasmosis*** and ***blastomycosis***.
- *Pneumocystis carinii.* ***Pneumocystis carinii*** is an infection almost exclusively associated with immunosuppressed patients, such as those with HIV/AIDS; people receiving cancer chemotherapy or immunosuppressive drugs to prevent the rejection of organ transplants; and those who don't have a functioning spleen.

Forms of pneumonia Each form of pneumonia may have a different presentation or set of cautions attached to it, so it's worthwhile to be familiar with the most common types.

- *Primary pneumonia* is relatively rare. In this case no predisposing factor has weakened the patient; it is simply an attack directly on the lungs.
- *Secondary pneumonia* is by the far the more common. In this a pathogenic assault on lung tissue is successful because the body's immune system is weakened by another disease. Even if the primary disease is viral, the accumulation of mucus is a perfect growth medium for bacteria, leaving the patient vulnerable to this complication.

Pneumonia may also be classified by the location of the infection:

- *Bronchopneumonia* starts as a bronchial inflammation and spreads into the lungs. It appears in a patchy pattern all over the lungs, not segregated to a specific area.
- *Lobar pneumonia* is restricted to one lobe of the lungs. Eventually the whole lobe may be affected.
- *Double pneumonia* affects both lungs. It can be bacterial or viral.

A final classification for pneumonia describes the source of the infectious agent.

- *Community-acquired pneumonia* is the most common form. It is usually a bacterial infection or a complication of flu.
- ***Nosocomial****, or hospital-acquired pneumonia* is an infection in a person who has been a hospital inpatient for at least 72 hours or within the previous 1 to 3 weeks. This is most common in intensive care units and in patients who require intubation, ventilation, or other interventions to help them breathe.

Signs and Symptoms

Signs and symptoms of pneumonia vary widely, depending on the causative factor and how much of the lung is affected. They include coughing, very high fever, chills, sweating, delirium, chest pains, cyanosis, thick and colored sputum, shortness of breath, muscle aches and pains, and pleurisy.

Pneumonia can have a sudden or gradual onset. Very often it follows the same course as flu, but instead of getting better, the respiratory symptoms get rapidly worse and are accompanied by fever up to 104°F (40°C).

Diagnosis

Pneumonia is usually diagnosed by clinical examination and a description of symptoms. Both viral and bacterial pneumonia have a sudden onset with rapid development of symptoms, while mycoplasma pneumonia may take weeks for symptoms to reach their peak. Different types of bacterial pneumonia produce different colors of sputum, from opaque green, to rust-colored, to currant jelly sputum, so these are often helpful diagnostic clues. Cultures of bacteria are rarely taken, as they take a long time to grow and are often inaccurate.

A diagnosis is sometimes confirmed with radiography, which shows where areas of the lungs have become pathologically dense. Again, different types of lung infections have particular patterns in radiographs, so this is another helpful diagnostic clue.

Other recommended tests include computed tomography (CT) of the thorax and an arterial blood gas test to analyze the efficiency of oxygen and carbon dioxide turnover in the lungs.

Treatment

Treatment depends entirely on what type of pneumonia is present. Bacterial and mycoplasma pneumonias generally respond well to antibiotics, but viral infections do not respond to these medications.

Symptomatic relief and supportive therapy include breathing humidified air, drinking ample fluids, and supplementing oxygen if necessary. If damage to the pleurae is extensive, surgery to drain the pleural space may be conducted.

Prevention

Two main methods prevent some of the most common types of pneumonia infections. Flu vaccines, if they are effective against the circulating viruses, prevent flu infections from complicating into viral or bacterial pneumonia. Pneumovax, a vaccine against pneumococcus, is also available. This vaccine is recommended for high-risk patients and for people who live or work in long-term care facilities or hospitals.

Prognosis

Considering the delicacy of the epithelium in the lungs, it is amazing that if a pneumonia infection is short-lived, it is completely reversible. The body can liquefy and absorb the consolidated matter in affected alveoli, as it can reabsorb the fluid from any inflamed part of the lung. A basically healthy patient can expect to recover fully within 2 weeks. Untreated pneumonia, however, has a mortality rate of about 30%. It can also complicate into meningitis, lung failure, and ***bacteremia*** (the presence of bacteria in the blood, a type of blood poisoning); these situations are nearly always fatal.

In long-standing cases with accumulation of fibrosis and scar tissue, permanent damage to the elasticity of the epithelial tissue may occur, or the freedom with which the lungs move in the pleural cavity may be compromised. This can raise the risk of future infections.

When people develop pneumonia as a complication of a more serious underlying disorder, this infection can be life threatening. Secondary pneumonia is an opportunistic disease. It kills more people every year than any other kind of infection because it takes advantage of low defenses. It is often the final complication of other serious diseases, even noninfectious ones. People who have had a stroke or who have heart failure, alcoholism, or cancer die of pneumonia more often than any other disease. People who are bedridden or paralyzed are susceptible too, because their cough reflex is often impaired; they cannot expel mucus easily. Having a preexisting chest problem such as flu, bronchitis, emphysema, or asthma is an open invitation. And finally, being immunosuppressed because of tissue transplant AIDS, sickle cell disease, steroid use, leukemia, or cytotoxic drug use makes a person particularly vulnerable to pneumonia.

Massage?

Pneumonia is a serious and complicated condition that frequently accompanies other serious disorders. Under the right circumstances postacute pneumonia can respond very well to the mechanical impact of percussive massage. Tapotement on the chest and back can help to move mucus from the alveoli into the bronchial tubes, where muscle action and the cough reflex can take over to expel it from the body. Massage therapists working with pneumonia patients would do well to be part of a well-informed health care team rather than working alone.

Modality Recommendations for Pneumonia	
Deep tissue massage	Systemically contraindicated while acute; during recovery work to increase thoracic mobility (respiratory muscles and fascias).
Lymphatic drainage	Systemically contraindicated while acute; otherwise supportive.
Polarity	S: Indicated. R: Supportive; determined by client's comfort. D: Avoid while acute.
PNF/MET/stretching	Systemically contraindicated while acute; otherwise supportive.
Reflexology	In subacute stage work throat, lungs, adrenals, diaphragm, back and chest, ileocecal valve, and lymphatic system points.
Shiatsu	Contraindicated while acute; then systemically: L, LI, TH. Locally: K, ST, SP in chest; BL in back. Palming on rib cage to warm lungs.
Swedish massage	Tapotement after infection subsides can assist with expectoration.
Trigger point therapy	Systemically contraindicated while acute; otherwise supportive.

See Chapter 1 for a brief description of each modality, including definitions of abbreviations.

Sinusitis

Definition: What Is It?

Sinusitis, as the name implies, is a condition in which the mucous membranes that line the sinuses become inflamed and swollen.

Sinusitis in Brief
Pronunciation: sy-nus-I-tis

What is it?
Sinusitis is inflammation of the paranasal sinuses from allergies, infection, or physical obstruction.

How is it recognized?
Signs and symptoms include headaches; tenderness over the affected area; runny or congested nose; facial or tooth pain; headache; fatigue; and, if it's related to an infection, thick, opaque mucus, fever, and chills.

Is massage indicated or contraindicated?
Acute infections contraindicate massage, but with chronic or noninfectious sinusitis bodywork can be appropriate as long as the client is comfortable on the table.

Demographics: Who Gets It?

Sinusitis rates are rising quickly. It is estimated that more than 37 million sinus infections occur in the United States each year, leading to 18 million doctor visits and $6 billion in medical expenses.

Etiology: What Happens?

Sinuses are hollow areas lateral to, above, and behind the nose (Figure 7.2). They provide resonance for the voice, and they lighten the weight of the head considerably. The mucous membranes lining sinuses are provided with cilia, tiny hairs that move the mucus along at about 16 beats per second, so that trapped pathogens and particulate matter can be swallowed and destroyed instead of reaching the lower respiratory system.

When the cilia break down or are paralyzed, often as a result of viral infection or environmental irritants, pathogen-laden mucus lingers over delicate epithelial cells, stimulating an inflammatory response. Soon the hollow areas fill with sticky, pus-filled mucus that cannot drain. This forms an ideal growth medium for bacteria that

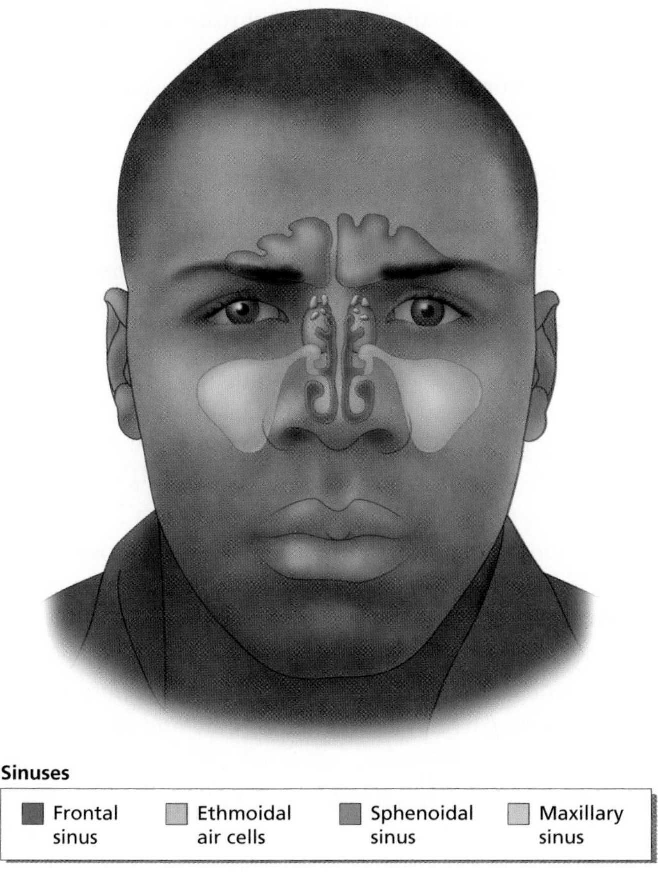

Figure 7.2. Sinusitis.

normally live in the sinuses. Inflamed, infected sinuses can be a source of tremendous pain and discomfort.

Alternatively, the cilia remain intact and highly functional, but the mucous membranes are stimulated to respond to oak pollen or cat dander as if they were life-threatening organisms. Inflammation ensues, with itchiness; production of huge amounts of thin, runny mucus; puffy, itchy eyes; and all of the symptoms associated with *allergic rhinitis*, or hay fever. This can also provide a hospitable environment for local bacteria, so a person with hay fever has a significantly higher than normal risk of intermittent sinus infections.

Sinusitis comes in two varieties, noninfectious and infectious. Noninfectious sinusitis is also called allergic rhinitis. Infectious sinusitis is a pathogenic invasion followed by an inflammatory response that creates a vicious circle: the body creates excessive mucus to help remove infectious agents, but the inflamed tissues make drainage of that mucus (which can harbor bacteria and other pathogens) difficult or impossible.

Noninfectious sinusitis Hay fever causes inflammation of the sinus membranes without underlying infection. Hay fever is often distinguished from infectious sinusitis by the lack of congestion and by the quality of the nasal discharge. It tends to be thin and runny rather than thick and sticky.

It is always a possibility that the irritation to sinuses caused by hay fever can open the door to a secondary bacterial infection, which makes the sinusitis infectious as well as allergic.

Infectious sinusitis In acute infectious sinusitis symptoms develop just as a respiratory infection subsides and continue to get worse for 6 to 8 weeks. The signs and symptoms of chronic sinusitis may be less severe but more prolonged: episodes of chronic sinusitis can last 8 weeks or more and can happen several times a year.

Many pathogens may contribute to infections in acute sinusitis, often in combinations. Some of the most common presentations include the following:

- *Viruses and bacteria.* The most common types of sinusitis begin as viral infections such as cold or flu. When defenses are low, the bacteria that normally colonize the skin and mucous membranes take advantage of the situation and begin to multiply. The bacteria most commonly associated with these infections are *Streptococcus pneumoniae* and *Haemophilus influenzae*. Dental work may very occasionally cause sinusitis if the content of an abscessed tooth is released into the nasal cavity.
- *Fungi and bacteria.* Some people with chronic sinusitis have significant amounts of fungal growth in their sinuses. One theory is that sensitivity to fungi stimulates an inflammatory response that allows naturally occurring bacteria to grow and cause a chronic infection. This is a problem particularly for persons with diabetes, HIV/AIDS, or other immunosuppressive disorders.
- *Structural problems.* A deviated septum or the growth of nasal polyps can obstruct the flow of mucus out of the sinuses. This is not an infection to begin with, but mucus held back from normal flow is a perfect growth medium for bacteria, so what begins as a simple structural anomaly can become a true infection.
- *Environmental irritants.* Exposure to cigarette smoke (first- or second-hand), indoor and outdoor pollutants, cocaine, or other irritants can destroy cilia and cause a high risk of infection.
- *Other conditions.* Acute or chronic sinusitis is frequently seen with other conditions. Severe dental caries (cavities) raises the risk of sinusitis, probably from the availability of local bacteria. Asthma is closely associated with sinusitis, as both conditions have to do with excessive mucus production and a hyperreactive inflammatory response.

Signs and Symptoms

Signs and symptoms of sinusitis vary according to the cause of the inflammation and which sinuses are involved. Severe headache is a key feature, especially upon waking. Bending over makes it much worse, because that position increases pressure on already stressed membranes. The affected area may be extremely painful to the touch, and swelling or puffiness around the eyes or cheeks may be visible. Fever and chills may accompany an acute bacterial infection. Sore throat, coughing (caused by postnasal drip), and congestion or runny nose may appear with any type of sinus irritation, and regardless of whether it's infectious or allergic, people with sinusitis are likely to experience fatigue and general malaise because the body is fighting hard to cast off an invader.

The mucus expressed with a sinus infection is likely to be streaked or opaque, in shades that range from pale green to yellow to brown. It tends to be thick and sticky. The mucus expressed with hay fever, on the other hand, tends to be thin, runny, and clear.

Treatment

Treatment for sinusitis begins with self-help measures: staying in humid air or breathing steam to help moisturize and liquefy the clogged mucus is an important step. Increasing daily water intake and reducing the use of alcohol, caffeine, and other diuretics may also help to soften and loosen thick, sticky mucus. Many experts recommend using a saline wash to rinse the sinuses regularly. Using air filters to remove irritating particles from the air can also help.

Drugs prescribed for this disorder begin with antibiotics if the infection is bacterial. Sinuses are difficult to access, and the bacteria associated with most cases of sinusitis tend to be drug resistant, so this condition often requires a long-term course of specialized antibiotics.

Decongestants are sometimes recommended to shrink the mucous membranes, but these are only appropriate for short-term use because they can create a terrible rebound effect when usage is stopped. Corticosteroids in nasal spray form can reduce swelling, but they can take several weeks to become effective.

In very extreme cases surgery is recommended. This involves inserting a tube through the nose and enlarging sinus passages, removing polyps, repairing a deviated septum, and doing anything else that may assist the mucus to drain freely. Using tiny balloons on catheters (***balloon sinusotomy***) is becoming more common, as this intervention tends to have fewer risks than the traditional endoscopy, and it can also be used with children.

Massage?

Massage is fine for allergic sinusitis because the client has no bacterial or viral infection to spread, catch, or complicate into a more serious condition. (It can be uncomfortable to be completely horizontal for extended periods, however.)

When a client has an acute sinus infection, however, and especially with aches and fever, circulatory bodywork is contraindicated.

Chronic sinus infections are probably safe for most types of bodywork as long as the client is comfortable. Clients may enjoy warm face packs, but face holes or cradles may put pressure on sensitive areas and exacerbate symptoms.

Modality Recommendations for Sinusitis

Modality	Recommendation
Deep tissue massage	Systemically contraindicated for infection; during recovery work suboccipitals, SCM, scalenes, jaw, trapezius.
Lymphatic drainage	Systemically contraindicated for infection.
Polarity	S: Indicated. R/D: avoid for infection; otherwise supportive determined by client's comfort.
PNF/MET/stretching	Systemically contraindicated for infection; otherwise supportive.
Reflexology	Contraindicated for infection; during allergies work sinuses, adrenals, lungs, lymphatic system points.
Shiatsu	Systemically: L, LI. Locally: face and head points, especially LI, ST, SI.
Swedish massage	Systemically contraindicated for infection; can be helpful to clear sinuses during allergic reactions.
Trigger point therapy	Systemically contraindicated for infection; otherwise supportive.

See Chapter 1 for a brief description of each modality, including definitions of abbreviations.

Tuberculosis in Brief
Pronunciation: tu-ber-kyu-LO-sis

What is it?
Tuberculosis (TB) is a bacterial infection that usually begins in the lungs but may spread to bones, kidneys, lymph nodes, central nervous system, or elsewhere in the body. It is a highly contagious airborne disease.

How is it recognized?
Infection with the TB bacterium may produce no initial symptoms. If the infection turns into the active disease, symptoms may include coughing, bloody sputum, fatigue, weight loss, and night sweats.

Is massage indicated or contraindicated?
Active TB disease contraindicates massage unless the client has been on consistent medication for at least 2 weeks and has medical clearance. Massage for clients with TB infection but no disease is fine, but these people should be under medical supervision as well.

Tuberculosis

Definition: What Is It?

Tubercle means *bump*, as in the greater tubercle of the humerus. Tuberculosis (TB) is a disease involving pus- and bacteria-filled *bumps*, usually in the lungs but sometimes in other places too.

Demographics: Who Gets It?

The World Health Organization reports that TB affects one-third of the world's population. Each year 8 million new infections occur, and 9 million people develop the infection in an active, contagious form. TB causes 2 to 3 million deaths each year; that's more than the deaths from AIDS, malaria, and all other tropical diseases combined.[13]

TB used to be considered conquered in the United States because in the 1940s a series of antibiotics was developed that finally managed to kill it. Its incidence steadily declined until 1986, when suddenly it began to rise again. Between 1986 and 1993 TB statistics in the United States rose alarmingly. When public health efforts became more focused, rates of new TB infection began to decline. However, 10 to 15 million Americans are infected with the disease, and about 14,000 have it in the contagious active phase.

The distribution of TB in the United States is not demographically even. It occurs in highest numbers among the poor, people of color, people with limited access to health care, people in prisons or homeless shelters, and recent immigrants.

Etiology: What Happens?

Tuberculosis is an airborne disease caused by *Mycobacterium tuberculosis.* This is a bacterium with a waxy coat that allows it to exist quite happily outside of a host. When a person with an active infection coughs or sneezes, about 3,000 infective droplets are released into the air.[14] The tiny bacteria, protected from drying out by their waxy covering, simply drift until another host comes along and takes a deep breath.

In most cases it takes prolonged exposure to pass TB bacteria from one person to another. This happens most readily when a person with active disease lives or works closely with other people. It has been documented to spread in some public settings, though, specifically airplanes on which a person with active disease shares space with others for 8 hours or more.[15]

Progression

Tuberculosis moves in the body in two phases:

- *Primary phase.* A person inhales some bacteria. The bacteria travel all the way to the alveoli, where they are engulfed by macrophages. Their waxy coating makes them resistant to the macrophages' digestive enzymes. Instead, the bacteria take up residence inside the macrophages and slowly build up whole colonies. Unable to expel these invaders, the body instead builds a protective fibrous wall around the site of infection: a tubercle. Tubercles are usually found in the lungs, but if some of the bacteria seep out into the bloodstream or lymph, they set up the same process elsewhere in the body. Kidneys, the spine, and the central nervous system are the most common other locations. A single undetectable capsule in the lung is where it all stops for most people. This is TB infection but *not* the active disease; it is also called a *latent infection.* Within 10 to 12 weeks T cells are activated, and a specific immune response ensues. The body produces antibodies that react to another contact with the bacillus, which is the mechanism behind the skin test that looks for past exposure. The inhaled bacteria remain stuck inside their tidy fibrous package. They may stay there forever unless something happens to set them free: this is usually a depression in immune system function.

- *Secondary phase.* About 10% of the people exposed to TB eventually develop the active disease. This usually happens within the first year after exposure, but it can be decades later. The bacteria escape and spread into other areas in the lungs or wherever else in the body they may be stationed. The body attempts to surround the new sites with bigger and bigger fibrous capsules, which can cause permanent scarring. Pleurisy, the scarring and sticking of the pleurae, is nearly always a complication of active TB. Inside the capsules, the bacteria destroy cells, and the tissue is necrotic, or dead (Figure 7.3).

New tubercles eventually erode enough lung tissue to impede function. A cough begins and gradually produces bloody sputum; this phlegm actually contains detached pieces of the bacteria-infested tubercles, which is why active TB is so very contagious. If several of the tubercles join together, their necrotic centers can cause a large cavity in the lung. Surrounding blood vessels may hemorrhage into the cavity, leading to coughing up blood, or ***hemoptysis***. Similar cavities can develop in the kidneys if the tubercles form there. Infections in the bones tend to destroy articular cartilage.

Risk Factors

The major risk factor for TB infection is any long-term exposure to someone with active disease. Travelers to parts of the world where TB is most common are at risk, as are people who spend time with immigrants from those areas, hospital workers, or residents of close living quarters where the disease may be rampant, such as prisons, nursing homes, and homeless shelters.

Once a person has been exposed to TB, the question is whether he or she will develop an active infection. Several risk factors for this process have been identified, including HIV status, socioeconomic standing, the use of injected illegal drugs, alcoholism, the presence of other immunosuppressive diseases or medications, age, and a history of not completing TB medication.

HIV and Tuberculosis HIV puts people very much at risk for active TB. In an otherwise healthy person, the bacterium enters the body and is controlled by the immune system. But if a person is coinfected with HIV and TB, each infection makes the other worse. The risk that latent TB will become active increases by 10% for each year that a person carries both infec-

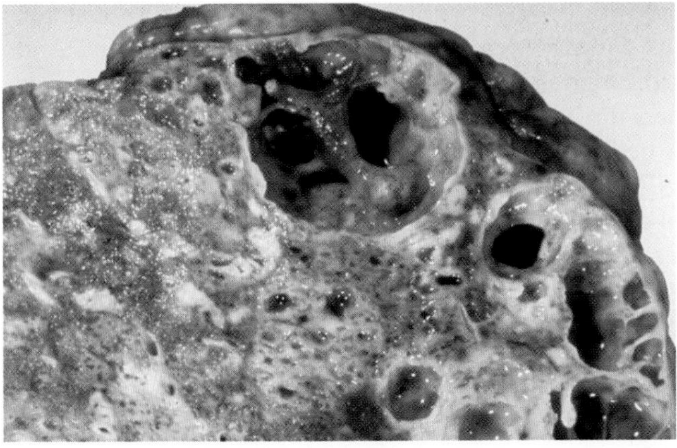

Figure 7.3. Tuberculosis: fibrous capsules surround necrotic tissue.

SIDEBAR 7.3: A TUBERCULOSIS VACCINE?

A vaccine against tuberculosis has been developed and is in use in some countries, but because of some inherit difficulties, it is not used in the United States. It is called the BCG, or *bacille Calmette-Guérin*, vaccine.

BCG vaaccine can reduce the risk of contracting TB, but it comes with some problems. It is most effective for infants and young children; it is only sporadically effective for adults. And because it initiates an immune response to TB, a person vaccinated with BCG shows positive on all TB tests. This means that if the vaccine fails and a person is truly infected, the infection is impossible to identify while it is still latent.[14]

Work on a more effective TB vaccine is under way. This, along with better means of delivering drugs, working with governments to educate patients and doctors, and many public outreach programs to limit the spread of TB around the globe, may eventually mean that this disease will be a thing of the past.[16]

tions.[14] Furthermore, having HIV and TB simultaneously can interfere with an accurate TB skin test, because a damaged immune system may not produce adequate antibodies to create a normal reaction.

It is estimated that worldwide about one-third of people with HIV are also infected with TB.

Signs and Symptoms

The primary phase of TB is so benign a person may never know about the exposure; the symptoms, if any develop at all, are the same as for a mild flu. But the active disease shows much more severe symptoms. They include fever, sweating, weight loss, and exhaustion. Chest pain and shortness of breath are common. A stubborn cough that starts dry and becomes productive of bloody or pus-filled phlegm is a cardinal sign. Other symptoms arise if other organs have been infected as well: bone pain, blood in the urine, or central nervous system symptoms, for instance.

Diagnosis

It isn't difficult to identify most people who have a latent TB infection. Within several weeks of exposure, enough antibodies to the pathogen are produced that a skin test creates a characteristic welt. Two issues make diagnosis at this stage difficult, however. Coinfection with HIV can interfere with a normal immune response, so a person may have to go through more intrusive testing to get an accurate result. Also, having been inoculated with the bacille Calmette-Guérin vaccine can create TB antibodies without an active or latent infection. For more information on the TB vaccine, see Sidebar 7.3.

When TB becomes active, it is surprisingly difficult to catch early because its symptoms mimic pneumonia, lung abscesses, and fungal infections. Radiography can reveal the tubercles in the lungs, but it is not until bacteria are expelled in bloody sputum that the disease can be reliably identified and the pathogens analyzed for which medications will be most effective.

Treatment

In the old days, wealthy TB patients were sent to sanitaria, where it was hoped that sunlight, rest, and good food would enable them to outlive their infection. Many of those facilities are now modern-day spas. Fresh air, rest, and good nutrition are still good ideas, but they work even better when they are combined with the right antibiotics. More than 90% of standard (not drug resistant) TB patients have full recovery if they complete their treatment. And in this country, at least, the cost of medication is not an issue: TB treatment is available free of charge to anyone in the United States through the U.S. Department of Health.[14]

Anyone who has standard TB, whether the infection is dormant or active, can successfully treat it, including people who are HIV positive. People identified with latent TB are recommended to treat it with a medication called isoniazid (INH). People with active TB need INH along with several other medications. Common side effects include sensitivity to sunlight and yellow or orange tears, sweat, and saliva. More serious side effects include liver damage, neuropathy, joint pain, dizziness, tinnitus, and other problems. These are most likely to develop if a person takes TB medication while consuming alcohol.

TB antibiotics must be taken with unfailing consistency for 6 to 12 months, but many patients do not take their medication as directed. This has led to a significant health threat in the form of drug-resistant TB.

Drug-resistant TB When patients don't take all of their TB medication properly, the bacterium may mutate into a form that some drugs can't affect. One form of this mutation is called multi–drug-resistant TB, or MDR-TB. MDR-TB is identified when the bacteria are resistant to two first-line therapies, so second-line therapies must be used to treat it. If a person has an active infection with MDR-TB, anyone who gets the infection from that person will also develop MDR-TB.

It costs about $250,000 to treat MDR-TB,[17] and it requires 18 to 24 months of intensive drug therapy that is highly toxic and has many unpleasant side effects. The mortality rate from treated MDR-TB is about the same as the death rate for *untreated* standard TB: 40% to 60%.[14]

The percentage of TB patients with the drug-resistant form is rising, even while rates of standard TB infection in the United States are declining. Standard TB has been reported in 47 states and the District of Columbia. At this writing, 128 people in the United States have been diagnosed with MDR-TB.[17] Worldwide, about 1% of the 2 billion TB infections are probably with the multi–drug-resistant form.[14]

Recently a new player has joined the field. This strain of TB can withstand treatment from virtually all known antibiotics. It is called *extensively drug resistant tuberculosis*, or XDR-TB. This form has been tracked in this country since 1993 and has so far claimed 74 American lives.[17] It is found all over the world but is most common in the former Soviet Union, parts of Asia, and among HIV-positive populations in South Africa.[18]

Massage?

TB can travel in the blood and lymph, and in the active form it is contagious; therapists won't do their clients much good if their own career is cut short by this condition. However, if a client has a latent infection, it is not contagious. Most experts agree that 2 weeks of antibiotic treatment limits the communicability of active TB, so if a client has an active infection but has been under medication, massage may be appropriate, with medical clearance to ensure that the risk of contagion has been eliminated.

Modality Recommendations for Tuberculosis

Modality	Recommendation
Deep tissue massage	Systemically contraindicated while acute or untreated; otherwise supportive.
Lymphatic drainage	Systemically contraindicated while acute or untreated; otherwise supportive.
Polarity	Systemically contraindicated while acute or untreated; otherwise S/R/D indicated.
PNF/MET/stretching	Systemically contraindicated while acute or untreated; otherwise supportive.
Reflexology	Systemically contraindicated while acute or untreated; otherwise work lungs, adrenals, lymphatic system points.
Shiatsu	Systemically contraindicated while acute or untreated; otherwise treat L, K, SP, TH, LI.
Swedish massage	Systemically contraindicated while acute or untreated; otherwise supportive.
Trigger point therapy	Systemically contraindicated while acute or untreated; otherwise supportive.

See Chapter 1 for a brief description of each modality, including definitions of abbreviations.

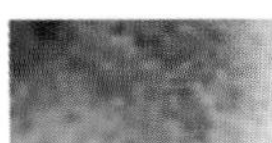

Chronic Obstructive Pulmonary Diseases

Asthma

Asthma in Brief

Pronunciation: AZ-muh

What is it?
Asthma is the result of spasmodic constriction of bronchial smooth muscle tubes in combination with chronic local inflammation and excessive mucus production.

How is it recognized?
Asthma attacks are sporadic episodes involving coughing, wheezing, and difficulty with breathing, especially exhaling.

Is massage indicated or contraindicated?
Massage is indicated for anyone with asthma who is not in the throes of an attack. Between episodes massage can be useful to reduce stress and deal with some of the muscular problems that accompany difficulty with breathing.

Definition: What Is It?

Asthma is a chronic disorder that may be triggered by external factors such as allergens or pollutants, but it is also linked to internal factors such as emotional stress. In asthma someone is exposed to a stimulus that causes a sympathetic reaction (causing bronchial dilation), which is followed by a parasympathetic overreaction (causing bronchial constriction).

Asthma is considered by some in the medical field to be part of a collection of lung problems called *chronic obstructive pulmonary disease* (COPD), because in some extreme cases it can cause structural changes in the lungs that open the door to two other COPD problems, chronic bronchitis and emphysema. In most cases, however, asthma does not cause irreversible damage to the lungs. Therefore, some professionals do not put it in the COPD category.

Demographics: Who Gets It?

Asthma affects some 20 million people in the United States; 9 million of them are under 18 years old. About 12.7 doctor visits and 2 million emergency department visits are made for this condition each year. Asthma is responsible for about 5,000 deaths per year. Direct and indirect health costs for asthma top $16 billion.

Asthma rates continue to climb: among children it went up 160% between 1980 and 1994. It is most common among African Americans: the incidence of asthma is 39% higher among this group,[19] and they tend to have more severe symptoms than other groups.[20]

Among children boys have asthma more often than girls, but among adults women with asthma outnumber men.

Etiology: What Happens?

All bronchioles are sensitive to foreign debris, but asthmatics' bronchioles are extremely irritable and hyperreactive. Furthermore, the bronchial tubes of a person with asthma appear to be in a state of chronic inflammation, always ready to begin an attack. When the right trigger comes along, an asthmatic person's bronchioles first dilate (a sympathetic reaction), and then the body overcompensates by sending the bronchioles into spasm (a parasympathetic reaction). The irritated membranes lining these tubes swell up and secrete extra mucus (Figure 7.4). People with asthma find it very difficult to breathe, especially to exhale, during an attack.

Rising asthma statistics over the past three decades have drawn a lot of attention to the quality of indoor air. As buildings become tighter to conserve energy, the amount of airborne irritants in them can accumulate to levels that are dangerous to some people. Specific substances such as pet-related allergens, cockroach wastes, cigarette smoke, and dust mites have been found to be especially potent asthma triggers. Other triggers include viral infections; breathing cold, dry air; and exercise.

Asthma is typically rated by severity and pattern.[21] These labels help to determine the best balance of treatment options to control symptoms.

- *Mild, intermittent asthma* means that episodes occur less than twice a week, and between episodes breathing is normal. This variety may have little impact on activity.

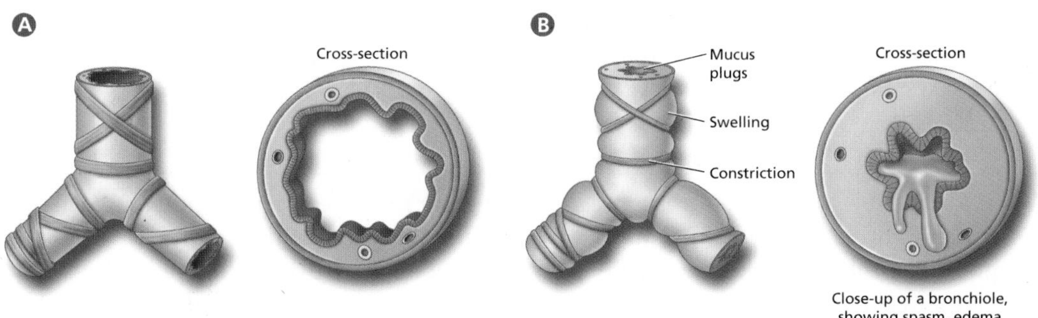

Figure 7.4. Asthma: Normal bronchiole **(A)** and bronchiole under attack **(B)**.

- *Mild, persistent asthma* means that episodes occur more often than twice a week, up to once a day. Nighttime episodes might happen once a month. Frequency and severity may affect activities.
- *Moderate, persistent asthma* is characterized by episodes every day and nighttime attacks at least once a week.
- *Severe, persistent asthma* means that attacks occur most days and nights, and activity is severely limited.

Signs and Symptoms

Symptoms of asthma include dyspnea (shortness of breath), wheezing (the sound of air moving through tightened and clogged bronchioles), and coughing that may or may not be productive. It feels especially difficult to *expel* air; the bronchioles are constricted, so the alveoli don't empty easily.

Asthma can show symptoms in several ways. *Bronchial asthma* is a typical episode with tight bronchioles and excessive mucus production and wheezing. *Exercise-induced* asthma occurs with physical exertion, sometimes hours later. *Silent asthma* shows no symptoms leading up to an episode, and then the patient suddenly is dangerously short of breath. *Cough variant asthma* shows coughing alone as its primary symptom.

If the symptoms are extreme and prolonged, the asthmatic person may start to feel panicky, adding sweating, increased heart rate, and anxiety to the list of symptoms. In emergencies the lips and face may take on a bluish cast (cyanosis) when access to oxygen is severely restricted.

Asthma attacks are sporadic, lasting anywhere from a few minutes to a few days. Between attacks the lungs are generally normal. Someone who has had asthma for a long time may develop structural changes in the lungs that raise the risk of other respiratory disorders, particularly chronic bronchitis and emphysema.

Diagnosis

Asthma is typically diagnosed by ruling out other lung infections or disorders and by measuring lung capacity and airflow through ***spirometry*** tests. A peak flowmeter measures the speed and force of exhalation; this can be used to identify when an attack is imminent.

Treatment

Treatment for asthma begins with managing the stimuli that are known to trigger attacks. Patients are also taught to recognize the warning signs of an attack so it can be treated as quickly as possible.

Medical intervention is available in several forms with two basic goals: immediate relief and long-term control. Short-term intervention is administration of beta agonist inhalers that act as bronchodilators. Inhaled or orally taken steroids can be used for long-term control.

When asthma attacks are directly related to a respiratory allergy, patients are often advised to take allergy medication and to consider immunotherapy, allergy shots to help desensitize the system to a particular allergen.

Massage?

A person who has asthma can derive great benefit from massage except during an attack. No one who is fighting for breath is comfortable on a massage table. Someone who struggles with this problem probably has a number of muscular reflections of it that massage can help with. Watch for hypertonic intercostals, scalenes, serratus posterior inferior, and diaphragm. These muscles of inspiration are often chronically tight for someone who doesn't breathe easily, and that tightness can further interfere with breathing.

Be aware, however, that many asthma patients have other allergies, including allergies to certain types of oils and perfumes. Clients with asthma typically derive the best benefit from the use of hypoallergenic lubricants.

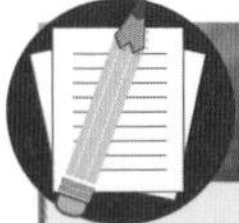

CASE HISTORY 7.1

A Smog Problem

Richard L., aged 52: "Asthma really limits my social life too. When someone asks us over to dinner, our first question has to be, `Do you have any pets?'"

I didn't contract asthma until I was 22, after I got back from Vietnam. I was living in Los Angeles, and I got real bad bronchitis. I was diagnosed then with just a common smog problem.

Then I moved to Corvallis, Oregon, and ran into the Willamette Valley crud: they have pollination 10 months of the year there. I saw an allergist who gave me skin tests, and I came up positive to 95% of the things he tested me for. I realized it wasn't just the smog; I had a lung problem.

At that time I started taking desensitization shots. I did that for about 5 years, but it didn't really help. I ended up quitting and just medicating myself with aspirin and over-the-counter decongestants and inhalants. I didn't have any really bad episodes that I couldn't handle, but I was working in construction, and I knew that I couldn't be sawing or working in a closed room because I would stop breathing; my lungs would just shut down.

Then I moved to Bellingham, Washington, and went into a roofing business. I was working with hot tar and this stuff called torch-down that's pretty fumy. A couple of times I ended up in the emergency room with breathing problems. They gave me a prescription inhalant and prednisone.

When I moved to Seattle, I wound up with an asthma specialist who's been really good for me. I've had a few bouts down here; one time a cold put me in the hospital for about a week. I work in a shipyard now. I can stay away from the worst of the fumes, but about once a year I get a bad attack and go on prednisone until it clears up.

I've been doing massage since the 1960s but just recently went to school and got licensed. I'm really sensitive to perfumes, and massage school students are 90% female, so I'd always choose where to sit away from anyone wearing perfume. But I never thought about massage oils until we got into it. I knew to stay away from oils and lotions that are scented at all. When I got a massage with almond oil I noticed my skin would turn really red, but it wasn't until someone worked on my chest and back that I noticed about an hour later my breathing was affected.

Asthma affects my life in all kinds of ways. My lung capacity is only about 65% of normal. I like to go listen to music, but the venues where the good bands play are always too smoky. I have to stay away from stale flower shops. It was almost impossible to go into a mall because you have to walk past the perfume counter to get through the big department stores, but that seems to be less of a problem now. Asthma really limits my social life too. When someone asks us over to dinner, our first question has to be, "Do you have any pets?"

As my massage clientele builds, I'm able to cut back at the shipyard. Eventually I'll be able to do massage full time. My focus now is on controlling my environment—keeping out the things I know will trigger an attack and trying to stay as healthy as possible.

Modality Recommendations for Asthma

Modality	Recommendation
Deep tissue massage	Between attacks work on intercostals, diaphragm, scalenes, SCM, trapezius, erector spinae, pectoralis major and minor, serratus muscles.
Lymphatic drainage	Supportive.
Polarity	S: Indicated between attacks. R: Gentle, determined by client's comfort. D: Supportive, determined by patient's comfort.
PNF/MET/stretching	Indicated: can improve muscle function between attacks; contraindicated during an episode.
Reflexology	Indicated: work lungs, adrenals, diaphragm, solar plexus points.
Shiatsu	Systemically: L, LI. Locally: K, ST, SP in chest; BL in back; L-1, GB-21, CV-22, GV-14 in shoulders and neck.
Swedish massage	Work between attacks: focus on intercostals, tracing the diaphragm, gentle cupping.
Trigger point therapy	Indicated to improve muscle function between attacks; avoid during an episode.

See Chapter 1 for a brief description of each modality, including definitions of abbreviations.

Chronic Bronchitis

Definition: What Is It?

Chronic bronchitis is part of a group of the closely connected lung problems called COPD. Chronic bronchitis, as its name implies, is long-term irritation of the bronchi and bronchioles, which may occur with or without infection. It is a progressive disorder that may be halted or slowed but not reversed. It often occurs simultaneously or as a predecessor to emphysema.

> **Chronic Bronchitis in Brief**
> Pronunciation: KRAWN-ik brong-KY-tis
>
> **What is it?**
> Chronic bronchitis is one of the lung disorders classified as chronic obstructive pulmonary disease (COPD). It involves long-term inflammation of the bronchi with or without infection, leading to permanent changes in the bronchial lining. Chronic bronchitis frequently occurs as a prelude to or simultaneously with emphysema.
>
> **How is it recognized?**
> Chronic bronchitis is diagnosed when a person has a productive cough that occurs most days for 3 months or more for at least 2 consecutive years. Other common signs are susceptibility to respiratory tract infections, cyanosis, and edema.
>
> **Is massage indicated or contraindicated?**
> Massage can be appropriate for chronic bronchitis patients as long as they are not fighting an acute respiratory infection at the time and as long as heart function is not compromised.

Demographics: Who Gets It?

About 9 million people in the United States have chronic bronchitis.[22] Men have it more often than women, and it appears more frequently in whites than any other racial group.

The leading risk factor for chronic bronchitis is cigarette smoking. Other contributors include exposure to occupational irritants, air pollution, and a history of severe respiratory infections during childhood. For more statistics on COPD, see Sidebar 7.4.

Etiology: What Happens?

Chronic bronchitis is the result of long-term irritation to bronchial tubes. When the delicate lining of the respiratory tract is chronically insulted with cigarettes (first-hand, second-hand, or sidestream smoke), air pollutants, industrial chemicals, or other contaminants, an inflammatory response ensues. Attacks against the bronchial lining destroy elastin fibers and cause overgrowth of mucus-producing cells, excessive production of mucus, and increased resistance to the movement of air in and out of the system. Eventually the damage to the bronchioles is permanent; chronic bronchitis is an irreversible progressive disorder.

As resistance to airflow in the bronchioles increases, less oxygen enters the body with each breath. The heart has to work harder to push enough blood into the lungs to supply the body with fuel. At the same time, red blood cell production may increase in an effort to provide more access to any oxygen that can seep into the capillaries. The blood may become thicker with excess erythrocytes (***polycythemia***), so the heart has to work even *harder* to push it through the pulmonary circuit. As oxygen levels in the blood drop, acidosis develops; this contributes to vasoconstriction in the pulmonary arteries and pulmonary hypertension. Eventually right-sided heart failure may develop and lead to edema, especially in the legs and ankles.

SIDEBAR 7.4: STATISTICS ON CHRONIC OBSTRUCTIVE PULMONARY DISEASE

It can be difficult to separate statistics for emphysema and chronic bronchitis, the two main conditions that make up the group called COPD, because many people have both conditions and many more have them in silent stages that aren't identified until their lungs have accrued extensive damage.

Collectively, the COPD statistics for this country are alarming both for their high numbers and for their upward trends.

By some estimates, 12 to 32 million Americans have some form of COPD.[22,23] It affects roughly 11% of the adult population, and that percentage is rising.[24]

The single greatest contributing factor to COPD is cigarette smoking; smoking causes 80% to 90% of COPD deaths.[22] About 15% of smokers eventually develop some form of COPD.[25]

While men with COPD outnumber women and have higher mortality rates than women, women are catching up fast: the death rate for women with COPD doubled between 1980 and 2000.[26]

COPD sends 1.5 million people to the emergency department each year and hospitalizes 726,000 of them.[26] It is responsible for some $37 billion in direct and indirect medical costs each year.[22]

COPD kills (usually with overwhelming infection and respiratory failure) about 120,000 people every year, making it the fourth leading cause of death in the United States.[22]

Signs and Symptoms

Signs and symptoms of chronic bronchitis develop slowly, often taking months or years before they are severe enough to attract attention. The process usually begins with a mild cough, perhaps following a typical flu or cold infection. But the cough lingers long after the infection has cleared. It is present most days for 3 months or more, producing thick, clear sputum. This pattern occurs for at least 2 years in a row.

The person may have to clear the throat very often, especially in the morning; this reflects the excessive production of mucus in the lungs. Shortness of breath progresses, and the chronic bronchitis patient becomes highly vulnerable to any respiratory infection on exposure.

Later in the process, the chronic bronchitis patient may develop signs of oxygen deprivation, including cyanosis and eventually edema related to right-sided heart failure.

Complications

Complications of chronic bronchitis are obvious. Bronchi that are chronically inflamed and producing a lot of mucus are highly vulnerable to viral or bacterial infection. A person with chronic bronchitis can develop pneumonia from cold or flu viruses much more easily than the general population.

The long-term risk of right-sided heart failure has already been discussed. This serious prognosis is the reason it's important to stop the progression of chronic bronchitis as soon as it can be recognized.

Diagnosis

Chronic bronchitis is diagnosed through a variety of methods, including history, physical examination, and pulmonary function tests that measure how quickly a person can exhale with and without the use of bronchodilators. Additional tests may be conducted to measure levels of oxygen and carbon dioxide in the blood. Chest radiography and/or CT may also be used to rule out other kinds of damage.

Treatment

People with chronic bronchitis are especially susceptible to viral and bacterial infections of the respiratory tract. If a bacterial infection arises, aggressive treatment with antibiotics may be recommended to prevent life-threatening pneumonia. Chronic bronchitis patients are encouraged to be vaccinated against pneumococcus pneumonia and to get yearly flu shots for the same reason.

Other than preventing worse infections, treatment for chronic bronchitis focuses on halting the progression of the damage and keeping the patient as comfortable as possible. Quitting smoking, if that is an issue, is the single most important step a chronic bronchitis patient can take. Patients should avoid polluted air and known triggers of bronchial spasm. Oxygen may be provided in a medical emergency, but most chronic bronchitis patients don't need to supplement oxygen on a regular basis.

Recent discoveries about the role of long-term inflammation in the development of chronic bronchitis have led to some new strategies for treatment of this irreversible disease. Balancing short-acting bronchodilators with longer-acting anti-inflammatories seems to lead to a better prognosis and overall function than has previously been seen. Ultimately, a combination of medication, education, and careful exercise to rehabilitate underused tissues may slow or even stop the progression of chronic bronchitis.

Massage?

If a person with chronic bronchitis has a healthy circulatory system and no current infections, massage, including circulatory massage, should probably be fine. Someone in an advanced stage of the disease may not be able to keep up with the internal changes to blood flow that circulatory modalities bring about; these clients need bodywork that does not move a lot of fluid, and they may have some special requirements for positioning to keep them comfortable.

Modality Recommendations for Chronic Bronchitis

Deep tissue massage	Can improve muscle function if symptoms are not severe; work respiratory muscles and fascias.
Lymphatic drainage	Supportive.
Polarity	S/R/D: Indicated.
PNF/MET/stretching	Indicated: can improve function for muscles of respiration.
Reflexology	Indicated: work lungs and adrenals; can include chest, solar plexus, back, diaphragm points.
Shiatsu	Palm thorax for warmth. Chest: L, K, ST, SP meridians; PC, HL, LI extensions. Back: BL meridian, assessment areas of L, H PC, SP, K.
Swedish massage	Can improve function for muscles of respiration; gentle cupping if well tolerated.
Trigger point therapy	Indicated to improve function for muscles of respiration.

See Chapter 1 for a brief description of each modality, including definitions of most abbreviations.
Assmt,

Compare and Contrast 7.2
Acute Bronchitis, Chronic Bronchitis, or Bronchiectasis: Which Is Which?

The lungs are particularly vulnerable to infection, stationed as they are at the receiving end of everything that enters the body through the nose. They have some structural features that make it easy to isolate sites of infection, and they are well stocked with stationary immune system cells to fight off incoming invaders, but they are susceptible to a variety of infectious disorders that can cause both short-term and long-term damage.

Acute bronchitis often accompanies upper respiratory infections or flu. This is a viral attack directly on the bronchi, although it can also complicate into a bacterial infection. Chronic bronchitis involves long-term irritation to the bronchial lining, all the way down to the terminal bronchioles. This irritation can cause the lining to become permanently thick with excessive mucus production that can make it difficult to breathe. Finally, bronchiectasis is a disorder brought about by repeated lung infections that cause structural changes to the bronchial tubes: they become permanently widened. When the bronchi become unable to move mucus out of the body, it pools in the lungs, creating a risk of further infection and more structural damage.

If a lung disorder is present, it is useful for the massage therapist to have a clear idea of the situation so that the client may be made as comfortable as possible on the table and so that the risk of spreading infection is minimized.

Characteristics	Acute Bronchitis	Chronic Bronchitis	Bronchiectasis
Cause	Viral attack on lungs; often accompanies cold or flu.	Long-term lung irritation, e.g., cigarette smoke, pollution, particles in air.	History of multiple lung infections, including acute bronchitis, pneumonia.
Symptoms	Productive cough with clear sputum (colored sputum: suspect secondary bacterial infection); fever, aches, pains.	Productive cough with clear sputum (colored sputum: suspect secondary bacterial infection). Excessive mucus production, frequent throat clearing. Susceptibility to lung infections. Wheezing, shortness of breath, cyanosis.	Frequent cough with green or yellow sputum, especially when lying down.
Prognosis	If basically healthy, full recovery with no long-term problems.	If irritation to lungs halts, may not progress but is not reversible. If it progresses, may develop into right-sided heart failure, respiratory failure, emphysema.	Patient must avoid lung irritants and possibility of further lung infections, which may further damage bronchi.
Implications for massage	Should not receive massage until infection resolves.	May receive massage if positioned on table so as not to exacerbate symptoms. Essential to rule out possibility of circulatory stress.	May receive massage if positioned on table so as not to exacerbate symptoms.

Emphysema

Definition: What Is It?

Emphysema, along with bronchial asthma and chronic bronchitis, is the third of a group of the classic COPD triad. The name *emphysema* means blown up (as in inflated, not exploded), and this is a very apt description of the disease process.

Demographics: Who Gets It?

About 3.6 million people have emphysema.[27] Most emphysema patients have smoked at least 20 cigarettes a day for at least 20 years.[28] Other cases develop from occupational hazards: working with grain dust, in coal mines, or in quarries can increase risk. A small number (less than 5%) of emphysema patients have a genetic lack of the protein ***a_1-antitrypsin***, which protects alveolar walls. These people generally develop the disease before they are 50 years old. For more information on COPD statistics, see Sidebar 7.4.

Emphysema in Brief

Pronunciation: em-fih-ZEE-mah

What is it?

Emphysema is a condition in which the alveoli of the lungs become stretched out and inelastic. They merge with each other, decreasing surface area, destroying surrounding capillaries, and limiting oxygen–carbon dioxide exchange.

How is it recognized?

Symptoms of emphysema include shortness of breath with mild or no exertion, a chronic dry cough, rales, cyanosis, and susceptibility to secondary respiratory infection.

Is massage indicated or contraindicated?

Emphysema indicates massage with caution for circulatory complications and secondary infection. It is also important to position the client for maximum comfort.

Etiology: What Happens?

During a normal breathing cycle, we contract muscles to increase the size of the thoracic cavity, and air rushes in to fill the vacuum. When we relax those muscles, elastin in the epithelium of the lung pulls them back to their smaller size. In this way, exhalation is mainly a passive process that doesn't require muscular contraction. If we want to expel *more* air from our lungs (this is called our expiratory reserve volume), we can contract our muscles (mostly the internal intercostals and transversus abdominus) to compress the thoracic cavity. Normal, healthy lungs can be compared to a new balloon: filled with air it is stretched tight, but when it is released the elastic walls compress and force air out. If we want that to happen faster or more completely, we can squeeze the balloon from the outside. But when the balloon gets old and stretched out, it doesn't snap back to its original size. Its elastic walls don't compress well, and air can linger inside and become stale. This is comparable to what happens to the alveoli in emphysema.

The lungs have 300 million alveoli that provide sites for oxygen–carbon dioxide exchange. Each one forms a tiny bubble with its own circulatory capillary to allow the exchange of oxygen and carbon dioxide. All healthy alveoli are supplied with α_1-antitrypsin, a protein that protects the delicate tissue from damage by environmental forces. Long-term exposure to cigarette smoke or other pollutants overcomes the protective abilities of α_1-antitrypsin, resulting in destruction of the alveolar elastin fibers. The alveoli become less elastic, and they fill up with mucus, which interferes with their ability to exchange oxygen and carbon dioxide. Instead of emptying and filling with every breath, they only partially empty or stay altogether full. This usually begins in a small area, but if the irritation continues, it spreads throughout the lung. The alveolar walls eventually break down and merge with each other, forming larger sacs, called ***bullae*** (Figure 7.5). These sacs have less volume and less surface area for gaseous exchange than the uninjured alveoli did. While most bullae remain smaller than 4 cm, some can become giant bullae and inflate enough to obstruct 30% of lung volume.

As the alveoli fuse and surface area for gaseous exchange is lost, the emphysema patient has to work much harder to move air in and out of the lungs. A person with healthy lungs expends about 5% of resting energy in the effort of breathing. A person with advanced emphysema puts closer to 50% of resting energy into this job and must do this every minute, 24 hours a day.

Less gaseous exchange means reduced oxygen levels in the blood, or ***hypoxia***, which is toxic to brain cells. It also causes the epithelial walls of the alveoli to thicken into tough fi-

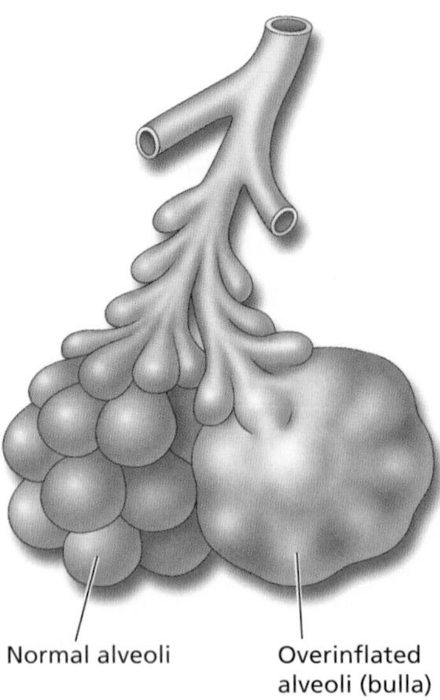

Figure 7.5. COPD/emphysema.

brous connective tissue, which allows even less diffusion. As breathing becomes more difficult (the emphysema patient must *consciously* exhale—it no longer happens passively), the respiration rate slows. This leads to even higher concentrations of carbon dioxide in the blood. The blood vessels supplying the damaged alveoli also sustain damage; it becomes harder to pump blood through the pulmonary artery. Hypoxia also leads to spasm of pulmonary blood vessels. All of these factors may contribute to pulmonary hypertension and right-sided heart failure, or ***cor pulmonale***. Eventually the untreated emphysema patient undergoes respiratory and circulatory collapse.

Signs and Symptoms

It can take many years for emphysema to advance to a stage at which a person seeks medical help. Because it usually affects people over 65 years of age, early symptoms are often assumed to be normal signs of aging. Symptoms of emphysema include pain with breathing, shortness of breath, a dry cough, and wheezing. Weight loss often occurs, as a person who must exert so much energy in breathing has little interest in eating. Rales, a characteristic bubbling, rasping sound of air moving through a narrowed passage, may occur. Difficulty in exhaling may also be reflected in a spirometry test. Exhalation takes longer, and the patient may develop a habit of pushing air out through pursed lips. This is an attempt to push against increasing back pressure in the lungs. Because the lungs no longer deflate normally with each breath, the diaphragm becomes permanently flattened. The emphysema patient often develops "barrel chest"; that is, the intercostals lock into a position that holds the rib cage out as wide as possible.

Complications

Emphysema patients are extremely vulnerable to influenza and pneumonia because they've lost much of the ability to resist secondary infection. Another complication occurs if the bullae rupture. This allows air into the pleural space (which is supposed to be a vacuum) and ends in total lung collapse, or ***pneumothorax***. And finally, the stress to the circulatory system is very great. The right ventricle, trying to pump blood through the partially collapsed pulmonary circuit, enlarges and eventually develops heart failure. The risk of blood clots forming in the circuit is also high, which results in pulmonary embolism.

CASE HISTORY 7.2

Emphysema

Roberta F., aged 68: "Emphysema makes it hard for Roberta to do anything . . . all daily routines have to be altered."

Roberta is 5'2" and weighs 100 lb. She started smoking in 1947 and quit in 1984. She first had pulmonary symptoms in the mid 1980s. She noticed that she was frequently short of breath, she had low energy, and she had consistent headaches on rising each morning. She was unable to walk far or fast. In an effort to catch her breath she hyperventilated easily, which only made matters worse. She had a lot of stress and frustration because breathing was so difficult and she could no longer accomplish the things she wanted to do.

Roberta's primary care physician diagnosed COPD and chronic bronchitis. She then saw a pulmonary specialist who diagnosed emphysema. This finding was based on a number of tests, including chest radiography, spirometry, an analysis of arterial blood gases, and measurement of the air volume she was able to expel.

Emphysema makes it hard for Roberta to do anything. The activities of daily living are difficult, and all daily routines have to be altered to accommodate the disease. Stairs and hills are especially challenging. Emphysema dulls the thinking by depriving the brain of oxygen. It reduces the appetite, and the lack of oxygen reduces the benefit from what food is eaten. It also strains the heart, because the heart has to work harder to push more blood, which contains less oxygen, through the body.

Roberta's radiography showed that she also has some degree of osteoporosis. This condition, in combination with her breathing difficulties, has significantly altered her posture. Her shoulders rise to her ears as she attempts to get more air. Also, the shoulders tend to roll forward. Because of the increased tension of trying to breathe, some muscle stiffness and pain were occasionally a problem.

Another aspect of Roberta's experience with emphysema is how it has seriously affected her resistance to disease. Some medicines Roberta takes to help her breathe weaken her immune system, so it is hard for her to ward off respiratory ailments. In March 1997 she had a crisis that hospitalized her for 10 days. At that time she began supplementing oxygen by nose. She was in a rehabilitation facility for 2 weeks, working with physical and occupational therapists, who taught her ways to accomplish more with less energy.

In June 1997 she had a bad cold, which put her in the hospital for 4 days.

In January 1998 Roberta contracted pneumonia, which was confirmed by chest radiography. She was in the hospital for 5 days. The pneumonia cleared up with antibiotics, and she returned home.

Roberta is now feeling improved. She still supplements oxygen, and her daily activities have become a little easier. She tries to keep up with her exercises, eat properly, and reduce stress. She also attends Better Breathing Club meetings sponsored by the American Lung Association to keep up with new information about techniques to deal with her disease, and she sees her pulmonary specialist regularly.

Author's note: Roberta passed away from pneumonia in 2002. Many thanks to her and her family for generously sharing her story.

Treatment

Emphysema is irreversible. If it is found and treated early, further damage can be avoided. But once the alveoli have begun to break down, they can't be rebuilt. The first course of action, of course, is to remove the irritating stimulus; usually this is cigarette smoke. Drugs may be administered to dilate the bronchi and take pressure off the alveoli, to remove mucus and edema from the lungs, and to ward off potential lung infections. Oxygen supplementation may be recommended during sleep or following exercise. Lung volume reduction surgery removes only damaged portions of the lung. This increases thoracic capacity for the diaphragm to work and improves circulation. Only a few emphysema patients are good candidates for this highly risky intervention, however. In rare cases a heart and lung transplant may be necessary.

Emphysema and other COPD patients are often strongly urged to be vaccinated against pneumococcus pneumonia and to get a yearly flu shot, since they are at higher risk for serious lung infections than the general population.

Massage?

If a client is in the early stages of this disease and the tissues are healthy and responsive (that is, the skin shows signs of normal blood flow by appropriate temperature and color changes with massage), and if the client has no heart problems or secondary infection, massage may be very beneficial. Back, neck, and chest massage may be especially helpful to help reduce any muscular resistance to the movement of air in and out of the body.

Advanced cases, with which a client has difficulty breathing and shortness of breath, may not be appropriate for rapid, vigorous strokes, but calming reflexive work may be excellent for dealing with anxiety and the stress of quitting smoking and the inevitable fatigue. Massage can also address the muscular contribution to barrel chest. Emphysema and other COPD patients often cannot tolerate lying completely prone or supine; they may be more comfortable receiving work in a reclining chair or on a massage chair.

MODALITY RECOMMENDATIONS FOR EMPHYSEMA	
Deep tissue massage	Can improve muscle function if symptoms are not severe; work respiratory muscles and fascias.
Lymphatic drainage	Supportive.
Polarity	S/R/D: Indicated per patient's comfort.
PNF/MET/stretching	Indicated: can improve function for muscles of respiration.
Reflexology	Indicated: short frequent sessions are preferable. Work lungs, adrenals, solar plexus, back, chest, diaphragm points.
Shiatsu	Chest: L, K, ST, SP meridians; PC, HL, LI extensions. Back: BL meridian, assessment areas of L, H PC, SP, K.
Swedish massage	Work gently on all muscles of respiration, anterior neck; gentle cupping if well tolerated,
Trigger point therapy	Indicated to improve muscle function if symptoms are not severe.

See Chapter 1 for a brief description of each modality, including definitions of most abbreviations.
Assmt,

OTHER RESPIRATORY DISORDERS

Cystic Fibrosis

Definition: What Is It?

Cystic fibrosis (CF) is an autosomal recessive genetic disorder. This means that a person must inherit one faulty gene from each parent. It affects exocrine glands, causing production of thick, viscous secretions. The digestive, integumentary, and reproductive system glands are all involved with this disease, but the greatest impact is on the respiratory system.

Demographics: Who Gets It?

CF is the most common lethal inherited disease of whites; it is rarer among other races. It occurs approximately once in 3,000 births in the United States.[29] Carriers of the CF genes are more common however; it is estimated that about 12 million people have the CF gene, although many don't know.[29]

About 30,000 people in the United States have CF.[30] It is usually diagnosed by a child's first birthday, but milder cases may not show until later. The life expectancy of CF patients is improving. Most patients who survive to adulthood make it to age 35, which is a marked increase over just a few years ago. Almost 40% of CF patients today are over 18 years old.[31]

Cystic Fibrosis in Brief

Pronunciation: SIS-tik fy-BRO-sis

What is it?

Cystic fibrosis (CF) is a congenital disease of exocrine glands that causes their secretions (mainly mucus, digestive enzymes, bile, and sweat) to become abnormally thick and viscous.

How is it recognized?

CF is a multisystem disease, but its effects on the respiratory system are typically the most common and most acute. Signs and symptoms include chronic lung infections, shortness of breath, productive cough, digestive difficulties, and failure to thrive in very young children.

Is massage indicated or contraindicated?

Persons with CF receive intensive physiotherapy to dislodge mucus from the lungs, and they are recommended to exercise within tolerance to build lung capacity and immune system resilience. Massage certainly doesn't tax the body any more than these measures, but day-by-day judgments must be made based on the client's health and the presence of acute or chronic infection.

Etiology: What Happens?

The genetic mutations that cause CF were isolated in 1989. Several hundred slightly different changes can happen, but the net result is that the transmembrane conductance regulator gene is altered so that cell membranes in secreting tissues can't conduct chloride. This leads to abnormally thick, sticky secretions in many exocrine glands but most particularly in the respiratory tract, digestive tract, skin, and reproductive tract.

- *Respiratory system.* CF usually has its most profound effects on the respiratory system. The changes in mucous membrane function cause mucus in the respiratory tract to become thick, gluey, and difficult to dislodge. This provides a rich growth medium for bacterial infection. Because of the genetic dysfunction, immune system action against pathogens reinforces the inflammatory response, which causes more damage and supports rather than suppresses the infection. A variety of bacterial agents may create chronic infection, but the one that is the most difficult to eradicate is *Pseudomonas aeruginosa*. Other respiratory system changes include the growth of nasal polyps and the development of chronic rhinitis.
- *Digestive system.* Digestive system dysfunction can affect both the gastrointestinal tract and the accessory organs. A warning sign for CF is a baby born with an intestinal obstruction; this happens because the mucus in the small and large intestines doesn't move well. Poor absorption in the small intestine also leads to failure to thrive. Poor access to vitamins produces symptoms as well. CF can interfere with the normal production of bile and drainage of bile into the small intestine, leading to an enlarged spleen, gallstones, portal hypertension, liver congestion, or cirrhosis. Poor secretion of bicarbonate and digestive enzymes from the pancreas can lead to peptic ulcers in the duodenum and pancreatitis.
- *Integumentary system.* CF affects sweat glands in the skin, leading to abnormally thick, salty perspiration and the risk of heat stroke and salt depletion, especially in infants.
- *Reproductive system.* Almost all men with CF are sterile. This occurs because the epididymis cannot secrete normally or because the vas deferens doesn't form completely. Women with CF often have normal reproductive systems and can have successful pregnancies.

Signs and Symptoms

Signs and symptoms of CF vary by the system that is affected most severely. Respiratory symptoms are most common. They include a dry or productive cough, shortness of breath, wheezing, chest pain, cyanosis, hemoptysis (coughing up blood), and clubbing of fingers, which occurs with oxygen deprivation in the extremities.

Symptoms affecting other systems are discussed in the etiology section.

Diagnosis

CF is usually diagnosed with a skin test to analyze the secretions of the sudoriferous glands. Other tests may be conducted to look for the specific defect in the affected genes or characteristic changes in the epithelial lining of the upper respiratory tract.

Complications

Complications of CF are related to the exocrine gland dysfunction of the affected system (Figure 7.6). Respiratory complications include chronic, intractable bacterial infection; **bronchiectasis**, the development of resistance in the pulmonary circuit; pneumothorax; and a risk of right-sided heart failure.

Digestive system dysfunction tends to be less severe than respiratory problems, but the complications are wide reaching. They include cirrhosis, gallstones, duodenal ulcers, intestinal obstruction with or without rectal prolapse, a risk of pancreatitis or diabetes from a damaged pancreas, and vitamin and mineral deficiencies from poor absorption. This can lead to osteoporosis in adults with CF.

Complications of CF for the integumentary system are discussed earlier. They include a risk of salt depletion or heat stroke. The group most at risk for these problems is infants.

The male reproductive system is more vulnerable to CF than the female system. As stated earlier, almost all men with CF are sterile.

Treatment

CF is not curable; treatment options focus on dealing with symptoms and complications. Devices to help break up congestion in the lungs, along with breathing exercises to maintain and improve function, are often suggested. Taking food in easily digestible forms and exercising to increase or maintain lung function are recommended for people who are not fighting

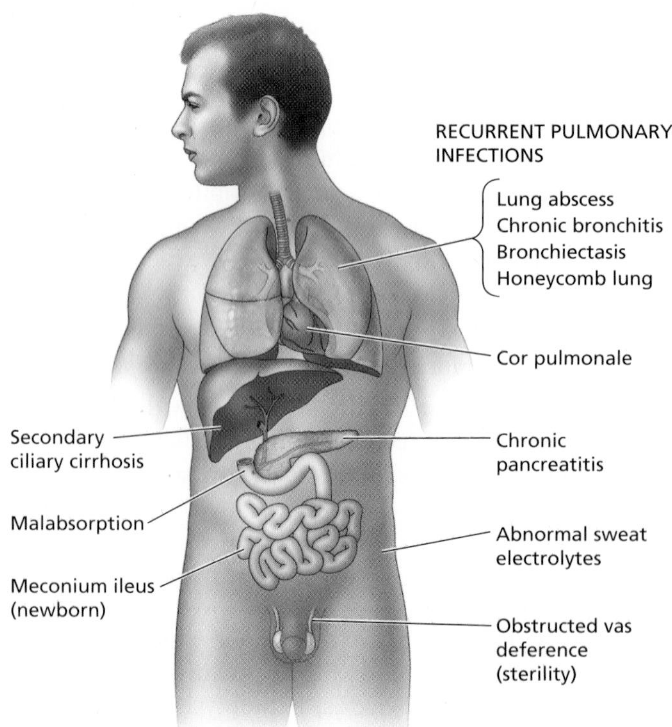

Figure 7.6. Complications of cystic fibrosis.

acute infection or intestinal blockages. Supplementing pancreatic enzymes and vitamins is usually recommended as well.

Bronchodilators, mucolytics (mucus-dissolving drugs), antibiotics to fight infection, and anti-inflammatories are typical interventions for CF patients. Patients with advanced cases may be good candidates for lung transplants, although this procedure has a high rejection rate.

Genetic therapists continue to explore ways to introduce healthy genes into the tissues of patients with CF. This field is in its infancy, but the future of CF treatment may lie in this direction.

Massage?

The role of massage for a client who has CF must be guided by the health and resilience of the client, which may vary greatly from one day to the next. Many children and adults with CF undergo intense physiotherapy to dislodge deposits of mucus in the lungs, and when no acute infection is present, they are recommended to exercise within tolerance to build stamina and strength. Massage is probably safe and appropriate under these circumstances as long as the therapist works with the rest of the health care team, is healthy, and doesn't share any virulent pathogens with the client.

Modality Recommendations for Cystic Fibrosis

Deep tissue massage	Supportive.
Lymphatic drainage	Supportive.
Polarity	S/R/D: Indicated per client's comfort.
PNF/MET/stretching	Supportive.
Reflexology	Indicated: work lungs, adrenals, lymphatic system points.
Shiatsu	Work for respiratory and immune strength with meridians, points, extensions, assessments of hara and back for L, LI, K, SP, Th, BL.
Swedish massage	Supportive; cupping can assist with expectoration.
Trigger point therapy	Supportive.

See Chapter 1 for a brief description of each modality, including definitions of abbreviations.

Lung Cancer

Definition: What Is It?

Lung cancer is the growth of malignant cells in the lungs. These cells eventually form tumors, but because they have extremely easy access to both the circulatory and lymph systems, they are capable of spreading before tumors are detectable.

Lung cancer is an example of epithelial cancer that tends to grow where tissue is vulnerable to repeated irritation and damage.

Demographics: Who Gets It?

Statistics in the United States vary, but it is estimated that 180,000 new cases of lung cancer are diagnosed and about 160,000 people die of this disease each year.[32] While it was once considered a men's disease, the social acceptability of women smoking has led to rising numbers of women being diagnosed with lung cancer, while statistics for men are beginning to fall off. The average lung cancer patient, therefore, is a man or a woman in the sixth to seventh decade of life who has smoked for 20 years or more.

Lung Cancer in Brief

What is it?
Lung cancer is development of malignant cells in the lungs. These cells have easy access to blood and lymph vessels and quickly spread to other organs in the body.

How is it recognized?
The early symptoms of lung cancer are virtually indistinguishable from normal irritation from cigarette smoke: a chronic cough, bloodstained sputum, shortness of breath, chest pain, and recurrent bronchitis or pneumonia.

Is massage indicated or contraindicated?
Sadly, most people diagnosed with lung cancer will not survive. Massage has a place in cancer recovery care, as well as in terminal care, but these situations call for specific adjustments to achieve maximum benefit with minimal risk.

Cancer in general is the second leading cause of death in the United States, and lung cancer accounts for nearly 30% of cancer deaths. Some statistics show that it is the cause of more deaths than breast, colon, and prostate cancers (the next three runners-up) combined.[33]

Etiology: What Happens?

Lung cancer occurs in epithelial cells that are chronically irritated by environmental contaminants. Although cigarette, pipe, and cigar smoke are responsible for 85% to 90% of cases of lung cancer,[34] other causes have also been identified. Exposure to radon, a naturally occurring radioactive gas that is released when rocks and soil are moved for construction, is another leading cause of lung cancer, along with exposure to asbestos, uranium, arsenic, air pollution, and other carcinogens.

When the epithelial cells that line the respiratory tract have a long history of exposure to highly toxic substances, their orderly pattern of replication and repair is eventually disrupted. Abnormal cells accumulate in uncontrolled and disorganized patches. A rich supply of blood and lymph vessels allows mutated cells to travel out of their immediate area before a detectable tumor appears; this is why lung cancer is seldom caught before metastasis.

The lymph nodes around the lungs and in the mediastinum are often the first site of metastasis for lung cancer. From there the cells have access to distant places in the body. The liver, bone tissue, skin, adrenal glands, and brain are frequently invaded.

Types of lung cancer Different types of lung cancer tend to grow at different rates and in different parts of the lung. Several types of lung cancer have been identified. They break down into two basic groups: small cell carcinoma and non–small cell carcinoma.

- *Small cell lung cancer.* This is also called "oat cell" carcinoma. It accounts for 15% to 25% of lung cancers. Small cell lung cancer grows fast, spreads quickly, and is rarely operable.
- *Non–small cell lung cancer.* This includes several types of cancers, depending on which cells they affect first. Non–small cell carcinomas account for 75% to 85% of lung cancers. They include squamous cell carcinoma, adenocarcinoma, large cell carcinoma, and several others (Figure 7.7). Most of these grow more slowly than small cell carcinoma, but the symptoms they produce are so subtle that diagnosis doesn't usually happen until long after the cancer has spread beyond its original area.
- *Other types of lung malignancies.* Small cell and non–small cell lung cancers account for most types of cancer, but a few cases of other types are identified as well. These include carcinoid tumors, adenoid cystic carcinoma, sarcomas, and others. ***Mesothelioma*** is a type of cancer that arises in the pleural sac that surrounds the lung; this is closely associated with asbestos exposure.

Risk Factors

The most obvious risk factor for lung cancer is smoking; close to 90% of cases can be linked to this habit.[34] Cigarette smoke contains more than 40 known carcinogens, and the tar in cigarettes holds the damaging chemicals close to the delicate linings of the lungs.

Lung cancer is also an occupational risk for people working with asbestos insulation, for coal miners, and for people who work with other toxic chemicals. Exposure to arsenic in water or to radon; radiation to the chest for breast cancer or other treatments; or a history of

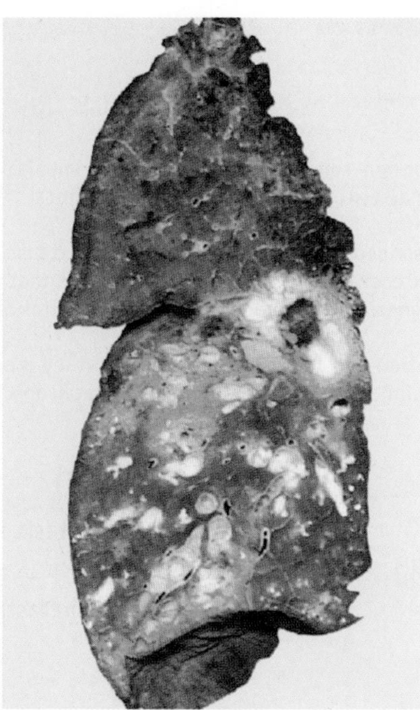

Figure 7.7. Lung cancer.

TB, COPD, or other lung infection can also increase risk, especially if the exposed person is also a smoker.

Every year about 15,000 people who were never smokers die of lung cancer. These cases are often linked to second-hand or sidestream smoke or other risk factors, but the potential for genetic predisposition is now being actively pursued through genetic research. This may eventually yield ways to identify people at particularly high risk for lung cancer, along with ways to identify it early and treat it more successfully.[35]

Signs and Symptoms

One of the biggest problems with lung cancer is that it is extremely difficult to identify early. The growth of abnormal cells in alveoli, bronchial linings, or mucous membranes stimulates virtually no changes in function or sensation. A persistent smoker's cough is one early sign, along with bloodstained phlegm, chest pain, wheezing, and possibly shortness of breath. None of these symptoms seems cause for alarm, since a smoker or someone who works with irritating chemicals often has them regardless of the health of their respiratory tract cells.

Later signs of lung cancer may be more revealing. If a tumor grows near the apex of the lung, it may put mechanical pressure on the brachial plexus, leading to symptoms that mimic thoracic outlet syndrome. A tumor that presses on the superior vena cava may cause facial swelling and dilated blood vessels in the neck and face; this is called ***superior vena cava syndrome***. If a tumor protrudes on the esophagus or larynx, a person may have chronic hoarseness. Tumors that press on the phrenic nerve can paralyze the diaphragm.

Diagnosis

Once a tumor has formed in the lung, it is not hard to find; any imaging technique, from radiography to CT to magnetic resonance imaging (MRI), can locate growths. An analysis of sputum might reveal abnormal cells, but then again it might not. Radiographic studies of bronchiole tubes can show where obstructions are growing, and needle biopsies of suspicious areas can help to pinpoint a diagnosis. The problem is that lung cancer often metastasizes *before* detectable tumors have grown. This makes it difficult to identify early enough to catch.

SIDEBAR 7.5: STAGING LUNG CANCER

The staging protocol for lung cancer depends on whether the diagnosis is for small cell or non–small cell lung cancer. It is important to stage any kind of cancer accurately to choose the best possible treatment options. Patients may also choose to volunteer for clinical trials to add to the body of knowledge about best options according to stage.

Small cell lung cancer, because it is so aggressive and is usually inoperable, is described as being either limited or extensive. Limited small cell lung cancer means that it is found in only one lung and local lymph nodes; extensive small cell lung cancer means that it is found in both lungs, multiple nodes, and in distant areas as well. It has a generally poor prognosis; the average life expectancy after diagnosis is 9 to 10 months,[35] and its 5-year survival rate is under 1%.[36]

Non–small cell lung cancer comes in several forms, but they are similar in presentation and treatment protocols, so they are all staged together using a combination of the TNM and stage 0 to IV classifications. These staging protocols are described in detail in Chapter 12. Here is a simplified version of non–small cell lung cancer staging:[36]

Tumor (T)	Node (N)	Metastasis (M)
T IS: cancer in situ, limited to endothelial cells	N 0: no nodes involved	M 0: no metastasis found
T X: positive findings on tests; no lesion found	N 1: some nodes involved near affected lung	M 1: distant metastasis found
T 1: tumor <3 cm in diameter	N 2: nodes in mediastinum on side of affected lung	
T 2: tumor >3 cm in diameter; may involve pleura	N 3: Nodes on opposite side of involved thorax	
T 3: tumor at apex of lung; one lung may collapse; extensions into nearby structures		
T 4: tumor invasion of mediastinal structures		

These delineations are then translated into stages 0 to IV in this way:

Stage	Tumor	Node	Metastasis	5-Year Survival Rate (%)
I A	T 1	N 0	M 0	75
I B	T 2	N 0	M 0	55
II A	T1	N 1	M 0	50
II B (option 1)	T 2	N 1	M 0	40
II B (option 2)	T 3	N 0	M 0	40
III A	T 1–3	N 2	M 0	10–35
III B	T 1–4	N 1–4	M 0	5
IV	T 1–4	N 1–4	M 1	<5

Diagnostic procedures for lung cancer are often problematic. Noninvasive options may miss small growths. They may wrongly identify growths, leading to false positives and unnecessary interventions. Other options can be highly intrusive, involving surgeries and associated risks. At this point no early screening program for lung cancer is considered effective, but as genetic research reveals more clues to how this disease works, that may change.

Treatment

Treatment for lung cancer depends on what kind of cancer is growing and how far it has progressed. For the lucky few who find non–small cell lung cancer while it is still local, surgery followed by radiation may be adequate. The surgery could involve the removal of a small section of lung tissue (a wedge resection), the removal of an entire lobe (a lobectomy) or even the removal of an entire lung (a pneumonectomy).

Small cell carcinoma grows so fast and spreads so quickly that it is generally treated with radiation and chemotherapy alone; surgery usually has no chance of containing the growth. While this can be successful in the short run, most small cell lung cancer patients have a recurrence within 2 years, and the cancer tends to become unresponsive to treatment.

New therapies for lung cancer are always in development. One of them is ***photodynamic therapy***, a process in which a laser-sensitive chemical is injected into the cancerous area, absorbed into abnormal cells, and then activated by a laser, which causes the chemicals to destroy the cancerous cells. Other options in development include drugs that interfere with the creation of new blood vessels or that suppress growth factors that stimulate the birth of new cells.

Massage?

Massage can be a useful stress reliever for a person undergoing cancer treatment; it stimulates immune system activity, reduces pain and fatigue, and generally adds to the quality of life. Of course, certain cautions must be observed when working with people who are receiving radiation therapy or chemotherapy or who have had recent surgery. For more details, see the discussion of cancer in Chapter 12.

If a client is dying, massage has a useful place in comfort care protocols. Even when a person is too fragile to receive most types of bodywork, energy work, gentle stroking of hands and feet, or simple laying on of hands can all contribute to feelings of peace and well-being. In these situations the massage therapist may want to teach family members and loved ones of the patient some simple techniques that may enrich their time together.

Modality Recommendations for Lung Cancer

Modality	Recommendation
Deep tissue massage	Supportive as part of health care team. Respect stage of recovery and treatment challenges.
Lymphatic drainage	Supportive, depending on stage; check with health care team in later stages.
Polarity	S/R/D: Indicated per client's comfort.
PNF/MET/stretching	Supportive as part of health care team; match to activity levels.
Reflexology	Indicated: work lungs, adrenals, lymphatic system, pituitary points.
Shiatsu	Work for respiratory and immune strength with meridians, points, extensions, assessments of hara and back for L, LI, K, SP, Th, BL.
Swedish massage	Supportive; depth depends on activity level.
Trigger point therapy	Supportive.

See Chapter 1 for a brief description of each modality, including definitions of abbreviations.

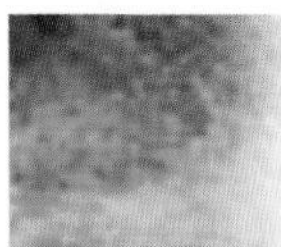

Chapter Review Questions: Respiratory System Conditions

1. How does the structure of the lungs work to limit the spread of infection?
2. What is the best defense against catching or spreading a cold virus?
3. Are antibiotics effective to shorten the duration of cold or flu? Why?
4. Why is asthma sometimes described as a chronic obstructive pulmonary disease?
5. Explain the sympathetic-parasympathetic swing that occurs with asthma.
6. What is MDR-TB? What is XDR-TB? How did these types of infection arise?
7. Why is cystic fibrosis associated with a high risk of lung infection?
8. What is the relationship between chronic bronchitis and acute bronchitis?
9. How does emphysema lead to right-sided heart failure?
10. Why is it difficult to find lung cancer in early stages?
11. A client has sinusitis. Her mucus is thick, opaque, and sticky. She has had a headache and a mild fever for several days. Is she a good candidate for massage? Why or why not?
12. Your client, a smoker, reports a mild cough and shortness of breath. She gets colds easily, and they often disable her for several days or even weeks. You notice that she clears her throat very frequently. What condition is probably present? What strategies might serve her best in a bodywork session?

References

1. Ong S. Bronchitis. © 1996–2006 by WebMD. http://www.emedicine.com/emerg/topic69.htm. Accessed autumn 2006.
2. Callahan C, Dittmer C. Bronchitis, Acute and Chronic. © 1996–2006 by WebMD. http://www.emedicine.com/ped/topic288.htm. Accessed autumn 2006.
3. The Common Cold. National Institute of Allergy and Infectious Diseases. http://www.niaid.nih.gov/factsheets/cold.htm. Accessed autumn 2006.
4. Common Cold (viral rhinitis). Centers for Disease Control and Prevention. http://www.intelihealth.com/IH/ihtPrint/WSIHW000/9339/9721.html?hide=t&k=basePrint. Accessed autumn 2006.
5. Common cold. © 1998–2006 Mayo Foundation for Medical Education and Research. All rights reserved. http://www.mayoclinic.com/health/common-cold/DS00056. Accessed autumn 2006.
6. Flu. National Institute of Allergy and Infectious Diseases. http://www.niaid.nih.gov/factsheets/flu.htm. Accessed autumn 2006.
7. Bird flu (avian influenza). © 1998–2006 Mayo Foundation for Medical Education and Research. All rights reserved. http://www.mayoclinic.com/health/bird-flu/DS00566. Accessed autumn 2006.
8. Key Facts about Avian Influenza (bird flu) and Avian Influenza A (H5N1) Virus. Centers for Disease Control and Prevention. http://www.cdc.gov/flu/avian/gen-info/facts.htm. Accessed autumn 2006.
9. Cumulative Number of Confirmed Human Cases of Avian Influenza A/(H5N1) Reported to WHO. © World Health Organization, 2006. All rights reserved. http://www.who.int/csr/disease/avian_influenza/country/cases_table_2006_09_14/en/index.html. Accessed autumn 2006.
10. Update on Avian Influenza in Animals (H5): 25 September 2006. © 2003 OIE World Organisation for Animal Health http://www.oie.int/downld/AVIAN%20INFLUENZA/A_AI Asia.htm. Accessed autumn 2006.

11. Pneumonia. © 1998–2006 Mayo Foundation for Medical Education and Research. http://www.mayoclinic.com/health/pneumonia/DS00135. Accessed autumn 2006.
12. Pneumonia Fact Sheet. © 2006 American Lung Association. All rights reserved. http://www.lungusa.org/site/pp.asp?c=dvLUK9O0E&b=35692. Accessed autumn 2006.
13. Fact Sheet. Centers for Disease Control and Prevention. http://www.cdc.gov/od/oc/media/pressrel/fs060323.htm. Accessed autumn 2006.
14. Li J, Brainard D. Tuberculosis. © 1996–2006 by WebMD. http://www.emedicine.com/emerg/topic618.htm. Accessed autumn 2006.
15. Tuberculosis. Travelers' Health: Yellow Book. Health Information for International Travel, 2005–2006. Centers for Disease Control and Prevention. http://www2.ncid.cdc.gov/travel/yb/utils/ybGet.asp?section=dis&obj=tb.htm. Accessed autumn 2006.
16. Questions and Answers about TB. Centers for Disease Control and Prevention. http://www.cdc.gov/nchstp/tb/faqs/pdfs/qa.psf. Accessed autumn 2006.
17. Robertson J. More Drug-resistant TB Seen in U.S. © 1999–2006 Imaginova Corp. http://www.livescience.com/humanbiology/060922_ap_TB_rise.html. Accessed autumn 2006.
18. Emergence of XDR-TB: WHO Concern over Extensive Drug Resistant TB Strains That Are Virtually Untreatable. © World Health Organization 2006. http://www.who.int/mediacentre/news/notes/2006/np23/en/index.html. Accessed autumn 2006.
19. Asthma Statistics. © 1996–2006. All Rights Reserved. American Academy of Allergy Asthma & Immunology. http://www.aaaai.org/patients/gallery/adultasthma.asp?item=1a. Accessed autumn 2006.
20. Asthma attacks more severe in blacks than whites. © 2006 Reuters Limited. All rights reserved. http://www.nlm.nih.gov/medlineplus/news/fullstory_38584.html. Accessed autumn 2006.
21. What Is Asthma? National Heart Lung and Blood Institute. http://www.nhlbi.nih.gov/health/dci/Diseases/Asthma/Asthma_All.html. Accessed autumn 2006.
22. Chronic Obstructive Pulmonary Disease (COPD) Fact Sheet. © 2006 American Lung Association. All rights reserved. http://www.lungusa.org/site/pp.asp?c=dvLUK9O0E&b=35020. Accessed autumn 2006.
23. Kleinschmidt P. Chronic Obstructive Pulmonary Disease and Emphysema. © 1996–2006 by WebMD. http://www.emedicine.com/emerg/topic99.htm. Accessed autumn 2006.
24. COPD—What is it? National Emphysema Foundation. http://emphysemafoundation.org/copdcbro.jsp#COPDWhat. Accessed autumn 2006.
25. Chronic Obstructive Pulmonary Disease (COPD) a.k.a. Chronic Obstructive Lung Disease (COLD). © 1996–2005 MedicineNet, Inc. All rights reserved. http://www.medicinenet.com/chronic_obstructive_pulmonary_disease_copd/article.htm. Accessed autumn 2006.
26. Chronic Obstructive Pulmonary Disease. National Heart, Lung, and Blood Institute. http://www.nhlbi.nih.gov/health/public/lung/other/copd_fact.pdf#search=%22Chronic%20bronchitis%20statistic%22. Accessed autumn 2006.
27. Emphysema. National Center for Health Statistics. http://www.cdc.gov/nchs/fastats/emphsema.htm. Accessed autumn 2006.
28. Sharma S. Chronic Bronchitis. © 1996–2006 by WebMD. http://www.emedicine.com/med/topic367.htm. Accessed autumn 2006.
29. What Is Cystic Fibrosis? National Heart, Lung and Blood Institute. http://www.nhlbi.nih.gov/health/dci/Diseases/cf/cf_all.html. Accessed autumn 2006.
30. Statistics about Cystic Fibrosis. © 2000-2005 Adviware Pty Ltd. All rights reserved. http://www.wrongdiagnosis.com/c/cf/stats.htm. Accessed autumn 2006.
31. Cystic fibrosis. © 2006, Lifespan. http://www.lifespan.org/adam/healthillustratedencyclopedia/1/000107.html. Accessed autumn 2006.
32. National Institutes of Health to Map Genomic Changes of Lung, Brain, and Ovarian Cancers. National Institutes of Health. http://www.nih.gov/news/pr/sep2006/nci-13.htm. Accessed autumn 2006.
33. Cancer—Lung Cancer Statistics. Centers for Disease Control and Prevention. http://www.cdc.gov/CANCER/lung/statistics/. Accessed autumn 2006.
34. Lung cancer. © 1998–2006 Mayo Foundation for Medical Education and Research. All rights reserved. http://www.mayoclinic.com/health/lung-cancer/DS00038. Accessed autumn 2006.
35. Sharma S. Cancer, Lung. 1996–2005 eMedicine.com, Inc. http://www.emedicine.com/aaem/topic84.htm. Accessed autumn 2006.
36. Hassan I. Lung Cancer, Staging. © 1996–2006 by WebMD. http://www.emedicine.com/radio/topic807.htm. Accessed autumn 2006.

8

Digestive System Conditions

Chapter Objectives

After reading this chapter, you should be able to . . .

- Name what structures are damaged with celiac disease.
- Name the most dangerous complication of gastroesophageal reflux disorder.
- Know the major differences between Crohn disease and ulcerative colitis.
- Identify the aggressive and defensive factors that contribute to peptic ulcers.
- Identify the precancerous condition associated with colorectal cancer.
- Explain why irritable bowel syndrome can also be called functional bowel syndrome.
- Name three possible complications of ulcerative colitis.
- List symptoms or complications of cirrhosis.
- Name the primary modes of communicability for hepatitis A, hepatitis B, and hepatitis C.
- Name three risk factors for liver cancer.

THE DIGESTIVE TRACT: STRUCTURE AND FUNCTION

The best way to discuss how the digestive tract works is to follow a piece of food through the system (Figure 8.1).

When the teeth grind a morsel of food, it is broken into small pieces so that the digestive enzymes in saliva and the rest of the gastrointestinal (GI) tract have access to the nutrients. The food moves from the mouth down the esophagus, through the lower esophageal sphincter, and into a wide place in the tube: the stomach. Here it is further pulverized by powerful muscular contractions while being exposed to more chemicals. When the former food, now referred to as ***chyme***, moves through the pyloric valve into the small intestine, the gallbladder and pancreas make their chemical contributions. By now the barrage of digestive enzymes has reduced the meal into its most primitive building blocks: sugars, fats, and proteins.

The secretion of digestive enzymes anywhere in the upper GI tract is largely a function of the vagus nerve, the biggest contributor to the parasympathetic nervous system. In this way the efficiency of digestion depends on whether a person is in a sympathetic or parasympathetic state.

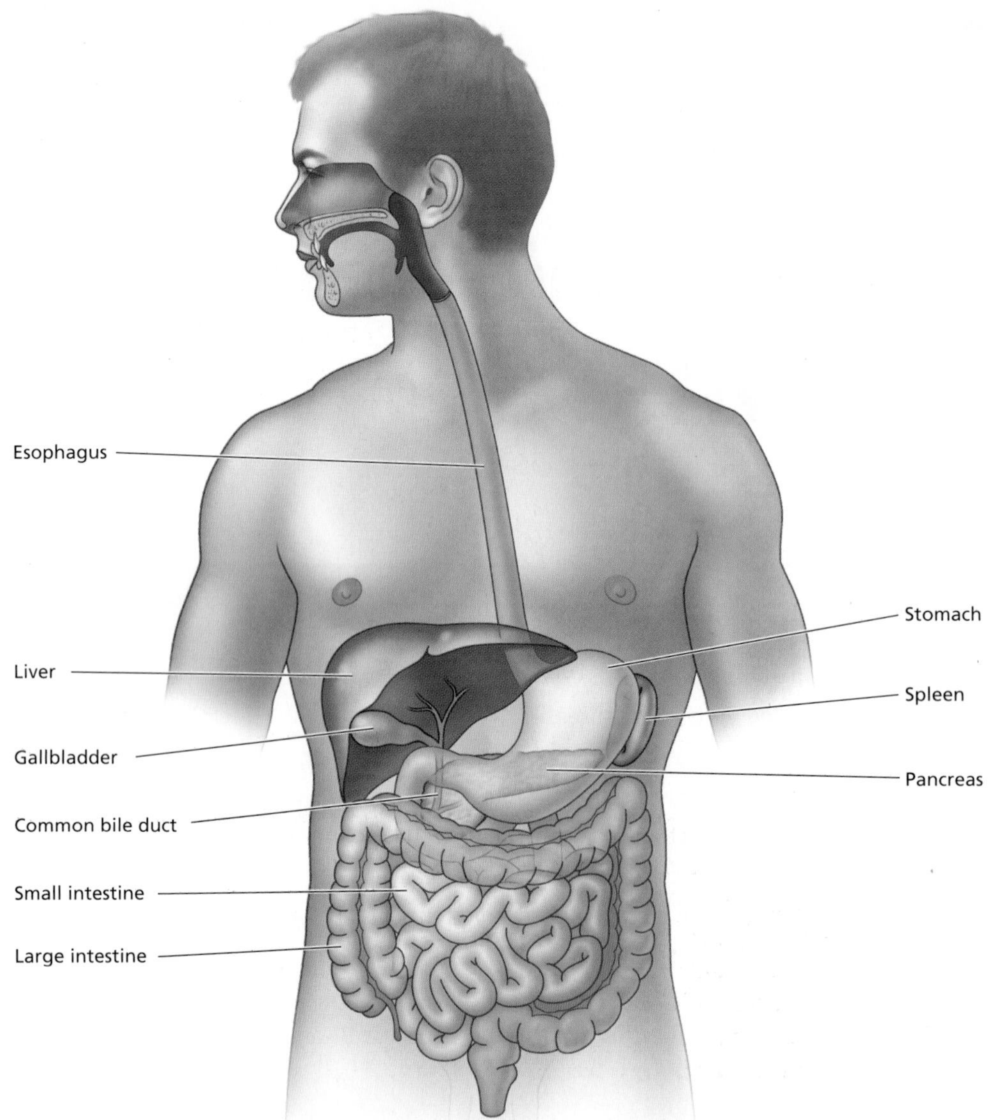

Figure 8.1. Overview of the digestive system.

The small intestine loops and twirls around the abdomen, secured by sheets of connective tissue membrane called the ***mesentery***, a part of the peritoneum. It is lubricated on the outside by other layers of the peritoneum, which allow it to move freely as a person twists, squirms, and changes positions. The inside of a healthy small intestine looks like velvet or velour, with millions of tiny ***villi***, each one supplied with blood and lymph capillaries for the absorption of nutrients and fats. Amino acids and glucose enter the bloodstream, and fats are drawn into the lymph system. Rhythmic waves of smooth muscle contraction gently ease the chyme along the tube until at the distal end of the small intestine the leftovers pass through the ileocecal valve, the entryway to the colon.

The colon is a much shorter and wider section of tubing than the small intestine, and it differs also in the absence of villi and the presence of anchoring pieces of connective tissue that bind the colon down at the four flexures, or corners, of the abdomen. A healthy colon has segments called ***haustra***. In this part of the tube water is squeezed out of the fecal matter and reabsorbed back into the body. This is also the site of vitamin K synthesis. The colon functions like a trash compactor; everything left of a meal that makes it this far is condensed and excreted.

The Accessory Organs: Structure and Function

The continuous tube that winds from mouth to anus is only one part of the digestive system; the *accessory organs* contribute to the process of turning food into energy or building blocks as well. These organs include the liver, gallbladder, and pancreas, each of which produces or releases chemicals into the digestive tract. Here is a brief review of each of these organs.

The Liver

The liver is an organ of immense complexity, with literally hundreds of functions. One of the things that makes the liver unique is its power of regeneration; hepatocytes are remarkably adaptable. Livers that have been partially removed can recover full functional size soon after surgery, and small pieces of liver that have been transplanted into other hosts can often grow to full function within a similar short period. The liver also has twice the blood supply of most other organs; between the hepatic artery delivering oxygen and the portal vein delivering fresh products of digestion from the small intestine, it's no wonder that this organ is hot and dark red. Although the internal blood pressure is relatively low, cellular activity in the liver is very high.

The liver is the largest organ in the body. It is the destination of the portal system detour, receiving all of the vitamins, amino acids, and glucose that are extracted from the small intestine and not immediately needed in the body. By storing glucose as glycogen until it is called for, the liver also acts as a sugar buffer, preventing the radical swings in blood glucose levels that would happen without an intermediate stop for sugar. The liver is also the site for much protein synthesis. Many of the enzymes that support cellular activity are made here, as are the blood proteins that regulate intracellular fluid and blood clotting.

Detoxification functions of the liver are well known. The liver alters many drugs into forms that are less toxic than the original, or that can be excreted. A functioning liver prevents many substances, including alcohol, from reaching toxic levels. It also processes the poisonous wastes generated by protein digestion, changing them to uric acid to be excreted by the kidneys.

In addition to these functions, the specialized leukocytes in the liver called ***Kupffer cells*** are constantly watching for any pathogens that they can eradicate. Finally, the liver helps to recycle the ***heme*** from dead red blood cells into ***bilirubin***, a major component of bile, which is vital for the digestion of fats. The liver produces up to 3 cups of bile each day. Bile leaves the liver via the cystic duct and enters the gallbladder.

The Gallbladder

The gallbladder is a small green sac that hangs off the liver about halfway along the right costal angle. Its function is fairly simple: it receives bile from the liver, stores it, and concentrates it. The gallbladder can hold up to 1 cup of bile at a time. On hormonal command it releases the bile into the duodenum via the common bile duct. There the bile helps to emulsify fats, that is, separate them into tiny separated globules to make them easier to digest. The gallbladder and its ducts are susceptible to dysfunction, which can have serious repercussions.

The Pancreas

The pancreas is a fascinating gland that holds the distinction of being both an exocrine gland, releasing digestive juices into the intestine via the pancreatic duct, and an endocrine gland, releasing hormones directly into the bloodstream. Its exocrine secretions are potentially corrosive. Any blockage in the pancreatic duct can lead to very serious tissue damage, as the pancreas is quite capable of digesting itself.

Digestive System Problems and Massage

Most of the digestive system problems that respond well to massage are related to autonomic imbalance; when a person is under stress, digestion is a low priority. If this state of affairs goes on for a long time, problems inevitably develop. The most common disorders of this type are spastic or flaccid constipation, indigestion, and gas.

The first concern, however, is to eliminate the possibility of more serious conditions that contraindicate circulatory massage. Massage practitioners are sometimes put in the position of deciding whether their work is going to help someone get over a stress-related stomachache or put the person in the hospital. Symptoms that are a red light for something very serious include severe local pain, bloody stools, anemia, bloating, and fever. A general rule is that if a new pattern persists for 2 weeks or more, it's time to visit the doctor.

Problems in the digestive system are impossible to pin down without diagnostic tests, which are outside the scope of practice of massage therapy. Massage should not be performed when the client has any unexplained or undiagnosed pain. Any relief that a massage provides may delay the client getting medical assistance for a serious and acute illness. Symptoms of simple, short-term problems are often indistinguishable from those of a serious illness. Although spastic constipation is not inherently dangerous, colon cancer is—and massage therapists are not equipped to tell the difference.

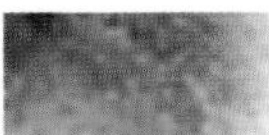

Digestive System Conditions

Disorders of the Upper Gastrointestinal Tract

Celiac disease
Crohn disease
Esophageal cancer
Gastroenteritis
Gastroesophageal reflux
Peptic ulcers
Stomach cancer

Disorders of the Large Intestine

Colorectal cancer
Diverticular disease
Irritable bowel syndrome
Ulcerative colitis

Disorders of the Accessory Organs

Cirrhosis
Gallstones
Hepatitis
Liver cancer
Pancreatic cancer
Pancreatitis

Other Digestive System Conditions

Candidiasis
Peritonitis

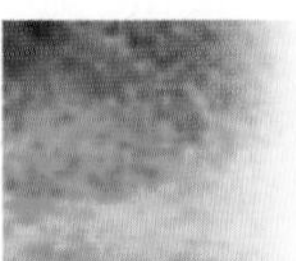

Disorders of the Upper Gastrointestinal Tract

Celiac Disease

Definition: What Is It?

Celiac disease is a condition in which the intestinal villi are flattened or destroyed altogether as part of an immune system reaction in the presence of ***gluten***, a group of proteins present in many types of grains. It is also known as *celiac sprue*, *nontropical sprue*, or *gluten-sensitive enteropathy*.

> **Celiac Disease in Brief**
> Pronunciation: SEE-le-ak dih-ZEZE
>
> **What is it?**
> Celiac disease is a condition in which an inflammatory response follows the consumption of any food with gluten. This leads to the destruction of intestinal villi and poor access to ingested nutrients.
>
> **How is it recognized?**
> Celiac disease can develop in childhood or adulthood, and its symptoms vary greatly from one person to another. Most symptoms are related to malabsorption (many nutrients are not absorbed and so pass through to the stools) or malnutrition (complications related to vitamin and nutrient deficiencies develop).
>
> **Is massage indicated or contraindicated?**
> Celiac disease is not directly affected by bodywork, although as with all intestinal discomfort, clients should be encouraged to seek a diagnosis if symptoms are persistent, even if massage provides temporary relief.

Demographics: Who Gets It?

The incidence of celiac disease in the United States is the topic of some controversy. Although it is diagnosed in 1 in about 3,000 people,[1] recent studies indicate that it may affect about 1 in 133 people.[2] It is most commonly diagnosed in people of northern European descent.

A genetic link for celiac disease is clearly demonstrable; it occurs in about 10% of first-degree relatives of diagnosed people. The fraternal twin of an affected person has a 30% chance of developing the disease, while an identical twin of an affected person has a 70% chance.[1] The exact location of the genetic mutation that leads to this condition is still under investigation.

Etiology: What Happens?

Some sources list celiac disease as an autoimmune disease, while others suggest it is an allergic reaction to the components of gluten. The truth is probably somewhere in the middle, and ongoing research continues to reveal clues about how this condition causes the problems associated with it.

Gluten is a group of proteins found in many grains, including wheat, rye, barley, spelt, and others. When gluten is consumed by a person without celiac disease, digestive enzymes break it down into small chains of amino acids that are absorbed into the intestinal villi and then used by the body. When celiac disease is present, gluten is broken into its component pieces, including a long chain of amino acids called ***gliadin***, but this substance resists any further enzyme action to break it into smaller pieces. For reasons that are not completely clear, gliadin is absorbed into the villi of people with celiac disease, where intracellular enzymes interact with it and trigger a mild or severe inflammatory response.

Eventually, repeated inflammatory attacks on intestinal villi cause them to degenerate, lie flat, or disappear altogether. The person then loses access to absorbable nutrition not only from sources of gluten but from other sources as well. Glucose from dairy products is often particularly difficult to digest, which leads to symptoms of lactose intolerance, although the problem isn't with the lactose itself but with the villi that are meant to absorb it. Fats become similarly unavailable, and they pass through the digestive system to be expelled in the stools. Poor uptake leads to signs of malabsorption and malnutrition, although the diet of a person with celiac disease may be identical to that of an average person.

New studies of the cells and chemicals that become active with celiac disease have revealed some hints that this condition may have an autoimmune component, with gluten and gliadin as the inflammatory triggers. Celiac disease frequently occurs concurrently with some other autoimmune disorders, which supports this theory. It is especially associated with type 1 diabetes, hypothyroidism, hyperthyroidism, lupus, and rheumatoid arthritis.

A genetic link in celiac disease is easy to trace, since the incidence within families is significantly higher than in the general population. Age at onset varies significantly, however. Some people develop symptoms in early childhood, and others develop symptoms after a significant stressful trigger in adulthood, such as surgery, childbirth, or trauma. Still others may go throughout life with symptoms so mild they are ignored or misdiagnosed as other GI disorders.

Some people with gluten sensitivity don't have significant GI symptoms, but they develop a painful, itchy rash on the elbows, neck, trunk, and buttocks. This skin condition is called ***dermatitis herpetiformis***. An indicator of celiac disease, it usually clears when gluten is eliminated from the diet.

Signs and Symptoms

Signs and symptoms of celiac disease typically center on malabsorption of nutrients and malnutrition. While some patients have pain or discomfort in the GI tract, many others have only the results of poor vitamin and nutrient uptake. Symptoms are somewhat determined by the section of the small intestine that is affected. Damage to the duodenum, for instance, results in different nutritional deficiencies from those of damage to the jejunum.

GI symptoms include gas, bloating, and diarrhea. Stools are often high-volume, pale, and foul-smelling, as they contain much of the fat and other material that would normally have been absorbed in the small intestines.

Related symptoms include weight loss (or failure to gain weight in children), anemia, irritability, depression, behavior changes, muscle cramps and weakness, poor stamina, tooth discoloration, and the dermatitis described previously.

Complications

The complications of celiac disease also have to do with malabsorption and malnutrition. Poor uptake of iron and vitamins leads to anemia, folic acid deficiency, and a high risk of miscarriage or neural tube defects in a growing fetus. Poor uptake of calcium leads to ***osteomalacia*** (weak bones) in children or osteoporosis in adults. Muscle weakness, chronic spasm, and joint pain may develop. Behavioral changes, irritability, peripheral neuropathy, and a risk of seizures can be linked to a vitamin B_{12} deficiency.

Young children with celiac disease have delayed growth and development and many never reach their projected height.

Constant irritation and inflammation of the GI tract raises a significant risk of adenocarcinoma or lymphoma in the small intestine. Non-Hodgkin lymphoma is a significant cause of death for persons whose celiac disease is never identified.

Diagnosis

The diagnosis of celiac disease recently became much easier, as the presence of certain antibodies in the blood can be traced with a blood test. A positive blood test is not definitive, however; a scope and a biopsy of the lining of the jejunum are typically conducted to confirm a diagnosis.

According to studies of the general population, celiac disease probably occurs more than 30 times more frequently in the United States than it is diagnosed. This discrepancy seems unreasonable: how could it go undiagnosed so often? The answer may lie in the fact that mild cases of celiac disease, while causing damage to the intestinal wall and raising the risk of serious complications, may never cause severe enough independent symptoms to warrant a directed search. Myriad other GI disorders may create the same symptoms, including irritable bowel syndrome and simple stress-related indigestion. To make matters more complicated, irritable bowel syndrome may coexist with celiac disease, making distinguishing between symptoms problematic.

Other disorders frequently confused with celiac disease include peptic ulcers, intestinal parasites, Crohn disease, ulcerative colitis, gastroenteritis, chronic fatigue syndrome, and depression.

Treatment

No treatment for celiac disease, except to avoid gluten in any form, is consistently successful. Gluten is present in many grains, including wheat, rye, barley, spelt, triticale, and kamut. Many (but not all) people with celiac disease are also sensitive to oats, although whether this grain actually contains gluten or is frequently contaminated with it is somewhat questionable. Gluten is also used in many other products, including vitamins and other pills, cosmetics (especially lipstick), and as a thickener in many processed foods.

Gluten is not present in corn, potatoes, beans, nuts, rice, or soy; flour made from these foods can frequently be substituted to help comprise a gluten-free diet. Other gluten-free foods include fruits, vegetables, and meats. It is possible to have a varied and well-balanced gluten-free diet, but eating processed foods or at restaurants may be problematic.

The majority of celiac disease patients who avoid all sources of gluten for months or years can heal completely, and achieve the complete rebuilding of their intestinal villi. However, this reconstruction can easily be undone if gluten-rich foods are consumed; a person with celiac disease must commit to a lifelong dietary adjustment.

Statistics show that people who don't manage their celiac disease, regardless of whether it creates debilitating symptoms, have a shorter lifespan than the general population. They are particularly susceptible to a variety of problems, including lymphoma and adenocarcinoma in the intestines, a high risk of miscarriage or birth defects, and nerve damage related to vitamin deficiency that may result in seizures or peripheral neuropathy.

Massage?

Massage has no impact on the health of intestinal villi. It can, however, temporarily relieve GI discomfort. While this is usually a benefit, it may lead to a delay in seeking a diagnosis. Celiac disease, like many other intestinal diseases, has the best prognosis when it is identified early. Consequently, if a client reports recurring symptoms that persist for more than a few days or weeks, that person should be referred to another medical professional as soon as possible.

A client who has been diagnosed with celiac disease and manages it successfully through dietary changes is a fine candidate for massage. Abdominal work should be conducted strictly within the comfort level of the client, of course.

Modality Recommendations for Celiac Disease

Modality	Recommendation
Deep tissue massage	Supportive: may relieve GI discomfort; work within comfort of client.
Lymphatic drainage	Supportive.
Polarity	S: Indicated. R/D: Avoid abdomen when symptoms are severe.
PNF/MET/stretching	Supportive.
Reflexology	Indicated. Work digestive tract; focus on liver and pancreas points.
Shiatsu	Supportive. Work SP, LI, SI. Add gentle ampuku, alarm points, hara assessment.
Swedish massage	Avoid abdomen when symptoms are severe; otherwise light abdominal touch and stroking can be helpful.
Trigger point therapy	Avoid the abdomen; otherwise supportive.

See Chapter 1 for a brief description of each modality, including definitions of abbreviations.

Crohn Disease

Definition: What Is It?

Crohn disease is a progressive inflammatory disorder that can affect any part of the GI tract, from the mouth to the anus. Advanced cases may also involve tissues outside the digestive system.

Crohn disease and ulcerative colitis are often described together under the umbrella term *inflammatory bowel disease* because of the way they affect tissues, but they are etiologically quite different. Although Crohn disease can and often does affect the large intestine as well as the upper GI tract, it is discussed in this section to help distinguish it from ulcerative colitis. For more information on how these two conditions are alike and dissimilar, see Compare and Contrast 8.1.

Demographics: Who Gets It?

Crohn disease affects about 500,000 Americans.[3] Men and women are affected more or less equally.[4] It is usually diagnosed in people aged 15 to 30, with another spike in diagnoses in people over 55 years old.

The geographic distribution of Crohn disease is fairly predictable. It is most common in urban areas in northern North America and Europe. Whites are most at risk for Crohn disease; it occurs among this population four times more commonly than among nonwhites.[3]

Crohn Disease in Brief

Pronunciation: krone dih-ZEZE

What is it?

Crohn disease is a progressive inflammatory condition that may affect any part of the GI tract. It is characterized by deep ulcers, blockages, and the formation of abnormal passageways (fistulas) around the small and large intestine.

How is it recognized?

The primary symptom of Crohn disease is abdominal pain, especially in the lower right quadrant (the distal end of the ileum). Cramping, diarrhea, and pain at the anus may also accompany active flares of this disease.

Is massage indicated or contraindicated?

Massage is appropriate for Crohn disease patients when their condition is in remission. During flares they may also benefit from reflexive or energetic work, but anything more challenging may be too intense.

Compare and Contrast 8.1
Crohn Disease and Ulcerative Colitis

Crohn disease and ulcerative colitis are two conditions linked under the description *inflammatory bowel disease*, or IBD. This may create the impression that these two disorders are slightly different manifestations of the same problem, but current research indicates that they are significantly different in etiology, progression, and long-term prognosis. Although differentiating between these conditions has little impact on a massage therapist's decision, it may have big impact on the life of the client.

CHARACTERISTICS	CROHN DISEASE	ULCERATIVE COLITIS
Area affected	Often begins in ileum but can spread to colon or to rest of small intestine.	Always begins in rectum. May spread up colon but never to small intestine.
Pattern of progression	Unpredictable, disconnected patches may appear anywhere along GI tract.	Contiguous connected series of lesions.
Depth of lesions	Ulcers may burrow through mucosa, into muscular or serous wall of GI tract. Perforation fairly common.	Ulcers penetrate only mucosa or submucosa of colon; seldom perforate.
Complications	Can lead to liver problems, skin and mouth ulcers, eye inflammation, peritonitis, bladder infections, colon cancer.	Significantly raises risk of colon cancer; other complications: liver inflammation, arthritis, skin rash, anemia.
Surgery	Surgery can remove affected areas, but disease often continues to attack healthy tissue; surgery often must be repeated.	Surgery to remove affected area is curative.

Genetic susceptibility is evidently part of the Crohn disease profile; about 20% of patients have a first-degree relative (parent, child, or sibling) who also has an inflammatory bowel disease.[3]

Etiology: What Happens?

Crohn disease involves the development of inflamed areas in the large and small intestine. Many cases begin in the distal portion of the small intestine, the ileum, but this progressive disease can affect upper regions of the GI tract, as well as the colon, and the anus.

One of the distinguishing features of Crohn disease is that the areas it affects are not contiguous; the inflamed regions appear in an unpredictable patchwork anywhere in the GI tract (Figure 8.2). These lesions may develop ulcers that affect deep layers of the intestinal wall, even to the point of perforation. Eventually these ulcers can cause accumulations of scar tissue that partially block the intestine, or they can stimulate the development of abnormal connecting tubes from the colon to other organs, for instance the bladder or even the surface of the skin. These tubes are called ***fistulas***, and they allow intestinal contents to exit the GI tract.

In some cases of Crohn disease, massive accumulations of scar tissue cause the GI tract to become dangerously narrow; this is called ***stenosis***. Stenosing Crohn disease can also lead to the formation of fistulas as the body tries to reroute digestive system contents past blockages.

Crohn disease is, so far, an idiopathic disease. It is considered to be a multifactorial problem, with aspects of pathologic invasion, genetic predisposition, immune system dysfunction, environmental influences, and dietary triggers. An inappropriate inflammatory response is part of the picture, but it is unclear whether that response is the cause or the result of the disease.

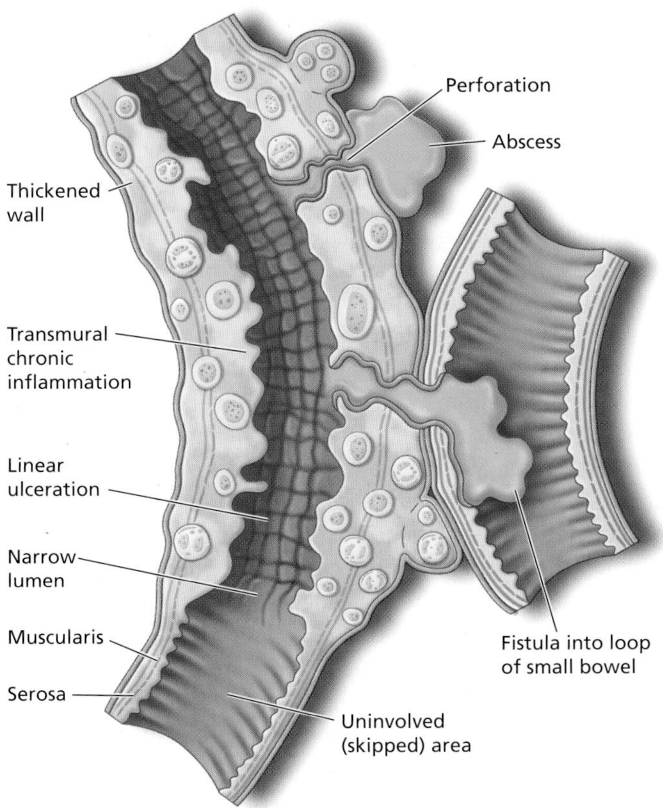

Figure 8.2. Crohn disease.

Some speculation about an initial exposure to a common pathogen, *Mycobacterium paratuberculosis*, is well accepted (Sidebar 8.1); this is the same pathogen that causes a similar condition called Johne's disease in animals.[5] Although this condition may be linked to bacterial exposure, it does *not* appear to be contagious.

Another factor in Crohn disease is immune system chemicals that are predominant in the patches of inflamed tissue during flares. Several cytokines that exacerbate the inflammatory response have been identified in higher-than-normal levels among Crohn disease patients. These discoveries continually yield new treatment options to limit the damage that Crohn disease can do.

Food sensitivities and stress have been seen to exacerbate Crohn disease symptoms, but they have not been identified as direct causes.

Regardless of the initial trigger, the development of Crohn disease depends on a genetic susceptibility to this kind of inflammatory response. Some genetic anomalies have already been identified; others are still being pursued.

Signs and Symptoms

Crohn disease occurs in periods of flare and remission, which implies an autoimmune component. During periods

SIDEBAR 8.1: HISTORY OF CROHN DISEASE

Throughout the twentieth century, descriptions of Crohn disease have gone through several incarnations. It has been called *granulomatosis enteritis* for the presence of white blood cell conglomerates called granulomas. It has been called *regional enteritis* for its patchy appearance throughout the small and large intestines. It has also been labeled *terminal ileitis* because it often begins at the distal end of the ileum.

One of the first researchers to document Crohn disease was a Scottish surgeon, Thomas Kennedy Dalziel (1861–1924). In 1913 he noted its similarity to certain inflammatory conditions found among livestock, and he proposed that it might be caused by the same pathogen—*Mycobacterium paratuberculosis*.

In 1932 a team of researchers, including physician Burrill Crohn (1884–1983), were unable to find significant signs of bacteria in the lesions, and so the theory of bacterial infection was dropped. Instead, the disease was studied as an immune system dysfunction involving inappropriate inflammatory attacks against digestive system tissue. It wasn't until 1959 that the disease was clearly distinguishable from the closely related ulcerative colitis.

In 1985 new tests revealed that particles of *M. paratuberculosis* can indeed be found in Crohn disease ulcers. Early treatment with the correct antibiotics shows promising results with many Crohn disease patients, although some of them require these antibiotics for a prolonged period.

M. paratuberculosis is a common pathogen that most people encounter early in life, when it usually causes a short-term bout of diarrhea. It seems that Crohn disease patients have a genetic susceptibility to creating a life-long inflammatory response to this pathogen that causes significant and extensive damage to the digestive tract.

CASE HISTORY 8.1

Crohn Disease

Karen, aged 41: "All I knew was, food hurt."

Karen was diagnosed with Crohn disease when she was a young adult, but she has had stomach pain as long as she can remember. "When I was a kid, my mother literally had to hold my head and put food in my mouth. She wasn't being mean, it's just what the doctors told her to do because I wouldn't eat. All I knew was, food hurt."

Karen's doctor was convinced that there was nothing wrong with her. "It's all in your head," he told her. The Thanksgiving she was 22, she collapsed on a trip to California. She had a fever of 105°F. She had formed an abscess on her intestine, and the infection had invaded her bloodstream: she had sepsis and was hospitalized in Los Angeles for a week. After the attack subsided, she had her first colonoscopy, and the evidence of Crohn disease was clear.

After her diagnosis Karen tried two medications to control the disease, but one gave her severe headaches and another, a sulfa drug, caused some breathing problems. Fortunately, she went into remission and had no problems for several years. Then in 1995 she developed severe stomach pain with diarrhea. Unable to absorb adequate nutrition from food, she developed bone pain, and her hair began to fall out. At this time she began treating her disease with stronger medication.

Karen's first surgery was conducted in 1997. Her small intestine was resected where a stricture had obstructed it; a fistula was repaired, adhesions between abdominal organs were released, and her appendix was taken out. She had remarkable relief after this, but it was short lived. "Most Crohn disease patients go about 4 years between surgeries; I go more like 2 years."

Karen's Crohn disease involves a tendency to build up scar tissue in the small intestine, leading to strictures, fistulas, and obstruction. She took infliximab (Remicade) to control symptoms, but several months ago it seemed to stop working. She finds that prednisone controls most of her symptoms, but she can use it only for about 6 weeks before developing serious side effects.

One of Karen's challenges is monitoring the progress of her disease. A colonoscopy goes only to the ileocecal valve, and a barium swallow shows problems only in the esophagus and stomach; Karen's problems are between the two points. She tried to use a new technology, a tiny camera in a pill-sized capsule, called a capsule endoscopy, that takes hundreds of pictures as it travels through the GI tract, but the camera got caught at an intestinal stricture, and she needed surgery to have it removed.

When she is in remission, Karen finds she doesn't have to be especially careful about her diet, but she doesn't tolerate caffeine well. When her disease is active she has to avoid any roughage; she needs a low-fiber diet. She takes vitamins to make up for some lost absorption in her small intestine.

Karen works out 4 days a week in a gym, which she says is very helpful for managing her stress. A massage therapist visits her office once a month. She enjoys this, but she reports that when her disease is active, she has a hard time receiving massage: "Obstructive pain is intense! The intestines are twisting and turning, trying to shove the stuff through. I get terrible spasms in my back, and the therapist says the muscles in my back are stiff as a board."

Karen had five surgeries between 1997 and 2006, and she says she now recognizes the symptoms of another stricture forming, just 6 months since her last surgery. She is hoping she can delay the next procedure until after a trip to Hawaii. She gets along well with her doctor, whom she calls GI Joe, and she enjoys interaction with other Crohn disease patients. She is happy to "share my agonies" with anyone who asks, and she does so with laughter and good will. "You have to laugh," she says. "What else are you gonna do?"

of remission a patient may have no symptoms at all, but during a flare the most common symptoms include abdominal pain, especially at the distal end of the ileum in the lower right quadrant, along with cramping, diarrhea (often with blood), and bloating. Weight loss, fever, joint pain, small ulcers in the mouth and throat, and characteristic lesions on the skin may also accompany acute flares. Many Crohn disease patients also have severe pain around the anus, along with anal fissures and abscesses.

Complications

Crohn disease disrupts normal digestion in several ways. Inflammation in the intestines means a patient is at risk for serious malnutrition. When Crohn disease occurs in young children, it can lead to stunted growth and delayed development.

This disease can cause bowel obstruction, at first by swelling and spasm and eventually by scar tissue strictures. Deep ulcers may bleed into the GI tract, or perforate, leading to peritonitis. Adhesions can form between layers of the peritoneum. Crohn disease can cause abscesses in the GI tract or around the anus. If fistulas into the bladder form, leaking fecal material can cause bladder infections. Chronic irritation to epithelial cells in the GI tract also increases the risk of colon cancer: this is the leading cause of death for people who die of Crohn disease.[4]

Crohn disease has been linked to problems outside the GI tract as well. It can cause inflammation at the bile duct, leading to cirrhosis, jaundice, and gallstones. It has been linked with kidney stones and acute inflammation affecting the liver, eyes, and joints. It can cause ulcers called ***aphthae*** in the mouth and characteristic lesions on the skin as well; these open sores most often appear around the ankles and lower legs.

Treatment

The damage to the whole length of the digestive system that Crohn disease can cause is significant, and so it is usually treated aggressively. Treatment during flares usually begins with steroidal anti-inflammatories and immunosuppressant drugs to quell the inflammatory reaction. Other drugs that inhibit the activity of inflammatory cytokines are proving useful as well. Most Crohn disease patients eventually have surgery to remove affected sections of intestine, but this surgery is not curative; new patches of inflamed tissue may arise in other places, requiring further surgery.

Crohn disease patients have to be extraordinarily careful about their diet, especially during flares. High-fiber, bulky foods can exacerbate symptoms and create obstructions if scar tissue has narrowed the passageway. Sometimes a high-calorie liquid diet is recommended during these episodes. In extreme cases the patient may take in all nutrients intravenously to give the whole system a break from the stress of digesting food.

Massage?

When Crohn disease is in remission and the digestive tract is not under inflammatory attack, massage is a supportive and appropriate choice. Deep abdominal work should probably be avoided, but anything that creates a parasympathetic response for increased efficiency of digestion and nutrient absorption would probably be useful.

During flares a client with Crohn disease will probably be uncomfortable on the table, and circulatory work may exacerbate symptoms. Other types of bodywork, however, may be welcome and helpful in the effort to reduce pain and distress.

Modality Recommendations for Crohn Disease	
Deep tissue massage	Locally contraindicated while acute. Between flares, work slowly to assist parasympathetic response.
Lymphatic drainage	Supportive.
Polarity	S: Indicated. R/D: avoid abdomen during flares.
PNF/MET/stretching	Supportive.
Reflexology	Indicated. Work digestive tract and abdominal points. Use light pressure and avoid crystals during flare.
Shiatsu	Supportive. Work SP, TH, K, SI meridian with extensions in legs. GV-20 and BL in low back for pain and diarrhea.
Swedish massage	Light touch on abdomen during and between flares can help create a parasympathetic response; watch for complications of steroid use.
Trigger point therapy	Avoid abdomen; supportive between flares.

See Chapter 1 for a brief description of each modality, including definitions of abbreviations.

Esophageal Cancer

Definition: What Is It?

Esophageal cancer is the development of malignant cells in the esophagus. It typically appears in either of two forms: cancer that grows in the thoracic area of the esophagus (squamous cell carcinoma) or cancer that grows at the distal end (adenocarcinoma).

> **Esophageal Cancer in Brief**
> Pronunciation: e-sof-uh-JE-ul KAN-sur
>
> **What is it?**
> Esophageal cancer is the growth of malignant cells in the esophagus. It is classified as either squamous cell carcinoma, which usually occurs in the thoracic portion of the esophagus, or adenocarcinoma, which occurs at the distal end, near the lower esophageal valve.
>
> **How is it recognized?**
> Esophageal cancer is rarely recognized in early stages. In later stages a growth may obstruct the esophagus, leading to a feeling of food or liquid "getting stuck" on the way to the stomach. Pain and difficulty swallowing, along with unintended weight loss, are the symptoms that usually prompt people to seek a diagnosis.
>
> **Is massage indicated or contraindicated?**
> As with other cancers, the guidelines for massage and esophageal cancer are determined largely by what stresses or complications cancer treatments may cause. Surgery, radiation therapy, chemotherapy, and other options all carry specific cautions and concerns for massage therapists.

Demographics: Who Gets It?

Worldwide, squamous cell esophageal cancer is quite common. In the United States the demographic group most at risk is mature African American men: it occurs roughly five times more often in this group than in any other.

Until the 1970s, squamous cell carcinoma was the most common form of esophageal cancer in the United States, accounting for 90% to 95% of cases. Since then, adenocarcinoma of the esophagus has been diagnosed more frequently. Indeed, it has the fastest-rising incidence of any cancer in the United States, increasing at about 2% per year.[6]

Regardless of whether esophageal cancer is squamous cell carcinoma or adenocarcinoma, men of all races with this diagnosis outnumber women by about 3 or 4 to 1.[6]

About 14,500 cases of esophageal cancer are diagnosed in this country each year, and about 13,700 people die of the disease annually.[7] The prognosis for esophageal cancer is usually poor; the overall 5-year survival rate is 20% to 25%. That said, new treatment options are proving effective, and the survival rate for esophageal cancer patients is expected to improve for those diagnosed after 2004.[8]

Etiology: What Happens?

The esophagus is a tube about 10 inches long. It runs from the throat to the lower esophageal valve, which opens into the stomach. It is composed of four layers of tissue: the mucous membrane, which lines the tube; the submucosa, which provides blood and lymph support for the active mucus-producing cells; the muscularis, which provides strong wavelike contractions to move a food bolus from the throat into the stomach; and the ***adventitia***, a connective tissue outer layer. The esophagus lacks a serous membrane covering.

When malignant cells grow in the upper or middle parts of the esophagus, they tend to appear in squamous epithelial cells; this is called *squamous cell carcinoma of the esophagus*. This condition is closely related to smoking or alcohol use; smoking in combination with alcohol use increases the risk of malignancies by a large margin.

When malignant cells grow in glandular tissue, the growth is called *adenocarcinoma*. This is the case when esophageal cancer originates at the distal end of the tube, close to the lower esophageal valve. A condition called ***Barrett esophagus*** is usually a predisposing factor for adenocarcinoma of the esophagus. Barrett esophagus, a complication of gastroesophageal reflux disease (GERD), is considered a precancerous state for esophageal cancer. While once rare, adenocarcinoma of the esophagus is now diagnosed more often than squamous cell carcinoma.

Malignant cells from esophageal cancer can invade other tissues by a number of routes. Because the esophagus has no serous membrane cover, any tumor that penetrates through all four layers of the esophagus may be able to spread easily to nearby structures. The trachea, diaphragm, aorta, vena cava, and laryngeal nerve are most susceptible. A generous supply of lymphatic capillaries in the esophageal submucosa means that lymphatic spread of the disease is also a risk. The lymph system can carry malignant cells to nearby nodes and other tissues, including the lungs, liver, and bones. Esophageal cancer can also spread through the bloodstream, although this appears to happen more rarely than other routes for metastasis.

Risk Factors

The primary risk factors for esophageal cancer are age, gender, and race, none of which are controllable. But several other risk factors *can* be controlled: use of tobacco products and use of alcohol have been seen to increase the risk for squamous cell carcinoma of the esophagus; this risk is multiplied when alcohol and tobacco use occur simultaneously.

The main risk factor for adenocarcinoma is damage to the esophageal lining when it is exposed to a chronic, repeated barrage of gastric juices. With this stimulus, cells of the esophageal mucosa change to resemble cells that line the stomach. This raises the risk of malignancy so significantly that many physicians recommend surgery or other interventions even before cancer is confirmed. Of patients who undergo endoscopy to diagnose GERD, 10 to 15% are also positive for Barrett esophagus.[9]

Other risk factors for esophageal cancer include obesity (this may contribute to GERD), a history of any other head or neck cancer, exposure to toxic substances (i.e., ingesting lye or other poisons), exposure to human papillomavirus in the throat, and a lifetime habit of drinking extremely hot beverages. Worldwide studies also reveal that a shortage of vitamins A, B, and C, beta carotene, and selenium are common among esophageal cancer patients.[10]

Signs and Symptoms

Early signs and symptoms of esophageal cancer are practically nonexistent, which is why this disease has such a high mortality rate; it is often undetected until a tumor is large enough to create a mechanical obstruction, and metastasis to other nearby organs and/or lymph nodes has already occurred.

SIDEBAR 8.2: STAGING ESOPHAGEAL CANCER

The staging of esophageal cancer is determined by how deeply the esophagus has been penetrated and by whether lymph nodes have been affected or metastasis has developed. Esophageal cancer is staged using both the TNM (tumor, node, metastasis) technique and numerical staging from 0 to IV.[8]

Tumor (T)	Node (N)	Metastasis (M)
T IS: cancer in situ, limited to superficial mucosa	N 0: no nodes involved	M 0: no metastasis found
T 1: mucosa and/or submucosa invaded	N 1: some nearby nodes involved	M 1a: distant lymph nodes involved
T 2: muscularis invaded		M 1b: distant organs involved
T 3: adventitia invaded		
T 4: nearby structures invaded		

These delineations are then translated into stages 0 to IV in this way:

Stage	Tumor	Node	Metastasis	5-Year Survival Rate (%)
0	T IS	N 0	M 0	52
I	T 1	N 0	M 0	41
II A	T2–3	N 0	M 0	26
II B	T 1–2	N 1	M 0	26
III (option 1)	T 3	N 1	M 0	13
III (option 2)	T 4	N 0–1	M 0	13
IV A	T any	N any	M 1a	3
IV B	T any	N any	M 1b	3

The symptoms that most often cause people to go to the doctor include dysphagia, a feeling of food or liquid "getting stuck" on its way to the stomach, pain with swallowing, hoarseness, and unplanned weight loss. A chronic cough, with or without blood, may also occur.

Diagnosis

The diagnostic procedure for esophageal cancer typically begins with a barium swallow. This test shows exactly where a lesion or tumor might have developed. Various depths and techniques of scopes may follow, along with positron emission tomography (PET), computed tomography (CT), or ultrasound to check for signs of lymphatic involvement. Staging protocols for esophageal cancer are provided in Sidebar 8.2.

Treatment

Treatment for esophageal cancer ranges from surgery to chemotherapy, radiation therapy, or other options. Photodynamic therapy is now often employed in this situation: special drugs are absorbed into cancerous cells and then activated by a laser to destroy the target cells.

Recovery from treatment for esophageal cancer is often problematic, since good nutrition is necessary to heal from such invasive procedures, and eating is often very difficult.

Massage?

The guidelines for massage and esophageal cancer are the same as for massage and any other type of cancer. Benefits and risks must be weighed in the context of the stresses brought about by cancer treatment as much as by the cancer itself. While massage can improve sleep and appetite, care must be taken not to overwhelm the system of a person undergoing an extraordinarily stressful process. For more information about massage in the context of cancer, see Chapter 12.

MODALITY RECOMMENDATIONS FOR ESOPHAGEAL CANCER

Deep tissue massage	Supportive as part of health care team. Respect stage of recovery and treatment challenges. Focus on erector spinae, thoracic outlet.
Lymphatic drainage	Supportive; use caution with submandibular work.
Polarity	S: Indicated. R: Supportive; determined by client's comfort. D: Avoid esophagus area.
PNF/MET/stretching	Supportive as part of health care team; match to activity levels.
Reflexology	Indicated. Work esophagus points, along with lymphatic, thymus, and pituitary areas.
Shiatsu	Support immune system with L, K, SP, TH meridians.
Swedish massage	Supportive; depth determined by activity level.
Trigger point therapy	Supportive.

See Chapter 1 for a brief description of each modality, including definitions of abbreviations.

Gastroenteritis

Definition: What Is It?

Gastroenteritis is inflammation of the GI tract, specifically the stomach or small intestine. By convention, gastroenteritis is usually discussed as a result of an infection with bacteria, viruses, or parasites. Noninfectious problems can also cause inflammation of the GI tract, however, and it can sometimes be difficult to identify the cause of a person's symptoms.

Demographics: Who Gets It?

Anyone of any age can get gastroenteritis, although it is most dangerous for the very young, the very old, and people whose immune systems are compromised. Because only a small minority of affected people seek medical consultation, it is difficult to calculate how common it is. Some estimates suggest that each year some 100 million cases of gastroenteritis occur in the United States. It is responsible for more than 210,000 hospitalizations of children and about 10,000 deaths each year.[11]

Worldwide, gastroenteritis is a much larger problem. It occurs about 500 million times per year. In underdeveloped countries gastroenteritis and its complications are a leading cause of death for children.[12]

Gastroenteritis in Brief

Pronunciation: GAS-tro-en-ter-I-tis

What is it?
Gastroenteritis is any form of GI inflammation.

How is it recognized?
The symptoms of gastroenteritis are nausea, vomiting, and diarrhea. Fever, blood in the stools, and other signs may be present, depending on the cause.

Is massage indicated or contraindicated?
Acute gastroenteritis contraindicates massage, especially when it is caused by an infectious agent. Clients with chronic disease may be appropriate for bodywork, as long as the etiology of the problem is clearly understood and the risk of infection is managed.

Etiology: What Happens?

Damage to the intestines can occur in a variety of ways. Some pathogens produce toxins that cause intestinal mucosa to secrete excess fluid. Others directly invade mucosal cells. When peristalsis is slowed or delayed, as can occur with diabetes and some other diseases, pathogens that would normally be quickly expelled can linger and overpower protective mechanisms. Some toxins, like those seen with shellfish from red tide areas, can damage intestinal cells as well.

When the GI tract is damaged or inflamed, absorption of nutrients and water is severely limited. This causes loss of both water and valuable electrolytes through diarrhea and vomiting. Gastroenteritis can have several causes:

- *Viruses.* The most common cause of GI inflammation among adults in the United States is with Norwalk virus (one of a group called ***noroviruses***). Among children, ***rotavirus*** infections are most common. Any of the hepatitis viruses can cause GI inflammation, as can any member of the ***enterovirus*** family. Viral gastroenteritis is highly communicable and can reach epidemic levels in environments like day care centers, where most infants have not yet developed antibodies against infection and the chance of fecal-oral contamination is very high. It is estimated that viruses cause anywhere from 50% to 70% of all cases of gastroenteritis in the United States.[12]
- *Bacteria.* Common bacterial pathogens include *Salmonella*, *Shigella*, *Campylobacter*, and several varieties of *Escherichia coli*. Bacterial gastroenteritis is usually spread through improperly stored or prepared food or contaminated water or ice. "Traveler's diarrhea" is almost always from *E. coli* or *Campylobacter jejuni*. One bacterial irritation is caused by *Helicobacter pylori*, the pathogen associated with gastric ulcers. Bacterial gastroenteritis accounts for 15% to 20% of all cases.[12] Another bacterial infection of the GI tract is particularly dangerous, as it produces toxins that can seriously damage the wall of the colon. It is sometimes called *necrotizing colitis* or ***pseudomembranous colitis***, and the pathogen is *Clostridium difficile*. It has become a common hospital-borne infection and is now being found in community settings. *C. difficile* is in most people's digestive tracts to begin with, and it becomes invasive when a person uses antibiotics that kill off other bacteria. *C. difficile* is a serious problem: along with the other discomforts of gastroenteritis, it can cause intestinal bleeding, perforation, sepsis, and even death.[13]
- *Parasites.* Microscopic animal parasites can invade the GI tract, causing typical symptoms of gastroenteritis. Among the most common are ***Giardia***, ***cryptosporidium***, and ***amebiasis***, which is infection with *Entamoeba histolytica*.
- *Others.* Other causes of inflammation in the GI tract include fungal infections, (i.e., candidiasis), toxins (i.e., poisonous mushrooms or shellfish, or seafood from red tide areas), dietary problems (i.e., food allergies), medications (i.e., antibiotics or magnesium-containing laxatives or antacids), and other conditions that interfere with absorption. These include celiac disease, appendicitis, Crohn disease, ulcerative colitis, irritable bowel syndrome, and diverticulitis. Weakness at the pyloric valve may allow contents of the duodenum to back up into the stomach, causing local irritation. This is called *bile reflux*.

Pathogenic forms of gastroenteritis are highly communicable. They can spread through an environment via oral-fecal contamination or via contaminated water or ice. Food prepared on contaminated surfaces can carry viruses or bacteria. For these reasons, travelers to places where gastroenteritis is common are counseled to use only bottled water for drinking and brushing teeth and to avoid raw fruits and vegetables that may have been rinsed in contaminated water.

Signs and Symptoms

Different causative factors of gastroenteritis can lead to various signs and symptoms, but the basic trio of intestinal inflammation includes nausea, vomiting, and diarrhea. These are appropriate responses to infection, as they are efficient methods of clearing out the GI tract, but several of these diseases are spread through oral-fecal contamination, so hygiene is critical when dealing with these symptoms.

Other signs that may develop with gastroenteritis include bloating, cramps, gas, and mucus or blood in the stools.

Complications

The most serious complication of gastroenteritis is dehydration from the massive fluid and mineral loss that goes along with diarrhea and vomiting. The loss of critical fluid and electrolytes can be fatal; gastroenteritis is a leading cause of death in many developing nations. In the United States the people most at risk for this extreme reaction are infants, immunocompromised persons, and the elderly, whose systems are not well able to cope with this extreme change in internal environment. Signs of dangerously progressed dehydration include sunken eyes, lack of urination, and skin tenting: when the skin is pinched it does not immediately go back to its original position.

Some gastroenteritis factors can cause other complications as well. *Campylobacter* has been linked with Guillain-Barré syndrome, and *Salmonella* can complicate into meningitis or blood poisoning. Some forms of *E. coli* are highly toxic and can lead to renal failure.

Diagnosis

Diagnosis of gastroenteritis is often a problem. Analyzing stool samples is the most efficient way to identify infectious agents, but this is a time-consuming and expensive process. On the other hand, treating bacterial infections with the wrong antibiotics can lead to more-extreme symptoms and more resistant pathogens. To complicate matters further, it is possible to continue carrying the infectious agents long after symptoms have subsided. This has serious repercussions for food handlers and child care and health care workers, who are in position to spread their infection to many other people.

Treatment

Gastroenteritis is usually an acute, self-limiting condition and is not generally treated with anything more sophisticated than rest and fluid and electrolyte replacement. Viruses do not respond to antibiotics, and antibiotics for bacterial infections may make intestinal inflammation worse. The use of antidiarrhea medications is often discouraged because the body is shedding pathogens, and interfering with that process may prolong the infection.

If administration of fluids by mouth aggravates vomiting, it may be necessary to use intravenous fluid replacement in a hospital setting.

Gastroenteritis is much easier to prevent than to treat. When gastroenteritis occurs in outbreaks, it is often due to some specific source of contamination: a shipment of infected meat, a contaminated well, or shellfish harvested from contaminated water. Since foodstuffs are now shipped quickly all over large areas, it is a constant public health challenge to track down the source of infection and to limit its spread among the rest of the population.

Prognosis

Most cases of gastroenteritis resolve within 2 or 3 days without medical intervention. If symptoms persist longer than 2 to 3 weeks, it is no longer considered an acute infection, but a chronic condition. This leads medical professionals to look for an underlying condition such as food allergy, irritable bowel syndrome, diverticulitis, Crohn disease, ulcerative colitis, hepatitis, or HIV/AIDS.

Massage?

Acute gastroenteritis contraindicates circulatory massage for several reasons: an infection may be exacerbated; an infection may be communicable; and the client is unlikely to be comfortable.

If a client has chronic digestive system irritation that is unrelated to infection, cancer, or other dangerous causes, bodywork could be helpful in producing a parasympathetic state that can improve efficiency and comfort.

MODALITY RECOMMENDATIONS FOR GASTROENTERITIS	
Deep tissue massage	Contraindicated while acute; otherwise work slowly to assist parasympathetic response.
Lymphatic drainage	Supportive.
Polarity	S: Indicated. R: Gentle especially at diaphragm. D: Avoid during acute infection.
PNF/MET/stretching	Supportive with no infection present.
Reflexology	Indicated. Work stomach and small intestine points; may progress to whole GI tract.
Shiatsu	Supportive. Work SP, TH to reduce inflammation. Treat hara, ampuku, alarm points for H, ST, GB, SP, LI, treat associated points for Middle Burner on back.
Swedish massage	Systemically contraindicated during acute infection; otherwise supportive.
Trigger point therapy	Systemically contraindicated during acute infection; otherwise supportive.

See Chapter 1 for a brief description of each modality, including definitions of abbreviations.

Gastroesophageal Reflux Disease

Definition: What Is It?

GERD is a condition involving damage to the epithelial lining of the esophagus when it is chronically exposed to digestive juices released from the stomach. It is usually associated with weak muscular action at the lower esophageal sphincter, but several other factors may contribute as well.

Demographics: Who Gets It?

Heartburn, the predecessor to GERD, is astonishingly common in this country. It is estimated that 8% to 10% of Americans have heartburn every day,[14] and up to 40% of Americans have it at least once a month.[15]

GERD is probably present in 40% to 60% of the people who report heartburn symptoms most days.[14] It is identified when heartburn is ongoing, especially in the presence of structural changes to the esophageal lining or lower esophageal sphincter. GERD can develop in any person at any age. It has been documented among infants, the elderly, and every age in-between, but it is most common among mature people.

Etiology: What Happens?

Most cases of GERD are connected to some combination of four problems: the lower esophageal sphincter is too relaxed; the lower esophageal sphincter doesn't allow appropriate clearing of acids in the esophagus; the diaphragmatic hiatus has trapped a portion of the stomach; or the stomach is slow to empty, adding to back-pressure at the lower esophageal sphincter.

Any one of these problems allows stomach contents, including highly corrosive hydrochloric acid (and occasionally bile and pancreatic enzymes that have backed up from a weak pyloric valve), to enter the esophagus, which lacks the thick layer of mucus that protects the stomach from acid exposure.

Chronic irritation of the esophageal lining can cause several reactions:

- *Respiratory injury* may occur if gastric secretions reach up to the larynx. It is fairly common for these substances to be aspirated into the lungs, especially by infants and young children. GERD is now being investigated as a risk factor for laryngeal cancer.
- *Decay of tooth enamel* may develop as acidic juices are increasingly present in the mouth.
- *Ulcers* may form in the esophagus. These lesions may become infected, or they may bleed into the GI tract.
- *A stricture* may form. This is a thickening of the esophageal wall with scar tissue in response to irritation (Figure 8.3). Strictures may make it difficult to swallow normally.
- *Barrett esophagus* may develop. This is a pathological change in the normal esophageal cells; they mutate into cells that resemble the stomach lining. Barrett esophagus has been identified as a possible precancerous condition, opening the door to adenocarci-

Gastroesophageal Reflux Disease in Brief

Pronunciation: gas-tro-e-sof-a-JE-ul RE-flux dih-ZEZE

What is it?

GERD is chronic splashing of acidic stomach secretions into the unprotected esophagus.

How is it recognized?

Most people occasionally have heartburn, the sensation of having corrosive gastric juices enter the esophagus. GERD is diagnosed when heartburn symptoms have been present long enough to cause structural changes to the esophageal lining, which can lead to serious complications.

Is massage indicated or contraindicated?

People with GERD often find that lying down exacerbates their symptoms, especially if it's within a couple of hours of eating. Further, massage and its influence on the parasympathetic state can increase gastric secretions. Clients may therefore wish to delay massage until at least 3 hours after eating. They often prefer to receive massage in a reclining or seated position, rather than lying flat on a table.

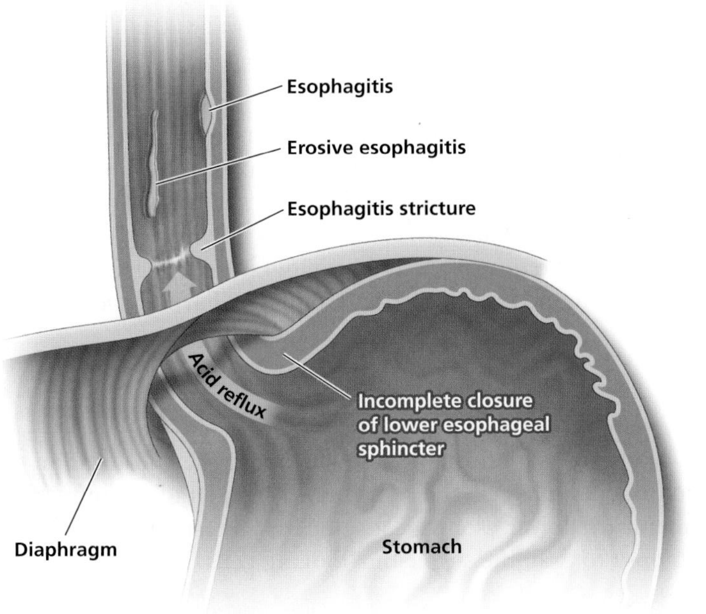

Figure 8.3. Gastroesophageal reflux disease.

noma, an increasingly common type of esophageal cancer. About half of GERD patients are at risk for developing Barrett esophagus.[14]

Risk Factors

A number of risk factors for developing GERD have been identified. Some of these are modifiable, which gives most GERD patients some influence over their disease process. Risk factors for GERD include the following:

- *Pregnancy.* Most pregnant women have some heartburn, especially when the baby is big enough to put mechanical pressure on the stomach. Some pregnant women go on to develop significant structural changes in the esophagus.
- *Obesity.* Being clinically overweight can cause the abdominal contents to put ongoing mechanical pressure on the diaphragm and esophageal sphincter.
- *Smoking.* Smoking has been seen to weaken and loosen the esophageal sphincter.
- *Diet.* A diet high in fatty or spicy foods or the ingestion of caffeine, alcohol, chocolate, and highly acidic foods can exacerbate GERD.
- *Connective tissue disease.* Disease such as lupus or scleroderma may result in inflammation and weakening of the lower esophageal sphincter.
- *Hiatal hernia.* A hiatal hernia (an enlargement of the opening in the diaphragm where the esophagus passes through to the stomach) may catch and irritate the superior part of the stomach. Most people with hiatal hernias have GERD, although not all GERD patients have hiatal hernias.
- *Delayed stomach emptying.* Some diseases, including diabetes, ulcers, and spinal cord injuries, cause reduced peristalsis and sluggish movement of substances through the GI tract. When stomach contents linger too long, the accumulation of pressure and gastric juices can cause them to put back-pressure on the esophagus.
- *Other risk factors.* These include exposure to radiation for chest tumors, infection of the esophagus, and certain medications, including progesterone, beta blockers, and calcium channel blockers.

Signs and Symptoms

Signs and symptoms of GERD are largely produced by the action of gastric juice on the delicate esophageal lining. A bitter taste, a feeling like some food has been regurgitated, gas, indigestion, bloating, and pain in the chest behind the sternum are common symptoms. It is fairly common for the pain of GERD to be mistaken for heart attack or angina. Symptoms are reliably aggravated by bending over or lying down.

Other GERD symptoms that occur less frequently include trouble swallowing, along with coughing, wheezing, and coughing up blood if ulcers in the esophagus have eroded into a blood vessel.

Diagnosis

Diagnostic tests for GERD reveal very precise information about the nature and location of structural changes to the stomach and esophagus. They include barium radiography, endoscopy, a test to measure pressure at the lower esophageal sphincter, a test for pH balance in the esophagus, and possibly a biopsy to examine suspicious-looking cells.

Treatment

Treatment for GERD falls into two categories: management and repair. Managing GERD so that it doesn't get worse includes strategies such as losing weight if the patient is overweight; eating smaller portions so the stomach doesn't get as full; not lying down within 2 hours after a meal; avoiding caffeine, alcohol, and nicotine; raising the bed about 6 inches at the head; loosening clothing that puts pressure around the waist; and putting a heating pad on the stomach when it is painful.

Medication for GERD can work in a variety of ways. Antacids neutralize stomach acid, but over-the-counter brands may also cause the stomach to expand with gas, putting more pressure on the esophageal valve. Other medications can block receptors in the stomach that stimulate acid production, increase stomach motility to assist in sluggish movement, and block the release of hydrogen ions that contribute to the stomach's acidic environment.

Surgery is reserved for Barrett esophagus. It usually focuses on strengthening the esophageal sphincter and taking pressure off the stomach. If the esophagus is limited by the development of a scar tissue stricture, this may be stretched and dilated. A portion of the stomach may be wrapped around the sphincter to give it external support in a procedure called a *fundoplication*. And of course if a hiatal hernia puts pressure on the stomach, surgery may be performed to correct it.

Massage?

Massage usually improves digestive function and efficiency through the parasympathetic response. With GERD patients, however, this may not be a benefit when gastric acid can splash back up into the esophagus. Therefore, it is important to work with clients who have GERD in a way that doesn't exacerbate symptoms. This may mean shorter, more frequent sessions; not working within 2 hours after the client eats; or working with a massage chair or with the client in a semireclined position. Although clients with GERD can benefit from bodywork, their special needs may require imaginative accommodations on the part of their massage therapist.

Clients who successfully control their GERD with medication are perfectly fine for massage, although work near the stomach should be conservative.

Modality Recommendations for Gastroesophageal Reflux Disease

Modality	Recommendation
Deep tissue massage	Contraindicated while acute; supportive if reflux is controlled. Work slowly with costal arch, diaphragm, scalenes.
Lymphatic drainage	Supportive.
Polarity	S: Indicated. R: Gentle around diaphragm. D: Supportive, determined by client's comfort.
PNF/MET/stretching	Supportive.
Reflexology	Indicated. Work esophagus, stomach, and diaphragm points; may progress to whole GI tract.
Shiatsu	Supportive: work Hara, ST, SP meridians; ST in neck.
Swedish massage	Supportive; do light abdominal work.
Trigger point therapy	Supportive.

See Chapter 1 for a brief description of each modality, including definitions of abbreviations.

Peptic Ulcers in Brief
Pronunciation: PEP-tik UL-surz

What are they?
Ulcers are sores that for various reasons don't heal normally; they remain open and vulnerable to infection. Peptic ulcers occur in the esophagus, stomach, or duodenum.

How are they recognized?
The symptoms of peptic ulcers include general burning or gnawing abdominal pain between meals that is relieved by taking antacids or eating. Other symptoms include bloating, burping, gas, and vomiting after meals.

Is massage indicated or contraindicated?
Specific work on the abdomen may exacerbate symptoms of peptic ulcers, so they are at least a local contraindication for mechanical types of bodywork. Other modalities and massage away from the upper abdomen are certainly indicated for ulcer patients.

Peptic Ulcers

Definition: What Is It?

Peptic ulcers of the esophagus, stomach, and duodenum are discussed in this section, but an ulcer is an ulcer, whether it's in the GI tract or on the skin. An ulcer is the result of tissue damage that never gets better because it is subject to constant irritation and/or because healing may be somehow impeded. Cells die and are sloughed off, and a crater intrudes into deep layers of tissue but doesn't crust over. An ulcer is a perpetually open sore and an invitation to infection. Skin ulcers, called *decubitus ulcers* or *bedsores*, are discussed in Chapter 2.

Demographics: Who Gets Them?

Peptic ulcers are a common malady in the United States, although their occurrence has recently begun to decline. It is estimated that about 10% of Americans will have at least one ulcer in their lifetime. About 25 million Americans have been diagnosed with ulcers at this time. Ulcers lead to about 630,000 hospitalizations per year, and complications of ulcers lead to about 6,500 deaths each year.[16]

Etiology: What Happens?

Ulcers in the esophagus, stomach, or small intestine are called peptic ulcers, named for pepsin, the protein-digesting enzyme that contributes to their development (Figure 8.4). Esophageal ulcers typically develop as a complication of gastroesophageal reflux disorder. The general understanding of how stomach and duodenal ulcers come about has undergone some radical changes in the past several years, and this process continues to be studied.

For as long as ulcers have been understood as sores on the stomach or intestinal wall, they have been treated with the assumption that they arise from too much stress and/or spicy food. Ulcer patients have historically been counseled to eat bland food and avoid getting upset or overly excited. Many found that their ulcers eventually healed but would recur later; ulcers were essentially a lifelong condition.

Contributing factor: stress It turns out that the link between stress and ulcers is a significant factor but probably not in the way that had always been assumed. Furthermore, the incidence of ulcers across the population doesn't follow demographics that are associated with high-stress situations, so some variables in stress coping mechanisms have evidently never been addressed.

The normal environment inside a stomach has some features that can be classified as *aggressive* and others that are *defensive*. Aggressive features include the production of hydrochloric acid and pepsin, which help to digest proteins. Defensive features include a generous blood supply to the stomach wall, which serves to help damaged cells regenerate quickly and stimulates mucus production; a lining that protects the stomach wall from acid and pepsin; and production of bicarbonate to neutralize acid. These aggressive and defensive mechanisms work best when they keep each other in balance.

Recall that when a person is in a sympathetic state, blood supply to the whole digestive tract is suppressed and blood is rerouted toward skeletal muscle to support the fight-or-flight reaction. Stomach activity is suspended during a sympathetic reaction. Lack of blood flow means that mucus production is slowed, but so is acid and pepsin production: the two mechanisms stay in balance. But when stress is lifted and a person shifts back into a relaxed, parasympathetic state, stomach secretions are stimulated again. The problem is that the stom-

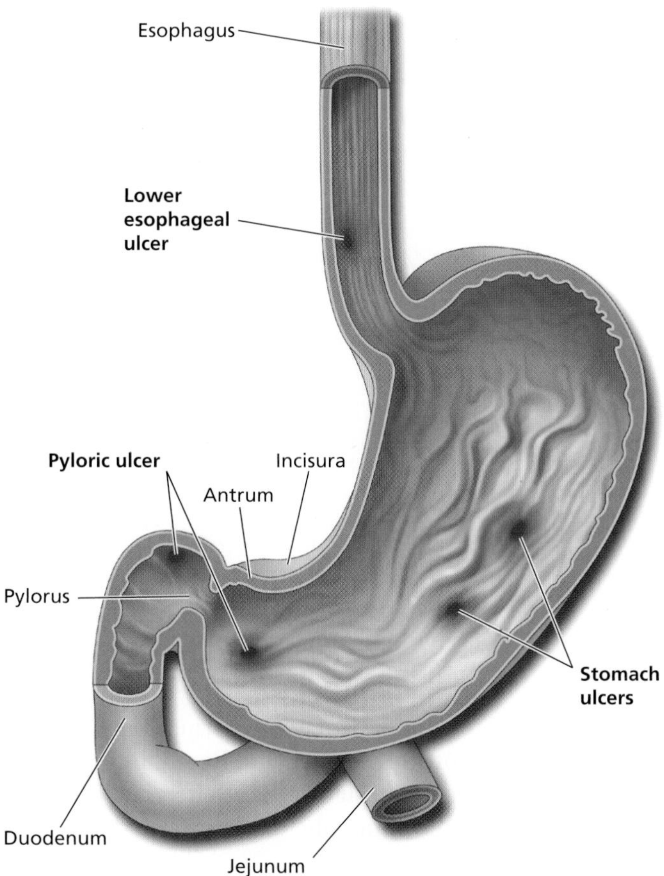

Figure 8.4. Sites of ulcers.

ach produces acid and pepsin much faster than it rebuilds a delicate mucus lining. This imbalance between aggressive and defensive features leaves the stomach wall vulnerable to damage. In other words, ulcers seem to be more related to the fluctuation between stress and relief than to the perception of stress alone.

Contributing factor: *H. pylori* Stress is only part of the ulcer picture, however. In 1984 a remarkable discovery revealed an unexpected phenomenon: a bacterium that can survive and thrive in the highly acidic environment of the stomach. This bacterium, *H. pylori*, is found in many biopsies of ulcers. It is an unusual bacterium, shaped like a bacillus (it can be rod shaped), but it also has spiral flagella (Figure 8.5). These organelles help drill into the stomach wall, allowing the bacterium to take up residence in the mucous lining of the stomach or duodenum. Identification of *H. pylori* led to the conclusion that imbalances in stomach chemistry can initiate tissue damage to the stomach wall, but bacterial infection makes the ulcer a long-term chronic problem. (For more information on *H. pylori*, see Sidebar 8.3.)

The presence of *H. pylori* in most ulcer biopsies led to a whole new understanding of how peptic ulcers develop and how to treat them. The addition of antibiotics to ulcer treatments leads to a successful, permanent solution for many ulcer patients. This finding was so conclusive that in 1994 the National Institutes of Health issued a statement asserting that up to 90% of peptic ulcers were related to *H. pylori* infection. A certain population, however, has ulcers that are unrelated to bacteria.

Contributing factor: NSAIDs The use of nonsteroidal anti-inflammatory drugs (NSAIDs) for everything from headaches to back pain to heart disease and stroke prevention has led to

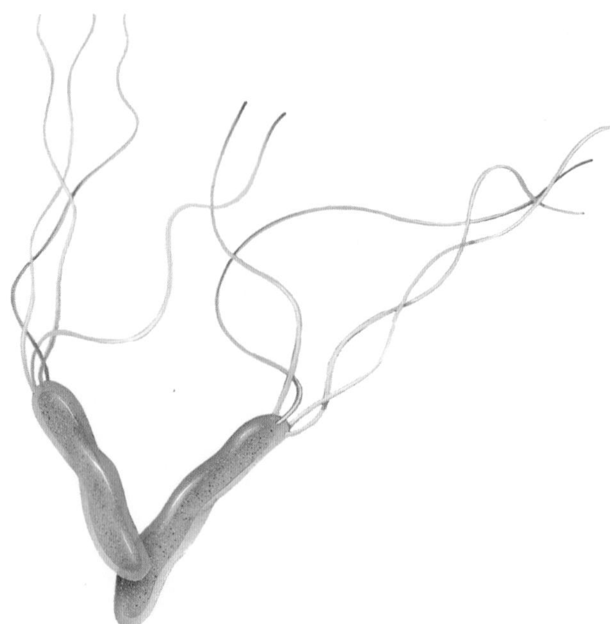

Figure 8.5. *Helicobacter pylori.*

some significant disruption of stomach function for many patients. Aspirin, ibuprofen, and naproxen sodium all interrupt the defensive aspects of stomach activity. By inhibiting the cyclooxygenase-1 pathway, they impede the production of prostaglandins that would otherwise support blood flow and healthy mucus production. (Acetaminophen, by contrast, does not affect stomach function.)

Other contributing factors Several other factors have been seen to exacerbate ulcers, although they are probably not causative. They include cigarette smoking (nicotine increases the amount and concentration of gastric acid); excessive alcohol consumption (alcohol can be absorbed through the mucous membrane directly into the bloodstream at the stomach); and other diseases, including Crohn disease, that may cause stomach dysfunction.

Signs and Symptoms

The primary symptom of peptic ulcers is a gnawing, burning pain in the chest or abdomen. It can last anywhere from 30 minutes to 3 hours. When the pain occurs in relation to eating varies greatly from one person to the next (it can depend on the location of the ulcer), but it is generally relieved by antacids or eating more food.

Other signs of ulcers can include nausea, vomiting, loss of appetite, and bleeding into the GI tract.

Complications

Complications of ulcers can be serious. When ulcers erode into capillaries, bleeding occurs, leading to anemia. If the eroded blood vessel is a larger arteriole or artery, hemorrhaging can lead quickly to shock and death if left untreated. Ulcers can also perforate, or eat all the way through the organ wall, releasing bacteria and partially digested food into the peritoneal space, leading to peritonitis. Perforation happens more often with duodenal than stomach ulcers. Ulcers can create a combination of scar tissue and inflammation that causes the pyloric valve to spasm, completely obstructing the digestive tract. If this is not quickly resolved, it can require surgery to reopen the digestive tract.

Finally, having a peptic ulcer raises the risk of developing stomach cancer by two to six times. Although stomach cancer is on the decline in the United States, it is still the second leading type of cancer worldwide. Another cancer, mucosal-associated lymphoid-type lymphoma, is also associated with *H. pylori* and a history of peptic ulcers.

Diagnosis

Blood tests for *Helicobacter* are a useful tool, but they don't indicate a stage of infection. Other tests include a stool examination for *H. pylori* remnants, a breath test that detects bacteria, a series of upper GI radiographs, and endoscopy, during which a biopsy sample may be taken, or bleeding ulcers can be cauterized.

Treatment

Treatment for most ulcers includes antibiotics for the *H. pylori*; bismuth, which protects the delicate stomach lining; and several medications that limit histamine release (H2 blockers) or acid production (proton pump inhibitors). When the treatment regimen is carefully followed for 2 weeks (this can involve taking up to 20 pills per day), ulcers are typically permanently healed.

Ulcers caused by the use of NSAIDs do not respond to antibiotic therapy. The only way to limit them is to suspend the use of the medications that damage the stomach lining.

Ulcers that don't heal satisfactorily or that continue to bleed, perforate, or cause strictures may be surgically corrected.

Massage?

Massage stimulates a parasympathetic response, which is usually a good thing. For a person with an ulcer, however, that may increase gastric secretions and possibly exacerbate symptoms. Clients with active ulcers may do better with shorter sessions and may be more comfortable not lying flat on a table. A semireclining position, body cushions, or a massage chair may be more appropriate.

SIDEBAR 8.3: WHAT IS *HELICOBACTER PYLORI*?

H. pylori is a bacterium that is admirably designed to withstand and even thrive in the corrosively acidic environment of the stomach. The bacterium has several anatomical features that allow it to infect the mucous membranes of the stomach wall.

Until 1984 it was never even considered that a bacterium could survive in the stomach. When pioneer researchers Barry Marshall and Robin Warren proposed the possibility, they were all but laughed offstage. But when biopsies of lesions consistently revealed the presence of *H. pylori*, the laughter quieted. And when ulcer patients found that combining appropriate antibiotics with other acid-limiting medications led to a permanent cure for their ulcers—something that was unheard of at the time—the approach to treating this common condition completely changed. In 1994 the National Institutes of Health issued a statement that it was clear that *H. pylori* does indeed cause most peptic ulcers and is also a contributing factor to stomach cancer and lymphoma.

So what is *H. pylori*, and where does it come from? Little is well understood about this pathogen. It is a short, microaerophilic gram-negative bacillus with spiraling flagella. Its presence can be easily determined by a blood test for antibodies, although this test does not indicate whether the infection is acute or longstanding. It is sensitive to common antibiotics such as tetracycline and amoxicillin. Worldwide, it is estimated that up to two-thirds of adults have been infected with *H. pylori*. In the United States most infections have been documented among older adults, African Americans, Hispanics, and people in lower socioeconomic classes.

The discovery of *H. pylori* and its role in peptic ulcers has raised as many questions as it has answered:

- How is the bacterium communicated? No one knows, but it could be through oral-fecal contamination or through salivary contact.
- How can it be prevented? It is impossible to prevent the spread of *H. pylori* without knowing how it gets from one person to another.
- If it is sensitive to common antibiotics, why isn't it eradicated when a person takes amoxicillin or tetracycline for something else? Antibiotics for *H. pylori* seem to work only when an ulcer has formed or when the infected person has acute gastritis from bacterial irritation.
- Does the presence of *H. pylori* contribute to general indigestion? It is unclear, but taking antibiotics for indigestion definitely doesn't clear up an *H. pylori* infection or relieve symptoms of dyspepsia.
- What diseases are associated with *H. pylori*? This one we know. This bacterium has been definitively associated with an assortment of serious conditions, including chronic active gastritis, stomach cancer, peptic ulcers, and lymphoma that begins in the stomach.

Modality Recommendations for Peptic Ulcers	
Deep tissue massage	Locally contraindicated while acute; otherwise slow work may assist with parasympathetic response.
Lymphatic drainage	Supportive.
Polarity	S: Indicated. R: Supportive, determined by client's comfort. D: Avoid abdomen.
PNF/MET/stretching	Supportive.
Reflexology	Indicated. Work upper GI tract and solar plexus points.
Shiatsu	Supportive. Work PC for blood supply, BL for stress, GB for digestive efficiency.
Swedish massage	Supportive; extra caution around abdomen.
Trigger point therapy	Avoid abdomen; otherwise supportive.

See Chapter 1 for a brief description of each modality, including definitions of abbreviations.

Stomach Cancer

Definition: What Is It?

Stomach cancer is the development of malignant tumors in the stomach that can block the passage of food through the digestive system, and can spread to other organs either through direct contact or through blood and lymph flow.

Stomach Cancer in Brief

What is it?
Stomach cancer is malignant tumors in the stomach that may metastasize directly to other abdominal organs or through lymph or blood flow to distant places in the body.

How is it recognized?
Symptoms of stomach cancer include a feeling of fullness after only a little food, heartburn, unintentional weight loss, anemia, blood in the stools, vague abdominal pain above the navel, and occasionally vomiting, constipation, or diarrhea.

Is massage indicated or contraindicated?
The prognosis for stomach cancer, which is rarely found before metastasis, is generally not promising. Most clients who know that they have stomach cancer will probably be undergoing a series of treatments including surgeries, chemotherapy, and radiation. Bodywork to alleviate the discomforts of cancer treatment may be appropriate as long as the risks involved with each type of intervention are respected.

Demographics: Who Gets It?

Stomach cancer used to be quite common in the United States. In much of the rest of the world, especially in Asia and South America, stomach cancer is still a major threat.

In the United States, about 23,000 people are diagnosed with stomach cancer every year, and about 14,000 people die. Most stomach cancer patients are in their 60s or 70s, and men with the disease outnumber women by almost 2 to 1.[17,18]

Most types of stomach cancer are declining in number, but cancers that occur at the *cardia*, or proximal end of the stomach, are seeing slight increases.[19]

Etiology: What Happens?

Although several types of cancer have been observed to grow from stomach cells, most stomach cancers are *adenocarcinomas*. It is not always clear what triggers the growth of these tumors, but a comparison of eating habits and the history of both refrigeration and antibiotic use yields some clues.

Stomach cancer rates in the United States began to decline in the 1930s, about the time that refrigeration became accessible for most Americans. The average diet shifted away from smoked, pickled, and salted foods and toward more fresh meats and fresh, canned, or frozen vegetables. In countries where stomach cancer is very prominent, the consumption of salted, smoked, or pickled foods is significantly higher than it is in the United States.

Most stomach cancer patients test positive for *H. pylori*. Indeed, the World Health Organization suggests that up to 50% of cases of stomach cancer worldwide are related to *H. pylori* infection.[18] This bacterium, which is associated with peptic ulcers, converts the nitrates and nitrites in high-risk foods (mainly cured meats) into carcinogens. Infection rates of this not-well-understood bacterium are relatively low in the United States.

Any situation that impedes the production of gastric digestive secretions increases the risk of stomach cancer. This can include a history of *H. pylori* infection, ***atrophic gastritis*** (long-term inflammation that destroys acid-producing cells), stomach surgery, pernicious anemia, and other factors. When the environment in the stomach is insufficiently acidic, ingested materials don't break down properly and many become carcinogenic.

As the stomach wall is assaulted with chronic exposure to carcinogenic substances, minute changes in the tissues may develop. These precancerous changes are virtually silent and are almost never detected. Malignant cells can grow into tumors large enough to obstruct the passage of food through the digestive tract, or they can invade and perforate the stomach wall, allowing them to spread to nearby abdominal organs.

By the time stomach cancer is detected, it has usually spread through the portal vein to the liver or into the lymph system. Adenocarcinomas account for 90% to 95% of stomach cancer diagnoses. Other types of cancers in the stomach include a type of non-Hodgkin lymphoma, carcinoid tumors that arise from hormone-producing cells, and stromal tumors, which can occur anywhere in the GI tract.

Risk Factors

The major risk factors for developing stomach cancer include the following:

- *H. pylori infection.* Most stomach cancer patients have *H. pylori* in their digestive tract. These bacteria have been seen to convert certain food products into carcinogens.
- *Diet.* Diets that are high in smoked food, salted fish and meats, and pickled vegetables increase the risk of developing stomach cancer. Nitrates used as food preservatives also contribute to this risk. Diets heavy in red meats (more than 13 portions per week) are seen to double stomach cancer risk. Diets that are high in fresh fruits, vegetables, and vitamin C, by contrast, may be protective against stomach cancer.
- *Tobacco and alcohol use.* These products have been associated with the development of stomach cancer, especially in the proximal portion of the stomach.
- *Other factors.* A wide variety of other factors increase stomach cancer risk, including having had previous stomach surgery, having type A blood, being male, being between 60 and 79 years old, and having the genes that have been associated with breast or colorectal cancer.

Signs and Symptoms

Signs and symptoms of stomach cancer are mostly related to having a physical obstruction in the digestive tract. They include a feeling of fullness after only a little food, vague abdominal pain above the navel, unintentional weight loss, heartburn and other ulcer symptoms, nausea and vomiting, and the development of ***ascites***: the accumulation of excessive fluid in the peritoneal space. Tumors may bleed slightly, leading to small amounts of blood in the stool. This is detected with a fecal occult blood test.

SIDEBAR 8.4: STAGING STOMACH CANCER

Stomach cancer is usually staged using a combination of the TNM (tumor, node, metastasis) and numerical (0–IV) protocols.[17]

Tumor Ratings	Node Ratings	Metastasis Ratings
T X: tumor can't be assessed.	N x: nodal involvement can't be assessed.	M x: metastasis can't be assessed.
T 0: no evidence of primary tumor.	N 0: no nodal involvement.	M 0: no metastasis.
T IS: in situ cancer, affecting mucosa only.	N 1: 1–6 nearby nodes invaded.	M 1: distant metastasis.
T 1: affects submucosal layer.	N 2: 7–15 nearby nodes invaded.	
T 2a: affects muscularis.	N 3: >15 nearby nodes invaded.	
T 2b: affects subserosa.-		
T 3: whole serosa affected; adjacent organs not involved.		
T 4: adjacent organs or blood vessels infiltrated.		

The TNM ratings are translated into stages 0 to IV:[20]

Stage	Tumor	Node	Metastasis				
0	T IS	NO	MO				
IA	T1	NO	MO				
IB	T1	N1	MO or T2a/b	MO	N 0	MO	
II	T1	N2	MO or T2a/b	MO or T3	N 0	M 0	
IIIA	T2a/b	N2	MO or T3	N1	MO or T4	NO	MO
IIIB	T3	N2	MO				
IV	T4	N1-3	MO or any T	any N	M1		

The complexities of the staging system for stomach cancer reveal the many growth patterns observed in different patients. The overall average 5-year survival rate is low but slowly improving. It has risen from 20% to 23% in the past 3 years.[19]

Diagnosis

Because the early changes that occur with stomach cancer are so subtle, in the United States it is very seldom identified before metastasis. In Japan, where it occurs about five times more frequently, mass screenings are conducted to try to find the cancer in earlier stages.

Diagnostic techniques for stomach cancer include endoscopy and biopsy; a barium wash of the upper GI tract, followed by radiographs; and an endoscopic ultrasound, CT scan, or MRI of the stomach wall to assist in staging. Staging protocols for stomach cancer are discussed in Sidebar 8.4.

Treatment

Stomach cancer is treated with the same arsenal of tools used against most cancers: chemotherapy, radiation therapy, and surgery. Undergoing a course of chemotherapy both before and after surgery has been seen to significantly improve the prognosis. Also, aggressive testing of nearby lymph nodes has been found to improve the accuracy of staging and therefore the success of treatment. The standard protocol is to test at least 15 of the hundreds of lymph nodes that lie close to the stomach.[21]

Massage?

If a client knows he or she has stomach cancer, that client is probably engaged in a combination of treatments to try to limit the spread of the disease, including chemotherapy, radiation therapy, and surgery. Cancer treatments can be extraordinarily harsh and taxing. Massage has a place in reducing pain, improving sleep, and generally supporting the process for cancer patients, as long as the cautions that accompany various cancer treatment options are respected. For more information about this topic, see Chapter 12.

Modality Recommendations for Stomach Cancer

Deep tissue massage	Supportive as part of health care team. Respect stage of recovery and treatment challenges.
Lymphatic drainage	Supportive.
Polarity	S: Indicated. R/D: Supportive, determined by client's comfort.
PNF/MET/stretching	Supportive as part of health care team; match to activity levels.
Reflexology	Indicated. Work stomach, lymphatic system, and pituitary points.
Shiatsu	Supportive. Work SP, TH meridians for immune support. Gentle generally.
Swedish massage	Supportive; depth determined by activity level.
Trigger point therapy	Supportive.

See Chapter 1 for a brief description of each modality, including definitions of abbreviations.

Disorders of the Large Intestine

Colorectal Cancer

Definition: What Is It?

Colorectal cancer is the development of tumors anywhere in the large intestine from the ascending right side to the rectum. Although the two conditions are linked, malignant colon or rectal cancer is not the same thing as the presence of *adenomas*, or colon polyps.

Demographics: Who Gets It?

Statistics on colon and rectal cancers vary, but most suggest that about 148,000 cases of these diseases are diagnosed each year, and they cause about 55,000 deaths each year.[22] This makes colorectal cancer the second leading cause of death by cancer in the United

Colorectal Cancer in Brief
Pronunciation: ko-lo-REK-tal KAN-sur

What is it?
Colorectal cancer is development of malignant tumors in the colon or rectum. Growths can block the bowel and/or metastasize to other organs.

How is it recognized?
Signs and symptoms of colorectal cancer depend on what part of the bowel is affected. The most obvious symptoms are changes in bowel habits, including diarrhea or constipation lasting more than 10 days. Other symptoms include blood in the stool, iron deficiency anemia, and unintentional weight loss.

Is massage indicated or contraindicated?
If a client is diagnosed with colon or rectal cancer in the early stages, some types of massage may be a useful supportive therapy to help deal with the side effects of cancer treatment. Colorectal cancer survivors are good candidates for massage, although the presence of a colostomy bag requires some adjustments.

States (only lung cancer is higher). That said, the death rate from colorectal cancer is on a decline, and about 1 million survivors live in the United States.[23]

Although it has traditionally been perceived as a men's disease, colorectal cancer affects men and women almost evenly. The leading demographic for developing these diseases is age: 90% of colorectal patients are over 50 years old.[23]

Etiology: What Happens?

The colon, or large bowel, is the last and widest section of the digestive tract. In this 6-foot long piece of tubing the remnants of food are compacted, water is reabsorbed into the body, and feces are stored in the rectum until they are expelled. The inner lining of the colon is composed of epithelium, which, as has been seen in other discussions of cancer, is particularly susceptible to uncontrolled cell growth.

Most colon cancers begin with the development of adenomas, small polyps in the bowel. Minor chromosome damage is believed to cause the formation of these polyps. The cells in the mucosa of the colon simply multiply without any reason and produce these small pile-ups of excess tissue (Figure 8.6). But if the polyps are present for a long period, two things happen: oncogenes are activated and tumor suppressor genes are inactivated. The net result is that cells on the surface of the colon mucosa continue to replicate and don't die off. They can invade the deeper layers of the bowel and even erode all the way through it. They can obstruct the movement of fecal matter through the GI tract (Figure 8.7). And they can metastasize through the lymph system to other places in the body, notably, the brain, liver, and lungs. This is the transition from polyps to colon cancer, and it generally happens silently, without warning.

No one knows what prompts common colon polyps, which occur in up to 50% of older Americans, to become malignant. Large polyps and ones that have been present for long periods are most likely to become cancerous (20% of polyps bigger than 2 cm have a high risk of becoming cancerous[24]), but what actually causes the shift is still a mystery. One theory is that high-fat foods linger in the colon longer than other types of food, and some of their byproducts are carcinogenic. This theory also suggests that diets that are high in fiber help

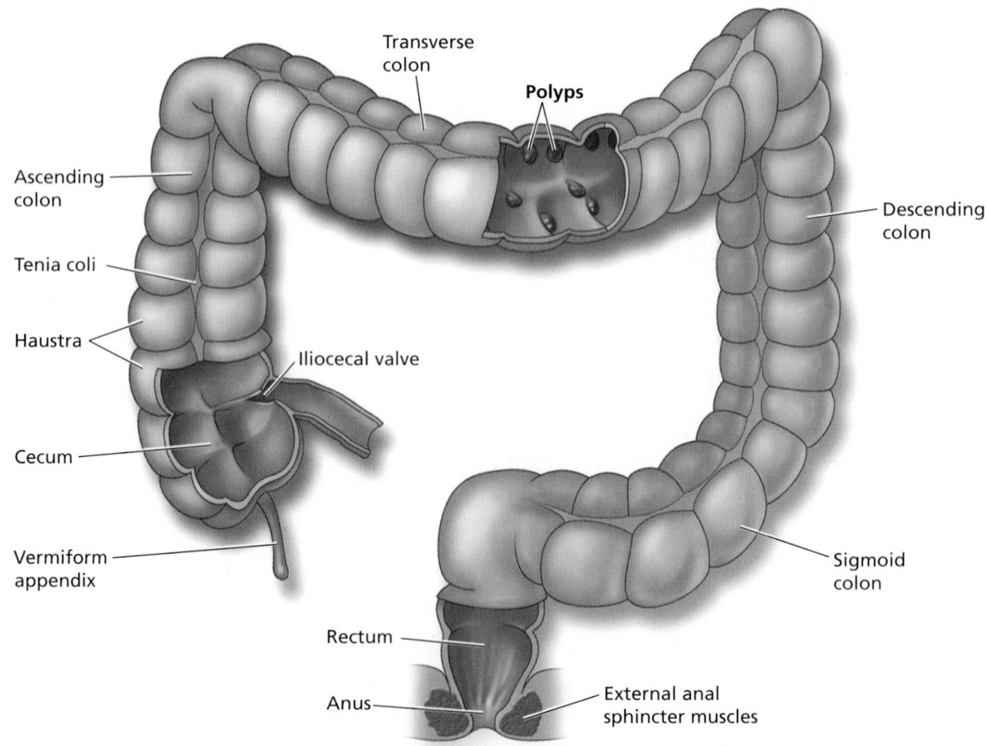

Figure 8.6. Colon polyps.

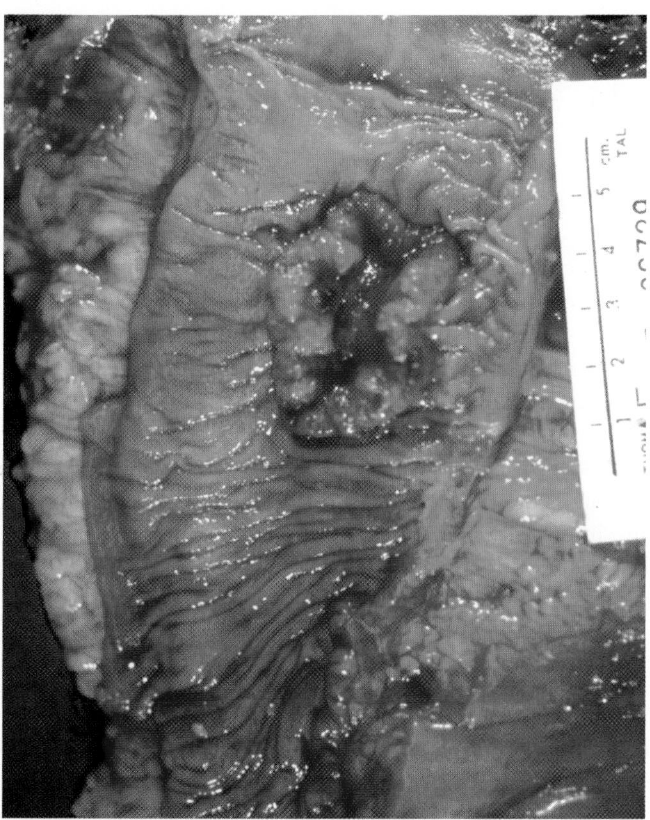

Figure 8.7. Adenocarcinoma of the colon. The opened colon contains an elevated, centrally ulcerated infiltrating mass.

material to move through the colon faster and more completely, "scrubbing" the bowel walls of damaging or irritating materials.

Research into the influence of diet and colon cancer is sometimes contradictory. General associations can be made between a high-fat, low-fiber diet and an increased risk of colorectal cancer, but when it comes to individual cases, other variables appear to influence the development of polyps and cancer, so diet is just one factor among many.

Risk Factors

As with many diseases, the risk factors for developing colorectal cancer include some that can be controlled and others that can't.

- *Obesity, sedentary lifestyle.* People who are obese have a relatively high chance of developing colon cancer. People who get little exercise are also prone to this disease; regular exercise has been shown to be protective against colorectal cancer.
- *Family history.* ***Familial adenomatous polyposis*** and ***hereditary nonpolyposis colorectal cancer syndrome*** are genetic conditions that predispose some people to the development of colorectal cancer. Familial adenomatous polyposis is sometimes known by its subgroup names, ***Gardner syndrome*** and ***Turcot syndrome***. Hereditary nonpolyposis colorectal cancer syndrome may also be called ***Lynch syndrome***. Although people with these genetic profiles have a 90% to 100% chance of developing the disease, they constitute only 5% of colorectal cancer patients. Most diagnoses are made in people who are not part of these high-risk groups.
- *Inflammatory bowel disease.* Ulcerative colitis and Crohn disease are very closely connected with colon cancer. The younger a person is when diagnosed with either of these problems, the greater the chances of eventually developing colon cancer. The risk is so

high that for some people preventive surgery to remove the whole colon is suggested before the cancer has a chance to develop.

- *Age.* The chances of having colon cancer rise with age; 90% of colon cancer patients are over 50 years of age.

Signs and Symptoms

Like so many other types of cancer, colon cancer doesn't often show distinctive symptoms until it has progressed to a dangerous stage. Symptoms vary according to where tumors grow. Cancer in the spacious ascending colon is often first manifested as unexplained anemia: tumors can bleed continuously into the colon, making less iron, and therefore less oxygen, available to body cells. Iron deficiency anemia, especially among men and postmenopausal women, is a warning sign for colon cancer.

Growths in the more constricted descending colon, however, are experienced as extreme constipation or narrowed stools. Other signs of colon cancer that a person may or may not be aware of are blood in the stools (sometimes it is obvious and bright red, sometimes it occurs in invisible, microscopic amounts), lower abdominal pain, a feeling that bowel movements are incomplete, and unintentional weight loss.

Diagnosis

Colorectal cancer isn't difficult to diagnose, but it requires some simple tests that many people choose to avoid, even though they aren't dangerous or painful. Because of this, many cases aren't found until the growths have invaded deeply into the colon wall. Nonetheless, aggressive public information campaigns, more consistent early testing, and better treatment options have resulted in a steady decline of colon cancer deaths in the past several years.

Basic screening for colon cancer for people with average risk factors begins with a yearly fecal occult blood test to look for signs of bleeding into the GI tract; this is recommended annually for people over age 40. A flexible sigmoidoscopy and/or a double-contrast barium enema are recommended every 5 years; and a full colonoscopy is suggested every 10 years after age 50.[25] A newer option, a variety of CT for the colon, continues to be refined.

Sigmoidoscopies and colonoscopies have the benefit that if polyps are found, they can be removed at the same time. (CT and barium enemas that show growths must be followed by an additional procedure to remove them.) If suspicious cells are found in a polyp, and especially if the cells are not surrounded by a margin of healthy tissue, more tests may be conducted to stage the extent of cancerous growth. For more information on colorectal cancer staging, see Sidebar 8.5.

These screening techniques sound to many people almost worse than having the disease itself. However, survival rates for people who are diagnosed early are significantly higher than for those who found their cancer late. This is a persuasive reason to follow the basic guidelines for colorectal cancer screening.

Treatment

Treatment for colon cancer depends on the stage at which it is identified. Stage I or II cancer is generally treated with surgery to remove the affected section of bowel. The remaining bowel may be sewn together if possible, or the healthy section may be connected to a colostomy bag for exterior storage and disposal of wastes.

Stage III colorectal cancer requires surgery to remove the affected length of bowel and chemotherapy to reduce the chance of metastasis through the lymph system.

Stage IV colorectal cancer is treated in much the same way as stage III but with more aggressive chemotherapy and radiation therapy to limit growths at distant sites.

The use of biologic mechanisms, specifically monoclonal antibodies, is beginning to find use in the context of colorectal cancers. These substances can inhibit the growth factors of cancer cells and have been shown to slow the growth of metastatic colorectal cancer.

SIDEBAR 8.5: STAGING COLORECTAL CANCER

The **TNM** classification system identifies the progress of tumors, lymph node involvement, and the extent of metastasis. The numerical classification is based on combinations of TNM staging, as follows:[26]

Tumor	Node	Metastasis
T x: can't be assessed	N x: can't be assessed	M x: can't be assessed
T 0: no evidence of tumor	N 0: no nodal involvement	M 0: no distant metastasis
T-IS: in situ tumor (affects mucosa only)	N 1: 1–3 nodes involved	M 1: distant metastasis
T 1: submucosa invaded	N 2: ≥4 nearby nodes involved	
T 2: muscularis invaded		
T 3: subserosa invaded		
T 4: serosa invaded; tumor may extend into other organs		

Stage	Tumor	Node	Metastasis Rate (%)	5-Year Survival
0	T-IS	N0	M0	
I	T-IS–T2	N0	M0	93
II A	T3	N0	M0	85
II B	T4	N0	M0	72
III A	T 1–T2	N1	M0	83
III B	T 3–T4	N1	M0	64
III C	T any	N2	M0	44
IV	Any	Any	M1	8

Prevention

While it has been difficult to prove specific diet and lifestyle *causes* of colorectal cancer, protective mechanisms have been somewhat easier to identify. The following habits are associated with a lower-than-average risk of developing this disease:[23]

- Eat at least five servings of fruits and vegetables every day; choose whole-grain foods.
- Reduce fats in the diet, especially saturated fats.
- Get recommended vitamins and minerals, particularly calcium, magnesium, vitamin B_6, and folate.
- Limit alcohol consumption to two drinks a day for men and one per day for women.
- Don't smoke.
- Be physically active and maintain a healthy weight.

Massage?

Clients who are fighting colorectal cancer need all the support they can get. Massage can be an important and useful addition to their therapy to help balance out the challenges of surgery, chemotherapy, and radiation therapy, as long as the cautions that accompany those treatments are respected (see Chapter 12).

Modality Recommendations for Colorectal Cancer

Modality	Recommendation
Deep tissue massage	Supportive as part of health care team. Respect stage of recovery and treatment challenges.
Lymphatic drainage	Supportive; use caution with inguinal region work.
Polarity	S: Indicated. R: Light; determined by client's comfort. D: Avoid abdomen.
PNF/MET/stretching	Supportive as part of health care team; match to activity levels.
Reflexology	Indicated. Work liver, gallbladder, pancreas, pituitary, lymphatic system, and GI tract points.
Shiatsu	Supportive. Work SP, TH for immune support.
Swedish massage	Supportive; depth determined by activity level; only light touch on abdomen.
Trigger point therapy	Locally contraindicated; otherwise supportive.

See Chapter 1 for a brief description of each modality, including definitions of abbreviations.

Colorectal cancer survivors are good candidates for massage. If they use a colostomy bag, adjustments may be needed for comfort and practicality. The best person to consult in this situation is the client.

Diverticulum

This is a Latin word from *deverto*, meaning to turn aside. Diverticula are byroads or detours in the large intestine

Diverticular Disease

Definition: What Is It?

Diverticular disease is a condition of the small intestine or colon in which the mucosal and submucosal layers of the GI tract bulge through the outer muscular layer to form a sac, or *diverticulum*. It happens most often in the descending section or sigmoid bend of the colon. These bulges may become infected, leading to diverticulitis.

Diverticular Disease in Brief

Pronunciation: dy-ver-TICK-yu-lar dih-ZEZE

What is it?
Diverticulosis is the development of small pouches that protrude from the colon or small intestine. **Diverticulitis** is the inflammation that happens when these pouches become infected. Collectively, these disorders are known as diverticular disease.

How is it recognized?
Diverticulosis is generally silent, or symptomless. It occurs much more often in the sigmoid colon than anywhere else. When inflammation (diverticulitis) is present, lower left side abdominal pain, cramping, bloating, constipation, or diarrhea may occur.

Is massage indicated or contraindicated?
Deep abdominal massage is locally contraindicated if the client knows diverticula have developed. Acute infection of diverticula systemically contraindicates circulatory massage.

Demographics: Who Gets It?

Diverticular disease is a common condition, affecting up to half of the U.S. population aged 60 to 80, and two-thirds or more of people over 85 years old.[27] Men and women are equally affected. It is diagnosed about 300,000 times each year, and about 2.5 million people in the United States are known to have diverticular disease in some form.[28]

Diverticular disease is most common in countries where diets are based on animal fats and processed grains. Interestingly, it was first documented in the early 1900s, just when new technology had been developed to remove the bran from wheat and the American diet shifted to rely heavily on low-fiber white flour.

Diverticular disease is rare in the rural parts of Asia and Africa, where the diet is built on whole grains, fruits, and vegetables.

Etiology: What Happens?

Research continues to reveal new aspects of diverticular disease. It is now considered a multifactorial condition involving a combination of inefficient colon ***motility***, changes in the strength of the colon wall, chronic low-grade infection, an imbalance in the types of bacteria present in the colon, and hypersensitivity of local neurons, leading to excessive and uncoordinated contractions in isolated areas.

Diverticula form during smooth muscle contraction in the large intestine. These contractions are very strong, but without adequate bulk (supplied by soluble and insoluble fiber) to press against, the pressure causes colon walls to bulge. This is especially problematic if the collagen matrix of the muscularis is impaired (as with Marfan syndrome or Ehlers-Danlos syndrome) or weakened by age. In this situation the mucosa and submucosa of the colon can herniate through the outer muscular layer to form small sacs, or diverticula. These sacs may be filled with fecal matter and bacteria, and the potential for infection is high (Figure 8.8). About 20% of the people diagnosed with diverticulosis eventually develop diverticulitis, or inflammation of the diverticula.[27]

Most diverticula form in the sigmoid flexure or descending colon, but they have been recorded throughout the alimentary canal, all the way up to the esophagus. They can range from about the size of a kernel of corn to the size of a walnut or even larger.

CASE HISTORY 8.2

Diverticulosis

Cathy S., aged 50: "Try warm prune juice."

My husband's mother had colon cancer. We knew what it was like to have to deal with this disease, so last August we all got checked. I had a colorectal scope that revealed a very large diverticulum. The doctor said it was big enough that he could double up the scope hose into it. I had no pain, and there was no infection. I didn't think much more about it.

For the past 10 years I've had problems with bowel movements, just being regular. I didn't think much of it. I had a hysterectomy 5 years ago and at that time I asked what would be the best way to become regular. I was told to take warm prune juice. I did it, and that took care of the problem for quite a while.

I didn't really know there was anything wrong until last April—Good Friday, as a matter of fact. It was worse than most days at work. I didn't have time to eat properly, so I snacked on graham crackers all day. By 2:00 I was just about bent over double—still charting patients, mind you, but bent over double. I just couldn't get any relief.

I continued to work until 6:00, at which point I was just about screaming (but of course not telling anybody). I went to the after-hours clinic, and they gave me prescription-strength Zantac [ranitidine] and an antibiotic. Within half an hour the pain went away—or at least resolved to the point where I could stand myself.

Having had that experience, I decided I'd better see a gastroenterologist. I had the upper and lower scope: a colonoscopy and endoscopy, and that's when they found the diverticulum again, although there was no longer any infection.

I was diagnosed with diverticulosis along with chronic inflammatory disease, which may go along with my generally hyperactive immune system.

These days I stick with a low-fat diet, and I drink *lots* of water—64 oz a day minimum. I eat small meals. I take Zantac every night, along with Relafen [nabumetone] for arthritis pain, and I've never had another episode. I receive massage regularly. Deep psoas work can often help to relieve my lower back pain, but I can't do it every time. Some days I'm just too tender.

Author's note: Cathy is a 50-year-old speech and language pathologist with a number of problems involving a hyperreactive immune system. She was recently diagnosed with multiple sclerosis. In addition to systemic arthritis, Cathy has spondylosis, a degeneration of the articular facets between L5 and S1 resulting in hypermobility of the low back, chronic pain, and a fragile state of balance that is easily disrupted by a minor force such as a cough or sneeze.

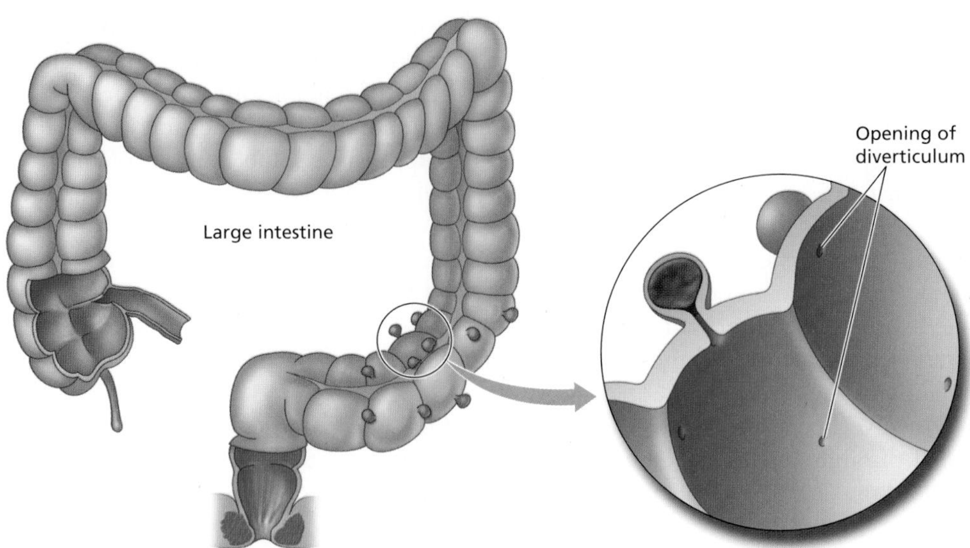

Figure 8.8. Diverticular disease.

Signs and Symptoms

Symptoms of diverticulosis may be nonexistent. When infection is present, however, symptoms include nausea, fever, cramping, and severe pain, usually on the lower left side of the abdomen. Diarrhea and or constipation may also occur. Symptoms of diverticulitis often have a sudden onset and become rapidly worse, but some people have several days of mild discomfort before severe infection sets in.

Complications

Complications of diverticulitis are rare, but they can be serious enough to become life threatening in a short amount of time. They can include the following:

- *Bleeding.* Sometimes capillaries get stretched over the dome of the protrusion, and they may tear open and bleed into the colon.
- *Abscess.* Infected diverticula may develop local collections of pus and dead white blood cells. If an abscess ruptures, its contents may be released into the peritoneum, causing peritonitis.
- *Perforation.* Diverticula may tear open and release their contents into the peritoneum. This is a medical emergency.
- *Blockage.* The accumulation of scar tissue where diverticula have formed and become infected may block the colon. A partial blockage requires medical attention but is not an emergency, but a total blockage requires immediate intervention.
- *Fistula.* Areas in the digestive tract that are damaged by inflammation have the potential to become abnormally joined to other abdominal or pelvic organs. Small passageways or ***fistulas*** may develop between the two organs, allowing the passage of fecal matter into spaces where it doesn't belong. Diverticula may connect the colon in this way with the urinary bladder, small intestine, or uterus.

Diverticular disease has not been associated with an increased risk of developing colorectal cancer, but this condition can make colon cancer more difficult to identify early. Therefore, diverticular disease patients need to take extra care to get regular screenings for colorectal cancer.

Treatment

Diverticular disease is more easily prevented than corrected. Daily fiber intake is recommended to be 25 to 30 g per day; the average American gets about 14 or 15 g per day. Without healthy amounts of soluble and insoluble fiber to create bulk in the colon, the smooth muscle has to work hard to compact fecal material and even harder to expel it from the body. The fact that vegetarians and people whose diets are built on whole grains, fruits, and vegetables seldom develop diverticular disease is an indication that healthy levels of dietary fiber can prevent this problem.

Treatment for diverticulosis alone isn't usually necessary because the symptoms are so mild or don't exist at all. Although the diverticula are not reversible, further growths can be prevented with changes toward a higher-fiber diet and exercise.

Treatment for diverticulitis starts with antibiotics and a strictly controlled diet. If substantial tissue damage has occurred, including a bowel obstruction, uncontrolled bleeding, perforation, large abscesses, or fistulas, surgery may be performed. Depending on the seriousness of the condition, surgery may involve a simple resection of the colon, removing the infected or damaged area, or it may require a temporary or permanent colostomy.

Massage?

A client probably won't know whether he or she has diverticulosis unless the colon has been scanned for some other reason. If the condition has already been diagnosed, conduct deep abdominal work with caution; the muscular wall of the colon is already structurally impaired. Acute infection of diverticula, identified by local pain with fever, chills, nausea, and diarrhea or constipation, systemically contraindicates circulatory bodywork.

Modality Recommendations for Diverticular Disease

Modality	Recommendation
Deep tissue massage	Locally contraindicated while acute; otherwise work slowly with hips, thoracolumbar fascia, distal psoas.
Lymphatic drainage	Supportive.
Polarity(S/R/D)	S: Indicated. R: Light when no pain, determined by client's comfort. D: Avoid abdomen.
PNF/MET/stretching	Locally contraindicated while acute; otherwise supportive.
Reflexology	Indicated. Work GI tract points.
Shiatsu	Supportive. Work meridians of GI tract, especially GB. Ampuku for hypogastric area.
Swedish massage	Gentle touch on abdomen can be soothing.
Trigger point therapy	Avoid abdomen always; reschedule if infection present; otherwise supportive.

See Chapter 1 for a brief description of each modality, including definitions of abbreviations.

Irritable Bowel Syndrome in Brief

What is it?
Irritable bowel syndrome (IBS) is a collection of signs and symptoms that indicate a functional problem with the digestive system, specifically the colon. Symptoms are aggravated by stress and diet.

How is it recognized?
The symptoms of IBS include abdominal pain along with constipation or diarrhea (or alternating between the two); bloating or abdominal distension; and a sensation of incomplete emptying with defecation.

Is massage indicated or contraindicated?
IBS indicates massage, as long as bodywork does not exacerbate symptoms.

Irritable Bowel Syndrome

Definition: What Is It?

Irritable bowel syndrome (IBS) is a recently acknowledged and little-understood condition involving digestive system dysfunction without structural changes. It has also been known as spastic colon, irritable colon, mucus colitis, and functional bowel syndrome.

Demographics: Who Gets It?

Statistics vary, but most agree that IBS is a relatively common condition. Some 10% to 20% of the U.S. population may have IBS symptoms at some point, although only a small fraction may seek medical help. Women are affected about three times more often than men. IBS accounts for some 5 million doctor visits each year.[29]

Etiology: What Happens?

In a normal colon, fecal matter is squeezed and compacted, while water and salts are reabsorbed into the bloodstream. Material moves back and forth through the colon, but eventually strong contractions move the formed stools into the rectum, where they are stored until another bout of strong colon contractions moves them out of the body altogether.

The development of IBS symptoms probably varies by individual, but some general observations have determined that the digestive tract as a whole and the colon in particular are hyperreactive in IBS patients. That is, small stimuli create major contractions for no discernible reason. Peristalsis, which should be smooth and rhythmic, becomes uncoordinated and irregular. People who have IBS tend to be particularly sensitive to pain and subtle changes in pressure inside the colon; this may become a diagnostic marker for this disorder.

Studies of the central nervous system of IBS patients compared with healthy individuals show that at least part of this syndrome may be connected to a dysfunction of the *brain-gut axis*, that is, the link of continuous feedback between GI tract sensation and motor response. Serotonin secretion and uptake are predictably changed in IBS patients. Interestingly, many people with IBS also have other smooth muscle tissue dysfunction, including a tendency toward neurally mediated hypotension, a condition noted in most chronic fatigue syndrome patients.[30] IBS frequently appears simultaneously with chronic fatigue syndrome and another chronic pain syndrome, fibromyalgia.

IBS very often goes hand in hand with anxiety and stress. Most people with this condition report flare-ups in conjunction with threatening situations: job interviews, examinations, major life changes, and so on. The development of IBS probably has little to do with the presence of stress per se and more to do with how the individual handles it. While some people lose sleep under stress, IBS patients lose coordinated bowel function.

Risk Factors

Many IBS patients have some factors in common, especially regarding gender and age at onset. Women with IBS outnumber men by 2 or 3 to 1, and most patients are diagnosed in adolescence to early adulthood. In addition, people who had low birth weight or any kind of prenatal compression in the uterus have a higher-than-normal risk of IBS.[31] Finally, IBS patients have a high incidence of some history of psychological trauma or abuse.[32]

CASE HISTORY 8.3

Irritable Bowel Syndrome

Debbie T., aged 29: "It's just something you ate."

I had my first attack of IBS in January 1991. I woke up out of a dead sleep. I thought I had appendicitis or something. I had diarrhea, I was throwing up, I had never hurt that bad. There was no warning, no buildup, it was just there. I hurt so bad I passed out. My husband called the ambulance and I went to the hospital. In the ambulance they asked about my sunburn—I was completely covered with a red rash. The rash only happened the first time.

At the hospital they gave me something through an IV [intravenous infusion] that was supposed to coat my stomach. They said I probably had food poisoning.

Then, 4 months later, it happened again. I woke up out of a dead sleep and ended up in the hospital. And 4 months later, there I was again. It was so painful I was really noisy, but I didn't care. They took a bunch of blood samples, but they didn't show anything. "It's just something you ate," they kept saying. It got to where they would recognize me coming in and knew exactly what to do.

When the attacks started happening more and more frequently, I finally went to see a gastroenterologist. He said, "Write down everything you eat, and call me from the hospital next time it happens." I knew it wasn't anything I was eating. I'd get attacks after a bowl of cereal! And I didn't want another attack to happen. People said it was lactose intolerance, but I have milk all the time, and my attacks didn't happen all the time.

The next time was 2 months later. I was in the hospital, and they decided to do a blood gas test. They have to stick the needle into an artery to do that. It is no fun. I couldn't have any medication, and I was supposed to lie completely still. Well, they couldn't get the needle in. My gastroenterologist said, "If you can't get the blood gas, I won't see you again." That's when I switched to a different doctor.

I told my new doctor what was happening, and he scheduled me for a colonoscopy right away. He looked at that; he was looking for ulcers or tumors or something, but there was nothing, and he diagnosed me with irritable bowel syndrome. He put me on 25 mg of amitriptyline, a mild antidepressant, and it cleared right up.

The only problem with the medicine was that I wanted to get pregnant again. I tried to go off it but found I couldn't go more than one day without another attack.

It was only after all this that I was finally told that IBS is a stress-related disease. I had sort of noticed a pattern: every time I had company, I would have an attack. Whenever my sister came to visit, she would stay with my son while my husband would take me to the hospital. Every time I went on vacation, I'd get so stressed because I didn't know where the hospital was, and sure enough, I'd need to go to one. My doctor said, "Get biofeedback." Well, I'd never even heard of biofeedback, and my insurance company wouldn't cover it. I didn't know what to do.

When I went through a divorce, I stopped taking the amitriptyline, and I didn't have any more major attacks. I went to counseling for a long time to help with other things, and now I'm taking a different antidepressant. I haven't seen my gastroenterologist in over a year.

These days I occasionally have a mild episode. Really greasy food tends to aggravate my stomach. I have found that if I can wake up before my stomachaches get really bad, and if I can make myself breathe slow and deep, I can make them go away—it takes about 20 minutes. But if I get all worked up and lose control, they just get worse and worse, and I have to go to the hospital. I haven't had to do that for a long time.

Signs and Symptoms

IBS can manifest in a variety of ways. Abdominal pain is a consistent symptom, along with cramps, gas, bloating, constipation and/or diarrhea, and a frequent need to defecate, although a feeling of incomplete evacuation is often present. Abdominal pain is usually relieved after bowel movements. This disorder is sometimes classified as IBS-D when diarrhea is the predominant symptom; IBS-C when constipation is the predominant symptom; or IBS-M or IBS-A (mixed or alternating) for people with both diarrhea and constipation.

The changes brought about by IBS are purely functional; no structural anomalies develop because of this disorder. For this reason, if a person with IBS develops a fever or has blood in the stool, IBS is *not* the cause, and symptoms should be reported to a physician.

Diagnosis

IBS can range from occasionally inconvenient to severely debilitating, but it is not a life-threatening disease. Its symptoms can mimic several serious digestive system conditions, however. In particular, diverticulitis, colon cancer, ulcerative colitis, and Crohn disease must be eliminated as possibilities. Other GI tract problems that mimic IBS include parasitic infestations (i.e., *Giardia*), celiac disease, food allergies, and chronic infections.

Some IBS patients develop long-term symptoms after a bout of acute gastroenteritis. Tissue studies of these patients reveal the possibility of low-grade inflammation, which may indicate the presence of infection. This is significant finding, as it suggests treatment options that are not successful with other IBS patients.

No definitive test identifies IBS; it is diagnosed in the absence of other conditions that may cause similar symptoms. Fortunately, this isn't difficult to do. A colonoscopy can confirm that no structural change or damage to the colon has occurred, and it may also show the characteristic uncoordinated contraction of the colon to aid in diagnosis.

Treatment

Treatment for IBS depends on the individual. The first recourse is to consider dietary and stress factors. Nicotine, caffeine, alcohol, the artificial sweetener sorbitol, and dairy products have been found to be particularly irritating, but no particular food or drink is a definitive trigger for IBS attacks for all patients. Some doctors recommend fiber supplementation; the addition of bulk to the diet can fill the colon more completely and help to limit spasm.

Some drugs have been developed specifically for IBS, but they have some potentially serious side effects and so are used only under close observation. Drug intervention usually involves antispasmodics, antidiarrheals, antacids, and antidepressants. Although these medicines may offer some relief, IBS is generally considered to be a lifelong condition, and so patients are encouraged to find their own best ways to cope by use of dietary changes, therapy, and relaxation techniques.

Alternative treatments for IBS have found some success. Acupuncture, peppermint, and the use of probiotics to restore normal intestinal bacteria have shown success with some patients.[33]

Massage?

Massage is useful for many IBS patients, if the individual welcomes this kind of stimulus. It is important to treat these clients very conservatively, especially with any mechanical work around the abdomen, but many of them respond well to the autonomic balancing that bodywork provides.

Modality Recommendations for Irritable Bowel Syndrome	
Deep tissue massage	Contraindicated while acute; otherwise supportive. Work slowly with side-lying pelvis, iliac crest, thoracolumbar fascia.
Lymphatic drainage	Supportive when not in flare.
Polarity	S: Indicated. R: Light when no pain; determined by client's comfort. D: Avoid abdomen.
PNF/MET/stretching	Supportive.
Reflexology	Indicated. Work intestinal tract; can progress to whole GI tract.
Shiatsu	Supportive. Work SP, LI meridians; TH, LI extensions, associated points from thorax to sacrum; clockwise ampuku.
Swedish massage	Do only gentle work if symptoms are present; avoid compression over abdomen.
Trigger point therapy	Avoid abdomen; otherwise supportive.

See Chapter 1 for a brief description of each modality, including definitions of abbreviations.

Ulcerative colitis

Definition: What Is It?

Ulcerative colitis is a disease involving inflammation and shallow ulcers in the colon. Ulcerative colitis and Crohn disease are sometimes referred to collectively as *inflammatory bowel disease*. The inflammation with ulcerative colitis is limited to the large intestine, however, which distinguishes it from Crohn disease. For more information on the connections between Crohn disease and ulcerative colitis, see Compare and Contrast 8.1.

Demographics: Who Gets It?

Ulcerative colitis affects men and women about equally. Most patients are diagnosed between ages 15 and 25 or ages 55 and 65. It is estimated that about 1 million Americans have some type of inflammatory bowel disease and that they are more or less evenly split between ulcerative colitis and Crohn disease.[34]

Etiology: What Happens?

The initial cause of ulcerative colitis is a subject of some debate. Although no definitive trigger has been identified, most researchers now agree that it is an autoimmune disease. Studies show that people with IBD have poor tolerance for antigens in the GI tract. An open question remains, however, about whether ulcerative colitis is an immune system attack against certain bacteria or viruses that damages the lining of the colon, or whether it involves an attack against the colon mucosa itself (or whether it starts as one and progresses to the other).

Ulcerative Colitis in Brief
Pronunciation: UL-ser-ah-tiv ko-LI-tis

What is it?
Ulcerative colitis is a condition in which the mucosal layer of the colon becomes inflamed and develops shallow ulcers.

How is it recognized?
Symptoms of acute ulcerative colitis include abdominal cramping pain, chronic diarrhea, blood and pus in stools, weight loss, and mild fever.

Is massage indicated or contraindicated?
Acute ulcerative colitis contraindicates circulatory massage at least locally. In subacute situations *gentle* abdominal massage may be helpful, but only within the tolerance of the client. Massage elsewhere is probably safe and appropriate.

Ulcerative colitis usually begins in the rectum when immune system cells attack the most superficial layer of the colon. The resulting inflammation kills tissue and results in the formation of shallow ulcers: open sores that may never fully heal. Colon function is extremely limited, and the patient has chronic bloody diarrhea. The sores may become infected, leading to the release of blood and pus in the stools.

Ulcerative colitis is classified by what part or parts of the colon are affected. Disease that is limited to the rectum is called *ulcerative proctitis*; *left-sided colitis* involves the descending colon; *pancolitis* describes inflammation of the entire colon. The most extreme and dangerous form of ulcerative colitis is *fulminant colitis*. In this condition the whole colon is acutely inflamed and ulcerated, and the risk of life-threatening complications is high.

Most people with ulcerative colitis undergo damage that reaches a relatively stable plateau. While some progress from limited disease to fulminant colitis, this is fairly rare. About half of ulcerative colitis patients have it in a mild form.

Signs and Symptoms

Symptoms of ulcerative colitis depend largely on how much of the bowel is affected: the greater the extent of inflammation, the worse the symptoms tend to be. Symptoms tend to run in cycles of flare and remission. During flares the primary symptom is painful chronic diarrhea with blood and pus in the stools. Abdominal cramping, loss of appetite, and mild fever may also occur during acute episodes.

The inflammatory nature of this disease often affects other systems in the body. A person with ulcerative colitis may also have inflammation of the liver or gallbladder ducts, arthritis, osteoporosis, anemia from blood loss, and kidney stones from the disruption in electrolyte balance and chronic dehydration that accompanies long-term diarrhea. ***Uveitis***, or inflammation of structures in the eye, may result in permanent vision loss if it is not treated. Some skin disruptions are also associated with ulcerative colitis; these may occur in connection with flares or may outlive a flare to be a chronic infection.

Between acute episodes the ulcerative colitis patient may have only minimal abdominal pain but must be careful to avoid any triggers of abdominal cramping or discomfort.

Diagnosis

Ulcerative colitis is diagnosed through a variety of tests. Blood tests show signs of anemia and inflammatory cells and chemicals; stool samples reveal whether rectal bleeding is taking place. A sigmoidoscopy or colonoscopy can show specific sites of ulcers, which may be sampled for biopsy to examine them for signs of infection or cancer.

It is important to reach a clear diagnosis of ulcerative colitis because the other two conditions that its symptoms sometimes mimic require different courses of treatment. The two conditions occasionally confused with ulcerative colitis are IBS and Crohn disease.

Complications

In addition to the disorders listed among symptoms, patients with ulcerative colitis that involves the whole colon are at significantly more risk for developing colorectal cancer than the general population. This risk goes up significantly 8 to 10 years after diagnosis of ulcerative colitis. In very rare situations the colon may swell to the point that it is in danger of rupture. This is called ***toxic megacolon***, and it is a medical emergency.

Treatment

Treatment options for ulcerative colitis begin with a class of medications that lessen the severity of flare-ups and prolong periods of remission. If these don't control the inflammation satisfactorily, corticosteroids may be prescribed for short periods. Immunosuppressive drugs and, surprisingly, nicotine patches have also been found to improve symptoms.

If a patient does not get relief with these options or if inflammation of the colon has progressed to a dangerous degree, surgery is the only permanent solution. Anywhere between 20 and 40% of ulcerative colitis patients eventually require surgery. Several surgical options have been developed, but all of them involve the removal of the entire bowel. External colostomy bags, internal colostomy bags, and the joining of the small intestine to the muscles of the rectum are options for replacing the main functions of the colon.

Massage?

Ulcerative colitis contraindicates local mechanical circulatory massage. Deep abdominal work is inappropriate for a client with ulcerative colitis in any stage. In periods of remission gentle massage to the abdomen may be useful within the client's tolerance, and any other work to balance the autonomic nervous system is highly called for.

Modality Recommendations for Ulcerative Colitis	
Deep tissue massage	Contraindicated while acute; otherwise slow work may assist with parasympathetic response.
Lymphatic drainage	Supportive when not in flare.
Polarity	S: Indicated. R: Light when no pain and to comfort of client. D: Avoid abdomen.
PNF/MET/stretching	Locally contraindicated while in flare; otherwise supportive.
Reflexology	Indicated. Work large intestine points.
Shiatsu	Supportive. Work GI meridians GB, LI, ST, SP. Ampuku, associated points from thorax through sacrum.
Swedish massage	Contraindicated during flare; gentle touch on abdomen is soothing between episodes.
Trigger point therapy	Avoid abdomen; don't work when fever is present. Otherwise supportive.

See Chapter 1 for a brief description of each modality, including definitions of abbreviations.

Disorders of the Accessory Organs

Cirrhosis

Definition: What Is It?

Cirrhosis is a result of a disease process rather than a disease itself. It consists of the crowding out and replacement of healthy liver cells with nonfunctioning scar tissue. Cirrhosis can interfere with virtually every function of the liver, with potentially fatal repercussions.

Demographics: Who Gets It?

Cirrhosis is difficult to track statistically because it is a result of many other liver problems. About 500,000 hospitalizations and about 26,000 deaths are attributed to cirrhosis each year.[35]

Cirrhosis

This Greek word is from the roots *kirrhos* (yellow) and *osis*, (condition). Thus it is easy to see the association between cirrhosis and a related condition, jaundice, which comes from the French word *jaune*, meaning yellow.

Cirrhosis in Brief
Pronunciation: sir-OH-sis

What is it?
Cirrhosis is a condition in which normal liver cells become disorganized and dysfunctional; many of them are replaced or crowded out by scar tissue. Cirrhosis is often the final stage of chronic or acute liver disease.

How is it recognized?
Early symptoms of cirrhosis include loss of appetite, nausea, vomiting, and weight loss. Later complications may include muscle wasting, jaundice, ascites, internal bleeding, vomiting blood, and mental and personality changes.

Is massage indicated or contraindicated?
Advanced cirrhosis is associated with difficulties with fluid flow in the body. Bodywork that challenges this function may not be appropriate. Some cirrhosis patients have muscle wasting as their ability to metabolize proteins diminishes. Exercise and physical therapy are recommended for these patients for maintenance of strength and function, and massage as part of a health care team may have a role in this process as well.

It is listed as the ninth leading cause of death in the United States[36] and it is estimated to shorten a normal lifespan by about 22 years.[37]

Etiology: What Happens?

The liver is composed of highly organized layers of epithelial hepatocytes: cells that produce a myriad of vital chemicals for metabolism and survival. The liver produces bile, which helps to metabolize fats, and other enzymes that metabolize proteins and carbohydrates. Clotting factors, proteins that maintain the proper balance of tissue fluid, and cells that help filter and neutralize toxins and hormones are all produced in the liver.

Under normal circumstances the liver is a remarkably forgiving organ with great powers of regeneration. But sometimes chronic long-term irritation or infection suppresses the regeneration of healthy, organized cells and stimulates the proliferation of extracellular matrix, that is, collagen and other substances that are meant to provide structural support for the active hepatocytes. When this happens the tiny channels that are meant to direct fluid flow to the appropriate vessels become blocked, and the liver, the largest gland in the body, becomes congested with blood, lymph, bile, and other fluids.

Cirrhotic deposits of scar tissue are interspersed with small nodules of functioning cells, giving the liver a characteristically knobby, bumpy appearance, hence the nickname hobnailed liver (Figure 8.9). In the early stages cirrhosis causes the liver to enlarge. But as the connective tissue contracts, the liver sometimes returns to normal or smaller size, although not to normal function.

Until recently alcoholism was considered to be the leading cause of cirrhosis in the United States. Now hepatitis C probably causes cirrhosis at least as often as long-term alcohol abuse. Cirrhosis can also arise from types B, D, drug-related, and autoimmune hepatitis.

A new discussion of risk factors for cirrhosis has arisen with the identification of another important contributor to liver damage. ***Nonalcoholic fatty liver disease*** (NAFLD) is now recognized as a significant contributor to cirrhosis. This condition is the result of deposition of fatty tissue in the liver, often as a complication of obesity, type 2 diabetes, and high triglycerides. The incidence of NAFLD is surprisingly high: experts suggest that 10% to 30% of American adults may have it in some form.[36,38] NAFLD progresses to another condition, ***nonalcoholic steatohepatitis*** (NASH) in 2% to 5% of adults. Steatohepatitis is inflammation of fatty tissue in the liver. Chronic inflammation is linked to the formation of excessive connective tissue, the hallmark of cirrhosis. The rising incidence of both NAFLD and NASH led researchers to predict that cirrhosis rates will continue to climb in this country.

Other causes for cirrhosis include any factor that can obstruct the bile duct, including gallstones, pancreatic tumors, and congenital malformation of the bile duct system. Long-term exposure to environmental toxins can contribute to cirrhosis, as can congestive heart failure and some congenital diseases.

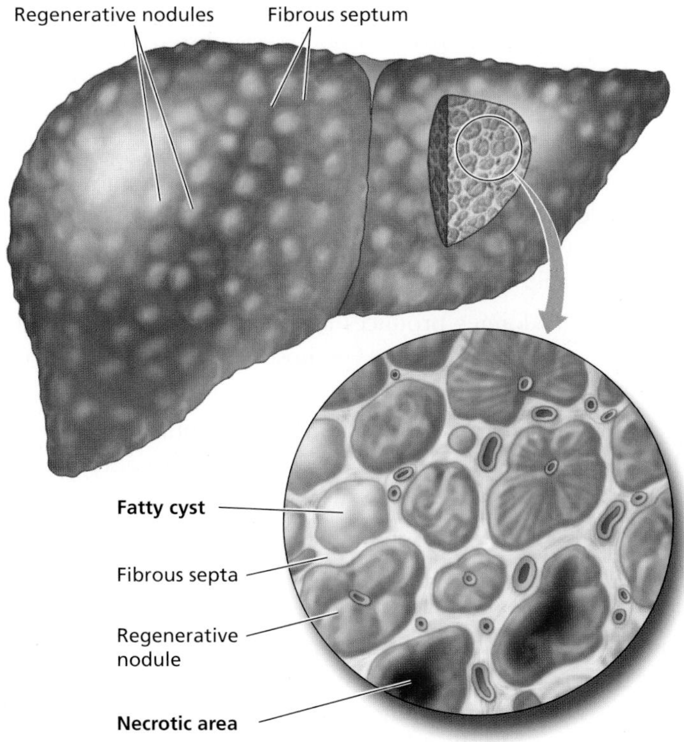

Figure 8.9. Cirrhosis: scarring of the liver.

Signs and Symptoms

Cirrhosis is often silent until it is quite advanced. Early symptoms are vague and can be attributed to any number of other common disorders. They include nausea, vomiting, weight loss, and the development of red or itchy patches on the skin. At this point in development, blood tests may be normal; no clear signs may point directly to cirrhosis. Later symptoms are usually identified by the complications discussed next.

Complications

As the liver loses more and more function, complications arise according to the parts of the liver affected and the speed of progression. The complications vary from one patient to another; it all depends on which part or parts of the liver are under attack. At the center of several complications is ***portal hypertension***. In this condition the liver becomes so congested that it cannot freely accept blood delivered from the digestive and accessory organs via the portal system, and pressure accumulates in the portal system veins. Other complications arise as the liver simply no longer produces enough vital blood components or inadequately filters and neutralizes hormones and toxic materials.

- *Splenomegaly (enlarged spleen).* The spleen enlarges because it can't drain through the portal vein. The danger with splenomegaly is that when fluid backs up in this organ, the risk of rupture and internal hemorrhage is high.

- *Ascites.* When pressure in the portal system increases, plasma seeps out of the veins and lymphatic vessels into the peritoneal space, causing the abdominal distension known as ascites (Figure 8.10). The bacteria that normally inhabit the GI tract may seep out to set up an infection in this fluid, causing spontaneous bacterial peritonitis, a life-threatening infection.
- *Internal varices.* Pressure in abdominal veins grows as fluid backs up through the system. This can lead to internal venous distensions and varicosities, especially in the esophagus and stomach. Varicose veins can hemorrhage during vomiting, leading to bloody vomit, internal bleeding, shock, or death.
- *Bleeding, bruising.* When the liver no longer produces adequate clotting factors, the ability to heal from minor injury is severely impaired. Cirrhosis patients may bruise extensively and bleed for abnormally long periods.
- *Osteoporosis.* The liver helps to process vitamin D. Without this function, it is impossible to absorb adequate calcium from the diet, so osteoporosis is likely to develop.
- *Muscle wasting.* When the enzymes that aid in protein metabolism are in short supply, a cirrhosis patient may undergo progressive atrophy, or wasting, of the skeletal muscles. Physical therapy and exercise are often recommended to patients with this problem to minimize permanent loss of bulk and function.
- *Jaundice.* Bilirubin (a byproduct of dead red blood cells) is produced in the spleen, and it is meant to be recycled in the liver to be a component of bile. When cirrhosis interferes with this process, water-soluble components of bilirubin accumulate in the bloodstream. Bilirubin is strongly pigmented, and it can turn the sclera of the eyes and skin a yellowish color. It can also cause rashes and itching, as some people have an extreme reaction to this unfamiliar chemical in their skin (Figure 8.11). Jaundice is discussed further in Sidebar 8.6.
- *Systemic edema.* One of the critical proteins for maintaining fluid balance in the body, ***albumin***, is significantly lowered in advanced cirrhosis. Without albumin, the body cannot maintain proper fluid levels, and edema accumulates systemically in all interstitial spaces.
- *Hormone disruption.* The liver of men with cirrhosis no longer inactivates their normal low levels of estrogen; feminizing characteristics such as breast development, loss of chest hair, impotence, and atrophy of the testicles soon follow. For women, hormonal changes include the cessation of periods, infertility, and the growth of body hair. Both men and women with cirrhosis can expect a decreased sex drive.

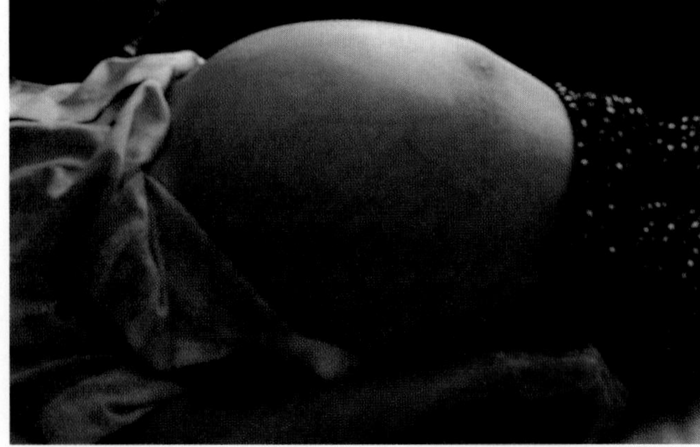

Figure 8.10. Cirrhosis leading to abdominal distension, or ascites.

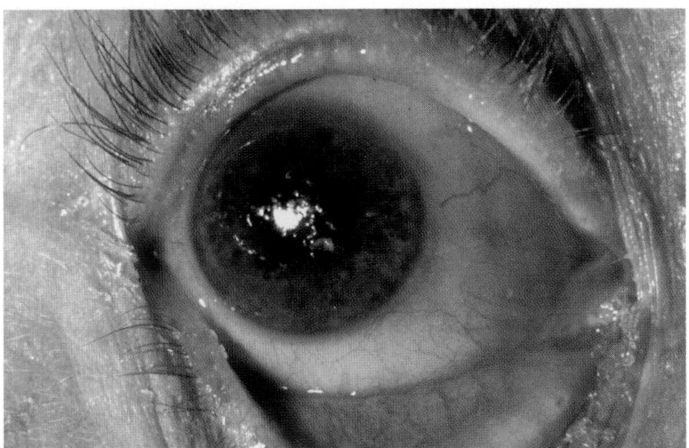

Figure 8.11. Yellowing sclera of the eye with jaundice.

- *Encephalopathy.* When cirrhosis is very advanced, the detoxifying agents in the liver are out of commission. Protection from the chemicals (ammonia, for instance) that are produced whenever protein is metabolized is no longer provided. Furthermore, the blood-brain barrier, which usually keeps the central nervous system safe, becomes much less effective with cirrhosis. Metabolic toxins accumulate in the blood and eventually cause brain damage. Symptoms include somnolence, confusion, tremors, hallucinations, even coma and death.
- *Kidney failure.* Advanced cirrhosis can reduce blood flow to the kidneys, resulting in kidney failure. ***Hepatorenal syndrome*** is an emergency that requires a liver transplant for survival.
- *Liver failure.* The progressive loss of liver function can lead to a failure of the liver to keep up with daily needs. A person with end-stage liver failure is a candidate for a liver transplant.
- *Liver cancer.* Chronic inflammation in the liver increases the risk of cellular mutation and liver cancer.

SIDEBAR 8.6: WHAT IS JAUNDICE?

Jaundice, from the French *jaune* (yellow), is also called *icterus*. It is not a disease in itself but a symptom of some underlying pathology.

One of the functions of the liver is to turn bilirubin into bile. (Bilirubin is the dark pigmented material recovered by the spleen from dead erythrocytes.) Bile drips from the liver to the gallbladder, which squirts it into the duodenum when fatty food is present. Bile helps hold particles of fat in suspension, so that fat-dissolving enzymes from the pancreas can break them down effectively. Eventually all bilirubin gets into the digestive tract, where it is a coloring agent for feces.

When dark reddish-brown bilirubin can't leave the liver for a variety of reasons, it accumulates in the bloodstream. Eventually it can visibly stain the skin, the mucous membranes, and the sclera of the eyes.

Several types of jaundice have been identified, each one categorized by the pathology that created the problem. *Neonatal jaundice* occurs in newborns when the liver is not mature enough to keep up with the turnover of fetal red blood cells. It takes a few days to catch up with this extra workload. Treatment is usually exposure to bili-lights, which stimulate liver activity. In *hemolytic jaundice*, red blood cells break down too fast, overwhelming the spleen and liver with too much material: this is seen with sickle cell disease, mismatched blood transfusions, and some infections. *Hepatic jaundice* is a result of internal liver dysfunction due to scar tissue, infection, or a congenital malfunction of enzyme systems. And *extrahepatic jaundice* is a result of a mechanical obstruction outside the liver. Gallstones, pancreatic tumors, or tumors in the GI tract are usually responsible.

A person with jaundice is most likely to have yellow-tinted skin, mucous membranes, and sclera of the eyes; while the urine commonly is dark. This reflects the accumulation of bilirubin in the bloodstream, some of which is removed by the kidneys. In contrast, stools tend to become light or clay-colored, because the bilirubin doesn't enter the GI tract.

Jaundice is an indication that the liver is overtaxed and unable to function normally. Massage in this situation must be adjusted to accommodate the fact that fluid flow in the abdomen (and consequently everywhere else) is impeded.

Treatment

The prognosis for someone in the early stages of cirrhosis caused by alcoholism is excellent *if* the damage can be stopped. That is the main treatment objective: *stop the damage*. Medication is sometimes administered to counteract the complications of the disease: diuretics for edema, antacids for intestinal discomfort, ***levulose***, an undigestible sugar, to bind with ammonia so that it can be excreted. Vitamins are recommended to guard against malnutrition. Cirrhosis due to hepatitis is treated with interferon as an antiviral measure. Steroids for inflammation due to autoimmune hepatitis are occasionally prescribed.

New options in medical interventions for cirrhosis are being aggressively pursued. A recent study showed that colchicine, a drug used to treat gout, can delay the progression of cirrhosis to liver cancer,[39] and investigation into a traditional herbal remedy for liver problems, milk thistle (*Silybum marianum*) has shown significant promise.[40]

In the short run, however, increasing numbers of people with cirrhosis are hoping for a liver transplant. In this country about 5,000 liver transplants are performed each year. About 18,000 people are on the waiting list, and 12% to 15% of those hoping for a liver die before one becomes available. The good news about liver transplants is that new procedures allow for living donors: 60% of a liver can be transplanted from a healthy donor to a recipient, and both donor and recipient can expect to have full-sized healthy livers within a short period.[36] This innovation, which has been available only since 1998, has brightened the outlook for many cirrhosis patients.

Massage?

Advanced cirrhosis contraindicates rigorous circulatory massage because the circulatory system is simply not equipped to handle the changes this work brings about. Noncirculatory work may be helpful and supportive, and massage with the goal of helping to maintain muscle health may also be appropriate. Bodywork for cirrhosis patients should be administered as part of an integrated health care effort.

Modality Recommendations for Cirrhosis	
Deep tissue massage	Systemically contraindicated in advanced stages.
Lymphatic drainage	Supportive.
Polarity	S: Indicated. R: Light, depending on toxicity. D: Avoid.
PNF/MET/stretching	Supportive.
Reflexology	Indicated with light touch and short sessions. Work liver points. Can add gallbladder, pancreas, lymphatic system.
Shiatsu	Supportive. Manage symptoms with work at lower rib cage, hypogastric, navel areas; base of skull; paraspinals mid thorax to mid lumbar.
Swedish massage	Only gentle work is appropriate; toxic balance is precarious.
Trigger point therapy	Supportive; light work in advanced stages.

See Chapter 1 for a brief description of each modality, including definitions of abbreviations.

Gallstones

Definition: What Are They?

The technical term for gallbladder is ***cholecyst***, because it is a cyst (holding tank) that collects, among other things, cholesterol. The formation of tiny crystals or stones in the gallbladder itself is called ***cholelithiasis***. Inflammation of the gallbladder from a stuck stone or other cause is called ***cholecystitis***. When stones become lodged in the common bile duct, the condition is called ***choledocholithiasis***. Inflammation of any of the ducts in the biliary system (the exocrine ducts of the liver, gallbladder, and pancreas) is called ***cholangitis***.

While these terms are fun to decipher, they actually have little to do with making a decision about massage for a client who has gallstones.

Demographics: Who Gets Them?

Gallstones are a fairly common condition, affecting some 42 million people in the United States. Not all people with gallstones have symptoms, however. Gallstones lead to about 800,000 hospitalizations and 500,000 surgeries each year.[41]

Women are far more prone to developing gallstones than men are; depending on age, they outnumber men by about 2 to 1. Some races show a predilection for gallstones; Native Americans and Mexican Americans all have higher incidences of gallstones than other population groups. Other contributing factors for developing gallstones are discussed shortly.

Gallstones in Brief

What are they?
Gallstones are crystallized formations of cholesterol or bile pigments in the gallbladder. They can be as small as a grain of sand or as large as a golf ball.

How are they recognized?
Most gallstones do not cause symptoms. When they do, pain that may last several hours develops in the upper right side of the abdomen. Pain may refer to the back between the scapula and the right shoulder. Gallstones stuck in the ducts of the biliary system may cause jaundice or pancreatitis.

Is massage indicated or contraindicated?
Silent (symptomless) stones have little impact on overall health and function, so massage for these clients is certainly appropriate, although draining strokes over the liver are contraindicated. A client with a history of gallstones but no present symptoms is fine for massage.

Etiology: What Happens?

Bile is produced in the liver and delivered to the gallbladder through the hepatic duct and the cystic duct (Figure 8.12). When a person eats a high-fat meal, hormonal commands cause the gallbladder to release its contents into the cystic duct. The bile flows into the common bile duct, and then into the small intestine. Pancreatic secretions also use the common bile duct for access to the small intestine.

The purpose of bile is to hold particles of fat in tiny, discrete pieces so that they can be absorbed into the lacteals, that is, lymphatic projections in the intestinal villi. Without bile, fat particles tend to stick together in indigestible clumps. This reduces access to important fat-soluble vitamins and nutrients.

Bile is primarily made up of water, bile salts (which help in fat digestion), bilirubin from recycled red blood cells, and cholesterol, which is filtered out of the bloodstream by the liver. When either cholesterol or bilirubin occurs in higher-than-normal concentrations in bile, they can precipitate out of the liquid to become tiny granules called "bile sludge", or larger stones (Figure 8.13).

Most gallstones (80%–90%) are composed of cholesterol. The others are made of bilirubin, the coloring agent for feces. Bilirubin stones are also called "pigment stones". They are usually a sign of some type of blood dysfunction that causes premature destruction of red blood cells, resulting in abnormally high levels of bilirubin in the blood and in the liver.

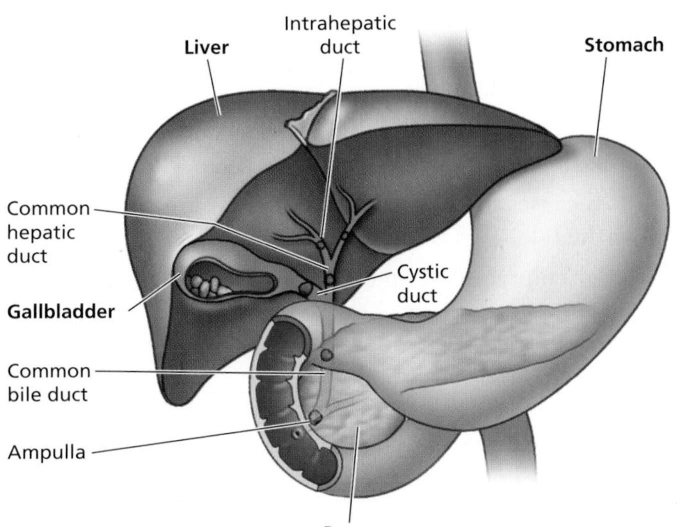

Figure 8.12. Gallstones may become lodged anywhere in the duct system.

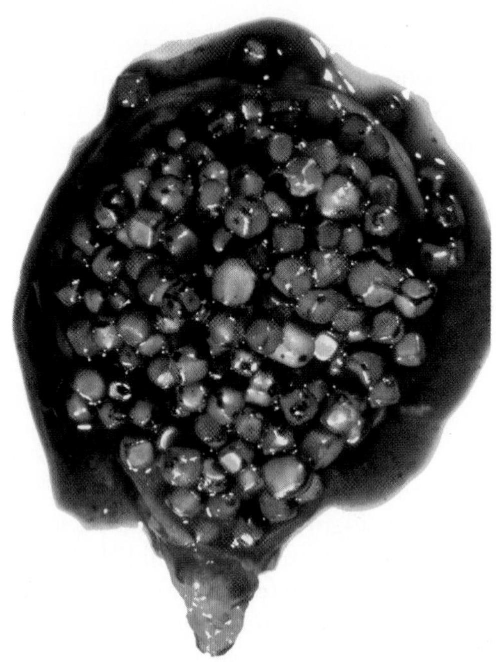

Figure 8.13. Gallstones.

Contributing factors Cholesterol stones are the most common type of gallstones. Several factors can increase the risk of developing cholesterol stones, including the following:

- *Obesity.* Obesity increases the amount of cholesterol manufactured by the liver and stored in the gallbladder.
- *Estrogen.* Estrogen tends to increase the amount of cholesterol in bile while decreasing gallbladder activity, which allows the cholesterol to crystallize. Estrogen levels may be related to pregnancy, birth control pills, or hormone replacement therapy.
- *Race.* Native Americans and Mexican Americans have the highest incidence of gallstones of any specific racial groups.
- *Gender.* Women age 16 to 60 with gallstones outnumber men by about 2 to 1.
- *Cholesterol-lowering drugs.* Drugs that are designed to lower blood cholesterol help to concentrate cholesterol in the gallbladder, increasing the risk of forming stones.
- *Diabetes.* Diabetics have high levels of triglycerides, which raises the risk for gallstones.
- *Rapid weight loss.* Rapid weight loss causes the liver to metabolize fat for fuel, resulting in higher levels of cholesterol in the bile.
- *Fasting.* Fasting reduces gallbladder emptying, so bile becomes concentrated and cholesterol precipitates out into stones.

Signs and Symptoms

Most people who have gallstones never have symptoms. The most common reason a person *does* have symptoms is that a stone has lodged in the hepatic duct, the cystic duct, or lower down in the common bile duct. The pain is excruciating and is referred to as biliary colic. (Colic is the spasmodic contraction of involuntary muscle, in this case in the common bile duct.) This extreme local pain often lasts for hours, building to a peak, and then gradually subsiding when the stone moves back into either the gallbladder or the duodenum. The pain may be intense enough to induce nausea and vomiting. If the stone gets immovably stuck, the patient may require hospitalization to have it surgically removed.

The gallbladder refers pain between the shoulder blades and over the right shoulder. Although most patients have pain in the upper right-hand quadrant of the abdomen, some feel it primarily in the back, where even the most gifted massage in the world won't relieve it.

Complications

Gallstones in themselves are not usually a serious threat, but they can create some unpleasant or even life-threatening complications. The most obvious is an obstruction of the cystic or hepatic duct, which can lead to jaundice. If the clog is distal to where the pancreas adds its secretions to the common bile duct, the pancreas can also sustain damage from a backup of its highly corrosive digestive juices; this is acute pancreatitis, and gallstones are the leading cause of this disorder. The pooling of stagnant bile can also lead to infection of the gallbladder, or cholecystitis. It is possible for an infected gallbladder to rupture, releasing its contents and causing peritonitis.

SIDEBAR 8.7: LOSE THE GALLBLADDER, KEEP THE FAT

Bile, manufactured in the liver and stored in the gallbladder, suspends consumed fats in tiny pieces so the body can absorb and digest them in the small intestine. A person who loses the gallbladder has less access to incoming fat and so absorbs less fat from the diet.

Why, then, do gallbladder surgery patients *not* lose a lot of weight after surgery? (We know they *don't*, because if they did, having one's gallbladder taken out would probably beat liposuction as the most popular form of elective surgery!)

It turns out that to *burn* fat that is stored in the body's lipid cells, we need to *consume* certain kinds of fats that will help to soften those lipid cells' membranes. When a person loses the gallbladder, hence access to incoming nutrition in the form of fats, it actually becomes *harder* to lose weight, because the body much more tenaciously retains whatever fat is in the lipid cells. Since obesity is a leading contributor to the formation of gallstones, losing one's gallbladder makes it doubly hard to resolve problems with being overweight.

Treatment

Surgery is the most common intervention to deal with gallstones. The whole gallbladder is removed, thereby preventing the formation of future gallstones. Recent advances in laparoscopic surgery have made it possible to remove the gallbladder using a series of very small incisions instead of open surgery. This minimizes general trauma to the body and radically reduces recovery time.

Another surgical intervention is ***endoscopic retrograde cholangiopancreatography***. This is a scope on a thin tube that is inserted through the mouth, down the esophagus, through the stomach, and into the small intestine and biliary duct system. It is often used as a diagnostic tool, but in some cases a device can be attached to the scope to remove or dislodge gallstones without removing the gallbladder.

A person whose gallbladder has been removed can still produce bile, but it is dripped into the duodenum in a steady stream rather than being saved for high-fat meals. The only real concern is that she may lose some access to important fat-soluble vitamins. Fortunately, digestive supplements can aid in the digestion of fats (Sidebar 8.7).

Massage?

Acute biliary colic, as seen with a gallbladder attack, contraindicates massage, especially if signs of an infection (fever, chills, sweating) are present. If a client *knows* he or she has gallstones but they are silent, consider the costal angle on the right side a local caution. Otherwise, people with gallstones, a history of gallstones or uncomplicated gallbladder surgery are fine for massage.

Modality Recommendations for Gallstones

Deep tissue massage	Contraindicated during acute inflammation. Supportive during recovery: work gently with costal arch, thoracolumbar fascia, diaphragm.
Lymphatic drainage	Supportive.
Polarity	S: Indicated. R: Avoid when symptoms present. D: Avoid area.
PNF/MET/stretching	Avoid local area when symptoms are present; otherwise supportive.
Reflexology	Indicated. Work liver, gallbladder, pancreas, pituitary points. Can add small intestines, lymphatic system if severe.
Shiatsu	Supportive. Work GB, LV, SP meridians. Ampuku to gallbladder area.
Swedish massage	Avoid jostling or compressing gallbladder area; otherwise supportive.
Trigger point therapy	Avoid local area when symptoms are present; otherwise supportive.

See Chapter 1 for a brief description of each modality, including definitions of abbreviations.

Hepatitis

Definition: What Is It?

Hepatitis means *inflamed liver.* It can be caused by drug reactions or exposure to certain toxins, but it is most often one of a variety of viral infections that can mildly or severely impair liver function. Seven types of viral hepatitis have been identified to date: hepatitis A through G. Hepatitis A, B, and C cause about 90% of cases in the United States; they are the primary focus of this discussion.

Demographics: Who Gets It?

Statistics on hepatitis are notoriously difficult to gather because some forms don't produce symptoms for weeks or even years after an initial infection. Consequently, the true number of new infections that occur each year is probably considerably higher than the statistics indicate. Estimates suggest that new hepatitis infections occur 500,000 to 750,000 times per year.[42] Aggressive vaccination programs and public health efforts have led to significant declines in viral hepatitis infections in the past decade.

Hepatitis in Brief
Pronunciation: hep-ah-TY-tis

What is it?
Hepatitis is inflammation of the liver, usually but not always due to viral infection.

How is it recognized?
All types of hepatitis produce the same symptoms, with variable severity. Symptoms, when any occur at all, include fatigue, abdominal pain, nausea, diarrhea, and jaundice.

Is massage indicated or contraindicated?
Acute hepatitis contraindicates circulatory massage. For clients with chronic hepatitis, the appropriateness of massage depends on their general health and resilience.

Etiology: What Happens?

Hepatitis A, B, and C all are viral attacks against liver cells. Each type of virus is unique, however. Exposure to one type of hepatitis does *not* impart immunity to any other type of hepatitis.

Methods of transmission and communicability of each type of virus are discussed in the individual headings. Once the virus has gained access to the body, however, it attacks liver cells and stimulates an immune system response. Hepatitis can be identified and diagnosed by the presence of antibodies in the blood, and also by the presence of enzymes that indicate liver damage.

Viral hepatitis of any kind may be described in four basic phases:

- *Phase 1.* New infection and viral replication. During this phase the virus attacks cells in the liver, but the liver keeps up with the damage, so no symptoms develop. Blood tests for indicator enzymes or antibodies are positive.
- *Phase 2.* Prodromal stage. Symptoms develop. Food aversion, nausea, vomiting, malaise, itchy skin rashes, and some chemical sensitivities may appear.
- *Phase 3.* Icteric stage. At this point the liver is significantly impaired. Signs of jaundice develop, including yellowing skin (***icterus***), pale stools, dark urine, and hepatomegaly. For more information on jaundice, see Sidebar 8.6.
- *Phase 4.* Convalescence. During this time the liver heals, jaundice resolves, enzymes return to normal levels, and health is restored.

The severity of symptoms varies widely from one person to another, depending on the phase of the infection, the general health of the patient, and the type of virus involved.

Hepatitis A

What Is It?

This used to be called *infectious hepatitis*. It is a short, acute infection that usually causes no lasting damage, and it creates lifelong immunity.

Demographics: Who Gets It?

Hepatitis A occurs among all age groups. Estimates suggest that about 90,000 people in the United States are infected every year, and most of them are young children who often don't show significant symptoms.[43] Up to 30% of Americans have antibodies to hepatitis A, showing that they've been exposed to this virus.

Risk groups for hepatitis A include travelers to places where water contamination is likely, day care workers, intravenous drug users, and people who have unprotected sex with hepatitis A patients.

Communicability of hepatitis A

Hepatitis A virus concentrates in the feces of an infected person; therefore it is most easily transmitted through oral-fecal contact, often in contaminated food or water. Hepatitis A is the reason for those ever-present signs about hand washing in restaurant bathrooms. Raw or undercooked shellfish grown in contaminated water can spread the disease to humans.

Oral-fecal contact is the most common transmission route for hepatitis A, but it can also be carried in the blood and body fluids, so shared drug needles or unprotected sex with hepatitis A patients can also spread the infection.

Signs and Symptoms

Symptoms of hepatitis A are similar to those of the rest of the hepatitis family, but they tend to be the most severe and the shortest in duration. They include weakness, nausea, fever, anorexia, and possible jaundice that is accompanied by dark urine and pale stools. This virus incubates for 2 to 6 weeks before symptoms appear, but it is contagious during this period. Once symptoms appear, the virus is present in the system for another 2 to 3 weeks, although a person may not feel fully restored to health for up to 6 months. In rare cases a person may have relapsing episodes of hepatitis A for several months.

Treatment

Treatment for hepatitis A is a combination of rest, fluids, and good sense. In some cases gamma globulin shots are recommended to provide short-term protection when a specific source of infection has been identified, such as a contaminated food source. A vaccine against this infection is available for people traveling, working, or living in places where the virus is prevalent.

Massage?

Acute hepatitis contraindicates circulatory massage. The liver is a keystone for fluid management in the body; to push more fluid through a system that is not functioning well could lead to some serious repercussions. Noncirculatory techniques, however, may be welcome and very supportive during a long recuperation.

Hepatitis B

What Is It?

Hepatitis B virus works very differently from hepatitis A. It causes chronic infections with much subtler symptoms. In this case the virus itself is not responsible for most liver injury; chronic inflammation is the cause of most of the damage. Hepatitis B carries risks and possible complications that are much more serious than those associated with hepatitis A.

Most adults who are exposed to hepatitis B recover fully. However, most infants and children who contract the disease and about 5% of exposed adults develop chronic infections. These individuals are long-term carriers of the virus. Within this group of patients the risk of developing other liver diseases later in life is higher than that of the general population.

Demographics: Who Gets It?

High-risk groups for hepatitis B include any person who comes in contact with someone else's body fluids. This includes people who live or work with hepatitis B patients, anyone who has unprotected sex with a hepatitis B patient, infants born to hepatitis B–positive mothers, immigrants from countries where hepatitis B is prevalent, and intravenous drug users.

About 78,000 new cases of hepatitis B are diagnosed each year in the United States, but because this infection may not cause symptoms right away, this number may be inaccurate. About 1.25 million Americans carry the virus as a chronic infection; all of them are capable of spreading the virus to others. Hepatitis B is a direct cause of death for 5000 to 6000 people each year.[43]

Communicability of hepatitis B

Hepatitis B is communicable primarily through body fluids. It does not appear to spread through the digestive system. Hepatitis B virus is most densely found in blood, semen, and vaginal fluid, but viral particles may also be found in saliva.

Unlike many pathogens, this virus is quite sturdy. It remains viable, outside the body for a week or more, and therefore is communicable through indirect contact.[44] Furthermore, it occurs in high concentrations, so limited exposure can cause an infection.[45] For this reason, it is especially important to sterilize any instruments that come in contact with human blood: tattoo needles, body piercing equipment, acupuncture needles, and professional medical and dental tools all fall into this category. Further, sharing household items that might contact blood, such as razors or toothbrushes, must be avoided.

Infants born to mothers with hepatitis B are at particularly high risk for infection; 90% of such infants become infected. If they are not treated immediately, most infants with hepatitis B develop chronic liver disease early in life.

Signs and Symptoms

Symptoms of hepatitis B are about the same as those of hepatitis A, but the onset is slower and they last for a much longer time. The incubation period is 2 to 6 months in this case (it is contagious during all that time), and it can stay in the system for months or years. The severity and duration of the viral attack are largely determined by the general health of the infected person. Long-term carriers of hepatitis B may have no symptoms at all.

Complications

About 5% of the adults who get hepatitis B develop chronic infections. (This figure is much higher for infants and children.) Chronic liver inflammation can lead to the development of varicose veins on the stomach and esophagus, which may rupture and bleed. Liver failure, cirrhosis, and liver cancer are other possible complications.

Treatment

Hepatitis B treatments are only sporadically successful. Interferon is effective slightly more than half the time, but it carries a lot of unpleasant and even dangerous side effects. Another antiviral agent, lamivudine, is better tolerated by most patients but tends to be less effective against viral activity.

Prevention

A vaccine series against hepatitis B has been developed. People who work in emergency response, hospitals, prisons, and long-term care facilities are often required to get it. People traveling to high-risk areas or people living with an infected person are also targeted. This vaccine is also recommended for children to guard against the spread of the disease from a hepatitis B–positive household member, or for when they become sexually active.

Massage?

Hepatitis B contraindicates circulatory massage in the acute stage, when the liver is already overtaxed. If a client has a chronic version of the disease, the decision about circulatory massage must be based on that person's overall health and resiliency. The benefits include improved immune system activity and restoration of autonomic balance, but the risks include the possibility of stressing a weak system that is incapable of adapting to the changes circulatory massage brings about. Noncirculatory massage may provide many of the benefits while minimizing the risks.

Clients who have recovered from hepatitis B infections with no other problems are fine for massage.

Hepatitis C

What Is It?

Before the viruses D, E, F, and G were discovered, hepatitis C virus was called "hepatitis non-A, non-B." Although it's been investigated since the late 1970s, the causative virus wasn't identified until 1989.

Like hepatitis B, hepatitis C causes chronic infections. Unlike hepatitis B, however, the percentage of hepatitis C patients who develop long-term problems is very high. Only 5% to 25% recover spontaneously; the other 75% to 95% percent of hepatitis C patients go on to experience chronic infection. Of those with chronic hepatitis C, about 70% are at risk for chronic liver disease, including cirrhosis, liver failure, and liver cancer.[46] The presence of other illnesses, specifically HIV, hepatitis B, or alcoholism, raises the risk of complications from long-term hepatitis C infections. Hepatitis C is estimated to cause about 10,000 to 20,000 deaths per year.[43]

Demographics: Who Gets It?

Hepatitis C is something of a silent epidemic; although many people have never heard of it, this virus is a common blood-borne infection in the United States. It is carried by more than 4 million Americans today, and about 3 million people have the disease as a chronic infection.[46]

The primary risk group for new hepatitis C infection is intravenous drug users. An estimated 26,000 new infections occur among this group every year. Happily, that number is on the decline; rates in the early 1990s were much higher.[43] That said, because hepatitis C virus can take a long time to develop symptoms, statistics for new infections can be misleading: some sources suggest that it infects up to 150,000 people each year.[42]

Another risk group for hepatitis C infection is people who received transfusions of blood or blood clotting factors before 1987. Since then improved screening techniques have made the public blood supply much safer.

Communicability

Blood-to-blood contact is the most reliable way to transmit hepatitis C, although in some cases the mode of transmission is unclear. Blood-to-blood contact can come about in the form of shared drug needles, accidental needle sticks in medical settings; and contaminated medical, tattoo, or body-piercing instruments. Hepatitis C virus may be transmitted through sexual activity, but this is not considered an efficient pathway for transmission.

Signs and Symptoms

Symptoms of hepatitis C are weakness, fever, nausea, and sometimes jaundice. In some cases these symptoms develop within a few weeks after exposure, but for 80% of patients symptoms don't develop until many years after infection. Many people never know that they've been infected with the hepatitis C virus until 20 or 30 years after exposure, when the liver can no longer compensate for the accumulated damage.

Treatment

Treatment of hepatitis C is good sense (rest, fluids, and good nutrition) and close monitoring to watch for signs of complications. No vaccine has been developed against this virus. Interferon and ribavirin may be prescribed separately or together to try to control the severity of the viral attack. Most liver transplants performed in the United States today are to treat hepatitis C infections.

Massage?

As with other hepatitis infections, circulatory massage is contraindicated in the presence of acute disease. When the infection is chronic, judgments must be based on the overall health and circulatory resiliency of the client.

Other Types of Hepatitis

Hepatitis may be caused by factors other than viruses A, B, and C. Hepatitis D is an incomplete virus that can work only in the presence of hepatitis B. Hepatitis E, F, and G are rare viruses that are uncommon in the United States.

It is also possible for other viruses to cause liver inflammation, often as a complication of a different primary infection. Epstein-Barr virus (seen with most mononucleosis infections) and cytomegalovirus are two examples.

Nonviral hepatitis has been seen as a reaction to certain medications or as an autoimmune disease launched against hepatocytes. Autoimmune hepatitis frequently accompanies other autoimmune diseases, including type 1 diabetes, Graves disease, and ulcerative colitis.

Massage?

The same rules apply here as for viral types of hepatitis: acute infection contraindicates circulatory massage, although energetic work may be supportive and helpful. Massage for clients with chronic disease must be determined by the overall health of the client and the ability to adapt to changes that bodywork brings about.

MODALITY RECOMMENDATIONS FOR HEPATITIS

Deep tissue massage	Systemically contraindicated, depending on type and severity.
Lymphatic drainage	Systemically contraindicated.
Polarity	S: Indicated. R/D: Systemically contraindicated when symptomatic; otherwise supportive.
PNF/MET/stretching	Systemically contraindicated when symptomatic; otherwise supportive.
Reflexology	Indicated. Work liver and gallbladder points.
Shiatsu	Support immune system with SP, TH meridians.
Swedish massage	Systemically contraindicated when symptomatic; otherwise supportive.
Trigger point therapy	Systemically contraindicated when symptomatic; otherwise supportive.

See Chapter 1 for a brief description of each modality, including definitions of abbreviations.

Liver Cancer

Definition: What Is It?

Primary liver cancer, also called ***hepatocellular carcinoma***, is cancer that originates in the liver. This is distinguished from secondary liver cancer, or metastatic liver disease, which is a result of cancer that originates elsewhere and leads to tumors in the liver.

Liver Cancer in Brief

What is it?
Primary liver cancer is the growth of malignant cells that starts among hepatocytes. Liver cancer is aggressive and usually silent in early stages, leading to late diagnoses and a generally poor prognosis.

How is it recognized?
Liver cancer is silent in early stages, but as tumors grow and interfere with function, signs and symptoms may include vague to intense abdominal pain, ascites, itchy rashes on the skin, psychological changes, muscle wasting, fever, unintended weight loss, and jaundice.

Is massage indicated or contraindicated?
A person with liver cancer may undergo extensive and intrusive treatment options; any bodywork must be adjusted to respect the challenges of these treatments. Liver cancer is often terminal, and massage may be an important and welcome comfort measure in this situation.

Demographics: Who Gets It?

Worldwide, liver cancer is one of the most common and most deadly forms of cancer. In the United States it is relatively rare, affecting about 18,000 people per year and causing about 16,000 deaths.[47] Unlike most cancers in the United States, liver cancer rates are on the rise. They doubled between 1980 and 1998, probably because of long-term infection with hepatitis C.[48] Asian immigrant populations have the highest rates of liver cancer in the United States, usually because of childhood infection with hepatitis B.

Men have liver cancer more commonly than women, by a ratio of about 3 to 1. In the United States most diagnoses are in people over 60 years old. In other countries where hepatitis B is more prominent, liver cancer is more common and often diagnosed at a younger age.

Etiology: What Happens?

Liver cancer develops when hepatocytes replicate out of control. A history of viral irritation, especially over several decades, alcoholism, and cirrhosis are all contributing factors to uncontrolled cellular activity. This is true especially when any combination of these factors affects a single person.

Liver cancer tumors may develop singly, or they may occur in several disconnected areas throughout the left and right lobes. They tend to be highly invested with blood vessels, which raises the risk for distant metastasis (usually to the lungs) before signs and symptoms lead to a diagnosis.

Risk Factors

Several risk factors for liver cancer have been identified. They are especially potent when they appear in combination.

- *Hepatitis B infection.* This virus has specifically been seen to *cause*, not just appear frequently with, a specific type of cancer. Genetic material from hepatitis B virus can be found in the malignant cells of liver cancer. Hepatitis B is an especially high risk for liver cancer when the infection is chronic and was contracted in childhood. Persons infected with hepatitis B as adults have a lower risk of developing liver cancer, although cirrhosis is still a strong possibility.
- *Hepatitis C infection.* The relationship between hepatitis C virus and liver cancer is not completely understood; some research indicates that the virus may actually cause the cancer, while other studies suggest that liver cancer develops indirectly through the cirrhosis associated with hepatitis C. Nonetheless, about 5% to 10% of people diagnosed with hepatitis C eventually develop liver cancer. Because Hepatitis C virus infects about 4 million people in the United States (with about 3 million in the form of chronic infections), liver cancer rates are expected to keep rising for the next several years.
- *Alcoholism.* Alcohol abuse, especially in combination with hepatitis B or C, greatly raises the risk of liver cancer. Interestingly, it appears that it is the cessation of alcohol use that triggers the cellular mutation: when a person stops drinking and the liver begins to regenerate, cells are more likely to become malignant.
- *Hemochromatosis.* This is a genetic blood disorder, production of too many red blood cells. Persons with untreated ***hemochromatosis*** are at high risk for cirrhosis and then may go on to liver cancer.
- *Cirrhosis.* This condition, the result of long-term liver damage, develops in the presence of chronic viral infection, alcoholism, or toxic exposure. It is possible for liver cancer to develop without cirrhosis, but it is not the usual presentation.
- *Aflatoxin B_1.* This is a chemical from a mold, *Aspergillus flavus*, that grows on peanuts and grains stored in hot, humid conditions. ***Aflatoxin B_1*** is an extremely potent carcinogen, responsible for many liver cancer cases in Asia and sub-Saharan Africa.

Signs and Symptoms

Tumors in the liver interfere with normal function. Because hepatitis and/or cirrhosis is probably also present, these signs may be missed or ignored. The most commonly reported signs and symptoms of liver cancer include vague abdominal pain that becomes increasingly intense, unintended weight loss and food aversion, muscle wasting, ascites (which may obscure signs of weight loss), fever, an abdominal mass, and if the bile duct is blocked, jaundice. Blood tests may reveal signs of liver dysfunction. One specific substance, **alpha fetoprotein**, is present in the blood about 60% of the time when liver cancer is present. Other blood tests may show unusual hormonal activity, as cancerous cells secrete chemicals usually restricted to other cells.

Diagnosis

Liver cancer is generally diagnosed by use of a combination of imaging techniques that include CT with or without contrast medium, ultrasound, and MRI, along with a biopsy of suspicious cells. One of the challenges of liver cancer diagnosis is that primary liver cancer cells appear similar to secondary liver cells that have metastasized from another location. These two problems require a different treatment approach, so it is important to distinguish between them.

For liver cancer staging patterns, see Sidebar 8.8.

SIDEBAR 8.8: STAGING LIVER CANCER

Staging protocols for liver cancer have several variations. The typical TNM classifications with numerical groupings follows this pattern:[48]

Tumor (T)

T 1: One tumor, no vascularization

T 2: One tumor with vascularization ***or*** multiple tumors < than 5 cm

T 3: Multiple tumors >5 cm ***or*** one tumor involving portal vein or hepatic artery

T 4: Multiple tumors with direct invasion of adjacent organs and/or perforation of visceral peritoneum

Node (N)

N 0: no nodes involved

N 1: regional nodes involved

Metastasis (M)

M 0: no metastasis found

M 1: tumors found outside the liver

These delineations are then translated into stages I to IV in this way:

Stage	Tumor	Node	Metastasis
I	T 1	N 0	M 0
II	T 2	N 0	M 0
III A	T 3	N 0	M 0
III B	T 4	N 0	M 0
III C	Any	N 1	M 0
IV	T any	N any	M 1

Liver cancer staging may be discussed in stages 0 through IV, as other cancers are, but it is also discussed in terms of best treatment options.

Localized resectable cancer indicates that a single tumor smaller than 2 cm without signs of spreading to blood or lymph vessels has been found.

Localized unresectable cancer means that although metastasis is not obvious, the liver is too damaged by cirrhosis or other factors to make surgery safe. These patients are often treated with alternatives.

Advanced cancer indicates that distant metastasis has occurred, and while chemotherapy and radiation may slow the progress, the cancer is probably not curable.

Recurrent cancer is cancer that returns after previous treatments.

Treatment

Even when liver cancer is caught in its earliest recognizable stages, survival for more than 5 years is rare. Most survivors of liver cancer surgery have a recurrence within several months. This cancer is aggressive and difficult to control, and most patients have serious underlying liver disease that makes them poor candidates for many types of surgery. Furthermore, liver cancer tends not to respond well to chemotherapy or radiation. Consequently, a number of treatment options have been developed that try to control the growth of the cancer without invasive surgery. These include techniques to burn or freeze tumors through laparoscopic or percutaneous instruments; injections of ethanol to destroy tumor cells; and the use of drugs or implements to block the blood vessels that supply tumors. No single treatment option shows outstanding promise for a long-term cure, however, and the 5-year survival rate is under 10%.

Surgery typically entails a resection of the liver (removing the portion or portions in which tumors are present) or liver transplant. The fact that many liver cancer patients have a long history of cirrhosis and/or hepatitis makes both resections and transplant surgeries difficult.

Massage?

A person who has been diagnosed with liver cancer is unlikely to survive the disease. If that person is undergoing therapy, side effects may make some types of bodywork uncomfortable or even dangerous; therapists should consult with the client's health care team to get information about any risks. If a person seeks massage as a comfort measure near the end of life, bodywork can be a wonderful, nurturing, and supportive experience. For more information about massage in the context of cancer and cancer treatments, see Chapter 12.

Massage therapists may wish to teach family members and friends some simple techniques to improve the quality of time spent between the dying person and the loved ones.

Modality Recommendations for Liver Cancer	
Deep tissue massage	Supportive as part of health care team. Respect stage of recovery and treatment challenges.
Lymphatic drainage	Depends on stage. Supportive in early stages; work with health care team in later stages.
Polarity	S: Indicated. R/D: Supportive, determined by client's comfort.
PNF/MET/stretching	Supportive as part of health care team; match to activity levels.
Reflexology	Indicated. Work liver and gallbladder points. In severe cases add lymphatic and pituitary points.
Shiatsu	Support immune system with SP, TH meridians. Add LV extensions in legs, K meridian.
Swedish massage	Supportive; depth determined by activity level.
Trigger point therapy	Supportive.

See Chapter 1 for a brief description of each modality, including definitions of abbreviations.

Pancreatic Cancer

Definition: What Is It?

Pancreatic cancer begins as mutation of certain genes that sponsor uncontrolled growth of cells in the pancreas. It usually grows in the exocrine ducts of this gland, but occasionally grows in the endocrine-producing cells. Pancreatic cancer is aggressive, metastasizes easily, and is difficult to detect in early stages; consequently it is the fourth leading cause of death from cancer in this country.[49]

Demographics: Who Gets It?

Pancreatic cancer is diagnosed about 34,000 times per year in the United States.[49] The average life expectancy after diagnosis is 4 to 6 months.[50] Consequently, it is the cause of about the same number of deaths every year.

Men get pancreatic cancer slightly more often than women, but in recent years that gender balance has been shifting; this may reflect an increasing number of women smokers who are now within the most common age range for a diagnosis of pancreatic cancer. African American men and women get pancreatic cancer slightly more frequently than whites. Other ethnic groups have a generally lower risk.

Pancreatic Cancer in Brief

Pronunciation: pan-kre-AT-ik KAN-sur

What is it?

Pancreatic cancer is the growth of malignant cells in the pancreas. It is usually a cancer of the exocrine cells, which normally produce digestive enzymes, but it occasionally grows in the islet cells, where hormones are produced.

How is it recognized?

Early signs of pancreatic cancer are subtle and not usually alarming: abdominal discomfort, unintended weight loss, and loss of appetite are frequently reported. Later signs may include jaundice, hepatomegaly or splenomegaly, ascites, and signs of distant metastasis, which vary according to location.

Is massage indicated or contraindicated?

Pancreatic cancer is almost always fatal within a few months of diagnosis. Massage is appropriate as a comfort measure, particularly as part of a health care team effort for pain relief and palliative effects.

Etiology: What Happens?

The pancreas is a small, spongy gland behind the stomach. It produces digestive enzymes that collect in an extensive duct system and eventually enter the duodenum. It also manufactures hormones for maintenance of blood sugar levels.

Pancreatic cancer has been studied extensively. Several exact mutations of specific genes in the exocrine ducts of the organ have been identified, all of which lead to the growth of invasive, aggressive, life-threatening tumors.

When these tumors arise in the exocrine ducts, they are ***adenocarcinomas***. When they grow in the islet cells, they are ***neuroendocrine*** tumors. In either case, the tumors tend to grow quickly and easily invade nearby tissues simply by spreading out. The duodenum, stomach, and peritoneal wall are often affected by these local extensions. When cells invade the abdominal lymph system or large blood vessels, the liver is often the first site of metastasis.

Risk Factors

Exact causes or triggers of pancreatic cancer have not been identified, but a number of risk factors have been seen to increase the chance that pancreatic genes will mutate. The primary risk factors for pancreatic cancer are as follows:

- Age (most diagnoses are among people 60–80 years old)
- Gender (men are diagnosed more often than women)
- Race (it occurs slightly more frequently among African Americans)
- A history of smoking (this may be responsible for up to 30% of genetic mutations)
- A history of type 2 diabetes
- Chronic pancreatitis due to alcohol abuse

Pancreatitis in Brief
Pronunciation: pan-kre-uh-TY-tis

What is it?
Pancreatitis is inflammation of the pancreas. It has an acute and a chronic form.

How is it recognized?
Constant or episodic pain high in the abdomen is the leading sign of pancreatitis. This pain often refers to the back. Other signs have to do with pancreatic dysfunction: poor absorption of food leading to weight loss, secondary diabetes mellitus, and jaundice are all possible signs of pancreatitis.

Is massage indicated or contraindicated?
Undiagnosed abdominal pain that persists for more than a few days necessitates medical attention. Massage is unlikely to make pancreatitis worse unless a therapist works deep high in the abdomen, but this is a potentially dangerous disease, so it is important that temporary relief of symptoms that massage might bring about not delay getting an accurate diagnosis. After an episode of pancreatitis has passed and the client, doctor, and therapist have a clear idea of the cause of symptoms, massage may be appropriate as long as it doesn't cause pain.

Pancreatitis

Definition: What Is It?

Pancreatitis is inflammation of the pancreas. Acute pancreatitis can be triggered by gallstones, toxic exposures, blunt trauma, or other factors; chronic pancreatitis is usually related to long-term abuse of alcohol.

Demographics: Who Gets It?

Each year about 80,000 people in this country are diagnosed with acute pancreatitis.[53] Numbers on chronic pancreatitis are more difficult to gather. It is most common among long-term alcoholics.

Etiology: What Happens?

The pancreas manufactures both endocrine and exocrine secretions. Its exocrine products are bicarbonate to neutralize material exiting the highly acidic stomach, and digestive enzymes that break down carbohydrates, proteins, and fats into absorbable particles. If the ducts in the pancreas are blocked or if the gland develops cysts or abscesses, these functions are lost, and the secretions may even turn back to destroy the pancreas tissue itself; this is called ***autodigestion***.

- *Acute pancreatitis.* In acute pancreatitis, a sudden onset of symptoms indicates that part of the extensive ductwork of the gland has been blocked. This can be brought about by alcohol use, blunt trauma, a congenital malformation of the pancreas, infection (usually with mumps or cytomegalovirus), gallstones lodged in the common bile duct, exposure to ethanol or other toxins, or cystic fibrosis. The net result is that the pancreatic secretions can't be released into the duodenum. Acute pancreatitis is usually mild and short-lived and has an uneventful recovery. But when it is severe, a number of complications may develop. These include cystlike pockets on the gland, abscesses, necrosis of pancreatic tissue, and the release of dangerous toxins into the bloodstream that can lead to circulatory shock, renal failure, or adult respiratory distress syndrome.
- *Chronic pancreatitis.* In chronic pancreatitis, long-term wear and tear leads to permanent damage to the delicate epithelial tissue of the gland. Chronic pancreatitis is almost always related to alcohol abuse. Ethanol can cause enzymes to be released prematurely, damaging the gland and forming protein plugs that may calcify to become pancreatic stones. Other causes of chronic pancreatitis include heredity, autoimmune dysfunction, and gallstones.

  The main complications of chronic pancreatitis include constant pain that begins in the abdomen but then penetrates to the back, malabsorption of nutrients (which can lead to ***steatorrhea***, or oily, foul-smelling stools), bleeding into the peritoneum, and secondary diabetes mellitus. The pain associated with chronic pancreatitis can be so persistent and extreme that addiction to opioid painkillers is a significant risk for these patients.

Signs and Symptoms

Upper abdominal pain is the leading symptom of acute and chronic pancreatitis. With acute pancreatitis the pain is extreme and has a sudden onset. It may appear with nausea, vomiting, fever, and rapid pulse.

With chronic pancreatitis the pain may be episodic, lasting for hours, days, or more and then subsiding until the next attack. Episodes get closer together until the pain is unremitting. Pancreatic pain often refers into the back, which is an issue of concern for massage therapists, of course.

Other symptoms indicate the loss of pancreatic enzymes and hormones: unintended weight loss, difficulties with the regulation of blood glucose, and the possibility of jaundice if the obstruction of the pancreatic duct also affects the common bile duct.

Diagnosis

Several varieties of imaging techniques can yield important information about pancreatitis, depending on whether the problem is in the head, neck, or tail of the organ. CT, MRI, radiography, and needle biopsy may all be used to identify the source of pancreatic pain. Blood tests may be conducted to look for heightened levels of amylase or other pancreatic enzymes in the blood.

Treatment

Pancreatitis is treated according to the cause. If it is related to gallstones, these are removed so the ducts can flow freely. If abscesses form, these are drained or removed. If tissue has died because of autodigestion, that is also removed. The pancreatic duct may be surgically reopened, or a stent may be inserted. Digestive enzymes may be taken orally to relieve the pancreas of the work of producing them. Finally, if the pain from chronic pancreatitis is unresponsive to any other interventions, surgery may be performed to sever the sensory nerves from the gland.

Massage?

Pancreatitis is a relatively rare condition that usually resolves without major complications. Sometimes, however, it can be life-threatening, and because it refers pain into the back, clients may not realize the source of the problem. This is an example of a situation in which undiagnosed abdominal discomfort or pain that persists for more than a few days should be referred to a physician.

A person undergoing treatment for pancreatitis may receive massage if he or she is comfortable on a table, but obviously abdominal work must be conducted with caution. A client with a history of pancreatitis but no symptoms or complications is a fine candidate for massage.

Modality Recommendations for Pancreatitis

Deep tissue massage	Supportive; may assist with parasympathetic response. Avoid deep work, especially upper psoas around navel.
Lymphatic drainage	Systemically contraindicated.
Polarity	S: Indicated. R/D: Supportive with no infection and to client's comfort.
PNF/MET/stretching	Supportive.
Reflexology	Indicated. Work pancreas points.
Shiatsu	Supportive. Work SP, ST, TH meridians.
Swedish massage	Only gentlest stroking when symptoms are present.
Trigger point therapy	Systemically contraindicated with infection; otherwise a local caution but supportive elsewhere.

See Chapter 1 for a brief description of each modality, including definitions of abbreviations.

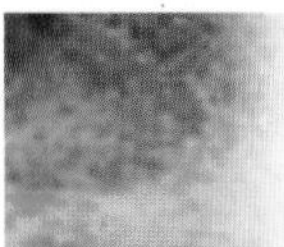

Other Digestive System Conditions

Candidiasis

Definition: What Is It?

Candida albicans is one type of many yeastlike fungi that inhabit the digestive tract, often from the mouth to the anus (Figure 8.14). They usually live in balance with other flora and fauna of the GI tract. Under certain circumstances that balance is upset and candida replicate too easily, leading to a variety of problems. This condition, having normal levels of candida grow out of control, is called candidiasis.

> **Candidiasis in Brief**
> Pronunciation: kan-dih-DY-ah-sis
>
> **What is it?**
> Candidiasis is a condition in which *Candida albicans* fungi that colonize the GI tract become invasive and disrupt normal function of the digestive system and other systems in the body. Other species of *Candida* can also cause a systemic fungal infection, but these are rare.
>
> **How is it recognized?**
> Signs and symptoms of candidiasis can be severe and acute, involving mouth and skin lesions as well as systemic blood infections, or subtle and chronic, involving fatigue, impaired mental ability, food and chemical sensitivities, and several other symptoms in varying degrees of severity.
>
> **Is massage indicated or contraindicated?**
> Chronic candidiasis indicates massage, but many acute candidiasis patients have compromised immune system function and so therapists should take care to protect clients from the threat of infection.

Demographics: Who Gets It?

Candidiasis affects different people in different ways, and its incidence as a health problem is largely a matter of opinion. Many medical professionals recognize an imbalance only in people who are extremely affected. These include groups whose immune system is generally weaker than normal, such as infants, AIDS patients, diabetics, organ transplant recipients, and the elderly.

Other researchers suggest that candidiasis affects a much broader population in a much more subtle way and that the symptoms of an imbalance are either too subtle to identify or attributed to other problems, such as allergies, chronic fatigue syndrome, hypothyroidism, and other disorders.

Etiology: What Happens?

Under normal circumstances, a balanced environment of flora (plantlike organisms) and fauna (animal-like organisms) peacefully coexist in the GI tract. The flora keep the fauna from replicating too much, and the fauna do likewise for the flora. These organisms live in symbiosis: a mutually beneficial relationship with their human hosts.

When a disruption in the balance of the GI tract occurs, either plants or animals can dominate. When bacteria are suppressed, candida in the GI tract convert from benign, helpful yeastlike organisms to more aggressive fungi. In the absence of balancing bacteria, the fungi have more opportunity to reproduce and spread. Because candida live in most people's digestive tract, the exact delineation between colonization and infestation is not always clear. Opinions vary about how extensive a candida colonization has to be before it causes symptoms (Sidebar 8.10).

Often the trigger for intestinal imbalance is use of antibiotics. These medications, designed to kill harmful bacteria, sometimes also kill beneficial bacteria. (This is why many health care providers recommend supplementing lactobacilli along with antibiotic prescrip-

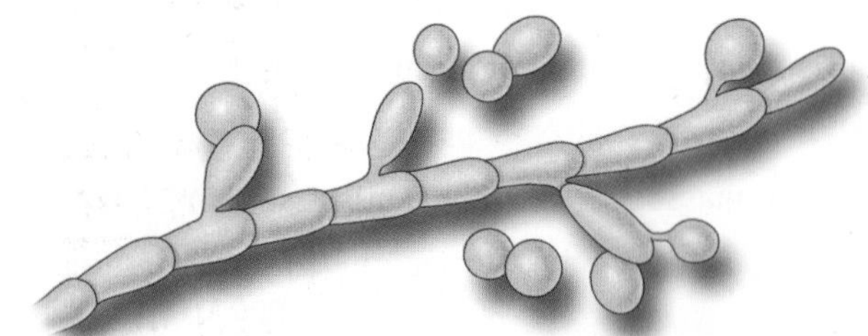

Figure 8.14. *Candida albicans*, the yeast that causes candidiasis.

tions.) Other well-accepted causes of candidiasis include genetic immune system dysfunctions, thymus tumors, and hormonal imbalances. Studies of patients with chronic candidiasis show that their immune system is often severely disabled and incapable of targeting this pathogen. When this occurs in women, it may be an early indicator of infection with HIV.

Some experts propose that candida overgrowth can also be a result of taking birth control pills or steroidal anti-inflammatories and having a diet that is high in simple sugars, wheat, and alcohol, all favorite foods for the growing fungi.

SIDEBAR 8.10: IS IT CANDIDIASIS?

Two schools of thought dominate the discussion of candidiasis. The more conservative allopathic approach generally assumes that the overgrowth of candida isn't a problem until very severe symptoms occur, which may involve the skin, mucous membranes, or invasive candidiasis, a systemic infection of the blood.

Many naturopathic and holistic practitioners propose that milder overgrowths of candida can also cause many chronic, low-grade symptoms. The fungi may grow and spread throughout the intestines, sinking rootlike structures into the walls. They produce waste products that can be highly irritating to the host. Invasion of the intestinal wall may also allow other substances to enter the bloodstream, where immune system responses launched against incompletely digested material may be extreme. Between losing access to nutrition because the fungi get it first, dealing with their metabolic wastes, and immune system responses against digestive contents, a person with chronic, low-grade candidiasis may develop a number of subtle or severe symptoms.

Practitioners who deal with candidiasis as a contributor to many other chronic disorders often report success when helping their patients change their diet and lifestyle in ways that restore balance to intestinal flora and fauna. This clinical evidence has yet to be reproduced in a formal research setting, however, which leads to resistance to the acceptance of candidiasis as a common, chronic disorder responsible for symptoms that range from fatigue to menstrual pain to food allergies.

Signs and Symptoms

Candida can show a variety of signs and symptoms, depending on the severity of the condition and the underlying health of the affected person:

- *Mouth lesions.* Thrush, an outbreak of whitish, usually painless lesions in the mouth, is one form that is commonly seen in infants and immunosuppressed people. Candidiasis may also create red, sore areas in the mouth and on the tongue.
- *Esophagitis.* Candida can develop deep in the throat, especially for HIV/AIDS and chemotherapy patients.
- *Anal lesions.* Babies with candida can develop painful and persistent diaper rash. In this case it's not irritation caused by exposure to the ammonia in urine but a skin reaction to the fungi colonizing the rectum and anus. Some forms of jock itch, a fungal infection of the groin, may also be candidiasis.
- *Intertrigo.* **Intertigo** is the development of a yeast infection at skin folds, for example around the groin, in the axilla, or under the breasts.
- *Other skin lesions.* Systemic candidiasis may affect fingernails and toenails, causing them to become thickened and discolored, often with edema around the cuticles. Lesions sometimes occur on the scalp, leading to baldness.
- *Vaginal infection.* Also called vulvovaginal candidiasis, this is the development of candida in and around the vagina. It is a common infection for women, affecting up to 75% of them at least once. Vulvovaginal candidiasis can cause itching and burning at the vagina, painful intercourse, and characteristic cottage cheese–like vaginal discharge.
- *Systemic symptoms (severe infection).* Fever and chills that do not respond to antibiotics may indicate invasive candidiasis, in which the organisms have directly entered the bloodstream through compromised capillaries in the intestines. Invasive candidiasis can be a very serious problem, as the organisms can affect and impair function in virtually any organ. The rise of invasive candidiasis has been cause for concern, since the introduction of powerful antibiotics and other immunosuppressants has made many people, especially those with compromised immune systems, susceptible to candida overgrowth.
- *Systemic symptoms (chronic, low-grade yeast infection).* If a person has an imbalance of fungi in the GI tract, he or she may have any combination of food and chemical sensitivities, headaches (including migraines), chronic vaginal and urinary tract infections, fatigue, reduced resistance to infection, acne, and many others.

Diagnosis

The sheer number and variety of symptoms that a candida imbalance can induce makes this condition a challenge to identify and treat. Many clinicians do not recognize that many common and persistent signs and symptoms may be caused by fungi, and many patients may read about candida symptoms and assume (rightly or wrongly) that this is the source of their problems. For all but the most extreme versions of the condition, it may be difficult to get an accurate diagnosis or successful treatment.

Diagnosis for extreme versions of candidiasis involves skin biopsy to examine obvious lesions for signs of fungal infection. For chronic cases of this condition, a stool sample is often examined to look for signs of intestinal imbalance. Not many facilities test for this kind of subtle problem, however, and the process can be time-consuming and expensive. Furthermore, no diagnostic criteria have been developed to distinguish between asymptomatic amounts of yeast that may normally appear in the stool and a symptomatic case of candidiasis.

Treatment

Various topical antifungal medications may be recommended for severe versions of candidiasis, along with treatment for whatever underlying conditions may be contributing to the disorder. The availability of antiyeast and antifungal medications without a prescription has given rise to concerns about people misdiagnosing their condition and taking unnecessary medication. Further, taking medication incorrectly may lead to development of more resistant strains of the pathogen.

For subtler versions of the disorder, internal antifungals are sometimes recommended, although these can take a long time to work and some people have severe reactions to them. Reestablishing internal flora to balance out the fungi is a high priority. Research is being conducted into inhibition of the transformation of the relatively passive yeast form of the organism into the more aggressive fungal form.

Massage?

A person with a severe candidiasis infection is likely to be under medical care for any of a variety of immunocompromising conditions. Massage in this situation depends on the health of the skin and whatever underlying disorders may be present.

Massage for someone who is trying to overcome a less severe chronic infestation of candida is appropriate and may support the process of ridding the body of yeast-related toxins.

MODALITY RECOMMENDATIONS FOR CANDIDIASIS	
Deep tissue massage	Contraindicated for severe infection; otherwise supportive.
Lymphatic drainage	Supportive.
Polarity	S: Indicated.
	R/D: Supportive with no acute infection and to client's comfort.
PNF/MET/stretching	Supportive.
Reflexology	Indicated. Work whole GI tract, circulatory system, neck, throat; add lymphatic system in severe cases.
Shiatsu	Supportive. Work SP, TH, K to reduce inflammation.
Swedish massage	Supportive when infection not overwhelming; may assist with toxin removal.
Trigger point therapy	Systemically contraindicated for acute infection; otherwise supportive.

See Chapter 1 for a brief description of each modality, including definitions of abbreviations.

Peritonitis

Definition: What Is It?

Peritonitis is an infection in the peritoneal space (Figure 8.15), where it is dark, moist, and just about 100°F (37.8°C), a perfect growth medium. Bacteria may also thrive in the peritoneal space because some key immune devices are absent: white blood cells have no direct access. Other irritants, including gastric juice from a perforated peptic ulcer or bile from the gallbladder or injured liver, may also cause inflammation of the peritoneum.

Peritoneum

This Latin word is derived from a Greek root. *Periteino* means to stretch over. This is an apt description of the peritoneum, which stretches over all the abdominal contents.

Etiology: What Happens?

The bacteria that cause peritonitis can gain access to the peritoneal space through a variety of sources:

- *Rupture of an organ* is one possibility. This is a complication of appendicitis (see Sidebar 8.11), perforated ulcers, and diverticulitis.
- *Pelvic or abdominal abscess,* such as those seen with ulcerative colitis or pelvic inflammatory disease, can release bacteria into the peritoneal space, leading to systemic infection.
- *Mechanical perforation* of the abdomen can introduce bacteria from the outside, with a knife wound, for instance. This is an occasional complication of intestinal or colon surgery, and the possibility of peritonitis is the reason behind the heavy doses of antibiotics that are prescribed before such surgeries.

Peritonitis in Brief

Pronunciation: per-ih-to-NY-tis

What is it?
Peritonitis is inflammation, usually due to bacterial infection, of the peritoneal lining of the abdomen.

How is it recognized?
Acute peritonitis usually shows the signs of systemic infection: fever and chills, along with abdominal pain, rigidity of abdominal muscles, distension, nausea, and vomiting.

Is massage indicated or contraindicated?
Acute peritonitis is a medical emergency that contraindicates massage.

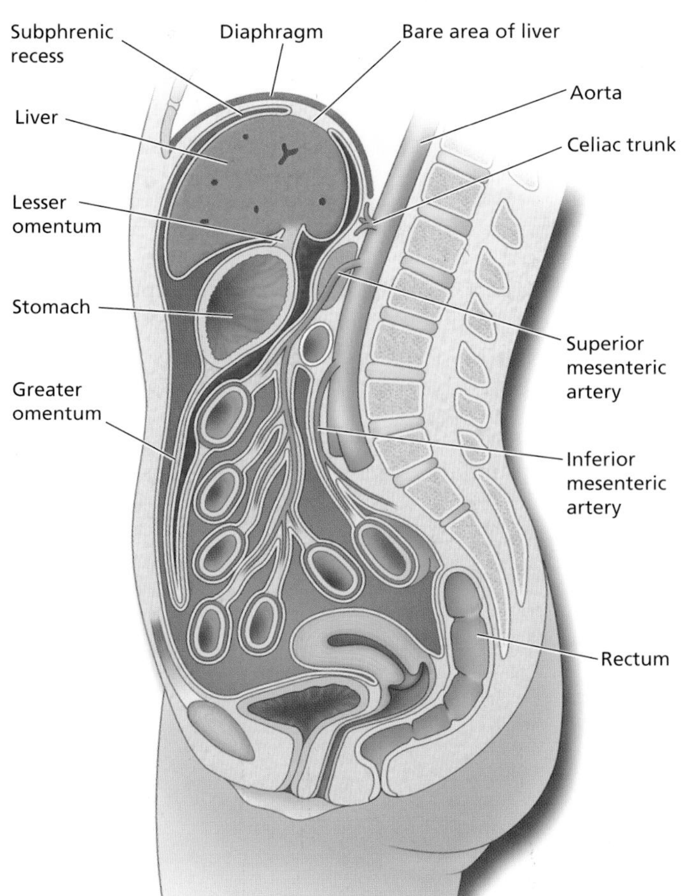

Figure 8.15. Peritonitis, an infection in the peritoneal space.

SIDEBAR 8.11: APPENDICITIS

Peritonitis develops when contents of the GI tract gain access to the warm, moist, dark environment of the abdominal cavity. One way this can happen is if the vermiform appendix is inflamed, infected, or ruptured. This is appendicitis, and it happens roughly 680,000 times per year.[54]

Inflammation of the appendix is generally related to an obstruction of the opening into the cecum. Many cases are related to the development of *fecaliths*, small petrified stools that block the connection between the appendix and the large intestine. When the appendix cannot drain appropriately, the risk of bacterial infection is very high. Once an infection begins, the appendix becomes inflamed and may develop internal or external abscesses. Left untreated, the infected appendix may reach the point of perforation or rupture, releasing bacteria and pus into the peritoneum.

Symptoms of appendicitis are notoriously variable. The classic symptoms are a combination of food aversion and general central abdominal pain, which eventually settles into severe pain in the right lower quadrant of the abdomen. This pain is especially severe during palpation and release: rebound pain. However, only about 50% of appendicitis patients report these symptoms. One of the challenges in appendicitis diagnosis is that the symptoms are similar to those of many other abdominopelvic disorders, including ovarian cysts, ectopic pregnancy, inflammatory bowel disease, diverticulitis, and kidney stones.

Acute abdominal pain with fever obviously contraindicates massage, but someone who has lost his or her appendix with no complications is perfectly safe to receive any kind of bodywork.

- *Spontaneous peritonitis* is an occasional complication of advanced cirrhosis and other liver diseases, because ascites, the seepage of plasma into the abdomen, may carry intestinal bacteria along with it.
- *Peritoneal dialysis* is a method of dialysis for people with advanced kidney failure. It uses the peritoneal membrane as a filter to clean the blood. One of the risks of peritoneal dialysis is contamination of the tubing that connects to the peritoneum, which can cause peritonitis.

Once bacteria establish residence in the peritoneal space, they promote the production of scar tissue. In other areas of the body this mechanism isolates infection and is a helpful response. In the peritoneum, however, it can lead to severe adhesions and cysts where bacteria can hide from white blood cell activity. In other words, the infection can become chronic and difficult to clear without intervention.

Signs and Symptoms

The symptoms of peritonitis vary, depending on the original cause. Abdominal pain is usually part of the picture. It tends to begin as diffuse pain, but it localizes at the original site of infection. Nausea and vomiting are usually present, and if the infection is untreated, severe dehydration may result. Many patients have reduced urine output and difficulty passing gas or bowel movements. After 2 or 3 hours the abdomen swells and pain may subside, but this is not a sign of improvement; rather, it is an indication that the intestines have gone into paralysis. At this point death is not far off unless the patient gets immediate hospital care.

Treatment

Treatment for peritonitis varies according to cause and severity. At the very least, antibiotics are needed. Emergencies require abdominal surgery to remove or repair the ruptured organ, and to wash out the peritoneal cavity as fully as possible. When peritonitis is caught early, it usually responds well to treatment, but if it is left too long, it can be deadly.

Massage?

Any form of acute peritonitis systemically contraindicates massage until all signs of infection have passed.

Modality Recommendations for Peritonitis	
Deep tissue massage	Systemically contraindicated for acute infection.
Lymphatic drainage	Systemically contraindicated for acute infection.
Polarity	Systemically contraindicated for acute infection.
PNF/MET/stretching	Systemically contraindicated for acute infection; otherwise supportive.
Reflexology	Contraindicated for acute infection.
Shiatsu	Contraindicated for acute infection.
Swedish massage	Systemically contraindicated for acute infection.
Trigger point therapy	Systemically contraindicated for acute infection.

See Chapter 1 for a brief description of each modality, including definitions of abbreviations.

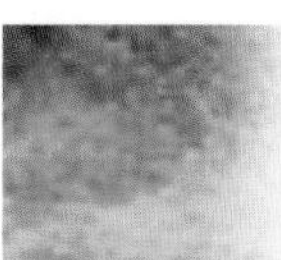

Chapter Review Questions: Digestive System Conditions

1. What is a caution for massage therapists and clients who have persistent gastrointestinal pain?
2. What are two types of esophageal cancer?
3. What is the most serious complication of gastroenteritis?
4. What is the leading causative factor for stomach cancer?
5. How can gallstones lead to pancreatitis?
6. What is the difference between diverticula and colon polyps?
7. What are some conditions that have significant overlap with irritable bowel syndrome?
8. Most people with gallstones never have symptoms. What finally causes symptoms to occur?
9. What is ascites? How can liver dysfunction cause it?
10. A client is recovering from a bout with hepatitis A. His skin has a yellowish tone, and the sclera of his eyes is yellow too. What condition is probably present? Is this client a good candidate for circulatory massage? Why?

References

1. Yang V. Celiac Sprue. © 1996–2006 by WebMD. http://www.emedicine.com/med/topic308.htm. Accessed autumn 2006.
2. Celiac Disease. © 1998–2006 Mayo Foundation for Medical Education and Research. All rights reserved. http://www.mayoclinic.com/health/celiac-disease/DS00319. Accessed autumn 2006.
3. Crohn's disease. © 1998–2006 Mayo Foundation for Medical Education and Research. All rights reserved. http://www.mayoclinic.com/health/crohns-disease/DS00104. Accessed autumn 2006.
4. Wu G, Raynor K. Crohn Disease. © 1996–2006 by WebMD. http://www.emedicine.com/MED/topic477.htm. Accessed autumn 2006.
5. Johne's Disease and Crohn's disease: Are they related? © 2003 by the National Academies. http://dels.nas.edu/dels/rpt_briefs/johnes_final.pdf. Accessed autumn 2006.

6. What Are the Key Statistics about Cancer of the Esophagus? © 2006 American Cancer Society, Inc. http://www.cancer.org/docroot/cri/content/cri_2_4_1x_what_are_the_key_statistics_for_esophagus_cancer_12.asp?sitearea=cri. Accessed autumn 2006.
7. Esophageal Cancer (PDQ): Screening. National Cancer Institute. http://www.cancer.gov/cancertopics/pdq/screening/esophageal/HealthProfessional. Accessed autumn 2006.
8. How Is Cancer of the Esophagus Staged? © 2006 American Cancer Society, Inc. http://www.cancer.org/docroot/CRI/content/CRI_2_4_3X_How_is_esophagus_cancer_staged_11.asp?site area=. Accessed autumn 2006.
9. Marco P, Tedesco P. Esophageal Cancer. © 1996–2006 by WebMD. http://www.emedicine.com/med/topic741.htm. Accessed autumn 2006.
10. Esophageal Cancer. © 1998–2006 Mayo Foundation for Medical Education and Research. All rights reserved. http://www.mayoclinic.com/health/esophageal-cancer/DS00500. Accessed autumn 2006.
11. Gastroenteritis. © The Cleveland Clinic 2006. http://www.clevelandclinic.org/health/health info/docs/3900/3901.asp?index=12418. Accessed autumn 2006.
12. Diskin A. Gastroenteritis. © 1996–2006 by WebMD. http://www.emedicine.com/emerg/topic 213.htm. Accessed autumn 2006.
13. Diff C. New Threat from Old Bug. © 2006 by WebMD. http://www.medicinenet.com/script/main/art.asp?articlekey=76890. Accessed autumn 2006.
14. Marco Fisichella, P. Gastroesophageal Reflux Disease. © 1996–2006 by WebMD. http://www.emedicine.com/med/topic857.htm. Accessed autumn 2006.
15. Scott M, Gelhot A. Gastroesophageal Reflux Disease: Diagnosis and Management. © 1999 by the American Academy of Family Physicians. http://www.aafp.org/afp/990301ap/1161.html. Accessed autumn 2006.
16. Statistics about Peptic Ulcer. © 2000–2005 Adviware Pty Ltd. All rights reserved. http://www.wrongdiagnosis.com/p/peptic_ulcer/stats.htm. Accessed autumn 2006.
17. Mehta V, Fisher G. Gastric Cancer. © 1996–2006 by WebMD. http://www.emedicine.com/med/topic845.htm. Accessed autumn 2006.
18. Stomach cancer. © 1998–2006 Mayo Foundation for Medical Education and Research. All rights reserved. http://www.mayoclinic.com/health/stomach-cancer/DS00301. Accessed autumn 2006.
19. What Are the Key Statistics about Stomach Cancer? © 2006 American Cancer Society, Inc. http://www.cancer.org/docroot/CRI/content/CRI_2_4_1X_What_are_the_key_statistics_for_stomach_cancer_40.asp?sitearea=. Accessed autumn 2006.
20. Staging of Stomach Cancer. © 2001–2006 The Doctors Lounge. http://www.thedoctorslounge.net/oncology/tnm/stomach.htm. Accessed autumn 2006.
21. McCoy K. Cancer Staging Affects Patients' Survival. © 2006 ScoutNews LLC. All rights reserved. http://www.nlm.nih.gov/medlineplus/news/fullstory_39108.html. Accessed autumn 2006.
22. What Are the Key Statistics for Colorectal Cancer? © 2006 American Cancer Society, Inc. http://www.cancer.org/docroot/CRI/content/CRI_2_4_1X_What_are_the_key_statistics_for_colon_and_rectum_cancer.asp. Accessed autumn 2006.
23. Colon cancer. © 1998–2006 Mayo Foundation for Medical Education and Research. All rights reserved. http://www.mayoclinic.com/health/colon-cancer/DS00035. Accessed autumn 2006.
24. Santoro M. Colon Polyps. © 1996–2005 MedicineNet, Inc. http://www.medicinenet.com/script/main/art.asp?articlekey=7761&pf=3&page=1. Accessed autumn 2006.
25. Colorectal Cancer: The Importance of Prevention and Early Detection. Centers for Disease Control and Prevention. http://www.cdc.gov/cancer/colorectal/pdf/about2004.pdf. Accessed autumn 2006.
26. How Is Colorectal Cancer Staged? © 2006 American Cancer Society, Inc. http://www.cancer.org/docroot/CRI/content/CRI_2_4_3X_How_is_colon_and_rectum_cancer_staged.asp. Accessed autumn 2006.
27. Kazzi A, Kazzi Z. Diverticular Disease. © 1996–2006 by WebMD. http://www.emedicine.com/emerg/topic152.htm. Accessed autumn 2006.
28. Digestive Diseases Statistics. National Institute of Diabetes and Digestive and Kidney Diseases. NIH Publication 06–3873. http://digestive.niddk.nih.gov/statistics/statistics.htm. Accessed autumn 2006.
29. Irritable bowel syndrome. © 1998–2006 Mayo Foundation for Medical Education and Research. All rights reserved. http://www.mayoclinic.com/health/irritable-bowel-syndrome/DS00106. Accessed autumn 2006.
30. IBS Patients Show Greater Brain Response to Subliminal Gut Stimuli. Reuters Health Information 2006. © 2006 Reuters Ltd. Gastroenterology 2006;130:26–33,267–269. http://www.medscape.com/viewarticle/523558. Accessed autumn 2006.

31. Inadequate fetal growth linked to irritable bowel. © 2006 Reuters Limited. All rights reserved. http://www.nlm.nih.gov/medlineplus/news/fullstory_39277.html. Accessed autumn 2006.
32. The Brain Gut Axis. IBS Research Update.org. http://www.ibs-research-update.org.uk/ibs/brain1ie4.html. Accessed autumn 2006.
33. Schoenfeld P. New Developments in the Treatment of Irritable Bowel Syndrome. Medscape Gastroenterology 2006;8(2) © 2006 by Medscape. http://www.medscape.com/viewarticle/540226. Accessed autumn 2006.
34. Ulcerative Colitis. National Institute of Diabetes and Digestive and Kidney Diseases. NIH Publication 06–1597. http://digestive.niddk.nih.gov/ddiseases/pubs/colitis/. Accessed autumn 2006.
35. Chronic Liver Disease/Cirrhosis. Centers for Disease Control and Prevention. http://www.cdc.gov/nchs/fastats/liverdis.htm. Accessed autumn 2006.
36. Wolf D. Cirrhosis. © 1996–2006 by WebMD. http://www.emedicine.com/med/topic3183.htm. Accessed autumn 2006.
37. Statistics about Cirrhosis of the Liver. © 2000–2005 Adviware Pty Ltd. All rights reserved. http://www.wrongdiagnosis.com/c/cirrhosis_of_the_liver/stats.htm. Accessed autumn 2006.
38. The American Liver Foundation Turns Its Attention to Fatty Liver Disease, a Serious Disease Affecting One Out of 10 Americans. © 2002–2006 American Liver Foundation. All rights reserved. http://www.liverfoundation.org/db/pressrelease/77. Accessed autumn 2006.
39. Gout Drug May Help Prevent Liver Cancer. © 2006 ScoutNews LLC. All rights reserved. http://www.nlm.nih.gov/medlineplus/news/fullstory_38476.html. Accessed autumn 2006.
40. Milk Thistle: Effects on Liver Disease and Cirrhosis and Clinical Adverse Effects. Summary, Evidence Report/Technology Assessment: Number 21, September 2000. Agency for Healthcare Research and Quality, Rockville, MD. http://www.ahrq.gov/clinic/epcsums/milktsum.htm. Accessed autumn 2006.
41. Dieting and Gallstones. National Institutes of Health. NIH Publication 02-3677. http://win.niddk.nih.gov/publications/gallstones.htm. Accessed autumn 2006.
42. Buggs A, Lim J. Hepatitis. © 1996–2006 by WebMD. http://www.emedicine.com/emerg/topic244.htm. Accessed autumn 2006.
43. Hepatitis and Liver Disease in the United States. © 2005 The American Liver Foundation. http://www.liverfoundation.org/cgi-bin/dbs/articles.cgi?db=articles&uid=default&ID=1008&view_records=1. Accessed autumn 2006.
44. O'Shea RS. Hepatitis B. © The Cleveland Clinic Foundation. http://www.clevelandclinicmeded.com/diseasemanagement/gastro/hepatitis_b/hepatitis_b.htm. Accessed autumn 2006.
45. Protect yourself against hepatitis A and hepatitis B . . . a guide for gay and bisexual men. Immunization Action Coalition. http://www.immunize.org/catg.d/p4115.htm. Accessed autumn 2006.
46. Hepatitis C Fact Sheet. Centers for Disease Control and Prevention. http://www.cdc.gov/ncidod/diseases/hepatitis/c/fact.htm. Accessed autumn 2006.
47. Cancer of the Liver and Intrahepatic Bile Duct. National Cancer Institute. http://seer.cancer.gov/statfacts/html/livibd.html. Accessed autumn 2006.
48. Stuart K, Stadler Z. Hepatic Carcinoma, Primary. © 1996–2006 by WebMD. http://www.emedicine.com/med/topic2664.htm. Accessed autumn 2006.
49. What Are the Key Statistics about Cancer of the Pancreas? © 2006 American Cancer Society, Inc. http://www.cancer.org/docroot/CRI/content/CRI_2_4_1X_What_are_the_key_statistics_for_pancreatic_cancer_34.asp?sitearea#. Accessed autumn 2006.
50. Erickson R. Pancreatic Cancer. © 1996–2006 by WebMD. http://www.emedicine.com/med/topic1712.htm. Accessed autumn 2006.
51. How Is Cancer of the Pancreas Staged? © 2006 American Cancer Society, Inc. http://www.cancer.org/docroot/cri/content/cri_2_4_3x_how_is_pancreatic_cancer_staged_34.asp?sitearea=cri. Accessed autumn 2006
52. Pancreatic cancer. © 1998–2006 Mayo Foundation for Medical Education and Research. All rights reserved. http://www.mayoclinic.com/health/pancreatic-cancer/DS00357. Accessed autumn 2006.
53. Pancreatitis. National Institute of Diabetes and Digestive and Kidney Diseases. NIH Publication 04–1596. http://digestive.niddk.nih.gov/ddiseases/pubs/pancreatitis/index.htm. Accessed autumn 2006.
54. Statistics about Peritonitis. © 2000–2005 Adviware Pty Ltd. All rights reserved. http://www.wrongdiagnosis.com/p/peritonitis/stats.htm. Accessed autumn 2006.

9

Endocrine System Conditions

Chapter Objectives

After reading this chapter, you should be able to . . .

- Describe why the pituitary gland is called the master gland.
- Identify the functions of the hormones calcitonin, parathyroid hormone, thyroxine, adrenaline, cortisol.
- List two risk factors for working with clients who have acromegaly.
- Identify two types of diabetes.
- List two emergencies associated with extremes in blood glucose levels.
- Identify a synonym for hypercortisolism.
- Name the major long-term risk for hyperthyroidism treatment.
- Name three types of thyroid cancer.
- Name three signs of hypothyroidism.
- Name five factors that contribute to metabolic syndrome.

INTRODUCTION

The endocrine system is a collection of glands that secrete hormones: chemical messages that instruct or stimulate other glands and tissues in the body to function in a variety of ways. Where the autonomic nervous system exerts electrical control over homeostatic body functions, the endocrine system exerts chemical control. Interestingly, the control center for both systems is the same structure, the hypothalamus.

The hypothalamus is a nondescript mass of tissue deep in the brain. It has a generous blood supply, which allows it to monitor functions of the body. The hypothalamus is primarily responsible for maintaining homeostasis, or a stable internal environment. It does so through electrical transmission to the brainstem to manage heart rate, blood pressure, temperature, and other functions and also through electrical and chemical transmission to the pituitary gland, the so-called master gland of the endocrine system. The hypothalamus is directly above and behind the pituitary, and it tells the pituitary what to secrete and when to secrete it. Sometimes the hypothalamus, via a stalk called the ***infundibulum***, sends out its own hormones to be released into the blood by the pituitary gland.

Chemicals released by the hypothalamus and pituitary travel to their target glands through the circulatory system. They stimulate those glands to release *their* hormones. When those secretions reach appropriate levels in the blood, the hypothalamus and pituitary stop sending out signals; most endocrine regulation is operated via a negative feedback loop.

The cycle of hormone stimulation and suppression usually works best when it occurs in gentle, rhythmic fluctuation. For example, when a person's blood sugar gets low, two things happen: he perceives that he is hungry, and his pancreas secretes glucagon, a hormone that stimulates the liver to release stored glucose. He eats, his digestive tract absorbs sugar from his meal, and his blood sugar rises. This stimulates the pancreas to release insulin to carry the sugar out of the blood and into cells, lowering blood sugar. When levels are low enough, the person gets hungry, beginning the cycle again. The blood sugar–insulin cycle takes place several times a day; it takes only a few hours to move from one state to another. Another endocrine cycle, the circadian rhythm, moves on a roughly 24-hour rotation. The menstrual cycle also depends on regular fluctuations, but this one lasts about 4 weeks. Other cycles, specifically those related to stress and perceived threat, depend on external circumstances to determine their frequency and duration.

Endocrine system glands secrete dozens of chemicals, each of which has specific target tissues and functions. Endocrine effects may also be determined by the frequency with which they are released into the bloodstream and the balance between each hormone and its antagonists.

Hormones fall into three chemical classes:

- ***Peptides*** are the most common type of hormones. They are made of chains of amino acids and are stored in various cellular holding tanks. Growth hormone, erythropoietin, and parathyroid hormone are peptide hormones.
- ***Amines*** are derived from a specific amino acid, ***tyrosine***. They are also stored in cellular deposits. Adrenaline and thyroxine are examples of amine hormones.
- ***Steroids*** are lipids. They are not stored; steroid levels are maintained through constant production. Cortisol and testosterone are steroid hormones.

Major Hormones

It is useful for massage therapists to be able to recognize the names of most hormones and their actions, since this is a key feature of physiology. But a few hormones are so strongly implicated in basic health issues that massage therapists may benefit from more than just passing familiarity:

- *Growth hormone* is released from the pituitary gland and stimulates conversion of fuel into new cells. Infants, children, and teenagers secrete massive amounts of growth hormone; adults secrete less. When a person has finished growing, the primary purpose of growth hormone is to stimulate regeneration and repair of damaged tissue, in other words, healing. Growth hormone is secreted primarily in stage IV sleep. Sleep disorders can lead to a shortage of this important chemical.
- *Adrenaline*, also called epinephrine, is a steroid hormone. It comes from the adrenal gland medulla, along with a very similar hormone, noradrenaline. It is associated with short-term, high-grade stress and acts to reinforce the reactions initiated by the sympathetic nervous system. An inefficient connection between the pituitary gland and the adrenal glands can cause a sluggish stress response system; this is discussed in the article on depression in Chapter 4.
- *Cortisol*, another steroid hormone, is one of a group of ***glucocorticoids*** secreted by the adrenal cortex. It influences the metabolism of proteins. It is the hormone secreted under long-term, low-grade stress, and it is measurable in the saliva. Cortisol is important for several reasons: It is a very powerful anti-inflammatory and is sometimes used systemically or locally for that purpose. It can damage connective tissues—people with systemically high levels of cortisol are prone to musculoskeletal injury and osteoporosis. It also suppresses immune system response to disease and infection. Chronically high levels of cortisol are a factor in many chronic stress-related disorders.
- *Mineralocorticoids* are adrenal cortex secretions that help to regulate electrolyte balance and control fluid retention. ***Aldosterone*** is a major mineralocorticoid.
- *Insulin and glucagon* work together to regulate blood glucose. Insulin decreases it, and glucagon increases it. Both are manufactured and released by the pancreas.
- *Thyroid hormones* are secreted by the thyroid gland in two molecular forms, triiodothyronine (T_3) and thyroxine (T_4). These hormones stimulate the metabolism of fuel into energy. Thyroid pathologies have to do with overproduction or underproduction of metabolic hormones.
- *Calcitonin*, another thyroid secretion, stimulates osteoblasts to extract calcium from the blood and add to bone density. In other words, it decreases blood calcium.
- *Parathyroid hormone* comes from the tiny parathyroid glands located deep to the thyroid gland. It is

the antagonist of calcitonin, stimulating osteoclast activity and pulling calcium off the bones to raise blood calcium.

- *Testosterone, estrogens, and progesterone* are steroid hormones released mainly by the gonads (testicles for men, ovaries for women). They have to do with secondary sexual characteristics, menstrual cycle, maintaining pregnancy, and a host of other issues. Anabolic steroid supplements increase muscle mass; this is why they are sometimes employed by athletes, often with unforeseen and dangerous results. The negative feedback loops in these hormone relationships seem to be especially precarious, possibly because environmental exposures to various types of hormones (in medications, dairy products, meat, plastics, pesticides, and other environmental toxins) overbalance the scales. A phenomenon called estrogen dominance is now being considered in the identification and treatment of symptoms relating to premenstrual syndrome, menopause, and other women's health issues. This is discussed further in Chapter 11.
- *Other hormones* have less implication for massage but a big impact on how well the body works. One is ***erythropoietin***, secreted by the kidneys. Erythropoietin stimulates the production of red blood cells. It can be artificially supplemented to increase oxygen-carrying capacity of the blood, but this may also increase the risk of blood clots. ***Thymosin*** is a hormone from the thymus; it is involved with the maturation of T-cells. ***Melatonin*** comes from the pineal gland and helps to regulate wake-sleep cycles. ***Prostaglandins*** are hormones produced by almost any kind of cell for local action. Prostaglandins produce a myriad of effects in the body, including smooth muscle contraction and increased pain sensitivity.

Endocrine glands release their secretions (often under direction of the pituitary-hypothalamus unit) directly into the blood. This distinguishes them from exocrine glands, which send their secretions into ducts for release into specific local areas. The hormones circulate systemically through the body but attach to specific receptor sites on their target tissues. Then they stimulate the target tissue to perform some function, such as making red blood cells (erythropoietin from the kidneys acting on bone marrow) or pulling calcium off the bones (parathyroid hormone acting on osteoclasts).

Most endocrine system disorders have to do with imbalances in the hormones being produced. Autoimmune attacks or tumors may stimulate or suppress certain glands, leading to problems with the negative feedback loop. When too much or too little of any hormone is present in the blood, symptoms can be felt throughout the body. Other endocrine disruptions occur when circulating hormone levels are normal but target tissues have developed resistance to their action.

Existing methods to measure and evaluate hormone balance are as accurate as scientists can make them, but it is likely that subtle dysfunctions are often missed in diagnosis, leading to chronic low-grade symptoms that may never successfully be resolved. Fortunately, most extreme endocrine problems are fairly rare and not exacerbated by massage. Most clients with endocrine disorders can receive great benefits from bodywork.

ENDOCRINE SYSTEM DISORDERS

Acromegaly
Addison disease
Cushing syndrome
Diabetes mellitus
Hyperthyroidism
Hypothyroidism
Metabolic syndrome

Acromegaly in Brief

Pronunciation: ak-ro-MEG-ah-le

What is it?

Acromegaly is a condition characterized by excessive secretion of growth hormone, often related to a benign tumor on the pituitary gland.

How is it recognized?

Acromegaly usually comes on in the 20s or 30s, when patients find that their hands, feet, and face have gradually grown and become distorted. Joint pain with bony deformation is common. Debilitating headaches, visual problems, or cranial nerve damage may occur if the tumor presses on sensitive tissue in the central nervous system. Ultimately, cardiovascular weakness develops as the enlarged heart struggles to pump blood to new tissues.

Is massage indicated or contraindicated?

The most serious risk for acromegaly patients is that their cardiovascular system cannot keep up with the demands of their suddenly growing body. High blood pressure, enlargement of the heart, and heart failure are common complications of this disorder. This population also has a higher-than-normal risk of diabetes and colorectal cancer. As long as those concerns are respected, massage may be appropriate for acromegaly patients, many of whom have bone and joint pain. Massage therapists should work with these clients as part of a well-informed health care team.

Acromegaly

Definition: What Is It?

Acromegaly is a disorder involving too much growth hormone. It is usually related to the development of a slow-growing benign tumor on the pituitary gland, although it can occasionally be connected to tumors elsewhere. It involves abnormal growth (*mega* is from the Greek for *large*) of many body parts, especially the hands and feet (*acro* refers to extremities). When a tumor on the pituitary occurs in an adult, the resulting disorder is called acromegaly. When it occurs in a child, the condition is called *gigantism*.

Demographics: Who Gets It?

Acromegaly is usually diagnosed among young adults. It affects men and women about equally. It is a relatively rare condition, affecting about 11,000 people in the United States. About 800 people are diagnosed each year.[1]

Etiology: What Happens?

Among the many jobs of the pituitary gland is the secretion of growth hormone under the command of the hypothalamus. The secretion of growth hormone in turn stimulates the release from the liver of *somatomedin C*, also known as insulinlike growth factor I (IGF-I). Growth hormone and IGF-I stimulate the metabolism of fuel into new cells for growth (in young people) and for repair (in older people).

When a tumor grows on the pituitary gland, excessive amounts of growth hormone are released, leading to excessive secretion of IGF-I. This stimulates production of masses of new tissues, resulting in bone enlargement, which can cause joint distortion and pain, and enlargement and weakening of the heart. In addition, the tumor itself can exert mechanical pressure in the central nervous system, causing a variety of problems unrelated to hormonal disruption. The type of tumor associated with acromegaly is benign, but dangerous for the symptoms it causes.

Signs and Symptoms

Often the earliest noticed symptoms of acromegaly are headaches and vision problems brought about by mechanical pressure inside the cranium. Excessive growth hormone secretion in adulthood leads to enlargement of the hands and feet and facial changes, including enlarged mandibles and spaces between teeth. Joint pain, fatigue, hyperhidrosis (excessive sweatiness) with body odor, and sleep apnea (probably related to an enlarged tongue) are frequent problems. Skin tags are common, as is a deepening voice. If a tumor grows to a significant size, other central nervous system symptoms may occur, including cranial nerve damage.

The onset of acromegaly is typically so slow that many years may elapse between the beginning of symptoms and a conclusive diagnosis.

Complications

Because the sudden growth of new tissues late in life puts a significant stress on the heart, many of the most serious complications of acromegaly have to do with cardiovascular stress. High blood pressure is a common complication, along with pathological enlargement of the heart. Eventually, untreated acromegaly patients may develop congestive heart failure.

Some acromegaly patients develop insulin resistance or diabetes mellitus. A higher-than-average risk of colorectal cancer has also been observed among this population. Women are more prone to uterine fibroid tumors as well.

Diagnosis

Acromegaly is diagnosed when abnormal growth is detected and when both growth hormone and IGF-I levels are elevated. These signs are confirmed with computed tomography (CT) or magnetic resonance imaging (MRI) that identifies a pituitary tumor.

Pituitary tumors often grow slowly, so the symptoms of acromegaly develop over a long period. More than 90% of diagnoses are made when the tumor is larger than 1 cm, which makes surgical removal difficult.[2]

Treatment

Surgery for acromegaly is most successful when the pituitary tumor is smaller than 1 cm, but only relatively few cases are diagnosed at this stage (Case History 9.1). Other therapies focus on attempts to rectify the growth hormone–IGF-I balance that is lost when the pituitary gland becomes hyperactive. Various medications inhibit growth hormone secretion or uptake in target tissues. If an acromegaly patient can begin treatment with these medications before developing circulatory problems, the disease can be manageable and not necessarily a life-shortening condition.

CASE HISTORY 9.1

My Dance with Acromegaly

Mark, aged "a very youthful 61": "The tips of my fingers showed tufting, not unlike the outline of mushroom caps; they were identical to the pictures of acromegaly in her orthopedic pathology text."

It's not uncommon, when new friends shake my hand, for them to react with surprise and to mention how large my hands are, as persons of my height don't usually have such large hands. I've gotten used to their shock and their unusually personal questions about my heritage and genetics and whether my hand size has anything to do with my 19 years as a massage therapist. I mention this as a reminder to bodyworkers to be respectful and to consider whether their questions are appropriate. It's not unlike asking an overweight person, "Are you so fat because of your genetics or because you eat too much and don't exercise?"

If my wife hadn't been a chiropractor, I likely would never have done anything about the gradual changes in my facial structure and hands. In 1991 she noticed subtle changes and decided to do some x-rays. The tips of my fingers showed tufting, similar to the outline of mushroom caps; they were identical to the pictures of acromegaly in her orthopedic pathology text. Subsequent blood tests showed abnormally high levels of human growth hormone, so I got an MRI of the cranium to see what was in there.

The cause turned out to be a benign 1-mm tumor on the pituitary, and it was stimulating excessive production of growth hormone. Surgery was scheduled; it's called a trans-sphenoidal adenectomy. The neurosurgeon drills a hole above the upper teeth, looks around inside the brain, and plucks out the tumor. After 4 days in intensive care and another few in the hospital, you're good as new.

About 10 years after the surgery I had another MRI that showed an undifferentiated mass of cells where the tumor had been, too small to call for surgery, so nothing was done about it. I've been taking a small dose of bromocriptine to control its growth and will likely do so for the rest of my life.

Today I live normally, more concerned about losing 10 lb and lowering my blood pressure than about my pituitary gland. The Pituitary Center continues to send me invitations to its pituitary support group for persons who suffer from acromegaly, but since I'm not suffering, I don't RSVP.

Massage?

High blood pressure, enlargement of the heart, and congestive heart failure are key complications of acromegaly. Swedish massage, sports massage, and other modalities that focus on moving a lot of fluid through the system may not be appropriate if these complications have developed.

Joint pain and arthritis are other common complications of acromegaly. Although bodywork cannot reverse these changes, it may be able to alleviate some of the musculoskeletal pain that they cause.

A massage therapist working with an acromegaly patient should be part of a well-informed health care team.

Modality Recommendations for Acromegaly

Modality	Recommendation
Deep tissue massage	Supportive if therapist acting as part of health care team. Work away from affected areas to release compression.
Lymphatic drainage	Supportive.
Polarity	S/R/D: Indicated.
PNF/MET/stretching	Supportive.
Reflexology	Work with health care team; focus on endocrine system, liver, kidney points.
Shiatsu	Indicated: treat endocrine function via the K meridian.
Swedish massage	Supportive with caution; match to client's activity level.
Trigger point therapy	Indicated.

See Chapter 1 for a brief description of each modality, including definitions of abbreviations.

Addison Disease in Brief

What is it?
Addison disease is a condition that inhibits secretions of the adrenal cortex. It is usually an autoimmune disease of the adrenal gland itself, but it can also be secondary to an infection or pituitary problem.

How is it recognized?
Signs and symptoms of Addison disease include muscle weakness, fatigue, weight loss, and low blood pressure. Depending on the source of the problem, salt craving, nausea, diarrhea, dehydration, and hyperpigmentation of isolated patches of skin may also occur.

Is massage indicated or contraindicated?
Addison disease often is accompanied by weakness and low blood pressure. Treatment entails taking steroids that carry important side effects. Massage therapists and other bodyworkers must respect these issues and make adjustments accordingly.

Addison Disease

Definition: What Is It?

Addison disease was first described in 1855 by Thomas Addison, who documented the consequences of adrenal cortex insufficiency. At that time tuberculosis infections of the adrenal glands were the most common cause; nowadays in industrialized countries Addison disease is usually an autoimmune condition that affects adrenal function. It can limit the secretion of any combination of cortisol, aldosterone, or androgenic hormones.

Demographics: Who Gets It?

Addison disease is relatively rare, affecting about 13,000 people in the United States.[3] It affects men and women about equally and is diagnosed most often between ages 30 and 50.[4]

Etiology: What Happens?

The adrenal glands are composed of two main regions: the medulla and the cortex. The adrenal cortex, or outer layer, produces several hormones in three main classes: glucocorticoids, mineralocorticoids, and androgens. Glucocorticoids, of which cortisol is the best known, produce appropriate stress responses; influence the metabolism of proteins, fats, and sugars; suppress immune system activity; and do several other important jobs. Mineralocorticoids (***aldosterone*** is the principal hormone in this group) help to maintain blood pressure by influencing water and salt retention at the kidneys. ***Androgens*** are male sex hormones; women secrete much of their androgens from the adrenal cortex, while men secrete most of theirs from the testes.

Primary Addison disease develops when the adrenal cortex doesn't produce enough of its characteristic hormones. About 70% of Addison disease cases are related to an autoimmune attack on the adrenal glands. When the adrenal glands are the only affected tissues, it is called *idiopathic adrenal insufficiency*. When the adrenal glands are damaged in conjunction with several other endocrine glands, it is called *polyendocrine deficiency syndrome*.

Tuberculosis infection of the adrenal glands can also cause primary Addison disease. Tuberculosis causes only about 20% of cases in the United States, but in undeveloped countries it is still a leading cause of Addison disease. Adrenal damage can also occur because of cancer metastasis, chronic fungal infection, local hemorrhage, and other more obscure reasons.

Secondary Addison disease is identified when pituitary secretions are abnormal. The pituitary typically stimulates the adrenal gland by secreting adrenocorticotropic hormone (ACTH). If ACTH levels drop, cortisol secretion also drops. This can occur when a person suddenly stops taking steroidal hormones (i.e., synthetic forms of cortisol) or when the pituitary is affected by a tumor or surgery.

Signs and Symptoms

Primary Addison disease usually affects secretion of all adrenal cortex hormones, so symptoms are indicative of cortisol depletion along with low levels of aldosterone and androgens. Secondary Addison disease affects cortisol secretion alone; aldosterone and androgen levels remain stable.

Signs and symptoms of cortisol depletion include muscle weakness and fatigue, low blood pressure, hypoglycemia, irritability, and depression. When aldosterone levels are low, salt craving and dehydration develop. Low androgen levels in women result in the loss of pubic and axillary hair; men, who secrete most of their androgens from the testes, are not affected in this way.

Chronically low cortisol levels stimulate the hypothalamus to release corticotrophin-releasing hormone (CRH), which tells the pituitary to release ACTH more frequently than normal. CRH has a chemical relation to melanocyte-stimulating hormone. Consequently, disruption in CRH levels can also lead to areas of hyperpigmentation, that is, darkened patches at skin folds and mucous membranes where melanocytes are overactive.

Complications

People with Addison disease are at risk for a sudden onset of extreme signs and symptoms that include sharp abdominal pain along with severe nausea, vomiting, and diarrhea. Low back pain and pain in the arms and legs may occur, along with dangerously low blood pressure and loss of consciousness. This describes an addisonian crisis, and it is a medical emergency.

Diagnosis

Addison disease is diagnosed with a variety of tests that measure cortisol levels in the blood, reactivity to certain hormones, and imaging (CT or MRI) of the adrenals and pituitary gland.

Adrenal cortex antibodies can be identified in blood tests. While adrenal cortex antibody levels can be higher than normal with no symptoms, this indicates a risk of developing Addison disease, so patients are advised to be vigilant about their adrenal health.

Treatment

Addison disease is highly treatable with oral doses of steroids, although finding the correct dosage to control symptoms without developing side effects can be challenging. Patients may take synthetic forms of cortisol, aldosterone, and androgens, depending on individual needs.

Massage?

Massage for a person with Addison disease is guided by the client's resilience, activities of daily living, and side effects of medication. Clients are likely to have hypotension, and many forms of bodywork lower blood pressure further, so strokes or techniques that stimulate rather than soothe the client are advised to conclude a bodywork session.

Modality Recommendations for Addison Disease

Deep tissue massage	Supportive: work to relax and release fascial tension.
Lymphatic drainage	Supportive.
Polarity	S/R/D: Indicated; can support immune system; pressure determined by client's comfort and resilience.
PNF/MET/stretching	Supportive.
Reflexology	Indicated with short, frequent sessions; work adrenals, solar plexus, brain, liver points.
Shiatsu	Indicated: treat adrenals via K meridian; immune system via TH, SP meridians and extensions.
Swedish massage	Indicated to facilitate homeostasis, if symptoms controlled with medication.
Trigger point therapy	Supportive.

See Chapter 1 for a brief description of each modality, including definitions of abbreviations.

Cushing Syndrome in Brief

What is it?
Cushing syndrome is a condition involving too much cortisol in the blood for long periods. It can be brought about by steroid use, pituitary tumors, or other tumors.

How is it recognized?
Leading signs and symptoms of Cushing syndrome include weight gain around the abdomen and thorax; fat deposits in the neck and face; thin, delicate skin that develops purplish stretch marks; weakness in arm and leg muscles; impaired immune system function; thinning bones; high blood pressure; and high blood glucose.

Is massage indicated or contraindicated?
Untreated Cushing syndrome is a dangerous condition involving weak bones and cardiovascular compromise; bodywork in this context must be conservative. Most patients with Cushing syndrome are able to minimize complications, however, so bodywork choices can be based on normal activity levels.

Cushing Syndrome

Definition: What Is It?

Cushing syndrome was first documented by American endocrinologist Harvey Cushing in 1932. It is a condition in which cortisol levels in the blood are excessively high for a long period (hypercortisolism), leading to tissue changes and possible death.

Demographics: Who Gets It?

Cushing syndrome has been diagnosed in 10 to 15 in 1 million people in the United States. This amounts to about 3,000 to 4,500 people who have Cushing syndrome at any given time.[5] One form of Cushing syndrome is more common in women than men; another form has the opposite pattern.

Etiology: What Happens?

Cortisol is the principal glucocorticoid hormone. It is secreted by the adrenal cortex, and it has many functions, including working with the stress response, immune system suppression, metabolism of food into energy, and balancing insulin activity. Cortisol production is controlled by the hypothalamus, which signals the pituitary gland when to release adrenocorticotrophic hormone (ACTH). ACTH stimulates the adrenal glands to release cortisol. When cortisol levels are dangerously high for too long, many tissues throughout the body are affected.

Hypercortisolism is often discussed as ***exogenous*** (coming from outside the body) or ***endogenous*** (from within the body) Cushing syndrome.

Patients who have autoimmune disease or who are organ transplant recipients may take cortisol-based steroid medications to control their disease or to prevent tissue rejection. These medications have serious side effects, including bone thinning, diabetes, mood swings, and high blood pressure. This is exogenous Cushing syndrome, and it is the most common form of hypercortisolism.

Endogenous Cushing syndrome develops when too much ACTH is secreted by the pituitary gland or other tissues, or when the adrenal glands themselves secrete too much cortisol. It is often discussed as one of these types:

- *Pituitary adenoma.* This is growth of a benign tumor on the pituitary that secretes abnormal levels of ACTH. Also called *Cushing disease*, this condition is five times more common in women than in men.
- *Ectopic ACTH syndrome.* This is secretion of ACTH from tissues outside the pituitary gland. Most often, these ACTH-secreting cells are cancer cells in the lung, pancreas, thymus, or thyroid gland. Ectopic ACTH syndrome is three times more common in men than in women.
- *Adrenal tumors.* In rare cases tumors grow on the adrenal glands themselves, and they secrete excessive cortisol. These can be benign adenomas or nodules, or they can be malignant growths on the adrenal glands.

Signs and Symptoms

Signs and symptoms of Cushing syndrome are produced by too much cortisol in the bloodstream. Because this hormone has so many functions, having it too much of it can cause many changes.

Perhaps the best-recognized sign of Cushing syndrome is the development of fatty deposits around the neck and face (giving rise to a "moon face" presentation) and around the abdomen and upper back. Arms and legs typically become quite thin and weak (Figure 9.1).

High levels of cortisol can damage supportive collagen. This is reflected in bone thinning, as the collagen matrix for calcium deposits is affected, and in the development of very thin, delicate skin, often with purple stretch marks. The superficial fascia loses much of its strength with this disease.

Other effects of hypercortisolism include high blood pressure; high blood glucose (with an increased risk of developing diabetes); mood changes that include irritability, anxiety, and depression; severe acne; slowed healing with suppressed immune system activity; the development of excessive body hair (hirsutism) and disrupted menstrual cycles for women; and decreased fertility, decreased sex drive, and erectile dysfunction for men.

Diagnosis

A number of tests have been developed to identify Cushing syndrome. Cortisol levels can be tracked over time in the blood, urine, or saliva. Once cortisol levels are established to be higher than normal, the next challenge is to determine where the dysfunction is. This is accomplished through a variety of hormone challenge tests or imaging, including CT or MRI of the adrenal glands and pituitary.

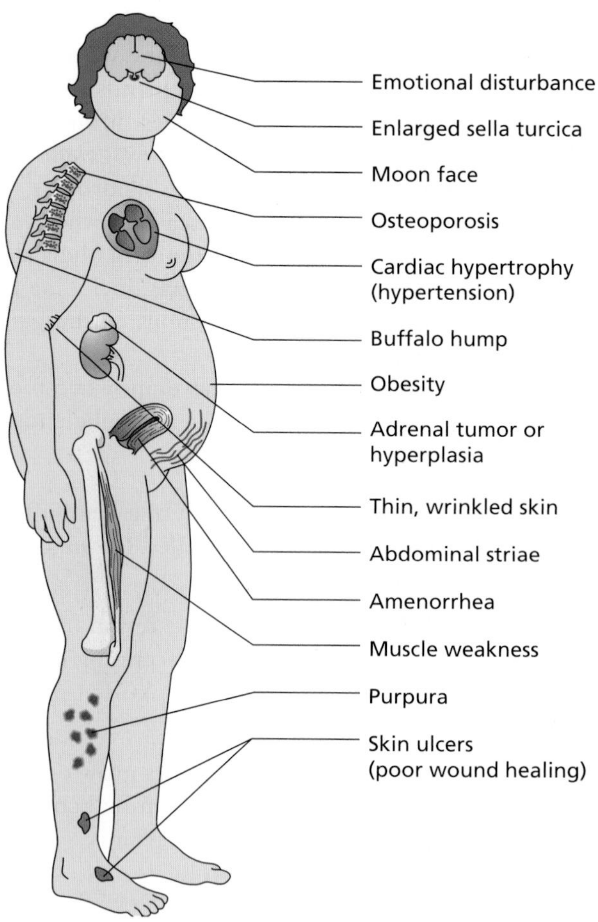

Figure 9.1. Systemic effects of Cushing syndrome.

Treatment

Cushing syndrome is treated according to its cause. Exogenous Cushing syndrome is treated by reevaluating the correct dose of corticosteroid drugs to achieve the best benefits with the least risk.

Pituitary adenomas are usually surgically removed, either through *transsphenoidal adenectomy* (a surgery conducted through the upper jaw or nose into the brain) or through *stereotactic radiosurgery*, in which multiple beams of radiation are aimed at the growth from different angles to kill the tumor without damaging nearby brain tissue.

Cushing syndrome brought about by cancer cells that secrete ACTH is treated by dealing with the cancer, but drugs that inhibit cortisol may also be used.

Massage?

The risks of bodywork for the client with Cushing syndrome are associated with high blood pressure, delicate bones, the possibility of diabetes, and a compromised immune system. As long as these issues are addressed, a massage therapist can provide a session that offers many benefits while effectively minimizing any risks.

Modality Recommendations for Cushing Disease	
Deep tissue massage	Supportive: work superficially to relax and release fascial tension.
Lymphatic drainage	Supportive.
Polarity	S/R/D: Indicated. Pressure determined by client's comfort.
PNF/MET/stretching	Supportive.
Reflexology	Indicated with short, frequent sessions; work adrenals, solar plexus, brain, liver points.
Shiatsu	Indicated: Treat K meridian and extension for endocrine function.
Swedish massage	Supportive with caution for fragile skin and bones; match massage to client's activity level.
Trigger point therapy	Supportive.

See Chapter 1 for a brief description of each modality, including definitions of abbreviations.

Diabetes Mellitus

Definition: What Is It?

Diabetes is not a single disease but rather a group of related disorders that all result in hyperglycemia, or elevated levels of sugar in the bloodstream. Two main varieties, type 1 and type 2 diabetes, are examined in this article. These account for about 98% of diabetes diagnoses.

Diabetes mellitus

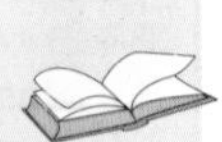

Diabetes comes from the Greek for "siphon" or to "pass through," referring to the tendency for diabetics to urinate very frequently. *Mellitus* is from Latin for *sweetened with honey*. Diabetes mellitus essentially means *sweet pee*.

Demographics: Who Gets It?

Diabetes is the sixth leading cause of death in the United States, contributing to about 224,000 deaths per year, although this is probably underreported.[6] Estimates vary, but most resources suggest that 18 to 21 million Americans have diabetes, although 5 million to 6 million people don't know it yet.[6,7] About 1.5 million people are diagnosed with diabetes each year.[6] Researchers credit an aging population along with higher numbers of obese young people and sedentary lifestyles for these alarming figures.

Diabetes, a largely treatable and even preventable disease, costs approximately $132 billion a year in direct medical costs and indirect costs of disability, lost wages, and premature mortality. It accounts for approximately 11% of health care costs.[8]

Type 2 diabetes occurs among all races but is most common among Native Americans, Alaskan, African American, Pacific Island, and Hispanic populations. Until recently, type 2 diabetes was a mature adult's disease; now many new diagnoses are among people under 25 years old.

Diabetes Mellitus in Brief

Pronunciation: di-ah-BE-tez meh-LY-tus

What is it?

Diabetes is a group of metabolic disorders characterized by disturbances in glucose metabolism.

How is it recognized?

Early symptoms of diabetes include frequent urination, thirst, and increased appetite along with weight loss, nausea, and vomiting. These symptoms are often subtle enough that the first signs of disease are the complications it can cause: neuropathy, impaired vision, kidney dysfunction, or other problems.

Is massage indicated or contraindicated?

Diabetes indicates massage as long as tissues are healthy and circulation is unimpaired. Many people with advanced or poorly treated diabetes have numbness, cardiovascular problems, and/or kidney failure. Circulatory massage in these situations is not appropriate, but less challenging forms of bodywork may be safer.

Etiology: What Happens?

Insulin is required to escort glucose into cells, where it can be consumed to produce energy; insulin also aids in the removal of fat from the blood into storage lipid cells. In diabetes glucose and fats accumulate in the blood, either because insulin is in short supply or because insulin receptor cells have developed resistance (or both). In the absence of insulin, the body cannot burn glucose, a remarkably

SIDEBAR 9.1: INSULIN RESISTANCE: SILENT AND DANGEROUS

Insulin resistance is a condition in which a given concentration of insulin does not have the expected effect on cellular uptake of blood glucose. It is typically related to decreased numbers of insulin receptors on cell membranes, often in conjunction with postreceptor problems inside the cell. Blood sugar levels climb, stimulating the production of more insulin. In this way, hyperglycemia and hyperinsulinemia (the presence of excessive insulin in the blood) occur simultaneously. This situation, along with excessive release of glucose from the liver, opens the door to type 2 diabetes mellitus.

Insulin resistance is also considered a causative factor for another disorder, *metabolic syndrome*, which is associated with a dangerously increased risk of many forms of heart disease.

Insulin resistance is directly connected to overloaded abdominal fat cells. These fat cells are metabolically different from subcutaneous fat cells; they produce many chemicals that have adverse affects on body functions. Losing 5% or more of overall fat storage can reduce the risk of insulin resistance and its associated diseases.[8]

Insulin resistance itself is often a silent disorder. Some patients develop a skin discoloration called **acanthosis nigricans**: velvety brown patches appear around skin folds, especially at the axilla. It is thought that excessive insulin interacts with skin cells to produce this sign. Episodes of hypoglycemia occasionally affect people with insulin resistance; this indicates that antibodies have destroyed damaged insulin receptor sites, temporarily causing a sudden uptake of blood glucose.

Insulin resistance may be identified by testing blood glucose and/or insulin after fasting, when levels should be low. Other experts suggest that a glucose tolerance test, which measures glucose in the blood 2 hours after a patient ingests 75 mg of sugar, is more indicative of the early stages of this disorder.

Statistics vary, but most suggest that about 3% of the general population has insulin resistance. That number is many times higher for target groups.[10]

clean fuel source, and must resort first to stored fat reserves and finally to proteins.

Several types of diabetes mellitus have been identified; the two most common varieties are considered here:

Type 1 diabetes mellitus Type 1 diabetes, formerly known as insulin-dependent diabetes mellitus (IDDM) is an autoimmune disorder. It can be brought about by a number of factors, including exposure to certain drugs and chemicals, or as a complication of some kinds of infections. Immune system cells of people with type 1 diabetes attack parts of the beta cells in the pancreas where insulin is produced. The destruction of these cells leads to a lifelong deficiency in insulin.

Type 1 diabetes usually shows symptoms before age 30, but one variety, called *latent autoimmune diabetes in adults* may not be identified until later. Type 1 diabetes is the rarer and more serious of the two basic types of diabetes. About 500,000 to 1 million people in the United States have it.[9] It accounts for 5% to 10% of diabetes in this country. It is most common in whites, but worldwide statistics for type 1 diabetes is on the rise.[10] Because type 1 diabetes requires self-administered doses of insulin to take the place of the constant steady production provided by a healthy pancreas, type 1 diabetics can go through extreme cycles of blood sugar levels—from high enough to cause ketoacidosis and diabetic coma to low enough to lead to insulin shock.

Type 2 diabetes mellitus This variety used to be called non–insulin-dependent diabetes mellitus (NIDDM), but that name is no longer accurate. It is slightly more common for women than men. Approximately 90% of people with type 2 diabetes are obese when they are diagnosed.[11] It is especially prevalent in African Americans, Hispanics, Pacific Islanders, and Native Americans.[12] Type 2 diabetes is usually controllable with diet, exercise, and possibly some antidiabetes drugs, depending on how far advanced it is when treatment begins, but many patients eventually benefit from supplementing insulin.

The exact cause of type 2 diabetes is uncertain and is probably different for different people. For some it seems clear that a lifelong habit of a high-carbohydrate diet simply wears out the pancreas and makes the insulin-producing cells less efficient. In others the insulin production may be at normal levels, but the incoming flood of glucose is too much to deal with. And for still others insulin production may be normal or even above normal, but the target cells have few receptor sites to receive the insulin. Insulin resistance is linked to several other diabetes risk factors, including metabolic syndrome, immune system problems, increased blood clotting, and impaired clot melting. Some researchers say that a combination of decreased insulin secretion and insulin resistance must be present for diabetes to develop. In any case the results are the same: frequent urination, excessive thirst, and excessive hunger, along with the possibility of dangerous accumulations of atherosclerotic plaques and other serious complications.

Other types of diabetes include gestational diabetes and secondary diabetes. Gestational diabetes occurs when a woman develops a transient case during pregnancy. Somewhere between 2% and 5% of pregnancies involve gestational diabetes. This condition can cause birth

CASE HISTORY 9.2

Diabetes

Maureen, aged 43: "A do-it-yourself project."

Maureen had gestational diabetes while pregnant with two of her three children. At age 42 she began having chronic yeast infections, unintentional weight loss, blurred vision, and unusual thirst. When she went for her annual checkup, she was not happy but also not surprised to be diagnosed with type 2 diabetes.

At first Maureen was intimidated by the glucose testing equipment she had to use, and she was terrified by the long-term complications that often develop with diabetes. But as she did more research, she came to the conclusion that diabetes is very much a do-it-yourself project. She found that proper control can be achieved through education, hard work, and stress reduction.

She tests her blood frequently and sees immediate relationships between her glucose levels and how much stress she's going through and how much exercise she gets. Since her diagnosis, Maureen's diabetes medication has been cut in half, and she is able to maintain reasonable glucose levels by being proactive about her health. Although she is still upset about her disease, she is thankful that she was diagnosed early enough to take control of her situation and change it for the better.

defects in the child, as well as changing fetal metabolism, which results in very high birth weights and a high incidence of cesarean sections. Women who have gestational diabetes and their babies also have an increased risk of developing type 2 diabetes later in life.

Secondary diabetes may develop with damage or trauma to the pancreas or as a symptom of some other endocrine disorder, such as acromegaly or Cushing syndrome. And ***diabetes insipidus*** is a dysfunction of the pituitary gland and insufficient production of antidiuretic hormone (ADH).

Signs and Symptoms

Three defining "polys" are common to all types of diabetes. ***Polyuria***, or frequent urination, results from elevated blood sugar, which acts as a diuretic; it pulls water from the cells in the body, and excess water is expelled in the urine. ***Polydipsia*** means excessive thirst, which accompanies the loss of water with polyuria. ***Polyphagia*** refers to increased appetite, since diabetics must get most of their energy from fats and proteins instead of carbohydrates, which are the most efficient kind of fuel. Other symptoms of diabetes include fatigue, weight loss, nausea, and vomiting.

Very often, signs of diabetes are missed until the disease has damaged other organs. These problems are discussed in the section on complications.

Diabetic Emergencies

People with diabetes are vulnerable to two classes of medical emergencies, both of which can be fatal if not treated promptly.

- *Ketoacidosis* is a critical *shortage* of insulin and lack of glucose in the cells in type 1 diabetics. The body partially metabolizes fats for fuel, and the acidic byproduct of that metabolism (ketones) dangerously changes the pH balance of the blood. ***Ketoacidosis*** is identifiable by a characteristic sweet or fruity odor to the breath. Diabetics can test themselves for ketoacidosis with test strips that look for signs of ketones in the urine. Ketoacidosis can be brought on by stress, infection, or trauma, and can lead to shock, coma, and death. It occurs only in people with type 1 diabetes.

- *Hyperosmolality* in type 2 diabetics is also related to high blood sugar. ***Hyperosmolality*** causes a change in the pH of the blood, which can lead to shock, coma, and death.
- *Insulin shock* is an emergency at the other end of the scale. In this case *too much* insulin is circulating, either because too much has been administered or because a skipped meal, sudden exertion, stress, infection, or trauma has resulted in the consumption of all available blood sugar. The consequence of having too much available insulin is a dangerously low blood sugar level, or ***hypoglycemia***. Symptoms of insulin shock include dizziness, confusion, weakness, and tremors. It too can lead to coma and death if not treated (with juice, milk, candy, or non-diet soda to replace blood sugar) quickly.

Complications

Complications of diabetes are many and serious and are often the first signs of the disease that cause a person to seek medical intervention.

- *Cardiovascular disease.* Diabetics are especially prone to these problems because high blood glucose and insulin resistance lead to chemical changes that damage endothelium, opening the door to atherosclerosis. Unlike many atherosclerosis patients, diabetics don't accumulate plaque just on coronary arterial walls but throughout the body. Diabetes increases the risk of stroke, hypertension, and aneurysm. Two-thirds to three-quarters of diabetes patients die of some form of cardiovascular problem.[8]
- *Edema.* This condition develops in the extremities because of sluggish blood return. It can also give rise to stasis dermatitis.
- *Ulcers, gangrene, and amputations.* Imagine what would happen if *all* of the body's blood vessels were caked with plaque. Even minor skin lesions don't heal well because of limited circulation. Ingrown toenails, blisters, or pressure spots on the feet can become life-threatening for diabetics: the tissue either dies of starvation or is infected with pathogens that are impossible to fight off, forming characteristic diabetic ulcers, usually on the feet (Figure 9.2). Diabetes leads to about 82,000 lower extremity amputations each year, or 60% of nontraumatic amputations.
- *Kidney disease.* Renal vessels get clogged with plaques very readily, since they are one of the first diversions from the descending aorta. Excessive blood glucose, which acts as a powerful diuretic, is also hard on the kidneys, causing reduced formation of glomerular filtrate and a thickening of the basement membrane in the Bowman capsule. Not surprisingly, then, diabetes is the leading cause of end-stage renal failure and of the need for kidney transplants.[8]
- *Impaired vision.* The capillaries of the eyes of diabetes patients can become abnormally thickened, depriving eye cells of nutrition. Diseased capillaries leak blood and proteins into the retina. Microaneurysms can form that also cut off circulation. All of these contribute to diabetic ***retinopathy***. Excessive glucose also binds with proteins in the lens, causing first cataracts, then blindness. This disease is the leading cause of new blindness among people 20 to 70 years old in the United States.[8]
- *Neuropathy.* Lack of capillary circulation and excessive sugar in the blood both contribute to nerve damage. Symptoms of peripheral neuropathy include tingling or pain and eventual numbness. Neuropathy of the autonomic motor system can lead to an inability to maintain postural blood pressure, delayed or inefficient emptying of the stomach, diarrhea, constipation, and sexual impotency. Neuropathy generally appears about 10 to 20 years after diabetes is diagnosed. About 30% of diabetes patients have some degree of neuropathy.[13]
- *Others.* Diabetes affects just about every body system in some way. It is linked to urinary tract infections, candidiasis, birth defects, a mold infection of the nose and sinuses

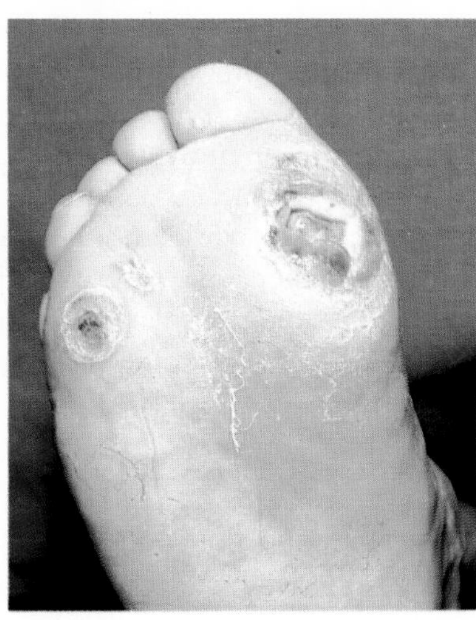

Figure 9.2. Diabetic ulcers.

called *mucormycosis*, aggressive ear infections that can invade the cranial bones (*malignant otitis externa*), and higher-than-normal rates of gingivitis and tooth loss.

Diagnosis

Normal fasting blood sugar (a measurement that is taken before eating in the morning) is 110 mg/dL of blood. Diabetes is diagnosed when fasting levels rise over 125 mg/dL for 2 or more consecutive days.

Another test, called the **hemoglobin A1c** test, measures how much sugar sticks to the hemoglobin in circulating erythrocytes. This is often considered a better long-term test, since it reflects general blood sugar levels for 3 months or more instead of in increments of several hours. A normal reading is 4% to 5.9%; diabetes is diagnosed when A1c tests show 8% or more glucose.

Treatment

Before the development of insulin in 1921, the diagnosis of diabetes was a death knell. Most people lived only a few years after the disease was identified. Now diabetes is a highly treatable disease, although not all diagnosed people treat it aggressively enough to prevent complications.

The goals for diabetes treatment are fourfold: to improve insulin production in the pancreas when possible, to inhibit the release of glucose from the liver, to increase the sensitivity of target cells to insulin, and to decrease the absorption of carbohydrates in the small intestines. In addition to these measures, special care of eyes and feet can reduce the risk of blindness and amputations associated with the disease.

Type 1 diabetes is treated primarily with insulin. New techniques for frequent administration of insulin have been developed to minimize the dangerous roller coaster ride of too much to too little blood sugar. These include insulin pens, which deliver a measured dose under the skin without a hypodermic needle; insulin pumps, which feed a steady drip into the body through a plastic tube; and inhalable insulin, which bypasses the need for needles.

Type 2 diabetes is first addressed with changes in diet and exercise, but many type 2 diabetes patients are eventually treated with insulin supplementation. Hypoglycemic agents may also be prescribed.

Many diabetes patients eventually develop renal insufficiency; their kidneys simply cannot keep up with their needs. ***Hemodialysis*** is a treatment in which the blood is routed through a filtering machine that removes excess water and waste products before returning the blood to the body. Dialysis of any kind is usually a stopgap measure while a person waits for a kidney to become available for transplant.

A kidney transplant may be recommended for people with advanced renal disease. Occasionally a kidney and pancreas are transplanted together for type 1 diabetics. Pancreas transplants have a high rejection rate, however. A new option, transplanting beta cells from a donor into the liver of the diabetic person, is being explored with some success, but it is not widely available.

Massage?

Massage may be appropriate for people with diabetes under the right circumstances. The main condition is that the client must have healthy, responsive tissue with good blood supply. For clients with advanced diabetes, kidney failure, and atherosclerosis, circulatory massage is probably out of the question, but energetic techniques are certainly appropriate.

Some researchers suggest that the best time to schedule a massage with a person who supplements insulin is *not* at the peak of insulin activity. Informal studies suggest that massage lowers blood sugar an average of 20 to 40 points,[14] so the risk of a hypoglycemic episode is significant. Diabetic clients who get regular massage would be well advised to measure their blood glucose before and after their sessions to determine whether they would benefit from eating a small meal before receiving massage. Massage therapists who have diabetic clients may want to keep high-sugar snacks (juice, milk, candy, sugared soda) available in case a client shows signs of hypoglycemia. Injection sites for insulin treatment should also be locally avoided.

Massage therapists should be aware that diabetic neuropathy can include lack of sensation. Someone with type 2 diabetes may be completely unaware of the condition until someone points out ulcers, which often occur on the feet.

Modality Recommendations for Diabetes Mellitus

Deep tissue massage	Contraindicated if advanced with tissue damage; otherwise supportive.
Lymphatic drainage	Supportive.
Polarity	S/R/D: Indicated. Pressure determined by client's comfort with caution for numbness.
PNF/MET/stretching	Supportive.
Reflexology	Work as part of health care team; focus on pancreas, solar plexus, liver, gallbladder, spleen, lymphatic system, kidneys, intestines points.
Shiatsu	Indicated. SP, GB meridians help stabilize condition when client works with diet and exercise.
Swedish massage	Indicated as long as client is healthy with no complications; massage can drop blood glucose levels.
Trigger point therapy	Supportive.

See Chapter 1 for a brief description of each modality, including definitions of abbreviations.

Hyperthyroidism

Definition: What Is It?

Hyperthyroidism is a condition in which the thyroid gland produces excessive amounts of hormones that stimulate metabolism of fuel into energy. Most cases of hyperthyroidism are related to autoimmune attacks against the whole thyroid gland. In these cases it may also be called *Graves disease* or *diffuse toxic thyroid*. More rarely, thyroid hyperactivity may be confined to one or a few nodes, or it may be due to thyroid inflammation.

Graves disease

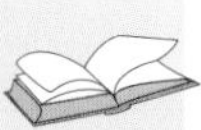

Graves disease is named after an Irish physician, Robert J. Graves (1796–1853). He first documented the relationship between an enlarged thyroid gland (goiter) and the symptoms it produces (excessive production of energy from fuel and bulging eyes).

Demographics: Who Gets It?

Hyperthyroidism is a common disorder affecting between 1 and 2% of people in the United States at some time in their lives. About 350,000 new cases are diagnosed every year. Women are affected more often than men, by a margin of about 8 to 1. Most cases are diagnosed between the ages of 20 and 40.[15]

A strong genetic link has been established in Graves disease; if one person has this disorder, it is likely that some kind of thyroid dysfunction will be present in some other first- or second-degree relative. In some families Graves disease shows as one of several problems that are known collectively as ***autoimmune polyglandular syndrome***. Related conditions in this syndrome include type 1 diabetes, systemic lupus erythematosus, pernicious anemia, and others.

Hyperthyroidism in Brief

Pronunciation: hy-per-THY-roid-izm

What is it?

Hyperthyroidism is a condition in which the thyroid gland produces too much of the hormones that stimulate the conversion of fuel into energy. It is usually related to an autoimmune attack against the whole thyroid gland, but it can also be caused by small hyperactive nodules or local inflammation.

What does it look like?

Signs and symptoms of hyperthyroidism arise from too much production of energy from available fuel. They include restlessness, sleeplessness, irritability, dry skin and hair, rapid heartbeat, tremor, unintended weight loss, and for women, irregularity of menstrual periods. Some hyperthyroid patients have eye problems or skin rashes. A severe and acute episode of hyperthyroidism can be life-threatening; this is called a thyroid storm.

Is massage indicated or contraindicated?

Most people with hyperactive thyroid glands respond well to massage, which may help, at least temporarily, to ameliorate some of their stress-related symptoms.

Etiology: What Happens?

Hyperthyroidism is usually caused by one of three things: an autoimmune attack against the thyroid gland that causes it to secrete excessive amounts of metabolic hormones, a nodule or group of nodules that become hyperactive for unknown reasons (this is called *toxic nodular* or *multinodular goiter*), or inflammation of the thyroid.

Autoimmune hyperthyroidism, or Graves disease, is by far the most common variety of this disorder, accounting for some 70% to 80% of cases. Antibodies called *thyroid-stimulating immunoglobins* attack the thyroid gland, causing it to grow to huge dimensions (this is called ***goiter***) and to secrete excessive levels of thyroid hormones, especially thyroxine.

Under normal circumstances, secretions of thyroid-stimulating hormone (TSH) from the pituitary controls thyroid activity. When Graves disease is well established, circulating levels of TSH drop significantly, but the thyroid produces much more hormone than normal. The result is that the conversion of fuel into energy increases by 60% to 100%.

While genetics clearly plays a major part in development of Graves disease, its onset often seems to be connected to a stressful trigger such as an accident or surgery, a death in the family, or a job change. Other risk factors for developing this disorder include exposure to x-rays and having taken antiviral medications such as interferon or interleukin.

Other forms of hyperthyroidism include toxic multinodular goiter; toxic adenoma, which is related to iodine deficiency; and thyroid inflammation, which can be related to recovery from a viral infection or a transient condition that follows childbirth (postpartum thyroiditis).

Signs and Symptoms

Signs and symptoms of hyperthyroidism are mostly related to the excessive secretion of thyroid hormones (Figure 9.3). They include anxiety, irritability, insomnia, rapid heartbeat,

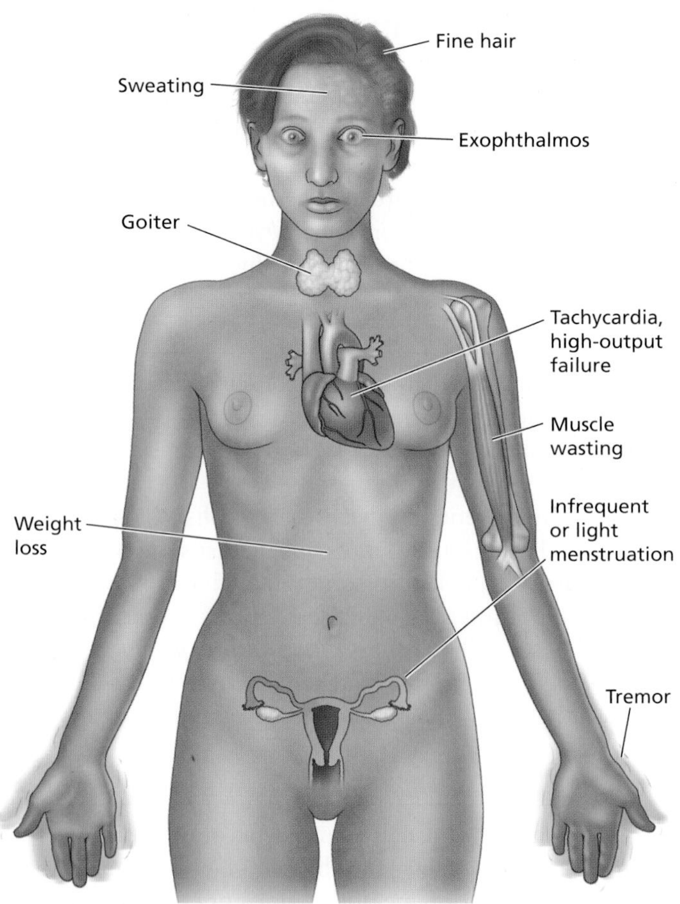

Figure 9.3. Systemic effects of hyperthyroidism.

tremor, increased perspiration, sensitivity to heat, frequent bowel movements, and unintentional weight loss. Skeletal muscles, especially in the upper arms and thighs, often become weak. Other symptoms may include light flow during menstrual periods, dry skin and brittle nails, and problems specifically with the skin and eyes, discussed in the section on complications. Many hyperthyroidism patients develop a goiter. That is, the thyroid becomes enlarged enough to create a visible painless swelling in the neck.

Complications

The thyroid is not the only tissue that may be attacked in Graves disease. Some other sites of tissue damage include the bones, the eyes, and the skin.

Osteoporosis is a risk for men and women with hyperthyroidism, because the thyroid and parathyroids together normally secrete hormones that influence bone density.

Hyperthyroidism can affect the eyes in a couple of ways. One fairly common condition is elevation of eyelids in a way that makes the eyes seem to bulge. Protrusion of the eyes is known as ***exophthalmos*** or ***proptosis*** (Figure 9.4).

Another eye problem related to Graves disease is a rare disorder called ***Graves ophthalmopathy***. This causes the eyeball to protrude beyond its protective orbit because tissues and muscles behind it swell. The front surface of the eye can dry out, causing light sensitivity, double vision, decreased freedom of movement within the orbit, pain, and excessive tearing.

Some Graves disease patients develop raised red patches of skin on their shins, feet, or elsewhere. These rashes, called ***pretibial myxedema***, are caused by deposition of ***mu-***

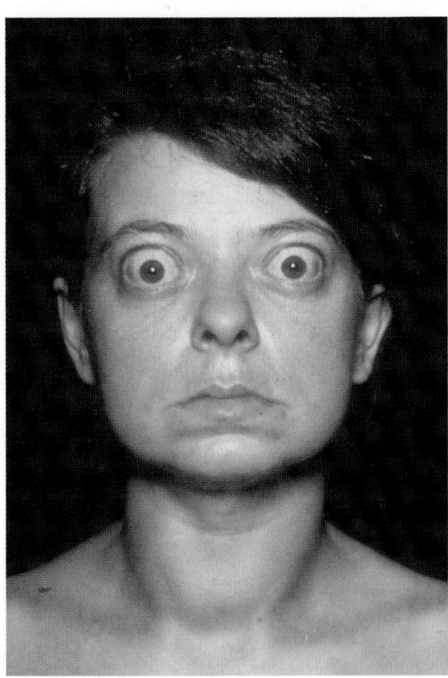

Figure 9.4. Hyperthyroidism: exophthalmos.

copolysaccharides in the dermis. They are generally not painful or dangerous. Another fairly rare complication is thyroid *acropachy*: the skin around the fingernails becomes swollen but is not typically painful.

In addition to eye and skin problems, some Graves disease patients have occasional episodes of especially high metabolism called *thyroid storms*. In these episodes symptoms suddenly become acute and may include rapid heartbeat, fever without infection, intolerance to heat, confusion, agitation, and finally shock. Thyroid storms can be medical emergencies and require immediate intervention to slow the heart and bring down the fever.

Diagnosis

Graves disease is usually diagnosed by physical examination, a blood test, and an examination of the way the thyroid takes up radioactive iodine. The physical examination concentrates on goiter, temperature, heart rate, muscle weakness, and tremor. Blood tests look for low levels of TSH combined with high levels of thyroid-stimulating immunoglobulins, along with abnormally high levels of T_4.

Ingestion of radioactive iodine shows how quickly the thyroid absorbs iodine (a primary component of thyroid hormones), along with which parts of the thyroid appear to be hyperactive. This test helps to delineate between Graves disease and nodular hyperthyroidism.

Treatment

Hyperthyroidism can be treated in a number of ways, depending on the underlying causes and the severity of the symptoms.

- *Radioactive iodine.* Although this is a diagnostic tool, radioactive iodine can also be used to kill off a portion of the hyperactive thyroid to bring levels of thyroid hormones within safe and normal standards. Many Graves disease patients find that their symptoms are abated with only one or two doses of radioactive iodine, although most develop signs of hypothyroidism in later months or years. Hypothyroidism is easier to manage than hyperthyroidism and so is considered the safer choice.

- *Beta blockers.* These medications can reduce heart rate and the feeling of palpitations. While they don't solve the problem of an overactive thyroid, they can ameliorate some of the symptoms.
- *Antithyroid medications.* Several classes of medications prevent the thyroid from producing too much T_4 or prevent T_4 from having major activity in the body. Sometimes these medications are used to prepare a patient for surgery or radioactive iodine treatment, but occasionally they are successful by themselves.
- *Surgery.* Patients who can't take antithyroid drugs or radioactive iodine may consider a thyroidectomy, a surgery in which most of the thyroid is removed. This is a risky procedure, however, because the parathyroids, which control calcium metabolism, are often damaged in the process, along with the vocal cords and laryngeal nerves. Surgery for hyperthyroidism is generally avoided if at all possible.

Massage?

As long as the person's skin is healthy and intact, massage of all kinds may be beneficial to clients with hyperactive thyroid glands. The calm, relaxed response that massage creates may provide a welcome change to the sympathetic-like symptoms of hyperthyroidism.

Modality Recommendations for Hyperthyroidism	
Deep tissue massage	Indicated for healthy tissue: work slowly for relaxation.
Lymphatic drainage	Supportive.
Polarity	S/R/D: Indicated.
PNF/MET/stretching	Supportive.
Reflexology	Indicated with gentle touch; work thyroid, solar plexus, throat, neck, eyes, shoulder points.
Shiatsu	Supportive.
Swedish massage	Supportive for soothing support of homeostasis.
Trigger point therapy	Supportive.

See Chapter 1 for a brief description of each modality, including definitions of abbreviations.

Hypothyroidism

Definition: What Is It?

Hypothyroidism is a condition in which circulating levels of thyroid hormones are abnormally low. This interferes with the body's ability to generate energy from fuel.

Demographics: Who Gets It?

Statistics on hypothyroidism are difficult to gather, but experts agree that this is the most common pathological hormone deficiency. Some surveys suggest that close to 5% of the U.S. population could be diagnosed with hypothyroidism based on blood tests, but only a small proportion of those cases produce significant symptoms.[16] Other sources claim that up to 8 million Americans have been diagnosed with hypothyroidism.[17] Women are diagnosed with hypothyroidism more often than men, by a margin of 2 to 8 to 1.[16]

Etiology: What Happens?

The thyroid gland produces thyroid hormone in two forms, T_3 and T_4. It does this under the direction of the pituitary gland, which releases TSH. When adequate amounts of T_3 and T_4 are circulating in the blood, secretion of TSH is suppressed. Thus, thyroid and pituitary secretions keep each other in balance.

The purpose of thyroid hormones is to stimulate the conversion of fuel (oxygen and calories) into energy. In hypothyroidism, inadequate amounts of thyroid hormones are produced, so incoming fuel is simply stored and never used. In a typical early case of hypothyroidism, the pituitary gland releases excessive TSH, but circulating levels of T_4 are converted to T_3 very quickly. Consequently, TSH levels are high, T_4 levels are significantly low, but T_3 levels are close to normal.

Several factors contributing to hypothyroidism have been identified:

- *Hashimoto thyroiditis.* This is an autoimmune attack against the thyroid gland that results in suppression of thyroid secretions (as opposed to the autoimmune attack that stimulates excessive thyroid secretions seen with Graves disease).
- *Complication of treatment for hyperthyroidism.* Most hyperthyroidism patients who use radioactive iodine to suppress thyroid activity eventually develop hypothyroidism.
- *Congenital birth defect.* Some babies are born with an abnormally small thyroid gland or none at all. If these children are not treated, they have stunted growth and mental retardation.
- *Postpartum hypothyroidism.* Some women have a transient episode of hypothyroidism after giving birth. This is especially common with type 1 diabetes.
- *Medications.* Some medications, specifically lithium (used to treat bipolar depression) and iodides (used as a form of iodine), can suppress thyroid function.
- *Exposure to radiation.* People who have been exposed to radiation in the neck for cancer treatment or in more general ways have a high risk of developing hypothyroidism.
- *Iodine deficiency.* Worldwide, this is the most common cause of hypothyroidism. In the United States, however, it is rare.
- *Idiopathic hypothyroidism.* Some cases of hypothyroidism don't seem to be related to any specific underlying disorder but simply arise without known cause. Because many patients exhibit the signs and symptoms of hypothyroidism without strongly indicative blood test confirmation, the identification and treatment of hypothyroidism for these patients is controversial.

Whatever the cause of hypothyroidism, the net result is that a person has difficulty turning fuel into energy. Changes in thyroxine-sensitive cells lead to decreased contractility of the heart muscle, heart enlargement, low cardiac output, and high levels of low-density lipoproteins (the atherosclerosis-promoting form of cholesterol). Other consequences include slow gastrointestinal activity (gastric stasis), delayed puberty, menstrual changes, and infertility.

Hypothyroidism in Brief

Pronunciation: hy-po-THY-roid-izm

What is it?

Hypothyroidism is a condition in which the thyroid gland produces an inadequate supply of the hormones that regulate metabolism of fuel into energy. Some cases of hypothyroidism are the result of an autoimmune attack on the thyroid gland, but others are related to the long-term complications of treatment for hyperthyroidism or other factors.

What does it look like?

Symptoms of hypothyroidism are subtle and often missed. They include fatigue, weight gain, depression, intolerance of cold, and, for women, heavy menstrual periods.

Is massage indicated or contraindicated?

One of the complications of hypothyroidism, especially in elderly patients, is the accelerated development of atherosclerosis and other forms of heart disease. As long as these complications are recognized and respected, massage can be a supportive and positive experience for hypothyroidism patients.

Signs and Symptoms

Signs and symptoms of hypothyroidism are often subtle but steadily progressive (Figure. 9.5). A person who cannot convert fuel into energy is likely to gain weight, feel fatigued and depressed, and have a sluggish digestive system with chronic constipation. She may have poor

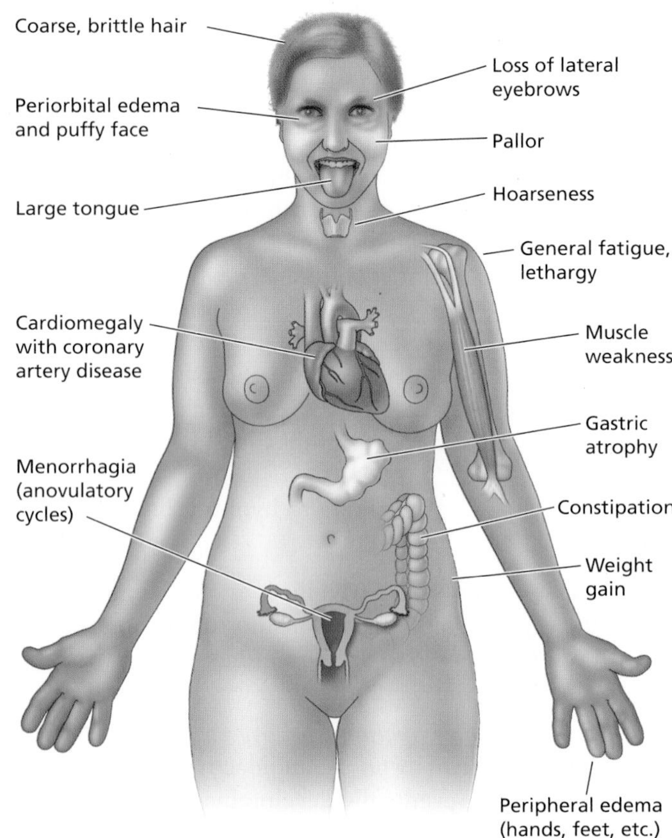

Figure 9.5. Systemic effects of hypothyroidism.

tolerance of cold, and her skin may be puffy but dry. Fluid retention in the extremities raises the risk of carpal tunnel syndrome and other nerve entrapment syndromes. Her hair becomes brittle and may even fall out. For some reason, this is especially common at the lateral aspect of the eyebrows. Menstrual periods tend to be heavy and long lasting. Some hypothyroidism patients develop goiter, a painless enlargement of the thyroid.

Very severe or untreated cases may cause a person to become so cold and drowsy that she becomes unconscious. This is called *myxedema coma*, and it is a rare but dangerous complication of hypothyroidism, especially among elderly patients.

Diagnosis

The leading indicator for hypothyroidism is a blood test for abnormally high TSH levels. This sign is considered to be more accurate and sensitive than tests for T_4 or T_3.

Physical examinations for hypothyroidism look for goiter along with a significantly slowed heart rate and low body temperature. Reflexes are often slow in hypothyroid patients.

It is especially important for pregnant women to be tested for thyroid function. Pregnancy can hide some symptoms of hypothyroidism, which can create serious repercussions for the unborn child. Most newborns are tested for thyroid function as a matter of course; early intervention in the rare cases when thyroid function is subnormal can prevent stunted growth and mental retardation.

The symptoms of hypothyroidism are general and often vague; it can resemble depression, fibromyalgia, chronic fatigue syndrome, and several other chronic conditions. Also, whether standard scales of "normal" blood tests are accurate for all women is controversial.

For these reasons the identification and treatment of mild cases of hypothyroidism may vary from one professional to another. Some experts suggest that early treatment can prevent heart disease associated with this condition, but others object to treatment without a firm diagnosis. Risks of overtreating hypothyroidism include stress to the heart, headaches, insomnia, and other signs of hyperthyroidism.

Treatment

The treatment for hypothyroidism is to supplement thyroid hormones, usually in the form of synthetic T_4, which most people can metabolize into adequate amounts of T_3. While many people find relief with this treatment, others must explore other options to find the right supplement for both T_3 and T_4. This can be in the form of synthetic versions of these hormones or as desiccated pig glands. Using animal products for hormone replacement is challenging, though, because the potency from one batch to another can vary greatly.

Massage?

Other than the risk of atherosclerosis (which is a risk for many mature clients regardless of thyroid function), massage is perfectly appropriate for hypothyroidism clients. Although it is unlikely to stimulate normal production of T_4, massage can certainly improve the quality of life of people who feel chronically drained and lethargic.

Modality Recommendations for Hypothyroidism	
Deep tissue massage	Supportive for relaxation: work slowly for relaxation.
Lymphatic drainage	Supportive.
Polarity	S/R/D: Indicated; pressure determined by client's comfort.
PNF/MET/stretching	Supportive.
Reflexology	Indicated with gentle touch; work thyroid, solar plexus, throat, neck, face, lymphatic system, liver, GI tract points.
Shiatsu	Supportive.
Swedish massage	Indicated if circulatory complications are controlled.
Trigger point therapy	Supportive.

See Chapter 1 for a brief description of each modality, including definitions of abbreviations.

Metabolic Syndrome

Definition: What Is It?

In the relatively short time that it has been studied, metabolic syndrome has been known by many names, including *syndrome X*, *dysmetabolic syndrome*, *insulin resistance syndrome*, *prediabetes*, and the *deadly quartet*. It is a collection of physical signs and symptoms that individually raise the risk of certain diseases but that when seen together increase that risk nearly to certainty.

Demographics: Who Gets It?

Estimates of the incidence of metabolic syndrome vary widely, but most agree that it affects some 47 million Americans. Latinos are affected more than other racial groups, and women have it more often than men.[18]

Metabolic Syndrome in Brief

Pronunciation: met-uh-BOL-ik SIN-drome

What is it?

Metabolic syndrome is a collection of signs that indicates a high risk of several serious diseases, including diabetes, heart attack, atherosclerosis, and stroke.

How is it recognized?

Metabolic syndrome is recognized by its combined associated conditions, including disruptions in cholesterol, hypertension, central obesity, and others.

Is massage indicated or contraindicated?

The appropriateness of massage for a person with metabolic syndrome depends on cardiovascular health. If exercise is recommended for weight loss and improved insulin function, massage is probably also safe. If, however, these conditions have led to severe cardiovascular problems, massage must be adjusted to accommodate circulatory weakness.

Etiology: What Happens?

Metabolic syndrome is identified as a cluster of five main features, including high triglycerides, low high-density lipoproteins (the "good" cholesterol), hypertension, central obesity (fat retention in the omentum more than in superficial fascia), and high fasting blood glucose levels. Other possible features in metabolic syndrome include a high risk of blood clotting, high levels of C-reactive protein (an indicator of inflammation), and polycystic ovary disease in women.

These factors are not particularly alarming when they appear alone, but in combination they set the stage for an extremely high risk of type 2 diabetes, atherosclerosis, heart attack, heart failure, aneurysm, and stroke. People with metabolic syndrome have a twofold risk of atherosclerotic cardiovascular disease and a fivefold risk of type 2 diabetes (which itself raises the risk of cardiovascular disease) compared with the general population.

The primary risk factors for metabolic syndrome are obesity and insulin resistance. Further, obesity tends to cause insulin resistance, and insulin resistance can cause obesity, forming a vicious circle.

Signs and Symptoms

Metabolic syndrome typically appears as central obesity (much of the body weight is carried around the abdomen in an "apple" rather than a "pear" shape), along with disruptions in cholesterol, hypertension, and blood glucose, as described earlier. Outside of excessive body weight, however, metabolic syndrome does not typically cause noticeable symptoms; its other components are silent.

Diagnosis

Metabolic syndrome is diagnosed when three of five risk factors are simultaneously present:

- High fasting blood glucose (over 100 mg/dL after 9 hours of fasting)
- Abdominal obesity (a waist measurement of over 35 inches for women or over 40 inches for men); this is somewhat flexible to allow for individual variations
- Elevated triglyceride levels (>150 mg/dL)
- Low levels of high-density lipoproteins (<40 mg/dL for men; <50 mg/dL for women)
- Hypertension (systolic blood pressure >130 mm Hg; diastolic >85 mm Hg)

Treatment

Treatment for metabolic syndrome is often divided into short-term and long-term goals. Short-term goals include lowering blood glucose and correcting cholesterol levels with medical intervention.

Long-term goals include increasing physical activity and losing weight. Reducing body weight by 5% to 7% (this is only 10–14 lb for a 200-lb person) significantly reduces the risk of complications due to insulin resistance, and exercise improves insulin action and decreases blood glucose. Limiting alcohol use and quitting smoking are other important steps.

Massage?

The appropriateness of massage in the context of metabolic syndrome depends entirely on the health and resilience of the client. If this person successfully controls the disease through diet and exercise adjustments, massage is probably safe and appropriate. If this person has developed any of the serious complications associated with these conditions, judgments must be made to accommodate possible weaknesses of the circulatory system.

Modality Recommendations for Metabolic Syndrome	
Deep tissue massage	Contraindicated.
Lymphatic drainage	Supportive.
Polarity	S/R/D: Indicated with very light pressure for cardiovascular problems.
PNF/MET/stretching	Supportive.
Reflexology	Locally contraindicated for cardiovascular problems; work endocrine and lymphatic systems, solar plexus points.
Shiatsu	Supportive.
Swedish massage	Indicated if client is healthy with no complications.
Trigger point therapy	Supportive.

See Chapter 1 for a brief description of each modality, including definitions of abbreviations.

Thyroid Cancer

Definition: What Is It?

Thyroid cancer is any type of cancer that originates in the thyroid gland. Three types of thyroid cells can become cancerous: follicular cells, C cells, and lymphocytes. Most varieties of thyroid cancer are slow-growing and easily treatable, but some forms are more aggressive.

Demographics: Who Gets It?

Thyroid cancer is relatively rare, diagnosed about 31,000 times per year in the United States. This figure has been rising, however, at a rate of about 2% per year. It affects women more than men, at a ratio of about 2 to 3 to 1.[19] Thyroid cancer causes about 1,500 deaths per year in this country. It has a very high cure rate, so close to 350,000 thyroid cancer survivors are alive.[20]

Etiology: What Happens?

The thyroid gland is composed of two main types of epithelial cells: follicular cells, which normally produce T_3 and T_4, and parafollicular cells, also called C cells, which produce calcitonin, a hormone that pulls calcium out of the blood to increase bone density.

Thyroid Cancer in Brief

Pronunciation: THY-royd KAN-ser

What is it?

Thyroid cancer is any type of cancer that arises from cells in the thyroid. It is derived from follicular cells that produce T_3 and T_4, from C cells that produce calcitonin, or from lymphocytes in the thyroid gland.

How is it recognized?

Most types of thyroid cancer cause enlargement of the gland, which may press on the trachea or esophagus, leading to hoarseness and difficulty with swallowing or breathing.

Is massage indicated or contraindicated?

The appropriateness of massage for clients with thyroid cancer, as with other types of cancer, is determined by what treatments the client is undergoing and how bodywork might challenge or support a person during a time of great stress. Because a common treatment for thyroid cancer is radioactive iodine, close contact with the patient must be avoided until this protocol is concluded.

Cancer develops when DNA in thyroid cells is damaged and cell growth becomes uncontrolled and disorganized. Thyroid cancer is often related to radiation exposure. People who were treated with radiation for acne, tonsillitis, or an enlarged thymus are at increased risk for this disease. Similarly, people exposed to radioactive fallout from nuclear testing or nuclear reactor accidents have a higher-than-normal risk for thyroid cancer; this is one of the long-term repercussions of the Chernobyl nuclear accident in 1986.

Radiation from standard neck or dental radiography is *not* associated with an increased risk of thyroid cancer.

Other forms of thyroid cancer are related to inherited genetic characteristics. Children of people with the genetic mutation for thyroid cancer have a 50% chance of developing the disease themselves. Inherited forms of thyroid cancer tend to be more aggressive and harder to treat than other forms, so when this condition is discovered, all family members, especially children, are recommended for genetic testing.

Types of thyroid cancer Thyroid cancer occurs in several varieties. While most cases are slow-growing and not particularly threatening, other types are highly aggressive and resistant to treatment.

- *Papillary thyroid cancer.* This is the most common type of thyroid cancer, accounting for 70% to 80% of diagnoses. Papillary cells look like fern leaves, with many tiny extensions; they arise from follicular cells. This type of cancer usually stays local, and while it may intrude on local lymph nodes, it is usually extremely stable and doesn't tend to grow or invade other tissues. In rare cases, it does metastasize through the lymph system to the bones or the lungs. Papillary thyroid cancer is usually diagnosed in women 30 to 50 years old.[19]
- *Follicular thyroid cancer.* This form of thyroid cancer also arises from follicular cells. It is less common than papillary thyroid cancer, accounting for about 10% of thyroid cancer diagnoses. Follicular thyroid cancer is more likely to metastasize than papillary thyroid cancer, particularly if it is diagnosed in someone over 50 years old. ***Hürthle cell carcinoma*** is a subtype of follicular thyroid cancer. It tends to have a poor prognosis because it is less responsive to treatment than other forms of thyroid cancer.
- *Medullary thyroid cancer.* This form of cancer arises from C cells. It is rarer but more aggressive than papillary or follicular thyroid cancer. Medullary thyroid cancer accounts for 3% to 5% of thyroid cancer diagnoses. Two subtypes of medullary thyroid cancer have been identified:
  - *Multiple endocrine neoplasia type IIA.* This is an inherited form of thyroid cancer. It is usually accompanied by benign tumors on the adrenal glands and/or parathyroid glands. Tumors on the parathyroid glands can increase calcium in the bloodstream. Adrenal tumors, also called ***pheochromocytomas***, can cause increased secretion of epinephrine and accompanying high blood pressure. It is important to check for adrenal tumors, as they can complicate surgeries.
  - *Multiple endocrine neoplasia type IIB.* This is also inherited, is characterized by adrenal tumors and multiple ***neuromas*** on the tongue, eyelids, and small intestines. It is an aggressive thyroid cancer that is usually diagnosed in young people.
- *Familial thyroid cancer.* This form is also inherited, but it affects only the thyroid: other glands are spared. It is slow growing, affecting mainly people 40 to 60 years old.
- *Anaplastic thyroid cancer.* Also called *undifferentiated thyroid cancer*, anaplastic thyroid cancer is highly aggressive, metastasizing easily to the mediastinal lymph nodes, trachea, lungs, and bones. It originates from benign or low-grade thyroid tumors and

usually affects people over 60 years old. Anaplastic thyroid cancer accounts for about 7% of thyroid cancer diagnoses.

- *Thyroid lymphoma.* Lymphocytes in the thyroid gland are also vulnerable to DNA mutation. This is most likely to happen along with hypothyroidism in the form of Hashimoto thyroiditis. Thyroid lymphoma accounts for about 4% of diagnoses.

Signs and Symptoms

Nonaggressive forms of thyroid cancer may be silent, especially in early stages. Later symptoms include painless enlargement in the throat. This may press on the esophagus or trachea, leading to problems with breathing, hoarseness, and difficulty with swallowing.

Later stages of aggressive thyroid cancers may include tumors in the lungs or on bones; symptoms may be related to these complications.

Diagnosis

Thyroid cancer is surprisingly difficult to diagnose accurately. This is because the thyroid gland is prone to benign tumors; only about 5% of the growths found in thyroid glands turn out to be malignant,[20] and imaging techniques cannot distinguish between benign and malignant growths. A biopsy or fine-needle aspiration of cells can yield more information, but thyroid cancer often cannot be fully staged until surgery.

Radioactive iodine may be used to identify areas of heightened thyroid activity: most tumors concentrate this chemical in easily identified areas. This technique may also be used to find and treat metastatic thyroid tumors in the lungs or elsewhere.

Genetic testing to identify the risk of inherited thyroid cancer is becoming more widely available. A person who is positive for the genes associated with thyroid cancer might be counseled to consider a prophylactic thyroidectomy. Thyroid hormones can be supplemented, and this procedure can prevent the most aggressive and untreatable forms of thyroid cancer.

Staging for thyroid cancer is determined by the type of cancer and the age of the patient. Staging protocols are discussed in Sidebar 9.2.

Treatment

Most cases of thyroid cancer are successfully treated with surgery to remove part or all of the thyroid gland. Of course, thyroid hormones must be supplemented after this procedure. Lymph nodes in the neck are often dissected to look for signs of metastasis.

Surgery may be followed with doses of radioactive iodine or external beams of radiation at tumor sites. This regimen is successful for most cases of thyroid cancer, even if it recurs after surgery.

Aggressive forms of thyroid cancer are typically treated with radioactive iodine and other forms of chemotherapy, but not surgery, since the chance of getting all of the cancer cells is negligible.

Massage?

As with other types of cancer, massage for thyroid cancer is based on the treatment options and the general resilience of the patient. One caution for this population is that someone undergoing treatment with radioactive iodine must be kept in isolation until the treatment is complete. This means massage must be delayed until the person is no longer "hot." Consulting with a client's health care team is particularly important in this context.

SIDEBAR 9.2: STAGING THYROID CANCER

Staging protocols for thyroid cancer are tied to the type of cancer, the age of the patient, and the best treatment options in the circumstances. As new ways to identify thyroid cancer early are developed, these staging protocols may continue to evolve.

As with other types of cancer, thyroid cancer is staged using the TNM system, which is then translated into stages I to IV, as follows:[21]

Tumor (T)

T X: tumor cannot be assessed

T 0: no evidence of primary tumor

T 1: tumor <2 cm

T 2: tumor 2–4 cm

T 3: the tumor is >4 cm; *or* the tumor has invaded nearby tissue

T 4a: tumor any size; has invaded anterior neck tissues

T 4b: tumor any size; has invaded posterior neck, spine, or large blood vessels

Node (N)

N X: nodes cannot be assessed

N 0: no nodes involved

N 1a: some nodes in neck involved

N 1b: some nodes in mediastinum involved

Metastasis (M)

M X: metastasis cannot be assessed

M 0: no metastasis found

M 1: distant metastasis to lymph nodes, organs, or bones

These delineations are translated into stages I to IV in this way:

For papillary or follicular thyroid cancer in patients **under** 45 years old:

Stage I any T, any N, M0
Stage II any T, any N, M1

For Anaplastic Thyroid Cancer

This cancer is so aggressive that diagnosis automatically puts it at stage IV.

Stage IVa T4a, any N, M0
Stage IVb T4b, any N, M0
Stage IVc any T, any N, M1

For papillary or follicular thyroid cancer in patients **over** 45 years old:

Stage I T1, N0, M0
Stage II T2, N0, M0
Stage III T1–3, N0–N1a, M0
Stage IVa T1–4a, N0–1b, M0
Stage IVb T4b, any N, M0
Stage IVc any T, any N, M1

For Medullary Thyroid Cancer

Same as for papillary or follicular in patients over 45 years old.

Modality Recommendations for Thyroid Cancer

Deep tissue massage	Supportive if therapist acting as part of a health care team. Respect stage of recovery and treatment challenges.
Lymphatic drainage	Supportive.
Polarity	S: Indicated; can support immune system.
	R/D: Supportive with light pressure.
PNF/MET/stretching	Supportive if therapist acting as part of health care team; match to activity level.
Reflexology	Supportive. Work thyroid, pituitary, lymphatic system points.
Shiatsu	Indicated to strengthen immune system via TH, SP, K meridians and extensions.
Swedish massage	Supportive if therapist acting as part of health care team; match massage to activity level.
Trigger point therapy	Locally contraindicated; otherwise supportive for light work.

See Chapter 1 for a brief description of each modality, including definitions of abbreviations.

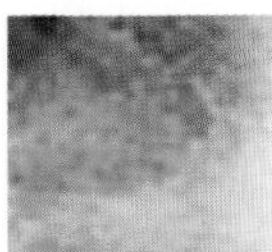

Chapter Review Questions: Endocrine System Conditions

1. Describe the negative feedback loop between insulin and glucagon.
2. What structure controls both the autonomic nervous system and the endocrine system?
3. What is the gland most often affected in acromegaly?
4. What is the name for adrenal cortex insufficiency?
5. What is the name for adrenal cortex hyperactivity?
6. How can diabetes contribute to heart disease? Kidney disease? Blindness?
7. What are two leading risk factors for thyroid cancer?
8. What are three symptoms of abnormally high levels of T_4?
9. Describe how successfully treating metabolic syndrome can prevent other serious health problems.
10. A 26-year-old client reports that she had papillary thyroid cancer 3 years ago. She had surgery to treat it and has had no further problems. What cautions might a massage therapist want to observe in this situation?

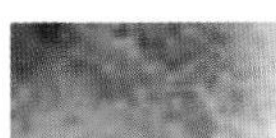

References

1. Statistics about Acromegaly. Copyright © 2000–2005 by Adviware Pty Ltd. All rights reserved. http://www.wrongdiagnosis.com/a/acromegaly/stats.htm. Accessed autumn 2006.
2. Acromegaly. © 1998–2006 by Mayo Foundation for Medical Education and Research. All rights reserved. http://www.mayoclinic.com/health/acromegaly/DS00478. Accessed autumn 2006.
3. Statistics by Country for Addison's Disease. Copyright © 2000–2005 by Adviware Pty Ltd. All rights reserved. http://www.wrongdiagnosis.com/a/addisons_disease/stats-country.htm. Accessed autumn 2006.
4. Addison's disease. © 1998 2006 by Mayo Foundation for Medical Education and Research. All rights reserved. http://www.mayoclinic.com/health/addisons-disease/DS00361. Accessed autumn 2006.
5. Cushing's Fact Sheet. National Institute of Diabetes and Digestive and Kidney Diseases. NIH Publication 02-3007. http://csrf.net/FactSheet.htm. Accessed autumn 2006.
6. National Diabetes Statistics. National Institute of Diabetes and Digestive Diseases. http://diabetes.niddk.nih.gov/dm/pubs/statistics/index.htm#11. Accessed autumn 2006.
7. Diabetes Statistics and Research. Centers for Disease Control and Prevention. http://www.cdc.gov/diabetes/faq/research.htm. Accessed autumn 2006.
8. Votey S, Peters A. Diabetes Mellitus, Type 2: A Review. © 1996–2006 by WebMD. http://www.emedicine.com/emerg/topic134.htm. Accessed autumn 2006.
9. Dushay J, Abrahamson M. Insulin Resistance and Type 2 Diabetes: A Comprehensive Review. Copyright © 2005 by Joslin Diabetes Center, Inc. All rights reserved. http://www.medscape.com/viewarticle/501569. Accessed autumn 2006.
10. Olatunbosun S, Dagogo-Jack S. Insulin Resistance. © 1996–2006 by WebMD. http://www.emedicine.com/med/topic1173.htm. Accessed autumn 2006.
11. Type 1 Diabetes Statistics. Centers for Disease Control and Prevention. http://www.angelfire.com/dragon2/coppelianohitsugi/statistics.html. Accessed autumn 2006.
12. Lamb W. Diabetes Mellitus, Type 1. © 1996–2006 by WebMD. http://www.emedicine.com/ped/topic581.htm. Accessed autumn 2006.
13. Diabetes: Neuropathies and Neuromuscular Disorders. © 2006 by Washington University School of Medicine. http://www.neuro.wustl.edu/neuromuscular/nother/diabetes.htm. Accessed autumn 2006.

14. Rose MK. Therapeutic Massage: Complementary Health Care for Diabetes. © Diabetes Self-Management. Diabetes Self-Management 17(6):111–112, 114. November-December 2000.
15. Racing the Engine – Hyperthyroidism. © 2004 by Thyroid Foundation of America. All Rights Reserved. http://www.tsh.org/disorders/hyperthyroidism/hyperthyroidism.html. Accessed autumn 2006.
16. Orlander P, Woodhouse W. Hypothyroidism. © 1996–2006 by WebMD. http://www.emedicine.com/med/topic1145.htm. Accessed autumn 2006.
17. The most common problem—Hypothyroidism. © 2004 by The Thyroid Foundation of America. All Rights Reserved. http://www.tsh.org/disorders/hyperthyroidism/hyperthyroidism.html. Accessed autumn 2006.
18. Metabolic Syndrome—Statistics. © 2006 by American Heart Association, Inc. All rights reserved. http://www.americanheart.org/downloadable/heart/1136819875357META06.pdf. Accessed autumn 2006.
19. Thyroid cancer. © 1998–2006 by Mayo Foundation for Medical Education and Research. All rights reserved. http://www.mayoclinic.com/health/thyroid-cancer/DS00492. Accessed autumn 2006.
20. Cancer of the Thyroid. National Cancer Institute. http://seer.cancer.gov/statfacts/html/thyro.html. Accessed autumn 2006.
21. Cancer of the Thyroid: Papillary & Follicular. © 2004 by Thyroid Foundation of America. http://www.tsh.org/disorders/nodules/cancer1.html. Accessed autumn 2006.
22. How Is Thyroid Cancer Staged? © 2006 by American Cancer Society, Inc. http://www.cancer.org/docroot/cri/content/cri_2_4_3x_how_is_thyroid_cancer_staged_43.asp?sitearea=&level=. Accessed autumn 2006.

10

Urinary System Conditions

Chapter Objectives

After reading this chapter, you should be able to . . .

- Name the basic functional unit of the kidneys.
- Name a hormone secreted by the kidneys.
- List four types of kidney stones and identify the most common type.
- Explain the difference between uncomplicated and complicated pyelonephritis.
- List the stages of chronic renal failure.
- Identify the most common early symptom of bladder cancer.
- Explain why women are more prone to urinary tract infections than men.
- Name the causative agent of most urinary tract infections and uncomplicated pyelonephritis.

URINARY SYSTEM INTRODUCTION

The urinary system is a relatively small system composed of the kidneys, ureters, bladder, and urethra.

The huge renal artery comes directly off the aorta and enters the kidneys. It rapidly decreases in diameter to form thousands of capillaries, terminating in tiny knots called ***glomeruli***. Each of these is surrounded by a ***Bowman capsule***, the entry point to the nephron. Blood pressure forces fluid from the glomeruli into the Bowman capsule. Nephrons and circulatory capillaries exchange water and waste products as they intertwine along the loop of Henle (Figure 10.1). By the time fluid enters the collecting tubules, any water, electrolytes, or other material the body needs has been reabsorbed, so that only waste products are left. This fluid is urine. The collecting tubules pour their contents into the renal pelvis; the renal pelvis empties into the ureters; they lead to the urinary bladder; and urine is excreted from the bladder through the urethra.

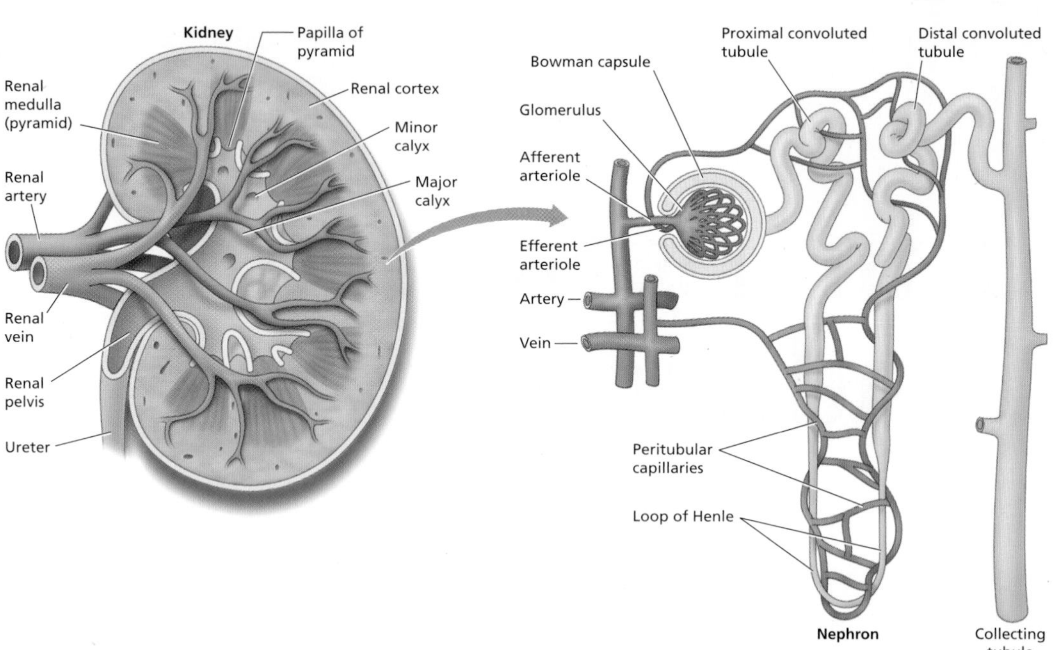

Figure 10.1. Overview of the urinary system.

The kidneys have another function that is not directly involved in the filtering of waste products from the blood. ***Erythropoietin*** (EPO), a hormone that stimulates red blood cell production, is produced in the kidneys. Damage to these delicate organs can therefore sometimes be identified by changes in red blood cell production.

Kidneys are constructed primarily of epithelial tissue, which makes them vulnerable to injury. This is why tapotement along the inferior edge of the rib cage is not recommended; it is unlikely but possible to injure the kidneys here. When the kidneys have been damaged, red blood cells leak from capillaries into the nephrons. This shows as blood in the urine (***hematuria***). It is evidence of trauma, infection, or another possibly dangerous condition in the kidneys.

Filtration, the movement of substances through a membrane by external mechanical pressure (in this case the blood pressure), is the mechanism that initially pushes waste-filled plasma into the kidneys. The speed with which this happens is called the ***glomerular filtration rate***, or GFR. Normal GFR is 120 mL/min: this adds up to 180 L of fluid moving through the kidneys each day! (Of course, most of the glomerular filtrate is reabsorbed into circulatory capillaries and put back into the bloodstream.) It is clear then, how carefully intertwined blood pressure and kidney health must be. If blood pressure is consistently too high, the kidneys sustain damage and become less efficient. Conversely, if the kidneys are not functioning adequately, the body accumulates excessive fluid, which raises blood pressure. Some of the conditions discussed in this chapter have to do with the complicated relation between the urinary and circulatory systems. Other conditions considered here are related to the vulnerability to infection of the urinary system organs.

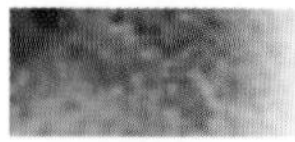

Urinary System Conditions

Kidney Disorders

Kidney stones
Pyelonephritis
Renal failure

Bladder and Urinary Tract Disorders

Bladder cancer
Interstitial cystitis
Urinary tract infection

Kidney Stones

Definition: What Are They?

Also called ***renal calculi*** or ***nephrolithiases***, kidney stones are crystals that sometimes develop in the renal pelvis. The size of kidney stones varies widely, depending on how long they have been developing and what they are made of. Most stones range between the size of grains of sand to about 1 inch in diameter. Some stones are much larger, growing into the cortex of the kidney, forming what is called a ***staghorn calculus*** (Figure 10.2).

Small stones may pass through the urinary tract with no symptoms, but larger ones may get stuck in the ureters. The technical name for them in this location is ***ureterolithiases***.

Kidney Stones in Brief

What are they?
Kidney stones are solid deposits of crystalline substances inside the kidney.

How are they recognized?
Small stones may cause no symptoms at all, but when larger stones enter the ureters, they can cause blood in the urine and extreme pain called renal colic. Renal colic may be accompanied by nausea and vomiting. Fever and chills indicate that infection is part of the problem. Pain may refer from the back into the groin.

Is massage indicated or contraindicated?
Acute renal colic contraindicates massage, although any kind of bodywork is appropriate for people with a history of stones but no symptoms.

Demographics: Who Gets Them?

Kidney stones usually form in the absence of adequate fluids. Thus, they are most common in tropical environments, where people tend to lose more liquid through sweat than they replace. Peak months for the diagnosis of kidney stones in the United States are June through August, for the same reason. The incidence of kidney stones appears to be rising in the United States, although the reasons for this are not clear.

Men with kidney stones outnumber women, and whites are affected more than other races. Every year about 1 million people in the United States pass a stone; this accounts for 600,000 emergency department visits per year. It is predicted that about 10% of all Americans will pass a stone at some time. Most people who are susceptible to kidney stones get their first one between 20 and 30 years old, and 75% of them will have at least one other stone sometime in their life.[1]

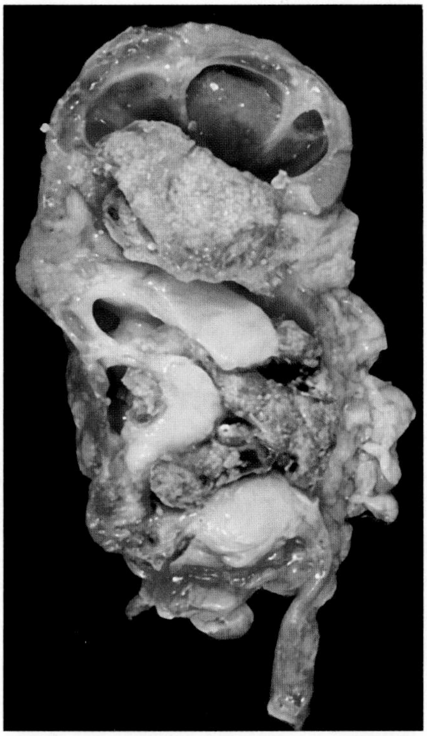

Figure 10.2. Staghorn calculus.

Etiology: What Happens?

Several genetic anomalies raise the risk of kidney stones, along with the use of certain medications, a history of surgery or inflammation in the gastrointestinal tract, and urinary tract infections (UTI) or blockages. Kidney stones can be composed of any of several substances, each one indicative of a different type of metabolic problem.

- *Calcium oxalate* or *calcium phosphate stones* account for about 75% of kidney stones. They are associated with parathyroid dysfunction (too much calcium is pulled off the bones into the bloodstream), too much vitamin D, abnormally high rates of calcium absorption in the gastrointestinal tract, abnormal leakage of calcium or phosphate into the nephrons, or other problems.
- *Struvite stones* are composed of magnesium and ammonia and are associated with chronic UTI. Approximately 10% to 15% of kidney stones are ***struvite*** stones. The number of diagnosed struvite stones has been decreasing, as urinary tract infections are being found earlier and treated more successfully.
- *Uric acid stones* form in the kidneys of people whose blood is abnormally acidic. Accounting for about 5% to 8% of all kidney stones, uric acid stones are associated with a diet high in meat and purines. People who have uric acid kidney stones are also at high risk for gout.
- *Cystine stones* are relatively rare, constituting less than 1% of kidney stones. They are directly related to a genetic dysfunction with the metabolism of ***cystine***, an amino acid.
- *Other stones* account for a tiny percentage of kidney stones. Genetic problems with metabolism and the use of protease inhibitors to treat HIV/AIDS are the primary causes of these stones.

Signs and Symptoms

Most kidney stones are completely silent; that is, they pass through the ureters without pain. When they get stuck or when they are large enough to scrape the delicate lining of the urinary tract, however, kidney stones cause a characteristic extreme grabbing pain. The ureters contract in irritation, causing ***renal colic***. The pain has a sudden onset, comes and goes in waves, and can be so severe that it causes nausea and vomiting as a sympathetic reaction. The pain often refers to the groin. Occasionally the stone may be caused by or may lead to an infection in the kidneys; in these instances, fever and chills accompany the severe pain.

Complications

Most kidney stones that are big enough to cause problems are excruciatingly painful but eventually pass into the bladder and out in the urine without causing long-lasting damage to the urinary system. Occasionally, however, a stone grows large enough to seriously disrupt kidney function. This may lead to chronic or acute renal failure.

Diagnosis

Many silent kidney stones are found during routine abdominal radiography. People reporting kidney stone pain may undergo several tests to rule out other disorders, such as gallstones, abdominal aneurysm, diverticular disease, and pancreatitis.

Tests to look for kidney stones include radiography, ultrasound, magnetic resonance imaging, and ***intravenous pyelography***, in which dye is injected and observed for how it moves through the kidneys.

CASE HISTORY 10.1

Kidney Stones

Walter B. aged 77: "Once you've had a kidney stone, you never forget it."

I've had kidney stone attacks since 1939, then in 1944, and so on and so forth. The first time I was 19 years old. I'd been horseback riding the day before, so when the pain started, we figured I had just thrown my back out somehow. The director of the hospital finally detected what it really was.

In 1944 I had an attack at night in bed. Once you've had a kidney stone attack, you never forget what it feels like. I knew immediately what was happening, and they rushed me via command car to the military hospital, 20 miles away from the Battle of the Bulge. The renal surgeon authorized an attempt to remove the stone with a uteroscopic tube. Back in those days the tube was metal, not flexible—hence the discomfort, which I've never forgotten. The procedure was unsuccessful because somehow I had already passed the stone.

The doctor said that I had "anomalous kidneys."

"What the hell does that mean?" I asked.

"It just means they're unlike any kidneys I've ever seen," he said.

After these two incidents I wasn't given any further treatment or medication. I was just told to drink plenty of liquids.

I had another attack in the 1960s. I was visiting a friend in Swampscott and had to try to drive 25 miles into Boston without killing myself or anyone else—quite an ordeal. But I never passed a whole stone; they all turned to gravel.

Then, in the blizzard of '78, I had my last attack. Boston was digging out from a huge snowstorm. No one was allowed to drive; the streets had to be clear for ambulances and fire trucks. The pain was God-awful, just unbearable. They always say it's like having a baby—you just wouldn't believe it. I couldn't get to the hospital right away, so the doctor told me to drink some whiskey to dull the pain. Finally, I was given special dispensation to take a taxicab to the hospital.

In the hospital they put a tube up the urethra to try to basket the stone. That was the only one they ever got. I remember, I was lying on my side with the sheet like a big tent draped over me. I just had a local anesthetic, and when the doctor finally got the stone, he dropped it on my sheet—it sounded just like a pebble dropping.

When the stone was basketed at the hospital, it was sent to the kidney stone lab, where it was identified as a calcium stone. The medication consisted of allopurinol tablets and hydrochlorothiazide pills taken daily. There's been no sign of an attack since then.

About 4 years ago I had another uteroscopic procedure as part of a regular examination. The urologist used a new flexible tube (not like the metal one from 1944!). The whole thing took about 4 minutes and involved a minimum of discomfort. Several of my friends, though, have had attacks within the past year or two, and their treatment and recovery seemed to be much more painful and prolonged than mine, in spite of all the new techniques available.

Treatment

The pain of kidney stones is so intense that long ago people operated on them without anesthesia: "cutting for stone" was considered worth the pain just to get rid of them. Nowadays several other options are available, and only a small percentage of kidney stone patients have to go through major surgery. If a person is unable to pass a stone without help, three main interventions are available. Which one is appropriate is determined by the stone's size and location and the general health of the patient.

- *Percutaneous nephrolithotomy* is a surgery conducted through a tiny tunnel in the back leading to the stone, which is either extracted or subjected to sonic waves that break it up.

- *Ureteroscopic stone removal* uses a flexible tube that is inserted into the urethra and snakes up to where the stone is lodged to remove it from the ureters.
- *Extracorporeal shockwave lithotripsy* is the use of sound waves to break up stones into a size that can be passed through the ureters with minimal risk of getting stuck. This procedure can leave the patient feeling bruised and battered from the extremity of the shock waves that are required to break up stones, but it can treat larger deposits than either of the other two options.

Preventive treatments for persons susceptible to kidney stones depend on what the stones are made of. This is why it is necessary for patients to catch their stones as they pass with the urine. The stones are then analyzed, as is the urine passed, for 24 hours after the stone passes. The treatment program is based on these findings.

Some interventions include surgery to remove the parathyroid glands, medication to regulate metabolism, dietary adjustments, and most important, adequate hydration. Kidney stone patients need to drink up to 1 gallon of water every day to keep stones moving through the system before they become big enough to cause problems. Patients are also frequently advised to limit caffeine, alcohol, and oxalate-rich foods (dark leafy vegetables, nuts, and chocolate) to reduce the risk of future stones.

Massage?

Massage for people with a history of kidney stones but no symptoms is perfectly appropriate. However, a person with or without a history of kidney stones who is having any signs or symptoms of renal colic is not a good candidate for vigorous massage.

Modality Recommendations for Kidney Stones

Deep tissue massage	Systemically contraindicated while acute; otherwise supportive.
Lymphatic drainage	Supportive.
Polarity	S/R/D: Indicated when no symptoms present.
PNF/MET/stretching	Systemically contraindicated while acute; otherwise supportive.
Reflexology	Indicated when no symptoms are present; work kidney and lymphatic points.
Shiatsu	Indicated: Treat K, SP, TH meridians and extensions for the urinary and immune systems.
Swedish massage	Systemically contraindicated while acute; otherwise supportive.
Trigger point therapy	Systemically contraindicated while acute; otherwise supportive.

See Chapter 1 for a brief description of each modality, including definitions of abbreviations.

Pyelonephritis

Definition: What Is It?

As the name implies, pyelonephritis is an infection of the nephrons in the kidney, although the renal pelvis may also be involved. Acute infections cause severe symptoms, but chronic infections may be silent while kidney function progressively diminishes.

Demographics: Who Gets It?

It is difficult to gauge how often kidney infections occur, since they are often silent complications of common UTI. However, about 250,000 cases of pyelonephritis are diagnosed each year, leading to about 190,000 hospitalizations.[2]

> **Pyelonephritis in Brief**
> Pronunciation: py-el-o-neh-FRY-tis
>
> **What is it?**
> Pyelonephritis is an infection of the kidney and/or renal pelvis.
>
> **How is it recognized?**
> Symptoms of acute pyelonephritis include burning pain with urination, back pain, fever, chills, nausea, and vomiting. Chronic infections may show no symptoms.
>
> **Is massage indicated or contraindicated?**
> Kidney infections systemically contraindicate circulatory massage until the infection has been eradicated.

Etiology: What Happens?

An uncomplicated kidney infection is one in which bacteria have moved from the lower urinary tract into the upper urinary tract. A complicated infection is one in which structural anomalies, urethral blockage, pregnancy, diabetes, a ***neurogenic bladder*** (a bladder that has no motor control and so empties passively into a bag), or simply being male are features. Contaminated surgical or medical instruments such as *cystoscopes* and catheters can also introduce pathogens into the urinary tract. The causative agent for uncomplicated infections is nearly always *Escherichia coli*, but in complicated situations the agents can be *Pseudomonas*, *Klebsiella*, *Citrobacter*, *Enterobacter*, *Enterococcus*, or other pathogens.

Signs and Symptoms

Acute pyelonephritis usually involves the rapid onset of symptoms that begin with a UTI and move deeper into the body. They include fever, burning and frequent urination, cloudy urine, extreme back pain, fatigue, nausea, and vomiting. Symptoms typically develop over a day or two.

Chronic pyelonephritis in adults is often related to an acute infection that was incompletely treated, and so bacterial invasion of the kidney continues but in a quieter fashion. Therefore, many chronic kidney infections are silent; they cause no symptoms, but damage in the kidney accumulates. When chronic pyelonephritis occurs in children, it is typically related to a structural anomaly at the vesicouretral valve. This condition, called ***vesicouretral reflux***, allows urine to back up into the kidney, which creates a high risk of long-term, silent, cumulative damage.

Complications

Whether pyelonephritis is chronic or acute, if it is recurrent, it can cause scarring and long-lasting kidney damage. Insufficient kidney activity leads to hypertension and renal failure. Another possible complication of a very acute infection is sepsis (blood poisoning from the infection leaking into capillaries). This can lead rapidly to dangerously low blood pressure and death.

Diagnosis

Urinalysis to look for signs of infection, combined with symptoms that describe pain higher and more extreme than that found with a typical UTI, is usually enough information for a diagnosis of kidney infection. If the infectious agent is something unusual, more tests may be needed. Computed tomography (CT) or intravenous pyelography is sometimes used to look for kidney stones or tumors that might be causing problems or abscesses on the kidneys that can cause similar symptoms.

Treatment

Most kidney infections clear up satisfactorily with antibiotic therapy. Some species of pathogens that invade the urinary tract are developing resistance to traditional antibiotics, so newer drugs are now being used to treat bladder and kidney infections. If the infection is extreme, the patient may need to be hospitalized to monitor processing of fluids. Some patients need to be monitored especially closely; these include people with diabetes, spinal cord injury survivors, and kidney transplant recipients.

Prevention

Acute pyelonephritis is most often caused by bacteria that enter the body at the urethral opening. Let this be a lesson, ladies: always wipe front to back.

Massage?

Acute kidney infections contraindicate circulatory bodywork. The risk of making the situation worse is matched only by the patient's inability to lie still, since the pain is so extreme. Chronic kidney infections are less dramatic, but the kidneys are still vulnerable to damage. The safest course is to avoid any circulatory work until the infection has been eradicated.

MODALITY RECOMMENDATIONS FOR PYELONEPHRITIS	
Deep tissue massage	Systemically contraindicated while acute; otherwise supportive.
Lymphatic drainage	Supportive.
Polarity	S: Indicated; can support immune system. R/D: Systemically contraindicated while acute otherwise supportive.
PNF/MET/stretching	Systemically contraindicated while acute; otherwise supportive.
Reflexology	Systemically contraindicated while acute; otherwise supportive.
Shiatsu	Indicated: Treat K, SP, TH meridians and extensions for the urinary and immune systems.
Swedish massage	Systemically contraindicated while acute; otherwise supportive.
Trigger point therapy	Systemically contraindicated while acute; otherwise supportive.

See Chapter 1 for a brief description of each modality, including definitions of abbreviations.

Renal Failure

Definition: What Is It?

Renal failure means that for various reasons the kidneys are not functioning adequately. If the kidneys slow down suddenly (e.g., in response to shock or systemic infection), it is *acute renal failure*. If they sustain cumulative damage over the course of many months or years, it is *chronic renal failure*. In either case, although the name implies that they have ceased functioning altogether, the truth is that the kidneys are still working but they are unable to keep up with the body's demands.

Demographics: Who Gets It?

Statistics for renal failure vary according to whether it is an acute or chronic problem. The main risk factors for chronic renal failure are chronic hypertension and diabetes. Race is also a determining factor: African Americans are far more likely to have both chronic high blood pressure and chronic renal failure than are whites.

Some researchers suggest that as many as 8 million Americans are in early stages of kidney disease, although at this stage it is silent, so it usually goes undiagnosed. Statistics for end-stage renal disease are also alarming. This serious condition is diagnosed about 102,000 times each year, and about 453,000 people in the United States live with it. About 324,000 kidney failure patients are in dialysis, and 65,300 are on the waiting list for a new kidney.[3]

Renal Failure in Brief

What is it?
Renal failure involves the inability of the kidneys to function at normal levels. It may be an acute or a chronic problem, and it can be life threatening.

How is it recognized?
Symptoms of acute and chronic renal failure differ in severity and type of onset, but some things they have in common are reduced urine output, systemic edema, and changes in mental state brought about by the accumulation of toxins in the blood.

Is massage indicated or contraindicated?
Acute and chronic renal failure systemically contraindicate circulatory massage.

Etiology: What Happens?

Although the kidneys are able to heal from most short-term abuse, any chronic or severe recurrent problems may eventually cause permanent damage to the delicate tissues, thereby interfering with kidney function. Fortunately, the human body is equipped with 2 million nephrons, about twice as many as it absolutely needs, so people can tolerate a lot of damage before problems develop.

Kidneys have several important functions: they produce EPO, the hormone that stimulates blood cell production; they manage electrolyte levels in the blood; they concentrate urine; and they manage overall fluid levels. Any of these functions may be lost during renal failure. This can lead to anemia; peripheral and pulmonary edema; pericarditis with fluid in the pericardial sac (***cardiac tamponade***); and dangerous changes in circulating levels of calcium, phosphorus, and potassium. This has important effects on bone density, digestive capabilities, the inflammatory process, and heart rhythms.

Kidney failure is classified as acute or chronic.

Acute renal failure Acute renal failure is identified when kidney function suddenly drops to 50% or less of normal levels; this may take place over several hours or days. Causes of acute renal failure usually fall into one of three categories:

- *Prerenal problems.* When something prevents blood flow into the kidneys, the glomeruli and nephrons essentially collapse from lack of fluid volume. Prerenal problems can include reduced blood volume, low blood pressure from septicemia or traumatic shock, extreme dehydration, or an embolism that blocks the renal artery.
- *Intrarenal problems.* These pathologies arise within the kidneys themselves, including ***glomerulonephritis*** (inflammation at the Bowman capsule), an embolism caught inside the kidney, an *E. coli* infection that produces tissue-damaging toxins (this is also called ***hemolytic uremic syndrome***), allergic drug reactions, and other problems.
- *Postrenal problems.* When fluid is prevented from leaving the kidneys, damage to the nephrons can accumulate to dangerous levels. Kidney stones, an enlarged prostate, or tumors can create this kind of problem.

Acute renal failure is generally a short-term problem that may become life threatening. Its mortality rate is usually connected to the general health and resiliency of the patient. It may last for days or weeks, but if the contributing factors are controllable, kidney function may be restored.

Chronic renal failure Chronic renal failure is an impairment in kidney function that may persist for months or years before it causes any symptoms. Kidney function is measured in terms of glomerular filtration rate (GFR), that is, how efficiently fluid moves from the glomeruli into the nephrons. Normal GFR is 120 mL/min. Renal failure is a progression along a continuum of lost function, and so may be discussed in the following stages:

- Stage I: Kidney damage is minor and GFR is close to normal, above 90mL per minute.
- Stage II: Mild reduction in function; GFR is 60 to 89 mL per minute.
- Stage III: Moderate reduction in function; GFR is 30 to 59 mL per minute.
- Stage IV: Severe reduction; GFR is 15 to 29 mL per minute.
- Stage V: End-stage renal failure; GFR is less than 15 mL per minute.

Diabetes mellitus is the most common cause of chronic renal failure, followed by chronic hypertension, glomerulonephritis, and other more obscure causes.

Signs and Symptoms

Because the kidneys have so many functions, symptoms of renal failure affect virtually every major organ system of the body. Symptoms include decreased urine output, systemic and pulmonary edema from salt and water retention, arrhythmia from potassium retention, anemia from the lack of EPO, and *osteomalacia* (bone thinning) from the lack of vitamin D, which is necessary for calcium metabolism. Rashes and skin discoloration arise from retention of toxic pigments in the blood. Other symptoms include lethargy, fatigue, headaches, loss of sensation in the hands and feet, tremors, seizures, easy bruising and bleeding, muscle cramps, and changes in mental and emotional states as the accumulation of wastes in the blood affects the brain.

Treatment

Treatment for acute and chronic renal failure is determined by whatever underlying pathologies caused the damage. Treatment goals are to control the symptoms, prevent further complications, and slow the progress of the disease. This often means aggressively controlling blood pressure and blood sugar levels (if diabetes is part of the picture). Medication to control potassium levels in the blood is important to avoid heart problems. Fluid and salt intake may be restricted until kidney function can keep up with the body's demands. Diuretics are sometimes prescribed to help the kidneys process fluids.

If a patient's kidneys are simply incompetent regardless of these interventions, dialysis may become necessary. This routes the blood through a machine or through the peritoneum to extract wastes.

Kidney transplants replace a damaged organ with a healthy kidney from an appropriate donor. They can be successful if the new tissue is not rejected. Unfortunately, the shortage of suitable donated organs means that among the 65,300 people waiting for kidney transplants this year, only 16,000 operations will be performed.[3]

Massage?

Any stage of renal failure contraindicates circulatory massage, although energy work may be supportive. If a client has a history of renal failure, the massage therapist should work with the client's health care team for the best outcome. Clients undergoing dialysis are vulnerable to infection at access points for the filtration system. Special care must be taken not to disrupt or contaminate these areas.

Massage for transplant recipients may be appropriate if it fits within the limits of normal activities of daily living. Therapists should be aware that organ transplant recipients commit to a lifetime of immunosuppressant medications, so they are at risk for some infections that the rest of the population doesn't have to worry about.

Modality Recommendations for Renal Failure	
Deep tissue massage	Contraindicated.
Lymphatic drainage	Supportive.
Polarity	S: Indicated. R/D: Supportive with light work within client comfort.
PNF/MET/stretching	Supportive.
Reflexology	Supportive with light work. Focus on kidney and lymph points, avoid crystals.
Shiatsu	Indicated: Treat K, SP, TH meridians and extensions for the urinary and immune systems.
Swedish massage	Systemically contraindicated.
Trigger point therapy	Supportive with light work.

See Chapter 1 for a brief description of each modality, including definitions of abbreviations.

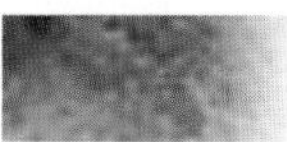

Bladder and Urinary Tract Disorders

Bladder Cancer

Definition: What Is It?

Bladder cancer is the growth of malignant cells in the urinary bladder. Transitional cells are most often affected: this may be called *transitional cell carcinoma* or *urothelial carcinoma*. Urothelial carcinoma is also the term used for transitional cell cancer in the renal pelvis, ureters, and urethra.

Demographics: Who Gets It?

Bladder cancer is a relatively common disease. It is the fourth leading cancer among men (following prostate, lung, and colorectal cancers) and the tenth leading cancer among women.[4] About 60,000 new cases are diagnosed each year, and it causes about 12,700 deaths each year in the United States. Rates of diagnosis of this disease increased by 33% per year between 1985 and 2000.[4] About 500,000 people in the United States live with or have had bladder cancer.[5]

Bladder cancer occurs in men about three times more often than in women. Bladder cancer is diagnosed in about 1 in 30 men and 1 in 90 women. It is usually a disease of mature people; the median age at diagnosis is 73 years.[6]

Etiology: What Happens?

Like most types of cancer, bladder cancer usually involves epithelial cells, in this case, the transitional epithelium that lines the urinary bladder. Constant repetitive damage to this epithelium causes the mature cells to die. This stimulates rapid replication in the basal layer, and soon new colonies of immature cells migrate to the sur-

Bladder Cancer in Brief

What is it?
Bladder cancer is the growth of malignant cells in the urinary bladder. Most bladder cancer starts in the superficial layer of transitional epithelium.

How is it recognized?
The earliest sign of bladder cancer is blood in the urine, which may be red or rust colored. Bladder cancer is painless at this point. In later stages the bladder may become irritable. Painful urination, reduced urination, or increased urinary frequency may all occur.

Is massage indicated or contraindicated?
As with most varieties of cancer, massage with parasympathetic effects and immune system support has a place in treatment. Bladder cancer has a high recurrence rate, and most patients undergo surgery at some point. As long as these issues are respected and the massage therapist works as part of a well-informed health care team, bodywork may be supportive for these patients. For more information about the role of massage for cancer patients, see Chapter 12.

face. These new cells are easily disrupted by genetic mutations and may become malignant growths that cause bleeding into the bladder.

Causes of bladder cancer vary according to medical history and geographic region. Persons who have undergone pelvic radiation for other problems are at an increased risk for developing bladder cancer, as are people who have had chronic infections, bladder stones, or catheter use. In Africa, Asia, and South America, bladder cancer is associated with a specific parasitic infestation, ***Schistosoma haematobium***.

In the United States and industrialized countries, most cases of bladder cancer are directly related to more controllable factors. The transitional epithelium of the bladder seems to be particularly susceptible to damage from environmental toxins. Several genetic mutations that limit the body's ability to inhibit tumor growth or invasion have been linked to bladder cancer. These mutations are frequently triggered by exposure to carcinogenic substances. Approximately half of bladder cancer cases are believed to be related to cigarette smoking. Other contributing factors include exposure to aromatic amines (chemicals used in dry cleaning fluid, hairdressing chemicals, and textile and rubber industries).[4]

The relation between bladder cancer and carcinogenic substances is one of the most clearly demonstrable links between environmental exposures and cancer. The good news is that bladder cancer is probably a completely preventable disease, if exposure to the carcinogenic substances is limited or eradicated.

Signs and Symptoms

The earliest and most dependable sign of bladder cancer is hematuria, or blood in the urine. The urine of a bladder cancer patient is often visibly reddened or rust colored, although the patient has no particular pain in the early stages of the disease. If the tumors continue to grow and invade deeper layers of the bladder, secondary symptoms may develop. These are the result of mechanical pressure, including bladder irritability (painful urination, increased urinary frequency, reduced urine output) and compression on the rectum, pelvic lymph nodes, and any other structures that happen to be in the way.

Diagnosis

If a man in his 60s or 70s has no pain, but his urine is bright red or rusty, the immediate conclusion most doctors will come to is that he has bladder cancer. Urine samples may be tested to look for shedding cancer cells, and a digital rectal examination (or pelvic examination if the patient is a woman) provides information about tumors. Other diagnostic techniques include using dye to stain the urine and make the bladder easy to radiograph; using a cystoscope, with which a physician visually examines the bladder through a tube inserted through the urethra; and performing local biopsies to examine abnormal tissue for signs of metastasis. For bladder cancer staging protocols, see Sidebar 10.1.

Specific markers for bladder cancer have recently been identified, but tests to find them are not yet consistently accurate or widely available. Continued development in this area, however, bodes well for the future of early detection and treatment of this disease.

Treatment

Bladder cancer treatment depends on the stage at diagnosis. Surgeons can use a small wire loop on the end of a cystoscope to remove abnormal tissue, or another tool may be used to burn the tumor away with electricity.

More invasive surgeries may remove part or all of the bladder, and if signs of pelvic metastasis are present, other tissues as well. Men may lose the prostate gland; women may lose the uterus, ovaries, and parts of the vaginal wall. Pelvic lymph nodes are also removed, leading to the risk of lymphedema in the legs. Urine flow may be routed out of the body through

SIDEBAR 10.1: STAGING BLADDER CANCER

Bladder cancer is staged with the traditional TNM classifications, which are translated to stages 0 to IV, as follows:[7]

Tumor (T)	Node (N)	Metastasis (M)
Ta: noninvasive papillary carcinoma	NX: nodes cannot be assessed	MX: metastasis cannot be assessed
TIS (cancer in situ): noninvasive flat cells	N0: no nodes involved	M0: no metastasis found
T1: cancer cells invaded urothelium but not muscle tissue	N1: one node involved; cells <2 cm	M1: distant metastasis to organs or bones
T2a: cancer cells invaded inner half of muscle layer	N2: 1 node with cells 2–5 cm; or multiple nodes with cells <5 cm	
T2b: cancer cells invaded outer half of muscle layer	N3: nodes have cells >5 cm	
T3a: microscopic invasion of fatty tissue outside bladder		
T3b: grossly observable invasion of fatty tissue outside bladder		
T4a: cells invaded prostate, uterus, or vagina		
T4b: cells invaded pelvic or abdominal wall		

These delineations are translated to stages 0 to IV in this way:

Stage 0a	Ta, N0, M0
Stage 0 IS	T IS, N0, M0
Stage I	T1, N0, M0
Stage II	T2 (a,b), N0, M0
Stage III	T3 (a,b) or T4, N0, M0
Stage IV	T4b, N0, M0; or any T, N1–3, M0; or any T, any N, M1

Bladder cancer is highly survivable, largely because most cases are found in stage 0 to II. The 5-year survival rates are as follows:

Stage 0	95%
Stage I	85
Stage II	55
Stage III	38
Stage IV	16

The overall 5-year survival rate is close to 81%.[6]

a *stoma*, or a variety of surgeries have been developed to form artificial bladders from parts of the large or small intestines.

In addition to surgery, radiation therapy and chemotherapy may be used to battle bladder cancer. Chemotherapy may be administered intravenously, orally with pills, or through a site-specific bladder wash to distribute the medication directly to the target tissues.

New procedures in bladder cancer treatment include the use of biological therapies. Specifically, introducing bacille Calmette-Guérin into the bladder has been seen to stimulate an immune response that inhibits the new growth of cancer cells. This therapy has some risks, but is finding success for many patients.

Prognosis

More than 70% of bladder cancer diagnoses are made when the cells affect only superficial layers of tissue. This is excellent news, of course, because the survival rate for cancers caught early is much better than for cancers caught in stage III or later. Nevertheless, bladder cancer has an unusual habit of growing in several places at the same time, so although it may be possible to catch one or two tumors, the invisible third, fourth, and fifth tumors may not become symptomatic for another several months. This means that the recurrence rate for bladder cancer is surprisingly high: up to 80% of patients have at least one recurrence.[4]

Massage?

The main issues of concern in working with bladder cancer patients are the high rates of recurrence and the frequency with which surgery is an early treatment intervention. Bladder cancer survivors may have stomas or medical devices that require the therapist to make adjustments.

The rules for massage and bladder cancer are the same as the rules for massage and any kind of cancer. While bodywork offers powerful benefits in the way of immune system strengthening, pain reduction, anxiety reduction, and general support, massage therapists must work as part of a team, sharing information and concerns with the rest of the client's health care staff.

Modality Recommendations for Bladder Cancer	
Deep tissue massage	Supportive as part of health care team. Respect stage of recovery and treatment challenges.
Lymphatic drainage	Supportive.
Polarity	S: Indicated for immune system support. R/D: Supportive within client comfort.
PNF/MET/stretching	Supportive as part of health care team; match to activity levels.
Reflexology	Indicated: Work lymphatic system, pituitary, urinary system points.
Shiatsu	Indicated: Treat K, SP, TH meridians and extensions for urinary and immune systems.
Swedish massage	Supportive as part of health care team; match massage to activity level.
Trigger point therapy	Supportive with light work.

See Chapter 1 for a brief description of each modality, including definitions of abbreviations.

Interstitial Cystitis

Definition: What Is It?

Interstitial cystitis (IC) is a condition in which the urinary bladder becomes small and inelastic. Because the diagnostic criteria for IC are still in development, it is sometimes referred to as IC/PBS (interstitial cystitis/painful bladder syndrome).

> **Interstitial Cystitis in Brief**
> Pronunciation: in-ter-STIH-shul sis-TY-tis
>
> **What is it?**
> Interstitial cystitis (IC) is a chronic inflammation of the bladder involving pain, scar tissue, stiffening, decreased capacity, pinpoint hemorrhages, and sometimes ulcers in the bladder walls.
>
> **How is it recognized?**
> Symptoms of IC are very much like those of urinary tract infections: burning, increased frequency, and urgency of urination; decreased capacity of the bladder; and pain, pressure, and tenderness.
>
> **Is massage indicated or contraindicated?**
> IC is a poorly understood condition that seems to be exacerbated by stress. Bodywork may be a helpful and supportive choice for IC patients, although it probably does not work to reverse the condition.

Demographics: Who Gets It?

Statistics on IC have been difficult to gather, but it is estimated that somewhere between 700,000 and 1 million Americans have it. Of those, 90% are women and 10% are men. IC is rare in children.[3]

Etiology: What Happens?

The bladder, a hollow organ, shrinks when it is empty and expands when it is full. A healthy bladder can hold 8 to 12 oz of urine. When the bladder is full, a signal is sent to the central nervous system that triggers the motor response to empty the bladder.

Normal urine is composed of water, excess salts and hormones extracted from the blood, nitrogenous wastes such as urea and uric acid, and other debris. It should not contain significant numbers of microorganisms. The bladder itself is shielded from the acidity of urine by a lining of protective mucous membrane.

IC occurs when the inner lining of the bladder no longer protects the organ from urine. Most IC patients develop tiny bleeding areas called pinpoint hemorrhages or ***glomerulations*** in the bladder wall. About 10% of patients develop a deeper lesion called a ***Hunner ulcer*** inside the bladder. As the problem progresses, the muscular walls of the bladder become fibrotic and inelastic; this is true most often for people with Hunner ulcers. Patients find that they have little capacity for storing urine, even if their bladder is a normal size. It is fairly common for IC patients to have to use the bathroom 16 to 60 times each day.[8]

The cause of IC is a mystery. One hypothesis is that this may be an autoimmune disease or allergy that weakens the protective mucous membrane in the bladder's epithelium. In this way, irritating chemicals from urine can infiltrate and damage the bladder wall. The presence of abnormal numbers of mast cells in some IC patients supports this idea. A pathological thinning of the mucous membrane on the bladder wall is another factor to consider. It is probably linked to a substance found in the urine of most IC patients called antiproliferative factor, which interferes with the normal growth of bladder-lining cells. Other researchers are investigating the possibility that the causative agent for IC is some pathological agent that has yet to be identified. IC does not respond to antibiotic therapy, so it is clear that no known strain of bacteria causes this problem. Other hypotheses postulate a neurological hypersensitivity to bladder fullness or problems with the perineum muscle that may refer pain into the pelvis.

As more is discovered about causes of severe pelvic pain with urinary symptoms, it may be determined that the condition IC is actually several problems with a similar profile.

Signs and Symptoms

Symptoms of IC include chronic pelvic pain, pain and burning on urination, increased urinary frequency and urgency, and painful intercourse. Symptoms are worst when the bladder is full, and they abate somewhat when the bladder is empty. Menstruation can exacerbate symptoms. Some patients find that symptoms occur in periods of flare and remission; others find that their daily experiences are all about the same.

Diagnosis

IC is diagnosed by a process of exclusion. Conditions that must be ruled out for a positive diagnosis include UTI, genital herpes, bladder cancer, kidney stones, urethral diverticula, cervical or uterine cancer, vaginitis and endometriosis for women, and prostate enlargement or prostatitis for men. Once other pathologies have been ruled out, a cystoscopic examination may be conducted to look for ulcers or bleeding spots, which can be seen only when the bladder is fully distended.

Treatment

Because this is a disease without a known cause, it is also without a known cure. IC treatment is generally aimed at symptomatic relief and the development of coping skills. Often the diagnostic tool of bladder distension can give relief, as can a distillation, or bladder wash. This is done with ***dimethyl sulfoxide*** (DMSO), which can pass into the bladder wall to act as an anti-inflammatory and block pain sensation. Lesions on the bladder wall may be removed with lasers or electrical wires. Oral medications to help rebuild the mucous lining have been developed. Aspirin and other painkillers may be recommended, as are exercise, smoking cessation, and dietary changes. Tricyclic antidepressants can be effective pain modulators. No single intervention is successful for all patients, however, and nothing has yet provided a permanent solution. IC may recur after months or even years of remission.

Some patients have such severe problems that surgery becomes an option. They may have a new bladder constructed from a segment of the colon, or they may have the bladder removed altogether and replaced with a stoma and external bag.

Massage?

Among the interventions IC patients may need to explore are options to reduce the stress and anxiety that accompany chronic, painful conditions. Acupuncture, hypnotherapy, biofeedback, and other therapies may be recommended. Massage can be a useful tool in this effort too, as long as the client's need for frequent urination can be met.

Modality Recommendations for Interstitial Cystitis	
Deep tissue massage	Supportive.
Lymphatic drainage	Systemically contraindicated while acute; otherwise supportive.
Polarity	S/R/D: Indicated for immune system and parasympathetic support.
PNF/MET/stretching	Supportive.
Reflexology	Indicated: Work lymphatic system, pituitary, and urinary system points.
Shiatsu	Indicated: Treat K, SP, TH meridians and extensions for the urinary and immune systems.
Swedish massage	Supportive as long as client is comfortable.
Trigger point therapy	Supportive.

See Chapter 1 for a brief description of each modality, including definitions of abbreviations.

Urinary Tract Infection

Definition: What Is It?

A urinary tract infection (UTI) is an infection that may occur anywhere in the lower urinary system. This section focuses on infections of the lower urinary tract, that is, the urethra (urethritis) and the bladder (cystitis).

Demographics: Who Gets It?

UTIs are the cause of about 8 million visits to the doctor every year. Estimates vary, but somewhere between 20 and 50% of women will have a UTI at least once.[3,9] It is almost always a women's disorder, because the female urethra is short and close to the anus, where bacteria that are harmless in the digestive tract can cause havoc if they gain access to the urinary tract.

Although women, particularly sexually active young women, are most at risk for UTIs, other populations may also have this problem. It is certainly possible for men to have a UTI; this is sometimes the warning sign of something that may be serious, like prostate problems or a sexually transmitted infection. People who must drain their bladder with a catheter are also at increased risk for UTI.

Urinary Tract Infection in Brief

What is it?
A urinary tract infection (UTI) is an infection usually caused by bacteria that live harmlessly in the digestive tract.

How is it recognized?
Symptoms of UTIs include pain and burning sensations during urination, increased urinary frequency and urgency, and cloudy or blood-tinged urine. Abdominal, pelvic, or low back pain may occur. In the acute stage, fever and general malaise may be present.

Is massage indicated or contraindicated?
Acute UTIs contraindicate circulatory massage, as do all acute infections. Massage may be appropriate in the subacute stage, although deep work on the abdomen is still a local caution until all signs of infection are gone.

Etiology: What Happens?

Under normal circumstances the environment in the bladder is sterile. The urine contains waste products to be expelled from the body, but no living microorganisms should be present. Furthermore, the bladder is lined with a protective mucus-producing layer of cells that works to prevent infectious or noxious agents from harming the bladder walls.

Sometimes foreign microorganisms are introduced into the urethra. If the circumstances are right, they can cling to the mucous lining of the urethra or the bladder and set up an infection that may stay local or may travel farther into the urinary system. New findings show that the bacteria that colonize the urethra are able to produce their own protective film; this opens new doors to treatments that can interfere with this process.[9]

E. coli are the causative agent behind close to 90% of UTIs. These strains of bacteria live normally and harmlessly in the digestive tract. Certain varieties of *Staphylococcus* cause a small percentage of UTIs, and other agents, including *Klebsiella*, *Chlamydia*, and *Mycoplasma* are behind a minority of infections. It is important to identify the correct causative agent, because not all of them respond to the same antibiotics.

Chronic irritation can also contribute to the development of UTIs. "Honeymoon cystitis" is inflammation and subsequent infection brought about by repeated irritation of the urethra from sexual activity.

The relation between stress and UTIs has much anecdotal support. Living in a sympathetic state may reduce blood flow to the bladder, which in turn may make it more susceptible to infection. However, clinical evidence shows that although stress may aggravate symptoms of UTIs, it has not been proved to cause them.

Risk Factors

Some women are more susceptible to UTIs than others, although the reasons for this are not completely clear; they may have to do with immune system differences and shortages of certain types of antibodies. Some factors, however, are reliable predictors of who is at risk for developing a UTI:

- *Spermicide use.* Spermicide foams and jellies used with a diaphragm or alone have been shown to raise the risk of UTIs in some women.
- *Diaphragm use.* Women who use a diaphragm show statistically higher rates of UTIs than women who do not.
- *Pregnancy.* Pregnant women do not necessarily get more UTIs than women who are not pregnant, but the risk of having a simple infection complicate into a more dangerous one is higher for these patients.
- *Diabetes.* Elevated sugar levels in the urine make a hospitable environment for bacteria to grow in the bladder.
- *Neurogenic bladder.* A bladder that has lost motor function does not empty as completely as a normal one. This raises the potential for infection, as does the presence of catheter tubes, which are used for people with limited bladder function.

Signs and Symptoms

The symptoms of UTIs are painful, burning urination; a frequent need to urinate; reduced bladder capacity; urinary urgency; and blood-tinged or cloudy urine. Pelvic, abdominal, or low back pain may also occur. Men with UTIs may have pain in the penis or scrotum. If severe flank or back pain and fever develop, a kidney infection should be suspected.

Complications

Bacteria that live in the digestive tract cause almost all UTIs. If the bacteria are able to travel up the system, they may set up an infection in the bladder. This is called cystitis, but it is not the same situation as interstitial cystitis, which is discussed elsewhere. If the infection remains unchecked, it may move all the way up the ureters and into the kidneys, causing a kidney infection, or pyelonephritis. Chronic UTIs may contribute to chronic renal failure. Untreated kidney infections can lead to the release of infectious bacteria in the blood and life-threatening septicemia.

Unfortunately, not all UTIs show symptoms, so they may be neglected, especially in children. It is possible for some people to have extreme complications of this type of infection that can easily lead to permanent kidney damage or even to death.

Treatment

The first step in self-treatment of a UTI is to drown it: radically increasing fluid intake gives the body the much needed opportunity to fully and frequently empty the bladder—not only of urine but of bacteria as well. Drinking highly acidic liquids such as blueberry or cranberry juice is helpful for many women, as an acidic environment inhibits bacterial growth. These berries also contain chemicals that limit the ability of bacteria to cling to bladder walls. It is important, however, to avoid sweetened juice; the amount of sugar it takes to make cranberry juice sweet may actually make the bladder a more hospitable environment for infection. In subacute infection, hydrotherapy in the form of hot and cold sitz baths may be recommended.

UTIs usually respond well to a short course of antibiotics. In this case, 3 to 5 days' worth of medication is more appropriate than 2 weeks' worth, because the body concentrates antibiotics in the urine. With bladder infections, as with all types of bacterial infections, it is especially important to take the full prescription of antibiotics. Stopping too soon may result in recurrent infections with more highly resistant bacteria.

People who have low-grade, chronic UTIs that do not clear up with normal treatments are sometimes successfully treated with long-term low doses of antibiotics. Structural problems with the way urine drains from the bladder may contribute to chronic infections; surgery may be recommended to correct these problems.

Prevention

Some basic precautions can help prevent UTIs, especially for women who are especially vulnerable to them. These include drinking lots of water and acidic juices; urinating whenever necessary rather than holding it for a more convenient time; wiping from front to back after a bowel movement to prevent the introduction of digestive bacteria into the urethra; taking showers rather than baths; emptying the bladder after sex; and avoiding feminine hygiene sprays and douches, which can aggravate the urethra.

Massage?

Acute UTIs are sometimes accompanied by fever, a systemic contraindication. A small but significant risk of spreading the infection to the kidneys should also be considered. Even in the postacute stage (after signs of acute infection have subsided), the lower abdomen is a local contraindication for massage until all signs of infection have been eradicated.

Modality Recommendations for Urinary Tract Infection	
Deep tissue massage	Systemically contraindicated while acute; otherwise supportive.
Lymphatic drainage	Systemically contraindicated while acute; otherwise supportive.
Polarity	S: Indicated. R/D: Locally contraindicated while acute; otherwise supportive.
PNF/MET/stretching	Systemically contraindicated while acute; otherwise supportive.
Reflexology	Indicated while subacute; work endocrine, lymphatic, urinary systems, lower back, hips, solar plexus, diaphragm points.
Shiatsu	Indicated. Treat K, SP, TH meridians and extensions for urinary and immune systems.
Swedish massage	Systemically contraindicated while acute; otherwise supportive.
Trigger point therapy	Systemically contraindicated while acute; otherwise supportive.

See Chapter 1 for a brief description of each modality, including definitions of abbreviations.

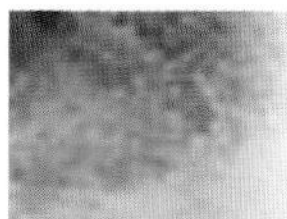

Chapter Review Questions: Urinary System Conditions

1. What forces fluid from the glomerulus into the Bowman capsule?
2. What happens to kidney function if blood pressure suddenly drops as a result of circulatory shock or loss of blood volume?
3. What is a normal GFR? What condition is rated according to declining GFR?
4. When do kidney stones cause pain?
5. What is the most common cause of bladder cancer in the United States?
6. What is the difference between a UTI and IC?
7. How can kidney dysfunction lead to anemia?

8. A client has IC and would like to receive massage. What are the benefits and risks? How might the practitioner adjust bodywork to meet this client's needs?
9. A client with chronic renal failure is on the wait list for a kidney transplant. He undergoes dialysis regularly. He would like to receive a massage for stress and pain relief. What are the benefits and risks? How might the practitioner adjust bodywork to meet this client's needs?
10. A client received a donated kidney 2 years ago. He would like to receive a massage for stress and pain relief. What are the benefits and risks? How might the practitioner adjust bodywork to meet this client's needs?

REFERENCES

1. Kidney Stones in Adults. National Institute of Diabetes and Digestive and Kidney Diseases. NIH Publication 05–2495. http://kidney.niddk.nih.gov/kudiseases/pubs/stonesadults/index.htm. Accessed autumn 2006.
2. Shoff W, Green-Mckenzie J. Pyelonephritis, Acute. © 1996–2006 by WebMD. http://www.emedicine.com/MED/topic2843.htm. Accessed autumn 2006.
3. Kidney and Urologic Diseases Statistics for the United States. National Institute of Diabetes and Digestive and Kidney Diseases. NIH Publication 06–3895. http://kidney.niddk.nih.gov/kudiseases/pubs/kustats/. Accessed autumn 2006.
4. Steinberg G, Kim H. Bladder Cancer. © 1996–2006 by WebMD. http://www.emedicine.com/med/topic2344.htm. Accessed autumn 2006.
5. What Are the Key Statistics for Bladder Cancer? © 2006 American Cancer Society, Inc. http://www.cancer.org/docroot/CRI/content/CRI_2_4_1X_What_are_the_key_statistics_for_bladder_cancer_44.asp?rnav=cri. Accessed autumn 2006.
6. Cancer of the Urinary Bladder. Surveillance Research Program, National Cancer Institute. http://seer.cancer.gov/statfacts/html/urinb.html. Accessed autumn 2006.
7. How Is Bladder Cancer Staged? © 2006 American Cancer Society, Inc. http://www.cancer.org/docroot/CRI/content/CRI_2_4_3X_How_is_bladder_cancer_staged_44.asp?rnav=cri. Accessed autumn 2006.
8. Urinary tract infection (UTI). © 1998–2006 Mayo Foundation for Medical Education and Research (MFMER). All rights reserved. http://www.mayoclinic.com/health/urinary-tract-infection/DS00286. Accessed autumn 2006.
9. Urinary Tract Infections in Adults. National Institute of Diabetes and Digestive and Kidney Diseases. NIH Publication 06–2097. http://kidney.niddk.nih.gov/kudiseases/pubs/utiadult/. Accessed autumn 2006.

11

Reproductive System Conditions

Chapter Objectives

After reading this chapter, you should be able to . . .

- List five uncontrollable factors in spontaneous abortion.
- Name a causative agent of cervical cancer.
- Identify the primary trigger for the genetic mutation that leads to uterine cancer.
- Name two main classes of uterine cancer.
- Name the two most common varieties of breast cancer.
- List three significant risk factors for the development of ovarian cancer.
- Identify a medical emergency associated with benign prostatic hyperplasia.
- List four classes of prostatitis; identify the most common version.
- List two classes of testicular cancer.
- List four pregnancy-related complications.
- List three bacterial sexually transmitted diseases.

INTRODUCTION

Massage therapists are often short-changed in their education about the reproductive system. This may be because of time constraints in the classroom or because of a tendency to skip over this system because of a residual stigma that confuses massage therapy with the sex industry. While massage is not a treatment of choice for most reproductive system diseases, many clients live with them, and the conditions themselves or their treatment options may have repercussions for bodywork choices.

Another stumbling block in the topic of reproductive system conditions is the perception that two perfectly normal, nonpathological states are often addressed as diseases: pregnancy and menopause. It is important for massage therapists (and other people too!) to understand that these conditions are *not* diseases but simply conditions that change the way the body functions, and for that reason we should know about them.

Terminology for structures in the reproductive system can sometimes be confusing. Many resources have moved toward labeling structures by their location or function rather than by their traditional names, which commonly refer to the physicians or anatomists who first recorded them. Thus, fallopian tubes, named for 16th century anatomist Gabriele Fallopio, may now be called *oviducts* or *uterine tubes*, which is more descriptive. Traditional names are still in common use, however. In this chapter structures will be referred to by both traditional and functional or locational names, so that practitioners educated in either terminology may feel at home.

Function and Structure of the Female Reproductive System

Most of the female reproductive structures are low in the pelvis. In a healthy, nonpregnant woman with no scar tissue or other anomalies, the ovaries are typically behind the upper corners where the pubic hair starts to grow. They are attached via the ovarian ligament to the uterus. The ovaries produce hormones, which are released into the bloodstream, and they produce eggs, usually one each month during ovulation, which are released into the peritoneal space. The ***fimbriae*** of the fallopian (uterine) tubes gently caress the ovaries, coaxing the released egg toward them. Once inside the tubes, the eggs make the 5-day journey to the uterus itself. If an egg is fertilized, it generally happens inside the uterine tube.

When the egg reaches the uterus, it is inside a hollow organ that is built of criss-crossed layers of muscle. The inside surface of the uterus, the ***endometrium***, is made of delicate epithelial tissue that holds vast billowy supplies of specialized capillaries to provide a nest for that fertilized egg (Figure 11.1). If the egg is not fertilized, the uterus sheds the tissue and egg with it in the menses. Then it begins to build a new nest for next month's candidate.

The timing of the ripening and release of eggs from the ovaries and the building and shedding of the endometrial nest is under the control of the endocrine system. Hormones secreted from the ovaries themselves and from the pituitary gland determine when and how these various events will happen. Birth control pills and other hormonal applications work by introducing artificial hormones into the blood. These trick the pituitary into believing that the woman is always pregnant, so she never ovulates.

The relation between the reproductive system and the endocrine system is extremely tight; the female reproductive cycle is under the control of hormone secretions. Several of the conditions discussed in this chapter could be considered endocrine system disorders, but the tissue changes occur in reproductive system organs, so they are discussed here (Sidebar 11.1).

Female reproductive conditions that have significance for massage therapists generally have to do with growths or local tenderness deep in the abdomen. Although deep work in the vicinity of the uterus or ovaries is not generally done, sometimes these conditions can displace internal organs, making them vulnerable in places they wouldn't ordinarily be found.

Function and Structure of the Male Reproductive System

The male reproductive system consists of the testes, the epididymis, the spermatic cord, other glands that contribute to the production of semen, and the urethra, which expels semen through the penis (Figure 11.2).

Sperm cells are among the smallest of human cells and the only ones equipped with flagella for locomotion. They are manufactured in specialized tubes in the testes, the ***seminiferous tubules***. Sperm cells grow and mature in the testes. The testes are suspended from the body in the scrotal sac, because sperm cells flourish best when the temperature is slightly lower than internal body temperature. Mature sperm cells are stored in the ***epididymis***, a long

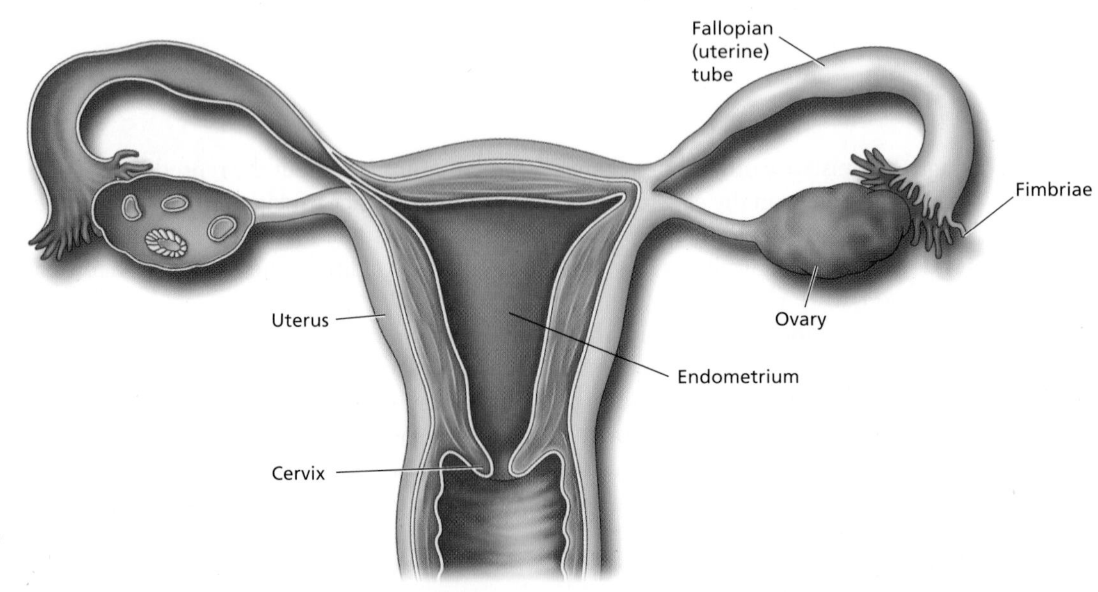

Figure 11.1. Overview of the female reproductive system.

SIDEBAR 11.1: WHAT IS THIS THING CALLED ESTROGEN?

Estrogen is not a single hormone but a group of closely related chemicals that includes ***estradiol***, ***estriol***, and ***estrone***. These chemicals are synthesized from cholesterol primarily in the ovaries during a woman's fertile years. After menopause they continue to be manufactured in peripheral tissues in much smaller amounts, using root chemicals secreted by the adrenal cortex.

Estrogens are received by target tissues all over the body. They are not only associated with sex organ function; they also influence the growth, health, and activity of many organs, including bones and the heart. They influence cell production and differentiation. Estrogens are also associated with mood swings and emotional responsiveness.

The liver makes estrogens chemically able to stimulate biological activity in their target cells. This metabolism can occur in a variety of ways, with great implications for long-term health. Some "bad" estrogen metabolites are associated with tissue proliferation (i.e., cancer) of the breast, uterus, cervix, ovaries, and thyroid. "Good" estrogen metabolites are associated with healthy bone maintenance and cardiovascular protection.

What determines which estrogen metabolites will be present in a woman's body? Two main factors are at work here: diet and estrogen exposure.

Diet

High-fat, low-fiber diets do several things to estrogen production. By providing excessive cholesterol, they allow the body to manufacture more estrogens than it otherwise would. By providing a minimum of fiber, they prevent the binding of excessive estrogens to the molecules that would inactivate them. And by disrupting the healthy balance of bacteria in the intestines, poor diet allows some estrogens to reenter the circulation.

Estrogen Exposure

People are exposed to estrogen from internal production (endogenous estrogens) and external sources (exogenous estrogens). Endogenous estrogens have already been discussed as a function of diet and estrogen metabolism. Endogenous estrogen exposure is also increased by obesity, as fat cells can contribute to estrogen production. Exogenous estrogen exposure is a topic that has only recently begun to be discussed. Oral birth control pills, hormone replacement therapy, and supplements in meat and dairy products, along with environmental chemicals such as pesticides, herbicides, plastics, and industrial solvents all contribute to cumulative endogenous estrogen exposure.

Excessive estrogen exposure and the metabolism of "bad" estrogens have been identified as contributing factors in several cancers of hormone-dependent tissues. In addition, estrogen dominance is being investigated as a factor in other reproductive system disorders, including premenstrual syndrome, endometriosis, uterine fibroids, and menopause. The good news is that estrogen exposure and metabolism can be influenced by diet and nutrition. Estrogen receptor sites in target tissues can bind with several estrogenlike substances (***phytoestrogens***, including soy, legumes, and other sources), and some nutritional supplements can help disable free estrogen metabolites before they influence cell proliferation or differentiation.

Ultimately these reproductive system disorders may be treated or even prevented by having patients take greater control over how much estrogen they are exposed to and how their bodies put that estrogen to use.

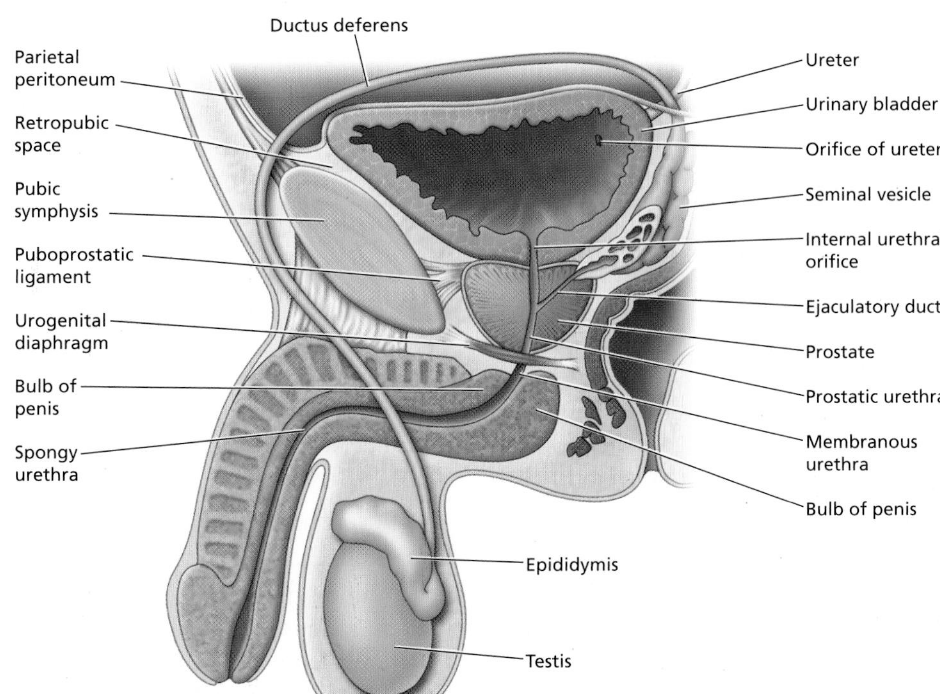

Figure 11.2. Overview of the male reproductive system.

tube that is coiled up behind the testes in the scrotum. Sperm cells leave the epididymis through the left and right *vas deferens*, which carries them through the inguinal ring into the abdomen. Along the way other glands, including the seminal vesicles and prostate, contribute to the fluid that suspends and nourishes the sperm on their long journey toward the ovum. The left and right vas deferens join together at the urethra, and sperm leaves the penis during ejaculation.

The most common disorders of the male reproductive system have to do with the prostate gland, which is in a position to obstruct the urethra during ejaculation or urination. While prostate massage is typically conducted by a urologist through the wall of the rectum during an examination (and is therefore outside the scope of practice of most massage therapists), prostate problems can seriously diminish a person's quality of life. Consequently, some clients seek bodywork as a coping mechanism while managing the disorder. Massage conducted to maximize the benefits of parasympathetic effect and improved immune system function can be safe and appropriate choice.

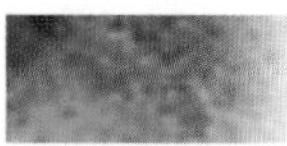

Reproductive System Conditions

Disorders of the Uterus

Abortion, spontaneous and elective
Cervical cancer
Dysmenorrhea
Endometriosis
Fibroid tumors
Uterine cancer

Disorders of Other Female Reproductive Structures

Breast cancer
Ovarian cancer
Ovarian cysts

Disorders of the Male Reproductive System

Benign prostatic hypertrophy
Prostate cancer
Prostatitis
Testicular cancer

Other Reproductive System Conditions

Pelvic inflammatory disease
Premenstrual syndrome
Pregnancy
Menopause
Sexually transmitted diseases

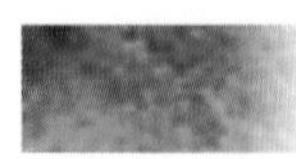

Disorders of the Uterus

Abortion, Spontaneous and Elective

Definition: What Are They?

An elective abortion is the intentional termination of a pregnancy; a spontaneous abortion is an unintentional termination. In either case the fetus and placenta are detached from the uterine wall and cannot continue to develop.

Etiology of Elective Abortion: What Happens?

A pregnancy can be terminated in various ways, depending on the stage. Within the first 12 weeks an elective abortion is usually conducted by vacuum suction. The walls of the cervix are dilated to allow a flexible tube into the uterus, and suction is applied to remove the fetal tissue. In the 13th to 15th weeks a D & C, or *dilation and curettage*, may be performed; this is a more complicated procedure and requires more anesthetic and sometimes a hospital stay. Later terminations are brought about by inducing premature labor. They can be very difficult and always require hospitalization.

A nonsurgical intervention for very early pregnancy has recently been approved for use in the United States. The "morning-after pill," when combined with carefully timed doses of prostaglandins, blocks cell division or counteracts the activity of progesterone, a hormone that supports the implantation of a fertilized egg.

Abortion, Spontaneous and Elective, in Brief

What are they?
Spontaneous and elective abortions are pregnancies that are ended, unintentionally or intentionally, before the fetus is born naturally.

How are they recognized?
General or pelvic pain may be present, along with vaginal bleeding. Often, however, no outward signs may show that a woman is recovering from a spontaneous or elective abortion.

Is massage indicated or contraindicated?
Deep abdominal work is locally contraindicated for women recovering from a recent spontaneous or elective abortion until her bleeding has stopped and she is free of any signs of infection. Bodywork elsewhere can be supportive and helpful.

Etiology of Spontaneous Abortion: What Happens?

Several factors may contribute to the unintentional disruption of a pregnancy. In many cases it can be hard to discover exactly what causes fetal development to fail, but many factors have been identified. Some of these are controllable, but many of them are not.

Controllable factors that may raise the risk of spontaneous abortion or miscarriage include smoking, untreated infections of the reproductive tract, untreated diabetes or thyroid disorder, and exposure to toxic chemicals, especially solvents. Another factor is progesterone deficiency in the early weeks of pregnancy, before the placenta has begun to secrete its own supply of this hormone that allows fetal implantation. An immune system response that causes blood in fetal vessels to clot can be controlled with low doses of aspirin or other blood thinners.

Factors over which a woman has no control include structural problems in the uterus (fibroid tumors or a weak cervix), fertilization of multiple eggs, age, autoimmune disease, an immune system rejection of fetal tissue, failure of the fetus to implant in the endometrium, and perhaps the most common cause of miscarriage: the fetus is simply missing key genetic information that would allow it to continue to develop. When the moment comes that the needed genes are missing, the fetus dies.

Miscarriages usually happen in the first 14 weeks of pregnancy, although the risk goes way down after the eighth week. If the fetus dies after the 20th week, the event is no longer called a miscarriage or spontaneous abortion; it's called a stillbirth, but the principles are the same.

Miscarriages are sometimes categorized in these ways:

- Inevitable (uterine bleeding with dilation of the cervix)
- Incomplete (some material is not expelled from the uterus)
- Complete (uterine bleeding, discharge, and pain are present)
- Missed (a nonviable fetus is retained without discharge; no material is expelled, but the fetus has died)

The frequency of spontaneous abortions is a subject of debate. It is estimated that up to 50% of fertilized eggs are expelled from the body for one reason or another before a woman may know that she's pregnant at all. Of recognized pregnancies, anywhere from 25% to 30% of fetuses are spontaneously aborted.[1]

Signs and Symptoms

When the endometrial lining of the uterus is disrupted in any way but a normal menses, the endometrium is traumatized. This is true for elective and spontaneous abortions and for childbirth. Symptoms of this trauma can include pain (local and referred), bleeding, and cramping. These are generally self-limiting; that is, the symptoms resolve with time unless complications develop.

Complications

Complications of abortions or miscarriages include infection from incomplete shedding of the uterine lining; damage to the uterus, bladder, or colon from surgical instruments; and hemorrhage. Depression and anxiety disorders are other frequent complications. The later the gestational age of the fetus, the higher the risk of complications from elective or spontaneous abortion.

Treatment

The best treatment for a woman recovering from an elective abortion, a miscarriage, or successful childbirth is tender loving care. If infection develops, or if the uterine lining has not been shed completely, a D & C or D & E (dilation and evacuation) and antibiotics may be necessary.

Massage?

Deep abdominal massage is locally contraindicated for women recovering from spontaneous or elective abortion and from childbirth, at least until the bleeding has stopped. Massage elsewhere is very much indicated, although the risk of blood clotting for pregnant women is quite high, so it is wisest to stick with noncirculatory modalities for the first weeks following a spontaneous or elective abortion.

Modality Recommendations for Abortion, Spontaneous and Elective	
Deep tissue massage	Supportive; avoid deep work in abdomen. Work slowly on feet and legs for grounding and reconnection.
Lymphatic drainage	Supportive.
Polarity	S: Indicated. R/D: Locally contraindicated; otherwise supportive.
PNF/MET/stretching	Supportive.
Reflexology	Indicated. Work uterus, ovaries, pelvic area, solar plexus, thyroid points.
Shiatsu	Indicated, but avoid leg stretches. Focus on SI leg extension to reduce physical and emotional trauma.
Swedish massage	Locally contraindicated until bleeding has stopped; otherwise supportive.
Trigger point therapy	Locally contraindicated; otherwise supportive with light work.

See Chapter 1 for a brief description of each modality, including definitions of abbreviations.

Cervical Cancer

Definition: What Is It?

Cervical cancer is the growth of malignant cells in the lining of the cervix. While some types of abnormal cells grow slowly and don't present a serious threat, other types are aggressive and invasive.

Demographics: Who Gets It?

Each year about 10,000 women in the United States are diagnosed with invasive cervical cancer, and this disease kills about 4,000 American women each year.[2] Rates of cervical cancer and deaths from it have been steadily declining at a rate of about 4% per year.[3] For more on the history of cervical cancer, see Sidebar 11.2.

The median age at diagnosis with cervical cancer is 48 years, but many cases are diagnosed in women who are significantly past menopause.[2]

Cervical Cancer in Brief

Pronunciation: SER-vih-kal KAN-ser

What is it?

Cervical cancer is the development of cancerous cells in the lining of the cervix. These may spread to affect the whole cervix, the rest of the uterus, and other pelvic organs.

How is it recognized?

Early stages of cervical cancer are virtually silent; this disease is detected by Pap (Papanicolaou) tests before symptoms develop. Later signs and symptoms include bleeding or spotting outside a normal menstrual period, vaginal discharge, and pelvic pain.

Is massage indicated or contraindicated?

Most cases of cervical cancer are caught and eradicated before the woman is in serious danger of metastasis. These patients are good candidates for any kind of bodywork. For a woman with advanced cervical cancer, the massage therapist must make adjustments for any radiation therapy, chemotherapy, or surgical procedures that she is receiving.

Etiology: What Happens?

Cervical cancer is a malignancy brought about directly by a viral infection, in this case with any of the 100 known varieties of the HPV family.

Statistics on the incidence of HPV are hard to gather because it can be silent, or symptoms may not develop for months or years after infection. Some estimates suggest that over 6 million people are infected with some type of HPV each year, and up to half of sexually active adults are exposed at some time.[4] Being infected with HPV is not a dependable indicator of cervical cancer, however; most of the viruses in this family are not associated with aggressive or invasive cancers.

When a woman is infected with HPV, the virus may trigger cellular changes in the lining of her cervix. Precancerous changes called ***dysplasia*** can be stimulated by both low-risk and high-risk types of HPV.

If a woman happens to be infected with a low-risk type of virus, her abnormal cells may spontaneously resolve, and she may never know anything had happened. But if she is infected with an aggressive form of HPV, cancerous cells may grow in the lining of the cervix and then may spread throughout the uterus, the vagina, and into the pelvic cavity, affecting the bladder, colon, and inguinal lymph nodes. Ultimately the cancer may travel to distant parts of the body.

HPV is a sexually transmitted disease, transferred by direct skin-to-skin touching. While condoms have been seen to reduce the risk of developing cervical cancer, they do not prevent the spread of all HPV, because skin still comes in contact during sexual activity.[5]

Risk Factors

Exposure to HPV is the central risk factor for developing cervical cancer. However, other factors may contribute to the likelihood of having abnormal cells become malignant. Sexual activity at an early age may increase the transmission rate of HPV, especially if a woman has multiple partners. Alternatively, if a woman has only one sexual partner but the partner has a history of multiple partners, her risk of cervical cancer is increased.

Smoking raises the risk of cervical cancer by roughly 100%.[2] Increased risk is also seen with women who are overweight and whose diet is low in fruits and vegetables.

Being the daughter of a woman who took ***diethylstilbestrol***, a drug prescribed to prevent miscarriage from 1940 to 1971, increases the possibility of cervical cancer, as does immune system suppression through HIV infection or immunosuppressant drugs. Co-infection with chlamydia also raises the risk. Finally, socioeconomic standing is a major factor, as this often determines whether a woman has adequate access to early detection and care.

Signs and Symptoms

Early stages of cervical cancer have no symptoms to speak of. The cancer must be significantly advanced before any signs appear. These usually include bleeding or spotting between menstrual periods or after menopause, vaginal discharge, and pelvic or abdominal pain.

SIDEBAR 11.2: CERVICAL CANCER: HISTORY OF A DISEASE

In the early part of the 20th century, cervical cancer was one of the leading causes of death by cancer for women in this country. This disease is virtually silent, causing no signs or symptoms until it has spread throughout the pelvic cavity and into the lymph system—by which time survival rates are very low.

Then from 1955 to 1992 a remarkable phenomenon occurred: rates of death by cervical cancer took a huge downswing, dropping by some 74%.

What made the difference? A simple examination: the *Papanicolaou test*, which makes it possible to detect precancerous cells in the cervix before they spread. Because of the Pap test, women could have abnormal cells detected and removed before they had a chance to become malignant, and women could find and remove malignancies before they had a chance to spread throughout the pelvic cavity. Consequently, the 5-year survival rate for cervical cancer is now over 95% for preinvasive cells and 71.6% overall.[2,3]

Today the recommended protocol for cervical cancer detection is to receive a traditional Pap test once a year or a liquid Pap test every 2 years. If a woman over 30 years old has three consecutive years without any sign of dysplasia, her doctor may recommend that she can have Pap tests less frequently. Higher mortality rates among nonwhite women and women of low socioeconomic status point out the fact that many at-risk women still do not have access to this inexpensive and highly useful test.

Cervical cancer has been largely controlled in the United States, but worldwide it is still a leading cause of death by cancer in countries where women don't have access to Pap tests. The recent development of a vaccine against the some types of human papillomavirus (HPV), however, promises that one day cervical cancer may be a completely preventable disease.

Diagnosis

The *Pap test* is the current standard for early cervical cancer detection. In this test a small scraping of cells and mucus from the cervix is extracted and analyzed. If abnormal cells are found, a follow-up visual examination of the cervix for suspicious changes (a *colposcopy*) may be conducted. A biopsy removes the affected part of the cervix; if more suspicious cells are found, further tests may be conducted to stage the cancer and determine the best possible treatment options.

Pap tests are fast, cost-effective, and only mildly uncomfortable, but if the tissue sample happens to miss some abnormal cells, false-negative results may be returned. A new variation on Pap tests is now available in some areas. In this version a liquid is used to remove cells from the cervix. These cells are preserved and fixed in a way that allows for more accurate test results.

If a test is positive for abnormal cells, tests for HPV DNA may be conducted. These tests are most accurate for women over 40, but they can give very specific information about what type of virus may be present. For specific information about cervical cancer staging, see Sidebar 11.3.

Prevention

A new option in prevention of cervical cancer has recently become available with the development of a vaccine for certain types of HPV. This vaccine, which is recommended for adolescent girls and young women before they become sexually active, prevents the transmission of HPV types 6 and 11 (the cause of some 90% of genital warts), and of HPV types 16 and 18 (the cause of about 70% of cervical cancers).

This vaccine, while a significant step forward in the management of this disease, is not a treatment and does not prevent cervical cancer in a woman who has already been exposed to the virus. Furthermore, while it prevents most cervical cancers, it does not protect against all aggressive forms of HPV. For this reason, a woman who has had the vaccine series still must undergo routine cervical cancer screening.

Treatment

Treatment for cervical cancer depends entirely on the stage at which it is diagnosed. Most cases are found in stage 0 or I, which means treatment can be limited to removing the abnormal cells and watching carefully for further changes. Surgical interventions to remove cervical dysplasia include cryotherapy, in which cells are frozen off; loop electrosurgical excision procedure, in which electricity is passed through a loop of thin wire to slice off the suspicious tissue; laser surgery; and cone biopsy.

Surgical procedures for cancer caught in later stages may range from full or partial hysterectomy (including a procedure that may preserve most of the uterus for the possibility of future childbearing) to full pelvic *exenteration*, in which virtually all of the pelvic organs are removed.

Radiation therapy and chemotherapy may also be employed with advanced cases of cervical cancer.

SIDEBAR 11.3: STAGING CERVICAL CANCER

The staging protocols for cervical cancer can be confusing, and as they are constantly under review, they change frequently. At this writing the recommendations for cervical cancer divide this disease into precancerous and cancerous stages.

Precancerous Staging

When abnormal cells are found in cervical cancer screening, they are classified into these four subgroups:

- **Atypical squamous cells.** Cells look abnormal, but infection or irritation may be the cause.
  - **Atypical squamous cells of unknown significance.** The patient may be told to repeat the test in several weeks or months.
  - **High-grade atypical squamous cells.** They look dangerous and should be removed for further study.
- **Squamous intraepithelial lesions.** These lesions may be classified as low-grade or high-grade, but they all need further study
- **Squamous cell carcinoma.** These cancerous cells must be staged and removed
- **Atypical glandular cells.** Mucus-producing cells are affected.

Cancer Staging

The staging protocol for invasive cervical cancer was developed by the *Fédération Internationale de Gynécologie et d' Obstétrique*, so it is sometimes called the FIGO system. The staging system for cervical cancer has been developed in great detail; a simplified version is included here:[3]

- Stage 0. Cancer cells are found only in the superficial layer of the cervix.
- Stage I. Cancer cells are found only in the cervix. Lesions can range from microscopic to 4 cm in width.
- Stage II. Cancer cells have moved from the cervix into the surrounding area, involving the upper vagina or tissue surrounding the uterus.
- Stage III. Cancer cells are found in the lower vagina and/or the pelvic wall. A growth may be big enough to block the flow of urine through the ureters. Pelvic lymph nodes may also be involved.
- Stage IV. Cancer cells are found in the bladder, rectum, or distant organs.

Massage?

Massage for a client who has cervical dysplasia is certainly fine, especially if she is receiving appropriate care. Clients who are dealing with advanced cases of cancer must cope not only with the disease process, but with the many complex and extremely unpleasant complications those treatments may involve. Carefully conducted bodywork that respects the many challenges of surgery, radiation, and chemotherapy can offer all of the benefits of massage while minimizing any possible risks. See more on this topic in Chapter 12.

Modality Recommendations for Cervical Cancer

Deep tissue massage	Supportive as part of health care team. Respect stage of recovery and treatment challenges.
Lymphatic drainage	Supportive.
Polarity	S/R/D: Indicated within client's comfort.
PNF/MET/stretching	Supportive as part of health care team; match to client activity.
Reflexology	Indicated. Work lymphatic system, ovaries, pituitary, pelvic area, uterus points.
Shiatsu	Supportive.
Swedish massage	Supportive as part of health care team; match to client's activity.
Trigger point therapy	Supportive with light work.

See Chapter 1 for a brief description of each modality, including definitions of abbreviations.

Dysmenorrhea in Brief
Pronunciation: dis-men-o-RE-ah

What is it?
Dysmenorrhea is the technical term for menstrual pain that is severe enough to interfere with and limit the activities of women of childbearing age. It may be a primary problem or secondary to some other pelvic pathology.

How is it recognized?
The symptoms of dysmenorrhea are dull aching or sharp severe lower abdominal pain preceding and/or during menstruation. Nausea and vomiting may accompany very severe symptoms. Secondary dysmenorrhea may cause pelvic pain outside normal periods as well.

Is massage indicated or contraindicated?
Massage is appropriate for primary dysmenorrhea, although the abdomen locally contraindicates deep work during days of heavy menstrual flow. The appropriateness of bodywork for secondary dysmenorrhea depends on the type of pathology involved, along with stage, severity, treatment, and other variables.

Dysmenorrhea

Definition: What Is It?

Dysmenorrhea is a technical term for painful menstrual periods. Generally a woman is said to have dysmenorrhea if she has to limit her regular activities or requires medication to function for one day or more every cycle.

Demographics: Who Gets It?

Most women have severe menstrual pain at least once in their life. The prevalence of dysmenorrhea is estimated to be 45% to 95% of fertile women.[6] Dysmenorrhea is a leading cause of lost time from school or work for women of childbearing age.

Etiology: What Happens?

Dysmenorrhea can be primary, that is, it starts within the first 3 years of menstruation in an otherwise healthy woman, or secondary to some underlying pathology.

Causes of primary dysmenorrhea Several factors can contribute to primary dysmenorrhea:

- ***Prostaglandins.*** These are chemicals produced all over the body, especially in the uterus. They cause smooth muscle contractions, but they also sensitize the body to pain. Prostaglandins are found in higher concentrations in women who have menstrual pain than in women who do not, and prostaglandin secretion is timed to increase at the beginning of the menstrual cycle.
- ***Pain-spasm cycle.*** When the uterus is in sustained contraction, oxygen cannot easily supply the muscle. Ischemia causes pain, which reinforces the spasm, and so on. This is often exacerbated by a shortage of calcium, which tends to make muscle spasms more tenacious.
- *Ligament irritation.* The uterine ligament, which anchors the uterus to the pelvic wall, can be pulled and irritated when the uterus is in spasm.

It is easy to see how physical or emotional stress fits into the picture of menstrual pain. Sympathetic reactions in the body exacerbate uterine ischemia, leading to pain, which reinforces the spasm. The emotional state of dreading the pain and discomfort of menstrual periods can then become a self-fulfilling prophecy: the stress of anticipating an unpleasant event works to make that event even more unpleasant.

Causes of secondary dysmenorrhea Secondary dysmenorrhea is a complication of some other pelvic disorder. Some of the most common problems that cause menstrual pain include pelvic inflammatory disease (PID), fibroid tumors, sexually transmitted diseases, and endometriosis. Pelvic adhesions, deposits of scar tissue from previous surgeries, or trauma may also contribute to menstrual pain.

Signs and Symptoms

Signs and symptoms of dysmenorrhea vary. They can include dull aches in the abdomen and low back or sharp pains and cramping in the pelvis and abdomen. These usually happen early in menstruation, but some women have symptoms during their whole period. Headaches, nausea, vomiting, diarrhea, and constipation are all possibilities, along with a frequent need to urinate.

Secondary dysmenorrhea may have other signs that indicate underlying pathology. Symptoms may not be limited to menstruation; menstrual flow may be irregular or abnormally heavy; pain medication is often not effective; and this condition is often accompanied by infertility.

Diagnosis

It is important to investigate ongoing debilitating menstrual pain, because it may indicate serious underlying problems. Diagnosis often involves a laparoscopy to check for endometriosis, which is a leading cause of secondary dysmenorrhea. Ultrasounds to look for fibroid tumors may be performed. Cultures of vaginal secretions may also be examined to look for signs of PID, chlamydia, syphilis, or gonorrhea. In the absence of these conditions, painful periods can be treated without fear of ignoring some important underlying causes.

Treatment

For most cases of dysmenorrhea, painkillers such as ibuprofen or naproxen work by inhibiting the secretion of prostaglandins.

For more serious dysmenorrhea, if painkillers, heat, and stretching don't affect the pain, more aggressive interventions may be considered. Low-dose birth control pills suppress ovulation, which in turn prohibits the secretion of prostaglandins in the uterus. If a structural condition, such as fibroid tumors, is at the root of the problem, surgery may be an option. And medications or laparoscopic surgery for endometriosis may alleviate symptoms if that is the source of the problem.

Dysmenorrhea is a common problem that seriously interferes with quality of life for millions of women. Fortunately, it is also frequently responsive to many alternative treatment options. A thorough nutritional analysis may reveal strategies for dealing with menstrual pain; this is a useful course for many women, but no specific nutritional supplements have been found to alleviate all cases of dysmenorrhea. Dietary changes to radically reduce fats and animal proteins while increasing fiber and calcium are often recommended. Exercise and stretches can also relieve the pain in the uterine ligament, which may be irritated by a uterus in spasm. One other new treatment option has been recently recognized for primary dysmenorrhea: the use of vitamin K injections at uterine acupuncture sites. The combination of acupuncture and this vitamin supplement has been seen to reduce perceived pain with a very high success rate.[7]

Massage?

A woman who is having a painful period probably will not welcome deep abdominal massage, but nurturing touch elsewhere is highly called for and beneficial. A woman who regularly has painful periods but who has no known pelvic pathologies is a good candidate for abdominal massage when she is not menstruating. This may help to relieve tension, take stress off the uterine ligament, and even minimize abdominal adhesions that may contribute to pain.

Modality Recommendations for Dysmenorrhea	
Deep tissue massage	Supportive when client is not menstruating. Work adductors, hip rotators, gluteals, and abdomen, including psoas.
Lymphatic drainage	Supportive.
Polarity	S: Indicated. R/D: Locally contraindicated while acute; otherwise supportive.
PNF/MET/stretching	Supportive.
Reflexology	Indicated. Work low back, hips, pelvic area, intestines, ovaries, uterus points.
Shiatsu	Indicated. Treat LV, SP, K, BL, GB, PC, SI meridians and extensions in the legs, abdomen, chest, back.
Swedish massage	Avoid abdomen during painful menstruation; otherwise indicated.
Trigger point therapy	Locally contraindicated while acute; otherwise supportive.

See Chapter 1 for a brief description of each modality, including definitions of abbreviations.

Endometriosis

Definition: What Is It?

Endometriosis is a condition in which cells from the endometrium, the inner lining of the uterus, implant elsewhere in the body. Growths usually begin in the pelvic cavity but may spread further into the abdomen and in rare cases above the diaphragm.

Endometriosis in Brief

Pronunciation: en-do-me-tre-O-sis

What is it?
Endometriosis is the implantation and growth of endometrial cells in the peritoneal cavity (and possibly elsewhere) that grow and then decay with the menstrual cycle.

How is it recognized?
Endometriosis may have no symptoms. When it does, they generally include heavy, painful menstruation; pelvic and abdominal pain; difficulties with urination or defecation; painful intercourse; and other problems, depending on which tissues are affected. Symptoms are worst just before and during menstruation. Infertility is a frequent complication of endometriosis.

Is massage indicated or contraindicated?
If a client knows she has endometriosis, deep abdominal or pelvic work may be painful, especially close to her menstrual period. The supportive effects of massage, however, can be an important part of the coping mechanisms women with this disorder must develop.

Demographics: Who Gets It?

Endometriosis is probably fairly common, but because it cannot be conclusively diagnosed without an invasive procedure, estimates for how many women are affected are largely speculative. Some resources suggest that 10% to 20% of women of childbearing age may have endometriosis (that's about 13.6 million women in the United States), but not all of them have symptoms or seek medical care.[8,9] Other resources suggest that 5.5 million women have been diagnosed with this disorder.[10]

Endometriosis affects girls as young as 9 years old and postmenopausal women, but most patients are diagnosed between ages 20 and 45. Most endometriosis patients are women who have heavy, long-lasting menstrual periods, whose cycles occur in fewer than 28 days, and who have never had children.

Etiology: What Happens?

Endometriosis is implantation and growth of endometrial cells anywhere outside the uterus. It was first described in 1921 by American gynecologist James Sampson, who noticed these growths in the peritoneal cavities of women undergoing abdominal surgery. He hypothesized that the endometrial cells got out of the uterus via retrograde backflow through the uterine tubes or through circulatory or lymphatic dissemination. These are still leading theories about the pathophysiology of this disorder, but other factors have also been identified.

Having endometrial cells outside of the uterus turns out to be a common phenomenon. In fact, up to 90% of women have some endometrial cells in the pelvic cavity during menstruation, but not all of those women have endometriosis.[11]

While the etiology of endometriosis is not precisely understood, some differences between women with this disease and women without it have been observed. These include immune system anomalies that promote inflammation and scar tissue without eradicating misplaced growths, unusually high levels of prostaglandins that contribute to pain and cramping, and the possibility of genetic predisposition. One newer theory looks at the phenomenon of ***metaplasia***, the transformation of one type of tissue into another type. It is possible that remnants of embryonic cells in the pelvic cavity undergo changes later in life to become outposts of endometrial cells in the pelvic cavity.

Endometrial growths usually become established on the uterine tubes, the broad ligaments, the ovaries, the bladder, or the colon (Figure 11.3). Rarely, growths have been found as far from the uterus as the lungs and even the brain. Wherever they land, they stimulate the growth of supplying blood vessels, and they proliferate in accordance with the hormonal commands in the body. But these growths cannot be shed with normal menstruation. Instead, they decay and accumulate in local areas, stimulating an inflammatory response. The body attempts to isolate them by surrounding the deposits with fibrous connective tissue. Eventually multitudes of fibrous "blood blisters" accumulate on whatever surfaces the endometrium can find.

Endometrial growths that are found early look like clear vesicles on the structures they have colonized. Later these vesicles become bright red. Over a course of 10 or more years they become thick, black, and scarred. Growths on ovaries that have darkened over time are sometimes called "chocolate cysts".

Signs and Symptoms

Very often infertility is the complaint that brings a woman with endometriosis to a doctor for a first diagnosis. Other signs and symptoms of endometriosis are often nonexistent, at least in the early stages, but premenstrual spotting, a sensation of urinary urgency with painful urination, and diarrhea and rectal bleeding during menstruation may occur. Some cases include se-

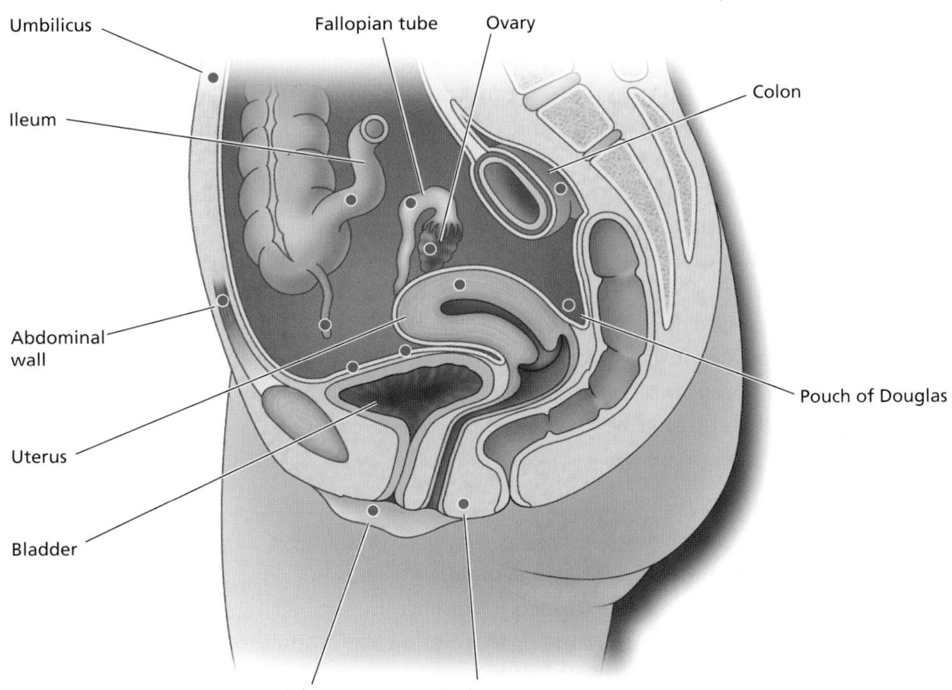

Figure 11.3. Sites of endometriosis.

vere dysmenorrhea before, during, and after periods. Interestingly, the amount of pain has little to do with the size of the endometrial growths; many women with microscopic growths report more pain than other women with advanced deposits.

Symptoms of endometriosis are cyclical, reaching a peak during menstruation. This feature has probably prevented a lot of women from seeking medical help, since traditionally it has been assumed that painful menstruation is a normal and expected part of the having "the curse." As women have become more proactive about health care, they have discovered that painful menstruation is not a given and have become more willing to explore the causes and possible solutions to their pain.

Complications

Accumulations of deposits and fibrous connective tissue can cause a lot of damage in the pelvic cavity. Scar tissue deposits can create adhesions in or on the uterine tubes and ovaries, which cause infertility or ectopic pregnancy. The collecting of blood in these deposits routes blood away from where it can be useful, resulting in anemia. Uterine ***hyperplasia*** is a condition that occasionally accompanies endometriosis; the normal endometrial lining becomes pathologically thickened, leading to excessive bleeding and further difficulties with fertility.

Diagnosis

Only one diagnostic test for endometriosis is definitive: laparoscopic surgery. While patients may describe characteristic symptoms that become worsen and peak during menstruation, only a laparoscopy specifically identifies the lesions.

Other tests for endometriosis are in development. At this point magnetic resonance imaging (MRI) and ultrasound are not accurate for this type of growth, and while some blood markers suggest a high likelihood of endometriosis, they are not definitive.

Treatment

Treatment for endometriosis depends on what outcome the woman desires. No permanent solution for this disorder has yet been developed; even a complete hysterectomy won't protect a patient from endometriosis if any remaining microscopic deposits are stimulated with hormone replacement therapy.

Because many women wish to treat endometriosis to become pregnant, treatment options are often geared toward limiting symptoms and progression long enough to allow fertilization to take place. Symptoms disappear during pregnancy, but they usually recur after a baby is born.

Four main goals are at the center of medical intervention for endometriosis. These are to relieve pain, to stop the progression of established growths, to prevent the establishment of any new growths, and to maintain or restore fertility if that is the patient's wish. Nonsteroidal anti-inflammatory drugs (NSAIDs) or other analgesics may be adequate for pain relief. Hormone therapy that disrupts the secretion of estrogen may be employed to limit growths. These may be used alone or as a preparation for surgery. Surgical intervention may include the use of lasers or ***electrocauterization*** to ***ablate*** (remove the top layer of tissue) or cut out visible growths and to reduce adhesions between pelvic organs.

Massage?

Endometriosis can displace the pelvic organs, as they are distorted with abnormal deposits and scar tissue. Consequently, deep abdominal massage is not appropriate for clients who know they have endometriosis, especially for those who are menstruating. The presence of inflammation and the threat that cells may break free and settle elsewhere in the pelvic cavity both make doing deep abdominal work problematic.

However, many women with endometriosis also live in a state of anxiety, stress, and frustration with their own body that may exacerbate their most painful symptoms. Massage therapy along with other relaxation techniques is frequently recommended for women who must learn to cope with the long-term consequences of a disorder that has no permanent cure.

Hysterectomy

This comes from the Greek root *hystera*, which means womb or uterus. The word hysteria comes from the same root. In the early days of medicine, hysteria was assumed to be a woman's complaint, associated with womb-related disturbances.

MODALITY RECOMMENDATIONS FOR ENDOMETRIOSIS	
Deep tissue massage	Locally contraindicated; otherwise supportive. Focus on fascial release.
Lymphatic drainage	Supportive.
Polarity	S: Indicated. R/D: Locally contraindicated while acute; otherwise supportive for light work.
PNF/MET/stretching	Locally contraindicated; otherwise supportive.
Reflexology	Indicated. Work hips, pelvic area, ovaries, uterus points.
Shiatsu	Indicated. Treat LV, SP, K, TH, BL, GB, PC, SI meridians and extensions in the legs, abdomen, back, sacrum.
Swedish massage	Locally contraindicated; otherwise supportive.
Trigger point therapy	Locally contraindicated; otherwise supportive for light work.

See Chapter 1 for a brief description of each modality, including definitions of abbreviations.

Fibroid Tumors

Definition: What Are They?

Fibroid tumors, or ***leiomyomas***, are benign tumors that grow in or around the uterus. They can grow within the smooth muscle walls, or, more rarely, they can be suspended from a stalk into the pelvic cavity or uterus (Figure 11.4). Some even hang down into the vagina. Fibroids can grow singly or in clusters, and they vary in size from microscopic to weighing several pounds and completely filling the uterus.

Demographics: Who Gets Them?

The number of women with fibroids is difficult to project, since fibroids are usually silent. Some estimates suggest that while they are found in up to 20% of fertile women, they may be present in up to 80%.[12] Growth of fibroids seems to be stimulated by estrogen; after menopause many shrink and ultimately disappear. Fibroids are more common in African American women than in other groups.[12]

Etiology: What Happens?

The pathophysiology of uterine fibroids is not well understood. While they sometimes run in families, they are not strictly genetically linked. Many experts believe that they arise as a combination of genetic, environmental, and hormonal factors.

Fibroids are typically classified by their location. Submucosal fibroids grow under the mucous lining of the uterus; they are the deepest type. Intramural fibroids grow within layers of the muscular

Fibroid Tumors in Brief

Pronunciation: FY-broyd TU-morz

What are they?
Fibroid tumors are benign growths in the muscle or connective tissue of the uterus.

How are they recognized?
Fibroid tumors are often asymptomatic. Some, however, cause heavy menstrual bleeding or put mechanical pressure on other structures in the pelvis.

Is massage indicated or contraindicated?
Large diagnosed fibroid tumors contraindicate deep abdominal massage. However, most fibroids are quite small and virtually silent, and massage has no effect on them at all. In these cases, massage is indicated for the benefit of the client, if not for the possibility of changing the state of her fibroid tumors.

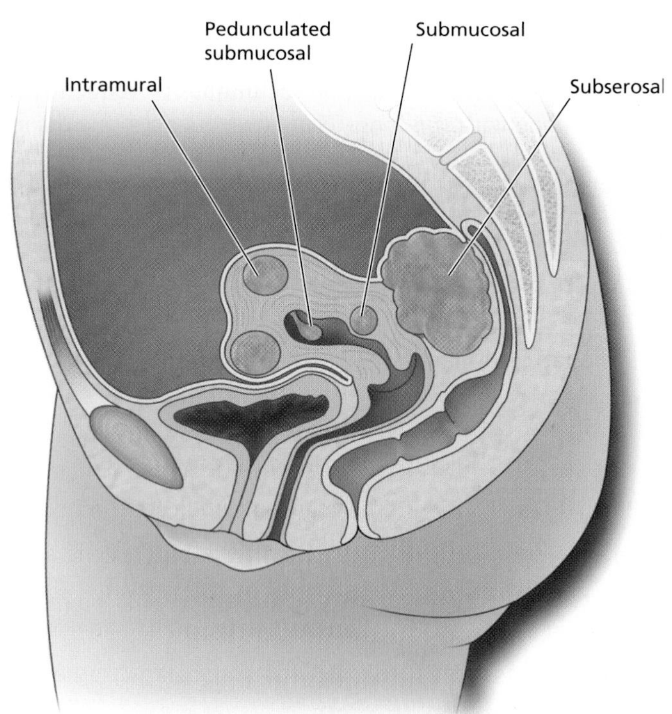

Figure 11.4. Leiomyomas (fibroid tumors).

wall of the uterus. Subserosal fibroids grow on the superficial aspect of the uterus but deep to the peritoneum.

One new line of research has found that the extracellular matrix of fibroid tumors lacks a key protein, and the collagen filaments are disorganized and not discretely formed. This is especially interesting because the same growth pattern has been observed in keloid scars. Both fibroids and keloids are about three times more common in African Americans than in the rest of the population.

Signs and Symptoms

Usually fibroids produce no symptoms at all. In extreme cases the fibroid may grow large enough to press on the sensory nerves inside the uterus. If they on nearby structures like the bladder, they can cause urinary frequency; if on the rectum, they can cause difficulties with defecation. If they press on the fallopian (uterine) tubes, they may interfere with pregnancy. They can also cause heavy menstrual bleeding and occasionally bleeding between menstrual periods.

Complications

Fibroids are very seldom serious, but they can lead to some troubling consequences. The heavy periods they cause sometimes lead to anemia from excessive blood loss. They can cause infertility by obstructing fallopian tubes or interfering with the implantation of a fertilized ovum. They can also interfere in pregnancies brought to term: if a fibroid is large enough, it can crowd the growing fetus or block the exit through the cervix. These problems can lead to premature births and cesarean sections.

Pedunculate fibroids, the type that dangle into the uterus or vagina, can twist on their stalk. This causes extreme pain and requires surgery for removal. It is also possible for very large fibroids to outgrow their blood supply. This leads to degeneration, in which tissue that is deprived of oxygen dies. The body slowly reabsorbs the necrotic mass, but it can be a long and painful process; more often, surgery is performed to remove the fibroid.

Diagnosis

Fibroids are generally found during a pelvic examination when it is noted that the uterus is enlarged or irregularly shaped. The diagnosis can usually be confirmed by ultrasound or MRI. However, occasionally it can be difficult to tell whether it is the uterus that is distended or if a cyst or tumor is growing on the ovaries, a potentially much more dangerous situation. If it is not clear what kind of growth is present, computed tomography (CT) or laparoscopy may be called for to rule out ovarian cancer.

Fibroids typically grow slowly, but occasionally they grow fast, doubling their size within a few months. In this situation a biopsy is recommended to rule out uterine malignancy.

Treatment

Fibroids seldom require treatment unless they cause pain and excessive bleeding or they interfere with pregnancy.

Hormone therapy can shrink them, but they grow back when medication is stopped. Other options include minimally invasive procedures to shrink the growths with liquid nitrogen (*cryomyolysis*) or blocking off the supplying arteries (uterine artery ***embolization***). Surgical possibilities include laser ablation, myomectomy (the removal of the tumor while preserving the rest of the uterus), or full hysterectomy. Fibroid tumors lead to about 180,000 hysterectomies in this country every year.[12]

Massage?

Diagnosed fibroids locally contraindicate deep abdominal work. Undiagnosed fibroids are not affected by massage to speak of, so massage is indicated for the benefit of the client, if not for the improvement of her condition.

MODALITY RECOMMENDATIONS FOR FIBROID TUMORS

Modality	Recommendation
Deep tissue massage	Locally contraindicated; otherwise supportive.
Lymphatic drainage	Supportive.
Polarity	S: Indicated. R/D: Supportive with pressure within client's comfort.
PNF/MET/stretching	Supportive.
Reflexology	Indicated. Work pelvic area, ovaries, uterus points.
Shiatsu	Indicated. Treat PC meridian and extension in legs and chest.
Swedish massage	Locally contraindicated if client knows she has them; otherwise supportive.
Trigger point therapy	Locally contraindicated; otherwise supportive for light work.

See Chapter 1 for a brief description of each modality, including definitions of abbreviations.

Uterine Cancer

Definition: What Is It?

Uterine cancer is the development of cancerous cells in the uterus. It is classified as *endometrial cancer* or *uterine sarcoma*.

Uterine Cancer in Brief
Pronunciation: YU-tah-rin KAN-ser

What is it?
Uterine cancer is the development of cancerous cells in the endometrium or other tissues of the uterus.

How is it recognized?
The most dependable symptom of uterine cancer is postmenopausal spotting or bleeding. Other signs can include spotting between periods for premenopausal women, vaginal discharge, pelvic pain, pain with sex, and unexplained weight loss.

Is massage indicated or contraindicated?
The guidelines for massage in the context of uterine cancer are the same as for other cancers. Modalities must accommodate whatever treatment options the client pursues, and the therapist is best working as part of a well-informed health care team.

Demographics: Who Gets It?

Uterine cancer is relatively common. It is diagnosed in about 41,000 American women each year. Mortality rates from uterine cancer are comparatively low however, at about 7,300 deaths per year. About 500,000 uterine cancer survivors are alive today.[13]

Uterine cancer is usually a disease of older women. Most patients are diagnosed between ages 45 and 74.[13] The average age at diagnosis is 60 years.[14] While it can occur in women younger than 40, these cases usually involve the most extreme forms of risk factors.

White women develop uterine cancer more often than other races, but African American women are far more likely to die of it. It is unclear whether this has to do with socioeconomic standing and access to health care, or whether other factors make uterine cancer more aggressive in African American women. This question is under investigation.[13]

Etiology: What Happens?

Uterine cancer begins, as all cancers do, with a mutation in the DNA of the affected cells. Most often these are cells in the endometrium, but uterine cancer can also develop in the connective tissue or muscle tissue of the uterus.

The primary trigger for many cases of uterine cancer appears to be exposure to excessive estrogen. That source can be endogenous (for instance if the ovaries or fat cells produce more estrogen than can be tolerated) or exogenous (with hormone replacement therapy or other sources). Other factors, including race, age, and history of other cancers, also influence a woman's chance of developing uterine cancer.

Types of Uterine Cancer

Uterine cancer is usually discussed as two main classes of cancer, with subtypes under each class.

Endometrial cancer This involves glandular endometrial cells. It can also be called adenocarcinoma. Endometrial cancer accounts for 95% of uterine cancer diagnoses.

- *Type 1 endometrial cancer* involves cells that resemble normal endometrial cells. It tends not to be aggressive.
- *Type 2 endometrial cancer* has cells that are markedly different from normal cells, with a higher risk of invasive characteristics. Type 2 endometrial cancer may be delineated into two versions:
    - Papillary serous adenocarcinoma
    - Clear cell adenocarcinoma
- *Adenosquamous carcinoma* involves squamous epithelial cells along with typical endothelial cells.

Uterine sarcoma This cancer originates from nonglandular tissues. While it progresses with essentially the same pattern as endometrial cancer, uterine sarcoma tends to be much more aggressive and has a poorer survival rate. These cancers account for only 5% of uterine cancers.

- *Stromal sarcoma* is cancer in the connective tissues of the uterus.
- *Leiomyosarcoma* involves muscle cells.

- *Malignant mixed mesodermal tumors* combine features of adenocarcinomas and sarcomas.

When a new growth develops in the uterus, it tends to be fragile and easily disrupted. This leads to vaginal bleeding or spotting, especially in postmenopausal women; this is the most dependable early symptom of the disease.

Uterine cancer is often slow growing and not aggressive. When it does spread, however, it can use any of four mechanisms to move outside the uterus. Direct contact can allow cells on the exterior of the uterus to become established on nearby organs, such as the bladder or the colon. Cells from the uterus can also float through peritoneal fluid to land elsewhere in the region and set up new growth sites. Finally, both the lymphatic and circulatory systems can be recruited to carry cancerous cells outside the pelvis to the lungs, bones, or other areas.

Risk Factors

Risk factors for uterine cancer have been extensively studied, and the most potent triggers all have to do with estrogen exposure. Evidently, when endometrial cells are exposed to excessive estrogen, they become more likely to develop mutations. A short-lived surge in uterine cancer diagnoses between 1973 and 1978 corresponded with an increase in prescriptions for estrogen replacement therapy that was not mitigated with progestin or progesterone. Now, when a woman considers hormone replacement therapy, she is counseled to use a combination of estrogen and progestin if she still has a uterus, to help prevent uterine cancer.[15]

Estrogen-related risk factors for uterine cancer include the following:

- Estrogen replacement therapy
- Obesity (fat cells produce estrogen)
- High-fat diet
- Never having had children
- Early menarche (before age 12), especially in combination with late menopause (after age 52)
- Polycystic ovarian syndrome or ovarian tumors
- Taking tamoxifen to lower the risk of breast cancer

Other risk factors for uterine cancer include age, race, and the genetic anomaly associated with a high risk of colorectal cancer. Type 2 diabetes is associated with uterine cancer; this is probably due to a tendency toward obesity, but the metabolic problems of diabetes itself may also have something to do with an increased risk of this disease.

Signs and Symptoms

Most women with uterine cancer are postmenopausal, so the most common early sign of this disease, vaginal spotting or bleeding, is easy to identify. While most women who have postmenopausal bleeding do not have uterine cancer, this early sign contributes to the excellent survival rates for this disease: it is found in stage I or II in up to 75% of cases.[16]

For women who still have a menstrual cycle, uterine cancer can be harder to identify early, but spotting between periods should be investigated.

Other signs and symptoms include vaginal discharge, pelvic pain, a pelvic mass, pain with sex, a change in bladder or bowel habits, and unintended weight loss.

Diagnosis

Uterine cancer is typically diagnosed with a combination of endometrial biopsy and transvaginal ultrasound. Chest radiography may be used to look for metastases to the lungs.

SIDEBAR 11.4: STAGING UTERINE CANCER

As with cervical cancer, the staging protocol for uterine cancer was developed by the *Fédération Internationale de Gynécologie et d' Obstétrique*, so it is sometimes called the FIGO system.

While growths are rated according to their aggressiveness with grades 1, 2, and 3, they are also staged by size and location. Staging for uterine cancer is done with postsurgical examinations of tissues. Endometrial cancer and uterine sarcomas are staged with essentially the same pattern.[17,18]

Stage		5-Year Survival (%)
IA	Only endometrium affected	91
IB	Endometrium, less than half of myometrium involved	90
IC	Endometrium, more than half of myometrium involved	81
IIA	Endocervical glands invaded	79
IIB	Cervical stroma invaded	71
IIIA	Serosa, adnexal (nearby) tissues invaded; possibly some cells in peritoneal fluid	60
IIIB	Vagina invaded	30
IIIC	Nearby lymph nodes invaded	52
IVA	Bladder and/or bowel invaded	15
IVB	Distant metastasis	17

Staging for uterine cancer is based on what is found as a result of surgery. Staging protocols are discussed in Sidebar 11.4.

Treatment

The mainstay of uterine cancer treatment is a hysterectomy, which is usually accompanied by the removal of the ovaries and uterine tubes as well. This may be followed by radiation and/or hormone therapy. Chemotherapy is used most often for uterine sarcomas rather than for endometrial cancer.

If a young woman is diagnosed with uterine cancer and wants to preserve her uterus for the possibility of childbearing, she may choose an intensive course of chemotherapy over surgery. This option carries a high risk of recurrence, however, so it must be followed by careful surveillance.

Massage?

Massage for a client with uterine cancer follows the same guidelines as massage for any kind of cancer. Accommodations must be made for cancer treatments, and any modality must stay within the limits of a client's activity levels.

MODALITY RECOMMENDATIONS FOR UTERINE CANCER

Modality	Recommendation
Deep tissue massage	Supportive as part of health care team. Respect stage of recovery and treatment challenges.
Lymphatic drainage	Supportive.
Polarity	S: Indicated. R/D: Locally contraindicated; otherwise supportive.
PNF/MET/stretching	Supportive as part of health care team; match to activity levels.
Reflexology	Indicated. Work lymphatic system, pituitary, uterus points.
Shiatsu	Supportive.
Swedish massage	Supportive as part of health care team; match to client activity level.
Trigger point therapy	Locally contraindicated; otherwise supportive for light work.

See Chapter 1 for a brief description of each modality, including definitions of abbreviations.

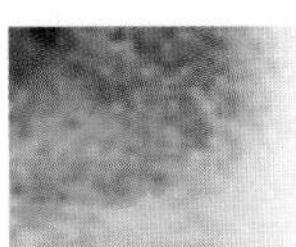

Disorders of Other Female Reproductive Structures

Breast Cancer

Definition: What Is It?

Breast cancer is the development of tumors in the epithelial or connective tissue of the breast. These growths may start out as nonmalignant, but may become invasive if neglected for a long period.

Breast Cancer in Brief

What is it?
Breast cancer is the growth of malignant tumor cells in breast tissue. These cells can invade skin and nearby muscles and bones. If they invade lymph nodes, they can metastasize to the rest of the body.

How is it recognized?
The first sign of breast cancer is a small painless lump or thickening in the breast tissue or near the axilla. The lump may be too small to palpate but may show on a mammogram. Later the skin may change texture, the nipple may change shape, and the nipple may produce a discharge.

Is massage indicated or contraindicated?
Breast cancer patients undergo treatments that are extremely taxing on general health as well as on physical and emotional well-being. If bodywork choices respect these challenges, massage can be a wonderful, supportive, important coping mechanism for many breast cancer patients.

Demographics: Who Gets It?

Breast cancer is the second most frequently diagnosed cancer in women (skin cancer is first). About 211,000 new cases of invasive breast cancer are diagnosed in women and about 1,700 cases in men each year in the United States. About 41,000 women and about 500 men die of this disease each year. Most women with breast cancer are mature; 77% of them are over 50 years old when diagnosed.[19]

Before 1980 the lifetime risk of contracting breast cancer was 1 in 11. Now it is 1 in 8. Some factors that may be driving that number up include women's increasing longevity (the chance of getting breast cancer increases significantly with age), and the fact that breast cancer is being found and diagnosed earlier than ever before.

Breast cancer diagnosis rates have recently shown a sudden drop. Since 2003 the number of women diagnosed with various types of breast cancer has declined by about 7%. While it is not yet fully clear why this has happened, most researchers suggest that the discovery that hormone replacement therapy can increase breast cancer risk led many women to stop using this drug regimen, and the drop in breast cancer diagnoses is a reflection of this shift.[20] For more information on the risks and benefits of hormone replacement therapy, see Sidebar 11.10.

Etiology: What Happens?

Breasts are constructed of 15 to 20 lobes where milk is produced in lactating women; ducts that deliver milk to the nipple; and the ***stroma***, or collagen, elastin, and fat cells that provide support and the bulk of breast tissue. The lobes and ducts are made of epithelial cells; the stroma is connective tissue and lipid cells. Although cancer may grow in any of these tissues, the lobes and ducts are by far the most likely to develop malignant cells.

- *Ductal carcinoma* is the most common type of breast cancer, accounting for 70% to 80% of diagnoses. It can occur ***in situ***, in which case cells affect only the epithelial lining of the ducts, or it can become invasive. Ductal carcinoma in situ (DCIS) is associated with the development of small calcified deposits in the breasts and a slightly increased risk for invasive breast cancer.
- *Lobular carcinoma* is less common than ductal carcinoma, accounting for 5% to 10% of tumors. It can be limited to the epithelial lining of the lobes (lobular carcinoma in situ, or LCIS), but this condition carries a significant risk of becoming invasive. Lobular carcinoma also has a higher incidence of appearing in both breasts than ductal carcinoma.

- *Other types of breast cancer* may develop, but collectively they account for only 10 to 15% of diagnoses. Inflammatory breast cancer is associated with edema, redness, and heat in the breast; this occurs because the tumors block lymphatic return. Inflammatory breast cancer usually has a poor prognosis. Paget disease of the breast affects specifically the nipple, and presents with specific eczema-like changes in the skin. Medullary breast cancer is a rare malignancy of the connective tissues in the breast.

Many types of breast cancer begin as in situ growths that eventually develop malignant characteristics. It can take a long time for a tumor to become large enough to notice; it is estimated that it takes several years for a growth to reach a diameter of 1 cm.

As tumors grow, the risk of some cells invading the circulatory or lymphatic system increases. The proximity of the axillary lymph nodes makes these a common site for the spread of malignant cells.

Breast cancer usually metastasizes to nearby lymph nodes in the axilla and thoracic cavity first; invasion of chest muscles, bones, and skin follows. Finally, distant metastatic sites include the liver, lung, and brain. If the cancer is not successfully treated, complications may include spinal cord pressure, bone fractures, pleural effusion, and bronchial obstruction.

Study of breast cancer tumors has revealed some distinguishing characteristics. Some breast cancer tumors are highly sensitive to estrogen and/or progesterone. Other tumors have proteins that promote cell division or are lacking in genes that inhibit cell division. All of these discoveries have created new avenues for carefully targeted treatment options, and an ever-improving prognosis.

Risk Factors

One of the most frustrating things about breast cancer is that no dependable profile of the women most likely to get it has ever been developed. Some cancers, such as lung, colon, and skin cancer, can be directly linked to diet or environmental factors; breast cancer cannot. Although some risk factors have been identified as increasing the chance that a woman may develop breast cancer, most women with these risk factors (outside of genetic predisposition) never develop the disease, and most breast cancer patients don't carry most of these risk factors (outside of age).

Age is the leading risk factor for breast cancer: most patients are diagnosed when they are over 50 years old. Prolonged estrogen exposure is another factor. Women who started having menstrual periods early in life; who had children after age 30 or not at all; who have late onset of menopause; who are obese, especially after menopause; or who use hormone replacement therapy are at greater risk than the general population. Women who have more than one alcoholic drink every day, who have a history of radiation treatments to the chest, or who have a history of lobular carcinoma in situ are more likely than the rest of the population to develop breast cancer.

Women with a family or personal history of breast cancer have a significantly increased risk of developing the disease. One reliable risk factor is the presence of two abnormal breast cancer genes, *BRCA 1* and *BRCA 2*. About 80% of women carrying these genes will develop breast cancer, but they account for only 5% to 10% of diagnosed patients. For the other 90% the only dependable risk factor is age.[21]

Signs and Symptoms

Early symptoms of breast cancer are subtle. Breast tissue is soft, so tumors have ample room to grow without causing pain. Sometimes self-examination can find hard spots or lumps before a mammogram can show them, and sometimes a mammogram reveals thickenings or minute calcifications that are too subtle to feel. Advanced cases of breast cancer show asymmetrical breast growth, inverted nipples that may have discharge, and sometimes a characteristic orange peel texture of the skin on the breast. Advanced cases may also cause symptoms in other parts of the body that are damaged by the growth of invasive tumors: bone pain, weight loss, spinal cord compression, and swelling in the arms may be the result of tumors far from the original site of the cancer. Specific protocols for breast cancer staging are discussed in Sidebar 11.5.

Diagnosis

Breast cancer is usually detected first by a woman who notices a change in her breast, and then confirmed by mammogram (Figure 11.5), ultrasound, and tissue biopsy. These procedures may rule out nonmalignant breast changes (Sidebar 11.6).

SIDEBAR 11.5: STAGING BREAST CANCER

Although the progression of cancer from stage to stage has been categorized for the sake of convenience, it is impossible to predict exactly how this disease will progress in each patient. Every person who develops breast cancer will undergo a unique disease process, unlike anybody else's.

At this writing the staging protocol for breast cancer uses the TNM classification for tumor, node, and metastasis to quantify the progression of the disease into stages 0 to IV.[22] This is a simplified version:

Tumor	Node	Metastasis
T0: no tumors found	N0: no nodes involved	M0: no metastasis
T-IS: cancer in situ; first layer of tissue involved	N1: 1–3 lymph nodes involved on affected side; not attached to each other or to other tissues	M1: distant metastasis
T1: $\geq$1 tumors, $<$2 cm in diameter	N2: 4–9 nodes on same side as tumor involved;nodes attached to each other or to surrounding tissues	
T2: $\geq$1 tumors 2–5 cm in diameter	N3: $\geq$10 axillary nodes involved, or nodes from other groups (e.g., infraclavicular, supraclavicular, internal mammary	
T3: $\geq$1 tumors $>$5 cm in diameter		
T4: Tumors invaded chest wall or skin		

Stage	TNM
Stage 0	T IS, N0, M0
Stage I	T 1, N0, M0
Stage IIA	T0-T2, N0-N1, M0
Stage IIB	T2-T3, N0-N1, M0
Stage IIIA	T0-T3, N1-2, M0
Stage IIIB	T4, Any, M0
Stage IIIC	Any, N3, M0
Stage IV	Any, Any, M1

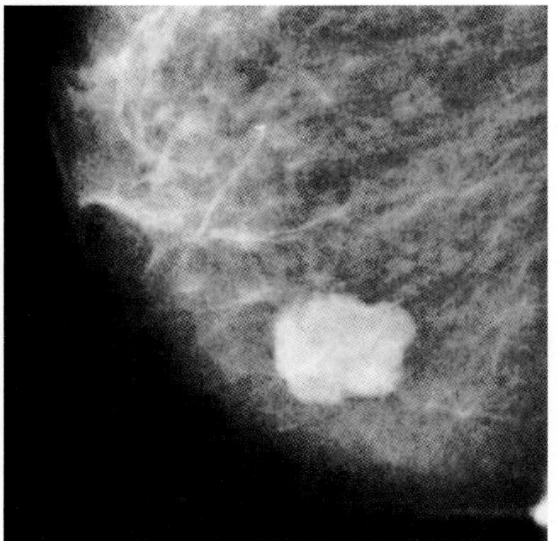

Figure 11.5. Mammogram of breast cancer (note the irregular shape and borders of the growth).

SIDEBAR 11.6: FIBROCYSTIC BREAST CHANGES

Not all breast growths are malignant. Most growths in breast tissue are cysts or benign tumors; many fall into the classification of what used to be called fibrocystic breast disease. It turns out these are so common (more than 50% of autopsied women show signs of fibrocystic breast growths) that this condition is no longer called a disease; it is now referred to as fibrocystic breast changes. Some of these growths carry a risk of eventually becoming malignant, but for the most part they are not serious conditions and can easily be distinguished from malignancies with testing procedures that include mammograms, fine-needle aspiration, ultrasound, or biopsy.

Gross cysts

In this situation *gross* means *large*, not ugly. Gross cysts are large enough to create a visible distortion of the breast. They grow most often in women in their 40s and can be reduced with fine-needle aspiration. They may recur, however, with the menstrual cycle.

Fibroadenomas

These are small cysts that may grow in clusters. They are most common in women in their 30s and 40s. Fibroadenomas are sensitive to estrogen; they tend to become enlarged and tender in the days that proceed a menstrual period, and then they subside until the following month.

Atypical Hyperplasia

Also called *proliferative breast disease*, atypical hyperplasia is characterized by changes in the epithelial lining of both ducts and lobes. When it grows in the ducts, it can be difficult to differentiate from ductal carcinoma in situ. Of all noncancerous breast changes, this one carries the highest risk of malignancy.

Fibrosis

Sometimes the connective tissue framework for breast tissue, called the stroma, becomes thick and dense with excessive connective tissue. These areas of fibrosis have a characteristic hard, rubbery texture. They are firm and painless.

Phyllodes Tumors

These are relatively rare growths of both epithelium and connective tissue. Most are benign, but phyllodes tumors carry a low risk of becoming cancerous.

Papillomas

These are tiny warts, each less than 1 cm in diameter, which may grow inside the ductal tissue.

Other Breast Pathologies

Breasts can also be affected by infection (called ***mastitis*** if a woman is lactating or ***ductal ectasia*** if she is not). Injury from trauma, surgery, or radiation may cause fat necrosis, a condition in which the fat cells that make up the bulk of breast tissue degenerate and die. Breast infections and ***fat necrosis*** can be serious, requiring medical intervention for the best outcomes.

If breast cancer is identified, it is staged. If lymph node involvement is suspected, a search for the "sentinel node" may be conducted. This means that a radioisotope is injected near the breast, and clinicians examine where the substance is taken up; most usually flows into a single lymph node before moving on to other nodes. This first stop is the sentinel node. If this lymph node is clear of cancer cells, the likelihood is that all of the lymph nodes are clear.

Prevention

Breast cancer is not a preventable disease. The two most dependable risk factors, age and genetics, are not controllable. Therefore, efforts for prevention are targeted at early detection, which significantly increases the life expectancy of the breast cancer patient. The three main courses for early detection are self-examination, breast examination by a professional, and mammograms, which use radiation to look for unusually dense masses in the breast tissue.

Recent studies have shown that breast self-examinations do not contribute to an improved diagnosis rate or prognosis, so their importance is being downplayed in women's health education.[21] Women are counseled, however, to become very familiar with the feel of their own breasts so that they can be alert to any changes.

Clinical breast examinations are recommended once every 3 years for women between 20 and 39 years old and annually for women 40 and older.

Opinions vary over how frequently mammograms should be performed. This stems from the fact that the breast tissue of many women is too dense to yield dependable results before age 40 or even later.

Women who have a personal or family history of breast cancer, who are positive for the breast cancer genes, or who are otherwise considered at high risk for this disease may be counseled to test earlier and more often than the general public.

A mammogram is not a definitive test for breast cancer. Mammogram interpretations vary widely, and mammograms may miss the subtle changes in breast tissue that only women who perform monthly self-examinations may notice. Therefore, an "all-clear" from a mammogram does not rule out breast cancer.

Treatment

Treatment for breast cancer depends entirely on the stage of the disease when it is found. Whatever treatment strategy is followed, every cancer patient should have access to support groups that will benefit her healing process.

Several options for treatment are often used in combination for best results.

- *Surgery.* Lumpectomies, partial mastectomies, total mastectomies, and modified mastectomies are surgical options for removing tumors and nearby lymph nodes. Lymph nodes are examined for signs of further metastasis.
- *Radiation therapy.* Radiation is aimed at tumors to slow or stop growth or to shrink tumors to make them easier to remove surgically. Radiation may be applied externally or internally, with radioactive pellets that are surgically placed around the tumors and removed later.
- *Chemotherapy.* Chemotherapy is treatment of cancer with highly toxic drugs that may slow or stop the growth of tumors. It may be used before surgery to reduce the size of a growth for a better chance of full removal, after surgery as a protective measure, or instead of surgery when tumors are determined to be inoperable.
- *Hormone therapy.* Some breast cancer tumors have been found to be sensitive to estrogen levels; they need access to this hormone to grow. Medications that bind up estrogen receptor sites or inhibit estrogen production (these include tamoxifen and aromatase inhibitors) are used to limit these growths.
- *Biological therapy.* A recent discovery that about 25% of breast cancer tumors are rich in proteins that promote cell division (called HER2) has led to the development of a biological therapy using a monoclonal antibody called trastuzumab (Herceptin). This substance is used to block the action of HER2 after surgery to reduce the risk of recurrence.[23]

Complications of Treatment

Cancer is a life-threatening disease that aggressively invades the body. Options to deal with cancer are similarly aggressive and often produce serious side effects. Though not as deadly as the disease itself, they can be temporarily debilitating.

Surgery to remove part of the breast tissue and lymph nodes can injure brachial plexus nerves, resulting in chronic pain in the shoulder and arm. If enough lymph nodes are removed, ***lymphedema***, the accumulation of protein-rich interstitial fluid in the arm, can be a serious problem. A variety of pumps and drainage devices have been developed to prevent or treat lymphedema, but all have limited success. Lymph drainage techniques can deal with this problem, but this is a very different approach from that of Swedish massage and it is not appropriate to practice it without rigorous training. Fortunately, as diagnosticians are refining their skills, generally fewer lymph nodes are taken for analysis than in the past; this means that the incidence of lymphedema as a complication of breast cancer is on the decline.

Radiation therapy can cause skin problems from drying and itchiness to burns and local ulcerations.

Chemotherapy drugs can kill cancer cells, but they also cause hair loss, nausea, mouth sores, and immunosuppression. Extremely high doses of chemotherapy can be successful at treating advanced cases of cancer but must be followed by bone marrow transplants to replace damaged tissue there as well.

Tamoxifen and other hormone-like drugs are effective at keeping hormone-sensitive tumors under control, but they are associated with several side effects, including symptoms resembling menopause, an increased chance of uterine cancer, and for some women a tendency to form blood clots leading to deep vein thrombosis, pulmonary embolism, or stroke.

For more information on cancer and cancer complications, see Chapter 12.

CASE HISTORY 11.1

Breast Cancer

Carol E., 60 years old: "When you have had breast cancer, the thought of possible recurrence is always with you. It makes you look at what is really important in life."

It was in July, right before my 57th birthday, when I found a lump in my left breast while doing a breast examination in the shower. We were just getting ready to leave on a vacation with friends, so I didn't say anything. My annual mammogram was already scheduled in about 3 weeks.

When I went in for my mammogram, I told the doctor about the lump. He said he couldn't feel it, and the mammogram was normal. A subsequent ultrasound did not reveal anything, and the technician also could not feel what I felt. So, even though I knew better, this gave me a sense of security that all was well.

Until January. I could still feel the lump and by now my husband could also, so I was not imagining it. I talked with our daughter, a registered nurse who worked in risk management. She said, "You could have a normal mammogram and ultrasound and still have breast cancer. You have to go by what you know is normal for you." So I made an appointment with a surgeon for the week I returned from a previously planned trip to Florida.

I returned on Valentine's Day, and my appointment was on February 16th. The surgeon not only felt what I had felt (which was a thickening, more than a lump), but in checking my previous mammogram, he found pinpoints of calcium in the right breast, which are sometimes indicators of cancer. Three days later I had bilateral biopsies.

During the biopsies, a frozen section was done on the thickening on the left side, which meant the pathologist could tell right away whether the tissue was malignant. (The tissue from the right breast biopsy went through routine pathology, and I had to wait for several days for those results.) So there I was, in the recovery room, when the doctor came in and told me that the left breast biopsy revealed a malignancy. Then he left to talk to my husband, and I was by myself. The greatest feeling I had was just incredible sadness. I don't know why I wasn't angry or anything else; I was just so sad. After a few minutes I was able to join my husband and we both cried.

When something like this happens to you, you begin by wondering, how bad is it? Are you going to die soon? Then you go home and do the waiting game again—for the results of the other biopsy—and this was absolutely incredibly stressful. You are already facing surgery on one breast, and now you are wondering if you will lose both breasts. After 3 days, the call came saying the second biopsy showed no malignancy. By that time I was thankful that only one breast had a malignancy. Strange thing for which to be thankful.

My diagnosis was a stage I infiltrated ductal carcinoma, upper medial quadrant, left breast. After I got a second opinion, surgery was scheduled for the following Monday. Before that, I had to have chest x-rays, a bone scan, and a radiation oncology consult, as I had opted to have conservative surgery (a lumpectomy followed by 6 weeks of radiation).

The surgeon performed a lumpectomy and also did an axillary dissection—removal of some lymph nodes in the armpit. It is during this surgery that a nerve in my armpit was either severed or damaged. This produces numbness in the underarm and inner upper arm that can be permanent. The lymph nodes removed (16 in my case) were tested for malignancy, and later I learned that they showed no cancer. Chances were that the cancer had been confined to the breast tissue. Good news indeed!

However, the next Thursday, the surgeon called and said that the margins of the tissue removed were not clean—meaning that there were still some cancer cells in the breast. So back to surgery the next Monday for another resection of the breast. My surgeon did not usually do this, but he felt that there was very little cancer left, and a mastectomy could still be avoided.

continued

Breast Cancer *continued*

After a few days of recuperation, the telephone rang and it was my surgeon again, saying (in a very upset and sad tone) that the margins on the last tissue sample still were not clean. He had spoken with the radiation oncologist and she thought she could kill the remaining cancer cells with radiation. However, the surgeon thought he could give me even better odds by performing a total mastectomy. Of course, I opted for the better odds against recurrence, and the following Monday again found me in surgery having a total mastectomy. Three major surgeries in 3 weeks with general anesthetic each time are a lot to cope with, but you do what you have to do.

Because I had a mastectomy, I did not have to have any radiation, and because my lymph nodes were negative for cancer cells, I also did not have to have chemotherapy. A big relief!

I do take tamoxifen, an anti–breast cancer drug used in certain circumstances to guard against recurrence. The standard commitment to this is 5 years. I also take amitriptyline, a mild antidepressant, to help break the cycle of chronic nerve pain that I have had in my left arm—an unusual and difficult complication. About 8 months ago I also started on Neurontin [gabapentin], an antiseizure drug that can also work on nerve pain, and in my case it has really helped. So after almost 2 years, the pain in my arm is under control. I have no lymphedema (swelling of the arm due to a compromised lymph system). However, this could happen at any time.

I do not feel that the doctors emphasize enough how vulnerable the affected arm is. Infections can develop very easily, and I have to be really careful, especially working in the garden. It seems that little burns and scratches take forever to heal. I should not lift more than 10 lb with the affected arm and should not have any needle sticks or have blood pressure taken on that arm. Once I awoke after minor surgery to find a blood pressure cuff on my left arm, and was I upset! I thought that I had taken enough precautions that this should not have happened. The prescription for medication post surgery had been clipped over the warning note! The next time I had an anesthetic, I wrote on my left arm with a surgical pen, and that did not come off!

When you have had breast cancer, the thought of recurrence is always with you. Breast cancer does not follow the 5-year rule; it can come back at any time. It is a lifelong commitment always to be on the watch and take really good care of yourself. This makes you look at what is really important in life. You try not to put off things that you want to say or do. Life is precious and I am glad to still have it!

Author's note: As a part of her recovery, Carol became active in several breast cancer support groups. One of the groups of Bosom Buddies that she helped to facilitate still meets every month to have fun and draw support from each other. Through Reach to Recovery, Carol does hospital and home visits to new breast cancer patients, teaching them about their options, telling them what they might expect, and giving them guidance in getting more information. She would like to see women become their own advocates as they deal with the complexities of this disease.

Massage?

For many years it was assumed that because Swedish massage increases circulation and lymph flow, it could contribute to cancer metastasis. Although research conducted specifically to explore this idea would be unethical, a closer look reveals some basic problems with this assumption. First, it takes years for tumors to reach palpable size; any tumor that is found after a massage has been in the making for a long time. Second, exactly how much massage increases blood and lymph movement and for how long are variables that have never been fully quantified. Does doing a 60-minute full-body Swedish massage move as much lymph or blood as taking a long, hot shower? How does it compare with a vigorous half-hour walk? Conversely, if massage promotes better sleep, improved appetite, and more efficient immune system function, do the benefits outweigh the risks?

Obviously, a massage therapist must locally avoid tumor sites, especially if they are close to the surface of the skin, but most of the other cautions that surround massage and breast cancer have to do with respecting the challenges brought about by the treatments these clients must deal with more than with the disease itself. Massage therapists can gauge their choices to provide the maximum benefit for cancer patients (anxiety and pain reduction, immune system strengthening, better appetite and sleep quality, along with general support and informed nurturing touch) while minimizing the risks of overchallenging a client who is already struggling to keep up with the demands of surgery, chemotherapy, radiation therapy, or all three.

If a decision is made to include massage as part of a treatment program for a cancer patient, certain cautions must be observed. Radiation and tumor sites are local contraindications. Chemotherapy compromises immune system reactions, making the client vulnerable to a variety of infections that may contraindicate massage. Changes in the health of the tissues may make clients susceptible to blood clots, bruising, or other damage that healthy people would not sustain. Because the severity of cancer treatment, symptoms vary widely, it is impossible to predict what is appropriate for all clients. Rather, the therapist should work as part of a well-informed health care team to provide the best care and support possible.

Modality Recommendations for Breast Cancer	
Deep tissue massage	Supportive as part of health care team. Respect stage of recovery and treatment challenges.
Lymphatic drainage	Indicated to deal with consequences of treatments.
Polarity	S: Indicated. R/D: Locally contraindicated; otherwise supportive with pressure to client's comfort.
PNF/MET/stretching	Supportive as part of health care team; match to activity levels.
Reflexology	Indicated. Work lymphatic system, pituitary, breast, chest, solar plexus points.
Shiatsu	Indicated after surgery to reduce side effects of treatment, support lymphatic system. Treat SP, TH, K, PC, L, GB, BL meridians and extensions.
Swedish massage	Supportive as part of health care team; match to client activity level.
Trigger point therapy	Locally contraindicated; otherwise supportive for light work.

See Chapter 1 for a brief description of each modality, including definitions of abbreviations.

Ovarian Cancer

Definition: What Is It?

Ovarian cancer is the growth of malignant tumors on the ovaries. Several varieties of ovarian cancer have been identified, but most of them begin in the epithelial cells of these organs. The tumors may take a long time to become established, but once they do, some types may grow quickly and metastasize readily to the peritoneum and other organs in the abdomen.

Demographics: Who Gets It?

Ovarian cancer can affect any woman of any age, but it is most common in women who are 60 years or older. The median age at diagnosis is 63.[24] Ovarian cancer is diagnosed in about 20,100 women each year. The incidence of ovarian cancer is slowly beginning to fall, but about 1 in 67 women in the United States will probably have this disease. Although the numbers of women with this disease is low compared to those of other cancers, its mortality rate is high: ovarian cancer kills about 15,000 women every year and is the fifth leading cause of death by cancer in women.[25]

The survivability of ovarian cancer is relatively low but improving. The overall 5-year survival rate is 44.7%. About 172,000 women with a history of ovarian cancer are alive in the United States today.[24]

> **Ovarian Cancer in Brief**
> Pronunciation: o-VARE-e-an KAN-ser
>
> **What is it?**
> Ovarian cancer is the development of malignant tumors on the ovaries that may metastasize to other structures in the pelvic or abdominal cavity.
>
> **How is it recognized?**
> Symptoms of ovarian cancer are generally extremely subtle until the disease has progressed to life-threatening levels. Early symptoms include a feeling of heaviness in the pelvis, vague abdominal discomfort, occasional vaginal bleeding, and weight gain or loss.
>
> **Is massage indicated or contraindicated?**
> As with all cancers, the appropriateness of massage depends on what treatment measures the client chooses. Massage therapists working with clients who have ovarian cancer should be part of a fully informed health care team.

Etiology: What Happens?

Three specific types of tumors have been found to grow on ovaries: tumors of germ cells, tumors of stromal cells, and tumors of epithelial cells. As with most types of cancers, epithelial tumors are the most common and often the most invasive. Epithelial tumors, or adenocarcinomas, comprise about 90% of ovarian cancers.

Epithelial tumors of the ovaries fall into several categories, each with different growth patterns and prognoses. Some of these tumors are slow growing and never become malignant. Early identification and removal of these growths may leave the reproductive system intact if the woman wishes to have more children. But many types of epithelial ovarian tumors aggressively invade not only the ovaries but other pelvic and abdominal organs as well. These tumors are life threatening, partly because they are so prone to metastasis, but also because they cause few (if any) noticeable symptoms in their early stages. Usually by the time a woman is concerned enough to consult a doctor, ovarian cancer has progressed to an advanced stage that is difficult or impossible to treat. Most diagnoses are made at stage III or IV.[26]

Ovarian cancer metastasizes through direct extension of tumors, or through the lymph or circulatory system. The most common route for the spread of ovarian cancer, however, is dissemination in peritoneal fluid. Cancer cells from a malignant tumor may land on other areas in the pelvis, directly on the peritoneum, or higher in the abdomen to colonize and invade other tissues. This is especially common in areas where peritoneal fluid tends not to move freely.

Risk Factors

Although the specific triggers for the growth of tumors on the ovaries are unknown, some of the most important risk factors for developing the disease have been identified:

- *Familial history.* A significant risk factor for ovarian cancer is having it in the family. Women who have a first-degree relative (mother, sister, or daughter) with ovarian cancer have a roughly 1 in 3 chance of developing the cancer themselves. Having a second-degree relative (grandmother, aunt, half-sister) with ovarian cancer also increases the chance of developing the disease. Families with a history of breast or colorectal cancer also have statistically higher rates of ovarian cancer than the general population. This is true especially if identified breast or colorectal cancer genes are present.
- *Reproductive history.* A woman who has never had a child or taken birth control pills, or who has had multiple miscarriages is at increased risk for developing ovarian cancer. This association points to the theory that ovarian cancer may be related to ovulation trauma: the ovaries must heal every time an egg is released, and this wear and tear may trigger genetic mutations in ovary cells. Women who never have a break in their menstrual cycle are at significantly increased risk for this disease. In addition, women who have taken fertility drugs without conceiving and bearing a child may also be at increased risk, although the statistics for these women have been inconsistent.
- *Hormone replacement therapy.* Women who have employed hormone replacement therapy have a higher chance of developing ovarian cancer than others. This is most likely when a woman who had a hysterectomy used estrogen alone for more than 10 years.[27]

- *Other.* Other risks include exposure to radiation or asbestos, the use of talcum powder on the genitals, a high-fat diet, and age; the chance of developing ovarian cancer goes up considerably between age 40 and 60.

Signs and Symptoms

The feature that makes ovarian cancer such a dangerous disease is that early symptoms are practically nonexistent or so subtle that they are easily passed over. When the cancer is finally identified, often it has already metastasized.

Symptoms of ovarian cancer include a feeling of heaviness in the pelvis; vague abdominal discomfort, including bloating, nausea, diarrhea, and constipation; urinary frequency or urgency; vaginal bleeding; a change in menstrual cycles; and weight gain or loss. Because the most common age for women to be affected by ovarian cancer is also the time when symptoms of perimenopause develop, these signals are easily ignored. Later symptoms can include a palpable abdominal mass, increased girth around the abdomen, and ascites—the accumulation of fluid in the peritoneum.

Diagnosis

Ovarian cancer is difficult to diagnose early. A pelvic examination may reveal unusual abdominal masses, but only a fourth of these turn out to be cancerous. Other tests that may be conducted include ultrasound tests conducted through the vagina, CT, and MRI. Barium enema and ***pyelography*** (a process that stains urine in the kidneys to see how it moves down the ureters into the bladder) may be conducted to look for structures pressing on other abdominal organs. A blood test called CA-125 looks for a particular tumor marker in the bloodstream. This has been useful in confirming a diagnosis, but it often yields false-positive or false-negative results, so it is not definitive. Ultimately, a ***laparotomy*** must be conducted to take a tissue sample from the ovaries for analysis.

For information on ovarian cancer staging protocols, see Sidebar 11.7.

SIDEBAR 11.7: STAGING OVARIAN CANCER

The *Fédération Internationale de Gynécologie et d' Obstétrique* has developed the most commonly used staging system for ovarian cancer. The tumors are described as being superficial or deep, and the capsule around the tumor is either intact or ruptured. A simplified version of the FIGO system follows:[26]

Stage	5-Year Survival Rate (%)	% of Patients at Diagnosis	Subdivisions of Stages
I: growth limited to ovaries	73	20	IA: one ovary affected; tumor deep; capsule intact; no ascites IB: two ovaries affected; tumors deep; capsules intact IC: tumor(s) superficial; capsule(s) ruptured; cancer cells in peritoneal fluid
II: one or both ovaries involved; extensions into pelvis	45	5	IIA: metastases to uterus and/or uterine tubes IIB: metastases to other pelvic organs IIC: metastases to uterus, tubes, other pelvic organs
III: One or both ovaries involved; cells in peritoneal fluid; possibly metastases in abdomen	21	58	IIIA: metastases limited to pelvis; no lymph nodes involved IIIB: tumors <2 cm outside pelvis; no lymph nodes involved IIIC: tumors >2 cm outside pelvis; lymph nodes may be involved
IV: Distant metastases	17	<5	Metastases in liver or lungs

Treatment

Ovarian cancer is generally treated with surgery and chemotherapy. Surgery removes the ovaries (***oophorectomy***) and often the uterine tubes and uterus as well. Surgical "debulking" is removal of as much cancerous tissue as possible. This may involve removing parts of the large or small intestines or other structures. Chemotherapy can be administered orally at home or intravenously in a hospital. One method delivers the cytotoxic drugs directly into the peritoneum, where it can have immediate access to malignant tumors.

Radiation therapy is not usually used for ovarian cancer.

Massage?

As with any kind of cancer, the appropriateness of massage for ovarian cancer is a matter of personal choice. A client who is recovering from ovarian cancer may find that massage can ameliorate the challenges of surgery and chemotherapy. If a client wishes to include massage in her treatment program, she and her massage therapist should consult with her oncologist and other health care team members for the best and safest results.

Modality Recommendations for Ovarian Cancer

Deep tissue massage	Supportive as part of a health care team. Respect stage of recovery and treatment challenges.
Lymphatic drainage	Supportive.
Polarity	S: Indicated. R/D: Locally contraindicated; otherwise supportive with pressure to client's comfort.
PNF/MET/stretching	Supportive as part of health care team; match to activity levels.
Reflexology	Indicated. Work lymphatic system, pituitary, ovaries points.
Shiatsu	Indicated after surgery to reduce the side effects of treatment. Treat SP, TH, K, GB, BL meridians and extensions.
Swedish massage	Supportive as part of health care team; match to client activity level.
Trigger point therapy	Locally contraindicated; otherwise supportive for light work.

See Chapter 1 for a brief description of each modality, including definitions of abbreviations.

Ovarian Cysts

Definition: What Are They?

A variety of cysts may grow on the ovaries. They may be related to endometriosis, or they may be types of precancerous growths that may develop into ovarian cancer. The cysts under discussion in this article, however, are functional cysts; that is, they arise from normal ovaries, usually as a result of hormonal imbalance or dysfunction.

Demographics: Who Gets Them?

Ovarian cysts have been found in females of all ages, from prenatal babies to elderly women. Most functional cysts are found in women between the onset of menstruation (***menarche***) and the onset of menopause. In other words, women who ovulate are most likely to have functional ovarian cysts.

Mittelschmerz

This term is derived from German for middle pain. It refers to the sensation some women have when the dominant follicle on an ovary ruptures and the egg is released into the pelvic cavity. It is called "middle" because it occurs precisely in the middle (about day 14) of the menstrual cycle.

> **Ovarian Cysts in Brief**
> Pronunciation: o-VARE-e-an SISTS
>
> **What are they?**
> Most ovarian cysts are fluid-filled growths on the ovaries. Some types of cysts are associated with ovarian cancer or other reproductive disorders, but the cysts under discussion in this article are benign.
>
> **How are they recognized?**
> Ovarian cysts may have no signs or symptoms, or they may cause a disruption in the menstrual cycle. Constant or intermittent pain in the pelvis, pain with intercourse, or symptoms similar to early pregnancy may arise from different types of ovarian cysts.
>
> **Is massage indicated or contraindicated?**
> Diagnosed ovarian cysts locally contraindicate massage.

When ovarian cysts are found in premenarchal girls or postmenopausal women, the chances of malignancy are much higher than among other patients. Abnormal growths in these populations are treated much more aggressively than in women of childbearing age.

Etiology: What Happens?

Each month a fertile woman develops several follicles (pockets where eggs are held) on one of her ovaries. As her cycle progresses, a single follicle becomes dominant and the others recede. At the appropriate hormonal signal, the follicle ruptures, releasing a mature egg, or ***oocyte***, into the pelvic cavity. From there the egg is drawn into the uterine tubes for the journey toward the uterus.

Every follicle that develops is a potential cyst. Sometimes the hormonal signal (a surge in luteinizing hormone) doesn't occur, and the follicle doesn't rupture completely. Consequently, a blister forms on the ovary. Sometimes the ruptured follicle (now called the ***corpus luteum***) seals up behind the discharged ovum, trapping the hormones that should flow freely from it. This kind of blister may eventually break and bleed into the pelvic cavity. Some other cysts arise in conjunction with abnormal pregnancies or as a result of hormonal imbalances that may begin in the pituitary gland.

Most ovarian cysts are not dangerous, but they have the potential to become large and painful, and they may develop dangerous complications.

Types of cysts Several types of cysts can form on the ovaries. Three of the most common kinds are discussed here:

- *Follicular cysts.* When a follicle that holds a mature egg doesn't rupture completely, a blister forms at the site. Follicular cysts rarely get bigger than 2 to 3 inches across, and they usually spontaneously recede within two menstrual cycles (Figure 11.6). Follicular cysts are the most common ovarian cysts.
- *Corpus luteum cysts.* Blisters can form over the corpus luteum, which blocks the hormones that should be secreted from the ovaries. Corpus luteum cysts delay subsequent ovulations and produce symptoms mimicking pregnancy (nausea, vomiting, breast tenderness) until they spontaneously resolve, usually within a month or two. Corpus luteum cysts are less common than follicular cysts, but they can be more serious, as they may cause bleeding into the peritoneal space.
- *Polycystic ovaries.* Also called ***Stein-Leventhal syndrome***, this condition is characterized by enlarged ovaries with multiple small cysts (Figure 11.7). The changes in hormone secretion that this condition produces may lead to loss of menstrual cycle, acne, and ***hirsutism*** (thickened body hair, especially on the face and legs). Polycystic ovary syndrome is also closely linked to poor use of insulin, high triglycerides, low high-density lipoproteins, and other signs associated with metabolic syndrome and an increased risk of diabetes and heart disease.

Other types of ovarian cysts include ***endometriomas*** (a result of endometriosis); ***cystadenomas***, which are usually benign tumors that can become cancerous; and ***dermoid cysts***, or ***teratomas***. In teratomas some primitive cells have been isolated from the rest of the body, and these develop into various types of tissues. Dermoid cysts may contain teeth, hairs, bone fragments, and other types of tissue. They are usually harmless in women. Men can develop them too, but for males teratomas are a much more serious condition that may lead to testicular cancer.

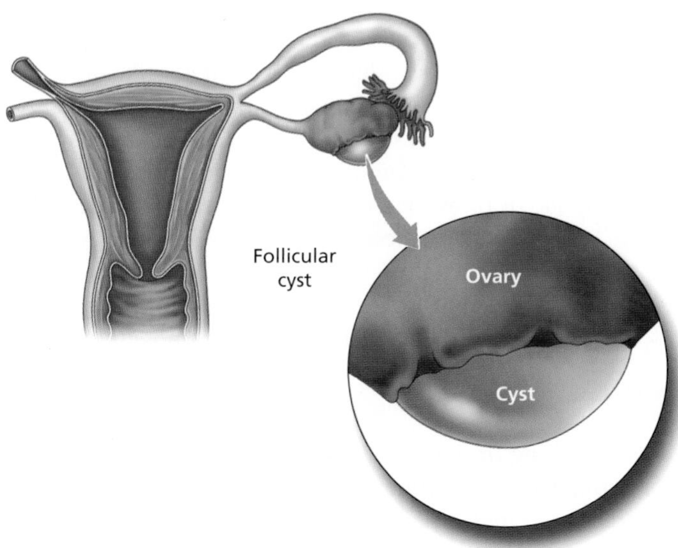

Figure 11.6. Ovarian cyst.

Signs and Symptoms

Most ovarian cysts have no symptoms until the cyst is injured in some way. Some women, however, have a dull ache in the lower abdomen on the affected side. A firm, painless swelling may develop in the pelvis, and occasionally an ovarian cyst causes pain with intercourse. Large cysts may cause low back pain, or, through pressure on the lumbar plexus, pain in the legs. Corpus luteum cysts and polycystic ovaries have symptoms of their own, which have been described. In the absence of these signs, a person might never know a cyst is there unless it grows big enough to interfere with other functions, or if it twists or ruptures.

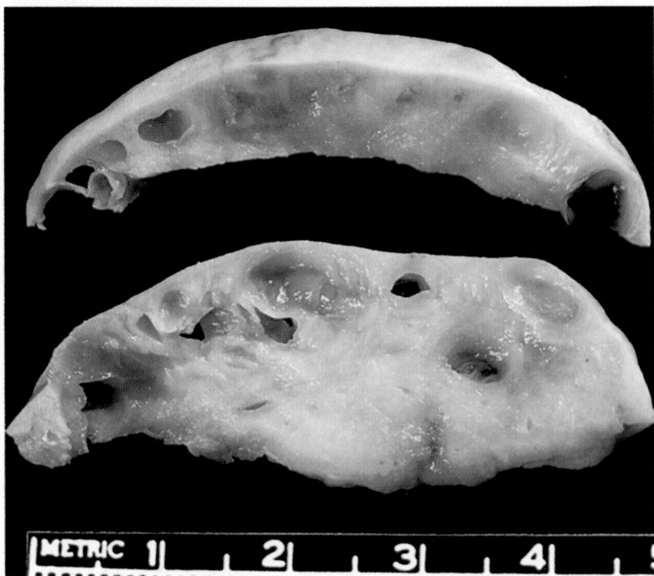

Figure 11.7. Polycystic ovary.

Complications

Size is the major factor that determines whether or not ovarian cysts cause any trouble. They can grow big enough to interfere with blood flow; they may also rest on the bladder. In rare cases they grow to incredible dimensions. An ovarian cyst that hangs from a stalk sometimes gets twisted; this is called ***torsion***. If that happens, acute abdominal pain, nausea, and fever develop; medical intervention is necessary, as the tissue may become necrotic. Similar symptoms are present if the cyst ruptures. The risk of peritonitis is high in this situation.

Perhaps the most serious complicating factor of ovarian cysts is that their early symptoms, subtle as they may be, mimic an *advanced* case of ovarian cancer. This is a threatening cancer that has few early symptoms. By the time a person can feel a firm, painless swelling in her pelvis, the disease is dangerously advanced. Therefore, if a client displays any of these symptoms but has not been examined, it is important for her to get more information as soon as possible.

Diagnosis

Ovarian cysts are frequently found as a swelling or mass during a routine pelvic examination. Ultrasound pictures generally confirm the diagnosis, although they may not delineate exactly what structures are involved. If the patient is at high risk for cancer or if the cyst looks to have a solid rather than liquid core, a laparoscopy may be performed to take a tissue sample for analysis. It is important to follow up on cystlike symptoms that last for more than 60 days, since follicular and corpus luteum cysts, the two most common and benign varieties, will usually have resolved within this period.

Treatment

Follicular and corpus luteum cysts are often treated with oral contraceptives. Birth control pills alter hormonal secretions and allow the cysts to recede completely or to shrink to a size that is easily removed. Ovarian cysts that don't spontaneously resolve may be aspirated, but more often surgery is performed to remove them. The affected ovary is usually taken too. In some cases, complete removal of the ovaries and uterus will be recommended because some types of cysts tend to recur and can develop into cancer.

Massage?

Ovarian cysts locally contraindicate massage. Ovarian cysts can also displace the pelvic contents, so deep abdominal work done where it would be safe on a woman without cysts may lead to bruising of the ovaries or even rupture of the cyst on someone who has this condition. Massage elsewhere on the body is appropriate.

Modality Recommendations for Ovarian Cysts

Modality	Recommendation
Deep tissue massage	Locally contraindicated; otherwise supportive.
Lymphatic drainage	Supportive.
Polarity	S: Indicated. R/D: Locally contraindicated; otherwise supportive.
PNF/MET/stretching	Locally contraindicated; otherwise supportive.
Reflexology	Indicated. Work lymphatic system, pituitary, thymus, ovaries points.
Shiatsu	Indicated. Treat K, BL, GB, LV, SP, PC meridians and extensions.
Swedish massage	Locally contraindicated; otherwise supportive.
Trigger point therapy	Locally contraindicated; otherwise supportive for light work.

See Chapter 1 for a brief description of each modality, including definitions of abbreviations.

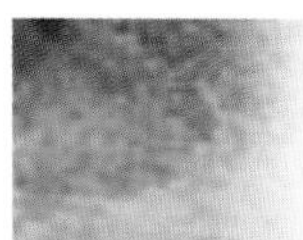

Disorders of the Male Reproductive System

Benign Prostatic Hyperplasia

Definition: What Is It?

Benign prostatic hyperplasia (BPH) is a condition in which the prostate gland of mature men becomes enlarged. This growth late in life is not related to prostate cancer, hence the name "benign".

Demographics: Who Gets It?

The single greatest risk factors for developing BPH are simply being a male and being mature. Although not all men with BPH experience symptoms, its incidence is remarkably high. Nearly 50% of men over 60 years old have some level of BPH; 70% of men over 70 have it; 80% of men over 80 have it, and so on.[28] Approximately 14 million men in the United States have been diagnosed with this condition.[29] Most men who have BPH don't have significant symptoms; Some resources suggest that while BPH leads to 4.5 million doctor visits per year,[30] only about 10% of men with it need treatment.[31]

Etiology: What Happens?

The prostate gland of a preadolescent male is very small. As a boy enters puberty, this pea-sized gland that wraps around the urethra just below the bladder grows approximately to the size of a walnut. It stays that size until a man is 25 to 40 years old, and then some prostates begin to grow again.

It is unclear why some prostate glands grow and others do not. Theories about triggers for late prostate growth involve hormonal changes with maturity. One possible factor may be the formation of ***dihydrotestosterone*** (DHT). This hormone is a form of testosterone that has been seen to increase prostate size. Another theory is that as men age, they produce less testosterone to balance out their normal levels of estrogen; this may lead to hyperplasia, as estrogen is also associated with prostate growth.

Regardless of the cause of prostate growth, BPH may lead to mechanical pressure on the urethra (Figure 11.8). This occurs for two reasons: the prostate is surrounded by a tough fascial capsule that does not allow it to expand outward, and the tissue usually affected by BPH is in the periurethral and transitional sections of the gland. (This helps to distinguish BPH from prostate cancer, which typically begins on the outer borders of the prostate.)

The extent of growth does not always correspond with the amount of pressure on the urethra; some men have advanced BPH with no urinary symptoms at all, while others have minimal amounts of prostate growth and severe urethral constriction.

Mechanical pressure on the urethra makes it difficult to expel urine from the body. Long-term consequences can include pathological changes in the bladder, which can become stiff, inelastic, and irritable. The risk of UTIs, pyelonephritis, and bladder stones is much higher in men who cannot urinate easily; these are common complications of BPH.

Signs and Symptoms

Signs and symptoms of BPH, when any develop at all, involve difficulties with urination. Weak flow, interrupted flow, frequency, and a feeling that the bladder is never completely emptied are often re-

> **Benign Prostatic Hyperplasia in Brief**
> Pronunciation: be-NINE pros-TAT-ik hi-per-PLA-zhah
>
> **What is it?**
> Benign prostatic hyperplasia (BPH) is a condition in which the prostate gland of a mature man begins to grow for the first time since the end of puberty. It is not related to cancer, which is why this condition is called "benign".
>
> **How is it recognized?**
> The primary symptoms of BPH have to do with mechanical obstruction of the urethra. This leads to problems with urination, including a feeling of frequency, difficulties with initiating flow, leaking, and the sensation that the bladder is never emptied. Many men with BPH never develop these symptoms, however. For them, BPH is a silent condition.
>
> **Is massage indicated or contraindicated?**
> BPH is a common condition among mature men, and it does not usually involve cancer or infection. Massage is perfectly appropriate for these clients, as long as no signs of urinary tract infection or kidney disorder are present.

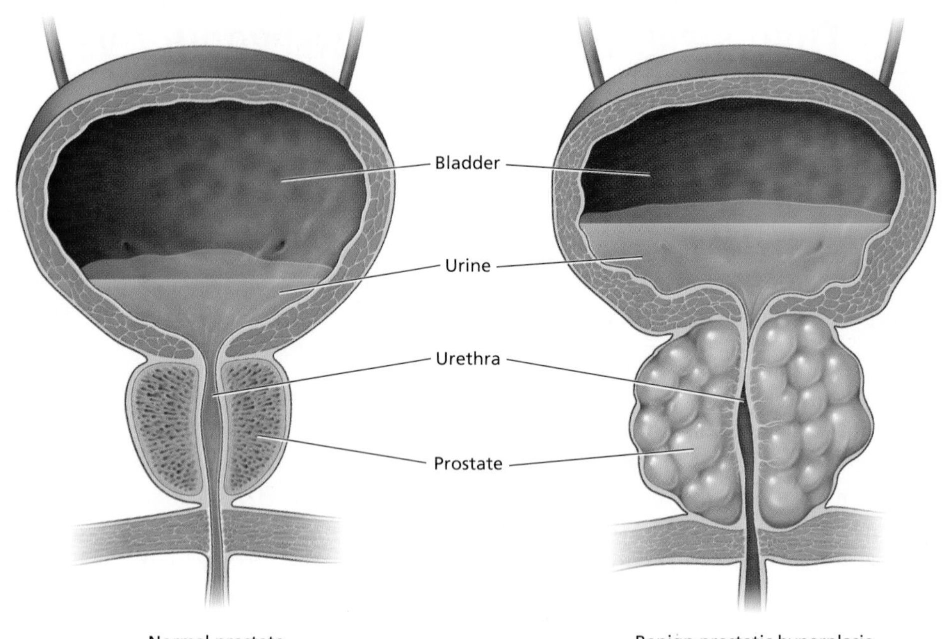

Figure 11.8. Benign prostatic hyperplasia.

ported. Leaking or dribbling urine between visits to the bathroom is common. Some men find it difficult to initiate urination, and they must strain or push to start their flow. Other men find that they need to urinate more frequently, especially at night. BPH does not typically cause pelvic pain, which distinguishes it from prostatitis.

One rare but serious sign of BPH is an abrupt obstruction of the urethra, called *acute urinary retention*. In this situation the urethra is suddenly completely obstructed and urine has no way to get out of the body. This is a medical emergency and must be treated in a hospital.

Diagnosis

BPH is diagnosed in a number of ways to identify exactly where and how seriously the urethra is obstructed. Palpation through the wall of the rectum yields information about the size and quality of the growths; BPH usually feels like overall enlargement or smooth, deep nodules, while prostate cancer involves harder, more superficial growths. Tests may measure the speed and completeness of urination, pressure in the bladder, or how much urine is left in the bladder after urination.

Because the symptoms of BPH are so similar to those of prostate cancer, part of any screening for BPH includes a ***prostate-specific antigen*** (PSA) blood test.

Treatment

BPH is treated according to severity. If it does not seriously affect a man's ability to urinate, it may be left untreated but closely monitored for signs of further growth. A number of options have been developed to limit prostate growth, including medications and a variety of surgeries.

Medications for BPH include drugs designed to lower levels of dihydrotestosterone, the testosterone derivative believed to stimulate prostate growth, and alpha-blockers. These are a group of medications originally developed to treat high blood pressure that help the prostate and bladder to relax. The side effects of these medications can be significant, however, including inability to achieve erection, lowered sex drive, lowered sperm counts, and others.

Surgical options for BPH include a variety of techniques that cut away, vaporize, burn, microwave, or otherwise remove small sections of the prostate gland to relieve pressure on the urethra. This field is rapidly expanding, since the American population is aging and many men may eventually need surgical intervention to help with BPH.

Tissue removed with prostate surgery is routinely examined for signs of cancer. About 10% of men who undergo surgery for BPH have developed early signs of prostate cancer, but they are usually slow-growing, nonaggressive types of cells that do not need immediate treatment.[30]

Massage?

Massage can have little (if any) impact on prostate growth, and the prostate itself is in an area that bodyworkers don't reach. Although massage won't improve this situation, it can certainly improve the quality of life of the patient; therefore, BPH indicates massage systemically, if not locally. If a client reports any symptoms of a urinary tract or kidney infection, however, it is important that he get appropriate care as soon as possible.

Modality Recommendations for Benign Prostatic Hyperplasia	
Deep tissue massage	Supportive within client's comfort. Work adductors, hip rotators and flexors, hamstrings, gluteals, and psoas/abdominal muscles.
Lymphatic drainage	Supportive.
Polarity	S/R/D: Indicated.
PNF/MET/stretching	Supportive.
Reflexology	Indicated. Work testes, pelvic area, prostate, ureters, bladder, hips, low back points.
Shiatsu	Indicated. Treat LV, K meridians, especially in upper thigh, and back K areas of Zen shiatsu system.
Swedish massage	Supportive.
Trigger point therapy	Supportive.

Prostate Cancer

Definition: What Is It?

Prostate cancer is the growth of malignant tumor cells in the prostate gland. This cancer often grows slowly, but some versions of it can be aggressive. Prostate cancer can metastasize to other parts of the body, most often the bladder, rectum, and bones of the pelvis.

Demographics: Who Gets It?

Each year about 234,000 cases of prostate cancer are diagnosed in this country, and about 27,000 men die of the disease. The lifetime risk of developing prostate cancer for all males in this country is about 1 in 6. Early detection and improved treatment options have combined to bring both diagnosis and death rates of prostate cancer down, but it is still the second most commonly diagnosed cancer in men (skin cancer is first) and the second leading cause of death by cancer in men (lung cancer is first).[32]

African American men are about twice as likely to develop prostate cancer as whites. They are also more likely to be diagnosed at an advanced stage, and they are about twice as likely as white men

Prostate Cancer in Brief

Pronunciation: PROS-tate KAN-ser

What is it?

Prostate cancer is the growth of malignant cells in the prostate gland, which may metastasize, usually to nearby bones or into pelvic or inguinal lymph nodes.

How is it recognized?

The symptoms of prostate cancer include problems with urination: weak stream, frequency, urgency, nocturia, and other problems arising from constriction of the urethra. Later symptoms include blood in the urine, painful ejaculation, and persistent bone pain.

Is massage indicated or contraindicated?

Prostate cancer patients may face any combination of surgery, radiation therapy, chemotherapy, and hormonal therapy. Bodywork that accommodates for these challenges while minimizing risks can be helpful and supportive, as long as the massage therapist is working as part of a fully informed health care team.

to die of this disease. Asians have the lowest rates of prostate cancer, both in the United States and worldwide.[32,33]

Etiology: What Happens?

The prostate is a doughnut-shaped gland that lies inferior to the bladder and encircles the male urethra. It produces the fluid that allows for the motility and viability of sperm. The prostate also controls the release of urine from the bladder. Some enlargement of the prostate in later years is almost a guarantee for men. Simple enlargement with no malignant cells is BPH. But sometimes the growth and thickening of the prostate gland is not benign; it indicates prostate cancer.

When cancerous cells begin to form a tumor in the prostate, they can exert direct pressure on the urethra. This can lead to a number of different problems, from difficulty in urinating to urgency, frequency, *nocturia*, painful ejaculation, and bladder infections. Because the symptoms of prostate cancer are so similar to those of BPH, these signs may be ignored until the urethra is seriously restricted. Prostate cancer grows slowly, and it can stay silent long enough for cells to metastasize before it is detected.

The precise genetic mutations that lead to prostate cancer are under intense scrutiny. At this point the disease seems to be related to several contributing factors: activation of oncogenes that stimulate the growth of new cells; inhibition of tumor suppressor genes that limit new growth; and absence of a key enzyme that works to bind up and neutralize free radicals that have been seen to damage prostate cells.

The triggers for prostate cancer are unknown. It has been observed, however, that for tumors to grow, they must have access to testosterone from fully functional testes. This disease is not seen in men who have been castrated, and removal of the testes shrinks cancerous tumors.

Men with prostate cancer in their immediate family are more likely than others to develop this disease. Likewise, men from families whose women have breast cancer evidently also have a higher risk. Heredity is estimated to account for about 5% to 10% of prostate cancer cases.[32]

Men whose diet is high in animal fats have higher rates of prostate cancer than others. And as discussed before, advanced age and being African American are risk factors for this disease. However, risk factors are only general tendencies. As with many other types of cancer, many prostate cancer patients do not fit the profile, and being free from these identified risk factors does not mean a person cannot get prostate cancer.

Signs and Symptoms

Signs of prostate cancer are exactly the same as those for BPH: an enlarged, hard prostate; obstruction of the urethra with resulting difficulty in urination; and susceptibility to urinary tract and kidney infections. In addition, men with prostate cancer may also have pain while urinating or ejaculating, blood in the urine, and an inability to maintain an erection. Low back pain and pain that refers into the upper thighs may follow as the growths become large enough to put mechanical pressure on pelvic nerves.

Diagnosis

Historically prostate cancer has been difficult to diagnose in the early stages, because its only signs and symptoms are so close to those of BPH, a disorder that is common in elderly men. But the advent of some early detection tests has made prostate cancer much easier to find before it has spread beyond the prostate (Compare and Contrast 11.1).

A digital rectal examination (DRE) is the first step in prostate cancer detection. Prostate cancer tends to grow first on the periphery of the prostate gland, in rough, palpable nodules; this feature distinguishes it from BPH, which tends to involve deeper and smoother nodules.

A blood test to look for PSA is another early detection device. Its usefulness is somewhat debatable, since many variables may cause PSA levels to rise or fall, but when levels are higher than normal, this blood test can serve as a warning sign to consider the possibility of prostate cancer. PSA tests can be further clarified to examine whether the PSA is "free" or "attached". Some research now associates free PSA with BPH, while PSA that is attached to blood proteins may indicate more aggressive forms of prostate cancer.

If the digital rectal examination and/or PSA turns up any specific concerns, further exploration is conducted through a transrectal ultrasound and biopsy of suspicious tissue.

Prostate cancer is staged by advancement and by the aggressiveness of the growths. Early detection methods have made it possible to find close to 91% of cases before the cancer has spread beyond the pelvis; the 5-year survival rate for these patients approaches 100%. For more information on staging prostate cancer, see Sidebar 11.8.

Treatment

Treatment options for prostate cancer include watchful waiting; radiation from internal or external sources; surgery to remove part or all of the prostate, seminal vesicles, or testes; and hormone therapy to counteract elevated levels of testosterone. Chemotherapy is generally reserved for very advanced cases. Most treatment options for prostate cancer cause serious complications, including incontinence, erectile dysfunction, and the development of feminine characteristics. Elderly men or men with other health problem who have slow-growing tu-

SIDEBAR 11.8: STAGING PROSTATE CANCER

Most specialists in the United States use the tumor, node, metastasis (TNM) staging system for prostate cancer, in combination with a cancer cell rating system, the Gleason scale. This looks at abnormal cells from a biopsy and rates them according to their appearance and aggressiveness. The Gleason ratings range from 2 to 10.

Prostate cancer, like some other cancers, sometimes cannot be fully staged until surgery is conducted and tissue is examined. The following is a combination of clinical staging (based on best estimates without surgery) and pathological staging (based on findings during or after surgery).[32]

Tumor	Tumor Substage	Node	Metastasis
T1: tumor cannot be palpated or found with transrectal ultrasound	T1A: tumor found with treatment for BPH; affects <5% of tissue	N0: no nodes involved	M0: no metastasis
	T1B: tumor found with treatment for BPH; affects >5% of tissue	N1: ≥1 regional nodes involved	M1: Distant metastasis
	T1C: tumor found with needle biopsy, elevated PSA levels		
T2: tumor palpable with DRE; confined to the prostate	T2A: <50% of one side is affected T2B: >50% of one side is affected T2C: both sides affected		
T3: tumors outside prostate and/or on seminal vesicles	T3A: tumors outside prostate but not on seminal vesicles T3B: tumors on seminal vesicles		
T4: tumors on other tissues, including bladder and wall of pelvis			

The TNM ratings are then combined with Gleason scores to stage prostate cancer from stage I to IV in this way:

Stage	Tumor	Node	Metastasis	Gleason score
I	T1A	N0	M0	2–4
II	T1–2	N0–1	M0	2–10
III	T3	N0	M0	2–10
IV	Any	N0	M0	2–10
IV	Any	Any	M1	2–10

mors may opt not to treat their disease because their quality of life would be so seriously affected.

Best-practice protocols for prostate cancer treatment are constantly in flux. Treatment choices are made on a case-by-case basis, weighing carefully the risks and benefits of treatment along with quality-of-life issues for mature and elderly patients. Several large-scale studies of prostate cancer patients and their treatment outcomes should yield more definitive guidelines soon.

Massage?

Massage therapists who have elderly men as part of their clientele inevitably have some clients who live with the threat of prostate cancer. It is important to know how the client keeps his condition under observation and what treatment options he chooses. Massage therapists working as part of a health care team can certainly improve the quality of these clients' lives by providing supportive, informed touch during a time of great stress and challenge.

Modality Recommendations for Prostate Cancer	
Deep tissue massage	Supportive as part of health care team. Respect stage of recovery and treatment challenges.
Lymphatic drainage	Supportive.
Polarity	S: Indicated. R/D: Supportive with pressure to client's comfort.
PNF/MET/stretching	Supportive as part of health care team; match to activity levels.
Reflexology	Indicated. Work lymphatic system, pituitary, pelvic area, prostate, ureters, bladder, hips, low back points.
Shiatsu	Supportive: treat immune system via SP, TH meridians and extensions, male reproductive system via K and LV.
Swedish massage	Supportive as part of health care team; match to client's activity level.
Trigger point therapy	Supportive.

See Chapter 1 for a brief description of each modality, including definitions of abbreviations.

Prostatitis

Definition: What Is It?

Prostatitis is a condition in which the prostate becomes painful and possibly inflamed. Unlike BPH, prostatitis usually involves significant pain throughout the pelvis and groin. While occasionally connected to a specific infection, it is often difficult to identify and treat the causes of prostatitis.

Demographics: Who Gets It?

Prostatitis is a common disorder; it is responsible for about 2 million doctor visits per year. It is estimated that 10% to 50% of men between 20 and 74 years old will have symptoms at least once.[34] That said, because prostatitis is defined in many ways, it is difficult to report statistics with any assurance of accuracy.

Etiology: What Happens?

The prostate is a walnut-sized gland that surrounds the urethra just distal to the urinary bladder of males. It is composed of ducts and channels into which epithelial cells secrete seminal fluid, a constituent of semen. The seminal fluid is expressed into the urethra during ejaculation.

The draining channels in the prostate are arranged in a basically horizontal plane around the periphery of the organ. This allows material to become stagnant within the gland if it is not frequently expelled. Furthermore, bladder reflux, in which urine collects in the prostate, can cause irritation or even direct bacterial exposure to these delicate epithelial tissues, leading to a risk of prostate stones and acute or chronic infection that may be difficult to treat.

Prostatitis is an umbrella term for four basic types of problems. These classes of prostatitis were outlined by the National Institute of Health in 1995 to create a framework for more efficient study of this often mysterious and difficult problem.[34]

- *Type 1.* Acute bacterial prostatitis is an acute infection of the prostate. This may be accompanied by an abscess, which requires surgery for removal.
- *Type 2.* Chronic bacterial prostatitis is a recurrent infection of the prostate.
- *Type 3.* Chronic nonbacterial prostatitis/chronic pelvic pain syndrome (CPPS) is prostate enlargement with no demonstrable infection. Another term for CPPS is *proctodynia*. Subgroups of this class include these:
  - *Type 3a.* Inflammatory chronic pelvic pain syndrome, in which white blood cells are found in the semen, expressed prostatic secretions, or urine
  - *Type 3b.* Noninflammatory chronic pelvic pain syndrome, in which white blood cells are not found in semen, expressed prostatic secretions, or urine
- *Type 4.* Asymptomatic inflammatory prostatitis has no subjective symptoms, but white blood cells are found in prostate secretions or in prostate tissue during an evaluation for other disorders.

Prostatitis in Brief
Pronunciation: pros-tah-TY-tis

What is it?
Prostatitis is inflammation or irritation of the prostate gland, either from pathogenic or nonpathogenic causes.

How is it recognized?
Symptoms of prostatitis vary according to their cause. Acute prostatitis involves fever, extremely painful urination, urinary frequency and urgency, and pain in the penis, testicles, perineum, and low back. Chronic prostatitis has similar signs and symptoms, but they tend to be less severe, and they don't include fever.

Is massage indicated or contraindicated?
Judgments about massage in the context of prostatitis should be made according to the causative factors. An acute bacterial infection contraindicates circulatory bodywork, but a low-grade, noninfectious chronic condition may not carry the same cautions. "Prostate massage" is a procedure performed by a doctor through the rectal wall and is not within the scope of practice of massage therapists.

When prostatitis is related to an acute or recurrent infection (type 1 or 2), the most common agent is *Escherichia coli*, although *Klebsiella* or *Proteus mirabilis* may be involved. It is not always clear how bacteria get into the prostate. Leading hypotheses suggest that they may move up the urethra following unprotected sexual intercourse or the use of a contaminated catheter, or they may migrate to the prostate through the circulatory or lymph systems.

Type 3 prostatitis, CPSS, is by far the most commonly reported condition, accounting for up to 90% of prostatitis diagnoses.[35] It is not well understood, because no specific causative factors have ever been identified. Some researchers suggest that it is indeed an infection, but the pathogens are of a type that don't culture on standard tests. Others have found that the pelvic pain that accompanies it may be due to chronic hypertonicity or even trigger point referral from the perineal muscle; this suggests that some cases may be related to myofascial pain.

Signs and Symptoms

Acute bacterial prostatitis has all of the signs and symptoms of a UTI: pain and burning with urination along with urinary frequency and urgency. In addition, pain in the pelvis, perineum, testicles, and penis may be present, along with penile discharge, painful ejaculation, low back pain, and fever. The prostate, felt through the wall of the rectum, is exquisitely painful and palpably hot.

Chronic bacterial prostatitis, which indicates recurrent low-grade infection, produces the same symptoms, but with less severity.

Chronic pelvic pain syndrome has the same profile without the element of fever, and palpation of the prostate often produces normal findings.

Complications

The most common complication of any type of prostatitis is the risk of urethral obstruction. If enough pressure is exerted deeply on the urethra, *acute urinary retention* may develop. This is a medical emergency, and it requires immediate intervention.

Diagnosis

The first goal in the diagnosis of prostate dysfunction is to rule out BPH and prostate cancer. Because prostatitis can raise PSA levels in the blood, it is sometimes confused with prostate cancer. In many cases of prostatitis, bacterial infection is assumed although seldom actually cultured.

Compare and Contrast 11.1
PROSTATE DYSFUNCTION

When the prostate gland becomes enlarged, symptoms are predictable: restriction of urinary flow, bladder irritation, and a risk of urinary tract infection that can complicate to pyelonephritis. The causes of prostate enlargement, however, are not so consistent. BPH can be hard to distinguish from prostate cancer, and prostatitis adds to the general confusion. Here are some general guidelines about similarities and differences with these conditions.

CHARACTERISTICS	PROSTATE CANCER	BENIGN PROSTATIC HYPERPLASIA	PROSTATITIS
Who gets it?	Usually affects men older than 50 but can occur in younger men with certain risk factors.	Very common in mature men; incidence increases with age.	Can occur in males of any age; leading cause of visits to urologist for young men.
Signs and symptoms	Restricted urinary flow; pain with pressure on other structures or bone damage; blood in urine possible	Restricted urinary flow, bladder irritation	Symptoms vary with causes, but usually significant pelvic pain.
Diagnosis	DRE, PSA tests, ultrasound to evaluate risk of prostate cancer; findings confirmed with biopsy.	DRE, PSA tests, tests to measure urinary flow usually confirm BPH.	DRE, examinations of urine, semen, prostate secretions to evaluate type of prostatitis.
Treatment	Determined by age of patient, stage of cancer. Options include surgery, chemotherapy, radiation, watchful waiting.	Medications to limit prostate growth may be prescribed; surgery to enlarge passageway for urethra may be performed.	Antibiotics for infections; otherwise treated symptomatically.
Implications for massage	Therapists must adapt to chosen treatment options (see Chapter 12).	Massage has no direct effect on BPH, is safe as long as no infection is present and client is comfortable on table.	After any infection is treated massage is safe. Some pelvic pain may be referred from trigger points.

Urologists who specialize in these disorders frequently conduct a series of tests to try to confirm the presence or absence of bacteria. Urine from three stages is analyzed: the initial stream (which may be contaminated with material from the urethra), midstream (where urine should be sterile), and after prostate massage, a procedure in which the prostate is manipulated through the rectal wall by a doctor to express fluid through the penis for examination. A semen sample may also be analyzed to look for bacteria or white blood cells that indicate inflammation in the urogenital tract.

Biopsy of prostate tissue is not recommended if infection is a possibility, to avoid the risk of inadvertently spreading any pathogens.

Treatment

Acute bacterial prostatitis (type 1) responds well to antibiotics. Unfortunately, type 2 (chronic bacterial prostatitis) does not. It may take 6 weeks or more of antibiotic therapy, and it frequently recurs.

If prostate stones are discovered, they are surgically removed, typically with laser surgery through the urethra.

Type 3 prostatitis is often treated with a short or long course of antibiotics just in case some bacteria were missed, and then dealt with symptomatically. Alpha-blockers relax the smooth muscle tissue in the bladder for easier urination; anti-inflammatories, frequent ejaculations, and *sitz baths* (a bath just for the pelvic area) to help relax the perineal muscle are also recommended. Antianxiety medications are sometimes prescribed. Biofeedback techniques to increase awareness of tightness in the perineal muscle have some success, as do some dietary supplements. For many men, however, chronic pelvic pain syndrome is a stubborn disorder with no simple answers; it can have a long-term and severe impact on their quality of life.

Massage?

Massage is only peripherally influential on prostate problems, since the gland is in an area that massage therapists do not reach. Nonetheless, when acute infection with fever and inflammation is present, massage is obviously inappropriate. For men who struggle with chronic problems, however, massage may be part of a useful coping mechanism as long as the client is comfortable on the table.

Modality Recommendations for Prostatitis	
Deep tissue massage	Supportive within client's comfort, as part of health care team. Work adductors, hip rotators and flexors, hamstrings, gluteals, psoas/abdominal muscles.
Lymphatic drainage	Supportive.
Polarity	S/R/D: Indicated.
PNF/MET/stretching	Supportive in absence of infection.
Reflexology	Indicated. Work lymphatic system, pituitary, prostate, ureters, bladder, kidney, hips, low back points.
Shiatsu	Indicated. Treat TH, SP, LV, K meridians and extensions, especially in upper thigh and torso, and back K areas of Zen Shiatsu system.
Swedish massage	Locally contraindicated for deep abdominal work while acute; otherwise supportive.
Trigger point therapy	Supportive.

See Chapter 1 for a brief description of each modality, including definitions of abbreviations.

Testicular Cancer in Brief

Pronunciation: tes-TIK-yu-lar KAN-ser

What is it?
Testicular cancer is the growth of malignant cells in the testicles, which may metastasize to the rest of the body.

How is it recognized?
Early signs of testicular cancer include a painless lump in the scrotum, a dull ache in the low abdomen or groin, a sense of heaviness in the scrotum, and enlarged or tender breasts.

Is massage indicated or contraindicated?
Guidelines about massage in the context of testicular cancer are the same as for other types of cancer. This particular variety of cancer usually has an excellent prognosis, and it responds well to radiation therapy or chemotherapy. Massage may be a useful adjunct to these therapies to improve tolerance and shorten recovery time, but it must be conducted within the client's tolerance as part of a fully integrated health care effort.

Testicular Cancer

Definition: What Is It?

Testicular cancer is growth of malignant cells in the testicles. These cells usually grow slowly, but they may metastasize through the lymph or blood systems.

Demographics: Who Gets It?

Testicular cancer accounts for 1% of male cancers. Although it is still comparatively rare, some research indicates that rates of testicular cancer have doubled in the past 40 years.[36]

Testicular cancer is diagnosed about 8,200 times per year and causes about 370 deaths per year in this country. It is significantly more common in whites than in other races. Testicular cancer is unusual in that it usually targets young men; it is the leading type of cancer among males 15 to 35 years old. It is a highly survivable form of cancer: the overall 5-year survival rate is 96%, and about 140,000 testicular cancer survivors are living today.[37]

Etiology: What Happens?

The causes or contributing factors of testicular cancer are not well understood. The only consistent risk factor is that males who were born with an undescended testicle (*cryptorchidism*) have a slightly higher risk of developing this disease. Other risk factors include other congenital abnormalities, age (it is most common in young men), race (whites are affected more than other groups), personal or family history of testicular cancer, and HIV status: men who are HIV positive have a slightly higher risk of testicular cancer than others.

Testicular cancer is typically discussed as germ cell tumors or stromal cell tumors.

Stromal cell tumors These are growths within the supportive tissue for the testicle. They are quite rare and account for only 5% or less of testicular cancers. They are called *Sertoli cell tumors* or *Leydig cell tumors*.

Germ cell tumors These are tumors that arise within the sperm and hormone-producing cells of the testicle. Germ cell tumors are further classified into *seminomas* and *nonseminomas*.

- *Seminomas.* Seminomas are the most common single variety of testicular cancer, accounting for 40% to 45% of diagnoses. They tend to grow slowly and are highly sensitive to radiation.
- *Nonseminomas.* These are several different types of testicular tumors, some of which are more aggressive than others. Some types of nonseminomas are diagnosed among young boys and are not classified as malignant, but they can change if neglected. *Embryonic carcinomas*, *yolk sac tumors*, and *teratomas* are growths in which tissues resemble the growth pattern of embryos. In teratomas the cells may even differentiate into tissue cells, including glands, nerve tissue, and bones. One type of nonseminoma is called *choriocarcinoma*. Of all of the types of testicular cancer, this one is the most aggressive and has the poorest prognosis.

Signs and Symptoms

Testicular cancer usually begins with a painless lump on the testicle. It may be accompanied by a feeling of fullness or heaviness or fluid in the scrotum. A dull ache in the low abdomen or groin may develop, along with enlargement and tenderness at the breasts. If any of these symptoms persist for more than 2 weeks, the person should consult his physician as soon as possible.

Diagnosis

The first step in diagnosing any testicular dysfunction is to rule out the possibility of infection or injury. Ultrasound tests may then be recommended; these are highly sensitive to growths in the testicles. Blood tests may show specific hormonal or enzyme markers of nonseminoma or stromal tumors. If a suspicious area is found, an ***inguinal orchiectomy*** (removal of the testicle and spermatic cord through the abdomen) is performed so the testicle can be examined for signs of cancer. This procedure is routed through the abdomen rather than through the scrotum to avoid the possibility of inadvertently spreading any malignant cells.

If cancerous cells are found in the testicle, they are identified for type, and deep abdominal lymph nodes may be extracted to look for signs of metastasis. For more information on testicular cancer staging, see Sidebar 11.9.

SIDEBAR 11.9: STAGING TESTICULAR CANCER

Testicular cancer is staged differently from most other cancers; instead of progressing from stage 0 to stage IV, it is usually discussed as stages 0 to III. Specialists use highly defined and detailed staging protocols to make appropriate treatment plans and prognoses. These often include measurements of cancer markers in the blood along with tumor, node, and metastatic progress. The following is a simplified version of testicular cancer staging:[38]

- Stage 0. This is cancer in situ: preinvasive germ cell cancer.
- Stage I. The testicle and spermatic cord are affected; no spread to lymph nodes; blood tests are normal.
- Stage II. Nearby lymph nodes are invaded.
- Stage IIA. The nodes show signs of microscopic invasion. This is sometimes called "nonbulky stage II".
- Stage IIB. The nodes are larger than 5 cm; this can be called "bulky stage II".
- Stage III. Distant lymph nodes and other tissues are invaded.
- Stage IIIA. Only lymph nodes are invaded, but growths are smaller than 2 cm (nonbulky stage III).
- Stage IIIB. Other tissues are invaded, usually the central nervous system and/or lungs. Lymph node metastases are larger than 2 cm (bulky stage III).

Treatment

The treatment options for testicular cancer begin with surgery to remove the affected testicle and any secondary tumors that are found. If the cancer is identified as a seminoma, radiation therapy follows surgery; these cancer cells are extremely sensitive to radiation, and this protocol is usually completely successful.

If the cancer was a mixed tumor or a nonseminoma, chemotherapy may be used following surgery. Recent new chemotherapeutic agents have significantly improved the prognosis of nonseminoma cancer.

Follow-up care after testicular cancer treatment is critical to make sure no metastases were missed. Furthermore, testicular cancer survivors have a small but significant risk of developing cancer in the other testicle.

The survival rate for testicular cancer is so high and the treatments available are so effective that no invasive early screening protocols for this disease have been developed or recommended. Nonetheless, many men are taught to conduct testicular self-examinations, just as women are taught to do breast self-examinations. In this way any changes in the tissue may be identified and investigated as quickly as possible.

Massage?

A person who is fighting testicular cancer is probably undergoing cycles of radiation therapy or chemotherapy. Massage may improve the tolerance for these demanding treatments, as long as the client is resilient enough to keep up with the changes massage brings about. Many testicular cancer patients are encouraged to exercise; this is a good sign that massage is appropriate as well. Massage may improve appetite and quality of sleep, two features that are especially important for patients undergoing treatment for cancer.

Massage therapists working with clients who have testicular cancer (or any other kind of cancer) must be sure to keep the rest of the client's health care team informed so that everyone can work together for the best possible outcome.

Modality Recommendations for Testicular Cancer	
Deep tissue massage	Supportive as part of health care team. Respect stage of recovery and treatment challenges.
Lymphatic drainage	Supportive.
Polarity	S: Indicated. R/D: Indicated with pressure determined by client's comfort.
PNF/MET/stretching	Supportive as part of health care team; match to activity levels.
Reflexology	Indicated. Work lymphatic system, pituitary, testes, pelvic area points.
Shiatsu	Supportive. Treat the immune system via SP, TH meridians and extensions, and male reproductive system via K and LV meridians.
Swedish massage	Supportive as part of health care team; match to client activity level.
Trigger point therapy	Locally contraindicated; otherwise supportive for light work.

See Chapter 1 for a brief description of each modality, including definitions of abbreviations.

Other Reproductive System Conditions

Menopause

Definition: What Is It?

Menopause is a specific event: the moment the ovaries permanently stop secreting enough hormones to initiate a menstrual cycle. The time leading up to this event and for a year after the last menstrual period is called ***perimenopause***, and many of the symptoms associated with declining hormone secretion occur during this period. Menopause itself is not conclusively identified until a full year after the last menstrual period.

It is important to point out that menopause is *not* a disease: it is a normal part of aging that every woman, if she lives long enough, will experience. Nevertheless, it can cause significant symptoms that can impair a woman's ability to function and her quality of life.

Menarche, menstruation, menses, menopause:

What are all these men doing in women's health ? The root word is mēn, which is Greek for "month".

- Menarche is *mēn* plus *arche*, or *beginning*.
- Menstruation is *mēn* plus *atus*, meaning *to be menstruant*.
- Menses is the plural for *mēn*, meaning *many months*.
- Menopause is *mēn* plus *pausis*, or *cessation*.

Demographics: Who Gets It?

The average age for the onset of perimenopausal symptoms is 47.5 years; the average age at which the transition is final is 51.4 years.[39] These average ages have not changed since records on menopause have been kept, but some factors, including cigarette smoking, living at high altitude, having an autoimmune disease, and genetic predisposition, are associated with an earlier onset of perimenopausal symptoms.[39,40]

It is estimated that about 46 million women in the United States are postmenopausal, and with the increasing number of mature Americans, about 50 million women will be postmenopausal by 2020.[39]

Etiology: What Happens?

In addition to ripening several eggs each month and releasing at least one for the possibility of fertilization, the ovaries secrete a variety of chemicals (mostly estrogen and progesterone) into the bloodstream. They do this under the control of hypothalamus and pituitary secretions of follicle-stimulating hormone (FHS) and luteinizing hormone (LH).

As ovaries age, they become less sensitive to these hormones. Consequently, they secrete less estrogen and progesterone. It is somewhat misleading to refer to estrogen and progesterone as only two hormones, as both of these substances are produced in various chemical forms, each of which is metabolized and used in different ways.

Estrogens and progesterones influence sex organs either to support a pregnancy or to shed the endometrial lining of the uterus. When the ovaries lose function, either as a normal part of aging or because their function has been interrupted by surgery, irradiation, or drugs (induced menopause) these processes come to a stop. When a woman no longer ovulates, she no longer grows an endometrial lining in her uterus, and she no longer sheds that lining during menstruation. But these ovarian hormones also work on many other tissues in the body in ways that are only just beginning to be explored.

- *Bone density.* The role of estrogens and progesterones in maintaining bone density is complex. It seems clear that estrogen inhibits osteoclast activity, that is, it helps to prevent the thinning of bone tissue. But some forms of progesterone are involved in maintaining bone density as well, stimulating osteoblast activity. In other words, estrogen prevents bone from being dissolved, while progesterone helps it to build up. When both of these are in short supply, women can lose a significant amount of bone mass (up to 20%) during the first years of hormonal fluctuation.[40]
- *Cardiovascular health.* As women age, the types of cholesterol in their blood change. Postmenopausal women have higher levels of low-density lipoproteins and triglycerides (the "bad" types of cholesterol) than other women. It seems clear that estrogen has some influence on cholesterol, but the exact mechanisms are not well understood. Researchers are exploring whether short-term estrogen supplementation at the onset of perimenopause could be protective against atherosclerosis.[41]
- *Protection from some types of cancer.* This is an extremely complex issue that reflects just how little is understood about the effects of different types of estrogens and progesterones on different types of tissues. High levels of some types of estrogen have a statistical link with lower rates of colon cancer but with higher rates of some other types of cancer, including breast and ovarian cancers. Ultimately it may be found that whether hormone levels are dangerous or protective depends on the chemical variation of the hormone, where it comes from, how it is metabolized, where it is used, and other variables that haven't even been considered yet.
- *Central nervous system functions.* Estrogen seems linked to mood, depression, and basic cognitive function. Supplementing low doses of estrogen has been seen to be effective for dealing with the mild depression, insomnia, and short-term memory loss that may accompany perimenopause, but it is not effective for more severe depressive disorders.

When the ovaries decrease hormonal production, a woman becomes dependent on other tissues to secrete enough hormones to provide for her daily function. Some fat cells and other tissues continue to produce estrogen after the ovaries atrophy, but at a fraction of previous levels. Further, while some estrogen production continues after menopause, most progesterone production does not. Combine this with exposure to exogenous estrogens, and the precarious balance between estrogens and progesterones is lost.

Menopause in Brief

Pronunciation: MEN-o-pawz

What is it?

Menopause refers to the moment when functioning ovaries become nonfunctioning ovaries. Although this usually happens as a normal part of aging, menopause can be induced through surgery, radiation, or medication.

How is it recognized?

The symptoms associated with a decline in ovarian function (perimenopause) include night sweats, hot flashes, insomnia, mood swings, decreased sex drive, vaginal itchiness or dryness, urinary incontinence, and poor concentration and memory. Longer-term changes include an increased risk of osteoporosis and cardiovascular disease.

Is massage indicated or contraindicated?

Bodywork is certainly indicated for a woman who is losing ovarian function. While for some women this is a liberating, exciting time, for others it involves radical and not always welcome changes in self-definition and self-perception. Massage gives powerful positive feedback about physical experience and can help to ameliorate some of the psychological and physical disruptions that menopause can bring about.

Signs and Symptoms

The symptoms of perimenopause are related to sudden changes in hormone secretion. Symptoms generally subside when hormone levels stabilize, but this may not happen until a year or more after a final menstrual period.

The signs and symptoms of menopause vary with each individual, but some of the most common ones are hot flashes (some women call them power surges or "my own personal summer"), night sweats, insomnia, mood swings, urinary urgency, loss of urinary continence, decreased sex drive, vaginal dryness or itchiness, confusion, short-term memory loss, and poor concentration. Some of these symptoms may be interrelated: for instance, insomnia may have to do with night sweats and hot flashes; depression and decreased sex drive may have to do with a change in self-perception as a woman becomes no longer fertile. But for some women the symptoms of perimenopause are directly linked to hormonal disruption, and taking steps to smooth out the hormonal shifts can alleviate a lot of discomfort.

The long-term consequences of menopause include pathological thinning of bones and decreased resistance to heart disease, although these phenomena are certainly controllable.

Treatment

Treatment options for the symptoms of perimenopause and the long-term consequences of reduced estrogen and pro gesterone secretion are many and varied. Estrogen replacement therapy provides supplements of various types of estrogens. This seems to be adequate for some women, but it doesn't address the lost balance between estrogens and progesterones that are implicated in many health issues. Further, it is appropriate only for women who have had a hysterectomy, because unopposed estrogen stimulates potentially dangerous endometrial growth.

Hormone replacement therapy supplements both estrogen and progesterone, in varying levels and in varying forms, but traditional hormone replacement therapy is also associated with increased risk of heart disease, stroke, and some types of cancer, especially if it is used for more than 2 years. Many ongoing studies are designed to determine how to get the best out of hormone supplementation while reducing possible risks (Sidebar 11.10).

If a woman decides not to supplement hormones to treat her menopausal symptoms, she may consider other options. Medications to support bone density and decrease the risk of heart disease are possibilities, as are a variety of herbal preparations. Many women report success with managing hot flashes, mood swings, and other perimenopausal symptoms, but controlled studies to date have not yielded conclusive information about their efficacy. Options include black cohosh (which should be avoided when other estrogen supplements are used), red clover, dong quai (which should not be used along with blood thinners), ginseng, wild yam, and kava (which has been associated with a risk of liver problems).[43] The long and short of herbal therapy for peri-

SIDEBAR 11.10: HORMONE REPLACEMENT THERAPY

Recently, a major research project called the Women's Health Initiative set out to study several long-term health trends in 161,809 postmenopausal American women between 50 and 79 years of age. The goal was to track these participants over 8 years to gather information about health trends for older women. One question they asked concerned the benefits and risks of the most common version of hormone replacement therapy: concentrated equine estrogens (Premarin) plus medroxyprogesterone acetate (progestin) for women who had not had a hysterectomy. This hormone supplement regimen has traditionally been prescribed to reduce perimenopausal symptoms like hot flashes and vaginal dryness and to reduce the risk of heart disease and osteoporosis.

After 5 years of following the study participants, researchers found some surprising results. While the relative risk of osteoporosis and colorectal cancer went down as expected, all other health concerns being tracked actually increased, as follows:[42]

Heart attack	Increased	29%
Breast cancer	Increased	26%
Stroke	Increased	41%
Blood clot in leg or lung	Increased	111%
Dementia	Increased	105%
Hip fractures (as measure of osteoporosis)	Decreased	33%
Colorectal cancer	Decreased	37%

The cardiovascular risks rose within 2 years of beginning hormone replacement therapy, and the increase in breast cancer risk was found after 4 years. Protection against osteoporosis was lost when therapy stopped. These findings were so significant that it was considered unethical to keep women on hormone replacement therapy without informed consent, and this branch of the study was concluded in July 2002.

Other branches of the study are continuing, including the use of estrogen replacement therapy (without progestin) in women who have had hysterectomies. Estrogen replacement is not appropriate for women who still have a uterus, because estrogen uncontrolled by progesterone stimulates endometrial growth and increases the risk of uterine cancer.

Since this study was published, researchers have continued to look at this issue. Current findings suggest that hormone replacement therapy for women at the onset of perimenopause may not only be helpful in managing symptoms but may also offer some cardiovascular protection. However, the general recommendation now is to encourage women to use the lowest possible dosage of hormones for the shortest period possible.[42]

menopausal symptoms is essentially that a woman should inform her health care team of any supplement she uses so as to avoid potentially dangerous interactions with other drugs.

Massage?

Bodywork is wonderful for a woman who has symptoms of perimenopause. This condition is not a disease; it is a natural process. While many women feel that entering this phase of life is a liberating, exciting time, others feel that their role in life changes so fundamentally that they lose touch with their own self-definition. Massage, because it involves supportive, nurturing, informed touch, can reinforce the positive aspects of a woman's physical experience and help her through what can be a difficult period.

Modality Recommendations for Menopause	
Deep tissue massage	Supportive with goals for relaxation.
Lymphatic drainage	Supportive.
Polarity	S/R/D: Indicated.
PNF/MET/stretching	Supportive.
Reflexology	Indicated. Work solar plexus, brain, and gland points, especially pituitary and thyroid.
Shiatsu	Indicated. Treat GB, BL, SP, PC, K, H, LI, especially legs, abdomen, back.
Swedish massage	Supportive.
Trigger point therapy	Supportive.

Pregnancy

Definition: What Is It?

Pregnancy, obviously, is the condition in which a woman carries a fetus. Most general information about pregnancy is skipped in this discussion, but it is worthwhile to look at some aspects of this condition as it relates to massage.

Signs and Symptoms

Pregnancy creates a wide array of signs and symptoms, and some of them have specific implications for massage. Here are some of the complaints of pregnant women that bodyworkers can influence:

- *Loose ligaments.* One of the hormones secreted during pregnancy is ***relaxin***. Its job is to loosen the ligaments so that the pelvis is elastic enough to allow the baby to emerge. But relaxin starts working very early in pregnancy, making all of the ligaments in the body looser and more mobile. This can cause numerous problems, from unstable vertebrae to asymmetrical sacroiliac joints. Muscles work to stabilize the joints, causing spasm and pain.

Pregnancy in Brief

Pronunciation: PREG-nan-se

What is it?
Pregnancy is the state of carrying a fetus.

How is it recognized?
The signs and symptoms of advanced pregnancy are obvious, but symptoms that specifically pertain to massage include loose ligaments, muscle spasms, clumsiness, and fatigue.

Is massage indicated or contraindicated?
All stages of uncomplicated pregnancy indicate massage, with specific cautions relating to each trimester.

- *Fatigue.* Pregnant women carry a lot of extra weight. The baby itself is only a fraction of the whole load, which includes the placenta, amniotic fluid, 40% more blood, and any extra fat she may accumulate during her pregnancy. In addition to carrying extra weight, a pregnant woman secretes hormones that signal her to get a lot of rest. This is a command that many pregnant women don't have the luxury of obeying, at least if they're trying to hold a job during the process.
- *Shifting proprioception.* Pregnant women change their size every day. This is true especially in the last trimester, when the baby grows at an astounding rate. The result is that a pregnant woman never knows exactly how much room she takes up. Her sense of where in space her body ends and the rest of the world begins is very shaky. This tends to make a pregnant woman clumsy and prone to injury. Massage provides an extraordinary sense of where bodies are in space. It can improve proprioceptive senses by giving continuous and positive feedback about boundaries.

Complications

In the vast range of things that can go wrong in a pregnancy, four conditions are especially important for massage therapists to watch out for: thromboembolism, gestational diabetes, pregnancy-induced hypertension, and ectopic pregnancy.

Thromboembolism This is a combination of deep vein thrombosis and pulmonary embolism, both of which are discussed in Chapter 6. Pregnant and newly postpartum women have approximately four times as much risk of blood clots as the nonpregnant population.[44] The risk increases as the pregnancy develops and is highest in the first few days after the baby is delivered. Identifying risk factors for thromboembolism may eventually lead to the use of prophylactic blood thinners during the postpartum period.

Gestational diabetes Pregnancy-related diabetes develops in about 4% of pregnancies, affecting some 135,000 women each year.[45] It is diagnosed with a glucose tolerance test, in which the woman drinks a sweet beverage, and then her urine is examined for elevated levels of glucose. Gestational diabetes is usually identified in the fifth or sixth month of pregnancy (between 24 and 26 weeks of gestation).

If diabetes develops during pregnancy, risks to the baby and mother are significant. The rerouting of nutrients in the blood can cause babies to grow abnormally large in a condition called ***macrosomia***, which may require a cesarean section. Babies born to women with gestational diabetes also have a high risk of respiratory distress syndrome, early hypoglycemia, and later obesity and type 2 diabetes.

A woman who develops gestational diabetes has a high risk of doing so again with subsequent pregnancies, and of developing type 2 diabetes later in life.

Pregnancy-induced hypertension This is a condition that generally starts mildly but can quickly become life-threatening both for the baby and the mother. It develops in about 5% of pregnancies. It occurs in three categories: hypertension alone; ***preeclampsia***, which is hypertension along with elevated proteins in the urine and possible systemic edema; and ***eclampsia***, which is the same condition along with convulsions or coma.[46]

Most cases of pregnancy-induced hypertension occur during a first pregnancy. Other women at risk include those who are obese prior to pregnancy, those who have a personal or family history of chronic high blood pressure, women under 20 or over 40 years old, women carrying multiple babies, and women who have an underlying disease that can affect the circulatory system, including diabetes, lupus, and scleroderma. Treatment includes medication to bring down the blood pressure, strict bed rest, and, where appropriate, cesarean section.

A complication of pregnancy-induced hypertension is ***HELLP*** syndrome, hemolysis with elevated liver enzymes and low platelet count. This disorder of damaged blood cells and impaired liver function can result in severe damage to the liver.

Complications of pregnancy-induced hypertension for mothers include renal failure, cerebral hemorrhage, liver damage, and retinal detachment leading to blindness. Risks to the baby include reduced growth from circulatory impairment and ***placenta abruptio***, a condition in which the placenta prematurely separates from the uterus.

Ectopic pregnancy An ectopic pregnancy is a fertilized egg that implants outside of the uterus. Most ectopic pregnancies develop in the fallopian tubes; some implant in the peritoneum, on the ovaries, or on the cervix. It is estimated that extrauterine implantation occurs in about 1% to 2% of pregnancies.[47]

Risk factors for ectopic pregnancy include intrauterine device use; a history of pelvic inflammatory disease, endometriosis, or sexually transmitted disease; and adhesions from previous abdominal surgeries. Ectopic pregnancies cannot come to term; the fallopian tube inevitably ruptures, killing the fetus and endangering the life of the mother. Ectopic pregnancies that are recognized early (usually by ultrasound and testing for hormone levels) may be terminated by medication or laparoscopic surgery, preserving the ovary and oviduct for the chance of another successful pregnancy.

Massage?

In pregnancies that are not complicated by diabetes, hypertension, or other disorders, massage is a wonderful gift for someone whose body doesn't quite belong to herself for a while.

Special training is available to learn pregnancy and prenatal massage, but for more general purposes, here are some guidelines and cautions to preserve the pregnant client's comfort and safety:

- *First trimester.* From the moment a woman knows she's pregnant to several days after she's delivered, deep abdominal work is contraindicated. The first and last trimesters are the times when the fetal attachment is most fragile, and massage therapists must respect that fragility. Practitioners of Eastern techniques would add that other cautions for massage in the first trimester include deep specific point work on the heels and Achilles tendons (reflexology abortion points), and on the *hoku* point in the web of the thumb.
- *Second trimester.* This is the safest, easiest part of the pregnancy. Very often a woman's energy levels are up and her nausea levels are down. She probably has not yet gained enough weight to be very uncomfortable. But connective tissue changes begin to show during this time: ligaments begin to loosen, and muscles may spasm in response. Massage at this stage centers on making sure the client is comfortable. Bolsters and other physical support tools are useful. Sometime in this trimester, often around week 22, she will no longer want to be face down; then the therapist is limited to doing work from the side or with the client supine unless extensive bolstering is employed.
- *Third trimester.* A midwife once said, "God invented the third trimester of pregnancy to make labor look like a pretty good deal." Massage therapists are more limited in what they do in this trimester than any other, but their work is more important than ever. Prone work is out of the question at this point, and supine work probably should be limited or modified, according to the mother's comfort. Being fully reclined allows the fetus to rest directly on the big abdominal blood vessels, which may either limit blood flow to the legs, leading to cramping in the gastrocnemius, or limit blood flow up the vena cava, leading to dizziness and unconsciousness (Figure 11.9). It may be best to do a lot of side work unless the client can be semireclined.

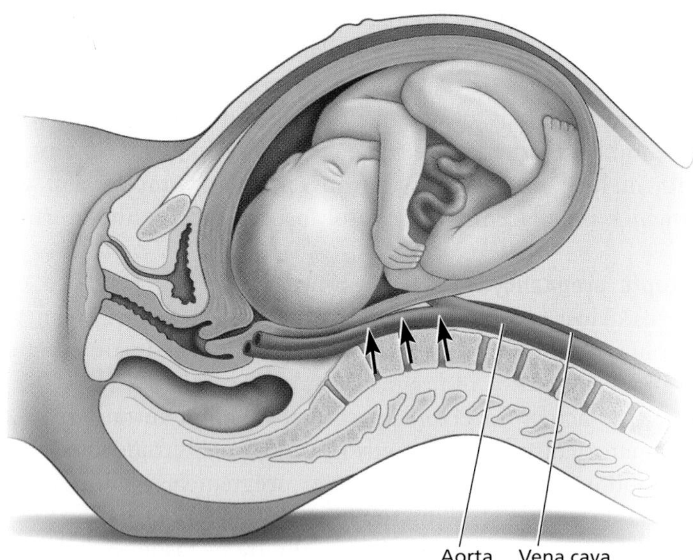

Figure 11.9. Pregnancy: a late-term fetus can obstruct blood flow through the iliac arteries or the vena cava.

Another caution for this stage is limited blood return from the legs, leading to edema. Watch for varicose veins, which, combined with long-standing edema and the increased number of red blood cells that is a normal part of being pregnant, can be an ideal environment for clot formation and deep vein thrombosis. Some people suggest that to be completely safe, the medial calf and thigh (in other words, the area around the great saphenous vein) should be a local contraindication for massage during the third trimester whether or not edema or varices are present.

If edema fever, dizziness, headache, and nausea are present, the client may be in preeclampsia and needs immediate medical attention.

Modality Recommendations for Pregnancy	
Deep tissue massage	Supportive after first trimester. Position client according to trimester. Work for adaptation and relaxation. Avoid deep work around abdomen, ankles, calves.
Lymphatic drainage	Supportive.
Polarity	S/R/D: Indicated. Avoid ovary and uterus points; pressure determined by client's comfort.
PNF/MET/stretching	Supportive.
Reflexology	Indicated, but avoid ovaries, uterus points. After 28 weeks work intestines, stomach, spine, neck, solar plexus/diaphragm, lymphatic system points.
Shiatsu	Indicated with caution. Avoid overstimulation, especially during first trimester. Be cautious around points contraindicated for acupuncture, especially GB21, SP6.
Swedish massage	Supportive with special training for contraindicated areas, proper positioning, and other skills.
Trigger point therapy	Locally contraindicated; otherwise supportive.

See Chapter 1 for a brief description of each modality, including definitions of abbreviations.

Premenstrual Syndrome

Definition: What Is It?

Premenstrual syndrome (PMS) is a collection of signs and symptoms that combine to interfere with a woman's ability to function normally during the luteal phase of the menstrual cycle: the time between ovulation and menstruation.

Demographics: Who Gets It?

Up to 75% of women between the onset of menarche and menopause report some symptoms of PMS.[48] While it can occur among ovulating women of any age, it is most common in women in their late 20s to early 40s.

Etiology: What Happens?

PMS is one of the most common and least well understood conditions that women experience. It has been described since ancient times; it was recognized as a specific pattern in 1931 and finally named in 1953. Nonetheless, the etiology of this condition remains mysterious. Several factors seem to contribute to it, and each woman's experience is unique. This makes it difficult to predict or treat, as no single approach is universally successful.

Some of the hypotheses for the causes or triggers of PMS include the following:

- *Hormonal imbalance.* During the luteal phase of the menstrual cycle, the body prepares to shed the endometrial lining that has accumulated for the implantation of a fertilized egg. Estrogen and progesterone levels rise as the lining thickens, and then just before menstruation begins, production of these hormones suddenly and rapidly drops. One theory behind PMS is that this precipitous drop in hormones is difficult to accommodate and that exposure to environmental estrogens (in animal fats and toxins) may cause the endometrial lining to become overactive, thus requiring an even more extreme fluctuation in hormonal levels. In addition to problems with estrogen and progesterone levels, some women with PMS report problems with adrenal function.
- *Nutritional deficiencies.* Some women with PMS are deficient in specific nutrients, notably calcium, vitamin B_6, and some essential fatty acids.
- *Neurotransmitter imbalance.* Plunging estrogen and progesterone levels have been seen to suppress the secretion of serotonin, a neurotransmitter that is strongly related to mood swings and depression. Opioid peptides are other brain chemicals that appear to be adversely affected by hormone disruption. These chemicals also help to determine mood.
- *Other factors.* Some factors that may contribute to PMS are more vague but definitely a part of the picture for many women. Genetic predisposition may be a factor, but no genetic mutation has been isolated for PMS; it's unclear whether it is passed on through heredity or the likelihood to seek help for it is passed on through environmental influence. Cultural expectations, general stress, and a number of unrelated disorders may also contribute to PMS. Recent studies have also suggested that many women who seek treatment for PMS are survivors of sexual abuse. They frequently also meet the diagnostic criteria for posttraumatic stress disorder. This finding creates some additional options for successful treatment.

Premenstrual Syndrome in Brief

Pronunciation: pre-MEN-stru-al SIN-drome

What is it?

Premenstrual syndrome (PMS) is a collection of many signs and symptoms that occur in the time between ovulation and menstruation and then subside after menstruation begins. It may have several causes and triggers.

How is it recognized?

Signs and symptoms of PMS are often divided into physical and emotional features. Physical symptoms include breast tenderness, bloating, digestive upset, fatigue, changes in appetite, backache, and many others. Emotional signs include irritability, anxiety, depression, mood swings, and other possible problems.

Is massage indicated or contraindicated?

Although the specific causes of PMS are not clearly understood, it is clear that it is not related to infection, structural problems, or neoplasm. Therefore, PMS indicates bodywork, which may help to reestablish balance in the endocrine and nervous systems.

Signs and Symptoms

More than 150 signs and symptoms have been documented among PMS patients. These have been loosely categorized into physical and emotional indicators of this disorder.

- *Physical manifestations.* The most common physical signs and symptoms associated with PMS include bloating, breast tenderness, acne, salt and sugar cravings (along with binge eating), headaches, backaches, insomnia, and digestive upset, that is, diarrhea and/or constipation. Less common physical manifestations include sinus problems, heart palpitations, dizziness, asthma, and seizures.
- *Emotional manifestations.* These include confusion, depression, anxiety, panic attacks, mood swings, and general irritability.

Another disorder, called ***premenstrual dysphoric disorder***, is essentially like PMS but with the added factor of extremely depressed mood and/or anxiety. It occurs cyclically, just as PMS does, but it is typically treated with antidepressants and antianxiety medications rather than with birth control pills.

Diagnosis

It seems clear that PMS has several causes and is a different experience for every woman who has it. The one constant in this condition is that symptoms appear after ovulation and subside when menstruation begins. The most important diagnostic test for PMS is a diary in which a woman records her experiences and finds that this pattern is consistent with her menstrual cycle.

Several other conditions have signs and symptoms that overlap with PMS. These include diabetes or hypothyroidism, eating disorders, depression, chronic fatigue syndrome, irritable bowel syndrome, or any combination of these disorders. Only PMS shows a different pattern of symptoms during and after menstruation, however.

Treatment

Since PMS is not understood as a distinct disease process, it is treated symptomatically. Women who consult allopathic physicians for this disorder may be prescribed low-dose birth control pills to control estrogen and progesterone levels, diuretics to control water retention, or antidepressants to address serotonin levels. One particular form of birth control pill has recently been approved specifically for treatment of premenstrual dysphoric disorder. Most women are also strongly advised to make sure that they get the best sleep they can muster during their difficult time and to exercise regularly.

Health professionals who focus on nutritional aspects of PMS often recommend that patients follow a low-fat vegetarian diet to avoid excessive estrogen exposure, and that they avoid salt, sugar, caffeine (specifically in soda, coffee, tea, and chocolate), and alcohol. Many herbal remedies have been reputed to help PMS; few of them have been accepted by the medical mainstream. Some of the more common herbal recommendations include borage or evening primrose (for essential fatty acids), black cohosh, and dong quai.

Ultimately PMS can usually be successfully managed so that a woman doesn't have to lose function for 10 days every month, but it is unlikely to spontaneously disappear until the onset of menopause.

Massage?

PMS is not related to circulatory dysfunction, neoplasm, structural problems, infection, or any other condition that might make bodywork inappropriate. PMS definitely indicates massage and other kinds of bodywork, which have been shown to reduce depression and anxiety and to help ameliorate some of the fluid retention that makes PMS so physically uncomfortable.[49]

Modality Recommendations for Premenstrual Syndrome

Deep tissue massage	Supportive for relaxation and relief from discomfort.
Lymphatic drainage	Supportive.
Polarity	S/R/D: Indicated.
PNF/MET/stretching	Supportive.
Reflexology	Indicated. Work pituitary, thyroid, ovaries, uterus, pelvic area, low back, hips, intestines, spine, brain, solar plexus points.
Shiatsu	Indicated. Treat SP, LV, GB, BL, K, PC, SI, LI meridians and extensions, especially in legs, abdomen, and back.
Swedish massage	Supportive.
Trigger point therapy	Supportive; lighter work may be necessary in the abdominal region.

See Chapter 1 for a brief description of each modality, including definitions of abbreviations.

Sexually Transmitted Diseases

Definition: What Are They?

Sexually transmitted diseases (STDs) are infections that spread through intimate contact. The primary mode of transmission is through vaginal, oral, or anal sex, although an infected mother carries a risk of infecting her baby either through the blood or through direct contact during birth.

Demographics: Who Gets Them?

Most STDs are diagnosed among adolescents and young adults. People aged 15 to 25 account for almost half of new infections.[49] As people tend to become sexually active at an earlier age and marry at a later age than in previous generations, the average number of sex partners a person has is increasing. This trend also increases the risk of exposure to many STDs, some of which can occur concurrently and many of which have dangerous and even life-threatening complications.

Statistics on STDs can be difficult to gather because it is generally accepted that only a fraction of these often-silent infections are diagnosed. Further, as diagnostic procedures become more readily available (some can now be identified through urinalysis instead of a full pelvic examination or culture of discharge), rates of diagnosis can shift, and it is unclear whether this means more infections are occurring or that more people are being diagnosed early.

The United States has the highest rate of STD diagnosis of all industrialized countries. It is estimated that some 19 million infections are diagnosed each year, at a cost of about $14 billion per year.[49] More information about the infection rates of specific STDs is included in the discussions that follow.

Types of STDs

More than 20 infectious diseases are spread through intimate contact. Several have been discussed elsewhere in this book; they include herpes simplex, HIV/AIDS, and hepatitis B and C. This

Sexually Transmitted Diseases in Brief

Pronunciation: SEKS-u-ah-le tranz-MIH-ted

What are they?

Sexually transmitted diseases (STDs) are contagious conditions that are spread through intimate contact. The three major diseases discussed here, chlamydia, gonorrhea, and syphilis, are all bacterial infections. Most other STDs, including genital herpes, *Molluscum contagiosum*, and genital warts, are viral infections.

How are they recognized?

The major bacterial STDs all share some signs when any signs are present at all. These include penile or vaginal discharge, painful urination, and painful intercourse. Other more specific symptoms vary by causative agent.

Is massage indicated or contraindicated?

Bacterial STDs are responsive to antibiotic therapy. Once an infection has been identified and controlled, massage is perfectly appropriate. Silent conditions that are untreated may lead to serious complications that contraindicate massage, depending on the severity of the infection.

discussion has been reserved for the most common bacterial STDs, chlamydia, gonorrhea, and syphilis, followed by a brief look at some others.

Chlamydia

Definition: What Is It?

Chlamydia is a bacterial infection with the agent *Chlamydia trachomatis.*

Demographics: Who Gets It?

Statistics on the rate of new infection with this bacterium are hard to gather. It is often completely asymptomatic in women, so it is difficult to project exactly how many people might be infected. The Centers for Disease Control and Prevention document that in 2005 new chlamydia infections were reported in more than 976,000 people,[49] but it may cause more than 3 million new infections each year.[50] The group with the highest rate of chlamydia infection is people 15 to 19 years old.[51]

Etiology: What Happens?

The bacteria that cause chlamydia have an affinity for columnar mucus-producing cells. These infections can develop at any site of sexual contact: the reproductive tract, the mouth and throat, and the anus.

The real danger with chlamydia is that while it is silently attacking columnar mucus cells in the reproductive tract, it can invade the uterus and uterine tubes, where a chronic low-grade infection and inflammatory response may lead to permanent scarring and infertility. This is one variety of pelvic inflammatory disease (PID) (Sidebar 11.11).

SIDEBAR 11.11: PELVIC INFLAMMATORY DISEASE

Pelvic inflammatory disease (PID) is an infection anywhere in the upper reproductive tract of women. Infection of the uterus (***endometritis***), infection of the uterine tubes (***salpingitis***), or abscesses on the ovaries (***oophoritis***) can all fall under the umbrella term of PID.

PID is usually the result of a bacterial infection that begins in the vagina. The infectious agent is often chlamydia or gonorrhea or both, but possible causes also include irritation from an IUD or incomplete elective or spontaneous abortion.

PID can be an acute or chronic infection. Acute PID is, as its name implies, a serious and severe condition. Its symptoms include abdominal pain; low back pain; fever; chills; nausea; vomiting; painful intercourse; heavy, irregular periods; and heavy, pus-laden vaginal discharge. Chronic PID has low-grade long-term symptoms that seldom flare up into an acute infection but that can ultimately cause the same kind of internal damage and complications as acute PID. Its symptoms include mild abdominal pain, backache, heavy menstrual periods, painful intercourse, and general lethargy.

Common complications of PID include infertility, ectopic pregnancy, and chronic pelvic pain. PID becomes dangerous when the infection backs up from the vagina to the uterus and into the fallopian tubes, where it can start growing in the open pelvic cavity. Occasionally PID causes the growth of tubo-ovarian abscesses. If an abscess ruptures, it releases infectious material into the pelvis. In either case, life-threatening peritonitis is the result.

PID is usually a fairly simple bacterial infection. Caught early, it responds well to antibiotics and bed rest, although some women need hospitalization and intravenous antibiotics. Sexual activity must be curtailed for several weeks, and the woman's sexual partner or partners should also be treated for gonorrhea or chlamydia if either of those is causing the infection.

Signs and Symptoms

Chlamydia is often silent; three-quarters of infected women and about half of infected men report no symptoms. When symptoms are present, they include vaginal or penile discharge, pain and burning during urination, and painful intercourse. If the infection invades the upper female reproductive tract, signs of PID (fever, abdominal and low back pain, inflamed lymph nodes) may be present.

Complications

The primary complication of a chlamydia infection for a woman is PID and the risk of ectopic pregnancy or lifelong infertility. An infection in a man may cause epididymitis, swelling of the testicles, and a risk of infertility for him too. A baby born to a woman with undiagnosed chlamydia has a risk of exposure in the birth canal that may lead to conjunctivitis or life-threatening pneumonia. A chlamydia infection also increases the rate of HIV transmission; the virus crosses from one partner to another more easily when a bacterial infection is present.

Diagnosis and Treatment

Chlamydia is typically diagnosed by taking a culture from the cervix or penis, but new tests allow for identification by urinalysis. If tests come back positive for an active chlamydia infection, a course of antibiotics is usually successful, as long as the person and all of his or her sex partners are treated completely. Chlamydia often appears with gonorrhea, which requires a different antibiotic treatment, so it is important to get a thorough diagnosis. Exposure and treatment for chlamydia does not impart immunity, so any future exposure to this pathogen can lead to a new infection that requires treatment.

Gonorrhea

Definition

Gonorrhea is infection with the bacterium *Neisseria gonorrhoeae*. This is a diplococcal bacterium, a spherical cell that tends to clump together in characteristic pairs.

Demographics: Who Gets It?

Gonorrhea is reported as a new infection about 339,000 times a year in this country,[49] but it may occur in up to 600,000 new infections.[52]

Etiology: What Happens?

Gonorrhea is spread through intimate contact. It can infect the throat, vagina, and rectum. It is rarely transmitted by any contact other than sex; it is unusual for a pregnant mother with gonorrhea to pass it to her child. Once inside the body, gonorrhea may infect other tissues than mucous membranes; it often affects joints in a condition called gonococcal arthritis, which can lead to permanent joint damage.

Signs and Symptoms

Like chlamydia, gonorrhea is often silent, especially in women. If symptoms do appear in a woman, they typically include vaginal discharge, urinary discomfort, and painful intercourse. An infection from oral sex may lead to sores in the mouth and a sore throat.

Male symptoms of gonorrhea include burning on urination, a yellow-white discharge from the penis, and *orchitis*, or swelling of the testicles.

Complications

Like chlamydia, gonorrhea has a high risk of developing into PID; this happens with 10% to 20% of women whose gonorrhea goes untreated.[52] As mentioned previously, gonorrhea can infect joints, causing septic arthritis. And as with chlamydia, the presence of gonorrhea increases the transmission rate of HIV.

Diagnosis and Treatment

Gonorrhea is diagnosed by a culture of mucus from the rectum, cervix, throat, or penis. It is responsive to antibiotics, although it has developed resistance to penicillin and is developing resistance to a number of other antibiotics. It frequently appears with chlamydia, which requires concurrent treatment with a different antibiotic.

A person with septic arthritis from gonorrhea may benefit from careful stretching and mobilization of the affected joints once the infection has been eradicated. Massage may be appropriate at this time as well.

Syphilis

Definition: What Is It?

Syphilis is an infection with a spirochetal bacterium, *Treponema pallidum*.

Demographics: Who Gets It?

Diagnosis rates of syphilis reached an all-time low in 2000 and have been slowly climbing ever since. It is identified about 8,700 times per year[49] but may actually infect up to 35,000 people each year.[53]

Etiology: What Happens?

Syphilis spreads through sexual contact and from mother to unborn child. This bacterium is very fragile outside a host and does not last when exposed to air or sunlight.

Syphilis moves through the system in specific stages. It is communicable only in the first two stages of infection. In the late stage, although it may cause very serious problems in the infected person, it is no longer contagious.

This bacterium is transmitted when an infected lesion comes in contact with microscopic openings in another person's skin. Syphilis travels through the blood and may affect joints, bones, blood vessels, and the central nervous system if it is untreated.

Signs and Symptoms

Primary syphilis is detectable 10 days to 3 months after exposure, when a characteristic ***chancre***, or open ulcer, appears. A chancre is usually not acutely painful, and if it appears inside the vaginal canal, a woman may not be aware of it. The tissue in chancres is very contagious. A typical chancre heals in 3 to 6 weeks.

Secondary syphilis takes the form of a rash of open brownish sores that appear several weeks after the chancre heals. This rash is often on the soles of the feet or palms of the hands, but it may be anywhere. These lesions are also highly infectious. The rash associated with secondary syphilis may come and go for 1 to 2 years before the infection becomes latent.

In some people syphilis becomes a silent infection after the secondary stage and may produce no further symptoms. No skin lesions appear, and the infection is no longer contagious. However, about one-third of people with secondary syphilis develop tertiary syphilis, a condition in which the bacteria invade other body systems. At this point the infection may attack the bones and joints, causing rheumatic pain, or the blood vessels, causing a risk of aneurysm. Most significantly, syphilis may attack the central nervous system, leading to a range of problems including blindness, loss of hearing, stroke, meningitis, or psychosis.

Complications

Like other bacterial STDs, syphilis significantly increases the transmission rate of HIV. A pregnant woman with syphilis, if she doesn't miscarry, has a nearly 100% chance of spreading the disease to her newborn through the bloodstream. Babies born with syphilis may not have symptoms immediately but may develop vision or central nervous system problems along with syphilitic rhinitis; their mucus secretions are highly contagious.

Other complications of tertiary syphilis have already been described.

Diagnosis and Treatment

The good news is that syphilis is simple to diagnose and to treat. It can be diagnosed by examining a scraping of a chancre or secondary rash or by a blood test. Syphilis is sensitive to penicillin, and a single dose is typically adequate. Treatment must be administered before organ damage takes place, however. Syphilitic damage to the central nervous system, blood vessels, and other structures is irreversible.

Other STDs

These STDs, although less of a concern than chlamydia, syphilis, and gonorrhea, warrant some discussion:

- ***Nongonococcal urethritis*** (NGU) is a bacterial infection of the urinary tract by an agent other than gonorrhea. It is often related to chlamydia, *Ureaplasma urealyticum*, or adenovirus. It is usually an STD but can also be related to prostatitis, UTI, or catheterization. If it is identified as a bacterial infection, it can be successfully treated with antibiotics.
- *Trichomoniasis* is a common infection, affecting up to 7.4 million men and women each year.[54] The infectious agent is a protozoan parasite that causes vaginal discharge, pain, itching, and an increased risk of HIV transmission. Trichomoniasis is treatable with medication.
- ***Molluscum contagiosum*** virus (MCV) is a generally benign condition that is commonly seen among children, in whom it is not an STD. It has increasing incidence among adults, however, as a result of skin-to-skin contact. It may also be transmissible through other surfaces; it may spread by contact with towels or other cloth or possibly even in water, as in a shared bath. When MCV appears as an STD, it appears on the thighs, buttocks, groin, external genitalia, and anus. It is treated by removing the growths with topical chemicals or cryotherapy.
- *Genital warts* are also called *Condylomata acuminata*. They affect more than 5 million people each year. They can grow on the vulva, the walls of the vagina, the perineum, or cervix of a woman or on the penis, scrotum, or anus of a man. Oral infections may grow in the mouth or throat. They have a high transmission rate; exposure leads to infection about two-thirds of the time.[55] Genital warts are typically small but can grow in large clusters. They may grow large enough to interfere with a pregnancy. Many types of human papilloma virus (HPV) can cause genital warts, and some of them are associated with cervical, penile, or vulvar cancer. Genital warts can be removed, but over-the-counter medications that treat common warts are inappropriate for these lesions, which grow on sensitive, delicate tissues.

Prevention

The transmission of STDs can be prevented, but the only completely consistent method is to practice abstinence. Having sex only with one partner who is known to be uninfected is of course highly recommended. Barrier methods of birth control (male or female condoms) provide protection from some but not all STDs: *Molluscum contagiosum*, genital warts, and syphilis may spread to areas not covered by condoms. And of course, other methods of birth control (spermicidal cream, birth control pills, and other hormonal applications) provide no protection from STDs.

Massage?

Most STDs are only spread through sexual contact, which makes communicability for massage therapists not an issue. Exceptions to this rule include *Molluscum contagiosum*, genital warts, and open syphilis lesions, which can travel by skin-to-skin contact and whose lesions may not be confined to the genitalia.

If a client knows he or she is positive for any type of STD, the first priority is to treat the infection. Since most of these clear within days of the administration of antibiotics, it is not a great hardship to postpone a massage until after the infection has resolved.

MODALITY RECOMMENDATIONS FOR SEXUALLY TRANSMITTED DISEASES	
Deep tissue massage	Systemically contraindicated while acute; otherwise supportive.
Lymphatic drainage	Systemically contraindicated while acute; otherwise supportive.
Polarity	S: Indicated. R/D: Contraindicated while acute; otherwise supportive with pressure determined by client's comfort.
PNF/MET/stretching	Supportive.
Reflexology	Contraindicated while acute; otherwise work lymphatic, endocrine, reproductive system points.
Shiatsu	Supportive.
Swedish massage	Contraindicated while acute; otherwise supportive with caution for open lesions away from genital region.
Trigger point therapy	Systemically contraindicated while acute; otherwise supportive.

See Chapter 1 for a brief description of each modality, including definitions of abbreviations.

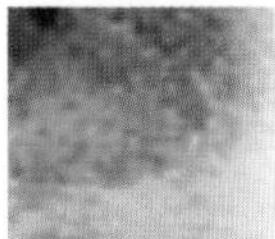

CHAPTER REVIEW QUESTIONS: REPRODUCTIVE SYSTEM CONDITIONS

1. Why have death rates from cervical cancer decreased in the past century? Why will they probably continue to decline?
2. Where are endometrial growths usually found?
3. What is the most common symptom of uterine fibroid tumors?
4. What is the lifetime risk for a woman in the United States to develop breast cancer?
5. Explain the significance of finding a sentinel node in the treatment of breast cancer.
6. Why does ovarian cancer have such a high death rate?
7. What is the difference between a follicular cyst and a corpus luteum cyst?
8. Why is it particularly easy for a man to ignore or discount the early symptoms of prostate cancer?
9. When is menopause identified?
10. A client has PMS. She is in the luteal phase of her cycle and would like to receive a massage. What are potential risks and benefits?

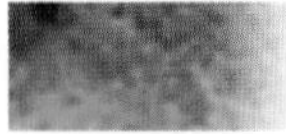

REFERENCES

1. Puscheck E, Pradhan A. First-Trimester Pregnancy Loss. © 1996–2006 by WebMD. http://www.emedicine.com/med/topic3310.htm. Accessed autumn 2006.
2. Cancer of the Cervix Uteri. National Cancer Institute. http://seer.cancer.gov/statfacts/html/cervix.html. Accessed autumn 2006.

3. Cervical Cancer. © 2006 by American Cancer Society, Inc. http://documents.cancer.org/115.00/115.00.pdf. Accessed autumn 2006.
4. FDA Approves First Cervical Cancer Vaccine. © 2006 Medscape. http://www.medscape.com/viewarticle/535778. Accessed autumn 2006.
5. HPV update: Condoms offer protection from HPV infection. © 1998–2006 Mayo Foundation for Medical Education and Research. All rights reserved. http://www.mayoclinic.com/health/hpv/WO00121. Accessed autumn 2006.
6. Edmundson L, Erogul M. Dysmenorrhea. © 1996–2006 by WebMD. http://www.emedicine.com/emerg/topic156.htm. Accessed autumn 2006.
7. Wang L, Cardini F, Zhao W, et al. Vitamin K Acupuncture Point Injection for Severe Primary Dysmenorrhea: An International Pilot Study. Medscape General Medicine. 2004;6(4):45. © 2004 Medscape. http://www.medscape.com/viewarticle/494022. Accessed autumn 2006.
8. Mounsey A, Wilgus A, Slawson D. Diagnosis and Management of Endometriosis. © 2006 by the American Academy of Family Physicians. http://www.aafp.org/afp/20060815/594.html. Accessed autumn 2006.
9. Statistics about Endometriosis. © 2000–2005 Adviware Pty Ltd. All rights reserved. http://www.wrongdiagnosis.com/e/endometriosis/stats.htm. Accessed autumn 2006.
10. Facts About Endometriosis. © 2006 by The Cleveland Clinic. http://www.clevelandclinic.org/health/health-info/docs/1100/1119.asp?index=5751. Accessed autumn 2006.
11. Saul T, Davé A. Endometriosis. © 1996–2006 by WebMD. http://www.emedicine.com/EMERG/topic165.htm. Accessed autumn 2006.
12. Fibroid Tumors Lack Crucial Structural Protein. National Institute of Child Health and Human Development. http://www.nichd.nih.gov/news/releases/fibroid_tumors.cfm. Accessed autumn 2006.
13. What Are the Key Statistics about Endometrial Cancer? © 2006 American Cancer Society, Inc. http://www.cancer.org/docroot/CRI/content/CRI_2_4_1X_What_are_the_key_statistics_for_endometrial_cancer.asp?sitearea=. Accessed autumn 2006.
14. Winter W, Gosewehr J. Uterine Cancer. © 1996–2006 by WebMD. http://www.emedicine.com/med/topic2832.htm. Accessed autumn 2006.
15. Endometrial Cancer (PDQ®): Prevention. National Cancer Institute. http://www.cancer.gov/cancertopics/pdq/prevention/endometrial/HealthProfessional/page2. Accessed autumn 2006.
16. Endometrial cancer. © 1998–2006 Mayo Foundation for Medical Education and Research. All rights reserved. http://www.mayoclinic.com/health/endometrial-cancer/DS00306. Accessed autumn 2006.
17. How Is Endometrial Cancer Staged? © 2006 American Cancer Society, Inc. http://www.cancer.org/docroot/cri/content/cri_2_4_3x_how_is_endometrial_cancer_staged.asp?sitearea=cri. Accessed autumn 2006.
18. How Is Uterine Sarcoma Diagnosed? © 2006 American Cancer Society, Inc. http://www.cancer.org/docroot/cri/content/cri_2_4_3x_how_is_uterine_sarcoma_diagnosed_63.asp?sitearea=cri. Accessed autumn 2006.
19. What You Need to Know about Breast Cancer. National Cancer Institute. http://www.cancer.gov/cancertopics/wyntk/breast/allpages. Accessed autumn 2006.
20. Gandey A. Sudden Decline in Breast Cancer Could Be Linked to HRT. © 2006 Medscape. http://www.medscape.com/viewarticle/549425. Accessed autumn 2006.
21. Breast Cancer. © 1998–2006 Mayo Foundation for Medical Education and Research. All rights reserved. http://www.mayoclinic.com/health/breast-cancer/DS00328. Accessed autumn 2006.
22. Breast Cancer Treatment Guidelines for Patients. © 2006 American Cancer Society, Inc. http://www.cancer.org/downloads/CRI/Breast_VIII.pdf. Accessed autumn 2006.
23. FDA Expands Use of Herceptin for Early Stage Breast Cancer After Primary Therapy. U.S. Food & Drug Administration. http://www.fda.gov/bbs/topics/NEWS/2006/NEW01511.html. Accessed autumn 2006.
24. Cancer of the Ovary. National Cancer Institute. http://seer.cancer.gov/statfacts/html/ovary.html. Accessed autumn 2006.
25. What Are the Key Statistics about Ovarian Cancer? © 2006 American Cancer Society, Inc. http://www.cancer.org/docroot/CRI/content/CRI_2_4_1X_What_are_the_key_statistics_for_ovarian_cancer_33.asp?sitearea=. Accessed autumn 2006.
26. Garcia A, Hamid O. Ovarian Cancer. © 1996–2006 by WebMD. http://www.emedicine.com/med/topic1698.htm. Accessed autumn 2006.
27. Hormone Therapy Ups Ovarian-Cancer Risk. © 2006 ScoutNews, LLC. All rights reserved. http://www.nlm.nih.gov/medlineplus/news/fullstory_39492.html. Accessed autumn 2006.

28. Benign Prostatic Hyperplasia (BPH). © 2005. All rights reserved. http://www.urologyhealth.org/content/moreinfo/bphtreatment.pdf. Accessed autumn 2006.
29. Leveillee R, Patel V. Prostate Hyperplasia, Benign. © 1996–2006 by WebMD. http://www.emedicine.com/med/topic1919.htm. Accessed autumn 2006.
30. Prostate Enlargement: Benign Prostatic Hyperplasia. National Institute of Diabetes and Digestive and Kidney Diseases. NIH Publication 06–3012. http://kidney.niddk.nih.gov/kudiseases/pubs/prostateenlargement/index.htm. Accessed autumn 2006.
31. Benign Prostatic Hyperplasia (BPH). © 1996–2005 MedicineNet, Inc. All rights reserved. http://www.medicinenet.com/benign_prostatic_hyperplasia/article.htm. Accessed autumn 2006.
32. Prostate Cancer. © 2006 American Cancer Society, Inc. http://documents.cancer.org/117.00/117.00.pdf. Accessed autumn 2006.
33. Prostate Cancer (PDQ®): Screening. National Cancer Institute. http://www.cancer.gov/cancerinfo/pdq/screening/prostate/patient/. Accessed autumn 2006.
34. Epidemiology and demographics of prostatitis. Andrologia, vol 35:5, 252, October 2003. http://www.blackwellsynergy.com/doi/full/10.1046/j.14390272.2003.00584.x?cookieSet=1. Accessed autumn 2006.
35. Henderson S, Magana R. Prostatitis. © 1996–2006 by WebMD. http://www.emedicine.com/emerg/topic488.htm. Accessed autumn 2006.
36. Testicular Cancer: Questions and Answers. National Cancer Institute. http://www.cancer.gov/cancertopics/factsheet/Sites-Types/testicular/print?page=&keyword Accessed autumn 2006.
37. What Are the Key Statistics About Testicular Cancer? © 2006 American Cancer Society, Inc. http://www.cancer.org/docroot/cri/content/cri_2_4_1x_what_are_the_key_statistics_for_testicular_cancer_41.as p?sitearea=&level=. Accessed autumn 2006.
38. How Is Testicular Cancer Staged? © 2006 American Cancer Society, Inc. http://www.cancer.org/docroot/cri/content/cri_2_4_3x_how_is_testicular_cancer_staged_41.asp?sitearea=ped. Accessed autumn 2006.
39. About Menopause. © 2007 The North American Menopause Society. All rights reserved. http://www.menopause.org/aboutmeno/04A.pdf. Accessed autumn 2006.
40. Curran D, Bachmann G. Menopause. © 1996–2006 by WebMD. http://www.emedicine.com/med/topic3289.htm. Accessed autumn 2006.
41. Expert Believes Early HRT Can Have Heart Benefits. © 2006 Reuters Limited. All rights reserved. http://www.nlm.nih.gov/medlineplus/news/fullstory_42930.html. Accessed autumn 2006.
42. Menopause: One Woman's Story, Every Woman's Story. National Institute on Aging, National Institutes of Health. http://www.niapublications.org/pubs/menopause/menopauseupdate2003.pdf. Accessed autumn 2006.
43. Do CAM Therapies Help Menopausal Symptoms? National Center for Complementary and Alternative Medicine. http://nccam.nih.gov/health/menopauseandcam/menopauseandcam.pdf. Accessed autumn 2006.
44. Evaluating the Risk for Pregnancy-Associated Venous Thromboembolism: A 30-Year Study. Ann Intern Med vol 143, 697–706. http://www.annals.org/cgi/content/full/143/10/I-12. Accessed autumn 2006.
45. Gestational Diabetes. © American Diabetes Association. http://www.diabetes.org/gestational-diabetes.jsp. Accessed winter 2007.
46. Shah AK. Preeclampsia and Eclampsia. © 1996–2207 WebMD. http://www.emedicine.com/neuro/topic323.htm. Accessed winter 2007.
47. Lozeau AM, Potter B. Diagnosis and Management of Ectopic Pregnancy. Am Fam Physician 2005;72:1707–1714, 1719–1720. © 2005 American Academy of Family Physicians. http://www.aafp.org/afp/20051101/1707.html. Accessed winter 2007.
48. Premenstrual syndrome (PMS). © 1998–2006 Mayo Foundation for Medical Education and Research. All rights reserved. http://www.mayoclinic.com/health/premenstrual-syndrome/DS00134. Accessed autumn 2006.
49. Trends in Reportable Sexually Transmitted Diseases in the United States, 2005. Centers for Disease Control and Prevention. http://www.cdc.gov/std/stats/05pdf/trends-2005.pdf. Accessed autumn 2006.
50. Chlamydia. © 2005 Planned Parenthood Federation of America, Inc. All rights reserved. http://www.plannedparenthood.org/sexual-health/std/chlamydia.htm. Accessed autumn 2006.
51. Morrow R, Smith C, Sutherland K. Chlamydia Screening of Young Adults. © 2006 Medscape. http://www.medscape.com/viewprogram/5570. Accessed autumn 2006.

52. Gonorrhea. © 2004 Planned Parenthood Federation of America, Inc. All rights reserved. http://www.plannedparenthood.org/sexual-health/std/gonorrhea.htm. Accessed autumn 2006.
53. Syphilis. © 2005 Planned Parenthood Federation of America, Inc. All rights reserved. http://www.plannedparenthood.org/sexual-health/std/syphilis.htm. Accessed autumn 2006.
54. Trichomoniasis—CDC Fact Sheet. Division of STD Prevention, Centers for Disease Control. http://www.cdc.gov/STD/Trichomonas/STDFact-Trichomoniasis.htm. Accessed winter 2007.
55. Genital Warts. © 1998–2007 Mayo Foundation for Medical Education and Research. http://www.mayoclinic.com/health/genital-warts/DS00087. Accessed winter 2007.

12

Principles of Cancer

Chapter Objectives

After reading this chapter, you should be able to . . .

- Describe the difference between a carcinoma and a sarcoma.
- Name two internal factors for cancer development.
- Name five infections associated with cancer risk.
- Name six early signs of cancer.
- Identify what TNM stands for.
- Name five treatment options for cancer.
- Name three complications or side effects of cancer treatment.
- Name three cautions for massage and cancer.
- Name three cautions for massage and cancer treatments.

PRINCIPLES OF CANCER

Cancer comprises more than 100 diseases that have one thing in common: normal body cells mutate slightly and begin to replicate uncontrollably. When the malignant cells begin in epithelial cells, the cancer is called **carcinoma**. When the original cells are muscle or connective tissue, the cancer is a type of **sarcoma**.

Many excellent resources are available for massage therapists and bodyworkers who want to explore working with cancer patients; these are listed in the bibliography on the Student Resource CD. The principles laid out here are designed to provide background information for the discussions that appear in this book, which include skin cancer; leukemia; myeloma; lymphoma; lung cancer; esophageal, stomach, colorectal, liver, and pancreatic cancer; thyroid cancer; bladder cancer; and cervical, uterine, breast, ovarian, prostate, and testicular cancer.

Cancer Statistics

About half of men and one-third of women in the United States will develop some sort of cancer in their lifetime. Cancer is diagnosed in about 1.4 million people and kills about 560,000 (about 1,500 per day) in the United States every year.[1] It is the second leading cause of death in the United States (heart disease is still the first).[2]

Survival rates from cancer continue to climb. From 1995 to 2001 the estimated 5-year survival rate for all types of cancer combined was 65%; this is up from 50% in the 1970s. However, the 5-year survival rate means only that the patient didn't die of cancer within 5 years of being diagnosed; it does not imply that a person is cancer free if he is alive 5 years after his or her cancer was first recognized.

Approximately 10.1 million people in the United States have had cancer. While deaths from cancer are generally dropping in this country, it is estimated that up to half of newly diagnosed cases of cancer could be prevented with lifestyle changes or interrupted through early screening.[3]

Skin cancer is the most common variety reported (and these statistics do not reflect the countless moles that are removed as a safeguard against melanoma development), but lung cancer is the leading cause of death by cancer for both men and women. Other leading causes of death include breast and ovarian cancer for women, prostate cancer for men, and cancer of the colon, rectum, and pancreas for both genders.[4]

Steps in Metastasis

It is still unclear exactly why or how a healthy cell changes into a malignant cell. One thing that all cancers have in common is that the DNA of a cell mutates so that the cell acquires certain growth properties. As researchers learn more about metastasis, new ways to interrupt the process and limit the ability of cancer cells to invade and destroy healthy tissue are being discovered.

The following is a simplified version of metastasis as it is understood at this writing:

- *Oncogene activation*. An **oncogene** is a gene that initiates malignant characteristics within a cell. Oncogene activation is the beginning of the changes that cause certain cells to become malignant. The trigger for activation may be toxic environmental exposures, diet, genetic predisposition, or some combination of them, but it is often not clear. Oncogenes are typically inhibited by the activity of tumor suppressor genes. Eventually it may be found that a lack of tumor suppressor genes (instead of or in addition to a surfeit of oncogenes) may be a significant factor in cancer risk.
- *Proliferation*. The mutated cells proliferate without control, often piling up into distinct masses called tumors. As they do this, they may secrete enzymes that allow them to survive a normal immune system attack. As masses of cells accumulate, they begin to lose the characteristics that define their tissue type. This lack of differentiation is associated with aggressiveness of the tumor.
- *Angiogenesis*. ***Angiogenesis*** is the growth of blood vessels to supply a tumor. Any growth of more than 1 or 2 cm^3 requires a dedicated blood supply. Some cancer cells seem well supplied with the chemical messengers that command the body to build new capillaries. The more highly invested a tumor is with blood vessels, the more likely it is to have metastasized.
- *Invasion*. As a tumor grows, it must convince the local extracellular matrix to make room for it without stimulating an inflammatory response. Again, special enzymes secreted by cancer cells are at the center of this process. These enzymes help to dissolve the connective tissue that provides the support for epithelium, where most cancers grow. This process doesn't stimulate a normal inflammatory response, which is partly why cancer is often silent in early stages.
- *Migration*. Cancer cells break off the primary tumor and travel to new areas. The circulatory or lymphatic system may be used as a transfer medium, but cancer cells can also spread through direct contact with other organs or in peritoneal fluid.

- *Colonization.* When cancer cells land in a new target tissue, they must begin the process over again, starting with proliferation. This requires that the cells be able to adhere to the new tissue and that they secrete the correct enzymes to suppress an immune system attack, create new blood vessels, and erode the new extracellular matrix. The first tumor that grows in the disease process is called the primary tumor; other tumors that grow from metastasis of the primary tumor are called secondary tumors. In other words, a tumor in the bladder that metastasized from the ovary is not bladder cancer. It is secondary ovarian cancer in the bladder.

It is unclear how often cells become malignant in an average human life. It may be a fairly common occurrence that simply is not successful as long as immune system mechanisms prevent the growth of abnormal new cells. This raises some interesting questions about the connections between cancer, stress, and immune system efficiency.

Causes

Triggers for oncogene activation vary by tissue type and individual case. Causes of cancer are slowly being narrowed to some identifiable factors. These are generally discussed as *internal* or *external* factors.

Internal Factors

Every cell in the body has a built-in capacity for self-destruction. This is a natural and healthy process called ***apoptosis***, or programmed cell death. A specific gene in some cancer cells has been found to inhibit apoptosis. Therefore, some cancers may be as much related to cells that refuse to die as it is to new cells coming to life.

Some cancers are brought about by or connected to inherited characteristics. This means an inherited gene is likely to cause cellular mutations sometime in the future. Such genes have been identified for a small percentage of breast and colon cancers. It may also mean that a person has a genetic susceptibility to environmental factors that would not be a threat to someone else.

Other internal factors may include hormonal activity (some hormones appear to stimulate malignant cell division) and immune system problems with the ability to recognize and fight off cancer cells.

External Factors

Carcinogens are chemical or environmental agents that have been identified as cancer causers. The National Institutes of Health lists 246 substances as carcinogens.[5] This list includes the hydrocarbons in cigarette smoke; compounds created when meats are grilled over high heat; and several substances found in dyes, inks, and paint. Radiation from the sun, radon gas, gamma rays, or excessive x-rays can cause cancer, as can exposure to asbestos, benzene, nickel, cadmium, uranium, and vinyl chloride.

In addition to environmental irritants and pollutants, some pathogens have been determined to cause certain types of cancer. Others simply have a strong statistical link with the development of various cancers, but the cause-and-effect relationship has not been defined. Cancer-related pathogens include viruses, bacteria, and animal parasites.

Viruses Some viral triggers for cancer include the following:

- *HTLV-1* (human T-lymphotrophic virus) resembles HIV; it is a retrovirus that is spread through intimate fluids. It can cause lymphocytic leukemia and non-Hodgkin lymphoma.

- *HPV* (human papillomavirus) is a large group of viruses associated with various types of warts. A few viruses in this group can cause cancer of the cervix, penis, anus, vagina, vulva, mouth, and throat. At this point it is not possible to tell from early cellular changes whether the HPV involved is dangerous, so all dysplastic cells are removed. Vaccines against some forms of HPV have recently become available.
- *HHV-8* (human herpesvirus 8) can cause Kaposi sarcoma, a type of skin cancer. HHV-8 is active only when the immune system is suppressed. Consequently, Kaposi sarcoma is an indicator disease for HIV infection.
- *HIV* (human immunodeficiency virus) is indirectly associated with cancer via suppressed immune system function that would otherwise protect against both HPV and HHV-8.
- *EBV* (Epstein-Barr virus) is another herpesvirus. It resides in B cells and usually causes mononucleosis in its first infection. EBV is associated with an increased risk of nasopharyngeal cancer, Burkitt lymphoma, Hodgkin lymphoma, and stomach cancer.
- *HBV* and *HCV* (hepatitis B and C viruses) open the door to liver cancer through chronic long-term inflammation that interrupts function in epithelial cells.

Bacteria These bacteria contribute to some cancers:

- *Helicobacter pylori*, which is also associated with peptic ulcers, has been seen to convert nitrites in foods to potential carcinogens. It is implicated in stomach cancer and lymphoma.
- *Others* include *Borrelia burgdorferi* (the spirochete that causes Lyme disease) and *Campylobacter jejuni*, which have both been associated with digestive tract lymphomas.

Animal parasites Some animal parasites are associated with an increased cancer risk:

- *Liver flukes* are associated with cancer in bile ducts. They are spread through the consumption of raw or undercooked fish. Liver flukes are not found in the United States.
- *Schistosoma haematobium* can cause cancer of the urinary bladder. They are spread through contaminated water. They are not found in the United States but may be carried by those who travel to areas where the parasites are common.

It is often a combination of external and internal factors that tips the scales in favor of developing cancer. Exposure to carcinogens in certain combinations can also be dangerous. For example, heavy smoking combined with excessive alcohol consumption is an especially potent combination for developing cancers of the mouth or upper gastrointestinal tract. Very often many years or even decades may pass between the initial exposure to a carcinogen and the development of distinguishable tumors. This makes it difficult to pin down precise causes of cancer that are consistent from person to person.

Signs and Symptoms

Signs and symptoms of cancer vary widely, depending on the site. One of the most insidious features of this disease is that it is often painless until it is far advanced. Tumors begin to cause pain when they press on nerve endings or when they cause a blockage in a tube or duct that in turn presses on nerve endings. A list of common signs that are red flags for the possibility of cancer includes the following:[1,6]

- A change in bowel or bladder habits
- A sore that does not heal, or that comes and goes in the same place
- Unusual bleeding or drainage

- Thickening or lump in the breast or elsewhere
- Indigestion or swallowing difficulty
- A change in a wart or mole
- Persistent cough or hoarseness
- Unexplained weight loss
- Fatigue, anemia
- Fever
- Skin changes, including darkening, yellowing, reddening, or sudden hair growth

Diagnosis

Cancers are found by a variety of methods, depending on the affected part of the body. Many cancers are found by either self- or clinical examinations; this is true for breast, cervical, colorectal, and prostate cancers. Other growths are found by imaging techniques such as radiography, computed tomography (CT), magnetic resonance imaging (MRI), endoscopy, and ultrasound. Barium swallows and barium enemas can reveal tumors in the gastrointestinal tract.

Cancer screening recommendations vary for types of cancer, risk factors, genetic history, and other issues. The most successful screening protocols aim to do two things: to find cancerous cells before symptoms develop, and to show that early detection eventually leads to an increased survival rate. Not all screening protocols accomplish these goals equally well, and some procedures carry risks themselves, including exposure to radiation, perforation of hollow organs, false-negative results, false-positive results, and overdiagnosis that may lead to anxiety and unnecessary therapy, including surgery, for the patient.[2,3] For more details on cancer screening recommendations, see Sidebar 12.1.

If suspicious changes are noted, tissue samples are taken and analyzed for the presence of malignant cells; this is called a biopsy. If these tests are positive, further examinations of the patient follow to determine how far the cancer has developed.

Staging

Most types of cancer develop in predictable enough patterns that they can be staged, or given a label that indicates how far the cancer has advanced. Staging is based on collected knowledge about how cancer grows and how readily various types of cancer may metastasize. Some variables include the location of the primary tumor, the size and number of tumors, lymph node involvement, the characteristics of cells in the examined tissue, and the presence or absence of distant growths.

The purpose of staging is to identify how far a cancer has progressed and to determine the best course of treatment. While individual cases vary, a reasonable prediction for survival can often be made with staging information.

Several staging protocols have been developed, but most cancers are rated by the TNM system, which may be translated into the stage 0 to IV system.[4] In addition, tumor cells may be rated by grade, which describes the appearance and aggressiveness of cancer cells.

- *TNM system.* The TNM system rates cancer progression by evaluations of *tumors*, *nodes*, and *metastasis*. These are further explained in Tables 12.1 to 12.3.
- *Stage 0 to IV system.* Some cancers are staged using the TNM system, which is translated to the more familiar stages 0 to IV. Cancers have varying growth patterns, though, so the exact translation from TNM to stages 0 to IV varies by type. The numerical staging system is explained in more detail in Table 12.4.

SIDEBAR 12.1: CANCER SCREENING: WHO, WHAT, WHERE, WHEN, WHY?

The science of early cancer detection is far from fully developed or universally accepted. A survey of several medical agencies yields significantly different guidelines for individuals to follow in the attempt to be vigilant against early signs of cancer. One of the concerns with making screening recommendations is the risk of false positives, or the identification as cancerous of nonthreatening growths. These findings may lead to unnecessary interventions and even dangerous surgeries. Screening recommendations are further complicated by differences for low-risk and high-risk populations.

The following is a brief synopsis of the leading recommendations for early cancer detection.[2] Any of these is subject to change as research reveals whether specific testing procedures actually reduce the mortality rate from the types of cancer they target.

Cancer Type	Low-risk Population Recommendations	High-risk Population Recommendations
Breast cancer	*Self-exam*. Monthly after age 20 onward. *Clinical exam*. Every 3 years from ages 20–39; annually from 40 onward. *Mammogram*. Opinions vary; most suggest exams every 1–3 years starting at age 40 or 50.	This includes women with the identified breast cancer genes, women who have 1st-degree relatives with breast cancer, or women who have had breast or other types of cancer before. Screening schedules are matched to individual cases.
Cervical cancer	When a woman becomes sexually active or reaches age 21 (whichever comes first), she should have an annual pelvic exam and Pap test; with three nomal tests in a row she can cut back to once every 3 years, or by her doctor's recommendation, for as long as she has a cervix. Some studies suggest that testing can be suspended after age 65.	This includes women who have shown signs of cervical dysplasia in pelvic exams or Pap tests. Screening should continue on a yearly basis until patients have three normal tests in a row. Screening can be discontinued if a patient has had a hysterectomy, *unless* the surgery was related to surgical cancer.
Skin cancer	Several agencies recommend a monthly self-exam for changes in skin, with a clinical visual exam every 3 years from age 20 to 40, and annually from age 40 onward.	This includes fair-skinned people, and anyone previously diagnosed with any type of skin cancer or precancerous condition; clinical exams should be scheduled on an as-needed basis.
Prostate cancer	A PSA test and digital rectal exam (DRE) are recommended yearly for men over 50 years old. Early screening for prostate cancer carries a high risk of false-positive results or over-diagnosis.	This includes African American men, and men with a father, brother, or son who have prostate cancer, testing should begin at age 40-45.
Colorectal cancer	Beginning at age 50: a fecal occult blood test (FOBT) or a fecal immunochemical test (FIT) should be conducted every year; a sigmoidoscopy or colonoscopy every 5–10 years.	This includes people with a history of colon polyps, inflammatory bowel disease, or a family history of hereditary colorectal cancer; screening should begin before age 50.
Lung, ovarian, and endometrial cancer	No effective noninvasive screening measures have been developed to detect these cancers in early stages. Post menopausal women with any vaginal bleeding or spotting should consult with their doctor.	Some screening techniques may find these cancers, but they tend to be invasive procedures that are reserved for patients with a high risk for developing them.

DRE, digital rectal examination; FOBT, fecal occult blood test; FIT, fecal immunochemical test; IBD, inflammatory bowel disease.

- *Grade*. Another predictor for how cancer grows is the grade of tumor cells. This refers to two issues: how well differentiated the cells are (the higher the differentiation, the better the prognosis), and the propensity for proliferation, or aggressiveness. Cancer grading is explained further in Table 12.5.[5]

Staging may be further qualified by the use of *A* and *B* designations to allow for differences in patterns of progression.

TABLE 12.1 T: Tumor

Tumor	Definition
Tx	Tumor cannot be evaluated.
T0	No evidence of primary tumor.
Tis	In situ: tumor has not spread to nearby tissue.
T1, T2, T3, T4	These refer to the size and extent of primary tumor.

TABLE 12.2 N: Node

Node	Definition
Nx	Node involvement cannot be evaluated.
N0	No cancer is found in nearby nodes.
N1, N2, N3	These refer to the number and extent of regional lymph nodes invaded by cancer cells.

TABLE 12.3 M: Metastasis

Metastasis	Definition
Mx	Metastasis cannot be evaluated.
M0	No distant metastasis can be found.
M1	Distant metastasis is found.

TABLE 12.4 Numerical Staging

Stage	Definition
0	Cancer in situ: cells have not penetrated tissue beyond original layers of affected tissue.
I, II, III	These refer to the size and extent of tumors, nodal involvement, and invasion of adjacent tissues.
IV	Cancer has spread to another organ. By convention stage IV often means metastasis to other side of diaphragm or into central nervous system.

CNS, central nervous system.

TABLE 12.5 Grading Cancer

Grade	Definition
Gx	Grade cannot be assessed.
G1	Cells are well differentiated (low grade).
G2	Cells are moderately well differentiated (intermediate grade).
G3	Cells are poorly differentiated (high grade).
G4	Cells are undifferentiated (high grade).

Not all cancers lend themselves to the TNM or 0 to IV staging systems. Leukemia and lymphoma do not involve primary tumors, so their staging systems refer to blood counts, symptoms, and grade of cancer cells. Some cancers may be discussed in other terms, such as whether the lesion is operable or whether it has reached nearby organs.

Treatment

Decisions on how to treat cancer depend on the stage it is in, the age and general health of the patient, and what kind of cancer is present. Within each tumor different kinds of cells may require different modes of attack. This makes successful treatment of cancer a matter of finding the correct combination of surgery, chemotherapy, hypothermia, radiation, hormones, and biologic therapies.

- *Surgery.* Cancer surgeries are performed to remove malignant tumors and a margin of healthy tissue around them when possible. A sample of nearby lymph nodes is often taken as well to examine them for signs of metastasis. If a sentinel node can be identified (this is a node through which most or all of the lymph entering an area passes before going on to other nodes), it can be taken alone for examination. This refinement has led to a reduction in some of the complications of cancer surgery.
- *Radiofrequency thermal ablation.* This is a procedure in which instruments are inserted through the skin to the depth of a targeted tumor, and an electrical current essentially "microwaves" cancerous material. It is used for tumors that are not easily accessible for traditional surgery, especially in liver cancer. It may find applications in treatment for kidney and prostate cancer as well.
- *Chemotherapy.* A variety of **cytotoxic** drugs have been developed for use in cancer treatment. These drugs specifically target any fast-growing cells in the body. Therefore, in addition to killing cancer cells they may attack the skin (resulting in hair loss), the gastrointestinal tract (leading to chronic nausea and mouth sores), and the blood cells (causing easy bruising and bleeding disorders as well as anemia and white blood cell suppression).
- *Autologous bone marrow transplant.* This is a procedure in which some healthy bone marrow is harvested from the patient and stored. Then a very extreme course of cytotoxic drugs is administered. This kills the cancer cells, but kills most white blood cells too. After chemotherapy, the stored bone marrow is replanted in the patient, where it replaces the immune system cells killed by chemotherapy. This procedure is for use only in very extreme cases; it has a number of dangerous side effects and serious complications, but it can be a lifesaver if nothing else works. *Allogenic bone marrow transplantation* is a similar procedure with use of the marrow of a closely matched donor.
- *Radiation therapy.* With this type of therapy, high-energy rays are focused on tumors to kill them or slow their growth. The radiation may be applied from an external machine, which requires daily outpatient visits for several weeks, or it may come from small radioactive pellets that are temporarily implanted close to the tumor.
- *Hormone therapy.* Breast and prostate cancer tumors both depend on certain hormones to grow. Therapies to limit the secretion of these hormones or to change the way they affect the body are used in the treatment of these cancers.
- *Hypothermia.* In some cases, specifically with precancerous cells on the skin or cervix, potentially malignant cells may be killed by freezing them off the affected structure.
- *Hyperthermia.* Raising the body's temperature has been seen to make some cancer cells more vulnerable to the effects of chemotherapy. Drugs are sometimes administered through warmed intravenous fluids or when the core temperature has been raised.
- *Biologic therapy.* Weaknesses and inefficiencies in metastasis have led to the development of more refined cancer treatments. These work to support the immune system in identifying and fighting cancer more aggressively. An exciting aspect of this research is that it targets *only* cancer cells, which could keep the side effects of treatment to a minimum. These highly specialized treatments may eventually reach the same prevalence as traditional cancer treatments. For more details on biologic therapy for cancer, see Sidebar 12.2.
- *Stem cell implantation.* The implantation of stem cells specifically for leukemia patients carries promise as an effective treatment. These cellular blanks have the potential to grow into whatever kinds of cells the body needs to replace.

Prevention

Most resources that study cancer publish a list of simple lifestyle choices that can reduce the risk of developing this disease. While different aspects are emphasized for different types of cancer, a basic approach includes these recommendations:

- Eat more fruit, vegetables, and whole grains, controlling dietary fat.
- Exercise regularly and control weight.
- Use sunscreen or clothing to protect the skin from ultraviolet radiation.
- Stop smoking and other tobacco use.
- Use alcohol moderately.
- Practice safe sex. (This is as a precaution against contracting HPV, which is associated with cervical cancer. However, barrier methods such as condoms do *not* reliably protect against the spread of this virus.[7] Therefore, "safe sex" in this context means to have relations only with an uninfected partner.)
- Use early cancer screening methods.

SIDEBAR 12.2: BIOLOGIC THERAPIES FOR CANCER

The options for cancer management today are broader than at any other time in history, with dozens of new possibilities in clinical trials at any given time. The day may come when we can look back on the three basic treatments that dominated the twentieth century (surgery, radiation therapy, chemotherapy) and say, "Aren't we glad those days are over?"

One of the most promising aspects of biologic therapies for cancer is that they target only the cancer cells and aim to minimize damage to healthy tissues that surround them. This may eventually reduce the debilitating side effects and collateral damage traditionally associated with cancer treatment.

Also known as immunotherapy, biotherapy, or biological response modifiers, biologic therapies involve several strategies. They aim to suppress cancer growth; to make cancer cells more recognizable to immune system cells; to boost the killing power of natural killer cells, killer T cells, and macrophages; to alter the growth pattern of new cells so they behave like healthy cells; to enhance healing; and to prevent the spread of suspect cells.

Several branches of biologic therapies are being pursued, including the use of interferons, interleukin-2, and factors that stimulate blood cell production; creation of antibodies against specific cancer cell membranes; vaccines against pathogens that can cause cancer; gene therapy; and many others.

Available forms of biological therapy do carry side effects, including inflammation at the site of injection, flulike symptoms, fatigue, bone pain, muscle aches, and fever.

Massage?

For many years it was assumed that circulatory types of massage carry the risk of aiding metastasis by boosting blood and lymph flow. Research shows, however, that cancerous growths can take years to become established before they are detectable by palpation. It seems far-fetched to suppose that a 60-minute massage could contribute to that process any more significantly than a brisk walk around the block or a long hot shower. Nonetheless, it is inappropriate to rub on a tumor or any undiagnosed swelling or thickening of tissue.

Massage for persons undergoing cancer treatment, however, has a vital and useful role. The five major symptoms of cancer and cancer treatment are pain, anxiety, nausea, fatigue, and depression.[8] In addition, constipation, poor body image, and poor sleep are problems that are well addressed by massage and bodywork. Massage in various forms is being researched in all of these contexts, with varying rates of efficacy. Perhaps most of all, massage provides for a basic human need: nurturing, caring, informed touch at a time when many cancer patients feel isolated and dehumanized. The benefits massage has to offer are so well accepted that many hospitals are now including massage treatments for their cancer patients.[9]

It is important to bear in mind the complications associated with cancer and various cancer treatments because they can have serious implications for the choice of bodywork modalities, especially when multiple treatments are employed. One way to clarify choices about massage for cancer patients is to determine whether certain cautions are brought about by the cancer itself or by cancer treatment.

Cancer Cautions

- *Tumor sites.* Massage should not disrupt any site where tumors or undiagnosed lesions are located close to the surface of the body. Further, a person with any kind of abdominal cancer is not a good candidate for deep abdominal work.

- *Bone involvement.* When cancer metastasizes to bones, they can become brittle and unstable. This can make a person extremely vulnerable to fractures.
- *Vital organ involvement.* A client who has cancer or metastasis in a vital organ (this includes the lungs, liver, brain, kidneys, and heart) may have compromised function of any of those organs. This should be evaluated for how well the patient can adapt to bodywork.
- *Deep vein thrombosis.* A potential complication of both cancer and cancer treatment, deep vein thrombosis is also a significant red flag for massage because of the risk of dislodgment and pulmonary embolism.

SIDEBAR 12.3: LYMPHEDEMA

Part of cancer staging is the removal and examination of local lymph nodes for signs of metastasis. If cancer cells are found, the remaining nodes may be treated with radiation therapy. Both the surgery to remove sample nodes and the treatment to kill cancer that might be growing in remaining nodes can lead to a serious complication called lymphedema.

Lymphedema describes the accumulation of protein-rich fluid in the interstitial spaces as a result of lymph system dysfunction. (This distinguishes it from simple edema, which is typically related to venous insufficiency or local trauma.) The chemistry of interstitial fluid is such that when it doesn't flow freely into nearby lymph vessels, it attracts water. That is, a small amount of fluid retention can become a significant problem in a short period.

Lymphedema can develop in the days or weeks after cancer surgery or radiation therapy, or it can suddenly appear decades later; all that is required is an insufficiency in lymph node function. Patients most at risk for this problem are those who have had nodes removed, had radiation therapy following surgery, who are overweight, and who are sedentary. Once the shift in tissue proteins occurs, the symptoms may subside, but the risk of recurrence is always high.

Signs and symptoms of lymphedema can include redness, heat, and pain; these signs indicate infection along with fluid retention. Often, however, it is simply the deep ache and loss of function of a limb that grows to huge proportions. Pitting edema is another indicator. Lymphedematous limbs are particularly vulnerable to bacterial and fungal infections and must be cared for very carefully.

Long-standing lymphedema can lead to fibrosclerotic changes in the interstitial spaces of the superficial fascia. As a result, the tissue and skin on the affected limb become indurated, or hardened. Once this stage is reached, it is very difficult to reverse.

Standard treatment options for lymphedema are limited. Compression machines, bandages, and supportive clothing are often unsatisfactory. Lymphedema is of particular relevance for massage therapists, because it would seem tempting to use Swedish massage, reputed to influence fluid flow, to help resolve it. However, because of the chemical imbalance in the interstitial spaces, any kind of work that compresses blood vessels only makes lymphedema worse. Various kinds of bodywork techniques have been developed to address lymphedema, but they are very light, and they employ extensive knowledge of the anatomy and physiology of the lymph system to maximize benefits while minimizing risks. Lymphatic techniques are highly specialized, and responsible use of them requires extensive training. Practitioners who learn these techniques, however, are likely to find an eager group of clients hoping to benefit from their work and acceptance in the medical community.

Clients with a history of lymphedema live with a lifetime risk of repeated episodes. While massage to the rest of the body may be safe, massage to the affected extremity must be conducted very conservatively.

Cancer Treatment Cautions

- *Surgery.* Several complications of cancer surgery can have implications for massage. Infection obviously contraindicates massage until the client is out of danger. Constipation is a frequent postsurgical complaint, but deep abdominal massage may be inappropriate, depending on the cancer site. Medical devices may be present after surgery, including ports, catheters, drains, or ostomies. These should be locally avoided, and the client must be positioned in ways that minimize the risk of their disruption. When regional lymph nodes are surgically removed for staging purposes, *lymphedema* may develop; see Sidebar 12.3 for details on this complication. (Figures 12.1 and 12.2)
- *Radiation therapy.* Radiation can affect several areas. When it is applied by an external machine, the skin at the entry and exit sites may become thin, red, and irritated. If radioactive pellets have been implanted, the patient may have to avoid contact with others until they have been removed. The gastrointestinal tract may be irritated, leading to nausea, vomiting, and diarrhea. Bone marrow suppression can lead to anemia, fatigue, poor clotting, and susceptibility to infection. Irradiated lymph nodes can be damaged, leading to a risk of lymphedema. Finally, externally or internally applied radiation can cause debilitating fatigue.
- *Chemotherapy.* Chemotherapeutic drugs may be administered orally or through intravenous drips. They often suppress bone marrow activity, leading to anemia, a risk of infection, and clotting problems. Gastrointestinal tract irritation, mouth sores, and hair loss are other side effects of drugs that kill fast-growing cells. Other complications of chemotherapy include neuropathy, constipation, skin rashes, and mood changes. Some varieties of chemotherapy are expressed through the skin. It may not be appropriate for a patient to be extensively touched during this process.
- *Other therapies.* Other cancer treatments may also hold cautions for massage. Hormone treatments may increase the risk of blood clots; biological therapies may cause fatigue and flulike symptoms; cryotherapy can leave irritated areas on the skin, and so on.

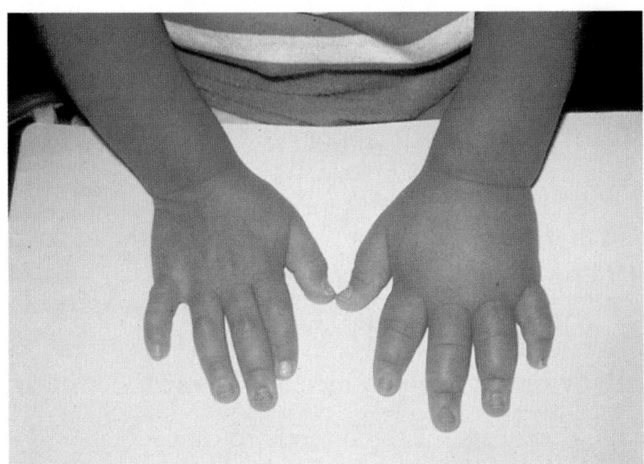

Figure 12.1. Lymphedema.

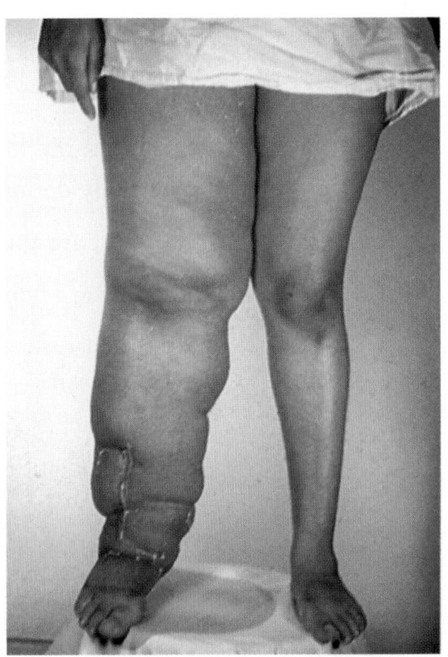

Figure 12.2. Extreme lymphedema.

No matter what kind of cancer or cancer treatments a person is going through, it is vital for his or her massage therapist to communicate with the rest of the health care team to provide the best benefits that bodywork has to offer with minimal risks. For more information on the role of massage and bodywork for cancer patients, please consult the works cited in the bibliography on the Student Resource CD.

Modality Recommendations for Cancer

Deep tissue massage	Can be supportive for people in recovery; work with health care team to increase client's comfort within limits of resilience.
Lymphatic drainage	Indicated, within client's tolerance.
Polarity	S: Indicated. R/D: Supportive within client's limits of activity.
PNF/MET/stretching	Supportive as part of health care team; match to activity levels.
Reflexology	Indicated. Work lymphatic system, pituitary points to increase T-cell production.
Shiatsu	Indicated, with respect for resilience of both client and practitioner. Focus on K, SP, TH meridians for immune support and those associated with affected organ systems.
Swedish massage	Supportive, within client's limits of activity.
Trigger point therapy	Supportive, within client's limits of activity.

See Chapter 1 for a brief description of each modality, including definitions of abbreviations.

Chapter Review Questions

1. Briefly define cancer.
2. Briefly define metastasis.
3. What are the two criteria for a successful cancer screening protocol?
4. Why are lymph nodes sometimes removed from cancer patients?
5. When cancer cells have been found but are limited to only one layer of tissue, what stage is it?
6. When cancer cells have been found in the central nervous system or on the other side of the diaphragm from the original growth, what stage is it?
7. What is the most commonly diagnosed form of cancer?
8. Which is the leading cause of death by cancer for both men and women?
9. What are three cautions for massage therapists related directly to cancer?
10. What are three cautions for massage therapists related to cancer treatments?

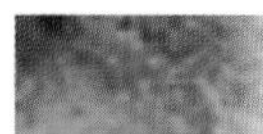

References

1. Signs and Symptoms of Cancer. © American Cancer Society. http://www.cancer.org/docroot/CRI/content/CRI_2_4_3X_What_are_the_signs_and_symptoms_of_cancer.asp?sitearea= .
2. Cancer Screening Overview (PDQ®). National Cancer Institute. http://www.cancer.gov/cancerinfo/pdq/screening/overview.
3. Guide to Clinical Preventive Services. Agency for Healthcare Research and Quality. http://www.ahrq.gov/clinic/cps3dix.htm. Accessed spring 2006.
4. Staging: Questions and Answers. National Cancer Institute. http://www.cancer.gov/cancer topics/factsheet/Detection/staging.
5. Tumor Grade: Questions and Answers. National Cancer Institute. http://www.cancer.gov/cancertopics/factsheet/Detection/tumor-grade/print?page=&keyword=.
6. Cancer: Questions and Answers. National Cancer Institute. http://www.cancer.gov/cancertopics/factsheet/Sites-Types/general.
7. Human Papillomavirus and Genital Warts. National Institute of Allergy and Infectious Diseases. http://www.niaid.nih.gov/factsheets/stdhpv.htm. Accessed spring 2006.
8. Walton T. Cancer and Massage Therapy: Essential Contraindications. Massage Therapy Journal, vol 45, no 2, summer 2006, pp 119–136.
9. Massage Benefits Hospitalized Cancer Patients. Massage Magazine. https://www.massagetherapyfoundation.org/or_article_massagemag105B.html.

Appendix A

Medications

Massage therapists are always encouraged to ask about what medications, prescription or otherwise, their clients are taking. Traditionally this has been to help discover what conditions a client might have that could influence the way massage should be conducted. But the possible interactions between bodywork and medications themselves are a related but separate topic.

The following is a *very* short descriptive list of classes of medications that are commonly prescribed for chronic conditions. Massage therapists must balance the effects of medications, medical interactions, all possible side effects, and the potential for bodywork to tip the scales in one direction or another. In many cases, a conversation with the primary care provider is in order—not so much to ask permission to do massage as to investigate whether the generally parasympathetic changes massage brings about carry any concern or risk in the presence of prescription drugs.

Recently some excellent resources about bodywork in the context of pharmaceuticals have been developed. I recommend these:

- Wible J. *Pharmacology for Massage Therapy*. Philadelphia: Lippincott Williams & Wilkins, 2005.
- Persad R. *Massage Therapy and Medications.* Toronto: Curties-Overzet, 2001.

In addition, massage offices would do well to have a general reference about medications on hand. In this way, when a client enters *doxercalciferol* on the intake form and neither of you is sure what it's for, you'll have a way to find out.

Two good options:

- *Springhouse Nurse's Drug Guide 2008*. Philadelphia: Lippincott Williams & Wilkins, 2008.
- Wible J. *Portable Pharmacology for Massage Therapists*. Philadelphia: Lippincott Williams & Wilkins, 2008.

The short list of medication classes under discussion here includes the following:

- Antianxiety drugs
- Antidepressants
- Anti-inflammatories and analgesics
- Autonomic nervous system drugs
- Cardiovascular drugs
- Cancer drugs

- Clot management drugs
- Diabetes management drugs
- Muscle relaxants
- Thyroid supplement drugs

With each description, the following information is provided:

- Examples of common name brands and some generic names. This information is perhaps the most changeable of all, and requires that every therapist get accurate and current information from every client. Generic names are in lowercase.
- Basic mechanism of the drug.
- Massage cautions and implications associated with the medication or the condition it treats.

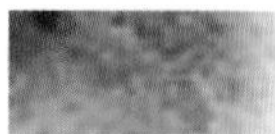

Antianxiety Drugs

These medications are used to alter the sympathetic flight-or-fight response that is so prevalent for many people with anxiety disorders. They act on the central nervous system (CNS), but their effects may be far-reaching. Common side effects of antianxiety medications include CNS depression, poor reflexes, dry mouth, and feeling unusually exhausted. All of these side effects influence decisions about bodywork. While most of the time side effects are mild and easily tolerated, they can become a medical emergency. Clients should be encouraged to report any troubling symptoms to their primary physician.

Classes of antianxiety drugs:

- Benzodiazepines
- Buspirone Hcl

Benzodiazepines

Common Examples

Valium, Ativan, Xanax, Loftran, Halcion, Dalmane, Restoril, Librium, Tranxene, Paxipam, Serax.

Basic Mechanism

It is believed that these medications mimic the inhibitory action of the neurotransmitter gamma-aminobutyric acid (GABA), making neurons harder to activate, and suppress the emotional component of anxiety in the limbic system. Benzodiazepines are used for short-term anxiety, seizures, insomnia, and convulsions. They are potentially addictive.

Implications for Massage

A person whose sympathetic response is suppressed is relatively prone to slide into a deep parasympathetic state. This is fine until the person tries to sit up and falls off the table because of orthostatic hypotension. Massage for a person under the influence of these drugs must be conducted conservatively to respect the client's reduced ability to adapt to external changes. Using extra stimulation throughout the massage will help the client to avoid dizziness and fatigue at the end of the session.

Buspirone HCl

Common Example

BuSpar

Basic Mechanism

The mechanism of this medication is not well understood. It appears to bind up serotonin and dopamine receptors in the brain, leading to calmer affect without the CNS side effects seen with benzodiazepines. It is less addictive as well. BuSpar is used for short-term anxiety and for chronic problems such as general anxiety disorder.

Implications for Massage

The systemic side effects of BuSpar are less than those of other antianxiety medications, but the rules are the same: clients should move carefully after a session because of sympathetic suppression, and extra stimulation throughout the session will aid in avoiding dizziness and fatigue.

Antidepressant Drugs

The exact causes of depression remain in dispute, and so do the exact working mechanisms of antidepressant medications. Three main classes have been developed: tricyclics, monoamine oxidase inhibitors (MAOIs), selective serotonin reuptake inhibitors (SSRIs), and some miscellaneous drugs. As a class these drugs prolong the availability of various types of neurotransmitters in synapses in the brain, although why exactly this makes a difference is still a matter of some contention. It takes time for the body to adapt to these changes, however; 4 weeks or more is often needed for the drugs to take effect.

Antidepressants all have some side effects, although these are usually temporary and mild. Agitation at the beginning of treatment is common, along with increased anxiety, headaches, and insomnia; these often fade quickly. Other side effects include dry mouth, constipation, reduced sexual function, bladder problems, increased heart rate, and dizziness. If these symptoms don't subside or if they become a significant issue, patients should consult with their prescribing doctor as soon as possible.

Two types of antidepressants are associated with significant health risks: MAOIs have dangerous interactions with decongestants and some food groups that lead to dangerously high blood pressure and a risk of stroke; and Serzone has been associated with liver toxicity.

Dizziness, drowsiness, and lightheadedness are common side effects to many antidepressants. Massage may exacerbate these symptoms, so the therapist should take care not to overtreat, especially when a client is just starting new course of drugs.

Classes of antidepressant medications:

- Tricyclics
- MAOIs
- SSRIs
- Others

Tricyclics

Common Examples

Imipramine/Tofranil, amitriptyline/Elavil, nortriptyline/Pamelor, desipramine/Norpramin, clomipramine/Anafranil, doxepin/Sinequan, protriptyline/Vivactil.

Basic Mechanism

Tricyclics block the reuptake of norepinephrine and serotonin at synapses; this leads to down-regulation and more nearly normal function of the postsynaptic receptors, but it may take 4 weeks or more before improvement is noticed.

Implications for Massage

Like other antidepressants, tricyclics may cause dizziness. Clients may need some gently stimulating strokes at the end of the session to come back to full alertness. Of all antidepressants, tricyclics tend to have the most extreme side effects.

Monoamine Oxidase Inhibitors

Common Examples

Nardil, Parnate, Marplan.

Basic Mechanism

MAOIs work by inhibiting monamine oxidase, an enzyme that breaks down the neurotransmitters. They are used less often than other antidepressants because of the risk of dangerous interactions with some substances, notably decongestants and tyramine-containing foods, such as aged cheeses, red wine, and pickles.

Implications for Massage

MAOIs and other antidepressants have the tendency to cause excessive drowsiness and dizziness; massage must be performed and concluded appropriately.

Selective Serotonin Reuptake Inhibitors

Common Examples

Prozac, Zoloft, Luvox, Paxil, Celexa, Lexapro.

Basic Mechanism

These drugs all work to keep serotonin in CNS synapses longer. The theory is that this will lead to a more nearly normal uptake of serotonin from presynaptic neurons and a decrease in symptoms. SSRIs are used to treat various types of anxiety disorders and eating disorders as well as depression.

Implications for Massage

SSRIs often have fewer side effects than other antidepressants, but therapists should be alert for signs of excessive dizziness or drowsiness and compensate appropriately.

Other Antidepressants

Common Examples

Effexor, Serzone, Wellbutrin, Remeron, Ludiomil, Desyrel, Symbyax.

Basic Mechanism

These drugs are similar to other antidepressants, although they focus on serotonin, norepinephrine, or dopamine uptake.

Implications for Massage

In addition to the general guidelines about massage and antidepressants, Serzone in particular is associated with a risk of liver toxicity. Clients with signs of jaundice, chronic nausea, or other abdominal discomfort should immediately consult their primary caregiver.

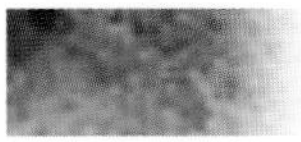

Anti-inflammatory and Analgesic Drugs

Inflammation is frequently a source of nerve irritation at acute or chronic sites of tissue damage. Consequently, many analgesics work to reduce pain sensation by reducing or inhibiting the inflammatory process. Other analgesics alter pain perception in the CNS and do not affect inflammation.

Regardless of the site of drug activity, analgesics and anti-inflammatories change tissue response. It is important to work extremely conservatively with clients who take these medications because information therapists gather about temperature, muscle guarding, local blood flow, and other signs will be altered, and overtreatment is a significant risk. Although it is inappropriate to suggest that clients skip or change their medication for massage, it is important to know when these drugs are at their peak of activity so that therapists can be prepared for the changes in tissue and the effects on clients.

Classes of drugs:

- Salicylates
- Acetaminophen
- Nonsteroidal anti-inflammatories (NSAIDs)
- Steroidal anti-inflammatories
- Opioids and mixed opioids

Salicylates

Common Examples

Aspirin, Bayer Aspirin, Empirin, Doan's Pills, Trilisate, Dolobid.

Basic Mechanism

Salicylates inhibit prostaglandin synthesis, which reduces pain sensitivity and inflammatory response. They also reduce fever by acting on the hypothalamus and promoting peripheral vasodilation. (They do not reduce a normal temperature.) In addition, aspirin works to inhibit platelet aggregation (see *anticoagulants*).

Implications for Massage

Reduced pain perception and inhibited inflammation mean that compromised tissue may not send a strong signal about pain; bodywork must be conservative to avoid overtreatment, and deep tissue massage must be used with caution. Also, the tendency for peripheral vasodilation raises the risk of hypotension (dizziness and lethargy) and chilling during and after a massage.

Acetaminophen

Common Examples

Tylenol, Anacin

Basic Mechanism

The mechanism for acetaminophen is not thoroughly understood. It is clear that these medications act on the heat-regulating center of the hypothalamus to reduce fever. These drugs reduce pain sensation, possibly both in the CNS and in the peripheral tissues, but they do *not* influence inflammation.

Implications for Massage

As with other pain medications, caution must be used to avoid overtreatment.

Nonsteroidal Anti-inflammatory Drugs

Common Examples

Celebrex, Lodine, Advil, Excedrin, Nuprin, Relafen, indomethacin/Indocin, Aleve, Ansaid, ketoprofen, Mobic, Clinoril.

Basic Mechanism

All of these medications work to inhibit prostaglandin synthesis at sites of tissue damage to reduce inflammation and the pain associated with it.

Implications for Massage

NSAIDs are effective for pain and inflammation, but they are also associated with stomach and kidney damage; clients need to consult their doctor if they have any discomfort. (Bear in mind that kidney pain may present as low back pain.) Regular use of Vioxx and Celebrex have been shown in some studies to increase the risk of cardiovascular disease, including heart attack and stroke.

Massage therapists carry the responsibility to avoid overtreatment, even if the client doesn't report feeling pain.

Steroidal Anti-inflammatories

Common Examples

Cortisone, Compound E, Beconase, Propaderm, H-Hydrocort, Hydrocortine, Depo-Medrol, Prednisol, prednisone, Decadron, methotrexate.

Basic Mechanism

These synthetic analogs to glucocorticoids produced in the adrenal cortex all work to undo the main symptoms of inflammation: they reduce pain, heat, redness, and edema in the short run. The mechanism by which they do this is not well understood, although some researchers suggest that they change local cellular activity, leading to suppressed production of prostaglandins, histamine, and other inflammatory substances.

Implications for Massage

Steroidal anti-inflammatories are powerful but have several serious side effects. In addition to altering tissue response (which requires extra caution with massage), they suppress immune system activity. Long-term use is associated with weakened connective tissues, fat deposition, muscle wasting, reduced bone density, fluid retention, hypertension, and easy bruising. Topical applications of steroid creams can lead to thinning skin. All of these features influence bodywork choices. Deep tissue massage should not be used when these drugs are used in the long term, and myofascial techniques should be used with great caution.

Steroidal anti-inflammatories may also be prescribed in inhalant form for treatment of asthma. While these medications specifically target the lung, long-term use may damage other tissues.

Opioids and Mixed Opioids

Common Examples

Codeine, Demerol, OxyContin, Darvon, Percocet, Lortab, Vicodin, fentanyl/Duragesic, Dilaudid, MS Contin, morphine.

Basic Mechanism

Opioids bind to opiate receptors in the brain to mimic the action of painkilling endorphins. This leads to a reduced sensation of pain without loss of consciousness, along with suppression of the cough reflex, and gastrointestinal tract sluggishness. Opioids are potentially addictive; mixed opioids were developed to minimize the risk of dependence, but they have proven to be addictive also.

Implications for Massage

A client taking these medications has a problem that is too extreme to be managed with less intrusive analgesics. Interference with pain perception is more complete, and appropriate caution is called for. Furthermore, clients taking opioid analgesics may be prone to mood swings and difficulties with accurate communication. Deep tissue massage should not be used, and stimulation during or at the end of the session is needed to prevent dizziness and fatigue. Avoid massaging around the area of transdermal patches.

Autonomic Nervous System Drugs

Autonomic nervous system drugs work to stimulate or block the action of the sympathetic or parasympathetic nervous system. They are used for a wide variety of diseases, including gastrointestinal, urinary, cardiac, and respiratory conditions. They can work directly on the receptors to stimulate or block them, or they can work to increase or decrease the associated neurotransmitters.

Classes of autonomic nervous system drugs:

- Cholinergic (increase parasympathetic nervous system actions)
- Anticholinergic (block the actions of the parasympathetic nervous system)
- Adrenergic (increase sympathetic nervous system actions)
- Adrenergic blockers (block sympathetic nervous system actions)

Cholinergics

Common Examples

Urecholine, Carbastat, pilocarpine, Aricept.

Basic Mechanism

These drugs mimic the action of the parasympathetic system.

Implications for Massage

Since these drugs do the exact thing that massage is usually meant to do (activate the parasympathetic nervous system), care should be taken not to overtreat. Stimulating forms of massage should be used throughout the session so the client is alert at the end rather than dizzy and in a deep parasympathetic lethargy.

Anticholinergic Drugs

Common Examples

Atropine, Transderm Scop, scopolamine, Anaspaz, Librax, Cogentin, Bentyl, Ditropan, Detrol, Artane.

Basic Mechanism

The actions of these drugs can vary. They are often organ specific and may suppress or stimulate parasympathetic nervous system receptors.

Implications for Massage

These drugs affect the parasympathetic response of the client and therefore the effects of massage. Looking up the drug, target organ, and side effects, as well as talking with the client about how the drug affects him or her, will help determine whether the parasympathetic response is stimulated or blocked. Massage can be given with these individual effects in mind.

Adrenergic Drugs

Common Examples

Dopamine, epinephrine, Isuprel, albuterol, terbutaline, Serevent, Neo-Synephrine.

Basic Mechanism

These drugs stimulate the sympathetic nervous system.

Implications for Massage

The goal of massage to induce a parasympathetic response is more difficult to achieve with the actions of these drugs. Longer, slower massages may be needed. Be cautious with strokes that stimulate, such as tapotement and friction.

Adrenergic Blockers

Common Examples

Cardura, Minipress, Flomax, Migranal, Coreg, Normodyne, Betagan, Corgard, Inderal, Betapace.

Basic Mechanism

These drugs block the action of the sympathetic nervous system at various receptor sites. They include alpha and beta blockers. They can be very specific to the target organ but may have systemic side effects.

Implications for Massage

Blocking the sympathetic nervous system means the client may be susceptible to a deep parasympathetic state with massage. Caution should be used to be certain the client is awake and not dizzy or experiencing other effects.

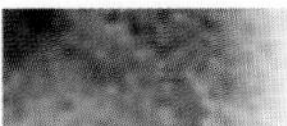

CARDIOVASCULAR DRUGS

Most of the drugs used to treat cardiovascular disease work in some way to minimize a sympathetic response or to dilate peripheral blood vessels. The overriding rule when a client uses these substances is that their slide into a parasympathetic state may be intensified by massage, leaving the client dizzy, fatigued, and lethargic. Ending a session with strokes that are more stimulating may help to ameliorate these effects, as long as they fit into a protocol that is suitable for a person with compromised cardiovascular health. Clients should be instructed to sit up and move slowly after their massage to minimize dizziness or discomfort.

Hydrotherapeutic techniques can present a greater challenge to maintain homeostasis than many other modalities. Many clients with cardiovascular diseases should avoid total immersion in favor of smaller, local hydrotherapy applications.

Classes of cardiovascular drugs:

- Beta blockers
- Calcium channel blockers
- Angiotensin-converting enzyme (ACE) inhibitors
- Digitalis
- Antianginal drugs
- Antilipemic drugs
- Diuretics

Beta Blockers

Common Examples

Inderal, Normodyne, Levatol, Corgard, Tenormin, metoprolol/Lopressor, Toprol, sotalol, Coreg, Betagan.

Basic Mechanism

These affect beta receptors at the heart, bronchi, blood vessels, and uterus. They lower blood pressure and cardiac output. They are used to treat angina, hypertension, anxiety, and some other disorders. Beta blockers may be selective for action on the heart only or nonselective for a more general effect.

Implications for Massage

Beta blockers can lead to excessively low blood pressure, especially when the client is in a relaxed state. Hydrotherapy is generally safer with local applications than systemic immersions in hot tubs, saunas, or other facilities.

Calcium Channel Blockers

Common Examples

Norvasc, Cardene, Isoptin, Procardia, Plendil, verapamil.

Basic Mechanism

These drugs block the movement of calcium ions in smooth and cardiac muscle tissue. The result is vasodilation and more efficient myocardial function. They are used for hypertension and long-term (not acute) angina.

Implications for Massage

Side effects of these drugs include flushing, dizziness, and hypotension. Massage should be conducted to minimize the risk of exacerbating these: little emphasis on big, draining strokes and more emphasis on smaller, less circulatory strokes is appropriate.

ACE Inhibitors

Common Examples

Lotensin, captopril, Vasotec, Monopril, Accupril, Altace, Zestril.

Basic Mechanism

ACE inhibitors work by limiting the action of an enzyme that is employed in the renin-angiotensin system, the loop between blood pressure and kidney function. They promote the excretion of sodium and water, reducing load on the heart. They are used to control hypertension and heart failure.

Implications for Massage

As with other drugs for cardiovascular disease, excessive hypotension is a possible side effect. Clients may experience fatigue, dizziness, and lethargy if gently invigorating strokes are not administered toward the end of the session.

Digitalis

Common Examples

Digitek, digoxin, Lanoxicaps, Lanoxin.

Basic Mechanism

Digitalis increases the force of the heartbeat by boosting calcium in cardiac muscle cells; it also slows the heartbeat through action in the CNS. It is used to treat arrhythmia and heart failure.

Implications for Massage

Clients who take any form of digitalis to control heart failure are not good candidates for rigorous circulatory massage. Invigorating strokes to conclude a session must be chosen to support alertness rather than circulatory flow.

Antilipemic Drugs

Common Examples

Locholest, Lopid, Prevalite, Questran, Lipitor, Lescol, Zocor, Crestor, Mevacor, Pravachol, Zetia, Lopid, Tricor, Niaspan, Vytorin.

Basic Mechanism

Cholesterol-lowering drugs work by sequestering bile or by inhibiting cholesterol synthesis. Bile-sequestering drugs promote the excretion of bile in stool, requiring the liver to use more cholesterol in bile manufacturing; this lowers blood cholesterol. Cholesterol synthesis inhibitors interfere with enzyme activity in the liver that leads to cholesterol synthesis. Both approaches lead to lower low-density lipoprotein levels.

Implications for Massage

A common side effect of all of these drugs is constipation, as they influence the gastrointestinal tract. Massage may help to relieve this, but if a client has abdominal pain and has had no bowel movement for several days, an acute bowel impaction is possible; this is a medical emergency.

Other side effects (which are not always listed) may include muscle soreness, cramping, and weakness. If a client taking an antilipemic drug has these problems, the prescribing doctor should be consulted before the massage therapist works to resolve them.

On rare occasions, these drugs can cause a life-threatening muscle wasting disease called rhabdomyolysis. Symptoms include worsening muscle pain and weakness. If your client has these symptoms, refer him or her to the physician immediately.

Diuretics

Common Examples

Thalidone, Kaluril, Lasix, Bumex, Lozide, Lozol, spironolactone/Aldactone, chlorthalidone, Demadex, Zaroxolyn, Dyazide, Maxzide, HCTZ (hydrochlorothiazide).

Basic Mechanism

Some diuretics prevent sodium from being reabsorbed in the kidney. As it is processed into urine, sodium pulls water along with it. Other medications target specific parts of the nephron to prevent water and salt reabsorption but can control the loss of other electrolytes more carefully.

Implications for Massage

Rigorously applied massage may put an extra load on the kidneys. Resting hypotension may also be a problem for people taking these medications. General diuretics may cause a loss of potassium that can contribute to muscle cramps. This must be addressed by a doctor rather than by a massage therapist.

Antianginal Medication

Common Examples

Apo-ISDN, Cedocard, IMDUR, Monoket, Nitrodisc, Nitrostat, Transderm-Nitro, nitroglycerin.

Basic Mechanism

Antianginal drugs reduce myocardial oxygen demand or increase the supply of oxygen to the heart, or both. Chronic angina is treated with beta blockers or calcium channel blockers, discussed elsewhere. Acute angina is typically treated with various nitrates. These cause vasodilation, especially of veins, leading to decreased load on the heart. They are typically dissolved under the tongue for fast action or applied with a skin patch or ointment for longer-lasting effect.

Implications for Massage

If a client has a transdermal patch for antianginal medication, that area and the adjacent tissue must be avoided, so that dosage is not influenced. Clients taking these medications have the same risk of hypotension, flushing, and dizziness seen with other cardiovascular drugs.

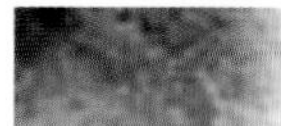

CANCER DRUGS

Cancer or chemotherapy drugs are a large group that act in a wide variety of ways on the body. While the goal is to attack the cancer cells, cancer drugs are generally toxic to the whole body. Newer drugs can target cancer cells more carefully, but they still tax the body as a whole. Massage should be applied very conservatively and circulatory massage minimized. Timing of the session should be related to excretion rates of the drug and discussed with the client's physician in detail.

Classes of drugs:

- Alkylating drugs
- Antimetabolite drugs
- Antibiotic antineoplastics
- Hormonal antineoplastics
- Natural antineoplastics
- Other antineoplastic drugs

Common Cancer Drugs

Common Examples

This is a limited list of the most commonly seen drugs: Cytoxan, dacarbazine/DIC, CCNU, TSPA, cisplatin, methotrexate, 5-fluorouracil, actinomycin, Tamofen, Teslac, vinblastine, vincristine, interleukin-2, interferon.

Basic Mechanism

These drugs target the cancer cells and kill them, block the growth of the cells, or block the vascular feeding of the cells.

Implications for Massage

Always consult with the physician. Massage application should be very conservative. Be aware of methods of excretion (some excrete through the skin) and take appropriate precautions. If radioactive elements are implanted in the body, check with the physician on any limits to the time that should be spent close to the client.

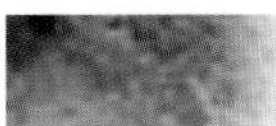

Clot Management Drugs

Medications to manage blood clots come in three basic forms: Anticoagulants prevent the formation of new clots by acting on clotting factors. Antiplatelet medications prevent the clumping of platelets to form new clots. Thrombolytics are used to dissolve preexisting clots. Thrombolytics are used only in emergencies (i.e., in early treatment for heart attack or ischemic stroke), and so are not discussed here. Other clot management drugs are used for chronic problems or to lower the risk of future clots.

Classes of drugs:

- Anticoagulants
- Antiplatelet drugs

Anticoagulants

Common Examples

Heparin, Lovenox, coumadin.

Basic Mechanism

Heparin and Lovenox are injected anticoagulants; coumadin is an oral medication. All of them alter the formation of clotting factors in the liver to prevent the formation of new clots, although they do not help to dissolve preexisting clots. These medications are used for people with atrial fibrillation or a high risk of deep vein thrombosis and for people using hemodialysis. Heparin may also be used in orthopedic surgery to reduce the risk of postsurgical deep vein thrombosis.

Implications for Massage

All blood-clotting medications carry a risk of bruising, even with relatively light massage. Furthermore, the need for these medications indicates a tendency to form blood clots that may contraindicate all but the lightest forms of bodywork. If a blood clot is present, massage should not be given.

Antiplatelet Drugs

Common Examples

Aspirin, Empirin, Pletal, Plavix.

Basic Mechanism

These drugs prevent platelets from clumping at the site where a clot might otherwise form.

Implications for Massage

Although these are typically less powerful than anticoagulants, the risk of bruising must still be respected for clients who take antiplatelet drugs.

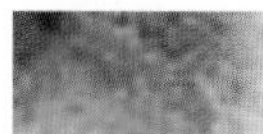

DIABETES MANAGEMENT DRUGS

Because type 2 diabetes is so prevalent in the United States, the chance that a massage therapist will have diabetic clients is high. When type 2 diabetes cannot be managed by diet and exercise alone, other interventions are used. They often start with diabetes management drugs and may eventually culminate with the supplementation of insulin in various forms. Type 1 diabetes is also fairly common and is managed with the use of insulin injections in various forms.

The implications for diabetes and massage therapists are many and complicated. While many diabetics manage their disease well and minimize their risk of secondary complications, others are prone to several problems that pose serious cautions for massage: systemic atherosclerosis, an increased risk of stroke, diabetic ulcers, and peripheral neuritis, to name a few.

Furthermore, massage lowers blood glucose. While this is an advantage to diabetic clients, this challenge to homeostasis can be overwhelming enough to trigger a hypoglycemic episode. Massage therapists with diabetic clients should be aware of signs of hypoglycemia and hyperglycemia, and should consult with those clients about how best to address their needs in an emergency.

Classes of drugs:

- Insulin
- Oral glucose management drugs

Insulin

Common Examples

Humulin, Humalog, Lantus, Novolog, Novolin.

Basic Mechanism

Insulin is a protein-based hormone that would be destroyed by digestive juices if taken orally. Consequently it is administered by injection, either by multiple daily injections or by an insulin pump. It decreases blood glucose by helping to deliver glucose to cells that need this clean-burning fuel to do their jobs.

Implications for Massage

Clients who supplement insulin vary their injection sites; these areas should be locally avoided so as not to interfere with normal uptake of the drug. Length of time for peak effect of the drug varies with the type of insulin, and it is best to avoid the injection area for at least that amount of time. If uncertain, avoid it for 24 hours.

Because blood glucose stability is an issue for diabetic clients, it is best for them to receive massage in the middle of their insulin cycle rather than at the end or at the beginning.

It might also be useful for a new client to check blood glucose before and after the session, so that if he or she needs to take in sugar in an easily accessible form, the therapist can plan ahead and have some juice, milk, or candy available.

Oral Glucose Management Drugs

Common Examples

Diabinase, Glucotrol, Glyburide, Glucophage, Precose.

Basic Mechanism

These drugs work in a variety of ways to inhibit production of sugar in the liver, to improve output of insulin in the pancreas, and to increase the sensitivity of insulin receptors on target cells.

Implications for Massage

Of these drugs, Glucophage may carry the least risk of setting up a hypoglycemic episode. Nonetheless, any clients who manage their diabetes with any combination of drugs and insulin must be monitored carefully for blood glucose stability. As with insulin, it is safest to work with these clients *after* the peak of drug activity.

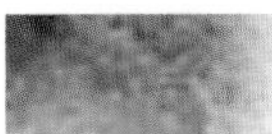

MUSCLE RELAXANTS

Muscle relaxants are prescribed to deal with acute spasms related to trauma or anxiety or to help with chronic spasticity from CNS damage as seen with multiple sclerosis, stroke, spinal cord injury, or cerebral palsy. They can act on the brain, the spinal cord, or in the muscle tissue itself.

A client who takes muscle relaxants is *not* inherently relaxed, although his or her tissues may seem that way. These drugs interfere with muscle protection reflexes, and so the risk of overtreatment with deep tissue work, range-of-motion exercises, or stretching is significant.

Classes of muscle relaxant drugs:

- Centrally acting skeletal muscle relaxants
- Peripherally acting skeletal muscle relaxants

Centrally Acting Skeletal Muscle Relaxants

Common Examples

Soma, Paraflex, Flexeril, Skelaxin, Norflex, baclofen, Valium, Robaxin, Zanaflex.

Basic Mechanism

These medications are CNS depressants. They suppress reflexes that would tighten muscles in response to stretching or damage. They are used to control painful acute spasms related to trauma or anxiety.

Implications for Massage

These drugs enforce a parasympathetic state, which may be intensified by massage. Therapists should take care that clients are not exhausted at the end of a session. In addition, the protective stretch reflex is inhibited under these medications; therapists should not try to increase range of motion while the client is in this altered state.

Peripherally Acting Skeletal Muscle Relaxants

Common Example

Dantrium.

Basic Mechanism

This drug interferes with calcium release at the sarcoplasmic reticulum of muscle cells, leading to weaker contractions. It is used to treat chronic spasticity associated with CNS damage, but the overall weakness that ensues makes it a questionable choice for patients whose strength is borderline.

Implications for Massage

A client taking Dantrium has a compromised stretch reflex and falsely hypotonic muscles; massage must be conducted conservatively.

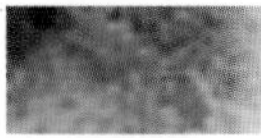

Thyroid Supplement Drugs

Hypothyroidism is typically treated with supplements to replace the thyroid secretions triiodothyronine (T_3) and thyroxine (T_4). Levothyroxine sodium is chemically identical to T_4 and is meant to be converted to bioactive T_3. While many hypothyroidism patients successfully treat their disease with levothyroxine sodium, some supplement T_3 instead of or in addition to T_4. This substance has traditionally been available in the form of desiccated animal glands, but a synthetic form of T_3 has recently become available.

Classes of drugs:

- Levothyroxine sodium
- Desiccated extract
- Liothyronine sodium

Levothyroxine Sodium

Common Examples

Synthroid, Eltroxin, levo-t, Levothroid, Levoxyl.

Basic Mechanism

Synthetic thyroid hormones mimic the action of naturally occurring thyroid hormones to boost protein synthesis in cells, promote the use of glycogen stores, increase heart rate and cardiac output, and increase urine output.

Implications for Massage

New users of synthetic thyroid supplements may go through a period of nervousness, agitation, and insomnia, which massage may help to improve. If these symptoms persist, the dosage may not be correct, and the person should consult with the prescribing physician.

Someone who has been taking synthetic thyroid supplements for a long time probably has no significant side effects and no implications for massage therapy.

Desiccated Extract

Common Examples

Armour Thyroid, Nature-Throid, thyroid USP, Westhroid.

Basic Mechanism

These forms of thyroid hormone have the same action as synthetic supplements: they mimic the action of naturally occurring thyroid hormones to boost protein synthesis in cells, promote the use of glycogen stores, increase heart rate and cardiac output, and increase urine output. The difference is that the potency of these drugs is more difficult to predict, so users may experience significant fluctuation of symptoms.

Implications for Massage

As with synthetic hormones, a new user may have increased anxiety, insomnia, or agitation, all of which indicate massage. If symptoms persist, the person needs to consult with the physician. Otherwise, massage is perfectly appropriate for clients who supplement thyroid hormones.

Liothyronine Sodium

Common Examples

Cytomel, Triostat.

Basic Mechanism

These synthetic forms of T_3 are prescribed for patients who don't have success with levothyroxine sodium. They are meant to mimic the action of naturally occurring thyroid hormones to boost protein synthesis in cells, promote the use of glycogen stores, increase heart rate and cardiac output, and increase urine output.

Implications for Massage

As with other hormone supplements, anxiety, insomnia, or agitation may occur until dosage is correctly gauged. If symptoms persist, the person needs to consult with the physician. Otherwise, massage is perfectly appropriate for clients who supplement thyroid hormones.

APPENDIX B

Research Literacy, Research Capacity

 "BUT WE'VE ALWAYS DONE IT THIS WAY"

Many people who were educated in massage therapy more than a few years ago learned about its physiological effects through revered but seldom-questioned lore, common sense, and educated guesses. Based on this tradition, massage therapists have been taught that "massage boosts circulation" without guidance for what kind of massage, for how long, and for whom. Many were taught that "massage spreads cancer" based on guesses about massage and fluid flow, but this claim turns out to be probably overstated. We have traditionally assumed that massage has its best applications for musculoskeletal issues, but our impact on the nervous and endocrine systems may be even more profound. What other traditions have we clung to out of loyalty rather than knowledge?

Every health care profession must have its beloved myths tested and analyzed. The justification of the traditional "we've always done it this way" approach doesn't always hold up under scrutiny. The process of testing and analysis is a reflection of a basic aspect of human nature: the drive to know the best possible way to go about achieving certain goals. Massage therapy is finally entering this world, and massage therapists must learn to read and interpret results: this is *research literacy*. Some practitioners must also learn to *conduct* research projects—otherwise, clinical trials will not accurately reflect what happens in a realistic massage setting. The ability to conduct credible research is *research capacity*.

Good research creates amazing opportunities: It supplies information to massage therapists and educators. It offers informed guidance to licensing and regulatory bodies. It provides a bridge to other health care practitioners. But, as Benjamin Disraeli wrote (and Mark Twain famously quoted), "There are three kinds of lies: lies, damned lies, and statistics." This can be true especially when highly individualized modalities, such as massage therapy, are studied with the intent to quantify the unquantifiable and where the practice of massage is often unique to each client-therapist relationship. This presents challenges to many traditional kinds of research design.

Fortunately, a number of invaluable resources have emerged to help massage therapists work their way through this jungle of observational studies, experimental studies, randomizing, blinding, confounds, and controls. This document is a grateful nod toward the pioneers who are working to make research literacy an attainable goal for massage therapists everywhere. These sources are listed with great appreciation and respect in the bibliography on the student resource CD.

Some vocabulary for research issues may be new to many readers. A brief definition of **boldface terms** is provided in Table B.1.

TABLE B.1	RESEARCH LITERACY VOCABULARY LIST: DEFINITION OF TERMS
Anecdotes	Informal stories, not rigorously analyzed.
Best practices	An example or guideline of a standard a profession recognizes as embodying the highest knowledge available.
Bias	Influence or error in a particular direction rather than objective evaluation of the evidence.
Case series	Multiple case studies for a particular condition or treatment.
Case study	A detailed rigorous observation and analysis of the effects of a treatment or a condition in one patient.
Confound	To interfere with or confuse the connection between treatment and outcome.
Control group	A group of subjects who do not receive the treatment being studied. Sometimes the control group receives a placebo treatment; other times it simply receives a different treatment from the one being studied.
Crossover study	A research study in which each subject receives, in random order, both the control treatment and the experimental treatment. In this way, each subject serves as his or her own control.
Descriptive study	A research study that describes the observed effects of treatments without forming a hypothesis or trying to find a cause for whatever effects were observed.
Double-blinded	A research study in which neither the researchers nor the study subjects know whether the subjects are getting the treatment being tested or a placebo. In other words, both the researchers and the study subjects are blinded to that information.
Empirical	Based on practical experimentation and observation.
Evidence-based	Medicine attaining to the highest standard of clinical care by medicine combining the best scientific evidence available with the practitioner's clinical judgment and experience and with respect for the patient's preferences.
Experimental/ explanatory study	A research study concerned not only with describing the effects of a treatment but also with discovering **how** and **why** it works or not—the relation between cause (treatment) and effect (outcome).
Likert scale	A scale in which a patient or a subject in a study indicates a level of agreement with statements that are arranged in order from more to less strong (or vice versa).
Power	A measurement of the number of study participants or subjects necessary to ensure that the study will reliably detect treatment effects.
Qualitative	Observations that are measured by qualities, or descriptive observations properties, rather than with numbers (e.g., soft, hard, easy, difficult, feels good, hurts, big, small, sad, happy).
Quantitative observations	Observations that are measured by numbers, such as 98.6°F, 120/80 blood pressure.

(continued)

TABLE B.1 RESEARCH LITERACY VOCABULARY LIST: DEFINITION OF TERMS *continued*

Randomization	A technique for lowering the opportunity for bias in a study by using chance to decide which group (treatment or control) the subjects of a study are assigned to.
Randomized controlled trial	A research study in which outcomes for a treatment group are compared with outcomes for a control group and the assignment of study subjects to one of the two groups is random.
Sham	A fake treatment, used to blind study subjects as to whether they are receiving the real treatment, so that their expectations cannot unconsciously bias the outcomes.
Single-blinded study	A study in which the researchers know whether the subjects are getting the treatment being tested or a placebo, but the subjects do not. In other words, **only** the study subjects are **blinded** to that information.
Validity	A measure of how well a study or experiment actually tests what it is intended to test.
Visual analog scale	A scale in which a patient or a subject in a study reports a subjective opinion of the intensity of a sensation. The visual analog scale is often used, for example, to report the degree of pain (i.e., from tolerable, or less intense, to intolerable, or very intense).

Traditionally, **quantitative** research has been held in higher regard than research on processes that cannot be quantified. For example, if a patient with high blood pressure gets a massage, her blood pressure may go from 145/95 to 130/85 mm Hg, a quantitatively measurable change. However, recent innovations have strengthened the acceptability of **qualitative** research, which focuses on describing process and experience, rather than on numbers. For example, **Likert scales** (Figure B.1) and **visual analog scales** (Figures B.2 and B.3) are validated methods by which measurement can be carried out qualitatively. In many ways these methods are better suited to track benefits of massage and bodywork, and as the results come in, we are discovering exciting, unexpected, and sometimes paradigm-shifting information.

Research in massage therapy is happening at an astonishing pace. As of this writing, a search for "Massage NOT cardiac NOT prostate" in the PubMed database of health sciences research articles (http://www.pubmed.com) yields more than 6,000 entries, each one an article describing some kind of research project in which massage was studied. The amount of information that is being generated today is dizzying—but how do we make sense of it and put it to use?

How interested are you in the topic of research literacy? (Circle one)

Very interested	Somewhat interested	Neutral	Not very interested	Not at all interested

Figure B.1. Likert scale.

SCIENCE AND THE SCIENTIFIC METHOD

Reading technical research reports on massage can feel intimidating at first, but a few principles make the process much more straightforward. Most research articles follow a basic framework, and all credible studies are grounded in science and the scientific method. This is simply a formalized way of observing and describing something about the natural world in a way that others can repeat.

Evidence from scientific studies is often referred to as **empirical**, meaning it is derived from experiments. People frequently assume that "doing science" requires lots of fancy machines or special training, but all it really means is making observations about the world that are well organized, unbiased, well documented, reproducible, and understandable to others.

The scientific method is a widely applicable set of steps that can be adjusted for any scientific study from physics to biology. For the context of massage, it can be described in the following steps:

1. Make an observation about the natural world.
2. Develop a testable theory about how massage or bodywork might influence that observation.
3. Make a prediction or hypothesis for what you expect to happen when you test your theory.
4. Carry out an experiment that tests your theory. Try to control the circumstances around your test so that you can accurately connect the experiment to the outcomes.
5. Observe and document your results. Did the test go as you expected or not?
6. Based on your results, decide whether your theory should be modified or successfully predicted what happened.

The scientific method can be much broader than what is presented here, but this model provides a good starting point for this discussion.

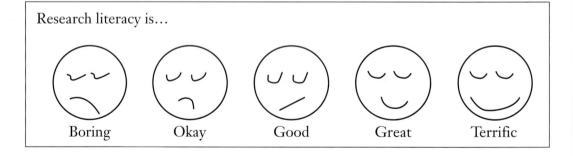

Figure B.2. Visual analog scale.

How much of an impact on your work has learning about research literacy had?

No effect ——————————————————— Huge effect

Figure B.3. Visual analog scale.

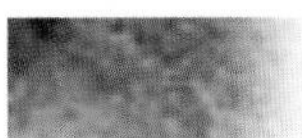

STRUCTURE OF A JOURNAL ARTICLE: IMRAD

In keeping with the scientific method, most research articles follow a standard format, which describes a project in an organized way. This allows other researchers to repeat the study to see if they get similar results. The format is sometimes called IMRAD, an acronym that stands for *introduction, methods, results, and discussion*. We'll use a study that tested whether massage could benefit the health of infants in an orphanage[1] to see how the parts of an article correspond to the scientific method.

I: *Introduction*

The *I* in IMRAD stands for *introduction*, which is the first part of the body of an article. The author uses the introduction to explain the importance of the research, to share an observation, and to offer a testable explanation and prediction of what is expected to happen in the study. In other words, the introduction covers steps 1 to 3 of the scientific process.

Step 1: Make an Observation about the Natural World

> *According to a recent World Health Organization report, during 2000 to 2003, diarrhea remained the second most common factor responsible for mortality of children younger than 5 years in the world . . . Diarrhea is quite common in institutions such as orphanages where infants come in close contact with each other for prolonged periods of time.*[1, p 314]

Step 2: Develop a testable theory about how massage or bodywork might influence that observation.

> *It is imperative that interventions with the potential to decrease the incidence of diarrhea be developed and tested to decrease the likelihood of diarrhea in infants and young children. Massage therapy is one intervention with such potential as it has been linked to positive health outcomes in a variety of populations.*[1, p 315]

Step 3: Make a prediction or hypothesis for what you expect to happen when you test your theory.

> *The purpose of this study was to determine whether infant massage would decrease the incidence of diarrhea and overall illness in infants living in orphanage settings.*[1, p 315]

M: *Methods*

The *M* in IMRAD stands for the *methods* section of the article. This segment describes exactly how the experiment is conducted. It needs to be especially clear, because the **validity** of the results depends mostly on the integrity of the methods.

Step 4: Carry out an experiment that tests your theory. Try to control the circumstances around your test so that you can accurately connect the experiment to the outcomes.

> *Infants in the experimental group received a 15-minute full-body (including the legs, stomach, chest, arms, face, and back) massage daily, usually in the morning, delivered by orphanage volunteers or staff, all of whom were trained in infant massage by a PhD-level, certified instructor using techniques endorsed by Infant Massage USA.*[1, p 316]

R: *Results*

The *R* in IMRAD stands for the *results* section of the article. This is where the researcher reports what happens, without interpretation. This may be done as a verbal description, and/or with charts or graphs to display data.

Step 5: Observe and document the results—did your prediction occur as expected, or not?

The prevented fraction for the target population was estimated to be 16%, indicating that by participating in the massage intervention, the incidence of diarrhea could possibly be reduced by 16% among similar populations of infants.[1, p 317]

AD: *And Discussion*

A stands for *and*, and *D* stands for the *discussion* section of the article. In this segment the researcher discusses the meaning of the results; whether the hypothesis was confirmed or not, and why; and what this means both for future research and in current applications.

Step 6: Based on your results, decide whether your theory needs to be modified, or if it really did successfully predict what happened.

Results of this experimental pilot project were promising in that infants who were massaged daily had significantly fewer days of diarrhea and slightly lower rates of overall illness than infants in the control group. As noted above, other studies have indicated that massage improves immune functioning, and there may have been increased immunity in the infants in the experimental group in this project. Another possibility is that massage improved infants' gastrointestinal functioning through stimulation of the vagus nerve. If massage can indeed decrease the incidence of diarrhea among orphaned infants, this avenue of intervention should be pursued, particularly given the high risk of mortality associated with this condition in developing countries.[1, p 317]

Understanding the structure of the scientific method and of research articles can help you to navigate the literature and decide what specific studies mean for you and your practice. But life is wonderfully complex, and this approach cannot be applied to all types of questions. Consequently, researchers have developed a wide array of designs to apply the scientific method to real-life circumstances that occur whenever we work with people. We'll discuss some of those approaches below, relating them to the steps we just went over, to keep them understandable in context.

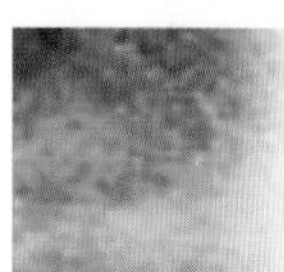

The Scientific Method and Massage: Strengths and Weaknesses

The scientific method often derives information about the natural world by separating components of a process and studying each piece independently of the others. Then that knowledge is reintegrated into a larger context. This is analysis (looking at individual pieces) followed by synthesis (putting ideas together).

An effective way to study how massage works is to isolate various aspects of the practice, which can later be reintegrated into larger pictures. This control of variables allows us to be more precise about how we link exposure to outcome, or cause to effect. For example, look at the following questions and identify which one is likely to yield the most reliable information about how massage affects human function.

Example A: What is the effect of massage therapy administered by parents on sleep disturbances in autistic children?
Example B: What is the effect of pétrissage administered by sports massage practitioners to marathon runners on postevent soreness in the gastrocnemius (calf) muscle?

Example B is the correct answer for several reasons: the scope of the research question is much narrower (one muscle versus the whole process of sleep). The population is much more similar to each other (highly trained athletes have more in common than does a diverse group of children with a poorly understood condition). The amount of time being studied is much shorter for the athletes (post event versus all night). There is much less variation in the one stroke (pétrissage) than in all of massage therapy. Finally, sports massage practitioners have more standardized training than do parents. All of these factors make a study of the effect of massage therapy administered by parents for sleep disturbances in autistic children much more challenging than a study of the effect of pétrissage administered by sports massage practitioners to marathon runners on postevent soreness in the gastrocnemius muscle. This does not mean that we can't study how massage affects the sleep patterns of autistic children, but we have to make some adjustments to the research design to do so.

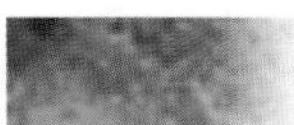

The Randomized Controlled Trial

A **randomized controlled trial** (RCT) is considered the gold standard of research study design, because it adheres as closely as possible to the ideal scientific method. A treatment group and a **control group** are studied, so that outcomes can be compared between them; this helps to isolate cause and effect and to eliminate **bias**. Participants are **randomized** into the two groups, so that any differences among the groups average out as much as possible and don't confuse or **confound** the outcome.

Other steps to reduce bias include blinding. The trial may be **single-blinded**, in which case the participants don't know whether they are receiving the treatment or not: in this way preconceived notions about effectiveness won't taint the outcomes. In blinded tests some participants receive a **sham** treatment, or participants could receive some different kind of intervention, such as a friendly visit or a relaxation tape, for instance, but not know which intervention is being studied. If the people analyzing the data don't know which participants received the real treatment, they work with the data exactly as it is generated, and expectations cannot creep in and taint their analysis. When analysts are blinded in this way as well, we say the trial is **double-blinded**.

You probably see some design challenges with this for massage already: if you're studying a drug, you can give the control group a sugar pill, and if you're studying acupressure, you can use a sham point instead of the real one as a placebo. But how do you give someone a placebo massage? That is one of the difficulties with carrying out RCTs in this context.

Another challenge is ethical. To carry out a full-fledged RCT, the study must have a large enough number of participants (sufficient **power**) to determine what is a real treatment effect and what is not. But it can be difficult and expensive to round up a significant number of participants and qualified therapists and analysts to conduct a large-scale study. In this case, two ethical imperatives compete against each other. On one hand, it is unethical to claim knowledge about massage that cannot be backed up with reliable evidence. On the other hand, if logistical problems interfere with the collection of information, is it right to deny patients the relief that massage may provide? In this situation, **evidence-based medicine** advises that we follow the **best practices** standard in the profession. It is our responsibility then to evaluate the effectiveness of massage to the best of our abilities and neither to overpromise what massage can do nor to deny patients the benefits of massage simply because it cannot meet the standards of an RCT.

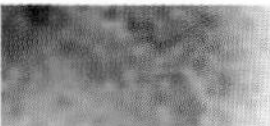

Beyond the Randomized Controlled Trial

It can be difficult or impossible to apply the RCT to some aspects of massage research, but other research designs may be a better fit. They can help identify best practices for massage, and they can provide research questions for later, methodologically stronger studies. For example, practitioners who work with catastrophic burn injuries or brain damage from oxygen deprivation can write up their work as case studies. Other practitioners with similar clients can use that work and write up their case studies in turn. And a university researcher can decide that several case studies indicate a trend that deserves further investigation and marshal the resources of the university and medical communities to design a larger RCT on the same research questions.

Researchers have created a hierarchy of evidence, ranging from the RCT at the strongest end to the **case study** and **anecdotes** (stories) at the weakest end. A **case series** is a collection of case studies that all address a similar question or make a similar observation. **Experimental** or **explanatory studies** allow the investigators to control the variables and to look for mechanisms or causes to explain results. **Descriptive** studies observe phenomena without attempting to explain cause and effect. In a **crossover study** each participant serves as the control, and the results of an intervention are measured twice: once when the subject gets no treatment and again when the subject receives the treatment. Each type of study is valuable in different situations.

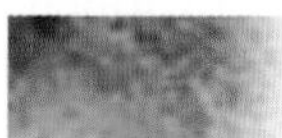

What Can One Massage Therapist Do?

The easiest and fastest way to begin moving from research literacy to research capacity is by conducting a case study. If you want to be part of a research team with funding to carry out studies on massage, a long journey of learning is probably ahead. But you can start along that path, and you can give back to others who would benefit from your experience by writing up interesting or unusual case reports from your practice. Most trade journals for massage dedicate space to research issues; consider submitting your report for publication. You may also consider participating in the Massage Therapy Foundation's student or practitioner case report contests. Visit http://www.massagetherapyfoundation.org/ for more information.

Remember the IMRAD structure as you document your experience.

- **I.** Write the introduction first. What is this patient's need? What is the larger context? What does the literature say about it? You can learn how to find articles related to your topic from databases such as PubMed, the Massage Therapy Foundation, and other sources. Explain your basis for thinking that massage would be a good treatment. The literature you refer to here will become your reference and/or bibliography section.
- **M.** Next comes the methods section: describe what you did to treat the patient. Be careful, clear, and detailed, so that an interested reader can reproduce your study.
- **R.** Report the outcome in your results section. This is a place just for the facts you have gathered; interpretation comes next.
- **D.** The discussion or conclusions section is the place to interpret or relate the meaning of your results to the larger context from your introduction and to recommend what you consider is the next step for other people to take.

Finally, write the abstract. An abstract is a very short summary that sketches out the entire article. Readers use it to decide whether your report is pertinent to their practice. If you have addressed an issue interesting to them, they can read the full text.

As a practicing massage therapist, you have a lot of knowledge to offer. Developing your research literacy and research capacity is a way of making an important contribution, both to other massage therapists and to the profession as a whole.

It is not an easy journey, but it is a wonderful one.

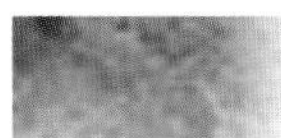

REFERENCE

1. Jump VK, Fargo JD, Akers JF. Impact of massage therapy on health outcomes among orphaned infants in Ecuador: Results of a randomized clinical trial. Family and Community Health. 2006 Oct-Dec;29(4):314–319.

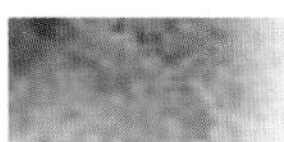

SUGGESTED READING

Dryden T, Achilles R. The Massage Therapy Research Curriculum Kit. Evanston, IL: Massage Therapy Foundation, 2004.

Hymel G. Research Methods for Massage and Holistic Therapies. Philadelphia: Mosby, 2005.

Menard MB. Making Sense of Research. Toronto: Curties-Overzet Publications, 2003.

Travillian RS. (working title) Massage Therapy: A Guide to Reading the Research Literature. Manuscript in preparation.

Glossary

Note: this glossary contains brief definitions of many terms found in *A Massage Therapist's Guide to Pathology*. Many entries also contain a reference to a particular condition where that term may be found: this is intended to direct readers to the body of the text. Thus, the definition of acne fulminans concludes with "See *acne vulgaris*" to indicate where this term is used in context.

Ablate (ah-BLATE): To remove or destroy function.

Abrasion (ah-BRA-zhun): A scrape involving injury to the epithelial layer of the skin or mucous membranes.

Absence seizure (AB-sens SE-zhur): A type of seizure characterized by lack of activity with occasional clonic movements.

Acanthosis nigricans (ak-an-THO-sis nig-rih-KANZ): An eruption of velvet warty benign growths and hyperpigmentation occurring in the skin of the axillae, neck, anogenital area, and groin; may be associated with endocrine disorders. See *metabolic syndrome*.

Acetaminophen (ah-set-ah-MIN-o-fen): A drug with antifever and analgesic effects similar to aspirin but with limited anti-inflammatory action.

Acetylcholine (ah-set-il-KO-lene): The neurotransmitter at cholinergic synapses. It causes cardiac inhibition, vasodilation, gastrointestinal peristalsis, and other parasympathetic effects.

Acne fulminans (AK-ne FUL-mih-nanz): Severe scarring acne with fever and joint pain; seen most often in teenage boys. See *acne vulgaris*.

Acral lentiginous melanoma (AK-ral len-TIH-jih-nus mel-ah-NO-mah): Pigmented lesions usually on the nailbed, fingers, palms, soles, or between toes. See *skin cancer*.

Acromegaly (ak-ro-MEG-ah-le): A disorder marked by progressive enlargement of peripheral parts of the body, linked to excessive secretion of growth hormone.

Acromioclavicular joint sprain (ah-KRO-me-o-klah-VIK-yu-lar joynt sprane): An injury to the ligaments that support the acromioclavicular joint.

Acropachy (AK-ro-pak-e, ah-KROP-ak-e): The swelling and clubbing of fingers associated with severe forms of hyperthyroidism.

Actinic cheilitis (ak-TIN-ik ki-LI-tis): Actinic keratosis lesions that appear on the lip. See *skin cancer*.

Actinic keratosis (ak-TIN-ik ker-ah-TO-sis): A premalignant warty lesion occurring on the sun-exposed skin of the face or hands in aged light-skinned persons. See *skin cancer*.

Acute (ah-KUTE): A stage of injury or infection that is short term and severe.

Acute exertional compartment syndrome (ah-KUTE eg-ZER-shun-al kom-PART-ment SIN-drome): A serious injury involving excessive swelling of muscles that may dangerously compress blood vessels and peripheral nerves. See *shin splints*.

Acute granulocytic leukemia (ah-KUTE gran-yu-lo-SIT-ik lu-KE-me-ah): Synonym for acute myelogenous leukemia. See *leukemia*.

Acute idiopathic polyneuritis (ah-KUTE ih-de-o-PATH-ik pol-e-nu-RI-tis): Synonym for Guillain-Barré syndrome.

Acute inflammatory demyelinating polyneuropathy (AIDP) (ah-KUTE in-FLAM-ah-tor-e de-MI-el-ih-na-ting pol-e-nu-ROP-ath-e): A form of Guillain-Barré syndrome.

Acute lymphoblastic leukemia (ah-KUTE lim-fo-BLAS-tik lu-KE-me-ah): Synonym for acute lymphocytic leukemia. See *leukemia*.

Acute lymphoid leukemia (ah-KUTE LIM-foid lu-KE-me-ah): Synonym for acute lymphocytic leukemia. See *leukemia*.

Acute myelocytic leukemia (ah-KUTE mi-el-o-SIT-ik lu-KE-me-ah): Synonym for acute myelogenous leukemia. See *leukemia*.

Acute myelogenous leukemia (ah-KUTE mi-el-OJ-en-us lu-KE-me-ah): Aggressive cancer of the myeloid class of blood cells. See *leukemia*.

Acute vestibular neuronitis (ah-KUTE ves-TIB-yu-lar nu-ro-NI-tis): Inflammation of the vestibular portion of cranial nerve VIII; a type of vestibular balance disorder.

Acyclovir (a-SI-klo-vir): An antiviral agent often used in the treatment of herpes simplex.

Adenocarcinoma (ah-den-o-kar-sih-NO-mah): A malignant neoplasm of epithelial cells in glandular or glandlike pattern.

Adenoma (ad-en-O-mah): A benign neoplasm, usually occurring in epithelial tissue. See *colorectal cancer*.

Adhesion (ad-HE-zhun): The joining or uniting of two surfaces. Layers of connective tissue may adhere, which limits movement and increases the risk of injury.

Adhesive capsulitis (ad-HE-siv kap-su-LI-tis): A condition involving inflammatory thickening of a joint capsule, usually at the shoulder, leading to loss of range of motion. Also known as frozen shoulder.

Adson test (AD-sun test): A test for thoracic outlet syndrome. The patient is seated with the head extended and rotated toward the affected side. With deep inspiration there is a diminution or total loss of radial pulse on that side.

Adventitia (ad-ven-TIH-shah): The outermost connective tissue layer that covers organs and vessels.

Aerobic metabolism (a-RO-bik meh-TAB-o-lizm): Metabolism that occurs in the presence of adequate oxygen, which reduces the overall production of toxic waste products.

Aflatoxin (AF-lah-tok-sin) B_1: A toxin produced by some strains of *Aspergillus flavus* that causes cancer in some animals. See *liver cancer*.

Agglutination (ah-glu-tin-A-shun): The process by which suspended red blood cells or other particles are caused to adhere and form clumps. See *chemical dependency*.

Agoraphobia (ah-gor-ah-FO-be-ah): A mental disorder characterized by an irrational fear of leaving the familiar setting of home or venturing into the open; often associated with panic attacks. See *anxiety disorders*.

Albumin (al-BYU-min): Any of several naturally occurring blood proteins, some of which contribute to blood clotting capacity.

Alcoholism (AL-ko-hol-izm): Chronic alcohol abuse, dependence, or addiction; chronic excessive drinking of alcoholic beverages resulting in impairment of health and/or social or occupational functioning and increasing adaptation to the effects of alcohol, requiring increasing doses to achieve and sustain a desired effect. See *chemical dependency*.

Aldosterone (al-DOS-ter-one): A hormone manufactured in the adrenal cortex. It helps to maintain appropriate fluid balance by influencing sodium reabsorption in the kidneys; the principal mineralocorticoid.

Alkaline phosphatase (AL-kah-lin FOS-fah-tase): A phosphatase with an optimum pH above 7.0, present in many tissues; low levels of this enzyme are seen in cases of hypophosphatasia. See *Paget disease*, *osteoporosis*.

Allergen (AL-er-jen): A substance that elicits an allergic reaction.

Allergic rhinitis (ah-LER-jik ri-NI-tis): Synonym for hay fever. See *sinusitis*.

Allodynia (al-o-DIN-e-ah): Condition in which a normally painless stimulus causes pain.

Allogenic transplant (al-o-JEN-ik TRANZ-plant): A graft transplanted between genetically different individuals of the same species.

Alpha-1-antitrypsin (AL-fah 1 an-te-TRIP-sin): A protein that protects the inner lining of alveoli. See *emphysema*.

Alpha-blockers (AL-fah BLOK-erz): A class of medications employed to help control hypertension.

Alpha-fetoprotein (AL-fah FE-to-pro-tene): An antigen present in the fetus, associated with neural tube defects. See *spina bifida*.

Alveolus, alveoli (al-VE-o-lus, al-VE-o-li): A small cavity or socket; specifically, the terminal epithelial structures in the lungs where gaseous exchange takes place.

Alzheimer disease (ALZ-hi-mer): Progressive mental deterioration manifested by losses of memory, ability to calculate, and visual-spatial orientation; confusion; disorientation.

Amantadine (ah-MAN-tah-dene): An antiviral agent sometimes used to treat influenza.

Ambulatory (AM-bu-lah-tor-e): Able to walk; not confined to bed or a wheelchair.

Amebiasis (am-e-BI-ah-sis): Protozoan infection, usually with *Entamoeba histolytica*.

Amenorrhea (ah-men-or-E-ah): Absence or abnormal cessation of menses.

Amine (AM-ene): A positively charged ion found only in association with negatively charged ions; amines combine with acids to form salts.

Amino acid (ah-ME-no AS-id): An organic acid in which one of the hydrogen atoms on a carbon atom has been replaced by NH_2, a type of ammonia. A building block of proteins.

Amniocentesis (am-ne-o-sen-TE-sis): Transabdominal aspiration of fluid from the amniotic sac for diagnostic purposes.

Amphiarthrosis, amphiarthroses (am-fe-arth-RO-sis): A joint in which the two bones are joined by fibrocartilage.

Amyloidosis (am-ih-loyd-O-sis): A disease characterized by extracellular accumulation of amyloid proteins in various organs and tissues. See *myeloma*.

Amyotrophic lateral sclerosis (am-e-o-TRO-fik LAT-er-al skler-O-sis): A disease of the motor tracts of the lateral columns and anterior horns of the spinal cord, causing progressive muscular atrophy, increased reflexes, fibrillary twitching, and spastic irritability of muscles. Also called Lou Gehrig disease.

Anaerobic metabolism (an-ah-RO-bik meh-TAB-o-lizm): Metabolism that takes place without adequate supplies of oxygen. It may result in excessive buildup of toxic waste products.

Anaphylaxis (an-ah-fil-AK-sis): An immediate, transient allergic reaction characterized by contraction of smooth muscle and dilation of capillaries.

Androgen (AN-dro-jen): A hormone that stimulates activity of sex organs.

Anergy (AN-er-je): Lack of ability to generate a sensitivity reaction to substances expected to be antigenic, immunogenic, or allergenic in that individual. See *HIV/AIDS*.

Aneurysm (AN-yur-izm): Circumscribed dilation of an artery or a cardiac chamber, in direct communication with the lumen, usually due to an acquired or congenital weakness of the wall of the artery or chamber.

Angina (an-JI-nah): A severe, often constricting pain. Usually refers to angina pectoris.

Angioedema (an-je-o-eh-DE-mah): Recurrent large circumscribed areas of subcutaneous edema of sudden onset, usually disappearing within 24 hours, frequently seen as an allergic reaction to foods or drugs. See *allergic reactions*.

Angiogenesis (an-je-o-JEN-eh-sis): Development of new blood vessels.

Angiogram (AN-je-o-gram): Radiograph of blood vessels after injection of contrast material.

Angioneurotic edema (an-je-o-nu-ROT-ik eh-DE-mah): Hives on the face and neck and swelling to the point that breathing becomes difficult.

Angioplasty (AN-je-o-plas-te): Recanalization of a blood vessel, usually by means of balloon dilation and/or the placement of a stent.

Ankle-brachial index (ANG-kel BRA-ke-al IN-dex): A comparison of blood pressure between the ankle and the arm, used to identify risk of peripheral artery disease. See *atherosclerosis*.

Ankylosing spondylitis (ANG-kih-lo-sing spon-dih-LI-tis): Arthritis of the spine; more common in the male, often with the rheumatoid factor absent and the human leukocyte antigen present. The strong familial aggregation suggests an important genetic factor.

Anoxia (an-OX-e-ah): Absence of oxygen.

Anterior knee pain syndrome (an-TE-re-or ne PANE SIN-drome): Synonym for patellofemoral syn-drome.

Antibody (AN-ti-bod-e): An immunoglobulin molecule produced by B cells and designed to react with specific antigens.

Anticholinergic (an-te-kol-ih-NER-jik): Antagonistic to the action of parasympathetic or other cholinergic nerve fibers, e.g., atropine.

Anticoagulant (an-te-co-AG-yu-lent): An agent that prevents or inhibits clotting of the blood.

Antidiuretic hormone (an-ti-di-ur-EH-tik HOR-mone): Also called vasopressin, a hormone that suppresses the output of urine.

Antigen (AN-tih-jen): Any substance that elicits an immune response on contact with sensitive cells.

Antigenic shift (an-tih-JEN-ik shift): The merging of genetic material that may occur when two subtypes of pathogens simultaneously coinfect a single host. See *influenza*.

Antinuclear antibody (an-ti-NU-kle-ar AN-ti-bod-e): An antibody showing an affinity for cell nuclei, demonstrated by exposing a cell substrate to the serum to be tested, followed by exposure to an anti–human globulin serum; found in the serum of a high proportion of patients with systemic lupus erythematosus, rheumatoid arthritis, and certain collagen diseases, in some of their healthy relatives, and in about 1% of normal individuals.

Antrectomy (an-TREK-to-me): Removal of the antrum (distal half) of the stomach in treatment of peptic ulcer.

Anular (AN-yu-lar): Ring shaped.

Anulus fibrosis (AN-u-lus fi-BRO-sis): Fibrous ring of tissue in an intervertebral disc.

Aphasia (ah-FA-zha): Impaired or absent comprehension or production of, or communication by, speech, writing, or signs; due to an acquired lesion of the dominant cerebral hemisphere. See *stroke*.

Aphtha, aphthae (AF-thah, AF-the): Small ulcer on a mucous membrane, usually in the mouth.

Aplastic (a-PLAS-tik): Referring to conditions characterized by defective regeneration, e.g., varieties of cancer.

Apnea (AP-ne-ah): Absence of breathing.

Aponeurosis (ap-o-nu-RO-sis): A fibrous sheet or flat expanded tendon giving attachment to muscular fibers and serving as the means of origin or insertion of a flat muscle; it sometimes serves as a fascia for other muscles.

Apoptosis (ap-op-TO-sis): Programmed cell death.

Arachinodonic acid (ah-rak-ih-DON-ik AS-id): An essential fatty acid associated with hypersensitivity reactions on the skin.

Arachnoid (ah-RAK-noyd): A delicate membrane of spider web–like filaments that lies between the dura mater and the pia mater.

Arrhythmia (ah-RITH-me-ah): Irregularity of the heartbeat.

Arteriogram (ar-TE-re-o-gram): Radiographic image of an artery after injection of a contrast medium.

Arteriole (ar-TE-re-ole): A minute artery continuous with a capillary network.

Arteriosclerosis (ar-TE-re-o-skler-O-sis): hardening of the arteries; types generally recognized are atherosclerosis, Mönckeberg arteriosclerosis, and arteriolosclerosis.

Arthrochalasia EDS (arth-ro-kah-LA-zha EDS): A type of Ehlers-Danlos syndrome involving easily dislocating hip joints.

Ascites (ah-SI-teze): The accumulation of serous fluid in the peritoneal cavity. See *cirrhosis*, *liver cancer*.

Aspergillosis (as-per-jil-O-sis): The presence of *Aspergillus*, a genus of fungi, in the tissues or on a mucous surface of humans and animals, and the symptoms produced thereby.

Asphyxia (as-FIX-e-ah): Impaired or absent exchange of carbon dioxide and oxygen in the respiratory system.

Ataxic (ah-TAX-ik): Unable to coordinate muscle activity for smooth movement.

Atelectasis (at-el-EK-tah-sis): Absence of gas from a part or whole of the lung; pulmonary collapse.

Atherosclerosis (ath-er-o-skler-O-sis): Hardening of the arteries characterized by the formation of lipid deposits in the intima of large arteries. Deposits lead to fibrosis, calcification, and a narrowing of the lumen.

Athetoid (ATH-eh-toyd): Referring to slow, writhing, involuntary movement of fingers and hands, sometimes of toes and feet.

Atopic (a-TOP-ic): Relating to an allergic reaction.

Atrial fibrillation (A-tre-al fib-rih-LA-shun): Fibrillation in which the normal rhythmical contractions of the cardiac atria are replaced by rapid irregular twitchings of the muscular wall. See *embolism*.

Atrium, atria (A-tre-um, A-tre-ah): A chamber or cavity connected to other cavities; specifically the superior chambers of the heart.

Atrophic (a-TRO-fik): Denoting tissue or organ wasting.

Atrophic gastritis (a-TRO-fik gas-TRI-tis): A condition in which long-term inflammation interferes with acid-producing cells in the stomach; a risk factor for stomach cancer.

Atrophy (AT-ro-fe): A wasting of tissues from a number of causes, including diminished cellular proliferation, ischemia, malnutrition, and death.

Auscultation (aw-skul-TA-shun): Listening to sounds made by various body parts as a diagnostic tool.

Autoantibody (aw-to-AN-ti-bod-e): Antibody occurring in response to antigenic constituents of the host's tissue; reacts with the inciting tissue component.

Autodigestion (aw-to-di-JES-chun): Enzymatic digestion of cells (especially dead or degenerate) by enzymes present within them. See *pancreatitis*.

Autogenic transplant (aw-to-JEN-ic TRANZ-plant): The transplant of a substance that originated within the patient's body, as in bone marrow cells. Also called autologous transplant.

Autoimmune (AW-to-ih-MUNE): Arising from and directed against the individual's tissues.

Autoimmune polyglandular syndrome (au-to-ih-MUNE pol-e GLAN-du-lar SIN-drome): A group term for conditions that frequently appear together or within families, including Graves disease, type 1 diabetes, systemic lupus erythematosus, and others.

Autologous transplant (aw-TOL-o-gus TRANZ-plant): Synonym for autogenic transplant.

Autonomic hyperreflexia (aw-to-NOM-ik hi-per-re-FLEX-e-ah): A syndrome occurring in some persons with spinal cord lesions and resulting from functional impairment of the autonomic nervous system. Symptoms include hypertension, bradycardia, severe headaches, pallor below and flushing above the cord lesion, and convulsions.

Avascular (a-VAS-ku-lar): Without blood or lymphatic vessels.

Avulsion (ah-VUL-zhun): A tearing away or forcible separation.

Axon (AK-son): The process of a nerve cell that conducts impulses away from the cell body.

Babesiosis (bah-be-ze-O-sis): An infection with a species of protozoan parasites, transferred to humans by tick bites.

Babinski sign (bah-BIN-ske sine): Extension of the great toe and abduction of the other toes instead of the normal flexion reflex to plantar stimulation, considered indicative of central nervous system injury.

Bacteremia (bak-te-RE-me-ah): The presence of viable bacteria in circulating blood.

Balloon sinusotomy (bah-LOON si-nus-OT-o-me): Procedure involving the use of tiny balloons on catheters to correct nasal sinus structural anomalies.

Barotrauma (BA-ro-traw-mah): Scuba diving injury involving a rapid change in pressure that can damage the inner ear. See *vestubular balance disorders*.

Barrel chest (BA-rel chest): An occasional symptom of emphysema, in which the intercostal muscles hold the rib cage out as wide as possible.

Barrett esophagus (BA-ret e-SOF-ah-gus): Chronic ulceration of the lower esophagus, often associated with gastroesophageal reflux disorder; sometimes a precursor to adenocarcinoma of the esophagus.

Basal ganglia (BA-sal GANG-le-ah): Large masses of gray matter at the base of the cerebral hemispheres.

Basal layer (BA-sal LA-er): Also called the stratum basale; the deepest layer of the epidermis.

Basophil (BA-so-fil): A phagocytic leukocyte.

Bell's law: The ventral spinal roots are motor, while the dorsal spinal roots are sensory.

Bence Jones proteins: Protein fragments found in association with multiple myeloma.

Benign (be-NINE): Denoting the mild character of an illness or nonmalignant character of a neoplasm.

Benign paroxysmal positional vertigo (be-NINE pah-rok-SIZ-mal po-SIH-shun-al VER-tih-go): A recurrent form of vertigo caused by otoliths outside of the vestibule. See *vestibular balance disorders*.

Benign prostatic hypertrophy (be-NINE PROS-tate hy-PER-tro-fe): A nodular hyperplasia of the prostate; the gland thickens in a way that may obstruct the urethra.

Benzene (BEN-zene): A highly toxic hydrocarbon from light coal tar oil, used as a solvent.

Benzodiazapine (ben-zo-di-AH-zah-pene): Any of a group of psychotropic drugs with sedative action; used as antianxiety drugs or sleeping aids. See *anxiety disorders*.

Beta amyloid (BA-tah AM-ih-loyd): A type of protein associated with formation of plaque in the brain. See *Alzheimer disease*.

Beta blocker (BA-tah BLOK-er): A type of drug that limits sympathetic reactions, specifically as they relate to the cardiovascular system.

Beta cell (BA-tah sel): Cell in the pancreas that secretes insulin.

Bile: Yellowish-brown or green fluid produced in the liver, stored in the gallbladder, and released into the duodenum to aid in the digestion of fats.

Biliary colic (BIL-e-a-re KOL-ik): Intense spasmodic pain in the right upper quadrant of the abdomen from impaction of a gallstone in the cystic duct.

Bilirubin (BIL-ih-ru-bin): A dark bile pigment formed from the hemoglobin of dead erythrocytes.

Biological response modifiers (bi-o-LOJ-ik-ul re-SPONS MOD-ih-fi-erz): Substances that alter the interaction between the body's immune defenses and cancer cells to boost, direct, or restore the body's ability to fight the disease.

Biophosphates (bi-o-FOS-fates): A group of medications that inhibit reabsorption of bone; often recommended in the treatment of osteoporosis.

Bipolar disease (bi-PO-lar): Synonym for manic-depressive psychosis.

Bismuth (BIZ-muth): A metallic element used in several medicines, specifically in those designed to affect stomach acidity.

Blastomycosis (blast-o-mi-KO-sis): A type of fungal infection that usually begins in the respiratory system. See *pneumonia*.

Blepharospasm (BLEF-ah-ro-spazm): Involuntary spasmodic contraction of the orbicularis oculi muscles. See *dystonia*.

Blood-brain barrier (blud-brane BA-re-er): A selective filter in a continuous layer of endothelial cells connected by tight junctions; prevents or inhibits the passage of ions or large compounds from the blood to the brain tissue.

Bolus (BO-lus): A masticated morsel of food or other substance ready to be swallowed.

Bone scan: A diagnostic test to look for bone cancer or infections, to evaluate unexplained pain, or to diagnose fractures.

Borrelia burgdorferi (bo-RE-le-ah burg-DOR-fer-i): A species of bacteria that causes Lyme disease; transferred to humans through tick bites.

Botulinum (BOT-yu-lin-um): A potent neurotoxin from *Clostridium botulinum*.

Bouchard nodes (boo-SHAR nodez): Enlargement of the proximal interphalangeal joints due to bone spurs associated with osteoarthritis.

Bovine spongiform encephalopathy (BO-vine SPUN-jih-form en-sef-ah-LOP-ath-e): A disease of cattle first reported in 1986 in Great Britain; characterized clinically by apprehensive behavior, hyperesthesia, and ataxia and histologically by spongiform changes in the gray matter of the brainstem; caused by a prion, like spongiform encephalopathies of other animals e.g., scrapie in cattle and Creutzfeldt-Jakob disease in humans. See *Alzheimer disease*.

Bowen disease (BO-wen): A form of intraepidermal carcinoma characterized by the development of slowly enlarging pinkish or brownish papules or eroded plaques covered with a thickened horny layer See *skin cancer*.

Bowman capsule (BO-man KAP-sule): The beginning of a nephron that surrounds the glomerulus.

Bradykinesia (brad-e-kin-E-se-a): A decrease in the spontaneity of movement.

Bronchiectasis (bronk-e-ek-TA-sis): Chronic dilation of the bronchi or bronchioles, often as a consequence of inflammatory disease or obstruction.

Bruxism (BRUK-sizm): Jaw clenching that results in rubbing and grinding of teeth, especially during sleep.

Buerger disease (BUR-ger): Inflammation of the intima of a blood vessel with thrombosis. See *Raynaud syndrome*.

Bulla, bullae (BUL-ah, BUL-ee): A bubblelike structure, specifically the air-filled blisters on the lung formed by fused alveoli in emphysema.

Burkitt lymphoma (BUR-kit lym-FO-mah): A form of malignant lymphoma frequently involving the submandibular and abdominal lymph nodes. Geographic distribution of Burkitt lymphoma suggests that it is found in areas with endemic malaria. It is primarily a B-cell neoplasm and is believed to be caused by Epstein-Barr virus, a member of the family Herpesviridae.

Bursectomy (bur-SEK-to-me): Surgical removal of a bursa.

Calcitonin (kal-sih-TO-nin): A hormone that increases the deposition of calcium and phosphate in bone.

Calcium channel blockers (KAL-se-um CHAN-el BLOK-erz): A class of medications that prevent the passage of calcium through membranes; used to treat hypertension, angina pectoris, and arrhythmia.

Calcium oxalate (KAL-se-um OK-sah-late): A sediment in urine and renal calculi. See *kidney stones*.

Calcium phosphate (KAL-se-um FOS-fate): Calcium salts of phosphoric acid.

Calcium pyrophosphate dihydrate (KAL-se-um pi-ro-FOS-fate di-HI-drate): Substance deposited in pseudogout, leading to acute attacks of joint inflammation. See *gout*.

Callus (KAL-us): A thickening of the keratin layer of the epidermis as a result of repeated friction or intermittent pressure.

Campylobacter jejuni (KAM-pih-lo-bak-ter jeh-JU-ni): A species that causes acute gastroenteritis of sudden onset with constitutional symptoms (malaise, myalgia, arthralgia, and headache) and cramping abdominal pain.

Campylobacter pylori (KAM-pih-lo-bak-ter pi-LOR-i): Synonym for *Helicobacter pylori*. See *ulcers*.

Candida albicans (KAN-di-dah AL-bih-kanz): A genus of yeastlike fungi.

Carbuncle (KAR-bunk-el): A group of local infections of hair follicles with connecting sinuses; a group of boils.

Carcinoma (kar-sih-NO-mah): Any of a variety of malignant neoplasms deriving from epithelial tissue.

Cardia of stomach (KAR-de-ah ov STUM-ak): Proximal end of the stomach.

Cardiac tamponade (KAR-de-ak TAM-po-nade): Pathological compression of the heart, related to increased volume of the pericardium.

Cardiomyopathy (kar-de-o-mi-OP-ath-e): Disease of the myocardium; a primary disease of heart muscle in the absence of a known underlying etiology.

Cataplexy (KAT-ah-plex-e): A transient attack of extreme generalized muscular weakness, often precipitated by an emotional state such as laughing, surprise, fear, or anger. See *sleep disorders*.

Catheter atherectomy (KATH-eh-ter ath-er-EK-to-me): Removal of atherosclerotic plaque through a catheter; usually applied to carotid arteries.

Cauda equina (KAW-dah e-KWI-nah): Bundle of spinal nerve roots that runs through the lumbar cistern; it comprises the roots of all the spinal nerves below L_1. From Latin: *horse tail*. See *ankylosing spondylitis, disc disease*.

Causalgia (kaw-ZAL-je-ah): Persistent severe burning sensation, usually following partial injury of a peripheral nerve, accompanied by trophic changes including thinning of skin, loss of sweat glands and hair follicles. See *complex regional pain syndrome*.

Celiac sprue (SE-le-ak spru): Chronic inflammation and atrophy of the mucosa of the small intestine, related to an allergy to gluten.

Cellular immunity (SEL-u-lar ih-MU-nih-te): Also called cell-mediated immunity. Immune responses that are initiated by T cells and mediated by T cells, macrophages, or both.

Cervical rib (SER-vih-kal rib): An abnormally wide transverse process of a cervical vertebra or a supernumerary rib that articulates with a cervical vertebra but does not articulate with the sternum. C7 is the vertebra most often affected.

Cervical spondylitic myelopathy (SER-vih-kal spon-dih-LIH-tik mi-el-OP-ath-e): Damage to the spinal cord due to osteophytic pressure. See *spondylosis*.

Chancre (KAN-ker): The primary lesion of syphilis, which begins at the site of infection after an interval of 10 to 30 days as a papule or area of infiltration, of dull red color, hard, and insensitive; the center usually becomes eroded or breaks down into an ulcer that heals slowly after 4 to 6 weeks. See *sexually transmitted diseases*.

Chemonucleolysis (ke-mo-nu-kle-OL-ih-sis): Injection of chymopapain into the nucleus pulposus of a herniated disc.

Chemotherapy (ke-mo-THER-ah-pe): The treatment of disease by chemical means, that is, drugs.

Childhood disintegrative disorder (child-hood dis-IN-teh-gra-tiv): A type of autism spectrum disorder involving a dramatic loss of vocabulary, motor, and communication skills.

Chimeric (ki-MER-ik): Any macromolecule fusion formed by two or more macromolecules from different species or from different genes. See *scleroderma*.

Chlamydia (klah-MIH-de-ah): A genus of bacteria that is a causative factor for pelvic inflammatory disease and other infections; the chief agent of bacterial sexually transmitted diseases in the United States.

Chlamydia trachomatis (klah-MIH-de-ah trak-o-MAH-tis): Spherical organism that causes a variety of infections, including conjunctivitis, pelvic inflammatory disease, and others.

Cholangitis (ko-lan-JI-tis): Inflammation of the bile duct or biliary tree.

Cholecyst (KO-leh-sist): Synonym for gallbladder.

Choledocholithiasis (ko-led-o-ko-lih-THI-ah-sis): Presence of a gallstone in the common bile duct.

Cholelithiasis (ko-leh-lih-THI-ah-sis): Presence of stones in the gallbladder or bile ducts.

Cholinesterase inhibitors (ko-lin-ES-ter-ase in-HIB-ih-torz): Class of drugs that improve myoneural function; used for myasthenia gravis, Alzheimer disease.

Chondroitin sulfate (kon-DROY-tin SUL-fate): One of

the substances in the extracellular matrix of connective tissue.

Chondromalacia patellae (kon-dro-mah-LA-she-a pah-TEL-a): Degenerative condition in the articular cartilage of the kneecap caused by abnormal compression or shearing forces at the knee joint; may cause patellalgia (knee pain).

Choriocarcinoma (KOR-e-o-kar-sih-NO-mah): A highly malignant neoplasm. Hemorrhagic metastases are found in the lungs, liver, brain, and vagina; choriocarcinoma may follow any type of pregnancy, especially hydatidiform mole, and occasionally originates in teratoid neoplasms of the ovaries or testes. See *testicular cancer*.

Christmas disease (KRIS-mas dih-ZEZE: Synonym for hemophilia B, involving a deficiency in clotting factor IX.

Chronic (KRON-ik): Having low intensity, lasting a long time; refers to a disease or disorder.

Chronic exertional compartment syndrome (KRON-ik eg-ZER-shun-al kom-PART-ment SIN-drome): The accumulation of fluid pressure in one or more of the tough fascial compartments of the lower leg. See *shin splints*.

Chronic granulocytic leukemia (KRON-ik gran-u-lo-SIT-ik lu-KE-me-ah): Synonym for chronic myelogenous leukemia. See *leukemia*.

Chronic myeloid leukemia (KRON-ik MI-eh-loyd lu-KE-me-ah): Synonym for chronic myelogenous leukemia. See *leukemia*.

Chronic venous insufficiency (KRON-ik VE-nus in-suh-FISH-en-se): A condition resulting from valve damage in veins that leads to permanent edema, skin discoloration or ulcers, and very slow healing in the affected area.

Chyme (kime): Semifluid mass of partly digested food in the stomach or small intestine.

Cilium, cilia (sil-e-um, sil-e-ah): Hairlike motile extension of the surface of certain epithelial cells.

Circadian rhythm (sir-KA-de-an RITH-em): Relating to biological variations or rhythms that last approxi-mately 24 hours. From Latin *circa* (*about*) and *dies* (*day*).

Cirrhosis (sir-O-sis): Progressive disease of the liver characterized by damage to hepatocytes and accumulation of scar tissue.

Clonic spasm (KLON-ik spazm): Alternating involuntary contraction and relaxation of a muscle.

Coagulability (ko-ag-yu-lah-BIL-ih-te): Ability to clot.

Cobalamine (ko-BAL-ah-mene): General term for compounds containing the nucleus of vitamin B_{12}.

Coccidioidomycosis (kok-sid-e-OY-do-mi-KO-sis): A potentially fatal fungal disease, usually of the respiratory tract.

Cognitive-behavioral therapy (KOG-nih-tiv be-HA-vyor-al THER-ah-pe): A technique in psychotherapy that uses guided self-discovery, imaging, self-instruction, and other elicited cognitions as the principal mode of treatment.

Colchicine (KOL-chih-sene): An alkaloid obtained from autumn crocus used for the treatment of gout.

Colic (KOL-ik): An abnormal contraction of smooth muscle, particularly in the digestive tract.

Collagen (KOL-ah-jen): A major protein forming the white fibers of connective tissue.

Collagenase (ko-LAJ-eh-nase): A proteolytic dissolving enzyme that acts on one or more of the collagens.

Colonoscopy (kol-o-NOS-ko-pe): A visual examination of the internal surface of the colon by means of a long fiberoptic endoscope.

Colostomy (ko-LOS-to-me): An artificial opening from the skin to the colon.

Colposcopy (kol-POS-ko-pe): Examination of the vagina and cervix by means of an endoscope.

Comedo (ko-ME-do): A dilated hair follicle filled with bacteria; the principal lesion of acne vulgaris. Plural, comedos, comedones.

Comminuted (KOM-ih-nu-ted): Broken into several pieces; denoting especially a fractured bone.

Comorbidity (ko-mor-BID-ih-te): Condition of having multiple pathologies simultaneously.

Complement (KOM-pleh-ment): A combination of many serum proteins that react with each other in various ways to disable antigens and assist immune system response.

Complex regional pain syndrome (KOM-plex RE-jun-al PAIN SIN-drome): A chronic pain syndrome; sometimes called *reflex sympathetic dystrophy syndrome*.

Condyle (KON-dile): A rounded articular surface at the extremity of a bone.

Condylomata acuminatum (kon-dih-LO-mah-tah ah-ku-min-AH-tum): A warty growth on the external genitals or at the anus, consisting of fibrous overgrowths covered by thickened epithelium showing koilocytosis, due to sexually transmitted infection with human papillomavirus; malignant change is associated with particular types of the virus. See *sexually transmitted diseases*.

Congenital (kon-JEN-ih-tal): Referring to mental or physical traits that exist at birth.

Congenital nevus (kon-JEN-ih-tal NE-vus): A benign local overgrowth of melanin-forming cells of the skin present at birth or appearing early in life.

Consolidation (kon-sol-ih-DA-shun): Solidification into a firm, dense mass, specifically with cellular exudate in the lungs during pneumonia.

Constriction (kon-STRIK-shun): A narrowed portion of a luminal structure.

Contact inhibition (KON-takt in-hih-BIH-shun): The tendency of basal cells involved in healing to stop reproducing when they encounter cells from the other side of the wound.

Contralateral (kon-trah-LAT-er-al): Relating to the opposite side, as when pain is felt or paralysis occurs on the side opposite to that of the lesion.

Cor pulmonale (kor pul-mo-NAL): Right-sided ventricular hypertrophy, often arising from disease of the lungs.

Corpus callosum (KOR-pus kal-LOS-um): The plate of nerve fibers interconnecting the cortical hemispheres.

Corpus luteum (KOR-pus LU-te-um): The site of egg release on follicles of the ovaries immediately after ovulation.

Corticosteroid injection (kor-tih-ko-STER-oyd in-JEK-shun): An injection of a specific steroid into an injured area for its anti-inflammatory and/or connective tissue–dissolving properties.

Cortisol (KOR-tih-sol): A glucocorticoid secreted by the adrenal cortex. It acts on carbohydrate metabolism and influences the growth and nutrition of connective tissue.

Cortisone (KOR-tih-sone): A form of cortisol that may be injected into specific areas to act as an anti-inflammatory or to help dissolve connective tissue.

Coup de sabre (koo deh SAHB): Linear scleroderma over the forehead.

Coup-contrecoup (koo-KON-treh-koo): Pattern of brain injury involving a primary impact on one side of the skull and a secondary impact as the brain bounces to the opposite side of the cranium. See *traumatic brain injury*.

COX-2 inhibitors: A class of nonsteroidal anti-inflammatory drugs that work by blocking COX (cyclo-oxygenase) 2 enzyme, which is involved in the inflammation pathway.

Coxsackievirus (kok-SAK-e-VI-rus): A group of viruses first isolated in Coxsackie, New York. They may be responsible for several human diseases, including meningitis and juvenile diabetes.

C-reactive protein: A beta-globulin found in the serum of various persons with certain inflammatory, degenerative, and neoplastic diseases. See *heart attack*, *atherosclerosis*.

Creatine kinase (KREE-ah-tene KI-nase): An enzyme used in muscle contraction that allows transformation of adenosine diphosphate into adenosine triphosphate and creatine; levels of creatine kinase are sometimes elevated following a heart attack. See *muscular dystrophy*.

Crepitus (KREP-ih-tus): A crackling sound resembling the noise heard on rubbing hair between the fingers.

CREST syndrome: *C*alcinosis, *R*aynaud phenomenon, *e*sophageal motility disorders, *s*clerodactyly, and *t*elangiectasia. See *scleroderma*.

Crisis (KRI-sis): A sudden change, usually for the better, in the course of an acute disease.

Cruciate ligament (KROO-she-ate LIG-ah-ment): Major ligaments that crisscross the knee in the anteroposterior direction, providing stability in that plane.

Crust (krust): A hard outer covering; a scab.

Cryomyolysis (kri-o-mi-OL-ih-sis): A procedure using liquid nitrogen to freeze uterine fibroid tumors.

Cryptococcus neoformans (KRIP-to-kok-us ne-o-FOR-manz): A species of yeastlike fungi that reproduce by budding. See *HIV/AIDS*.

Cryptorchism (krip-TOR-kizm): Failure of one or both of the testes to descend. See *testicular cancer*.

Cryptosporidium (krip-to-spor-IH-de-um): A genus of sporozoans that are common parasites of humans with impaired immunity. See *gastroenteritis*.

Cyanosis (si-ah-NO-sis): A bluish or purplish coloration of the skin and mucous membranes due to deficient oxygenation of the blood. See *Raynaud syndrome*, *anemia*.

Cyclo-oxygenase-2 (si-klo-OX-ih-jen-ase): See COX-2 inhibitors.

Cystadenoma (sist-ah-den-O-ma): A benign neoplasm derived from glandular epithelium. See *ovarian cysts*.

Cystine (SIS-tene): A type of acid that can form deposits of crystals in the urine or in the kidneys.

Cystoscope (SIS-to-skope): A lighted tubular endoscope for examining the interior of the bladder.

Cytokine (SI-to-kine): Hormonelike proteins secreted by many cells and involved in cell-to-cell communication.

Cytomegalovirus (si-to-MEG-ah-lo-vi-rus): A group of viruses in the Herpesviridae family infecting humans and animals.

Cytotoxic drug (si-to-TOX-ik drug): A drug that is detrimental or destructive to certain cells.

Dactylitis (dak-tih-LI-tis): Inflammation of the fingers.

De Quervain tenosynovitis (deh kare-VA ten-o-sin-o-VI-tis): Inflammation of the tendons of the first dorsal compartment of the wrist, which includes the extensor pollicis brevis and the abductor pollicis longus.

Debridement (da-brede-MONH): Excision of dead tissue and foreign matter from a wound.

Decubitus ulcer (de-KU-bih-tus UL-ser): Focal ischemic necrosis of skin and underlying tissues at sites of constant pressure or recurring friction in persons confined to bed or immobilized by illness.

Degeneration (de-jen-er-A-shun): A retrogressive pathological change in tissues, in consequence of which their functions may be impaired or destroyed.

Degenerative joint disease (de-JEN-er-ah-tiv JOYNT): Synonym for osteoarthritis.

Dementia (de-MEN-sha): The loss, usually progressive, of cognitive and intellectual functions without impairment of perception or consciousness.

Dendrite (DEN-drite): The process of a nerve cell that carries impulses toward the cell body.

Dermabrasion (der-mah-BRA-zhun): Procedure to remove acne scars or pits from the skin using sandpaper, rotating wire brushes, or other abrasive materials.

Dermatitis herpetiformis (der-mah-TI-tis her-pet-ih-FOR-mis): A chronic disease of the skin marked by a symmetrical itching eruption of vesicles and papules that occur in groups; relapses are common; associated with gluten-sensitive enteropathy. See *celiac sprue*.

Dermatome (DER-mah-tome): The area of skin supplied by cutaneous branches from a single spinal nerve.

Dermatophyte (der-MAT-o-fite): A fungus that causes superficial infections of the skin, hair, and nails.

Dermatophytosis (der-mat-o-fi-TO-sis): An infection of the hair, skin, or nails caused by any one of the dermatophytes. The lesions are characterized by erythema, small papular vesicles, fissures, and scaling. See *fungal infections*.

Dermatosparaxis EDS (der-mat-o-spah-RAK-sis): A type of Ehlers-Danlos syndrome involving loose, sagging skin even in young children, and ligament laxity.

Dermographia (der-mo-GRAF-e-ah): A form of urticaria in which wheals develop where the skin has been stroked.

Dermoid cyst (DER-moyd SIST): A tumor consisting of displaced ectodermal structures along lines of embryonic fusion, the wall being formed of epithelium-lined connective tissue, including skin appendages and containing keratin, sebum, and hair. See *testicular cancer*, *ovarian cysts*.

DEXA: Dual-energy x-ray absorptiometry. Use of low-dose x-radiation of two different energies to measure bone mineral content at different anatomic sites.

Dextroamphetamine (dex-tro-am-FET-ah-mene): A medication for central nervous system stimulation.

Diabetes insipidus (di-ah-BE-teze in-SIP-ih-dus): Chronic excretion of very large amounts of pale urine of low specific gravity, causing dehydration and extreme thirst; ordinarily results from inadequate output of pituitary antidiuretic hormone.

Diaphoresis (di-ah-for-E-sis): Perspiration.

Diaphysis (di-AH-fih-sis): The shaft of a long bone.

Diarthrosis, diarthroses (di-arth-RO-sis, di-arth-RO-seze): Also called synovial joint. A joint in which articulating surfaces are covered by articular cartilage and held together by a capsular ligament, which is lined with a synovial membrane. Some degree of freedom of movement is possible with diarthrotic joints.

Diastole (DI-ah-stole): Normal postsystolic dilation of the heart cavities, during which they fill with blood.

Diethylstilbesterol (di-eth-il-stil-BES-ter-ol): An estrogenic compound that used to be used to prevent miscarriage; it is associated with a risk of cervical cancer in the daughters of women who took it.

Diffuse axonal injury (dih-FUSE AK-so-nal IN-jur-e): Injury to white matter in the central nervous system that is frequently associated with a persistent vegetative state. See *traumatic brain injury*.

Diffuse idiopathic skeletal hyperostosis (DISH) (dih-FUSE id-e-o-PATH-ik SKEL-eh-tal hi-per-os-TO-sis): A common condition involving the deposition of calcium deposits along the anterior longitudinal ligament of the spine.

Diffuse large cell lymphoma (dih-FUSE larj sell lim-FO-mah): A type of intermediate-grade lymphoma.

Diffuse mixed cell lymphoma (dih-FUSE mixt sell lim-FO-mah): A type of intermediate-grade lymphoma.

Diffuse scleroderma (dih-FUSE skler-o-DER-mah): A form of systemic scleroderma characterized by sudden onset and early involvement of internal organs.

Diffusion (dih-FU-zhun): Random movement of small particles in solution to a uniform distribution within a closed space.

Dihydrotestosterone (DHT) (di-hi-dro-tes-TOS-ter-one): An androgenic hormone with the same uses and actions as testosterone. Elevated levels are associated with an increased risk of benign prostatic hyper-plasia.

Dilation (di-LA-shun): The enlargement of a hollow structure or opening.

Dilation and curettage (di-LA-shun and ku-reh-TAHJH): Dilation of the cervix and scraping of the endometrium.

Dimethyl sulfoxide (DMSO) (di-METH-il sul-FOX-ide): A penetrating solvent enhancing absorption of therapeutic agents through the skin.

Dioxin (di-OX-in): A contaminate in some herbicides; associated with toxicity, some forms of cancer, and birth defects.

Diphtheria (dif-THE-re-ah): A highly infectious bacterial disease that begins in the nose and throat; can resemble mononucleosis.

Diplegia (di-PLE-je-ah): Paralysis of corresponding parts on both sides of the body.

Discoid lupus erythematosus (DIS-koid LU-pus eh-rih-them-ah-TO-sis): Autoimmune disease involving lesions on the skin. See *lupus*.

Discectomy (dis-KEK-to-me): Excision of part or all of an intervertebral disk. See *disc disease*.

Diuretic (di-u-REH-tik): A chemical agent that increases urine output.

Diverticulum, diverticula (div-er-TIK-u-lum, div-er-TIK-u-lah): A pouch or sac opening from a tubular or saccular organ, e.g., the colon or urinary bladder.

DMARDs: Disease-modifying antirheumatic drugs. Agents that apparently alter the course and progression of rheumatoid arthritis; other substances (not DMARDs) suppress inflammation and decrease pain but do not prevent cartilage or bone erosion or progressive disability.

DOMS: Delayed-onset muscle soreness.

Dopamine (DO-pah-mene): A neurotransmitter in the basal ganglia.

Double crush syndrome (DUB-el KRUSH SIN-drome): Irritation of peripheral nerves at multiple sites, leading to confusing signs and symptoms. See *carpal tunnel syndrome*.

Ductal ectasia (DUK-tal ek-TA-zha): Inflammation of the ducts of the breast. See *breast cancer*.

Dupuytren contracture (du-pwe-TRAH kon-TRAK-cher): A disease of the palmar fascia resulting in thickening and shortening of fibrous bands on the palmar surface of the hand and fingers resulting in a characteristic flexion deformity of the fourth and fifth digits.

Dura mater (DU-rah MA-ter): A tough, fibrous membrane forming the outer covering of the central nervous system.

Dural ectasia (DUR-al ek-TA-zha): Stretching and weakening of the dura mater with age; associated with Marfan syndrome.

Dysarthria (dis-ARTH-re-ah): Disturbance of speech related to paralysis or spasticity. See *stroke*.

Dyshidrosis (dis-hi-DRO-sis): A skin eruption with blisters and itching that usually appears on the volar surface of the hands or feet.

Dysmobility (dis-mo-BIL-ih-te): Inefficient or uncoordinated peristalsis in the gastrointestinal tract. See *scleroderma*.

Dyspepsia (dis-PEP-se-ah): Upset stomach: pain, burning, nausea, and gas.

Dysphagia (dis-FA-je-a): Difficulty in swallowing.

Dysplasia, dysplastic (dis-PLA-zha, dis-PLAS-tik): Abnormal tissue development.

Dysplastic nevus (dis-PLAS-tik NE-vus): Atypical mole associated with an increased risk of developing into malignant melanoma. See *skin cancer*.

Dyspnea (disp-NE-ah): Shortness of breath.

Dysthymia (dis-THI-me-ah): Chronic mood disorder involving long-term, low-grade depression.

Dystonia (dis-TO-ne-ah): A state of abnormal (too much or too little) muscle tone.

Dystrophic (dis-TRO-fik): Relating to progressive changes that may result from defective nutrition of a tissue or organ.

Dystrophin (dis-TRO-fin): A protein found in the sarcolemma of normal muscle tissue; it is missing in individuals with some forms of muscular dystrophy.

E. coli, *Escherichia coli* (E-KO-li, esh-er-IK-e-ah KO-li): A species of bacteria linked with infections of the gastrointestinal or urinary tracts.

EAST: Elevated arm stress test. See *thoracic outlet syndrome*.

Ecchymosis (ek-ih-MO-sis): A purplish patch caused by blood leaking into the skin; a bruise.

Echocardiogram (ek-o-KAR-de-o-gram): The record obtained by the use of ultrasound in the investigation of the heart and great vessels and diagnosis of cardiovascular lesions.

Eclampsia (e-KLAMP-se-ah): One or more convulsions not attributable to other cerebral conditions. In this case, related to pregnancy-induced hypertension.

Ecthyma (ek-THI-mah): A form of streptococcal infection of the skin. See *impetigo*.

Eczema (EG-zeh-mah): Generic term for inflammatory conditions of the skin, particularly with blistering in the acute stage, often accompanied by sensations of itching and burning.

Edema (eh-DE-mah): An accumulation of an excessive amount of watery fluid in cells, tissues, or serous membranes.

Ehrlichiosis (er-lik-e-O-sis): A tickborne bacterial infection of humans and dogs. See *Lyme disease*.

Elastin (e-LAS-tin): A yellow, elastic fibrous protein that contributes to the connective tissue of elastic structures.

Electrocauterization (e-lek-tro-kaw-ter-i-ZA-shun): Cauterization by passage of high-frequency current through tissue or by metal that has been electrically heated.

Electroencephalogram (EEG) (e-lek-tro-en-SEF-ah-lo-gram): A recording of electrical potentials of the brain, derived from electrodes attached to the scalp.

Electrolyte (e-LEK-tro-lite): Any compound that in solution conducts electricity and is decomposed by it.

Electromyography (EMG) (e-lek-tro-mi-OG-raf-e): A recording of electrical activity in muscle tissue.

Electronystagmogram (e-lek-tro-nis-TAG-mo-gram): A test to measure the extent of horizontal or vertical nystagmus. See *vestibular balance disorders*.

ELISA: Enzyme-linked immunosorbent assay. In vitro binding assay in which an enzyme and its substrate (rather than a radioactive substance) serve as the indicator system; in positive results, the two yield a colored or other easily recognizable substance. See *HIV/AIDS*.

Embolization (em-bo-li-ZA-shun): Therapeutic introduction of various substances into the circulation to occlude vessels, either to arrest or prevent hemorrhaging or to devitalize a structure or organ by occluding its blood supply.

Embryonic carcinoma (em-bre-ON-ik kar-sih-NO-mah): A type of testicular cancer.

Emery-Dreifuss muscular dystrophy (EM-er-e DRI-fus MUS-ku-lar DIS-tro-fe): A generally benign type of muscular dystrophy that typically begins in the shoulder girdle and then spreads distally; an X-linked inherited disorder.

Emollient (e-MOL-i-ent): An agent that softens or soothes the skin.

Empyema (em-pi-E-mah): Pus in a body cavity; usually refers to the thorax. See *pneumonia*.

Encephalitis (en-sef-ah-LI-tis): Inflammation of the brain.

Endarterectomy (en-dar-ter-EK-to-me): Excision of the diseased layers of an artery along with atherosclerotic plaques.

Endemic (en-DEM-ik): Present in a community or among a group of people; said of a disease prevailing continually in a region.

Endo- (EN-do): A prefix indicating within, inner, absorbing, or containing.

Endocarditis (en-do-kar-DI-tis): Inflammation of the the innermost tunic of the heart.

Endogenous (en-DOJ-en-us): Originating or produced within the organism or one of its parts.

Endolymph (EN-do-limf): The fluid in the membranous labyrinth of the inner ear.

Endometrioma (en-do-me-tre-O-mah): Mass of abnormal tissue in the endometrium. See *ovarian cysts*.

Endometritis (en-do-meh-TRI-tis): Inflammation of the endometrium.

Endometrium (en-do-ME-tre-um): The inner layers of the uterine wall.

Endomysium (en-do-MI-ze-um): The connective tissue sheath surrounding muscle fibers.

Endoscopic retrograde cholangiopancreatography (ERCP) (en-do-SKOP-ik RET-ro-grade ko-lan-je-o-pan-kre-ah-TOG-raf-e): A diagnostic procedure to detect problems in the liver, gallbladder, bile ducts, or pancreas. See *gallstones*.

Endoscopy (en-DOS-ko-pe): Examination of the interior of a hollow area by means of a special instrument, an endoscope.

Endosteum (en-DOS-te-um): A layer of cells lining the inner surface of the central medullary cavity of long bones.

Endovascular (en-do-VAS-kyu-lar): Referring to procedures conducted within blood vessels.

Enterovirus (EN-ter-o-vi-rus): Any of a diverse group of viruses that attack the intestines.

Enzyme (EN-zime): A protein that acts as a catalyst to induce chemical changes in other substances while remaining unchanged itself.

Eosinophil (e-o-SIN-o-fil): A class of phagocytic white blood cells with antiparasitic functions.

Ephelis, ephelides (eh-FE-lis, eh-FE-lih-deze): Freckles.

Epi- (EP-e): Prefix indicating upon, following, or subsequent to.

Epicondylitis (ep-ih-kon-dih-LI-tis): Infection or inflammation of an epicondyle.

Epidermis (ep-ih-DER-mis): The superficial epithelial portion of the skin.

Epidermophyton (ep-ih-der-MOF-ih-ton, ep-ih-der-mo-FI-ton): A genus of fungi whose macroconidia are clavate and smooth walled. The only species, *Epidermophyton floccosum*, is a common cause of tinea pedis and tinea cruris. See *fungal infections*.

Epididymis (ep-ih-DIH-dih-mus): A tube on the posterior aspect of the testes in which sperm mature.

Epimysium (ep-ih-MIS-e-um): The connective tissue membrane surrounding a skeletal muscle.

Epinephrine (ep-ih-NEF-rin): The chief hormone of the adrenal medulla; a potent stimulant of the sympathetic response.

Epistaxis (ep-ih-STAK-sis): Profuse bleeding from the nose.

Epitenon (ep-ih-TEE-non): Sheath that wraps around tendons; also a synonym for tenosynovial sheath.

Epithelium (ep-ih-THE-le-um): A purely cellular avascular layer covering all free surfaces including skin, mucous, and serous glands.

Epstein–Barr virus (EP-stine BAR VI-rus): A herpesvirus that causes infectious mononucleosis and is implicated in Burkitt lymphoma.

Ergot (ER-got): The resistant, overwintering stage of the parasitic ascomycetous fungus *Claviceps purpurea*. Ergot induces uterine contractions, controls bleeding, and alleviates certain localized vascular disorders, such as migraine headaches.

Ernest syndrome (ER-nest SIN-drome): A condition involving a weakened and irritated stylomandibular ligament; frequently mistaken for temporomandibular joint disorder. See *temporomandibular joint disorder*.

Erysipelas (er-ih-SIP-eh-lus): A specific acute, cutaneous inflammatory disease caused by beta-hemolytic streptococci and characterized by hot, red, edematous, brawny, and sharply defined eruptions; usually accompanied by severe constitutional symptoms. See *cellulitis*.

Erythema (er-i-THE-mah): Redness of the skin due to capillary dilation.

Erythema migrans (er-i-THE-mah MI-granz): A type of rash, usually seen as an early symptom of Lyme disease.

Erythrocyte (e-RITH-ro-site): A mature red blood cell.

Erythrodermic psoriasis (e-rith-ro-DER-mik so-RI-ah-sis): A generalized form of psoriasis that can cover 85% or more of the body.

Erythropoietin (EPO) (e-rith-ro-POY-eh-tin): A hormone secreted by the kidneys and possibly other tissues that stimulates the formation of red blood cells.

Essential (e-SEN-shal): Of unknown etiology, specifically in reference to hypertension.

Estradiol (es-tra-DI-ol): The most potent naturally occurring estrogen in mammals.

Estriol (ES-tre-ol): Estrogenic metabolite of estradiol; usually the predominant estrogenic metabolite found in urine, especially during pregnancy.

Estrogen (ES-tro-jen): A group of hormones secreted by the ovaries, placenta, testes, and possibly other tissues. Estrogens influence secondary sexual characteristics and the menstrual cycle.

Estrogen replacement therapy (ERT) (ES-tro-jen re-PLASE-ment THER-ah-pe): A treatment for the prevention or slowing of osteoporosis by replacing some of the hormones that are lost or diminished with the onset of menopause.

Estrone (ES-trone): A metabolite of estradiol.

Exenteration (ek-sen-ter-A-shun): Removal of internal organs and tissues, usually to ablate cancer.

Exogenous (eg-ZOJ-en-us): Originating or produced outside the organism.

Exophthalmus (ex-of-THAL-mus): Protrusion of one or both eyeballs.

External scar tissue (ex-TER-nal SKAR TISH-u): Scar tissue that develops outside of the injured structure, often binding that structure to other nearby structures in adhesions.

Extracorporeal shockwave lithotripsy (ex-trah-kor-POR-e-al SHOK-wave LITH-o-trip-se): Breaking up of renal or ureteral calculi by focused ultrasound energy.

Extramedullary plastocytoma (ex-trah-MED-u-la-re plas-to-si-TO-mah): Growth of myeloma tumors outside of bone tissue.

Exudate (EK-su-date): Any fluid that has seeped out of a tissue or its capillaries because of inflammation or injury.

Facioscapulohumeral dystrophy (FASH-e-o-SKAP-u-lo-HU-mer-al DIS-tro-fe): A relatively benign, slowly progressive type of muscular dystrophy involving the muscles of the face, shoulders, and arms.

Familial adenomatous polyposis (fah-MIL-e-al ad-en-O-mah-tus pol-e-PO-sis): An inherited trait characterized by formation of epithelial polyps in the colon; may be associated with an increased risk of colorectal cancer.

Fascicle, fasciculi (FASH-i-kel, fah-SHIK-u-li): A band or bundle of fibers, specifically muscle fibers.

Fasciculation (fash-ik-u-LA-shun): Involuntary contractions or twitchings of fasciculi.

Fat necrosis (fat nek-RO-sis): The death of fat cells, often in the breast.

Fecalith (FE-kah-lith): A hard mass composed of solidified or petrified feces. See *diverticular disease*.

Festinating gait (FES-tin-a-ting GATE): Gait in which the trunk is flexed, legs are stiff but flexed at the knees and hips, and the steps are short and progressively more rapid.

Fetal alcohol syndrome (fe-tal AL-ko-hol SIN-drome): A specific pattern of fetal malformation and health problems among offspring of mothers who are chronic alcoholics.

Fibrillation (fib-ril-A-shun): Exceedingly rapid contractions or twitching of muscular fibrils.

Fibrillin (FIB-ril-in): A protein of connective tissue. See *Marfan syndrome*.

Fibrin (FI-brin): An elastic filamentous protein that aids in coagulation of the blood.

Fibrinogen (fi-BRIN-o-jen): A globulin of the blood plasma that is converted into fibrin by the action of thrombin in the presence of ionized calcium to produce coagulation of the blood.

Fibroadenoma (fi-bro-ad-en-O-mah): A benign neoplasm of glandular epithelium, in which fibroblasts and other connective tissue proliferate. See *breast cancer*.

Fibroblast (FI-bro-blast): A cell capable of forming collagen fibers.

Filtration (fil-TRA-shun): The process of passing a liquid or gas through a filter.

Fimbria, fimbriae (FIM-bre-ah, FIM-bre-a): Any fringe-like structure. Ovarian fimbriae extend over the ovaries.

Fistula, fistulae (FIS-tu-lah, FIS-tu-le): An abnormal passage from one epithelial surface to another.

Fixation (fik-SA-shun): The condition of being firmly attached or set. In regard to the spine, being excessively limited in movement between individual vertebrae.

Flaccid paralysis (FLAK-sid pah-RAL-ih-sis, FLAS-id pah-RAL-ih-sis): Paralysis with a loss of muscle tone, although sensation is present.

Focal dystonia (FO-kal dis-TO-ne-ah): A movement disorder that affects only one region of the body.

Folate (FO-late): A form of folic acid.

Folic acid (FO-lik AS-id): Member of the vitamin B complex necessary for the normal formation of red blood cells.

Follicular cleaved cell lymphoma (fo-LIK-u-lar kleved sell lim-FO-mah): A type of low-grade lymphoma.

Follicular large cell lymphoma (fo-LIK-u-lar larj sell lim-FO-mah): A type of intermediate-grade lymphoma.

Follicular mixed cell lymphoma (fo-LIK-u-lar mixt sell lim-FO-mah): A type of low-grade lymphoma.

Folliculitis (fo-lik-u-LI-tis): Inflammatory reaction in hair follicles leading to papules or pustules.

Fragile X syndrome (FRAJ-il X SIN-drome): Genetic anomaly associated with developmental disability and one form of autism spectrum disorder.

Frozen shoulder (FRO-zen SHOL-der): See *adhesive capsulitis*.

Fulminant (FUL-mi-nant): Occurring suddenly, with great intensity or severity.

Fulminant colitis (FUL-mi-nant ko-LI-tis): Sudden and extreme onset of colon inflammation seen with ulcerative colitis.

Fundoplication (fun-do-plih-KA-shun): Suture of the fundus of the stomach around the esophagus to prevent reflux with hiatal hernia.

Furuncle (FYU-runk-el): A local bacterial infection in a hair shaft. A boil.

Gamma globulin (GAM-ah GLOB-u-lin): A preparation of proteins of human plasma containing the antibodies of normal adults.

Gamma-aminobutyric acid (GABA) (GAM-ah ah-me-no-bu-TIR-ik AS-id): A principal inhibitory neurotransmitter.

Gardner syndrome (GARD-ner SIN-drome): A type of familial adenomatous polyposis; a genetic risk factor for colorectal cancer.

Gastritis (gas-TRI-tis): Inflammation, especially mucosal, of the stomach.

Gastrostomy (gas-TROS-to-me): Establishment of a new opening into the stomach.

Geniculate ganglion (jen-IK-u-late GANG-le-on): A ganglion of the fibers conveyed by the facial nerve, located within the facial canal, containing the sensory neurons innervating the taste buds on the anterior two-thirds of the tongue and a small area on the external ear.

Geste antagoniste (jhest an-tag-o-NEEST): The habit of repeatedly touching an area affected with dystonia to reduce the severity of local contractions.

Giardia (je-AR-de-ah): A genus of parasitic flagellates that colonize the gastrointestinal tract of many mammals.

Gigantism (JI-gan-tizm): A condition of abnormal size or overgrowth of the entire body or of any of its parts. See *acromegaly*.

Gliadin (GLI-ah-din): A class of protein, separable from wheat and rye glutens. See *celiac sprue*.

Globus pallidus (GLO-bus PAL-id-us): The inner and lighter gray portion of the lentiform nucleus. See *Parkinson disease*.

Glomerular filtration rate (glo-MARE-yu-lar fil-TRA-shun RATE): The amount of fluid that passes from the glomeruli to the nephron within a given amount of time.

Glomerulations (glo-mare-yu-LA-shunz): Pinpoint hemorrhages of the bladder wall, seen with some cases of interstitial cystitis.

Glomerulonephritis (glo-MARE-yu-lar nef-RI-tis): Inflammation of the glomerulus and Bowman capsule.

Glomerulus (glo-MARE-yu-lus): A tuft of capillary loops surrounded by the Bowman capsule at the beginning of each nephric tubule in the kidney.

Glucagon (GLU-kah-gon): A hormone secreted by the pancreas; elevates blood sugar concentration.

Glucocorticoid (glu-ko-KOR-ti-koyd): Any steroidlike compound capable of influencing metabolism; also exerts an anti-inflammatory effect. Cortisol is the most potent of the naturally occurring glucocorticoids.

Glucosamine sulfate (glu-KO-sah-mene SUL-fate): An amino sugar used to support cartilaginous repair in osteoarthritis.

Glutamate (GLU-tah-mate): A salt or ester of glutamic acid, an amino acid that occurs in proteins; the sodium salt is monosodium glutamate. See *amyotrophic lateral sclerosis*.

Gluten (GLU-ten): The insoluble protein constituent of wheat and other grains.

Gluten-sensitive enteropathy (GLU-ten SEN-sih-tiv en-ter-OP-ath-e): Synonym for celiac sprue.

Glycogen (GLI-ko-jen): A substance found primarily in the liver and muscles that is easily converted into glucose.

Goiter (GOY-ter): Chronic enlargement of the thyroid gland not due to a neoplasm. May be related to both hyperthyroidism and hypothyroidism.

Golfer's elbow (GOL-ferz EL-bo): Synonym for medial epicondylitis.

Golgi tendon organ (GOL-je TEN-don OR-gan): A proprioceptive sensory nerve ending embedded in tendon fibers. It is activated by changes in tendon tension.

Grand mal seizure (grand MAL SE-zhur): Also called generalized tonic-clonic seizure. Characterized by a sudden onset of tonic contraction of the muscles, giving way to clonic convulsive movements.

Granulation tissue (gran-u-LA-shun TISH-u): Vascular connective tissue that forms on the surface of a healing wound.

Granulocyte (GRAN-u-lo-site): A mature granular leukocyte.

Granuloma (gran-u-LO-mah): A nodular inflammatory lesion; includes epithelial cells along with phagocytes, macrophages, and lymphocytes. See *inflammation*.

Granulomatosis enteritis (gran-u-lo-mah-TO-sis en-ter-I-tis): A term that was once used to refer to Crohn disease.

Graves disease (Graves): An organ-specific autoimmune disease of the thyroid gland. See *hyperthyroidism*.

Graves ophthalmopathy (graves of-thal-MOP-ath-e): Exophthalmos caused by increased water content of retroocular orbital tissues; associated with thyroid disease, usually hyperthyroidism.

Greater omentum (GRA-ter o-MEN-tum): A fold of peritoneum holding fat cells that hangs like an apron in front of the intestines.

Growth hormone (GH) (growth HOR-mone): See *somatotrophin*.

Guaifenesin (gwi-FEN-ih-sen): An expectorant that reduces the viscosity of sputum; sometimes recommended in the treatment of fibromyalgia syndrome.

Guillain-Barré syndrome (ge-YAH bar-RA SIN-drome): A self-limiting demyelinating syndrome related to autoimmune dysfunction, surgical complication, some vaccines, Hodgkin disease, and some types of drug reactions. Motor and/or sensory dysfunction begins in the extremities and moves proximally, sometimes leading to respiratory failure, before function is restored within weeks or months.

Guttate psoriasis (GUT-ate so-RI-ah-sis): A type of psoriasis that appears in round small patches, often following streptococcal infections.

HAART: Highly active antiretroviral therapy. *See HIV/AIDS*

Haemophilus influenzae (he-MOF-ih-lus in-flu-EN-za): A species in the respiratory tract that causes acute respiratory infections including pneumonia, acute conjunctivitis, bacterial meningitis, and purulent meningitis in children, rarely in adults.

Hallux valgus (HAL-lux VAL-gus): A deviation of the great toe toward the lateral side of the foot; bunion.

Hashimoto thyroiditis (hah-shih-MO-to thi-royd-I-tis): Diffuse infiltration of the thyroid gland with lymphocytes, resulting in diffuse goiter, progressive destruction of the parenchyma, and hypothyroidism. See *hypothyroidism*.

Haustrum, haustra (HAW-strum, HAW-strah): One of a series of sacs or pouches, as seen in the colon.

Heberden nodes (HE-ber-den nodez): Small bone spurs that form on the distal phalanges of the hands in association with osteoarthritis.

Helicobacter pylori (hel-ik-o-BAK-ter pi-LOR-i): Species of bacteria associated with peptic ulcers.

HELLP: A mnemonic for *h*emolysis, *e*levated *l*iver enzymes, *l*ow *p*latelet count; associated with pregnancy-induced hypertension.

Hemagglutinin (hem-ah-GLU-tih-nin): A type of protein found in the outer coating of influenza and other antigens; it causes the agglutination of red blood cells.

Hematoma (he-mah-TO-mah): A localized mass of extravasated blood that is relatively or completely confined within an organ or tissue, a space, or a potential space; the blood is usually clotted, and depending on how long it has been there, may manifest various degrees of organization and decolorization.

Hematuria (he-mah-TYU-re-ah): Any condition in which the urine contains blood or red blood cells.

Heme (hēm): The oxygen-carrying, color-bearing group of hemoglobin.

Hemiplegia (hem-ih-PLE-je-ah): Paralysis of one side of the body.

Hemo- (HE-mo): A prefix denoting blood.

Hemochromatosis (he-mo-kro-mah-TO-sis): A genetic disorder characterized by the absorption of too much iron in the blood; sometimes associated with liver cancer.

Hemodialysis (he-mo-di-AL-ih-sis): Dialysis of soluble substances and water from the blood by diffusion through a semipermeable membrane.

Hemoglobin (HE-mo-glo-bin): Red protein of erythrocytes which binds to oxygen.

Hemoglobin A1c test: A test of blood glucose that reflects trends over a 3-month period. See *diabetes*.

Hemolysis (he-MOL-ih-sis): Destruction of blood cells.

Hemolytic (he-mo-LIH-tik): Destructive to blood cells.

Hemolytic uremic syndrome (he-mo-LIH-tik u-RE-mik SIN-drome): Hemolytic anemia and thrombocytopenia with acute renal failure.

Hemophilia (he-mo-FELE-e-ah): An inherited disorder of blood coagulation characterized by a permanent tendency to hemorrhages, spontaneous or traumatic, due to a defect in the blood coagulating mechanism.

Hemophilic arthritis (he-mo-FIL-ik arth-RI-tis): Joint damage and inflammation associated with bleeding into joint cavities seen with hemophilia.

Hemoptysis (he-MOP-tis-is): Expectoration of blood derived from the lungs or bronchi as a result of pulmonary or bronchial hemorrhage.

Hemorrhage (HEM-or-aj): An escape of blood through ruptured vessels.

Hemorrhoid (HEM-or-oyd): A varicose condition of the external or internal rectal veins causing painful swellings at the anus.

Hepatocellular carcinoma (hep-at-o-SEL-u-lar kar-sih-NO-mah): A carcinoma derived from parenchymal cells of the liver. See *liver cancer*.

Hepatorenal syndrome (hep-AT-o-RE-nal SIN-drome): Occurrence of acute renal failure in patients with disease of the liver or biliary tract, apparently due to decreased renal blood flow.

Hereditary nonpolyposis colorectal cancer syndrome (her-ED-ih-ta-re non-pol-ih-PO-sis KO-lo-rek-tal KAN-ser SIN-drome): A genetic condition that predisposes some people toward the development of colorectal and other cancers.

Herniated disc (HER-ne-a-ted DISK): Protrusion of a degenerated or fragmented intervertebral disk into the intervertebral foramen with potential compression of a nerve root or into the spinal canal with potential compression of the cauda equina in the lumbar region or the spinal cord at higher levels. See *disc disease*.

Heterophile (HET-er-o-file): A neutrophilic leukocyte. See *mononucleosis*.

Heterotopic ossification (het-er-o-TOP-ik os-if-ih-KA-shun): The formation of calcium deposits in soft tissues, particularly seen with spinal cord injury patients. See *myositis ossificans*, *spinal cord injury*.

Hidradenitis suppurativa (hi-drad-en-I-tis SUP-per-a-tee-va): Chronic suppurative folliculitis of apocrine sweat gland–bearing skin, producing abscesses with scarring. See *boils*.

High-density lipoprotein (HDL) (hi-DEN-sih-te LI-po-pro-tene): A compound in plasma containing both lipids and proteins; HDLs are associated with a reduced risk of cardiovascular disease.

Hip dysplasia (hip dis-PLA-jhah): A type of hip dislocation.

Hirsutism (HIR-zu-tizm): Presence of excessive bodily and facial terminal hair in a male pattern, especially in women; may develop in children or adults as the result of androgen (male hormone) excess due to tumors, drugs, or medications. See *ovarian cysts*.

Histamine (HIS-tah-mene): A secretion of some cells that is a powerful stimulant of gastric secretion, a constrictor of bronchial smooth muscle, and a vasodilator.

Histoplasmosis (his-to-plaz-MO-sis): An infectious disease caused by *Histoplasma capsulatum*, usually acquired by inhalation of fungal spores, and manifested by a primary lung infection.

Hobnailed liver (HOB-naled LIV-er): Characteristically knobby, bumpy appearance of a liver with advanced cirrhosis.

Homans sign (HO-manz sine): A pain at the back of the knee or calf when the ankle is slowly dorsiflexed with the knee bent. This test indicates incipient or established thrombosis in the veins of the leg.

Homeostasis (ho-me-o-STA-sis): A state of equilibrium in the body with respect to various functions and the chemical compositions of fluids and tissues.

Human herpesvirus 6 (HU-man HER-pez-vi-rus): A herpesvirus found in certain lymphoproliferative disorders. See *mononucleosis*.

Human papillomavirus (HPV) (HU-man pap-il-O-mah vi-rus): Class of DNA viruses that cause genital and cutaneous warts.

Human T-cell lymphotropic virus (HU-man T-sell lim-fo-TRO-fik VI-rus): A group of viruses (subfamily Oncovirinae, family Retroviridae) that are lymphotropic with a selective affinity for the helper/inducer cell subset of T lymphocytes and that are associated with adult T-cell leukemia and lymphoma.

Humoral immunity (HU-mor-al ih-MU-nih-te): Immunity associated with circulating antibodies, as opposed to cellular immunity.

Hunner ulcer (HUN-er UL-ser): A focal and often multiple star-shaped lesion involving all layers of the bladder wall; a sign of interstitial cystitis.

Hürthle cell carcinoma (HUR-tel sel kar-sih-NO-mah): A type of thyroid tumor; may be benign or malignant.

Hyaluronic acid (hi-al-yur-ON-ik AS-id): A gelatinous material in tissue spaces that acts as a lubricant and shock absorbant.

Hydrocephalus (hi-dro-SEF-ah-lus): A condition marked by an excessive accumulation of cerebrospinal fluid resulting in dilation of the cerebral ventricles and raised intracranial pressure; may also result in enlargement of the cranium and atrophy of the brain. See *cerebral palsy*.

Hyper- (HI-per): A prefix denoting excessive, above normal.

Hyperacusis (hi-per-ah-KU-sis): Abnormal acuteness of hearing due to irritability of sensory nerves. See *Bell palsy*.

Hyperalgesia (hi-per-al-JE-ze-ah): Extreme sensitivity to painful stimuli. See *peripheral neuropathy*.

Hyperglycemia (hi-per-gli-SE-me-ah): An abnormally high concentration of glucose in the circulating blood.

Hyperkinesia (hi-per-kin-E-ze-ah): Excessive muscular activity.

Hyperosmolality (hi-per-oz-mo-LAL-ih-te): Increased concentration of a solution expressed as osmoles of solute per kilogram of serum water. See *diabetes*.

Hyperplasia (hi-per-PLA-zha): An increase in the number of cells in a tissue or organ, outside of tumor formation.

Hyperreflexia (hi-per-re-FLEX-e-ah): A condition in which the deep tendon reflexes are exaggerated.

Hypersensitivity (hi-per-sen-sih-TIV-ih-te): An exaggerated response to the stimulus of a foreign agent.

Hyperthermia (hi-per-THER-me-ah): High body temperature; fever.

Hypertonic (hi-per-TON-ik): Having an increased degree of tension.

Hypertrophic scar (hi-per-TRO-fik SKAR): An elevated scar resembling a keloid but that does not spread into surrounding tissues.

Hypertrophy (hy-PER-tro-fe): General increase in bulk of a part or organ, due to increase in size but not in number of the individual tissue elements.

Hyperuricemia (hi-per-ur-ih-SE-me-ah): Enhanced blood concentrations of uric acid.

Hypnagogic hallucination (hip-nah-GOJ-ik hah-lu-sih-NA-shun): Vivid hallucination that occurs on waking from sleep; occurs with narcolepsy. See *sleep disorders*.

Hypnic myoclonia (HIP-nik mi-o-KLO-ne-ah): The startling sensation that a person is about to fall; it often occurs while nearly asleep.

Hypo- (HI-po): A prefix denoting deficient, below normal.

Hypoglycemia (hi-po-gli-SE-me-ah): An abnormally low concentration of glucose in circulating blood.

Hypokinesia (hi-po-kih-NE-zha): Diminished or slowed movement.

Hypothermia (hi-po-THER-me-ah): In humans a body temperature significantly below 98.6°F (37°C).

Hypotonic (hi-po-TON-ik): Having a reduced degree of tension.

Hypoxia (hi-POX-e-ah): Below-normal levels of oxygen in the body.

Ichthyosis (ik-the-O-sis): Congenital disorders of keratinization characterized by noninflammatory dryness and scaling of the skin, often associated with other defects and with abnormalities of lipid metabolism.

Icterus (IK-ter-us): Synonym for jaundice, a yellowish staining of the skin, sclerae, and mucous membranes that occurs with cirrhosis and other liver diseases.

IDDM: Insulin-dependent diabetes mellitus. Obsolete term for type 1 diabetes mellitus.

Idiopathic (id-e-o-PATH-ik): Denoting a disease of unknown cause.

Idiopathic endolymphatic hydrops (id-e-o-PATH-ik en-do-lim-FAT-ik HI-drops): Synonym for Ménière disease.

Idiopathic environmental intolerance (id-e-o-PATH-ik en-vi-ron-MEN-tal in-TOL-er-ans): Synonym for multiple chemical sensitivity syndrome. See *allergic reactions*.

Imatinib (im-ah-TIN-ib): Drug used to suppress cellular replication for one type of leukemia.

Immunoblastic lymphoma (im-u-no-BLAS-tik lim-FO-mah): A type of high-grade lymphoma.

Impetigo (im-peh-TI-go): A contagious superficial pyoderma caused by *Staphylococcus aureus* or group A streptococci; begins with a superficial flaccid vesicle that ruptures and forms a thick yellowish crust, most commonly on the face of children.

In situ (in SI-tu): At the site only; refers to early stages of cancer development.

Incision (in-SIH-zhun): A cut or surgical wound.

Indomethacin (in-do-METH-ah-sin): A nonsteroidal analgesic agent used in the treatment of various types of arthritis.

Induction (in-DUK-shun): The introduction of chemotherapeutic drugs into the central nervous system.

Infantile paralysis (IN-fan-tile pah-RAL-ih-sis): Synonym for polio.

Infarction (in-FARK-shun): Sudden insufficiency of arterial or venous blood supply due to emboli, thrombi, vascular torsion, or necrosis.

Inflammatory bowel disease (in-FLAM-mah-tor-e BOW-el): Umbrella term for Crohn disease and ulcerative colitis.

Infundibulum (in-fun-DIB-u-lum): Funnel-shaped structure or passage; the link between the pituitary gland and the hypothalamus.

Inguinal orchiectomy (ING-wih-nal or-ke-EK-to-me): Removal of one or both testes through the abdominal cavity. See *testicular cancer*.

Insulin (IN-su-lin): A hormone secreted by beta cells in the pancreas that promotes the utilization of glucose in tissue cells.

Integumentary (in-teg-u-MEN-tar-e): Relating to the skin.

Interferon (in-ter-FE-ron): A class of proteins with antiviral properties.

Interleukin-1 (IN-ter-lu-kin): A cytokine that enhances the proliferation of T helper cells and the growth and differentiation of B cells.

Intermittent claudication (in-ter-MIT-ent klaw-dih-KA-shun): Condition caused by transient ischemia, usually of calf muscles, brought on by walking.

Internal scar tissue (in-TER-nal SKAR TISH-u): Scar tissue that accumulates within an injured structure, e.g., tendon, muscle, or ligament.

Interstitial (in-ter-STIH-shal): Relating to spaces within a tissue or organ but excluding such spaces as body cavities or potential space.

Intertrigo (in-ter-TRI-go): A cutaneous yeast infection that grows in skin folds around the groin, axilla, and under the breasts.

Intrathecal pump (in-tra-THE-kal pump): Device for introducing drugs directly into the central nervous system. See *complex regional pain syndrome*.

Intravenous pyelography (in-trah-VE-nus pi-el-O-grah-fe): Radiological study of the kidney, ureters, and usually the bladder, performed with the aid of a contrast agent injected intravenously.

Intrinsic factor (in-TRIN-zik FAK-tor): A mucoprotein in the stomach necessary for the absorption of vitamin B_{12}.

Inverse psoriasis (IN-verse so-RI-ah-sis): Psoriasis in which lesions are red, thickened, and clustered around skin folds.

Iritis (i-RI-tis): Inflammation of the iris of the eye.

Ischemia (is-KE-me-ah): Local anemia due to a mechanical obstruction of the blood supply.

IUD: Intrauterine device. A plastic or metal device to be inserted into the uterus for contraception.

Ixodes (ik-SO-dez): A genus of hard ticks, many of which are parasitic to humans and which may be the vector for the spread of some diseases. See *Lyme disease*.

Joint mice: Freely floating bits of cartilage inside joint capsules, usually at the knee or talotibial joints.

Jumper's knee: Synonym for patellofemoral syndrome.

Kaposi sarcoma (kah-PO-seze sar-KO-mah): A malignant neoplasm occurring in the skin and sometimes in lymph nodes or viscera; clinically manifested by cutaneous lesions consisting of reddish-purple to dark-blue macules, plaques, or nodules; seen most commonly in men over 60 years of age and in AIDS patients.

Keloid scar (KE-loyd skar): A nodular mass of scar tissue that may occur after surgery, a burn, or cutaneous diseases.

Keratin (KER-ah-tin): A substance present in cuticular structures, e.g., hair, nails, and horns.

Keratinocyte (ker-AT-in-o-site): A cell of the epidermis that produces keratin.

Ketoacidosis (ke-to-as-id-O-sis): Acidosis caused by enhanced production of ketonic acids.

Ketogenic (ke-to-JEN-ik): Giving rise to ketones in metabolism.

Ketone (KE-tone): A potentially toxic product of metabolism; the most widely recognized ketone is acetone.

Kinin (KI-nin): Any of a variety of chemicals with physiological effects on cell activity, including visceral muscle contraction along with vascular muscle relaxation, which leads to vasodilation.

Klebsiella (kleb-se-EL-ah): A genus of bacteria that may or may not be pathogenic, depending on the individual type.

Kupffer cells (KUP-fer selz): Phagocytic cells found in the liver.

Kyphosis (ki-FO-sis): A deformity of the spine characterized by extensive flexion. See *postural deviations*.

Labyrinthitis (lab-ih-rin-THI-tis): Inflammation of the labyrinth of the inner ear; may be associated with vertigo and/or hearing loss. See *vestibular balance disorders*.

Laceration (las-er-A-shun): A torn or jagged wound.

Lactobacillus (lak-to-bah-SIL-us): A genus of bacteria that are part of the normal flora of the mouth, intestinal tract, and vagina.

Lamivudine (lah-MIH-vu-dene): A reverse transcriptase inhibitor used to treat HIV and hepatitis B.

Lanugo (lah-NU-go): Fine, soft, lightly pigmented hair, associated with fetal development and advanced anorexia nervosa.

Laparoscopy (lap-ah-ROS-ko-pe): Examination of the abdominal contents with a scope passed through the abdominal wall.

Laparotomy (lap-ah-ROH-to-me): Incision into the abdominal wall.

Lavage (lah-VAJH): The washing out of a hollow cavity by repeated injections and rejections of fluid.

Ledderhose disease (LED-er-hoze): A condition similar to Dupuytren contracture that develops on the plantar surface of the foot. Also called *plantar fibromatosis*.

Legg-Calve-Perthes disease (leg KAHL-va PER-tez): Epiphysial necrosis of the upper end of the femur. See *avascular necrosis*.

Leiomyoma (li-o-mi-O-mah): A benign neoplasm derived from smooth muscle tissue. See *fibroid tumors*

Lentigo (len-TI-go): A brown macule or spot resembling a freckle.

Leprosy (LEP-ro-se): A chronic bacterial infection caused by *Mycobacterium leprae* affecting the cooler body parts, especially the skin, peripheral nerves, and testes. Leprosy is classified into two main types, lepromatous and tuberculoid, representing extremes of immunological response. Also called Hansen disease.

Lesion (LE-zhun): A wound or injury; a pathogenic change in tissues.

Letrozole (LET-ro-zole): A medication used to reduce the risk of recurrent breast cancer.

Leukocyte (LU-ko-site): A type of blood cell formed in several types of tissues, involved in immune reactions. A white blood cell.

Leukoplakia (lu-ko-PLA-ke-ah): A white patch of oral mucous membrane which cannot be wiped off and cannot be diagnosed clinically; biopsy may show malignant or premalignant changes. See *skin cancer*.

Levodopa (lev-o-DO-pah): The biologically active form of dopa; a precursor of dopamine.

Levulose (LEV-yu-lose): Fructose; fruit sugar.

Lewy body disease (LU-we BOD-e): A degenerative cerebral disorder of elderly people characterized by progressive dementia or psychosis; can resemble Alzheimer disease and Parkinson disease.

Leydig cell tumor (LI-dig sel TU-mor): A type of testicular cancer.

Lhermitte sign (ler-METE sine): Sudden electric-like shocks extending down the spine on flexion of the head. See *muscular dystrophy*, *multiple sclerosis*.

Ligamenta flava (lig-ah-MEN-tah FLAH-vah): A pair of yellow elastic fibrous structures that bind the laminae of adjoining vertebrae.

Limb-girdle dystrophy (lim GIR-del DIS-tro-fe): One of the less well-defined types of muscular dystrophy; characterized by weakness and wasting, usually symmetrical, of the pelvic girdle muscles, the shoulder girdle muscles, or both, but not the facial muscles.

Limbic system (LIM-bik SIS-tem): A group of brain structures and their connections that exert important influence on the endocrine and autonomic nervous systems. The limbic system is associated with motivational and mood states.

Limited systemic scleroderma (LIM-ih-ted sis-TEM-ik skler-o-DERM-ah): A form of scleroderma that carries a relatively low risk of internal organ involvement.

Linea alba (LIN-e-ah AL-bah): Fibrous band that runs vertically from the xiphoid process to the pubis; site of attachment for abdominal muscles.

Lipoprotein (lip-o-PRO-tene): Complexes or compounds containing lipid and protein. Plasma lipoproteins are characterized as very low density (VLDL), intermediate density (IDL), low density (LDL), high density (HDL), and very high density (VHDL). Levels of lipoproteins are important in assessing the risk of cardiovascular disease.

Lithium (LITH-e-um): An element of the alkali metal group used to treat depression and other mood disorders.

Lithotripsy (LITH-o-trip-se): The crushing of a stone in the renal pelvis, ureter, or bladder by mechanical force or sound waves.

Lordosis (lor-DO-sis): A deformity of the spine characterized by excessive extension. See *postural deviations*.

Low-density lipoprotein (LDL) (lo-DEN-sih-te lip-o-PRO-tene): A compound in plasma containing both lipids and proteins; associated with an increased risk of cardiovascular disease.

Lumen (LU-men): The space in the interior of a tubular structure.

Lymphadenitis (lim-FAD-en-I-tis): Inflammation of a lymph node or nodes.

Lymphadenoma (lim-FAD-en-O-mah): Enlarged lymph node; may be associated with cancer.

Lymphangion (lim-FAN-je-on): A lymphatic vessel.

Lymphedema (lim-feh-DE-mah): Swelling as a result of obstruction or damage to lymph nodes.

Lymphoblastic lymphoma (lim-fo-BLAST-ik lim-FO-mah): A type of high-grade lymphoma.

Lymphocyte (LIM-fo-site): A white blood cell formed in lymphatic tissues.

Lymphocytic lymphoma (lim-fo-SIT-ik lim-FO-mah): A type of low-grade lymphoma.

Lymphokines (LIM-fo-kinez): A group of hormonelike substances that mediate immune responses; released by lymphocytes.

Lynch syndrome (LINCH SIN-drome): A synonym for hereditary nonpolyposis colorectal cancer syndrome, a genetic risk factor for colorectal cancer.

Macrophage (MAK-ro-fahj): A type of phagocytic white blood cell.

Macrosomia (mak-ro-SO-me-ah): Condition in which a fetus grows abnormally large as a consequence of gestational diabetes.

Magnetic resonance imaging (MRI) (mag-NET-ik REZ-o-nans IM-ah-jing): A diagnostic modality in which the magnetic nuclei of a patient are aligned in a strong, uniform magnetic field. The signals they emit are converted into images that permit three-dimensional reference to soft tissues.

Malaise (mah-LAZE): A feeling of general discomfort or uneasiness.

Malar rash (MA-lar rash): A rash of the cheeks or cheekbones, often associated with lupus or erysipelas.

Malignant (mah-LIG-nant): Having the property of locally invasive and destructive growth and metastasis.

Malignant hypertension (mah-LIG-nant hi-per-TEN-shun): Severe hypertension that runs a rapid course, causing necrosis of arteriolar walls in kidney and retina, hemorrhages, and death most frequently due to uremia or rupture of a cerebral vessel.

Malocclusion (mal-o-KLU-zhun): Any deviation from a physiologically acceptable contact of opposing dentitions.

Mast cell: A white blood cell found in connective tissue that contains heparin and histamine.

Mastitis (mas-TI-tis): Infection of the breast.

Matrix (MA-trix): The intercellular substance of a tissue.

Medial tibial stress syndrome (ME-de-al TIB-e-al STRES SIN-drome): Pain at the posteromedial border of the tibia that occurs in conjunction with exercise. See *shin splints*.

Meige syndrome (MEZH-eh SIN-drome): A type of dystonia that combines blepharospasm and oromandibular dystonia.

Melanin (MEL-ah-nin): Dark brown to black pigment formed in the skin and some other tissues.

Melanocyte (mel-AN-o-site): A pigment-producing cell in the basal layer of the epidermis.

Melatonin (MEL-ah-to-nin): A substance secreted by the pineal gland that suppresses some glandular function; associated with circadian rhythm.

Menarche (men-AR-ke): A woman's first menstrual period.

Meningitis (men-in-JI-tis): Inflammation of the membranes of the brain or spinal cord.

Meniscus (men-IS-kus): A crescent-shaped fibrocartilaginous structure of the knee, involving the acromioclavicular, sternoclavicular, and temporomandibular joints.

Menses (MEN-seze): Periodic hemorrhage from the uterine mucosa; usually preceded by ovulation but not by fertilization.

Mesangial glomerulonephritis (mes-AN-je-al glo-MARE-yu-lo-nef-RI-tis): A type of glomerulonephritis associated with immune system abnormalities and the loss of erythrocytes into the urine.

Mesentery (MES-en-ter-e): A double layer of peritoneum attached to the abdominal wall and enclosing a portion of the abdominal viscera.

Mesothelioma (mes-o-the-le-O-mah): A malignant neoplasm derived from cells of the pleura or peritoneum.

Metabolite (meh-TAB-o-lite): Any product of metabolism, especially catabolism.

Metaplasia (met-ah-PLA-zhia): Abnormal transformation of adult, fully differentiated tissue into another type of tissue. See *endometriosis*.

Metastasis (met-AS-tah-sis): The spread of a disease process from one part of the body to another, as with the spread of cancer.

Methicillin-resistant *Staphylococcus aureus* (MRSA) (METH-ih-sil-in re-ZIS-tant staf-ih-lo-KOK-us OR-e-us): Common infective bacterium that does not respond to methicillin, a standard treatment.

Methylphenidate (meth-il-FEN-ih-date): A central nervous system stimulant often used to treat attention deficit hyperactivity disorder.

Microaerophilic (mi-kro-air-o-FIL-ik): Referring to a type of bacteria that requires oxygen, although less than is available in the air.

Microbe (MI-krobe): Any very minute organism.

Micrographia (mi-kro-GRAF-e-ah): Handwriting that grows progressively smaller and more cramped. See *Parkinson disease*.

Microsporum (mi-kro-SPOR-um): A genus of pathogenic fungi causing dermatophytosis. See *fungal infections*.

Mineralocorticoid (min-er-al-o-KOR-tih-koyd): One of the steroids from the adrenal cortex that influence salt metabolism.

Mitochondrion (mi-to-KON-dre-on): An organelle of the cell cytoplasm; the principal energy source of the cell.

Mittelschmerz (MIT-el-shmertz): Abdominal pain occurring at the time of ovulation.

Molluscum contagiosum (mo-LUS-kum kon-ta-je-O-sum): A contagious disease of the skin caused by proliferation of a virus of the family Poxviridae and characterized by the appearance of small, pearly epidermal growths. In adults it typically occurs on or near the genitals and is sexually transmitted. See *sexually transmitted diseases, warts*.

Monoamine oxidase inhibitor (MAOI) (MON-o-ah-mene OX-ih-dase in-HIB-ih-tor): A class of antidepressants that inhibit the breakdown of certain neurotransmitters.

Monoclonal immunoglobulins (MON-o-klo-nal im-u-no-GLOB-u-linz): A type of antibody produced by B cells affected by myeloma. Also called M proteins.

Monocyte (MON-o-site): A relatively large leukocyte; normally comprises 3% to 7% of the leukocytes in circulating blood.

Mononeuropathy (mon-o-nur-OP-ath-e): Disorder involving a single nerve.

Mononucleosis (mon-o-nu-kle-O-sis): Presence of abnormally large numbers of mononuclear leukocytes in the circulating blood, especially with reference to forms that are not normal.

Motility (mo-TIL-ih-te): The power of spontaneous movement.

Movie-goer's knee: Synonym for *patellofemoral syndrome*.

MRSA: See *methicillin-resistant* Staphylococcus aureus.

Mucolytic (myu-ko-LIT-ik): Capable of dissolving, digesting, or liquefying mucus.

Mucopolysaccharide (myu-ko-pol-e-SAK-ah-ride): Protein-polysaccharide complex, obtained from proteoglycans. See *hyperthyroidism*.

Mucormycosis (myu-kor-mi-KO-sis): A fungal infection associated with genera of the class Zygomycetes. Also called zygomycosis. See *diabetes*.

Mucosal-associated lymphoid-type lymphoma (myu-KO-sal ah-SO-se-a-ted LIM-foyd tipe lim-FO-mah): A type of cancer associated with *Helicobacter pylori*. See *ulcers*.

Mucous cyst (MYU-kus SIST): A type of ganglion cyst most often seen on the distal interphalangeal joint of older people.

Multiple system atrophy (MUL-tih-pel SIS-tem AT-ro-fe): A central nervous system disorder leading to stiffness, rigidity, loss of balance, poor coordination, and other symptoms. See *tremor*.

Muscle spindle (MUH-sel SPIN-del): Proprioceptor that wraps around specialized muscle fibers to relay information about the relative length of the muscle fibers.

Myalgic encephalomyelitis (mi-AL-jik en-sef-ah-lo-mi-el-I-tis): Inflammation of the brain and spinal cord characterized by muscle pain. See *chronic fatigue syndrome*.

Myasthenia gravis (mi-as-THE-ne-ah GRAV-is): Immunological disorder of neuromuscular transmission, marked by fluctuating weakness, especially of the oculofacial muscles and the proximal limb muscles.

Mycobacterium (mi-ko-bak-TE-re-um): Genus of bacteria that causes tuberculosis in humans.

Mycoplasma (mi-ko-PLAZ-mah): A specialized type of bacteria that do not possess a true cell wall but are bound by a three-layered membrane.

Mycosis (mi-KO-sis): Any disease caused by a fungus.

Myelin (MI-eh-lin): A membrane composed of fat and protein molecules that surrounds nerve fibers.

Myelodysplastic anemia (mi-el-o-dis-PLAS-tik ah-NE-me-ah): A primary neoplastic stem cell disorder characterized by peripheral blood cytopenias and prominent maturation abnormalities in the bone marrow; evolves progressively and may transform into leukemia.

Myeloid cell (MI-el-oyd sel): Any cell that develops into a granulocyte of blood; also refers to any bone marrow cell.

Myocardial infarction (mi-o-KAR-de-al in-FARK-shun): Synonym for *heart attack*.

Myoclonic (mi-o-KLON-ik): Related to one or a series of shocklike contractions of a group of muscles; of variable regularity, synchrony, and symmetry, generally due to a central nervous system lesion.

Myofibril (mi-o-FI-bril): One of the fine longitudinal fibrils in skeletal or cardiac muscle fiber.

Myopia (mi-O-pe-ah): Optical condition in which only rays from a finite distance from the eye focus on the retina; nearsightedness. See *Marfan syndrome*.

Myositis ossificans (mi-o-SI-tis OS-ih-fih-kanz): Ossification of inflammatory tissue within a muscle, usually at the site of a hematoma due to blunt trauma.

Myotonia (mi-o-TO-ne-ah): Delayed relaxation of a muscle after a strong contraction.

Myrmecia (mir-ME-she-ah): Synonym for deep palmoplantar warts.

Myxedema coma (mik-seh-DE-mah KO-mah: A state of profound unconsciousness related to extreme hypothyroidism.

NAFLD: Nonalcoholic fatty liver disease. See *cirrhosis*.

Nailfold capillaroscopy (nale fold kap-il-ah-ROS-ko-pe): A diagnostic test to look for signs of arteriole distortion seen with Raynaud syndrome.

Narcolepsy (NAR-ko-lep-se): A sleep disorder characterized by recurring episodes of sleep during the day and interrupted sleep at night.

Necrosis (nek-RO-sis): Pathological death of one or more cells or of a portion of tissue or organ.

Needle aponeurotomy (NE-del ap-o-nur-OT-o-me): A procedure to treat Dupuytren contracture with tiny punctures to release the palmar aponeurosis.

Neisseria gonorrhoeae (ni-SE-re-a gon-o-RE-a): A species that causes gonorrhea and other infections in humans; the type species of the genus *Neisseria*.

Neisseria meningitidis (ni-SE-re-a men-in-JIH-tih-dis): A bacterial species found in the nasopharynx; the causative agent of meningococcal meningitis.

Neoplasm (NE-o-plazm): An abnormal tissue that grows by cellular proliferation more rapidly than normal and continues to grow after the stimuli that initiated the new growth cease.

Nephrolithiasis (nef-ro-lih-THI-ah-sis): Presence of renal calculi.

Nephron (NEF-ron): A long convoluted tubular structure; the functional unit of the kidney.

Nerve growth factor: A protein that helps to control the development of sympathetic neurons and other nerve tissue; associated with heightened pain sensitivity.

Neuralgia-inducing cavitational osteonecrosis (NICO) (nur-AL-je-a in-DU-sing kav-ih-TA-shun-al os-te-o-nek-RO-sis): Tissue death at the site of extracted teeth that causes pain in the face. Also called *osteomyelitis*.

Neuraminidase (nur-am-IN-ih-daze): One of a group of proteins found on the external surface of influenza viruses.

Neurilemma (nur-ih-LEM-mah): A cell that enfolds one or more axons of the peripheral nervous system.

Neuroendocrine (nur-o-EN-do-krin): Descriptive of cells that release hormones in response to a neural stimulus. See *pancreatic cancer*.

Neurofibrillary tangle (nur-o-FIB-rih-la-re TANG-el): Intraneural accumulations of filaments with twisted, contorted patterns; associated with Alzheimer disease.

Neurogenic bladder (NUR-o-jen-ik BLAD-er): Bladder dysfunction that originates with nervous system damage.

Neuroma (nur-O-mah): General term for any neoplasm derived from cells of the nervous system, especially Morton neuroma. See *pes planus*, *pes cavus*.

Neuron (NUR-on): The functional unit of the nervous system; consists of the nerve cell body, the dendrites, and the axon.

Neuropeptide (nur-o-PEP-tide): Any of a variety of peptides found in neural tissue; e.g., endorphins, enkephalins.

Neurotrophic factors (nur-o-TRO-fik FAK-torz): Chemicals that support the health of nerve cells; they may be absent in amyotrophic lateral sclerosis.

Neutrophil (NU-tro-fil): A type of mature white blood cell formed in the bone marrow.

Neutrophilic (nu-tro-FIL-ik): Characterized by the presence of neutrophils.

Nevus, nevi (NE-vus, NE-vi): A malformation of the skin colored by hyperpigmentation or increased vascularity.

NIDDM: Non–insulin-dependent diabetes mellitus. Obsolete term for type 2 diabetes mellitus.

Nit: The ovum of a head or body louse.

Nociceptor (no-si-SEP-tor): A peripheral nerve organ or mechanism for the reception and transmission of painful or injurious stimuli.

Nocturia (nok-TUR-e-ah): Urinating at night.

Nodular (NOD-u-lar): having nodes or knotlike swellings.

Nonalcoholic steatohepatitis (NASH) (non-al-ko-HOL-ik ste-AT-o-hep-ah-TI-tis): Inflammation of fatty tissue in the liver not associated with alcohol abuse.

Non-Burkitt lymphoma (non-BUR-kit lim-FO-mah): A type of high-grade lymphoma.

Nongonococcal urethritis (non-gon-o-KOK-al u-re-THRI-tis): Urethritis not from gonococcal infection; *Chlamydia trachomatis* is the most common agent. See *sexually transmitted diseases*.

Nonseminoma (non-sem-ih-NO-mah): A type of testicular cancer.

Nonsteroidal anti-inflammatory drug (NSAID) (non-ster-OYD-al AN-te-in-FLAM-ah-tor-e drug): Any collection of anti-inflammatory drugs that do not include steroidal compounds. Examples include aspirin, acetaminophen, ibuprofen, and naproxen.

Nontropical sprue: Synonym for celiac sprue.

Noradrenaline (nor-ah-DREN-ah-lin): See *norepinephrine*.

Norepinephrine (nor-ep-ih-NEF-rin): A hormone produced in the adrenal medulla; secreted in response to hypotension and physical stress.

Norovirus (NOR-o-vi-rus): Genus name for the group of viruses provisionally described as Norwalk-like viruses.

Nosocomial (no-so-KO-me-al): Of a disease acquired while being treated in a hospital; specifically applied to some varieties of pneumonia.

Noxious (NOK-shus): Injurious, harmful.

Nucleus pulposus (NU-kle-us pul-PO-sus): The soft fibrocartilage central portion of an intervertebral disk.

Numb-likeness: A condition characterized by reduced sensation but not total numbness.

Nummular eczema (NUM-u-lar (EG-zeh-mah): Discrete coin-shaped patches of eczema.

Nystagmus (nis-TAG-mus): Involuntary rhythmic oscillation of the eyeballs.

Occult (o-KULT): hidden; concealed; not manifest.

Oculopharyngeal muscular dystrophy (ok-u-lo-fah-RIN-je-al MUS-ku-lar DIS-tro-fe): An inherited progressive form of muscular dystrophy that often involves ptosis and problems with swallowing.

Oligodendrocyte (ol-ih-go-DEN-dro-site): One of the three types of glial cells, the other two being astrocytes and microglia, that together with nerve cells compose the tissue of the central nervous system.

Olivopontocerebellar atrophy (OL-ih-vo-PON-to-ser-ah-BEL-ar AT-ro-fe): A central nervous system movement disorder that is part of multiple system atrophy. See *tremor*.

Oncogene (ONK-o-jene): Any of a family of genes that may foster malignant processes if mutated or activated by certain viruses.

Onycholysis (on-ih-KOL-ih-sis): Loosening of the nails, beginning at the free border and usually incomplete. See *psoriasis*.

Onychomycosis (on-ih-ko-mi-KO-sis): Fungal infection of the nails.

Oocyte (o-o-site): The female sex cell.

Oophorectomy (o-o-for-EK-to-me): Surgical removal of the ovaries.

Oophoritis (o-o-for-I-tis): Inflammation of an ovary.

Orchiectomy (or-ke-EK-to-me): Removal of one or both testes.

Orchitis (or-KI-tis): Inflammation of the testes.

Orthotics (or-THOT-iks): The science of making and fitting of orthopedic appliances. Also used to refer to orthopedic appliances that are made to adjust the alignment and weight-bearing stress in the feet.

Os coxae (oz KOK-se): The fused unit containing the ilium, ischium, and pubis.

Oscillation (os-il-A-shun): A to-and-fro movement. See *tremor*.

Osgood-Schlatter disease (OZ-good SHLAT-er): Inflammation or partial avulsion of the tibial tuberosity due to traction forces.

Osteitis deformans (os-te-I-tis de-FOR-manz): Synonym for *Paget disease*.

Osteoblast (OS-te-o-blast): A bone-forming cell.

Osteoclast (OS-te-o-klast): A cell functioning in the absorption and removal of osseus tissue.

Osteomalacia (os-te-o-mah-LA-shah): A disease characterized by progressive softening and bending of the bones.

Osteomyelitis (os-te-o-mi-el-I-tis): Inflammation of the bone marrow and adjacent bone tissue.

Osteonecrosis (os-te-o-nek-RO-sis): The death of bone en mass, as distinguished from caries ("molecular death") or relatively small foci of necrosis in bone.

Osteopenia (os-te-o-PE-ne-ah): Pathological thinning of bones; may be a precursor to osteoporosis.

Osteophyte (OS-te-o-fite): A bony outgrowth or protuberance.

Osteotomy (os-te-OT-o-me): The cutting of bone, usually using a saw or chisel.

Ostomy (OS-to-me): Artificial opening (stoma) into the trachea, urinary tract, or gastrointestinal tract.

Otolith (O-to-lith): Tiny ear stone of hardened material found in the vestibule of the inner ear.

Overuse syndrome (O-ver use SIN-drome): Synonym for patellofemoral syndrome.

Oxygen free radical (OX-ih-jen fre RAD-ih-kal): An atom or atom group carrying an unpaired electron and no charge. They may promote heart disease, cancer, Alzheimer disease, and other progressive disorders.

Pain-spasm-pain cycle: Self-perpetuating cycle of pain, which causes spasm, which increases pain, ad infinitum.

Palliative (PAL-le-ah-tiv): Denoting alleviation of symptoms without curing the underlying disease.

Palmar fasciitis (PAL-mar fash-I-tis): Synonym for Dupuytren contracture.

Palpable (PAL-pah-bel): Perceptible to touch.

Palpitation (pal-pih-TA-shun): Forcible or irregular pulsation of the heart perceptible to the patient, usually with an increase in frequency or force, with or without an irregularity in rhythm.

Pancolitis (pan-ko-LI-tis): Inflammation of the entire colon. See *ulcerative colitis*.

Pap test: Microscopic examination of cells scraped usually from the uterine cervix and stained with Papanicolaou stain to look for signs of cancer.

Paraplegia (pare-ah-PLE-je-ah): Paralysis of both lower extremities and generally the lower trunk.

Parathyroid hormone (PTH) (pare-ah-THI-royd HOR-mone): A hormone secreted by the parathyroid glands that raises serum calcium levels by causing bone resorption.

Parenchyma (pare-en-KI-mah): The distinguishing or specific cells of a gland or organ, contained within a connective tissue framework stroma.

Paresis (pah-RE-sis): Partial or incomplete paralysis.

Paresthesia (pare-es-THE-zha): An abnormal sensation, such as burning, prickling, tickling, or tingling.

Parkinsonism (PAR-kin-son-izm): A neurological syndrome that has signs and symptoms of Parkinson disease.

Patellar tendinitis (pah-TEL-ar ten-din-I-tis): Injury to the insertion of the quadriceps group.

Patellofemoral syndrome (pa-TELL-o-fem-o-ral SIN-drome): Anterior knee pain as a result of a structural or functional malfunction between the patella and distal femur.

Pathogen (PATH-o-jen): Any virus, microorganism, or substance causing disease.

Pediculosis (ped-ik-yu-LO-sis): The state of being infested with lice.

Pediculus (ped-IK-yu-lus): A genus of parasitic lice that live in the hair and feed periodically on blood. Important species include *Pediculus humanus* var. *capitis*, the head louse of humans; *Pediculus humanus* var. *corporis*, also called *Pediculus corporis*, the body louse or clothes louse, which lives and lays nits in clothing and feeds on the human body.

Pedunculate (peh-DUNK-u-late): Having a pedicle; suspended by a stalk.

Peptide (PEP-tide): A compound of two or more amino acids.

Percutaneous nephrolithotomy (per-ku-TA-ne-us nef-ro-lith-OT-o-me): Incision through the skin directly to the kidney for the removal of a renal calculus.

Percutaneous transluminal coronary angioplasty (PCTA) (per-kyu-TA-ne-us trans-LU-min-al KOR-o-na-re AN-je-o-plast-e): A surgical procedure for enlarging a narrowed coronary vessel by inflating and withdrawing through the narrowed region a balloon on the tip of a catheter.

Perforation (per-for-A-shun): Abnormal opening in a hollow organ.

Perfusion (per-FU-zhun): The forcing of fluid to flow through the vascular bed of a tissue or through the lumen of a hollow structure.

Peri- (PER-ih): Prefix denoting *around*, *about*, or *near*.

Pericarditis (per-ih-kar-DI-tis): Inflammation of the pericardium.

Perilymph fistula (PER-ih-limf FIS-tu-lah): An abnormal portal that allows fluid to move between the inner ear and the middle ear. See *vestibular balance disorders*.

Perimenopause (per-ih-MEN-o-pawz): The 3- to 5-year period before the final cessation of the menstrual cycle, during which estrogen levels begin to drop.

Perimysium (per-ih-MI-se-um): The fibrous sheath enveloping each of the primary bundles of skeletal muscle fibers.

Periodic limb movement disorder (PLMD): A disorder characterized by periodic episodes of repetitive and highly stereotyped limb movements that occur during sleep. See *sleep disorders*.

Periosteum (per-e-OS-te-um): The thick fibrous membrane covering every surface of a bone except the articular cartilage.

Periostitis (per-e-os-TI-tis): Inflammation of the periosteum. See *shin splints*.

Peripheral vascular disease (per-IF-er-al VAS-ku-lar dih-ZEZE): Condition related to the consequences of atherosclerosis in the extremities, especially the legs; can include blood clots, stasis dermatitis, skin ulcers, and infections.

Pervasive development disorders: Synonym for autism spectrum disorders.

Pes cavus: Condition characterized by increased height of the foot's medial longitudinal arch.

Pes planus: A condition in which the longitudinal arch is broken down, the entire sole touching the ground. Flatfoot.

PET: Positron emission tomography; use of nuclear medicine and digital imaging to observe chemical and electrical activity in living tissue.

Petit mal (peh-TE MAL): A brief seizure characterized by arrest of activity and occasional clonic movements.

Peyronie disease (pa-ro-NE): A condition in which the

skin on the shaft of the penis becomes thickened and scarred. Can be associated with Dupuytren contracture.

Phalen maneuver (FA-len mah-NU-ver): Maneuver in which the wrist is maintained in flexion for 60 seconds or more; the sensation of paresthesia or other symptoms may indicate carpal tunnel syndrome.

Pheochromocytoma (fe-o-kro-mo-si-TO-mah): Benign adrenal tumor that can cause increased secretion of epinephrine. Associated with a form of thyroid cancer.

Phlebectomy (fleb-EK-to-me): Excision of a segment of a vein, especially to treat varicose veins.

Phlegm (flem): Abnormal amounts of mucus, especially as expectorated from the mouth.

Photodynamic therapy (fo-to-di-NAM-ik THER-ah-pe): A treatment option that destroys some types of cancer cells through the use of a fixed-frequency laser light in combination with a photosensitizing agent.

Photosensitivity (fo-to-sen-sih-TIV-ih-te): Abnormal sensitivity to light, especially of the eyes.

Phyllodes tumor (FIL-odez TU-mor): A low-grade, rarely metastasizing form of breast neoplasm. See *breast cancer*.

Phyto- (FI-to): Having to do with plants.

Phytoestrogen (fi-to-ES-trah-jen): Plant-based chemical with an estrogenic effect on the body.

Pia mater (PI-ah MA-ter, PE-ah MA-ter): A delicate fibrous membrane firmly adherent to the brain and spinal cord.

Pilonidal cyst (pi-lo-NI-dal sist): An abscess in the sacral region containing hair, which may act as a foreign body leading to chronic inflammation. See *boils*.

Pinna (PIN-na): A feather, wing, or fin—used to describe the ear.

Pitting edema (PIT-ing eh-DE-mah): Edema that retains for a time the indentation produced by pressure.

Placenta abruptio (plah-SEN-tah ab-RUP-te-o): Premature separation of the placenta.

Plantar fibromatosis (PLAN-tar fi-bro-mah-TO-sis): A condition similar to Dupuytren contracture, appearing on the foot. Also called Ledderhose disease.

Plaque (plak): A small differentiated area on a surface; atheromatous plaques form well-defined yellow areas or swellings on the intimal surface of an artery.

Plasmapheresis (plaz-mah-fer-E-sis): Removal of whole blood from the body, separation of its cellular elements, and reinfusion of them suspended in saline or another plasma substitute.

Plastocytoma (plas-to-si-TO-mah): A collection of proliferating cancerous immature B cells found outside bone tissue. See *myeloma*.

Platelet (PLATE-let): An irregularly shaped fragment of a megakaryocyte that aids in blood clotting.

Pleurisy (PLU-rih-se): Inflammation of the pleurae.

Plexus (PLEK-sus): A network or interjoining of nerves, blood vessels, or lymphatic vessels.

Pneumococcus (nu-mo-KOK-us): Synonym for *Streptococcus pneumoniae*.

Pneumocystis carinii pneumonia: Former name for *Pneumocystis jiroveci* pneumonia.

Pneumocystis jiroveci pneumonia: Pneumonia resulting from infection with *Pneumocystis carinii*, frequently seen in the immunologically compromised, such as persons with AIDS, or steroid-treated individuals, the elderly, or premature or debilitated babies. A protozoan infection of the lungs associated with impaired immunity. Formerly called *Pneumocystis carinii* pneumonia.

Pneumothorax (nu-mo-THOR-ax): The presence of air or gas in the pleural cavity.

Poliomyelitis (pol-e-o-mi-el-I-tis): An inflammatory process involving the gray matter of the spinal cord.

Poly- (POL-e): Many; multiplicity.

Polyarteritis nodosa (pol-e-ar-ter-I-tis no-DO-sah): A disease involving segmental inflammation and necrosis of medium-size and small arteries.

Polycythemia (pol-e-si-THE-me-ah): An increase above normal in the number of red cells in the blood.

Polydipsia (pol-e-DIP-se-ah): Excessive thirst that is relatively prolonged. See *diabetes*.

Polyendocrine deficiency syndrome (pol-e-EN-do-krin de-FISH-en-se SIN-drome): An autoimmune condition associated with Addison disease in which the adrenal glands, along with other endocrine structures, are impaired.

Polyneuropathy (pol-e nu-ROP-ath-e): A disease process involving a number of peripheral nerves.

Polyphagia (pol-e-FA-je-ah): Excessive eating. See *diabetes*.

Polysomnography (pol-e-som-NOG-raf-e): Continuous monitoring of normal and abnormal physiological functioning during sleep.

Polyuria (pol-e-U-re-ah): Excessive excretion of urine. See *diabetes*.

Popliteal cyst (pop-LIT-e-al sist, pop-lit-E-al sist): Synonym for Baker cyst.

Popliteal fossa (pop-LIT-e-al fos-ah, pop-lit-E-al fos-ah): The diamond-shaped space posterior to the knee bounded superficially by the diverging biceps femoris and semimembranosus muscles above and inferiorly by the two heads of the gastrocnemius muscle.

Portal hypertension (POR-tal hi-per-TEN-shun): Elevation of pressure in the hepatic portal circulation due to cirrhosis or other fibrotic change in liver tissue.

Postherpetic neuralgia (post-her-PET-ik nu-RAL-je-ah): A pain that lasts after the lesions related to herpes zoster have healed.

Posturography (pos-tur-OG-raf-e): A measurement of

postural stability under varying visual and proprioceptive inputs. See *vestibular balance disorders*.

Prednisone (PRED-nih-zone): An analog of cortisol; used as a steroidal anti-inflammatory.

Preeclampsia (pre-e-KLAMP-se-ah): Development of hypertension with proteinuria or edema, or both, due to pregnancy.

Premenstrual dysphoric disorder (PMDD) (pre-MEN-stru-al dis-FOR-ik dis-OR-der): A pervasive pattern occurring during the last week of the luteal phase in most menstrual cycles for at least a year and remitting within a few days of the onset of the follicular phase; the symptoms are comparable in severity to those seen in a major depressive episode, distinguishing this disorder from the far more common premenstrual syndrome.

Pretibial myxedema (pre-TIB-e-al mik-seh-DE-mah): A rash that occurs in the tibial region, specifically associated with hyperthyroidism.

Priapism (PRI-ah-pizm): Persistent erection of the penis, accompanied by pain and tenderness.

Prion (PRI-on): Small infectious proteinaceous particle on nonnucleic acid; the causative agent for bovine spongiform encephalopathy, Creutzfeldt-Jacob disease, kuru, and others.

Prodromic (pro-DRO-mik): Relating to the early or premonitory symptom of a disease, especially herpes simplex.

Progestin (pro-JEST-in): A hormone of the corpus luteum.

Proliferants (pro-LIF-er-ants): Injected substances that are designed to stimulate the growth of new collagen fibers, which with appropriate stretching and exercise, lie down in alignment with the original fibers.

Prophylaxis (pro-fil-AK-sis): Prevention of a disease or of a process that can lead to a disease.

Proprioceptor (pro-pre-o-SEP-tor): Sensory end organs that relay information about position and muscle tension.

Proptosis (prop-TO-sis): Protruding eyes; exophthalmos. See *hyperthyroidism*.

Prostadynia (pros-tah-DIN-e-ah): Synonym for chronic pelvic pain syndrome; associated with prostate pain.

Prostaglandins (PROS-tah-glan-din): Substances in many tissues with effects such as vasodilation, vasoconstriction, and stimulation of smooth muscle tissue.

Prostate-specific antigen (PSA) (PROS-tate speh-SIF-ik AN-tih-jen): A glycoprotein found in normal seminal fluid and produced in prostate epithelial cells. Elevated levels of PSA are associated with prostatic enlargement and an increased risk of prostate cancer.

Protease inhibitor (PRO-te-aze): A group of AIDS drugs that work to interrupt the maturing phase of the virus.

Pruritis (pru-RI-tis): Itchiness.

Pseudogout (SU-do-gowt): Acute episodes of synovitis caused by calcium pyrophosphate crystals as opposed to urate crystals, as in true gout.

Pseudohypertrophy (SU-do-hy-PER-tro-fe): Increase in size of an organ or a part, due not to increase in size or number of the specific functional elements but to that of some other tissue, fatty or fibrous. See *muscular dystrophy*

Pseudomembranous colitis (su-do-MEM-brah-nus ko-LI-tis): Intestinal inflammation due to infection with *Clostridium difficile*; often related to prolonged antibiotic therapy.

Pseudomonas aeruginosa (su-do-MO-nah ah-ru-jin-O-sah): Species of aerobic bacteria that sometimes infect humans, especially when the host is otherwise compromised. See *cystic fibrosis*.

Psoralen (SOR-ah-len): A phototoxic drug used in the treatment of psoriasis.

Psoriasis (sor-I-ah-sis): A common inherited condition characterized by the eruption of reddish, silvery-scaled maculopapules, predominantly on the elbows, knees, scalp, and trunk.

Psychodynamic therapy (si-ko-di-NAM-ik THER-ah-pe): Therapy based on the psychological forces that underlie human behavior.

Psychoneuroimmunology (si-ko-nur-o-ih-myu-NOL-o-je): Study of emotional or other psychological states that affect the immune system, rendering an individual susceptible to a disease or the course of a disease.

Pthirus pubis (THI-rus PU-bis): A species of pubic or crab lice.

Ptosis (TO-sis): A sinking down or prolapse of an organ, specifically the eyelid. See *myasthenia gravis*.

Pugilistic parkinsonism (pu-jih-LIS-tik PAR-kin-son-izm): A disorder of professional boxers who receive multiple blows to the head and in whom symptoms progress even after they stop fighting. See *Parkinson disease*.

Pustular psoriasis (PUS-tyu-lar so-RI-ah-sus): Psoriasis with pustule formation in normal and psoriatic skin.

Pustule (PUS-tyule): A small, circumscribed elevation of the skin containing purulent material.

PUVA: Oral administration of *p*soralen and subsequent exposure to long-wavelength *u*ltra*v*iolet-*A* light; used to treat psoriasis.

Pyelogram (PI-el-o-gram): A radiograph of the kidneys and ureters following the injection of a contrast medium.

Pyelography (pi-el-OG-rah-fe): Radiological study of the kidneys, ureters, and bladder.

Pyrogen (PI-ro-jen): A fever-inducing agent.

Q-angle: The angle formed by the line of traction of the quadriceps tendon on the patella and the line of traction of the patellar tendon on the tibial tubercle. See *patellofemoral syndrome*.

Quadriplegia (kwoh-drih-PLE-je-ah): Paralysis of all four limbs.

Quercetin (KWER-seh-tin): A bioflavonoid with antihistamine and anti-inflammatory properties. See *prostatitis*.

Radiation (ra-de-A-shun): The sending forth of light, short radio waves, ultraviolet or x-rays, or any other waves for treatment, diagnosis, or other purpose.

Radicular pain (rah-DIK-u-lar pane): Pain felt along the pathway of a spinal nerve.

Radiculopathy (rah-dik-u-LOP-ath-e): Any disorder of the spinal nerve roots.

Radioimmunotherapy (ra-de-o-ih-my-no-THER-ah-pe): The use of radiation with medication to target specific tumor cells.

Radioisotope (ra-de-o-I-so-tope): An isotope that changes to a more stable state by emitting radiation.

Rales (RALE-ez): Term for an extra sound heard on auscultation of breath sounds.

Ramsay-Hunt syndrome type 1: Facial paralysis, ear pain, and herpes zoster resulting from viral infection of the seventh cranial nerve and geniculate ganglion.

Raynaud syndrome (ra-NO SIN-drome): Idiopathic bilateral cyanosis of the digits due to arterial and arteriolar contraction.

Reduction (re-DUK-shun): The restoration, by surgical or manipulative procedures, of a part to its normal anatomic relation.

Reed-Sternberg cells: Large transformed lymphocytes, indicative of Hodgkin disease.

Regional enteritis (RE-joh-nal en-tur-I-is): Synonym for Crohn disease.

Reiter syndrome (RI-tur sin-drome): A combination of symptoms, including urethritis, cutaneous lesions, arthritis, and diarrhea. One or more of these symptoms may recur at intervals, but the arthritis may be persistent.

Relaxin (re-LAK-sin): A hormone secreted during pregnancy that allows the softening and lengthening of the pubic symphysis, along with other connective tissues.

Renal calculus (RE-nal KAL-kyu-lus): A stone or pebble formed in the kidney collection system. See *kidney stones*.

Renal colic (RE-nal KOH-lik): Severe pain caused by the impaction or passage of a calculus in the ureter or renal pelvis.

Renin (REN-in): An enzyme produced by the kidneys that is involved in vasoconstriction and hypertension.

Repetitive stress injury (re-PET-ih-tiv STRESS IN-jur-e): Any injury related to wear-and-tear brought about by repeated, especially percussive, movements. See *carpal tunnel syndrome*.

Restenosis (re-sten-O-sis): Recurrence of stenosis after corrective surgery on the heart valve; narrowing of a structure, usually a coronary artery, following the removal or reduction of a previous narrowing.

Restless leg syndrome: A sense of uneasiness, twitching, or restlessness that occurs in the legs after going to bed. See *sleep disorders*.

Reticulocyte (reh-TIK-u-lo-site): An immature red blood cell.

Retinoin (RET-ih-no-in): A class of keratolytic drugs derived from retinoic acid and used for treatment of severe acne and psoriasis.

Retinopathy (ret-ih-NOH-path-e): Noninflammatory degenerative disease of the retina.

Retrovirus (RET-ro-vi-rus): A virus in the family Retroviridae. They possess RNA, which serves as a template for synthesis of DNA in the host cell.

Rett syndrome: A progressive and severe form of autism found mainly in girls.

Rheumatoid spondylitis (RU-mah-toid spon-dih-LI-is): See *ankylosing spondylitis*.

Rhinitis (ri-NI-tis): Inflammation of the nasal mucous membrane.

Rhinophyma (ri-no-FI-mah): Hypertrophy of the nose with follicular dilation, resulting from hyperplasia of sebaceous glands with fibrosis and increased vascularity. See *acne rosacea*.

Rhupus (RU-pus): Term for a common comorbidity of lupus and rheumatoid arthritis.

Rickettsia rickettsii (rih-KET-se-ah rih-KET-se-i): The agent of Rocky Mountain spotted fever and its geographic variants; transmitted by infected ixodid ticks, especially *Dermacentor andersoni* and *D. variabilis*. See *Lyme disease*.

Rimantadine (ri-MAN-tah-dene): An antiviral agent that closely resembles amantadine but is often better tolerated.

Ringworm: A fungal infection of the keratin component of hair, skin, or nails.

Rodent ulcer (RO-dent UL-ser): A slowly enlarging ulcerated basal cell carcinoma, usually on the face. See *skin cancer*.

Rotavirus (RO-tah-vi-rus): A group of RNA viruses, some of which cause human gastroenteritis. These viruses are major causes of infant diarrhea throughout the world.

Rotoscoliosis (ro-to-sko-li-O-sis): Combined lateral and rotational deviation of the vertebral column.

Rubella (ru-BEL-ah): An acute exanthematous disease caused by the rubella virus *Rubivirus*, with enlargement of lymph nodes but usually with little fever or constitutional reaction; a high incidence of birth defects in children results from maternal infection during the first several months of fetal life (congenital rubella syndrome). See *mononucleosis*.

S-adenosyl-methionine (SAM) (S-ah-DEN-o-sil meh-THI-o-nine): An amino acid associated with mood improvement. See *depression*.

Salmonella (sal-mo-NEL-ah): A group of bacteria associated with gastrointestinal tract infections and food poisoning.

Salpingitis (sal-pin-JI-tis): Inflammation of the fallopian (uterine) tube.

Sarcoidosis (sar-koyd-O-sis): A systemic granulomatous disease of unknown cause, especially involving the lungs with fibrosis.

Sarcolemma (sar-ko-LEM-ah): The plasma membrane of a muscle fiber.

Sarcoma (sar-KO-mah): A neoplasm of connective tissue.

Sarcomere (SAR-ko-mere): The segment of a myofibril between Z lines; the functioning contractile unit of striated muscle.

Sarcoptes scabiei (sar-KOP-teze SKA-be-i): The itch mite, varieties of which are distributed worldwide and affect humans and many animals. The mite burrows into the skin and lays eggs within the burrow; intense itching and rash develop near the burrow in about a month.

Scheuermann disease (SHOY-er-mahn): Epiphysial osteonecrosis of adjacent vertebral bodies in the thoracic spine. See *postural deviations*.

Schistosoma haematobium (skis-to-SO-ma he-mah-TO-be-um): The vesical blood fluke, a species that occurs as a parasite in the portal system and mesenteric veins of the bladder, causing human schistosomiasis; found throughout Africa and the Middle East; See *bladder cancer*.

Schwann cells (shwahn selz): Cells forming a continuous envelope around each fiber of peripheral nerves.

Sclerodactyly (skler-o-DAK-tih-le): Stiffness and tightness of the skin of the fingers, with atrophy of the soft tissue and osteoporosis of the distal phalanges of the hands and feet; a limited form of progressive systemic sclerosis. See *scleroderma*.

Scleroderma (skler-o-DER-mah): Thickening and induration of the skin caused by new collagen formation; either a manifestation of progressive systemic sclerosis or localized morphea.

Scoliosis (sko-le-O-sis): Abnormal lateral curve of the vertebral column.

Seasonal affective disorder (SAD) (SE-zon-al ah-FEK-tiv dis-OR-der): A depressive disorder that is exacerbated by short days and less sunlight; subsides in spring and summer.

Sebaceous gland (seh-BA-shus gland): Gland in the dermis that usually opens into hair follicles and secretes an oily semifluid; sebum.

Seborrheic (seb-o-RE-ik): Relating to overactivity of the sebaceous glands resulting in an excessive amount of sebum. See *eczema*.

Seborrheic keratosis (seb-o-RE-ik ker-ah-TO-sis): Superficial benign skin lesions of proliferating epithelial cells.

Sebum (SE-bum): The secretion produced by sebaceous glands.

Second impact syndrome: Exacerbation of a head injury by another before the first has fully healed.

Selective estrogen receptor modulators (SERMs) (seh-LEK-tiv ES-tro-jen re-SEP-tur MOD-u-la-terz): A group of medications developed to reduce the risk of some recurrent cancers; can also be used for osteoporosis.

Selective serotonin reuptake inhibitors (SSRIs) (seh-LEK-tiv SER-o-to-nin re-UP-take in-HIB-ih-torz): A class of drugs used in the treatment of depression that selectively prevent the reuptake of serotonin in the brain.

Self-limited disease: A disease that resolves spontaneously with or without treatment.

Seminiferous tubules (sem-ih-NIF-er-us TU-byulez): The glandular part of testicles that contains the sperm-producing cells.

Seminoma (sem-ih-NO-mah): A type of germ cell tumor. See *testicular cancer*.

Sentinel lymph node (SEN-tih-nal LIMF node): The first lymph node to receive lymph drainage from a malignant tumor; if it is found clear of metastasis, all of the other nearby nodes are clear also.

Septicemia (sep-tih-SE-me-ah): Systemic disease caused by the spread of microorganisms and their toxins in the circulating blood. See *cellulitis*, *lymphangitis*.

Seronegative (ser-o-NEG-ah-tiv): Denoting the absence of specific antibodies in serum.

Serotonin (ser-o-TO-nin): A chemical found in many tissues. In the brain it is a neurotransmitter associated with mood disorders; in the body it can be a vasoconstrictor, can stimulate smooth muscle contraction, and can inhibit gastric secretion.

Sertoli cell tumor (ser-TO-le sel TU-mor): A testicular tumor containing Sertoli cells, which may cause feminization. See *testicular cancer*.

Severe acute respiratory syndrome (SARS): A highly contagious respiratory illness caused by a type of coronavirus.

Shigella (shih-GEL-ah): A genus of bacteria associated with gastrointestinal infection.

Shoulder-hand syndrome: Synonym for complex regional pain syndrome.

Shy-Drager syndrome (SHI-DRA-ger SIN-drome): A progressive central nervous system disorder involving tremor, muscle wasting, hypotension, and other symptoms. See *tremor*.

Sigmoidoscopy (sig-moid-OS-ko-pe): Endoscopic inspection of the sigmoid flexure of the colon.

Sine scleroderma: An unusual form of systemic scleroderma with significant organ involvement and minimal effect on the skin.

Sinoatrial node (si-no-A-tre-al node): The mass of specialized cardiac fibers that act as the pacemaker for the heart.

Sitz bath: Immersion of only the perineum and buttocks, with the legs being outside the tub.

Sjögren syndrome (SHOR-gren SIN-drome): An autoimmune disorder with a collection of signs and symptoms, including conjunctivitis, dryness of mucous membranes, and bilateral enlargement of the parotid glands. See *rheumatoid arthritis*, *lupus*, *scleroderma*.

Sleep paralysis (slepe pah-RAL-ih-sis): Brief episodic loss of voluntary movement that occurs when falling asleep (hypnagogic sleep paralysis) or when awakening (hypnopompic sleep paralysis). See *sleep disorders*.

Sodium urate (SO-de-um YUR-ate): Uric acid.

Somatomedin C (so-mat-o-ME-din C): A peptide that stimulates growth in bone and cartilage. See *acromegaly*.

Somatotrophin (so-mat-o-TRO-fin): A hormone produced in the anterior pituitary that promotes body growth, fat mobilization, and inhibition of glucose utilization.

Sonogram (SON-o-gram): A diagnostic technique that uses ultrasound waves to create a computer image.

Spastic paralysis (SPAS-tik pah-RAL-ih-sis): Central nervous system damage resulting in permanent muscle contraction; combines aspects of hypertonia, hypokinesia, and hyperreflexia.

Spasticity (spas-TIS-ih-te): A state of increased muscle tone with exaggerated muscle tendon reflexes. See *cerebral palsy*, *spinal cord injury*.

Specific immunity (speh-SIF-ik ih-MYU-nih-te): The immune state in which an altered reactivity is directed solely against the antigens that stimulated it.

Specific muscle weakness: Degeneration and weakening of muscles supplied by specifically damaged motor neurons; as opposed to general muscle weakness, which may not be related to nerve damage.

Sphincter (sfink-tur): A muscle that encircles a duct, tube, or orifice.

Sphygmomanometer (sfig-mo-man-OM-eh-ter): Blood pressure cuff.

Spigelian hernia (spih-JE-le-an HER-ne-ah): A bulge at the lateral aspect of the rectus abdominus.

Spina bifida meningocele (SPI-nah BIF-ih-dah men-ING-go-sele): Protrusion of the membranes of the brain or spinal cord through a defect in the skull or vertebral column.

Spina bifida myelomeningocele (SPI-nah BIF-ih-dah mi-el-o-men-ING-go-sele): Protrusion of the spinal cord and its membranes through a defect in the vertebral column.

Spina bifida occulta (SPI-nah BIF-ih-dah o-KUL-tah): Spina bifida in which there is a spinal defect but no protrusion of the cord or its membrane, although there is often some abnormality in their development.

Spirochete (SPI-ro-kete): A type of bacteria shaped like undulating spiral rods. See *ulcers*, *Lyme disease*, *syphilis*.

Spirometry (spi-ROM-et-re): A test to measure respiratory gases using a spirometer.

Splenomegaly (splen-o-MEG-ah-le): Enlargement of the spleen. See *mononucleosis*, *anemia*.

Spondyloarthropathy (spon-dih-lo-arth-ROH-path-e): Group name for dysfunction or disease at spinal joints.

Spondylolisthesis (spon-dih-lo-lis-THE-sis): Forward movement of the body of one of the lumbar vertebrae on the vertebra below it or on the sacrum.

Spondylolysis (spon-dih-lo-LI-sis): Degeneration of the articulating part of the vertebra.

Spondylosis (spon-dih-LO-sis): Stiffening of the vertebra; often applied nonspecifically to any lesion of the spine of a degenerative nature.

Sporadic (spor-AD-ik): Occurring irregularly, haphazardly.

Sputum (SPYU-tum): Expectorated matter, especially mucus or mucopurulent matter expectorated in diseases of the air passages.

Squamous (SKWA-mus): Relating to or covered with scales.

St. Anthony's fire: Any of several inflammatory infections of the skin, especially erysipelas. See *cellulitis*.

Staghorn calculus (STAG-horn KAL-kyu-lus): A calculus occurring in the renal pelvis, with branches extending into the calices. See *kidney stones*.

Staging (STA-jing): The classification of distinct phases or periods in the course of a disease.

Stapedius (stah-PE-de-us): Muscle that connects the eardrum (tympanum) to the stapes.

Staphylococcus (staf-ih-lo-KOK-us): A genus of bacteria formed of spherical cells that divide to make irregular clusters.

Starling equilibrium (star-ling ek-wih-LIB-re-um): Also called Starling hypothesis (hi-POTH-eh-sis): The principle that the amount of fluid squeezed out of circulatory capillaries should be almost equal to the amount drawn back in; leftovers form interstitial fluid.

Status epilepticus (STAT-us ep-ih-LEP-tih-kus): Repeated

seizure or a seizure prolonged for at least 30 minutes; may be convulsive tonic-clonic, nonconvulsive absence, complex partial, partial epilepsia partialis continuans, or subclinical electrographic status epilepticus. See *seizure disorders*.

Steatorrhea (ste-at-o-RE-ah): Passage of large amounts of feces due to failure to digest and absorb nutrients, especially fats. Often linked to absence of bile salts in the gastrointestinal tract.

Stein-Leventhal syndrome (stine LEV-en-thal SIN-drome): Synonym for polycystic ovary disease. See *ovarian cysts*.

Stenosis (sten-O-sis): A stricture or narrowing of any canal.

Stent: A device to hold tissue in place or provide support.

Steroids (STER-oydz): A large group of chemical compounds including some hormones and drugs of a particular molecular composition. Some steroids include gonadal and adrenal hormones.

Stoma (STO-mah): An artificial opening between two cavities or between a hollow area and the surface of the body.

Stomatitis (sto-mah-TI-tis): Inflammation of the mucous membrane of the mouth.

Strabismus (strah-BIS-mus): A lack of parallelism in the visual axes of the eyes. See *cerebral palsy*.

Stratum basale (STRAT-um bah-SAL): The deepest layer of the epidermis, composed of dividing stem cells and anchoring cells.

Streptococcus (strep-to-KOK-us): A genus of bacteria formed of spherical cells that occur in pairs or in long or short chains.

Streptococcus pneumoniae (strep-to-KOK-us nu-MO-ne-a): A species diplococci frequently occurring in pairs or chains. Normal inhabitants of the respiratory tract and the cause of lobar pneumonia, otitis media, meningitis, sinusitis, and other infections.

Striatonigral degeneration (stro-at-o-NIH-gral de-jen-ur-A-shun): A movement disorder that may appear with Shy-Drager syndrome and olivopontocerebellar atrophy in a condition called multiple system atrophy. See *tremor*.

Stroma (STRO-mah): The framework, usually made of connective tissue, of an organ, gland, or other tissue.

Stromal cell tumor (STRO-mal sel TU-mur): A tumor that arises from connective tissue stroma rather than epithelium. See *breast cancer*.

Struvite (STRU-vite): A compound of magnesium ammonium phosphate found in some renal calculi. See *kidney stones*.

Subacute (sub-ah-KYUTE): Between acute and chronic, denoting medium duration or relatively mild severity.

Subacute cutaneous lupus (sub-ah-KYUTE kyu-TA-ne-us): A group of skin disorders related to lupus erythematosus; may progress to systemic lupus.

Subcutaneous (sub-kyu-TA-ne-us): Beneath the skin.

Subluxation (sub-luk-SA-shun): An incomplete dislocation; although a relationship is altered, contact between joint surfaces remains.

Substance P: A neurotransmitter that is primarily involved in pain transmission and is one of the most potent compounds affecting smooth muscle tissue. See *fibromyalgia*.

Substantia nigra (sub-STAN-te-ah NIG-rah): A large mass composed of pigmented cells in the brainstem. The site of dopamine synthesis.

Sudeck atrophy (SU-dek AT-ro-fe): Synonym for *complex regional pain syndrome*.

Superficial fascia (su-per-FISH-al FASH-a): A loose fibrous envelope of connective tissue under the skin containing fat, blood vessels, and nerves.

Superior vena cava syndrome (su-PE-re-or VE-na KA-va SIN-drome): Obstruction of the superior vena cava by benign or malignant lesions that cause engorgement of the blood vessels of the face, neck, and arms. See *lung cancer*.

Sympathectomy (sim-pa-THEK-to-me): Excision of a section of a sympathetic nerve or one or more of the sympathetic ganglia. See *complex regional pain syndrome*.

Synarthrosis, synarthroses (sin-ar-THRO-sis, sin-ar-THRO-sez): A fibrous joint, sometimes said to be immovable.

Syncytial (sin-SIH-shal): Relating to a mass formed by the secondary union of originally separated cells.

Syndesmophyte (sin-DEZ-mo-fite): A bone spur attached to a ligament.

Syndrome X: A synonym for *metabolic syndrome*.

Synkinesis (sin-kin-E-sis): Involuntary movement that follows a voluntary one. See *Bell palsy*.

Synovectomy (sin-o-VEK-to-me): The excision of part or all of the synovial membrane of a joint.

Synovial joint (sin-O-ve-al joynt): A diarthrosis, or freely movable joint.

Systemic lupus erythematosus (sis-TEM-ik LU-pus eh-rih-the-mah-TO-sus): An inflammatory connective tissue disease with variable features including fever, weakness and fatigability, joint pains or arthritis resembling rheumatoid arthritis, and diffuse erythematous skin lesions on the face, neck, or upper extremities.

Systole (SIS-tole): The contraction of the heart, specifically of the ventricles.

Tachycardia (tak-e-KAR-de-a): Rapid heartbeat, usually applied to rates greater than 100 beats per minute.

Tamoxifen (tah-MOX-ih-fen): An antiestrogen agent used in the treatment of breast cancer.

Tau (tow): A protein that helps to maintain the structure of the cytoskeleton; found in the plaques of persons with Alzheimer disease.

Telangiectasia (tel-an-je-ek-TA-ze-ah): Dilation of previously existing small vessels, most commonly in the skin. Also called *spider veins*. See *scleroderma*, *varicose veins*, *acne rosacea*.

Tender point: One of many predictable bilateral pairs of points that produce a painful response with a minimum of pressure 4 kg; used to help diagnose fibromyalgia.

Tendinosis (ten-din-O-sis): The condition of chronic tendon injury without inflammation. See *tendinopathies*.

Tennis elbow (TEH-nis EL-bo): A synonym for *lateral epicondylitis*.

Tenosynovitis (ten-o-sin-o-VI-tis): Inflammation of a tendon and its enveloping sheath.

TENS, transcutaneous electrical nerve stimulation: A device to control pain with electrical stimulation applied through the skin to the nerves.

Teratoma (ter-ah-TO-mah): A neoplasm that contains tissues not normally found in the tissue in which it arises; usually found as benign ovarian cysts in women and malignant testicular growths in men. See *testicular cancer*; *ovarian cysts*.

Terminal ileitis (TER-min-al il-e-I-tis): Synonym for *Crohn disease*.

Testosterone (tes-TOS-teh-rone): A naturally occurring androgen found in testes and other tissues.

Tetraplegia (tet-rah-PLE-je-a): Quadriplegia.

Thalassemia (thal-ah-SE-me-ah): Any of a group of inherited disorders of hemoglobin metabolism.

Thenar (THE-nar): Referring to the fleshy mass on the lateral side of the palm; the ball of the thumb.

Thermal capsulorraphy (THER-mal kap-su-LOR-ah-fe): The use of heat to shrink and repair a joint capsule, specifically at the shoulder, to prevent future dislocations.

Thermography (ther-MOG-raf-e): The making of a regional temperature map of the body, obtained by using an infrared sensing device.

Thrombocyte (THROM-bo-site): Platelet.

Thrombocytopenia (throm-bo-si-to-PE-ne-ah): Decreased number of thrombocytes.

Thrombosis (throm-BO-sis): Formation or presence of a clot.

Thrush: Infection of the oral tissues with *Candida albicans*; often an opportunistic infection in persons with AIDS or other conditions that depress the immune system. See *HIV/AIDS*, *Candida*.

Thymoma (thi-MO-ma): A neoplasm originating in the thymus; usually benign. See *myasthenia gravis*.

Thymosin (THI-mo-sin): A hormone that restores thymus function.

Thyroxin (thi-ROK-sin): Tetraiodothyronine (T_4); a secretion of the thyroid gland.

Tibial tuberosity apophysitis (TIB-e-al tu-ber-OS-ih-te ap-of-ih-SI-tis): Inflammation of the tibial tuberosity; synonym for *Osgood-Schlatter disease*.

Tic douloureux (tik doo-lo-ROO): A synonym for *trigeminal neuralgia*.

Tinea (TIN-e-ah): A fungal infection of the keratin component of hairs, skin, or nails.

Tinea barbae (TIN-e-ah BAR-ba): Tinea of the beard, occurring as a follicular infection or as a granulomatous lesion; the primary lesions are papules and pustules. See *fungal infections*.

Tinea capitus (TIN-e-ah KAP-ih-tus): A common fungus infection of the scalp caused by various species of *Microsporum* and *Trichophyton* on or within hair shafts. See *fungal infections*.

Tinea corporis (TIN-e-ah KOR-por-is): A well-defined, scaling, macular eruption of dermatophytosis that frequently forms annular lesions and may appear on any part of the body. See *fungal infections*.

Tinea cruris (TIN-e-ah KRU-ris): A form of tinea imbricata occurring in the genitocrural region, including the inner side of the thighs, the perineal region, and the groin. See *fungal infections*.

Tinea manus (TIN-e-ah MAN-us): Ringworm of the hand, usually referring to infections of the palmar surface. See *fungal infections*.

Tinea pedis (TIN-e-ah PED-is): Dermatophytosis of the feet, especially of the skin between the toes, caused by one of the dermatophytes, usually a species of *Trichophyton* or *Epidermophyton;* the disease consists of small vesicles, fissures, scaling, maceration, and eroded areas between the toes and on the plantar surface of the foot. See *fungal infections*.

Tinea unguium (TIN-e-ah UNG-we-um): Ringworm of the nails due to a dermatophyte. See *fungal infections*.

Tinea versicolor (TIN-e-ah VER-sih-koh-lor): An eruption of tan or brown branny patches on the skin of the trunk, often appearing white, in contrast with hyperpigmented skin after exposure to the summer sun; caused by growth of *Malassezia furfur* in the stratum corneum with minimal inflammatory reaction. See *fungal infections*.

Tinel sign (te-NEL sine): Distally radiating pain or tingling caused by tapping over the site of a superficial nerve, indicating inflammation or entrapment of that nerve; a test used to help identify carpal tunnel syndrome.

Tinnitus (TIN-ih-tus, tin-I-tus): A sensation of noises ringing, whistling, or booming in the ears.

Tissue plasminogen activator (tPA) (TISH-u plaz-MIN-o-jen AK-tiv-a-tor): A genetically engineered protein that acts as a powerful thrombolytic clot-busting agent.

Titer (TI-ter): The standard of strength of a volumetric test solution; the assay value of an unknown measure by volumetric means.

Tonic spasm (TON-ik SPAZ-em): Continuous involuntary spasm of skeletal muscle.

Tonic-clonic seizure (TON-ik KLON-ik SE-zher): The sudden onset of tonic contraction of muscles, giving way to clonic convulsive movements. Synonym for grand mal seizure.

Tophus, tophi (TO-fus, TO-fi): Deposits of uric acid and urates in tissue around joints and other areas; seen with gout.

Topical immunomodulators (TINs) (TOP-ih-kal im-u-no-MOD-u-la-torz): A class of anti-inflammatory ointments used as an alternative to steroidal applications in the treatment of atopic dermatitis. See *eczema*.

Torsion (TOR-shun): A twisting of a structure along its long axis.

Torticollis (tor-tih-KOL-is): A contraction, often spasmodic, of the muscles of the neck, chiefly those supplied by the spinal accessory nerve; the head is drawn to one side and usually rotated so that the chin points to the other side.

Toxic megacolon (TOK-sik MEG-ah-ko-lon): Acute nonobstructive dilation of the colon.

Toxoplasma gondii (TOX-o-plaz-mah GON-de-i): A widespread parasitic species of sporozoan; may cause mononucleosis.

Transcriptase (tran-SKRIP-tase): An enzyme that converts RNA to DNA in the AIDS virus.

Transcutaneous (tranz-kyu-TA-ne-us): Denoting the passage of substances through unbroken skin.

Treponema pallidum (trep-o-NE-mah PAL-ih-dum): A species of spirochetal bacteria that causes syphilis in humans.

Trichophyton (trih-KOF-ih-ton): A genus of pathogenic fungi that cause dermatophytosis in humans and animals. See *fungal infections*.

Tricyclic antidepressants (tri-SIK-lik an-te-de-PRES-ants): A chemical group of drugs that share a three-ringed nucleus, e.g., amitriptyline, imipramine.

Trigger point: A small area in which muscle fibers have been injured and not healed normally. Pressure on a trigger point elicits moderate to severe pain in specific referring patterns.

Triiodothyronine (tri-I-o-do-THI-ro-nene): T_3, a secretion of the thyroid gland. See *hypothyroidism*.

Trophic (TRO-fik): Relating to or dependent on nutrition; resulting from interruption of nerve supply.

Trophic ulcer (TRO-fik UL-ser): Ulcer resulting from cutaneous sensory denervation.

Tubercle (TU-ber-kel): A nodule or bump; may refer to bony prominences, elevations on the skin or other tissues, or to the lesions caused by infection with *Mycobacterium tuberculosis*.

Tumor (TU-mor): Any swelling, usually denoting a neoplasm.

Tumor necrosis factor (TU-mur nek-RO-sis fak-tor): A polypeptide hormone produced by activated macrophages; can initiate fever.

Tunica intima (TU-nih-kah IN-tih-mah): The innermost coat of a blood or lymphatic vessel.

Tunica media (TU-nih-kah ME-de-ah): The middle, usually muscular coat of a blood vessel or lymphatic vessel.

Turcot syndrome (tur-KO SIN-drome): A subgroup of a genetic predisposition to colorectal cancer; part of familial adenomatous polyposis.

Tyrosine (TI-ro-zene): An amino acid present in most proteins.

Unilateral (u-nih-LAT-er-al): Confined to one side only.

Ureaplasma urealyticum (u-re-ah-PLAZ-mah u-re-ah-LIH-tih-kum): A species of bacteria that cause infections in the genitourinary tract. See *sexually transmitted diseases*.

Uremia (yu-RE-me-a): An excess of urea and other nitrogenous waste in the blood.

Ureterolithiasis (u-re-ter-o-lith-I-ah-sis): A kidney stone lodged in the ureter.

Ureteroscopic stone removal (u-re-ter-o-SKOP-ik STONE re-MU-val): Removal of a calculus in the mid to lower ureters with a ureteroscope.

Urogram (YUR-o-gram): Radiographic record of any part of the urinary tract.

Urticaria (ur-tih-KA-re-ah): An eruption of itching wheals; synonym for hives.

Uveitis (yu-ve-I-tis): Inflammation of the uveal tract: iris, ciliary body, and choroid of the eye. See *ulcerative colitis*.

Vagotomy (va-GOT-o-me): Division of the vagus nerve.

Valgus (VAL-gus): Laterally deviated.

Vapocoolant (VA-po-koo-lant): A topical anesthetic aerosol spray used for pain relief and stretching of muscles affected by trigger points. See *myofascial pain syndrome*.

Varicocele (VAR-ih-ko-sele): A condition manifested by abnormal dilation of the veins of the spermatic cord,

caused by incompetent valves in the internal spermatic vein and resulting in impaired drainage of blood into the spermatic cord veins when the patient assumes the upright position.
Varix, varices (VAR-ix, VAR-ih-sez): A dilated vein.
Varus (VAR-us): Medially deviated.
Vas deferens (vas DEF-er-enz): The secretory duct of the testicle, running from the epididymis to the prostatic urethra, where it terminates as the ejaculatory duct.
Vasculitis (vas-ku-LI-tis): Inflammation of a blood or lymphatic vessel.
Venography (ve-NOG-rah-fe): A radiographic demonstration of a vein after the injection of a contrast medium.
Ventricle (VEN-trih-kul): A normal cavity, specifically in the brain or heart.
Venule (VEN-yule, VE-nyule): A venous branch continuous with a capillary.
Verruca (veh-RU-ka): A wart composed of a thickened keratin layer of the epidermis.
Vesicle (VES-ih-kul): A small, circumscribed fluid-filled elevation of the skin; a blister.
Vesicoureteral reflux (VES-ih-co-u-RE-tul RE-flux): Backward flow of urine from bladder into ureter.
Villus, villi (VIL-us, VIL-i): A projection from the surface, especially of a mucous membrane.
Virchow triad (FERE-kow TRI-ad): A description of precipitating factors for clot formation; injury to endothelium, hypercoagulability, and venous stasis.
Viremia (vih-RE-me-ah): The presence of a virus in the bloodstream.
Virulent (VIR-u-lent): Extremely toxic, denoting a markedly pathogenic microorganism.
Von Willebrand disease (fon vil-eh-BRAHNT): A disease characterized by the tendency to bleed primarily from the mucous membranes and prolonged bleeding time.

Wernicke-Korsakoff syndrome (VER-nih-ke KOR-sah-kof SIN-drome): A combination of conditions related to prolonged alcohol abuse and thiamin deficiency, including tremor, psychosis, confusion, memory loss, and delirium tremens.
Wheal (wele): A reddened, itchy, changeable edematous area of the skin that is caused by exposure to an allergenic substance in a susceptible individual.
Wolff law (volf law): A law stating that every change in the form and/or function of a bone is followed by changes in internal and external architecture of the bone.
Wright test (rite test): A thoracic outlet syndrome test in which the hand is placed over the head and the head is turned toward the affected side. If this exacerbates symptoms or reduces the strength of the pulse of the affected side, impingement to the axillary artery and lower brachial plexus nerves is suspected.

Xeroderma (ze-ro-DER-mah): Excessively dry skin; a mild form of ichthyosis.
Xeroderma pigmentosum (ze-ro-DER-mah pig-men-TO-sum): A genetic disorder that impedes the ability to heal from overexposure to ultraviolet radiation.
Yolk sac tumor: Malignant neoplasm occurring in the gonads. See *testicular cancer*.
Yuppie flu: Vernacular for a set of signs and symptoms that may be diagnosed as chronic fatigue syndrome.

Zygapophyseal joint (zi-gah-po-FIZ-e-al): Relating to a zygapophysis or articular process of a vertebra.

Illustration Credits

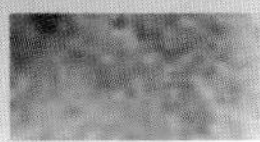

Chapter 1

1.1 Public Images Library, Centers for Disease Control and Prevention. http://phil.cdc.gov/phil.detail.?id52170.
1.2 McClatchey KD. Clinical Laboratory Medicine, 2nd ed. Philadelphia: Lippincott Williams & Wilkins, 2002.
1.3 Public Images Library, Centers for Disease Control and Prevention. http://phil.cdc.gov/phil.detail.?id52170.
1.4 Koneman EW, Allen SD, Janda WM, Schreckenberger PC, Winn WC, Jr. Color Atlas and Textbook of Diagnostic Microbiology, 5th ed. Philadelphia: Lippincott Williams & Wilkins, 1997.
1.5 Sun T. Parasitic Disorders: Pathology, Diagnosis, and Management, 2nd ed. Baltimore: Lippincott Williams & Wilkins, 1999.
1.6 Public Images Library, Centers for Disease Control and Prevention. James Gathany, Photographer.
1.7 Goodheart HP. Goodheart's Photoguide of Common Skin Disorders, 2nd ed. Philadelphia: Lippincott Williams & Wilkins, 2003.
1.8 Volk WA et al. Essentials of Medical Microbiology, 5th ed. Philadelphia: Lippincott-Raven, 1996.

Chapter 2

2.2 Barankin Dermatology Collection, © Stedman's 2006.
2.3 Rubin E, Farber JL. Pathology, 3rd ed. Philadelphia: Lippincott Williams & Wilkins, 1999.
2.4 Goodheart HP. Goodheart's Photoguide of Common Skin Disorders, 2nd ed. Philadelphia: Lippincott Williams & Wilkins, 2003.
2.5 Rubin E, Gorstein F, Schwarting R, Strayer DS. Rubin's Pathology: Clinicopathologic Foundations of Medicine, 4th ed. Philadelphia: Lippincott Williams & Wilkins, 2005.
2.6 Barankin Dermatology Collection, © Stedman's 2006.
2.7 Goodheart HP. Goodheart's Photoguide of Common Skin Disorders, 2nd ed. Philadelphia: Lippincott Williams & Wilkins, 2003.
2.8 McClatchey KD. Clinical Laboratory Medicine, 2nd ed. Philadelphia: Lippincott Williams & Wilkins, 2002.
2.9 Sutton DA, Fothergill AW, Rinaldi MG. Guide to Clinically Significant Fungi. Baltimore: Williams & Wilkins, 1998.
2.10 Goodheart HP. Goodheart's Photoguide of Common Skin Disorders, 2nd ed. Philadelphia: Lippincott Williams & Wilkins, 2003.
2.11 Goodheart HP. Goodheart's Photoguide of Common Skin Disorders, 2nd ed. Philadelphia: Lippincott Williams & Wilkins, 2003.
2.12 Public Images Library, Centers for Disease Control and Prevention. http://phil.cdc.gov.

2.13 Goodheart HP. Goodheart's Photoguide of Common Skin Disorders, 2nd ed. Philadelphia: Lippincott Williams & Wilkins, 2003.
2.14 Reprinted with permission from Goodheart HP. A Photoguide of Common Skin Disorders: Diagnosis and Management. Baltimore: Lippincott Williams & Wilkins, 1999: 90.
2.15 Smeltzer SC, Bare BG. Textbook of Medical-Surgical Nursing, 9th ed. Philadelphia: Lippincott Williams & Wilkins, 2000.
2.16 Goodheart HP. Goodheart's Photoguide of Common Skin Disorders, 2nd ed. Philadelphia: Lippincott Williams & Wilkins, 2003.
2.19 Goodheart HP. Goodheart's Photoguide of Common Skin Disorders, 2nd ed. Philadelphia: Lippincott Williams & Wilkins, 2003.
2.20 Fleisher GR, Ludwig S, Baskin MN. Atlas of Pediatric Emergency Medicine. Philadelphia: Lippincott Williams & Wilkins, 2004.
2.21 Reprinted with permission from Goodheart HP. A Photoguide of Common Skin Disorders: Diagnosis and Management. Baltimore: Lippincott Williams & Wilkins, 1999: 310.
2.22 Reprinted with permission from Rassner G. Atlas of Dermatology, 3rd ed. Philadelphia: Lea & Febiger, 1994: 46.
2.23 Goodheart HP. Goodheart's Photoguide of Common Skin Disorders, 2nd ed. Philadelphia: Lippincott Williams & Wilkins, 2003.
2.25 Goodheart HP. Goodheart's Photoguide of Common Skin Disorders, 2nd ed. Philadelphia: Lippincott Williams & Wilkins, 2003.
2.26 Sauer GC, Hall JC. Manual of Skin Diseases, 7th ed. Philadelphia: Lippincott-Raven, 1966.
2.27 Goodheart HP. Goodheart's Photoguide of Common Skin Disorders, 2nd ed. Philadelphia: Lippincott Williams & Wilkins, 2003.
2.28 Barankin Dermatology Collection, © Stedman's 2006.
2.29 Goodheart HP. Goodheart's Photoguide of Common Skin Disorders, 2nd ed. Philadelphia: Lippincott Williams & Wilkins, 2003.
2.30 Reprinted with permission from Goodheart HP. A Photoguide of Common Skin Disorders: Diagnosis and Management. Baltimore: Lippincott Williams & Wilkins, 1999: 44.
2.31 Goodheart HP. Goodheart's Photoguide of Common Skin Disorders, 2nd ed. Philadelphia: Lippincott Williams & Wilkins, 2003.
2.33 Rubin E, Gorstein F, Schwarting R, Strayer DS. Rubin's Pathology: Clinicopathologic Foundations of Medicine, 4th ed. Philadelphia: Lippincott Williams & Wilkins, 2005; 1217.
2.34 Reprinted with permission from Goodheart HP. A Photoguide of Common Skin Disorders: Diagnosis and Management. Baltimore: Lippincott Williams & Wilkins, 1999: 49.
2.35 Goodheart HP. Goodheart's Photoguide of Common Skin Disorders, 2nd ed. Philadelphia: Lippincott Williams & Wilkins, 2003.
2.36 Barankin Dermatology Collection, © Stedman's 2006.
2.37 Courtesy of the American Cancer Society, Inc., Atlanta, GA.
2.38 Tasman W, Jaeger E. The Wills Eye Hospital Atlas of Clinical Ophthalmology, 2nd ed. Philadelphia: Lippincott Williams & Wilkins, 2001.
2.39 Barankin Dermatology Collection, © Stedman's 2006.
2.40 Smeltzer SC, Bare BG. Textbook of Medical-Surgical Nursing, 9th ed. Philadelphia: Lippincott Williams & Wilkins, 2000.
2.41 Rubin E, Farber JL. Pathology, 3rd ed. Philadelphia: Lippincott Williams & Wilkins, 1999.
2.42 Goodheart HP. Goodheart's Photoguide of Common Skin Disorders, 2nd ed. Philadelphia: Lippincott Williams & Wilkins, 2003.

2.43 Rubin E, Gorstein F, Schwarting R, Strayer DS. Rubin's Pathology: Clinicopathologic Foundations of Medicine, 4th ed. Philadelphia: Lippincott Williams & Wilkins, 2005; 1253.
2.44 Nettina SM. The Lippincott Manual of Nursing Practice, 7th ed. Lippincott, Williams & Wilkins, 2001.
2.45 Barankin Dermatology Collection, © Stedman's 2006.
2.46 Barankin Dermatology Collection, © Stedman's 2006.
2.47 Fleisher GR, Ludwig S, Baskin MN. Atlas of Pediatric Emergency Medicine. Philadelphia: Lippincott Williams & Wilkins, 2004.
2.48 Reprinted with permission from Willis MC. Medical Terminology: The Language of Health Care. Baltimore: Williams & Wilkins, 1996: A5.
2.49 Rubin E, Gorstein F, Schwarting R, Strayer DS. Rubin's Pathology: Clinicopathologic Foundations of Medicine, 4th ed. Philadelphia: Lippincott Williams & Wilkins, 2005.

Chapter 3

3.6 Yochum TR, Rowe LJ. Essentials of Skeletal Radiology, 2nd ed. Baltimore: Lippincott Williams & Wilkins, 1996.
3.13 Reprinted with permission from Roentgen EJ. Diagnosis of Diseases of Bone, 3rd ed. Baltimore: Williams & Wilkins, 1981;2:841.
3.14 Rubin E, Gorstein F, Schwarting R, Strayer DS. Rubin's Pathology: Clinicopathologic Foundations of Medicine, 4th ed. Philadelphia: Lippincott Williams & Wilkins, 2005: 1336.
3.15 Reprinted with permission from Agur AMR, Lee MJ. Grant's Atlas of Anatomy, 10th ed. Baltimore: Lippincott Williams & Wilkins, 1999:251.
3.16 Reprinted with permission from Brant WE, Helms CA. Fundamentals of Diagnostic Radiology, 2nd ed. Baltimore: Lippincott Williams & Wilkins, 1999: 1058.
3.18 Porth CM. Pathophysiology: Concepts of Altered Health States, 7th ed. Philadelphia: Lippincott Williams & Wilkins, 2005.
3.21 Reprinted with permission from Baker CL. The Hughston Clinic Sports Medicine Book. Baltimore: Williams & Wilkins, 1995: 365.
3.22 Reprinted with permission from Rubin E, Gorstein F, Schwarting R, Strayer DS. Rubin's Pathology: Clinicopathologic Foundations of Medicine, 4th ed. Philadelphia: Lippincott Williams & Wilkins, 2005; 1374.
3.23 Rubin E, Gorstein F, Schwarting R, Strayer DS. Rubin's Pathology: Clinicopathologic Foundations of Medicine, 4th ed. Philadelphia: Lippincott Williams & Wilkins, 2005.
3.24 Reprinted with permission from Koneman EW, Allen SD, Janda WM, Schreckenberger PC, Winn WC Jr. Color Atlas and Textbook of Diagnostic Microbiology, 5th ed. Philadelphia: Lippincott Williams & Wilkins, 1997; Figure E.
3.25 Sanders CV, Nesbitt LT Jr. The Skin and Infection: A Color Atlas and Text. Baltimore: Williams & Wilkins, 1995. Figure 9.1.
3.27 Reprinted with permission from Harris JH Jr, Harris WH, Novelline RA. The Radiology of Emergency Medicine, 3rd ed. Baltimore: Williams & Wilkins, 1993; 440.
3.28 Reprinted with permission from MacNab I, McCulloch J. Neck Ache and Shoulder Pain. Baltimore: Williams & Wilkins, 1994: 45.
3.29 Reprinted with permission from MacNab I, McCulloch J. Neck Ache and Shoulder Pain. Baltimore: Williams & Wilkins, 1994: 45.

3.31 Rubin E, Farber J. Pathology, 3rd ed. Philadelphia: Lippincott Williams & Wilkins, 1999.
3.32 Reprinted with permission from Barker LR, Burton JR, Zieve PD. Principles of Ambulatory Medicine, 4th ed. Baltimore: Williams & Wilkins, 1995: 946.
3.33 Reprinted with permission from Barker LR, Burton JR, Zieve PD. Principles of Ambulatory Medicine, 4th ed. Baltimore: Williams & Wilkins, 1995: 946.
3.35 Barankin Dermatology Collection, © Stedman's 2006.
3.37 Moore KL, Dalley AF II. Clinically Oriented Anatomy, 4th ed. Baltimore: Lippincott Williams & Wilkins, 1999.
3.40 Reprinted with permission from Yochum TR, Rowe LJ. Essentials of Skeletal Radiology, 2nd ed. Baltimore: Williams & Wilkins, 1996;2;1291, Figure 13-59B.
3.43 Goodheart HP. Goodheart's Photoguide of Common Skin Disorders, 2nd ed. Philadelphia: Lippincott Williams & Wilkins, 2003.

Chapter 4

4.3 Reprinted from Rubin E, Strayer DS. Rubin's Pathology: Clinicopathologic Foundations of Medicine, 5th ed. Philadelphia: Lippincott Williams & Wilkins, 2008.
4.5 Fleisher GR, Ludwig W, Baskin MN. Atlas of Pediatric Emergency Medicine. Philadelphia: Lippincott Williams & Wilkins, 2004.
4.9 Courtesy of Robert Schwarzmann, MD, Philadelphia, PA.
4.13 Reprinted with permission from Yochum TR, Rowe LJ. Essentials of Skeletal Radiology, 2nd ed. Baltimore: Williams & Wilkins, 1996, 1:398.
4.18 Adapted from Smeltzer SC, Bare BG. Brunner & Suddarth's Textbook of Medical-Surgical Nursing, 9th ed. Philadelphia: Lippincott Williams & Wilkins, 2000.

Chapter 5

5.1 Cohen BJ, Wood DL. Memmler's The Human Body in Health and Disease, 9th ed. Philadelphia: Lippincott Williams & Wilkins, 2000.
5.5 Reprinted with permission from Rubin E, Farber J. Pathology, 3rd ed. Philadelphia: Lippincott Williams & Wilkins, 1999.
5.8 Reprinted with permission from Rubin E, Farber J. Pathology, 3rd ed. Philadelphia: Lippincott Williams & Wilkins, 1999.
5.12 Courtesy of the nonprofit International Scleroderma Network, www.sclero.org.
5.14 Moore KL, Dalley AF II. Clinically Oriented Anatomy, 4th ed. Baltimore: Lippincott Williams & Wilkins, 1999.

Chapter 6

6.2 Rubin E, Gorstein F, Schwarting R, Strayer DS. Rubin's Pathology: Clinicopathologic Foundations of Medicine, 4th ed. Baltimore: Lippincott Williams & Wilkins, 2005.
6.3 Reprinted with permission from Fitzpatrick J, Aeling J. Dermatology Secrets in Color, 2nd ed. Philadelphia: Hanley & Belfus, 2000: 191.

6.4 Reprinted with permission from Bickley LS. Bates' Guide to Physical Examination and History Taking, 7th ed. Baltimore: Lippincott Williams & Wilkins, 1999: 660.
6.5 Neville B et al. Color Atlas of Clinical Oral Pathology. Philadelphia: Lea & Febiger, 1991. Used with permission.
6.6 DeVita VT Jr, Hellaman S, Rosenberg S, Durran J, Essex M, Fauci AS. AIDS: Etiology, Diagnosis, Treatment, and Prevention, 4th ed. Philadelphia: Lippincott-Raven, 1997.
6.7 Goodheart HP. Goodheart's Photoguide of Common Skin Disorders, 2nd ed. Philadelphia: Lippincott Williams & Wilkins, 2003.
6.8 Reprinted with permission from Porth CM. Essentials of Patholophysiology: Concepts of Altered Health States, 2nd ed. Philadelphia: Lippincott Williams & Wilkins, 2007.

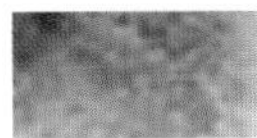

CHAPTER 7

7.3 Rubin E, Farber J. Pathology, 3rd ed. Philadelphia: Lippincott Williams & Wilkins, 1999.
7.7 Moore KL, Dalley AF II. Clinically Oriented Anatomy, 4th ed. Baltimore: Lippincott Williams & Wilkins, 1999.

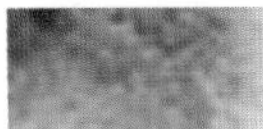

CHAPTER 8

8.5 Asset provided by Anatomical Chart Co.
8.7 Rubin E, Farber JL. Pathology, 3rd ed. Philadelphia: Lippincott Williams & Wilkins, 1999.
8.10 Sun T. Parasitic Disorders: Pathology, Diagnosis and Management, 2nd ed. Baltimore: Lippincott Williams & Wilkins, 1999.
8.11 Rubin E, Farber J. Pathology, 3rd ed. Philadelphia: Lippincott Williams & Wilkins, 1999.
8.13 Rubin E, Farber J. Pathology, 3rd ed. Philadelphia: Lippincott Williams & Wilkins, 1999.

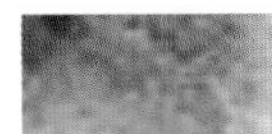

CHAPTER 9

9.1 Reprinted with permission from Porth CM. Essentials of Patholophysiology: Concepts of Altered Health States, 2nd ed. Philadelphia: Lippincott Williams & Wilkins, 2007.
9.2 Smeltzer SC, Bare BG. Textbook of Medical-Surgical Nursing, 9th Ed. Philadelphia: Lippincott Williams & Wilkins, 2000.
9.3 Rubin E, Farber J. Pathology, 3rd ed. Philadelphia: Lippincott Williams & Wilkins, 1999.
9.4 Weber J, Kelley J. Health Assessment in Nursing, 2nd ed. Philadelphia: Lippincott Williams & Wilkins, 2003.

CHAPTER 10

10.2 Rubin E, Gorstein F, Schwarting R, Strayer DS. Rubin's Pathology: Clinicopathologic Foundations of Medicine, 4th ed. Philadelphia: Lippincott Williams & Wilkins, 2005.

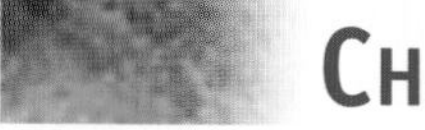

CHAPTER 11

11.5 Reprinted with permission from Mitchell GW. The Female Breast and Its Disorders. Baltimore: Williams & Wilkins, 1990: 140.

11.7 Rubin E, Gorstein F, Schwarting R, Strayer DS. Rubin's Pathology: Clinicopathologic Foundations of Medicine, 4th ed. Philadelphia: Lippincott Williams & Wilkins, 2005.

CHAPTER 12

12.1 Gold DH, Weingeist TA. Color Atlas of the Eye in Systemic Disease. Baltimore: Lippincott Williams & Wilkins, 2001.

12.2 Rubin E, Gorstein F, Schwarting R, Strayer DS. Rubin's Pathology: Clinicopathologic Foundations of Medicine, 4th ed. Philadelphia: Lippincott Williams & Wilkins, 2005.

INDEX

Page numbers followed by an "f " designate figures; page numbers followed by a "t" designate tables; (*see* and *see also*) designate related topics or more detailed subentries

A

Abdomen, mechanical perforation of, peritonitis due to, 551
Abdominal abscess, peritonitis due to, 551
Abdominal radiography, in kidney stones diagnosis, 590
Ablate, defined, 711
Ablation, for endometriosis, 620
Abrasion, defined, 711
Abscess(es)
  abdominal, peritonitis due to, 551
  diverticular disease and, 518
  pelvic, peritonitis due to, 551
Absence seizures, 325
  defined, 711
Absorption
  calcium, osteoporosis and, 116
  skin in, 24
ABT. *See* Asian bodywork therapy (ABT)
Abuse, chemical dependency—related, 265
Acanthosis nigricans, defined, 711
Accessory organs
  of digestive tract, 484–485, 484f
  disorders of, 525–547. *See also specific disorders and* Digestive disorders, of accessory organs
Accident(s), motor vehicle, SCI due to, 297
ACE inhibitors, 692
Acetaminophen, 688
  defined, 711
Acetylcholine (ACh), myasthenia gravis and, 210
Acetylcholine (ACh), defined, 711
ACh. *See* Acetylcholine (ACh)
Achiness, Parkinson disease and, 240
Acid(s)
  amino, defined, 755
  arachidonic, defined, 756
  fatty, deficiency of, eczema due to, 56
  folic, defined, 768
  gamma-aminobutyric, defined, 769
  hyaluronic
    defined, 772
    in ganglion cysts, 177
  salicylic, for psoriasis, 64
Acne, boils vs., 54
Acne fulminans, 53
  defined, 711
Acquired immunodeficiency syndrome (AIDS). *See also* HIV/AIDS
  defined, 427
Acral lentiginous melanoma, 71, 72f
  defined, 711
Acromioclavicular (AC) joint, injuries of, 152
Acromioclavicular joint sprain, defined, 711
Acropachy
  defined, 711
  hyperthyroidism and, 575
ACTH syndrome, ectopic, 565
Actinic cheilitis, defined, 711
Actinic keratosis, 66–67, 67f, 74
  defined, 711
Action tremor, 243
Activity(ies)
  cellular, inflammation and, 14–15
  vascular, inflammation and, 13, 14f
Acute, defined, 6t, 711
Acute chest syndrome, sickle cell disease and, 363
Acute compartment syndrome, 104, 349
Acute exertional compartment syndrome, defined, 711
Acute granulocytic leukemia, defined, 711
Acute idiopathic polyneuritis, defined, 711
Acute infectious disease, anemia and, 343
Acute inflammatory demyelinating polyneuropathy (AIDP), 314
  defined, 711
Acute lymphoblastic leukemia, defined, 711
Acute lymphocytic leukemia, 353
Acute lymphoid leukemia, defined, 711
Acute motor axonal neuropathy, 314
Acute motor-sensory axonal neuropathy, 314
Acute myelocytic leukemia, defined, 711
Acute myelogenous leukemia, 353
  defined, 711
Acute renal failure
  causes of, 595
  defined, 594
Acute stage of healing, 15
Acute urinary retention, 642
Acute vestibular neuronitis, 331
  defined, 711
Acyclovir, defined, 711
Addiction. *See also* Alcoholism; Chemical dependency
  types of, 267
Addison, Thomas, 562
Adenectomy, transsphenoidal, in Cushing syndrome, 566
Adenocarcinoma(s), 495, 508, 543
  defined, 711
Adenoma(s), 511
  defined, 711
  pituitary, 565
Adenomatous polyposis, familial, colorectal cancer due to, 513
Adenosquamous carcinoma, 624
S-Adenosyl-methionine (SAM), defined, 736
S-Adenosyl-methionine (SAM-e), for depression, 275
ADHD. *See* Attention deficit hyperactivity disorder (ADHD)
Adhesion(s)
  defined, 712
  strains and, 109–110
Adhesive capsulitis, 152
  defined, 712
Adjustment disorder, 272
Adolescence, acne vulgaris during, 53
Adrenal insufficiency, idiopathic, 563
Adrenal tumors, 565
Adrenaline, 558
Adrenergic blockers, 690–691
Adrenergic drugs, 690
Adson test
  defined, 712
  in thoracic outlet syndrome diagnosis, 214
Adventitia, 495
  defined, 712
Aerobic metabolism, 87
  defined, 712
Aflatoxin, defined, 712
Aflatoxin B_1, liver cancer due to, 540
Aftercare, in chemical dependency treatment, 269
Agglutination, defined, 712
Agoraphobia, 256
  defined, 712
AIDP. *See* Acute inflammatory demyelinating polyneuropathy (AIDP)
Albumin
  cirrhosis effects on, 528
  defined, 712
Alcohol
  body system effects of, 268–269
  familial effects of, 269
Alcohol consumption
  excessive, peptic ulcers due to, 506
  high, stroke due to, 305
  stomach cancer due to, 509
Alcohol-based hand rub, defined, 10
Alcoholic families, 269
Alcoholism
  causes of, 266
  death related to, 266
  defined, 712

Alcoholism—*continued*
liver cancer due to, 540
signs and symptoms of, 267–268
treatment of, 269
Aldosterone, 563
defined, 712
Alfa-fetoprotein, 296
Alkaline phosphatase, 121
defined, 712
Allergen(s), defined, 712
Allergic rhinitis, 455
defined, 712
Allergy(ies), stress and, 59
Allodynia
defined, 712
peripheral neuropathy and, 235
Allogenic transplant, defined, 712
Alpha fetoprotein
defined, 712
in liver cancer, 540
Alpha-1-antitrypsin, defined, 712
Alpha-blockers, defined, 712
ALS. *See* Amyotrophic lateral sclerosis (ALS)
Alveolus(i), defined, 712
Amantadine
defined, 712
for influenza, 449
Ambulatory, defined, 712
Amebiasis, 498
defined, 712
Amenorrhea, defined, 712
American Academy of Dermatology, 66
American College of Rheumatology, criteria for FMS, 93
American Rheumatology Association, in rheumatoid arthritis diagnosis, 146
Amine(s), 558
defined, 712
Amino acid, defined, 712
Amniocentesis, defined, 712
Amphiarthrosis(es), 87
defined, 712
Amputation(s), diabetes mellitus and, 570, 571f
Amyloidosis, 360
defined, 712
Anaerobic metabolism, 87
defined, 712
Anal lesions, candidiasis and, 549
Analgesic(s), 687–689
Anaphylaxis, 419
defined, 713
Anaplastic thyroid cancer, 582–583
Androgen(s), 563
defined, 713
Anecdotes, 708
defined, 702
Anencephaly, 293
Anergy, defined, 713
Angina
defined, 713
stable, heart attack and, 389–390
unstable, heart attack and, 390
Angina chest pain, features of, 393
Angina pectoris, 373
atherosclerosis and, 376
heart attack and, 389
Angioedema, 61–62, 419, 420, 420f
defined, 713
Angiogenesis
defined, 713
in metastasis, 672
Angiogram
in atherosclerosis diagnosis, 376
defined, 713
Angioneurotic edema, defined, 713
Angioplasty
for atherosclerosis, 376–378
defined, 713
percutaneous transluminal coronary, defined, 781
Angular stomatitis, 37
Animal parasites, 8, 9
cancer due to, 674
Ankle sprains, 152
Ankle-brachial index, 376
defined, 713
Annulus fibrosus, 204, 204f
Anorexia nervosa
causes of, 278
complications of, 280–281
defined, 277
diagnosis of, 281
prevalence of, 277
signs and symptoms of, 279
Anoxia, defined, 713
Anoxic brain injury, TBI due to, 308
Anterior knee pain syndrome, 142–144
defined, 713
Antianginal medication, 693–694
Anti-anxiety drugs, 684–685
for anxiety disorders, 248
Antibiotic(s)
for boils, 26
for cellulitis, 20
prophylactic, for Marfan syndrome, 162
Antibody(ies)
antinuclear, defined, 713
defined, 713
Anticholinergic, defined, 713
Anticholinergic drugs, 690
Anticoagulant(s), 695
defined, 713
for Guillain-Barré syndrome, 315
for thrombophlebitis/deep vein thrombosis, 366
Antidepressant(s), 685–687
for anxiety disorders, 258
for depression, 274
MAOIs, 686
SSRIs, 686
tricyclic, 686
for anxiety disorders, 248
defined, 792
for depression, 274
Antidiuretic hormone, defined, 713
Antigen(s)
defined, 713
prostate-specific, defined, 734
Antigenic shift, 450
defined, 713
Antihistamine(s)
for eczema, 59
for hives, 61
Anti-inflammatory drugs, 687–689
nonsteroidal (NSAIDs), 688
for Alzheimer disease, 225
defined, 731
for osteoarthritis, 141
peptic ulcers due to, 505–506
steroidal, 688–689
Antilipemic drugs, 693
Antimicrobial soap, defined, 10
Antinuclear antibody, defined, 713
Antiplatelet drugs, 695
Antisepsis, defined, 10
Antithyroid medications, for hyperthyroidism, 576
Antrectomy, defined, 713
Anular, defined, 713
Anxiety disorders, 254–258
causes of, 255–256
defined, 254, 255
demographics of, 254–255
GAD, 254
limbic system and, 255
massage for, 255, 258
OCD, 257
panic disorder, 254
prevalence of, 254
PTSD, 254
signs and symptoms of, 257
social phobias, 257
treatment of, 257–258
types of, 256–257
Aphasia
defined, 713
stroke and, 306
Aphtha(ae), 37, 493
defined, 713
Aplastic, defined, 713
Aplastic anemia, 343
Apnea, 328
defined, 713
Aponeurosis, defined, 713
Aponeurotomy, needle
defined, 730
for Dupuytren contracture, 176
Apophysitis, tibial tuberosity, defined, 739
Apoptosis, 673
defined, 299, 713
SCI and, 299
Appendicitis, 552
Appendix, vermiform, defined, 2
Arachidonic acid, defined, 713
Arachnoid, defined, 713
Arnold-Chiari malformation, 293
Arrhythmia(s)
atherosclerosis and, 376
defined, 713
Arterial embolism, 347
Arterial wall muscle, congenitally weak, aortic aneurysm due to, 369
Arteriogram, defined, 713
Arteriole(s), 339, 340f
defined, 713
Arteriosclerosis, defined, 713

Artery(ies), 339, 340f
Arthritis
 asymmetric, 64
 DIP, 64
 hemophilic, 351
  defined, 724
 psoriatric, 64
 rheumatoid. *See* Rheumatoid arthritis
 symmetric, 64
Arthritis mutilans, 64
Arthrochalasia Ehlers-Danlos syndrome, 159
 defined, 713
Arthropod(s), 8
Arthroscopy, for osteoarthritis, 141
Ascites
 cirrhosis and, 528, 528f
 defined, 714
 stomach cancer and, 509
Asian bodywork therapy (ABT), 20
Asperger syndrome, 263
Aspergillosis, defined, 714
Aspergillus flavus, liver cancer due to, 540
Asphyxia, defined, 714
Asymmetric arthritis, 64
Ataxic, defined, 714
Ataxic cerebral palsy, 287
Atelectasis, defined, 714
Atherectomy, catheter, defined, 716
Athetoid, defined, 714
Athetoid cerebral palsy, 287
Athlete's foot, 32, 32f
Atopic, defined, 714
Atopic dermatitis, eczema and, 57, 57f
ATP energy crisis, 97
Atrial fibrillation, 347
 defined, 714
 heart attack and, 391
 stroke due to, 305
Atrium(a), 339
 defined, 714
Atrophic, defined, 714
Atrophic gastritis, 509
 defined, 714
Atrophy
 defined, 714
 in hippocampus, depression due to, 271
 multiple-system, 243
 olivopontocerebellar, 243
  defined, 731
 Sudeck, 289–292, 291f. *See also* Complex regional pain syndrome (CRPS)
  defined, 738
Attachment trigger point, 97
Atypical face pain, 312
Auscultation, defined, 398, 714
Autism, high-functioning, 264
Autistic disorder, 263
Autoantibody(ies), defined, 714
Autodigestion, 546
 defined, 714
Autogenic transplant, defined, 714
Autoimmune, defined, 714
Autoimmune polyglandular syndrome, 573
 defined, 714
Autologous bone marrow transplant, in cancer management, 678
Autologous transplant, defined, 714
Autonomic hyperreflexia
 defined, 714
 SCI and, 300
Autonomic nervous system, drugs for, 689–691
Autosomal dominant inheritance, 162
Autosomal recessive inheritance, 162
Avascular, defined, 714
Avascular osteonecrosis, 111–113, 112f. *See also* Avascular necrosis
Avian flu, 450
Avulsion(s)
 defined, 714
 Osgood-Schlatter disease and, 182, 182f
Axon(s), 220, 221f
 defined, 714
Axonal injury, diffuse, defined, 764

B
B cells, 405–406
Babesiosis, 137
 defined, 714
Babinski sign, 227
 defined, 714
Bacillus(i), 7
Bacteremia, 453
 defined, 714
Bacteria
 cancer due to, 674
 gastroenteritis due to, 498
 pneumonia due to, 451
 sinusitis due to, 456
Bacterial activity, acne vulgaris due to, 53
Bacterial meningitis, 249
Baker cysts, 168–169, 169f
Balloon sinusotomy
 defined, 714
 for sinusitis, 457
Bandage(s), liquid, 11
Barotrauma, 331
 defined, 714
Barrel chest, defined, 714
Barrett esophagus, 495
 defined, 714
 GERD and, 501–502
Basal ganglia, defined, 714
Basal layer, defined, 714
Basilar impression, osteogenesis imperfecta and, 167
Basilar invagination, osteogenesis imperfecta and, 167
Basophil(s), 339f, 405
 defined, 714
Bath(s), Sitz, defined, 737
Becker muscular dystrophy, 164
Bedsore(s), 77–79, 78f
Bell, Charles, Sir, 283
Bell's law, defined, 714
Bence Jones proteins
 defined, 714
 myeloma and, 359
Benign, defined, 714
Benign neglect, defined, 49
Benign paroxysmal positional vertigo, 331
 defined, 715
Benign prostate hypertrophy, defined, 715
Benzene, defined, 715
Benzodiazepine(s), 684
 for anxiety disorders, 248
 defined, 715
Berry aneurysm, 369, 370f
Best practices, defined, 702
Best practices standard, 707
Beta amyloid, 223
 defined, 715
Beta blockers, 691
 for anxiety disorders, 248
 defined, 715
 for hyperthyroidism, 576
Beta cell, defined, 715
Bias, 707
 defined, 702
Bile, 531–534
 defined, 715
Biliary colic, defined, 715
Bilirubin, 485
 defined, 715
 in gallstones, 531
Bilirubin stones, 531
Binge eating
 causes of, 278–279
 complications of, 281
 defined, 277
 diagnosis of, 281
 prevalence of, 278
 signs and symptoms of, 279
Biological response modifiers, defined, 715
Biological therapy, in cancer management, 678, 679
 breast, 631
Biophosphate(s), defined, 715
Bipolar disorder, 273
 defined, 715
Birth control pills, high-estrogen
 stroke due to, 305
 thrombophlebitis/deep vein thrombosis due to, 365
Birth defect, congenital, hypothyroidism and, 577
Birth trauma, cerebral palsy due to, 287
Bismuth, defined, 715
Bisphosphonate(s), for osteoporosis, 118
Blackheads, acne vulgaris and, 54
Bladder, neurogenic, 593
 defined, 730
 UTIs and, 604
Bladder disorders, 597–606
 bladder cancer, 597–600
 interstitial cystitis, 601–602
 UTIs, 603–605
Blastomycosis, defined, 715
Bleeding. *See also* Hemorrhage
 cirrhosis and, 528
 diverticular disease and, 518
 excessive, SCI and, 299
Blepharospasm, 237
 defined, 715
Blister(s), herpes zoster and, 247
Blockage, diverticular disease and, 518
Blood cancers, 360
Blood cells, 340

Blood components, 338–339, 339f
Blood disorders, 341–368
  anemia, 341–344
  embolism, thrombus, 345–348, 345f, 346f
Blood disorders—*continued*
  hematomas, 348–349
  hemophilia, 350–352
  leukemia, 352–356
  malaria, 356–358
  myeloma, 359–361
  sickle cell disease, 361–363
  thrombophlebitis/deep vein thrombosis, 364–368, 366f
Blood poisoning, lymphangitis and, 410
Blood pressure, high
  atherosclerosis due to, 374, 375
  stroke due to, 304
  types of, 379–380, 379t
Blood vessel pressure, spondylosis and, 150
Blood vessels, 339–340, 340f
Blood–brain barrier, defined, 715
Body lice, 44
Body ringworm, 31, 31f
Bodywork modalities, 17–22, 21t
Bolus, defined, 715
Bone(s), 86
  cancer metastasis to, 680
  function of, 86
  structure of, 86
Bone density
  menopause and, 653
  optimal, recommendations for, 118–119
  osteoporosis and, 116–117, 117f
Bone disorders
  avascular necrosis, 111–113, 112f
  fractures, 113–115, 114f
  osteoporosis, 115–119, 117f
  Paget disease, 119–122, 120f
  postural deviations, 122–124, 123f
Bone loss, osteoporosis due to, 116–117, 117f
Bone marrow transplants
  autologous, in cancer management, 678
  for leukemia, 355
Bone scan, defined, 715
Borrelia burgdorferi
  Bell palsy and, 285
  cancer due to, 674
  defined, 715
  Lyme disease due to, 134, 135
Botox injections, for cerebral palsy, 288
Botulinum, defined, 715
Bouchard nodes, defined, 715
Bovine spongiform encephalopathy
  defined, 715
  permanent memory loss due to, 225
Bowen disease, defined, 715
Bowman capsule, 587, 588f
  defined, 715
BPH. *See* Benign prostatic hyperplasia (BPH)
Bradykinesia
  defined, 715
  Parkinson disease and, 240
Brain attack, 302–307. *See also* Stroke
Brain injury, anoxic, TBI due to, 308
Breast(s), fibrocystic changes to, 630
Bronchiectasis
  characteristics of, 468
  defined, 715
Bronchiole(s), 442, 442f
  of asthmatics, 462, 463f
Bronchopneumonia, 452
Bronchus(i), anatomy of, 441–442, 442f
Bruise(s), defined, 348
Bruising, cirrhosis and, 528
Bruxism, 155
  defined, 759
  TMJ disorders and, 156
Buerger disease, defined, 715
Bulge(s), nucleus pulposus due to, 206
Bulimia nervosa
  causes of, 278
  complications of, 281
  defined, 277
  diagnosis of, 281
  non—purge-type, 279
  prevalence of, 277
  purge-type, 279
  signs and symptoms of, 279
Bulla(ae), 469, 470f
  defined, 715
Bullous impetigo, 38
Burkitt lymphoma, defined, 715
Bursectomy, 174
  defined, 715
Buspirone HCl, 685
Butcher's warts, 48

C
C cells, in thyroid cancer, 581
Calcinosis, scleroderma and, 190
Calcitonin, 558
  defined, 715
Calcium
  absorption of, osteoporosis and, 116
  in bone density maintenance, 118–119
  loss of, osteoporosis and, 116
Calcium channel blockers, 692
  defined, 716
Calcium oxalate, defined, 716
Calcium oxalate stones, 590
Calcium phosphate, defined, 716
Calcium phosphate stones, 516
Calcium pyrophosphate dihydrate, defined, 716
Calcium pyrophosphate dihydrate deposition (CPDD), gout vs., 132
Calculus(i)
  renal, 589–592, 589f. *See also* Kidney stones
    defined, 735
  staghorn, 589, 589f
    defined, 737
Callus, 24
  defined, 716
  plantar warts vs., 48
Camphor, for osteoarthritis, 141
Campylobacter
  C. jejuni
    cancer due to, 674
    defined, 716
  C. pylori, defined, 716
Cancer. *See also specific types, e.g.,* Cervical cancer
  bladder, 597–600. *See also* Bladder cancer
  blood, 360
  breast, 627–634, 629f
  causes of, 673–674
  cervical, 612–615
  colorectal, 511–516, 512f, 513f
  diagnosis of, 675
  esophageal, 494–497. *See also* Esophageal cancer
  incidence of, 671–672
  liver, 539–542. *See also* Liver cancer
  lung, 475–479, 477f. *See also* Lung cancer
  massage for, 679–681, 681f
  metastasis of, steps in, 672–673
  ovarian, 634–637
  pancreatic, 543–545
  prevalence of, 671
  prevention of, 679
  principles of, 671–682
  prostate, 643–646
  signs and symptoms of, 674–675
  skin, 66–74, 672. *See also specific types and* Skin cancer
  staging of, 675–677, 676t, 677t
  statistics related to, 671–672
  stomach, 508–511
  survival after, 672
  testicular, 650–652
  thrombophlebitis/deep vein thrombosis due to, 365
  thyroid, 581–584. *See also* Thyroid cancer
  treatment of, 677–678
    cautions related, 680–681, 681f
    chemotherapy in, 680
    drugs in, 694
    radiation therapy in, 680
  uterine, 623–626. *See also* Uterine cancer
Candida albicans, defined, 548, 548f, 716
Canker sores, 37
Capillaroscopy, nailfold, 383
  defined, 730
Capillary(ies), 339–340, 340f
  in lymph system, 403–404, 404f
Capsaicin, for osteoarthritis, 141
Capsule(s), Bowman, defined, 715
Capsulitis, adhesive, 152
  defined, 712
Capsulorrhaphy, thermal
  defined, 739
  for dislocations, 129
Carbuncle, defined, 716
Carcinogen(s), cancer due to, 673
Carcinoma(s). *See also specific types and* Cancer(s)
  adenosquamous, 624
  defined, 671, 759
  ductal, 627
  embryonic, 650
    defined, 766
  hepatocellular, defined, 724
  Hürthle cell, 582
    defined, 725
  lobular, 627
  urothelial, 597–600. *See also* Bladder cancer
  verrucous, 48
Cardia
  defined, 508

of stomach, defined, 716
Cardiac tamponade, defined, 716
Cardiomyopathy, defined, 716
Cardiovascular disease
case example, 394
diabetes mellitus and, 570
SCI and, 300
Cardiovascular drugs, 691–694
ACE inhibitors, 692
antianginal, 693–694
antilipemic drugs, 693
beta blockers, 691
calcium channel blockers, 692
digitalis, 692
diuretics, 693
Cardiovascular health, menopause and, 653
Cardiovascular system
alcohol effects on, 268
lupus effects on, 436
Marfan syndrome effects on, 161
Carotid artery disease, 307
Carpal tunnel, 200, 200f
Case series, 708
defined, 702
Case study, 708
defined, 702
Cataplexy, 329
defined, 716
Catheter atherectomy, defined, 716
Cauda equina, 208
defined, 716
Causalgia, 289, 290
defined, 716
CDC. *See* Centers for Disease Control and Prevention (CDC)
Celiac sprue, 486–489. *See also* Celiac disease
defined, 716
Cell(s)
beta, defined, 715
blood, 340
C, in thyroid cancer, 581
chimeric, in scleroderma, 190
endothelial, inflammation and, 14
epithelial, in thyroid cancer, 581
follicular, in thyroid cancer, 581
Kupffer, 485
defined, 727
mast
defined, 728
inflammation and, 14
myeloid, defined, 730
parafollicular, in thyroid cancer, 581
Reed-Sternberg, 413
defined, 735
Schwann, defined, 736
T, 405–406
imbalance and dysfunction of, eczema due to, 56
Cell body, 220, 221f
Cellular activity, inflammation and, 14–15
Cellular immunity, defined, 716
Centers for Disease Control and Prevention (CDC), in chronic fatigue syndrome, 421
Central nervous system (CNS)
components of, in chronic fatigue syndrome, 422
function of, menopause and, 653
Central sleep apnea, 328
Central trigger point, 97
Centrally acting skeletal muscle relaxants, 697
Cerebral thrombosis, stroke due to, 303
Cerebrovascular accident (CVA), 302–307. *See also* Stroke
Cervical misalignment, thoracic outlet syndrome vs., 213
Cervical rib
defined, 716
in thoracic outlet syndrome, 212–213
Cervical spondylitic myelopathy, 150
defined, 716
Cervical vertebrae
chronic misalignment of, TMJ disorders and, 157
misaligned, whiplash and, 197
Chair(s), care of, 12
Chancre, defined, 716
Cheilitis, actinic, defined, 711
Chemical balance, circulatory system in, 338
Chemical headaches, 316, 319
Chemical mediators, inflammation and, 15
Chemonucleolysis
defined, 716
for disc disease, 208
Chemotherapy
in cancer management, 678, 680
breast, 631
defined, 716
for leukemia, 355
for lymphomas, 414
for ovarian cancer, 637
Chest, barrel, defined, 714
Chest pain
angina, features of, 393
features of, 393
heart attack, features of, 393
pulmonary embolism, features of, 393
types of, 393
Childbirth, thrombophlebitis/deep vein thrombosis due to, 365
Childhood disintegrative disorder, 263
defined, 716
Children
asthma in, 462
school-age, ADHD in, 259
Chimeric, defined, 716
Chimeric cells, in scleroderma, 190
Chlamydia, 662–663
Chlamydia
C. trachomatis, defined, 716
defined, 760
Cholangiopancreatography, endoscopic retrograde, for gallstones, 533
Cholangitis, defined, 530, 716
Cholecyst(s), defined, 530, 716
Cholecystitis, defined, 530
Choledocholithiasis, defined, 530, 716
Cholelithiasis, defined, 530, 716
Cholesterol
described, 375
in gallstones, 531–532
high levels of
atherosclerosis due to, 374
stroke due to, 304
Cholesterol stones, 532
Cholesterol-lowering drugs, cholesterol stones due to, 532
Cholinergic(s), 690
Cholinergic hives, 61
Cholinesterase inhibitors
for Alzheimer disease, 225
defined, 716
Chondroitin sulfate, 88
defined, 716
for osteoarthritis, 141
Chondromalacia patellae, defined, 717
Chorea, language of, 243
Choriocarcinoma, 650
defined, 717
Christmas disease, 350
defined, 717
Chronic, defined, 6t, 717
Chronic compartment syndrome, 104
Chronic degenerative disorders, 223–236. *See also* Degenerative disorders, chronic
Chronic exertional compartment syndrome, defined, 717
Chronic fatigue immune dysfunction syndrome, 421
Chronic granulocytic leukemia, defined, 717
Chronic illness, as factor in depression, 272
Chronic myelogenous leukemia, 353
Chronic myeloid leukemia, defined, 717
Chronic obstructive pulmonary disease (COPD)
asthma, 462–465, 463f
bronchitis, chronic, 465–467
emphysema, 469–472, 470f
Chronic renal failure
causes of, 595–596
defined, 594
Chronic venous insufficiency
defined, 717
thrombophlebitis/deep vein thrombosis and, 366
Chyme, 483
defined, 717
Cilium(a), defined, 717
Circadian rhythm, 327
defined, 717
Circadian rhythm disruption, 329
Circulation, reduced, thrombophlebitis/deep vein thrombosis due to, 364
Circulatory system conditions, 337–401
blood components, 338–339, 339f
blood vessels, 339–340, 340f
general function of, 338–340, 339f, 340f
heart, 339, 340f
heart attack, 388–395, 390f
heart conditions, 388–399
in homeostasis maintenance, 338
Classic Ehlers-Danlos syndrome, 159
Claudication, intermittent, 376
defined, 726
Clonic spasm, defined, 717
Clotting
circulatory system in, 338
management of, drugs in, 695
Cluster headaches, 319
Coagulability, defined, 717

Coal tar, for psoriasis, 64
Cobalamine, defined, 717
Coccidioidomycosis, defined, 717
Coccus(i), 7, 7f, 8f
Cochicine, for gout, 130
Cognitive function, loss of, MS and, 232
Cognitive-behavioral therapy
  defined, 717
  for depression, 274
Colchicine, defined, 717
Cold
  common, 445–447. *See also* Common cold
  intolerance to, anemia and, 344
Cold rocks, care of, 12
Colic
  biliary, defined, 715
  defined, 717
  renal, defined, 590, 735
Colitis
  fulminant, defined, 524, 723
  left-sided, defined, 524
  pseudomembranous, 498
    defined, 734
  ulcerative, 523–525. *See also* Ulcerative colitis
Collagen, defined, 717
Collagenase, defined, 717
Colon
  adenocarcinoma of, 512, 513f
  motility of, 516
Colon polyps, 511, 512f
Colonization, in metastasis, 673
Colonoscopy, defined, 717
Colostomy, defined, 717
Colposcopy
  in cervical cancer diagnosis, 614
  defined, 717
Coma, myxedema, 578
  defined, 730
Comedo, defined, 717
Comedone(s)
  closed, acne vulgaris and, 54
  open, acne vulgaris and, 54
Comminuted, defined, 717
Comminuted fractures, 113, 114f
Communication, verbal, nervous system problems with, 222
Community-acquired pneumonia, 452
Comorbidity, defined, 422, 761
Complement, defined, 717
Complex partial seizures, 324
Complication, defined, 6t
Compound fractures, 113
Compression, spinal cord effects of, 297
Compression fractures, 113
Concussion
  spinal cord effects of, 297
  TBI due to, 308
Condyle, defined, 762
Condylomata acuminata, 665
  defined, 762
Confound, defined, 702
Congenital, defined, 717
Congenital birth defect, hypothyroidism and, 577
Congenital heart problems, 392
Congenital muscular dystrophy, 164
Congenital nevus, defined, 717
Congenital torticollis, 238
Congestion, liver, acne vulgaris due to, 53
Connective tissue(s)
  problems associated with, 89–90
  types of, 87–90, 88f
Connective tissue bands, in thoracic outlet syndrome, 213
Connective tissue disorders, 168–199
Connective tissue fibers, 89
Consolidation, defined, 717
Constraint-induced movement therapy, for stroke, 307
Constriction, defined, 718
Contact dermatitis
  causes of, 57
  signs and symptoms of, 58, 59f
Contact inhibition, 80
  defined, 718
Contractility, impaired, strains and, 109
Contracture(s)
  Dupuytren, 174–176, 175f. *See also* Dupuytren contracture
  SCI and, 300
Contraindicated, defined, 6t
Contralateral, defined, 718
Control group, 707
  defined, 702
Contusion(s)
  spinal cord effects of, 297
  TBI due to, 308
COPD. *See* Chronic obstructive pulmonary disease (COPD)
Cor pulmonale, 396, 470
  defined, 718
Coronary artery disease, 372, 373f
Corpus callosum, defined, 718
Corpus luteum, 638
  defined, 718
Corpus luteum cysts, 638
Corticosteroid(s), for eczema, 59
Corticosteroid injection, defined, 718
Cortisol, 558, 563
  in Cushing syndrome, 564–565
  defined, 718
  for eczema, 59
  stress and, 59
Cortisone
  defined, 718
  in scar tissue management, 81
Cot(s), finger, 11
Cough variant asthma, 463
Coup de sabre, 189
  defined, 718
Coup-contrecoup, defined, 718
COX-2 inhibitors, defined, 718
Coxsackievirus, defined, 718
CPDD. *See* Calcium pyrophosphate dihydrate deposition (CPDD)
C-reactive protein
  atherosclerosis due to, 374–375
  defined, 718
  stroke due to, 305
Creatine kinase
  defined, 718
  in muscular dystrophy diagnosis, 165
Crepitus
  defined, 718
  patellofemoral syndrome and, 143
CREST syndrome, 189, 190, 190f
  defined, 718
Creutzfeldt-Jakob disease, permanent memory loss due to, 225
Crisis, defined, 718
Crossover study, 708
  defined, 702
CRPS. *See* Complex regional pain syndrome (CRPS)
Cruciate ligament ruptures, 152
Cruciate ligament sprains, 152
  defined, 718
Crust, defined, 718
Cryomyolysis, 623
  defined, 718
Cryptococcus neoformans, defined, 718
Cryptogenic stroke, 303
Cryptorchidism, 650
  defined, 718
Cryptosporidium, 498
Cryptosporidium, defined, 718
Crystal(s)
  care of, 12
  gout due to, 131, 131f
Cushing, Harvey, 564
CVA (cerebrovascular accident), 302–307. *See also* Stroke
Cyanosis, defined, 718
Cyclo-oxygenase-2, defined, 718
Cyst(s)
  acne vulgaris and, 53
  Baker, 168–169, 169f
  corpus luteum, 638
  dermoid, 638
    defined, 719
  follicular, 638, 639f
  ganglion, 177–178, 177f
  gross, of breast, 630
  mucous, 177
    defined, 778
  ovarian, 637–640, 639f. *See also* Ovarian cysts
  pilonidal, 26
    defined, 733
  popliteal, defined, 733
Cystadenoma(s), 638
  defined, 718
Cystic warts, 48
Cystine, 590
  defined, 718
Cystine stones, 590
Cystitis, interstitial, 601–602
Cystoscope(s), 593
  defined, 718
Cytokine, defined, 718
Cytomegalovirus
  defined, 718
  HIV/AIDS and, 430
Cytotoxic drugs
  in cancer management, 678
  defined, 718

D

Dactylitis, defined, 718
DASH (Dietary Approaches to Stop Hypertension) diet, for NHLBI, 381
D&C. *See* Dilation and curettage (D&C)
de Quervain tenosynovitis, 194
  defined, 718
Deadly quartet, 579–581
Débridement, defined, 718
Decongestant(s)
  nasal, dependency issues related to, 267
  for sinusitis, 457
Deep palmar plantar warts, 48, 49f
Deep tissue massage/myofascial release, 18
Deep vein thrombosis, 364–368, 366f. *See also* Thrombophlebitis/deep vein thrombosis
  cancer-related, 680
  SCI and, 300
Deer tick, Lyme disease spread by, 134, 134f, 135
Degeneration
  defined, 718
  mental, Parkinson disease and, 241
  striatonigral, defined, 738
Degenerative disc disease, 206
Degenerative disorders, chronic, 223–236
  ALS, 226–229
  Alzheimer disease, 223–226, 224f
  MS, 230–234, 234t
  peripheral neuropathy, 235–236
Degenerative joint disease, defined, 718
Dementia(s)
  defined, 719
  Lewy body, permanent memory loss due to, 225
  vascular, permanent memory loss due to, 225
Demographic, defined, 6t
Dendrite(s), 220, 221f
  defined, 719
Dependency(ies). *See also specific types, e.g.,* Chemical dependency
  chemical, 265–270
Dermabrasion, defined, 719
Dermatitis herpetiformis, 487
  defined, 719
Dermatome, defined, 719
Dermatophyte(s), 30
  defined, 719
Dermatophytosis, 30
  defined, 719
Dermatosparaxis, defined, 719
Dermatosparaxis Ehlers-Danlos syndrome, 159
Dermographia, defined, 719
Dermoid cysts, 638
  defined, 719
DES. *See* Diethylstilbestrol (DES)
Descriptive study, 708
  defined, 702
Desiccated extract, 698
Desmodus rotundus salivary plasminogen activator (DSPA), for stroke, 306
Detoxification, in chemical dependency treatment, 269
Deviation(s), postural, 122–124, 123f. *See also* Postural deviations
DEXA (dual-energy x-ray absorptiometry), defined, 719
Dextroamphetamine, defined, 719
DHT. *See* Dihydrotestosterone (DHT)
Diabetes insipidus, 569
  defined, 719
Diabetic emergencies, 569–570
Diabetic retinopathy, 570
Diagnosis, defined, 6t
Diagnostic and Statistical Manual of Mental Disorders (DSM-IV-TR)
  in anorexia and bulimia diagnosis, 281
  in depression, 272–273
Dialysis, peritoneal, peritonitis due to, 552
Diaphoresis, defined, 719
Diaphragm(s), UTIs due to, 604
Diaphysis, 86
  defined, 719
Diarthrosis(es), 87
  defined, 719
Diastole, defined, 379, 719
Diet
  estrogen production and, 609
  GERD and, 502
  high-fat, uterine cancer due to, 625
  stomach cancer due to, 509
Dietary Approaches to Stop Hypertension (DASH) diet, for NHLBI, 381
Diethylstilbesterol (DES), defined, 719
Diethylstilbestrol (DES), cervical cancer and, 613
Diffuse axonal injury
  defined, 719
  TBI due to, 308
Diffuse idiopathic skeletal hyperostosis (DISH), 148–149
  defined, 719
Diffuse large cell lymphoma, defined, 719
Diffuse mixed cell lymphoma, defined, 719
Diffuse scleroderma, 189
  defined, 719
Diffuse toxic thyroid, 573
Diffusion, defined, 338, 719
Digestive system, 483–555
  alcohol effects on, 268
  cystic fibrosis effects on, 473
  disorders of, 486–555. *See also* Digestive disorders
  MS effects on, 233
  overview of, 483–484, 484f
  problems related to, overview of, 485
Digestive tract. *See also* Digestive disorders; Digestive system
  accessory organs, 484–485, 484f
  structure and function of, 483–484, 484f
Digitalis, 692
Dihydrotestosterone (DHT)
  BPH due to, 641
  defined, 719
Dilation, defined, 719
Dilation and curettage (D&C), defined, 719
Dimethyl sulfoxide
  defined, 719
  for interstitial cystitis, 602
Dioxin, defined, 719
DIP arthritis. *See* Distal interphalangeal predominant (DIP) arthritis
Diphtheria, defined, 719
Diplegia
  defined, 719
  spastic, 298
Diplococcus(i), 7, 7f
Disability(ies), learning, nonverbal, 264
Disc(s)
  damaged, whiplash and, 197
  herniated, defined, 725
  problems associated with, 205–206
Discectomy
  defined, 719
  transcutaneous, for disc disease, 208–209
Discoid lupus erythematosus (DLE), 433–434, 433f, 434f
  defined, 719
Disease-modifying antirheumatic drugs (DMARDs), defined, 720
DISH. *See* Diffuse idiopathic skeletal hyperostosis (DISH)
Disinfection, defined, 10
Dissecting aneurysm, 369–370, 369f
Distal interphalangeal predominant (DIP) arthritis, 64
Diuretic(s), 693
  defined, 719
Diverticulosis, case example, 517
Diverticulum(a)
  defined, 516, 719
  described, 517, 518f
DLE. *See* Discoid lupus erythematosus (DLE)
DMARDs (disease-modifying antirheumatic drugs), defined, 720
Dopamine, defined, 720
Double crush syndrome, defined, 720
Double pneumonia, 452
Double-blinded study, 707
  defined, 702
Drainage, lymphatic. *See* Lymphatic drainage
Drug(s). *See* Medication(s)
DSM-IV-TR. *See Diagnostic and Statistical Manual of Mental Disorders (DSM-IV-TR)*
DSPA (*Desmodus rotundus* salivary plasminogen activator), for stroke, 306
Dual-energy x-ray absorptiometry (DEXA), defined, 720
Duchenne muscular dystrophy, 164
Ductal carcinoma, 627
Ductal ectasia, 630
  defined, 765
Dura mater, defined, 720
Dural ectasia, 161
  defined, 720
Dysarthria
  defined, 720
  stroke and, 306
Dyshidrosis
  defined, 720
  eczema and, 58, 58f
Dysmetabolic syndrome, 579–581
Dysmobility, defined, 720

Dysmotility, esophageal, scleroderma and, 190
Dyspepsia, defined, 720
Dysphagia, 370, 420, 420f
  defined, 720
Dysphonia, vocal, 237
Dysplasia, 613
Dysplasia (dysplastic)
  defined, 720
  hip, defined, 725
Dysplastic nevus, defined, 720
Dyspnea
  anemia and, 344
  defined, 720
Dyssomnia(s), 327
Dysthymia, 272
  defined, 720
  gender predilection for, 237
  generalized, 237
  massage for, 237–239
  multifocal, 237
  oromandibular, 237
  prevalence of, 237
  segmental, 237
  signs and symptoms of, 238
  treatment of, 238
Dystonic cerebral palsy, 287
Dystrophic, defined, 720
Dystrophin, 163–164
  defined, 720
Dystrophy(ies)
  facioscapulohumeral, 164
    defined, 722
  limb girdle, 164
    defined, 728
  muscular, 163–165. *See also* Muscular dystrophy

E

Ear pain, TMJ disorders and, 156
EAST (elevated arm stress test), defined, 720
EAST test, in thoracic outlet syndrome diagnosis, 214
EBV (Epstein-Barr virus)
  cancer due to, 674
  defined, 721
Ecchymosis, defined, 348, 720
Echocardiogram, defined, 720
Eclampsia, 656
  defined, 720
ECT. *See* Electroconvulsive therapy (ECT)
Ectasia
  ductal, 630
    defined, 720
  dural, 161
    defined, 720
Ecthyma, 38–39
  defined, 720
Ectopic ACTH syndrome, 565
Ectopic pregnancy, 657
Eczema herpeticum, 37
EEG. *See* Electroencephalogram (EEG)
Ehrlichiosis, 137
  defined, 720
Elastin, defined, 720
Elbow
  golfer's, defined, 723
  student's, 172
  tennis, defined, 739
Elderly, seizure disorders in, 323
Elective abortion
  methods of, 610–611
  defined, 610, 611
Electrocauterization
  defined, 720
  for endometriosis, 620
Electroconvulsive therapy (ECT), for depression, 275
Electroencephalogram (EEG), defined, 720
Electrolyte(s), defined, 720
Electromyography (EMG), defined, 720
Electronystagmogram
  defined, 720
  in vestibular balance disorders diagnosis, 332
Elevated arm stress test (EAST), defined, 720
ELISA (enzyme-linked immunosorbent assay)
  defined, 720
  in HIV/AIDS diagnosis, 431
Embolization
  defined, 720
  uterine artery, 623
Embryonic carcinoma, 650
  defined, 721
Emery-Dreifuss muscular dystrophy, 164
  defined, 721
EMG. *See* Electromyography (EMG)
Emollient, defined, 721
Empirical, defined, 702, 704
Empyema, defined, 721
Encephalocele, 293
Encephalomyelitis, myalgic, 421
  defined, 729
Encephalopathy(ies)
  bovine spongiform
    defined, 715
    permanent memory loss due to, 225
  cirrhosis and, 529
Endarterectomy
  for atherosclerosis, 376–378
  defined, 721
Endemic, defined, 6t, 721
Endo-, defined, 721
Endocarditis, defined, 721
Endocrine glands, 559
Endocrine system, 557–586
  described, 557
  disorders of, 560–584. *See also* Endocrine disorders
  glands of, 558
Endogenous, defined, 565, 766
Endolymph, 321, 321f
  defined, 721
Endolymphatic hydrops, idiopathic, 322
  defined, 726
Endometrial cancer, 623–626. *See also* Uterine cancer
  screening for, 676
Endometrioma(s), 638
  defined, 721
Endometritis, defined, 721
Endometrium, 608, 608f
  defined, 721
Endomysium, 87, 87f
  defined, 721
Endoscopic retrograde cholangiopancreatography (ERCP)
  defined, 721
  for gallstones, 533
Endoscopy, defined, 721
Endosteum, 86
  defined, 721
Endothelial cells, inflammation and, 14
Endothelial damage, atherosclerosis due to, 372
Endothelium, 339
Endovascular, defined, 721
Enteritis
  granulomatosis, 491
    defined, 724
  regional, 491
    defined, 735
Enteropathy(ies), gluten-sensitive, 486–489
  defined, 723
Enterovirus, 498
  defined, 721
Environment, massage, care of, 13
Environmental factors
  in chemical dependency, 266
  in depression, 271
Environmental intolerance, idiopathic, defined, 726
Environmental irritants, sinusitis due to, 456
Enzyme(s), defined, 721
Enzyme-linked immunosorbent assay (ELISA)
  defined, 720
  in HIV/AIDS diagnosis, 431
Eosinophil(s), 339f, 405
  defined, 721
Ephelis (ephelides), defined, 721
Epi-, defined, 721
Epicondylitis, 152
  defined, 721
Epidemic, defined, 6t
Epidermis, defined, 721
Epidermophyton, defined, 721
Epididymis, 608–610, 609f
  defined, 721
Epigastric hernia, 179
Epimysium, 87, 87f
  defined, 721
Epinephrine, 558
  defined, 721
Epistaxis, defined, 351, 721
Epitenon, 194
  defined, 721
Epithelial cells, in thyroid cancer, 581
Epithelial tumors, of ovaries, 635
Epithelium(a), 339
  defined, 721
  healing of, 24
Epsom salt baths, for psoriasis, 64
Epstein-Barr virus (EBV)
  cancer due to, 674
  defined, 721
Equipment, care of, 11–13
ERCP. *See* Endoscopic retrograde cholangiopancreatography (ERCP)
Ergot, defined, 721
Ernest syndrome, 157
  defined, 721

ERT. *See* Estrogen replacement therapy (ERT)
Erysipelas, defined, 721
Erythema, defined, 721
Erythema migrans, 135
  defined, 721
Erythrocyte(s), 338
  defined, 721
Erythrodermic psoriasis, 64
  defined, 722
Erythropoietin, 338, 343, 559
  defined, 722
Escherichia coli, defined, 720
Esophageal dysmotility, scleroderma and, 190
Esophageal lining, chronic irritation of, reactions to, 501
Esophagitis, candidiasis and, 549
Esophagus, Barrett, 495
  defined, 714
  GERD and, 501–502
Essential, defined, 722
Essential tremor, 243
Estradiol, defined, 722
Estriol, defined, 722
Estrogen, 559
  cholesterol stones due to, 532
  defined, 722
  described, 609
  dietary effects of, 609
  exposure to, 609
Estrogen replacement therapy (ERT)
  defined, 722
  uterine cancer due to, 625
Estrone, defined, 722
Evidence-based medicine, 707
  defined, 702
Excitotoxicity, SCI and, 299
Excretion, skin in, 24
Exenteration
  for cervical cancer, 614
  defined, 722
Exercise
  asthma induced by, 463
  in bone density maintenance, 119
  muscle cramping due to, 106
  for osteoarthritis, 141
Exhaustion, heat, 425
Exogenous, defined, 565, 722
Exophthalmos
  defined, 722
  hyperthyroidism and, 574, 575f
Experimental studies, 708
Experimental/explanatory study, defined, 702
Explanatory studies, 708
Extensively drug-resistant tuberculosis, 461
External scar tissue, defined, 722
Extracorporeal shockwave lithotripsy
  defined, 722
  for kidney stones, 592
Extramedullary plastocytoma, 359
  defined, 722
Extrusion(s), nucleus pulposus due to, 206
Exudate, defined, 722
Eye disorders, Marfan syndrome effects on, 161–162

F

Fabrics, care of, 11–12
Face pain, atypical, 312
Facet joint capsules, damaged, whiplash and, 197
Facial flushing, acne rosacea and, 51
Facial nerve, 283, 283f
Facioscapulohumeral dystrophy, 164
  defined, 722
Fall(s), SCI due to, 298
Familial adenomatous polyposis
  colorectal cancer due to, 513
  defined, 722
Family(ies), alcoholic, 269
Family history
  colorectal cancer and, 513
  ovarian cancer and, 635
  thyroid cancer and, 582
Fascia, superficial, defined, 738
Fascicle (fasciculi), 87
  defined, 722
Fasciculation(s), defined, 227, 722
Fasciitis
  palmar, 174–176, 175f. *See also* Dupuytren contracture
    defined, 732
  plantar, 186–188, 187f. *See also* Plantar fasciitis
Fasting, cholesterol stones due to, 532
Fat necrosis, 630
  defined, 722
Fatigue
  anemia and, 344
  fibromyalgia and, 91–92
  MS and, 233
  Parkinson disease and, 240
  pregnancy and, 656
Fatty acids, deficiency of, eczema due to, 56
FDA. *See* Food and Drug Administration (FDA)
Fecaliths, 552
  defined, 722
Femoral hernia, 180
Festinating gait, 241
  defined, 722
Fetal alcohol syndrome, defined, 722
Fetoprotein, alpha
  defined, 712
  in liver cancer, 540
Fiber(s), connective tissue, 89
Fibrillation(s)
  atrial, 347
    defined, 714
    heart attack and, 391
    stroke due to, 305
  defined, 722
  ventricular, 389
    heart attack and, 391
Fibrillin, defined, 722
Fibrin, defined, 722
Fibrinogen, defined, 722
Fibroadenoma(s)
  of breast, 630
  defined, 722
Fibroblast(s)
  defined, 722
  inflammation and, 15
Fibromatosis, plantar, 175
  defined, 733
Fibromyalgia syndrome, myofascial pain syndrome vs., 94
Fibrosis(es)
  annulus, defined, 713
  of breast, 630
  cystic, 472–475, 474f. *See also* Cystic fibrosis
Fibrotic build-up, carpal tunnel syndrome due to, 201
Filtration, defined, 588, 722
Fimbria(ae), defined, 722
Finger cot, 11
First-degree burns, 75, 75f
Fish oil, omega-3, for depression, 275
Fistula(ae), 490
  defined, 768
  diverticular disease and, 518
  perilymph, defined, 732
Fixation, defined, 722
Flaccid paralysis, defined, 298, 722
Flat warts, 49
Flea(s), 8, 9f
Flu, 447
  Avian, 450
  history of, 448
  yuppie, defined, 741
Fluke(s), animal, cancer due to, 674
Flushing, facial, acne rosacea and, 51
Foam cells, atherosclerosis due to, 373
Focal dystonia, 237
  defined, 768
Folate, defined, 722
Folic acid, defined, 722
Folic acid deficiency anemia, 342
Follicular cells, in thyroid cancer, 581
Follicular cleaved cell lymphoma, defined, 722
Follicular cysts, 638, 639f
Follicular large cell lymphoma, defined, 722
Follicular mixed cell lymphoma, defined, 723
Follicular thyroid cancer, 582
Folliculitis, 26, 27f
  defined, 769
Food and Drug Administration (FDA), in influenza, 449
Food sensitivities, Crohn disease and, 491
Foot (feet)
  architecture of, 183
  athlete's, 32, 32f
Fossa(ae), popliteal, defined, 733
Fragile X syndrome, 262
  defined, 723
Freckle(s), 71
Free radical activity, SCI and, 299
Frozen shoulder, 152
  defined, 723
Fulminant, defined, 723
Fulminant colitis, defined, 524, 723
Fundibulum, 557
Fundoplication
  defined, 723
  for GERD, 503
Fungus(i), 8
  pneumonia due to, 452
  sinusitis due to, 456

Furuncle(s), 26–28, 27f. *See also* Boil(s)
  defined, 723
Fusiform aneurysm, 369, 369f

G
GABA. *See* Gamma-aminobutyric acid (GABA)
GAD. *See* General anxiety disorder (GAD)
Gait
  festinating, 241
    defined, 722
  shuffling, Parkinson disease and, 240–241
Gallbladder
  defined, 530
  overview of, 484f, 485
  removal of, fat retention after, 533
Gamma globulin, defined, 723
Gammaaminobutyric acid (GABA), defined, 723
Ganglion(a)
  basal, defined, 714
  geniculate, defined, 723
Ganglion cysts, 177–178, 177f
Gangrene, diabetes mellitus and, 570, 571f
Gardner syndrome
  colorectal cancer due to, 513
  defined, 723
Garrod's nodes, 175
Gastritis
  atrophic, 509
    defined, 714
  defined, 723
Gastrointestinal tract, upper, disorders of, 486–511. *See also specific disorders and* Digestive disorders, of upper gastrointestinal tract
Gastrostomy, for ALS, 229
Gender
  as factor in ADHD, 259
  as factor in Alzheimer disease, 223
  as factor in aortic aneurysm, 368
  as factor in atherosclerosis, 374
  as factor in avascular necrosis, 111
  as factor in bladder cancer, 597
  as factor in cholesterol stones, 532
  as factor in CRPS, 290
  as factor in depression, 277–278
  as factor in dystonia, 237
  as factor in gallstones, 531
  as factor in hemophilia, 350
  as factor in stroke, 305
  as factor in trigeminal neuralgia, 310
  as factor in UTIs, 603
Gene(s), described, 162
General anxiety disorder (GAD), 254
Generalized dystonia, 237
Generalized seizures, 324–325
Genetic(s), 162
  in atherosclerosis, 373
  in celiac disease, 486–487
  in chemical dependency, 266
  in Crohn disease, 490
  in depression, 271
  thyroid cancer due to, 582
Genetic musculoskeletal disorders, 158–167. *See also* Musculoskeletal disorders, genetic
Geniculate ganglion, defined, 723
Genital warts, 49, 665
GERD. *See* Gastroesophageal reflux disease (GERD)
Germ cell tumors, 650
Gestational diabetes, pregnancy and, 656
Geste antagoniste, 238
  defined, 723
GFR. *See* Glomerular filtration rate (GFR)
Giardia, 498
  defined, 723
  protozoa and, 8, 9f
Gigantism, defined, 723
Gliadin, 487
  defined, 723
Globus pallidus, defined, 723
Glomerular filtration rate (GFR), 588
  defined, 723
Glomerulation(s), 601
  defined, 723
Glomerulonephritis, 595
  defined, 723
  mesangial, defined, 729
Glomerulus(i), 587, 588f
  defined, 723
Glossopharyngeal neuralgia, 312
Glucagon, 558
  defined, 723
Glucocorticoid(s), 558, 563
  defined, 723
Glucosamine
  in ganglion cysts, 177
  for osteoarthritis, 141
Glucosamine sulfate, defined, 723
Glutamate
  ALS and, 227
  defined, 723
Gluten. *See also* Celiac disease
  defined, 723
  described, 486–488
Gluten sensitivity, 487
Gluten-sensitive enteropathy, 486–489
  defined, 723
Glycogen, defined, 723
Goiter
  defined, 573, 723
  multinodular, 573
  toxic nodular, 573
Golfer's elbow, defined, 723
Golgi tendon organ, defined, 723
Gonorrhea, 663
Grand mal seizure, defined, 723
Granulation tissue, defined, 723
Granulocyte(s)
  defined, 723
  inflammation and, 14
Granuloma, defined, 723
Granulomatosis enteritis, 491
  defined, 724
Graves disease, 573
  defined, 724
  language of, 573
Graves ophthalmopathy
  defined, 724
  hyperthyroidism and, 574
Greater omentum, defined, 724
Greek word parts, 3t–5t
Greenstick fractures, 113, 114f
Grinding teeth, 155
  TMJ disorders and, 156
Grippe, 447
Gross cysts, of breast, 630
Growth hormone, 558
  defined, 724
Guaifenesin, defined, 724
Gunshot wounds, SCI due to, 297–298
Guttate psoriasis, 64
  defined, 724

H
HAART. *See* Highly active antiretroviral therapy (HAART)
  defined, 724
Haemophilus influenzae
  defined, 724
  sinusitis due to, 456
Haemophilus influenzae type B (HiB) vaccine, for meningitis, 251
Hallucination(s), hypnagogic, 329
  defined, 726
Hallux valgus, 169–171, 171f. *See also* Bunion(s)
  defined, 724
Hand care, 11
Hand rub, alcohol-based, defined, 10
Hand washing, 10–11
Handwriting, changes in, Parkinson disease and, 241
Hashimoto thyroiditis
  defined, 724
  hypothyroidism and, 577
Haustrum(a), 484
  defined, 724
HDL. *See* High-density lipoprotein (HDL)
Head injuries, 331
Head ringworm, 32, 32f
Healing, stages of, 15
Hearing loss, Ménière disease and, 322
Heart, 339, 340f
  congenital problems of, 392
  enlarged, hypertension and, 380
  hypertrophy of, 392
  infectious diseases of, 392
Heart conditions, 388–399
  heart attack, 388–395, 390f
  heart failure, 395–399, 397f, 398f
Heart disease, in U.S., statistics for, 374
Heart murmurs, 392
Heartbeat, rapid, anemia and, 344
Heartburn, as predecessor to GERD, 500
Heat cramps, 425
Heat exhaustion, 425
Heat stroke, 425
Heberden nodes, defined, 724
Helicobacter pylori
  cancer due to, 674
  defined, 724
  peptic ulcers due to, 505, 506f, 507
  stomach cancer due to, 509
HELLP syndrome, 657
  defined, 724
Helminth(s), 8

Hemagglutinin, 450
 defined, 724
Hematochromatosis, defined, 724
Hematuria, 588
 in bladder cancer, 598
 defined, 351, 724
Heme, 485
 defined, 724
Hemidystonia, 237
Hemifacial spasm, 312
Hemiparesis, stroke and, 306
Hemiplegia
 defined, 724
 spastic, 298
 stroke and, 306
Hemo-, defined, 724
Hemochromatosis
 defined, 724
 liver cancer due to, 540
Hemodialysis
 defined, 724
 for diabetes mellitus, 572
Hemoglobin, 338
 defined, 724
Hemoglobin A1c test, defined, 724
Hemolysis, defined, 724
Hemolytic, defined, 724
Hemolytic anemia, 342
 malaria and, 357
Hemolytic uremic syndrome, 595
 defined, 724
Hemophilic arthritis, 351
 defined, 724
Hemoptysis, 347
 defined, 724
Hemorrhage. *See also* Bleeding
 defined, 724
 intracerebral, stroke due to, 304
 subarachnoid, stroke due to, 304
 TBI due to, 309
Hemorrhagic anemias, 342
Hemorrhagic stroke, 303, 304f
Hemorrhoid, defined, 724
Hepatocellular carcinoma, defined, 724
Hepatorenal syndrome, 529
 defined, 724
Hereditary nonpolyposis colorectal cancer syndrome
 colorectal cancer due to, 513
 defined, 724
Herniated disc, defined, 725
Herpes gladiatorum, 37
Herpes whitlow, 36–37, 36f
Herpesvirus 6, human, defined, 725
Herpetic sycosis, 37
Heterophile(s), 416
 defined, 725
Heterotopic ossification, 100
 defined, 725
 SCI and, 300
HHV-8 (human herpesvirus 8), cancer due to, 674
Hiatal hernia, 180
 GERD and, 502
Hidradenitis suppurativa, 26
 defined, 725
High-density lipoprotein (HDL)
 defined, 725
 described, 375
High-estrogen birth control pills, thrombophlebitis/deep vein thrombosis due to, 365
High-functioning autism, 264
Highly active anti-retroviral therapy (HAART)
 defined, 724
 for HIV/AIDS, 431
Hip dysplasia, defined, 725
Hippocampus, atrophy in, depression due to, 271
Hirsutism, 638
 defined, 725
Histamine, defined, 725
Histoplasmosis, defined, 725
HIV (human immunodeficiency virus)
 cancer due to, 674
 tuberculosis due to, 459–460
Hobnailed liver, defined, 725
Hodgkin disease, language of, 412
Hodgkin lymphoma
 demographics of, 412
 described, 413, 414f
Homans sign, defined, 725
Homeostasis
 circulatory system, 338
 defined, 725
 skin in, 24
Homocysteine, atherosclerosis due to, 375
Hormonal imbalance
 acne vulgaris due to, 53
 depression due to, 271
 PMS due to, 659
Hormone(s)
 antidiuretic, defined, 713
 classes of, 558
 growth, 558
  defined, 724
 parathyroid, 558–559
  defined, 732
 stimulation and suppression of, cycle of, 557–558
 thyroid, 558
 types of, 558–559
Hormone disruption, cirrhosis and, 528
Hormone replacement therapy (HRT)
 described, 654
 in menopause, 654
 for osteoporosis, 118
 ovarian cancer due to, 635
 stroke due to, 305
 thrombophlebitis/deep vein thrombosis due to, 365
Hormone therapy, in cancer management, 678
 breast, 631
Hospital-acquired pneumonia, 452
Hot compress, for boils, 26–27
Hot rocks, care of, 12
Housemaid's knee, 172
HPA axis. *See* Hypothalamic-pituitary-adrenal (HPA) axis
HPV. *See* Human papillomavirus (HPV)
HRT. *See* Hormone replacement therapy (HRT)
HSV. *See* Herpes simplex virus (HSV)
HTLV-1 (human T-lymphotrophic virus), cancer due to, 673
Human herpesvirus 6 (HHV-6), defined, 725
Human herpesvirus 8 (HHV-8), cancer due to, 674
Human immunodeficiency virus (HIV). *See also* HIV/AIDS
 cancer due to, 674
 defined, 427
 response to, 429–430
Human papillomavirus (HPV)
 cancer due to, 673, 674
 cervical cancer due to, 613
 defined, 725
 warts and, 47
Human T-lymphotrophic virus (HTLV-1)
 cancer due to, 673
 defined, 725
Humoral immunity, defined, 725
Hunner ulcer, 601
 defined, 725
Huntington disease, 243
 permanent memory loss due to, 225
Hürthle cell carcinoma, 582
 defined, 725
Hyaluronic acid
 defined, 725
 in ganglion cysts, 177
Hydrocephalus, 250
 defined, 725
 spina bifida and, 296
Hydrops, endolymphatic, idiopathic, 322
 defined, 726
5-Hydroxytryptophan, for depression, 275
Hygienic practices, 9–13
 applications for massage therapists, 10–13
 hand care, 11
Hyper-, defined, 725
Hyperactivity, ADHD and, 260
Hyperacusis, 284
 defined, 725
Hyperalgesia
 defined, 725
 peripheral neuropathy and, 235
Hypercortisolism, 565
Hyperglycemia, defined, 725
Hyperkinesia, defined, 298, 725
Hyperkyphosis, 124
Hyperlexia, 264
Hyperlordosis, 124
Hypermobility Ehlers-Danlos syndrome, 159
Hyperosmolality
 defined, 725
 in type 2 diabetes, 570
Hyperplasia
 atypical, of breast, 630
 benign prostatic, 641–643, 642f. *See also* Benign prostatic hyperplasia (BPH)
 defined, 725
 uterine, 620
Hyperreflexia
 autonomic
  defined, 714
  SCI and, 300
 defined, 725
 SCI and, 298–299

Hypersensitivity, defined, 725
Hypersensitivity reactions
  type I, massage oil and, 406
  type(s) of, 406
Hyperthermia
  in cancer management, 678
  defined, 725
  malignant, 425
  types of, 425
Hypertonia, defined, 298
Hypertonic, defined, 725
Hypertrophic scar, 80
  defined, 725
Hypertrophy
  benign prostatic, defined, 715
  defined, 201, 726
  of heart, 392
Hyperuricemia
  defined, 726
  gout and, 131
Hypnagogic hallucination, 329
  defined, 726
Hypnic myoclonia, 327
  defined, 726
Hypo-, defined, 726
Hypoglycemia, 570
  defined, 726
Hypokinesia, defined, 298, 726
Hypotension, neurally mediated, chronic fatigue syndrome and, 422
Hypothalamic-pituitary-adrenal (HPA) axis
  anxiety disorders and, 255
  depression due to, 271
Hypothalamus, 557
Hypothalamus-pituitary-adrenal (HPA) axis, dysfunction of, chronic fatigue syndrome and, 422
Hypothermia
  in cancer management, 678
  defined, 726
Hypotonia, defined, 298
Hypotonic, defined, 726
Hypoxia, 469
  defined, 726
Hypoxic brain injury, TBI due to, 309
Hysterectomy, 621

I

Ichthyosis, defined, 726
Icterus, defined, 726
IDDM. *See* Insulin-dependent diabetes mellitus (IDDM)
Idiopathic, defined, 6t, 726
Idiopathic adrenal insufficiency, 563
Idiopathic anemia, 341
Idiopathic endolymphatic hydrops, 322
  defined, 726
Idiopathic environmental intolerance, defined, 726
Idiopathic hypothyroidism, 577
Idiopathic polyneuritis, acute, defined, 711
IgE. *See* Immunoglogulin(s), IgE
Ileitis, terminal, 491
  defined, 739
Imatinib, defined, 726
Imbalance
  hormonal
    acne vulgaris due to, 53
    depression due to, 271
    PMS due to, 659
  muscle, in thoracic outlet syndrome, 213
Immobility, thrombophlebitis/deep vein thrombosis due to, 365
Immune system
  alcohol effects on, 268
  conditions of, 418–438
  function of, 405–406
  mistakes made by, 406
  response to HIV, 429
Immune system activity, SCI and, 299
Immunity
  cellular, defined, 716
  humoral, defined, 725
  specific, defined, 788
Immunoblastic lymphoma, defined, 726
Immunoglobulin(s)
  for Guillain-Barré syndrome, 315
  monoclonal
    defined, 729
    myeloma and, 359
  thyroid-stimulating, 573
Immunoglogulin(s), IgE, eczema due to, 57
Immunomodulator(s), topical
  defined, 740
  for eczema, 59
Impacted fractures, 113
Impetigo contagiosa, 38, 39f
Impulsivity, ADHD and, 260
IMRAD, 705–706
In situ, defined, 726
Inattentiveness, ADHD and, 260
Incidence, defined, 6t
Incision(s), defined, 726
Incisional hernia, 180
Incomplete fractures, 113
Indication, defined, 6t
Indomethacin, defined, 726
Induction, defined, 726
Infant torticollis, 238
Infantile paralysis, 251
  defined, 726
Infarction(s)
  defined, 362, 726
  myocardial, defined, 730
Infection(s)
  local, thrombophlebitis/deep vein thrombosis due to, 364
  respiratory, SCI and, 299
  sickle cell disease and, 362
  UTIs, 300
Infectious agents, 2, 5–8, 7f–9f
  animal parasites, 8, 9
  bacteria, 7, 7f, 8f
  care of surfaces and equipment, 11–13
  fungi, 8
  hand washing, 10–11
  prions, 5
  viruses, 6
Inflammatory bowel disease
  colorectal cancer due to, 513
  defined, 489, 726
Inflammatory process, 13–17, 14f
Inflammatory rosacea, acne rosacea and, 51, 51f
Infundibulum, defined, 726
Inguinal hernia, 179, 179f
Inguinal orchiectomy
  defined, 726
  for testicular cancer, 651
Inheritance
  autosomal dominant, 162
  autosomal recessive, 162
Inherited diseases, variations of, 162
Inhibition, contact, 80
  defined, 718
Injury(ies), TBIs due to, 308–309
Insomnia, 327–328
Insulin, 558, 696
  defined, 726
Insulin resistance, 568
Insulin resistance syndrome, 579–581
Insulin shock, 570
Insulin-dependent diabetes mellitus (IDDM), 568
  defined, 726
Integumentary, defined, 726
Integumentary system, 23–83. *See also* Skin
  cystic fibrosis effects on, 473
  lupus effects on, 435
Intention tremor, 243
Interferon, defined, 726
Interferon betas, for MS, 233
Interleukin(s), IL-1, 425
  defined, 726
Intermittent claudication, 376
  defined, 726
Internal disc disruption, 206
Internal scar tissue, defined, 726
Interpersonal therapy, for depression, 274
Interstitial, defined, 726
Interstitial cystitis, 601–602
Interstitial fluid, in lymph system, 404
Intertrigo
  candidiasis and, 549
  defined, 726
Intolerance, environmental, idiopathic, defined, 726
Intracerebral hemorrhage, stroke due to, 304
Intrathecal pumps
  for CRPS, 292
  defined, 726
Intrauterine devices (IUDs), defined, 726
Intravenous pyelography
  defined, 726
  in kidney stones diagnosis, 590
Intrinsic factor, 342
  defined, 726
Invasion, in metastasis, 672
Inverse psoriasis, 64
  defined, 726
Iodine, radioactive, for hyperthyroidism, 575
Iodine deficiency, hypothyroidism and, 577
Iritis, defined, 727
Iron deficiency anemia, 341–342
Irritant(s), environmental, sinusitis due to, 456
Irritation(s), ligament, described, 205

Ischemia
cramps and, 106, 107f
defined, 727
Ischemic stroke, 303, 303f
Isometric tremor, 243
Isoniazid, for tuberculosis, 460
Itch, jock, 33, 33f
IUDs (intrauterine devices), defined, 727
Ixodes, defined, 727

J
Jackhammerer's shoulder, 172
Jaundice
cirrhosis and, 528, 529f
described, 529
Jaw, popping in, TMJ disorders and, 156
Jaw pain, TMJ disorders and, 156
Job's Body, 221
Jock itch, 33, 33f
Joint(s), 87–90, 88f
function of, 88
injuries of, 152
lavage and débridement of, for osteoarthritis, 141
locking of, TMJ disorders and, 156
structure of, 88, 88f
synovial, defined, 738
zygapophyseal, 213
defined, 741
Joint disorders, 125–158
Joint mice, defined, 727
Joint replacement surgery, for osteoarthritis, 141
Journal article, structure of, 705–706
Jumper's knee, 142–144
defined, 727

K
Kaposi sarcoma
defined, 727
HIV/AIDS and, 430, 430f
Keloid scar, 80, 80f
defined, 727
Keratin, defined, 727
Keratinocyte(s), 24
defined, 727
Keratosis(es)
actinic, 66–67, 67f, 74
defined, 711
seborrheic, 71
defined, 736
solar, 66–67, 67f, 74
Ketoacidosis, 569
defined, 727
Ketogenic, defined, 727
Ketone, defined, 727
Kidney(s)
failure of. *See* Renal failure
functions of, 587–588
Kidney disorders, 589–597
anemia and, 343
atherosclerosis and, 374
diabetes mellitus and, 570
hypertension and, 380
kidney stones, 589–592, 589f
pyelonephritis, 592–594
renal failure, 594–597
Kidney failure. *See* Renal failure
Kinin(s), 15
defined, 727
Klebsiella, defined, 727
Knee(s)
housemaid's, 172
jumper's, 142–144
defined, 727
movie-goer's, 142–144
defined, 729
Knuckle pads, 175
Kupffer cells, 485
defined, 727
Kyphoscoliosis Ehlers-Danlos syndrome, 159
Kyphosis, defined, 727

L
Labyrinthitis, 331
defined, 727
Laceration(s)
defined, 727
spinal cord effects of, 297
Lactobillus, defined, 727
Lamivudine, defined, 727
Lanugo, defined, 727
Laparoscopy, defined, 727
Laparotomy
defined, 727
in ovarian cancer diagnosis, 636
Large intestine, disorders of, 511–525. *See also* Digestive disorders, of large intestine
Latent autoimmune diabetes, in adults, 568
Latin word parts, 3t–5t
Lavage, defined, 727
Law(s)
Bell's, defined, 714
Wolff, defined, 741
LDL. *See* Low-density lipoprotein (LDL)
Learning disabilities, nonverbal, 264
Ledderhose disease, 175
defined, 727
Left ventricle, heart attacks affecting, 388, 390f
Leftsided colitis, defined, 524
Legg-Calvé-Perthes disease, defined, 727
Leiomyoma(s), 621–623, 622f. *See also* Fibroid tumors
defined, 727
Leiomyosarcoma, 624
Lentigine(s), 71
Lentiginous melanoma, acral, defined, 711
Lentigo, defined, 727
Lentigo melanoma, 71, 72f
Leprosy, defined, 727
Lesion(s)
anal, candidiasis and, 549
defined, 6t, 727
mouth, candidiasis and, 549
scabies, 41, 41f
skin, candidiasis and, 549
Letrozole, defined, 727
Leukocyte(s), 338, 339f
defined, 727
Leukoplakia, defined, 727
Levodopa (L-dopa)
defined, 727
for Parkinson disease, 241–242
Levothyroxine sodium, 698
Levulose, 529
defined, 727
Lewy body dementia, permanent memory loss due to, 225
Lewy body disease, defined, 727
Leydig cell tumor, 650
defined, 727
Lhermitte sign
defined, 727
MS and, 233
Lichenification, 57
Lifestyle, sedentary
atherosclerosis due to, 374
colorectal cancer due to, 513
stroke due to, 305
Ligament(s)
injuries of, 152
irritation of
described, 205
dysmenorrhea due to, 616
laxity of, sprains and, 154
loose, pregnancy and, 655
sprains of, whiplash and, 197
Ligamenta flava, 149
defined, 728
Light therapy, for depression, 274
Likert scales, 703, 703f, 704f
defined, 702
Limb girdle dystrophy, 164
defined, 728
Limbic system
anxiety disorders and, 255
defined, 728
Limited systemic scleroderma, 189
defined, 728
Linea alba, defined, 728
Linear scleroderma, 189
Liothyronine sodium, 699
Lipodystrophy, HIV treatment and, 432
Lipoprotein(s), 375
1, 776
high-density, defined, 725
low-density
defined, 728
described, 375
Liquid bandage, 11
Liquid nitrogen, for squamous cell carcinoma, 69–70
Literacy, research, 701–709
defined, 701
Lithium
defined, 728
for depression, 274
Lithotripsy
defined, 728
shockwave
extracorporeal
defined, 722
for kidney stones, 592
for plantar fasciitis, 188
Liver
described, 526

Liver—*continued*
  function of, 526
  hobnailed, defined, 725
  overview of, 484f, 485
  scarring of, 526, 527f
Liver congestion, acne vulgaris due to, 53
Liver failure, cirrhosis and, 529
Liver flukes, cancer due to, 674
Lobar pneumonia, 452
Lobular carcinoma, 627
Lordosis, defined, 728
Lou Gehrig disease, 226–229. *See also* Amyotrophic lateral sclerosis (ALS)
Low-density lipoprotein (LDL)
  defined, 728
  described, 375
Lumen, defined, 728
Lung(s), structure of, 442
Lymph
  defined, 404
  flow of, mechanisms in, 404
  origin of, 404, 404f
Lymph nodes, sentinel, defined, 736
Lymph system
  conditions of, 407–418
  function of, 404–405
  structure of, 403–404, 404f
Lymphadenitis, 410
  defined, 728
Lymphadenoma, defined, 728
Lymphangion, 409
  defined, 728
Lymphatic drainage, 18
Lymphedema, 631, 680, 681f
  defined, 728
Lymphoblastic lymphoma, defined, 728
Lymphocyte(s), 339f, 405
  defined, 728
  inflammation and, 15
Lymphocytic leukemia
  acute, 353
  chronic, 353
Lymphocytic lymphoma, defined, 728
Lymphokine(s), 425
  defined, 728
Lynch syndrome
  colorectal cancer due to, 513
  defined, 728

M
Macrophage(s)
  atherosclerosis due to, 372
  defined, 728
  inflammation and, 14–15
Macrosomia, 656
  defined, 728
Magnetic resonance imaging (MRI)
  defined, 728
  in musculoskeletal system evaluation, 85
Major depressive disorder, 272
Malaise, defined, 728
Malar rash, 433, 434f
  defined, 728
Malignant, defined, 728
Malignant hypertension, 379
  defined, 728
Malignant hyperthermia, 425
Malignant mixed mesodermal tumors, 625
Malignant otitis externa, 571
Malocclusion, 155
  defined, 728
Malunion fractures, 114
Mammogram, of breast cancer, 629, 629f
Manic depression, 273
MAOIs. *See* Monoamine oxidase inhibitors (MAOIs)
Massage chairs, care of, 12
Massage oil, type I hypersensitivity reactions and, 406
Massage tables, care of, 12
Mast cells
  defined, 728
  inflammation and, 14
Mastitis, 630
  defined, 728
Matrix, defined, 728
MCS syndrome. *See* Multiple chemical sensitivity (MCS) syndrome
Mechanical perforation, of abdomen, peritonitis due to, 551
Medial tibial stress syndrome, 104
  defined, 728
Medication(s), 683–699
  ACE inhibitors, 692
  acetaminophen, 688
  adrenergic blockers, 690–691
  adrenergic drugs, 690
  analgesics, 687–689
  antianginal, 693–694
  anti-anxiety, 684–685
  anticholinergic drugs, 690
  anticoagulants, 695
  antidepressants, 685–687
  anti-inflammatory, 687–689
    steroidal, 688–689
  antilipemic drugs, 693
  antiplatelet, 695
  autonomic nervous system, 689–691
  benzodiazepines, 684
  beta blockers, 691
  buspirone HCl, 685
  calcium channel blockers, 692
  cancer-related, 694
  cardiovascular drugs, 691–694
  cholinergics, 690
  in clotting management, 695
  desiccated extract, 698
  in diabetes management, 696–697
  digitalis, 692
  diuretics, 693
  hypothyroidism and, 577
  insulin, 696
  levothyroxine sodium, 698
  liothyronine sodium, 699
  MAOIs, 686
  muscle relaxants, 697
  nervous system problems with, 222
  NSAIDs, 688
  opioids, 689
  oral glucose–related, 696–697
  salicylates, 687–688
  skeletal muscle relaxants
    centrally acting, 697
    peripherally acting, 697
  SSRIs, 686
  stroke due to, 305
  thyroid supplement, 698–699
  tricyclics, 686
Medullary thyroid cancer, 582
Megacolon, toxic, 524
  defined, 740
Meige syndrome, 237
  defined, 728
Melanin, defined, 728
Melanocyte(s), 24
  defined, 728
  described, 70
Melanoma(s)
  lentiginous, acral, 71, 72f
    defined, 711
  lentigo, 71, 72f
  malignant, 70–74, 72f. *See also* Malignant melanoma
  nodular, 71, 72f
  superficial spreading, 71, 72f
Melatonin, 559
  defined, 728
Menarche, 637
  defined, 728
  early, uterine cancer due to, 625
Meningocele(s), spina bifida, 294
  defined, 737
Meniscus, defined, 729
Meniscus tears, 152
Menses, defined, 729
Mental degeneration, Parkinson disease and, 241
Mental illness, as factor in chemical dependency, 266
Menthol, for osteoarthritis, 141
Mesangial glomerulonephritis, defined, 729
Mesentery, 484
  defined, 729
Mesothelioma, 476
  defined, 729
Metabolic gout, 131
Metabolism
  aerobic, 87
    defined, 712
  anaerobic, 87
    defined, 712
Metabolite, defined, 729
Metaplasia, 619
  defined, 729
Metastasis(es)
  to bone, 680
  defined, 729
  steps in, 672–673
Methicillin-resistant *S. aureus* (MRSA)
  boils due to, 26
  defined, 729
Methylphenidate, defined, 729
Microaerophilic, defined, 729
Microbe(s), defined, 729
Micrographia, 241
  defined, 729
Microsporum, defined, 729

Middle ear, sense of fullness in, Ménière disease and, 322
Middle pain, 637
Migraine(s), 318–319
Migration, in metastasis, 672
Miller-Fisher syndrome, 314
Mineralocorticoid(s), 558, 563
  defined, 729
Misalignment(s)
  cervical, thoracic outlet syndrome vs., 213
  rib, thoracic outlet syndrome vs., 213
Mitochondrion(a), defined, 729
Mittelschmertz, 637
  defined, 729
Mixed cerebral palsy, 287
Mixed connective tissue disease, 437
MMS. *See* Mohs micrographic surgery (MMS)
Mohs micrographic surgery (MMS), for squamous cell carcinoma, 69–70
Mole(s), 71
Molluscum contagiosum, 49, 665
  defined, 729
Monoamine oxidase inhibitors (MAOIs), 686
  for anxiety disorders, 258
  defined, 729
  for depression, 274
Monoclonal immunoglobulins
  defined, 729
  myeloma and, 359
Monocyte(s), 339f, 405
  atherosclerosis due to, 372
  defined, 729
  inflammation and, 14–15
Mononeuropathy, 235
  defined, 729
Morbidity, defined, 6t
Morphea scleroderma, 189
Mortality, defined, 6t
Mosquitoes, 8
Motility
  colon, 516
  defined, 729
Motor neuron disease, 226–229. *See also* Amyotrophic lateral sclerosis (ALS)
Motor neurons, 220, 221f
Motor vehicle accidents, SCI due to, 297
Mouth lesions, candidiasis and, 549
Mouth sores, 37
Movement disorders, 236–244. *See also specific disorders, e.g.,* Dystonia
  dystonia, 236–239
  Parkinson disease, 239–242, 241f
  tremors, 243–244
Movement therapy, constraint-induced, for stroke, 307
Movie-goer's knee, 142–144
  defined, 729
MRI. *See* Magnetic resonance imaging (MRI)
MRSA
  boils due to, 26
  defined, 729
MS. *See* Multiple sclerosis (MS)
Mucolytic, defined, 729
Mucopolysaccharide(s)
  defined, 729
  hyperthyroidism and, 574–575
Mucormycosis, 571
  defined, 729
Mucosal-associated lymphoid-type lymphoma, defined, 729
Mucous cyst, 177
  defined, 729
Multifocal dystonia, 237
Multinodular goiter, 573
Multiple chemical sensitivity (MCS) syndrome, 419
Multiple endocrine neoplasia
  type IIA, 582
  type IIB, 582
Multiple myeloma, 359
Multiple system atrophy, 243
  defined, 729
Murmur(s), heart, 392
Muscle(s), 86–87, 87f
  function of, 87
  structure of, 86–87
Muscle cramp, exercise-associated, 106
Muscle energy technique, 18
Muscle imbalance, in thoracic outlet syndrome, 213
Muscle relaxants, 697
  dependency issues related to, 267
  skeletal
    centrally acting, 697
    peripherally acting, 697
Muscle spindle, defined, 729
Muscle wasting, cirrhosis and, 528
Muscle weakness
  disc disease and, 207
  specific, defined, 737
Muscular disorders, 90–111
Musculoskeletal disorders, 90–215
Musculoskeletal system, 85–218
  bones of, 86
  evaluation of, MRI in, 85
  joints of, 87–90, 88f
  lupus effects on, 435
  Marfan syndrome effects on, 161
  muscles of, 86–87, 87f
  musculoskeletal disorders of, 90–215
Myalgic encephalomyelitis, 421
  defined, 729
Mycobacterium
  defined, 729
  M. paratuberculosis, Crohn disease due to, 491
  M. tuberculosis, tuberculosis due to, 458
Mycoplasma, 7
  defined, 729
  pneumonia due to, 451
Mycosis(es), 30
  defined, 730
Myelin, 220, 221f
  defined, 730
Myelodysplastic anemia, 343
  defined, 730
Myelogenous leukemia
  acute, 353
  chronic, 353
Myeloid cell, defined, 730
Myelomeningocele, spina bifida, 294
  defined, 737
Myelopathy(ies), cervical spondylitic, 150
  defined, 716
Myocardial infarction, 388–395, 390f. *See also* Heart attack
  defined, 730
Myoclonia, hypnic, 327
  defined, 726
Myoclonic, defined, 730
Myoclonic seizures, 325
Myofascial release, 18
Myofiber(s), 86–87
Myofibril(s), defined, 730
Myopia, defined, 730
Myositis ossificans traumatica, 100
Myotonia, 164
  defined, 730
Myotonic muscular dystrophy, 164
Myrmecia, 48, 49f
  defined, 730
Myxedema, pretibial
  defined, 734
  hyperthyroidism and, 574–575
Myxedema coma, 578
  defined, 730

N

NAFLD. *See* Nonalcoholic fatty liver disease (NAFLD)
Nailfold capillaroscopy, 383
  defined, 730
Narcolepsy, 328–329
  defined, 730
Nardil, for depression, 274
Nasal decongestants, dependency issues related to, 267
NASH. *See* Nonalcoholic steatohepatitis (NASH)
National Commission for the Certification of Acupuncture and Oriental Medicine (NCCAOM), 20
National Heart Lung and Blood Institute (NHLBI), DASH diet of, 381
National Institutes of Health, in carcinogena, 673
National Sleep Foundation, 329
National Survey on Drug Use and Health Issues, in chemical dependency, 266
NCCAOM. *See* National Commission for the Certification of Acupuncture and Oriental Medicine (NCCAOM)
Neck pain, TMJ disorders and, 156
Necrosis(es)
  avascular. *See also* Avascular necrosis
  defined, 730
  fat, 630
    defined, 722
Needle aponeurotomy
  defined, 730
  for Dupuytren contracture, 176
Neglect, benign, defined, 49
Neisseria
  N. gonorrhoeae, defined, 730
  N. meningitidis, defined, 730

Neonatal lupus, 433
Neoplasm(s), defined, 730
Nephrolithiasis, 589–592, 589f. *See also* Kidney stones
  defined, 730
Nephrolithotomy, percutaneous
  defined, 732
  for kidney stones, 591
Nephron, defined, 730
Nerve(s). *See also specific types, e.g.*, Peripheral nerves
  described, 219
Nerve damage, terminology related to, 298
Nerve growth factor, 92
  defined, 730
Nerve pain, spondylosis and, 150
Nervous system
  alcohol effects on, 268
  described, 219
  function of, 219–221, 220f, 221f
  injuries of, 283–313. *See also specific injury and* Nervous system conditions
  lupus effects on, 435–436
  Marfan syndrome effects on, 162
  problems associated with, cautions for massage therapists, 222
  structure of, 219–221, 220f, 221f
Nervous system conditions, 219–336, 283–313
Neural tube defects, 293
Neuralgia(s)
  glossopharyngeal, 312
  occipital, 157
  postherpetic, 312
    defined, 733
  trigeminal, 157, 310–313, 311f. *See also* Trigeminal neuralgia
Neuralgia-inducing cavitational osteonecrosis (NICO), defined, 730
Neuraminidase, 450
  defined, 730
Neuraminidase inhibitors, for influenza, 449
Neurilemma, 220, 221f
  defined, 730
Neuritis, optic, MS and, 232
Neurodermatitis, 58
Neuroendocrine, defined, 730
Neuroendocrine tumors, 543
Neurofibrillary tangle
  in Alzheimer disease, 223, 224f
  defined, 730
Neurogenic bladder, 593
  defined, 730
  UTIs and, 604
Neurological problems, general, 221–222
Neurological symptoms, whiplash and, 197
Neuroma, defined, 730
Neuromuscular disorders, 200–215. *See also specific disorders, e.g.*, Carpal tunnel syndrome
  carpal tunnel syndrome, 200–203, 200f, 201f
  disc disease, 204–209, 204f, 207f
  myasthenia gravis, 209–211
  thoracic outlet syndrome, 211–215, 212f
Neuron(s)
  defined, 730
  function of, 219–220
  motor, 220, 221f
  parts of, 220, 221f
  in peripheral nervous system, 220, 221f
  sensory, 220, 221f
Neuronitis, vestibular, acute, 331
  defined, 711
Neuropathy(ies)
  acute motor axonal, 314
  acute motor-sensory axonal, 314
  diabetes mellitus and, 570
  peripheral, 235–236. *See also* Peripheral neuropathy
Neuropeptide, defined, 730
Neurotransmitter(s)
  anxiety disorders and, 256
  imbalance of, chronic fatigue syndrome and, 422
Neurotransmitter imbalance
  depression due to, 271
  PMS due to, 659
Neurotrophic factors, defined, 730
Neutrophil(s), 339f, 405
  defined, 779
Neutrophilic, defined, 730
Nevus(i), 71
  congenital, defined, 717
  defined, 730
  dysplastic, defined, 720
NHLBI. *See* National Heart Lung and Blood Institute (NHLBI)
NICO. *See* Neuralgia-inducing cavitational osteonecrosis (NICO)
NIDDM. *See* Non-insulin–dependent diabetes mellitus (NIDDM)
Nit(s), 43, 43f
  defined, 730
Nitrogen, liquid, for squamous cell carcinoma, 69–70
Nociceptor(s), 87
  defined, 730
Nocturia, 644
  defined, 731
Node(s)
  Bouchard, defined, 715
  Garrod's, 175
  Heberden, defined, 724
  lymph, sentinel, defined, 736
  sinoatrial, defined, 738
Nodular, defined, 731
Nodular melanoma, 71, 72f
Nonalcoholic fatty liver disease (NAFLD), 526
  defined, 730
Nonalcoholic steatohepatitis (NASH), 526
  defined, 731
Non–Burkitt lymphoma, defined, 731
Nongonococcal urethritis, 665
  defined, 731
Non-Hodgkin lymphoma, 412–415, 414f
  demographics of, 412
  described, 413, 414f
  HIV/AIDS and, 430
Non–insulin-dependent diabetes mellitus (NIDDM), 568
  defined, 731
Nonseminoma(s), 650
  defined, 731
Non–small cell lung cancer, 476, 477f
Nontropical sprue, 486–489
  defined, 731
Nonverbal learning disabilities, 264
Noradrenaline, defined, 731
Norepinephrine, defined, 731
Norovirus(es), 498
Norovirus, defined, 731
Nosocomial, defined, 731
Nosocomial pneumonia, 452
Noxious, defined, 731
NSAIDs. *See* Anti-inflammatory drugs, nonsteroidal (NSAIDs)
Nucleus pulposus, 204, 204f
  defined, 731
  herniated, 206, 207f
Numb-likeness, defined, 731
Numbness
  disc disease and, 208
  nervous system problems with, 222
  SCI and, 300
Nummular eczema, 58, 58f
  defined, 731
Nutrient(s), delivery of, circulatory system in, 338
Nutrition, cramps and, 106
Nutritional anemias, 341–342
Nutritional deficiencies, PMS due to, 659
Nutritional supplements, for osteoarthritis, 141
Nystagmus, Ménière disease and, 322

O

Oatmeal, for psoriasis, 64
Obesity
  cholesterol stones due to, 532
  colorectal cancer due to, 513
  GERD and, 502
  stroke due to, 305
  uterine cancer due to, 625
Oblique fractures, 114, 114f
Obsessive-compulsive disorder (OCD), 257
Obstructive sleep apnea, 328
Obturator hernia, 180
Occipital neuralgia, 157
Occult, defined, 731
OCD. *See* Obsessive-compulsive disorder (OCD)
Oculopharyngeal muscular dystrophy, 164
  defined, 731
Oligodendrocyte(s), 230
  defined, 731
Olivopontocerebellar atrophy, 243
  defined, 731
Omega-3 fish oil, for depression, 275
Oncogene(s)
  activation of, 672
  defined, 731
Onycholysis, 63
  defined, 731
Onychomycosis, 32
  defined, 731
Oocyte(s), 638
  defined, 731

Oophorectomy
defined, 731
for ovarian cancer, 637
Oophoritis, defined, 731
Ophthalmopathy, Graves
defined, 724
hyperthyroidism and, 574
Opioid(s), 689
mixed, 689
Optic neuritis, MS and, 232
Oral glucose management drugs, 696–697
Orchiectomy
defined, 731
inguinal
defined, 726
for testicular cancer, 651
Orchitis, defined, 731
Oromandibular dystonia, 237
Orthopedic injuries, types of, 152
Orthotic(s), defined, 731
Os coxae, defined, 731
Oscillation, defined, 731
Ossification, heterotopic
defined, 725
SCI and, 300
Osteitis deformans, 119–122, 120f. *See also* Paget disease
Osteoblast(s), 86
defined, 731
Osteoclast(s), 86
defined, 731
Osteomalacia, 596
celiac disease and, 487
defined, 731
Osteomyelitis, 157
defined, 731
Osteonecrosis
avascular, 111–113, 112f. *See also* Avascular necrosis
defined, 731
neuralgia-inducing cavitational, defined, 730
Osteopenia, 115
defined, 731
Osteophyte, defined, 731
Osteotomy, defined, 731
Ostomy, defined, 731
Otitis externa, malignant, 571
Otolith(s), 331
defined, 731
Ovary(ies), polycystic, 638, 639f
Overuse syndrome, 142–144
defined, 731
Oxygen
defined, 731
delivery of, circulatory system in, 338

P

Pain
chest. *See* Chest pain
disc disease and, 207
ear, TMJ disorders and, 156
face, atypical, 312
fibromyalgia and, 92
jaw, TMJ disorders and, 156
middle, 637
neck, TMJ disorders and, 156
nerve, spondylosis and, 150
radicular
defined, 735
whiplash and, 198
SCI and, 300
shoulder, TMJ disorders and, 156
Painkillers, dependency issues related to, 267
Pain-spasm-pain cycle
defined, 732
dysmenorrhea due to, 616
Palliative, defined, 732
Pallor, anemia and, 344
Palmar fasciitis, 174–176, 175f. *See also* Dupuytren contracture
defined, 732
Palpable, defined, 732
Palpitation, defined, 732
Palsy(ies), Bell, 283–286. *See also* Bell palsy
Pancolitis, defined, 524, 732
Pancreas, overview of, 484f, 485
Pandemic, defined, 6t
Panic disorder, 254
Pap test
in cervical cancer diagnosis, 614
defined, 732
Papillary thyroid cancer, 582
Papilloma(s), of breast, 630
Parafollicular cells, in thyroid cancer, 581
Paralysis
defined, 298
flaccid, defined, 298, 722
infantile, 251
defined, 726
sleep, 329
defined, 737
spastic, defined, 298, 737
Paraplegia
defined, 732
spastic, 298
Parasite(s)
animal, 8, 9
cancer due to, 674
gastroenteritis due to, 498
Parasomnia(s), 327
Parate, for depression, 274
Parathyroid hormone (PTH), 558–559
defined, 732
Paraumbilical hernia, 180
Parenchyma
defined, 732
encephalitis infections effects on, 245
Paresis, defined, 298, 732
Paresthesia(s)
defined, 298, 732
disc disease and, 207
MS and, 232
Parkinson, James, 239
Parkinsonism
defined, 140, 732
pugilistic, defined, 734
Partial seizures
complex, 324
simple, 324
Patellar tendinitis, 143, 152
defined, 732
Patent foramen ovale, 303, 346, 365
Pathogen(s)
defined, 732
protection from, circulatory system in, 338
Pathology
bodywork modalities, 17–22, 21t
fundamental concepts in, 1–22
hygienic practices, 9–13
infectious agents, 2, 5–8, 7f–9f
inflammatory process, 13–17, 14f
terminology related to, 2, 3t–6t
Pediculosis, defined, 732
Pediculus, defined, 732
Pediculus
P. humanus capitis, 42–44, 42f
P. humanus humanus, 44
Pedunculate, defined, 732
Pedunculate fibroids, 622
Pelvic abscess, peritonitis due to, 551
Pelvic inflammatory disease (PID), 662
Penetrating injury, TBI due to, 308
Peptide(s), 558
defined, 732
Percutaneous nephrolithotomy
defined, 732
for kidney stones, 591
Percutaneous transluminal coronary angioplasty (PTCA)
defined, 732
for heart attack, 392–393
Perforation
defined, 732
diverticular disease and, 518
mechanical, of abdomen, peritonitis due to, 551
Perfusion, defined, 732
Peri-, defined, 732
Pericarditis, defined, 732
Perilymph, 321, 321f
Perilymph fistula, defined, 732
Perimenopause, 652
defined, 732
symptoms of, age of onset of, 652
Perimysium, 87
defined, 732
Periodic limb movement disorder (PLMD), 328
defined, 732
Periosteum, defined, 732
Periostitis, 104
defined, 732
Peripheral circulatory damage, atherosclerosis and, 376
Peripheral nerves
composition of, 220
location of, 220–221
vulnerability of, 220
Peripheral nervous system, neurons in, 220, 221f
Peripheral vascular disease, 376, 377f
defined, 732
Peripherally acting skeletal muscle relaxants, 697
Peritoneal dialysis, peritonitis due to, 552
Peritoneal space, infection in, 551–553, 551f
Pernicious anemia, 342
Personality traits, as factor in depression, 271

Pervasive developmental disorder, not otherwise specified, 263
Pervasive developmental disorder(s), 261–265. *See also* Autism spectrum disorders
  defined, 732
PET scan, defined, 732
Petit mal, defined, 732
Peyronie disease, 175
  defined, 732
Phalen maneuver
  in carpal tunnel syndrome diagnosis, 202
  defined, 733
Pheochromocytoma(s), 582
  defined, 733
Phlebectomy, defined, 733
Phlegm, defined, 733
Phobia(s)
  social, 257
  specific, 257
Photodynamic therapy
  defined, 733
  for lung cancer, 479
Photosensitivity, 435
  defined, 733
Phototherapy, for psoriasis, 64
Phyllodes tumors
  of breast, 630
  defined, 733
Physical hives, 61
Physical trauma, thrombophlebitis/deep vein thrombosis due to, 364
Phyto-, defined, 733
Phytoestrogen, defined, 733
Pia mater, defined, 733
Pigment stones, 531
Pilonidal cyst, 26
  defined, 733
Pimple(s), acne vulgaris and, 53
Pinna, defined, 733
Pitting edema, 407–408, 408f
  defined, 733
Pituitary adenoma, 565
Placenta abruptio, 657
  defined, 733
Plain soap, defined, 10
Plane warts, 49
Plantar fibromatosis, 175
  defined, 733
Plantar warts
  callus vs., 48
  deep palmar, 48, 49f
Plaque(s)
  in Alzheimer disease, 223
  defined, 733
Plaque psoriasis, 63, 63f
Plasmapheresis
  defined, 733
  for Guillain-Barré syndrome, 314
  for MS, 234
  for myasthenia gravis, 211
Plastocytoma(s), 359
  defined, 733
  extramedullary, 359
    defined, 722
Platelet(s), 338–339
  atherosclerosis due to, 373
  defined, 733
  inflammation and, 14
Pleurisy, defined, 733
Plexus, defined, 733
PLMD. *See* Periodic limb movement disorder (PLMD)
PMDD. *See* Premenstrual dysphoric disorder (PMDD)
PMS. *See* Premenstrual syndrome (PMS)
Pneumococcus, defined, 733
Pneumocystis
  P. carinii pneumonia, 452
    defined, 733
    HIV/AIDS and, 430
  P. jiroveci pneumonia, defined, 733
Pneumothorax, 470
  defined, 733
PNF. *See* Proprioceptive neuromuscular facilitation (PNF)
Poison ivy, 420
Poison oak, 420
Poison sumac, 420
Poisoning, blood, lymphangitis and, 410
Polarity, 19
Polio, language of, 251
Poliomyelitis, defined, 733
Poliovirus, 251–254, 253f
  causes of, 252, 253f
  defined, 251, 252
  demographics of, 251–252
  described, 252
  prevention of, 253–254
  signs and symptoms of, 252
  treatment of, 253
Poly-, defined, 733
Polyarteritis nodosa, defined, 733
Polycystic ovarian syndrome, uterine cancer due to, 625
Polycystic ovary(ies), 638, 639f
Polycythemia, 466
  defined, 733
Polydipsia, 569
  defined, 733
Polyendocrine deficiency syndrome, 563
  defined, 733
Polyneuritis, idiopathic, acute, defined, 711
Polyneuropathy(ies), 235
  acute inflammatory demyelinating, 314
    defined, 711
  defined, 733
Polyp(s), colon, 511, 512f
Polyphagia, 569
  defined, 733
Polyposis, adenomatous, familial
  colorectal cancer due to, 513
  defined, 722
Polysomnography, defined, 733
Polyuria, 569
  defined, 733
Popliteal cyst, defined, 733
Popliteal fossa, defined, 733
Port wine stains, 71
Portal hypertension
  cirrhosis and, 527
  defined, 733
Postacute stage of healing, 15
Postherpetic neuralgia, 312
  defined, 733
Postmenopausal women, prevalence of, 652
Postpartum depression, 273
Poststroke depression, 306
Posttraumatic stress disorder (PTSD), 254–255
Postural reflexes, poor, Parkinson disease and, 240
Postural tremor, 243
Posturography
  defined, 733
  in vestibular balance disorders diagnosis, 332
Power, defined, 702
Prediabetes, 579–581
Prednisone, defined, 734
Preeclampsia, 656
  defined, 734
Premenstrual dysphoric disorder (PMDD), 660
  defined, 734
Pressure
  blood vessel, spondylosis and, 150
  spinal cord, spondylosis and, 150
Pressure sores, 77–79, 78f
Pretibial myxedema
  defined, 734
  hyperthyroidism and, 574–575
Prevalence, defined, 6t
Priapism
  defined, 734
  sickle cell disease and, 363
Prion(s), 5
  defined, 734
Proctitis, ulcerative, defined, 524
Prodromic, defined, 734
Progesterone, 559
Progestin, defined, 734
Prognosis, defined, 6t
Programmed cell death, 673
Proliferant(s)
  defined, 734
  for dislocations, 129
Proliferation, in metastasis, 672
Prophylaxis, defined, 734
Proprioception, shifting, pregnancy and, 656
Proprioceptive neuromuscular facilitation (PNF)/MET/stretching, 19
Proprioceptor, defined, 734
Proptosis, 574, 575f
  defined, 734
Prostadynia, defined, 734
Prostaglandin(s), 559
  defined, 734
  dysmenorrhea due to, 616
Prostate-specific antigen (PSA)
  for BPH, 642
  defined, 734
Protease inhibitor, defined, 734
Protection, skin as, 24
Protein(s)
  Alzheimer-related, 223, 224f
  Bence Jones
    defined, 714
    myeloma and, 359

C-reactive
atherosclerosis due to, 374–375
defined, 718
stroke due to, 305
Protozoa, 8, 9f
Protrusion(s), nucleus pulposus due to, 206
Prozac, for depression, 274
Pruritus
defined, 734
pancreatic cancer and, 544
Pseudogout
defined, 734
gout vs., 132
Pseudohypertrophy
defined, 734
muscular dystrophy and, 164
Pseudomembranous colitis, 498
defined, 734
Pseudomonas aeruginosa, defined, 734
Psoralen, defined, 734
Psoriatric arthritis, 64
Psychiatric disorders, 254–282
Psychodynamic therapy
defined, 734
for depression, 274
Psychoneuroimmunology, defined, 734
Psychotherapy
for anxiety disorders, 248
for depression, 274
PTCA. *See* Percutaneous transluminal coronary angioplasty (PTCA)
PTH. *See* Parathyroid hormone (PTH)
Pthirus pubis, 44–45, 45f
defined, 734
Ptosis, defined, 734
PTSD. *See* Posttraumatic stress disorder (PTSD)
Pubic lice, 44–45, 45f
Pugilistic parkinsonism, defined, 734
Pulmonary embolism, 346–347, 346f
case example, 367
complications of, 347
prevention of, 347
risk factors for, 346–347
SCI and, 300
signs and symptoms of, 347
sources of, 346, 346f
treatment of, 347
Pulmonary embolism chest pain, features of, 393
Pump(s), intrathecal, defined, 726
Purine(s), gout due to, 131
Pustular psoriasis, 64
defined, 734
Pustule(s)
acne vulgaris and, 54
defined, 734
PUVA
defined, 734
for psoriasis, 65
Pyelography
defined, 734
intravenous
defined, 726
in kidney stones diagnosis, 590
in ovarian cancer diagnosis, 636
Pyrogen, 426
defined, 734

Q
Q angle
defined, 734
exaggerated, patellofemoral syndrome due to, 143
Quadriplegia
defined, 735
spastic, 298
Qualitative observations, defined, 702
Qualitative research, 703
Quantitative observations, defined, 702
Quantitative research, 703
Quercetin, defined, 735

R
Race/ethnicity
asthma and, 462
cholesterol stones and, 532
as factor in gallstones, 531
as factor in hypertension, 378
as factor in MS, 230
as factor in sickle cell disease, 361
as factor in spina bifida, 293
as factor in stroke, 305
Radiation
defined, 735
exposure to
hypothyroidism and, 577
thyroid cancer due to, 582
Radiation therapy
in cancer management, 678, 680
breast, 631
for lymphomas, 414
Radicular pain
defined, 735
whiplash and, 198
Radiculopathy, defined, 735
Radioactive iodine, for hyperthyroidism, 575
Radiofrequency thermal ablation, in cancer management, 678
Radiography, in kidney stones diagnosis, 590
Radioimmunotherapy, defined, 735
Radioisotope, defined, 735
Radiosurgery, stereotactic, in Cushing syndrome, 566
Rales, defined, 735
Ramsay-Hunt syndrome, type 1, 247
defined, 735
Randomization, defined, 703
Randomized, 707
Randomized controlled trial (RCT), 707
beyond, 708
defined, 703
Range of motion, limited, TMJ disorders and, 156
Rash(es), malar, 433, 434f
defined, 728
Raynaud disease, Raynaud syndrome due to, 383
Raynaud phenomenon
defined, 382
Raynaud syndrome due to, 383
scleroderma and, 190
RCT. *See* Randomized controlled trial (RCT)
Recombinant tissue plasminogen activator, for stroke, 306

Red blood cells (erythrocytes), 338
defined, 721
Reduction, defined, 735
Reed-Sternberg cells, 413
defined, 735
Reflex(es), postural, poor, Parkinson disease and, 240
Reflex arc, 220, 220f
Reflex sympathetic dystrophy syndrome (RSDS), 289
Reflexology, 20
Reflux, vesicoureteral, 593
Regional enteritis, 491
defined, 735
Reiki, 19
Reiter syndrome, defined, 735
Relaxant(s), muscle, dependency issues related to, 267
Relaxin, 655
defined, 735
Relenza, for influenza, 449
Renal calculus, 589–592, 589f. *See also* Kidney stones
defined, 735
Renal colic, 590
defined, 735
Renal gout, 131
Renin, defined, 380, 735
Repetitive stress injury, defined, 735
Reproductive conditions, 610–669
Reproductive history, ovarian cancer due to, 635
Reproductive system, 607–669
alcohol effects on, 268–269
cystic fibrosis effects on, 473
female
disorders of, 610–640. *See also specific condition and* Reproductive conditions
function and structure of, 608, 608f
overview of, 608, 608f
lupus effects on, 436
male
disorders of, 641–652. *See also* Reproductive conditions, male
function and structure of, 608–610, 609f
overview of, 608–610, 609f
Research
qualitative, 703
quantitative, 703
Research capacity, 701–709
defined, 701
Research literacy, 701–709
defined, 701
Respiratory disorders, 462–479
Respiratory injury, GERD and, 501
Respiratory system, 441–481
conditions of, 441–481. *See also* Respiratory disorders
cystic fibrosis effects on, 473
function of, 442
lupus effects on, 436
overview of, 441, 442f
structure of, 441–442, 442f
Restenosis, defined, 376, 735
Resting tremor, 243
Parkinson disease and, 240

Restless leg syndrome, 328
  defined, 735
Reticulocyte(s)
  anemia and, 342
  defined, 735
Retinoin, defined, 735
Retinopathy
  defined, 735
  diabetic, 570
Retrovirus, defined, 735
Rett syndrome, 263
  defined, 735
Rheumatic fever, 392
Rheumatoid spondylitis, 125
  defined, 735
Rhinitis
  allergic, 455
    defined, 712
  defined, 735
Rhinophyma
  acne rosacea and, 51, 51f
  defined, 735
Rhupus, defined, 735
Rhythm(s), circadian, 327
  defined, 717
Rib(s)
  cervical
    defined, 716
    in thoracic outlet syndrome, 212–213
  misalignment of, thoracic outlet syndrome vs., 213
Rickettsia rickettsii, defined, 735
Rigidity, Parkinson disease and, 240
Rimantadine
  defined, 735
  for influenza, 449
Ringworm, 30
  case example, 31
  head, 32, 32f
RMSF. *See* Rocky Mountain spotted fever (RMSF)
Rocky Mountain spotted fever (RMSF), 136
Rodent ulcer, defined, 735
Rosacea, vascular acne roacea and, 51
Rotational vertigo, Ménière disease and, 322
Rotator cuff injuries, 152
Rotavirus, defined, 735
Rotavirus infections, 498
Rotoscoliosis, 122
  defined, 735
Roundworms, 8
RSDS. *See* Reflex sympathetic dystrophy syndrome (RSDS)
Rubella, defined, 735
Rupture(s)
  cruciate ligament, 152
  nucleus pulposus due to, 206

S

Saccular aneurysm, 369, 369f
Salicylate(s), 687–688
Salicylic acid, for psoriasis, 64
Salk vaccine, 254
Salmonella, defined, 736
Salpingitis, defined, 736
SAM-e. *See* S-Adenosyl-methionine
San Joaquin fever, 452
Sanitation, defined, 10
Sarcoidosis, defined, 736
Sarcolemma, 210
  defined, 736
Sarcoma(s)
  defined, 671, 736
  Kaposi
    defined, 727
    HIV/AIDS and, 430, 430f
  stromal, 624
  uterine, 623–626. *See also* Uterine cancer
Sarcomere(s), 87
  defined, 736
Sarcoptes scabei, 40, 40f
  defined, 736
Satellite points, 97
S-beta thalassemia sickle cell disease, 362
Scabies, case example, 46
Scabies lesions, 41, 41f
Scabies mite, 40, 40f
Scabiosis, 46
Scar(s)
  hypertrophic, 80
    defined, 725
  keloid, 80, 80f
    defined, 727
Scheurmann disease, defined, 736
Schistosoma haematobium
  cancer due to, 674
    bladder, 598
  defined, 736
School-age children, ADHD in, 259
Schwann cells, defined, 736
SCI. *See* Spinal cord injury (SCI)
Scientific method, 704
  massage and, 706–707
  strengths and weaknesses of, 706–707
Sclerodactyly
  defined, 736
  scleroderma and, 190
Sclerosis(es)
  amyotrophic lateral. *See* Amyotrophic lateral sclerosis (ALS)
  tuberous, 262
Scoliosis, 123–124
  defined, 736
Seasonal affective disorder (SAD), 273
  defined, 736
Sebaceous gland, defined, 736
Seborrheic, defined, 736
Seborrheic eczema, 58
Seborrheic keratosis, 71
  defined, 736
Sebum, defined, 736
Second impact syndrome, defined, 736
Second World Congress on Fibromyalgia and Myofascial Pain, criteria for FMS, 93
Secondary anemias, 343
Second-degree burn, 75, 75f
Sedentary lifestyle
  atherosclerosis due to, 374
  colorectal cancer due to, 513
  stroke due to, 305
Segmental dystonia, 237
Seizure(s)
  absence, 325
    defined, 711
  generalized, 324–325
  grand mal, defined, 723
  myoclonic, 325
  partial
    complex, 324
    simple, 324
  static, 325
  tonic-clonic, 325
    defined, 740
Selective estrogen receptor modulators (SERMs)
  defined, 736
  for osteoporosis, 118
Selective serotonin reuptake inhibitors (SSRIs), 686
  for anxiety disorders, 258
  defined, 736
  for depression, 274
Self-limited disease, defined, 736
Semantic pragmatic communication disorder, 264
Semicircular canals, 321, 321f
Seminiferous tubules, 608, 609f
  defined, 736
Seminoma(s), 650
  defined, 736
Sensation
  changes in, MS and, 232
  reduced, disc disease and, 207
Sensitivity, gluten, 487
Sensory envelope, skin as, 24
Sensory neurons, 220, 221f
Sentinel lymph node, defined, 787
Septicemia
  defined, 736
  lymphangitis and, 410
Sequestration, 206
SERMs. *See* Selective estrogen receptor modulators (SERMs)
Seronegative, defined, 736
Seronegative spondyloarthropathy, 125
Serotonin, defined, 736
Serotonin norepinephrine reuptake inhibitors (SNRIs), for depression, 274
Sertoli cell tumors, 650
  defined, 736
Severe acute respiratory syndrome (SARS), defined, 736
Sexual dysfunction, MS and, 232
Sham, defined, 703
Sham treatment, 707
Shiatsu, 20
Shigella, defined, 736
Shingles, 246–249, 248f. *See also* Herpes zoster (shingles)
Shock
  heart attack and, 391
  insulin, 570
Shockwave lithotripsy, for plantar fasciitis, 188
Shoulder(s)
  frozen, 152
    defined, 769
  jackhammerer's, 172

Shoulder pain, TMJ disorders and, 156
Shoulder-hand syndrome, 289–292, 291f. *See also* Complex regional pain syndrome (CRPS)
  defined, 736
Shy-Drager syndrome, 243
  defined, 737
Sickle cell crises, sickle cell disease and, 362
Sigmoidoscopy, defined, 737
Sign, defined, 6t
Silent asthma, 463
Silent killer. *See* Hypertension
Simple fractures, 113
Simple partial seizures, 324
Sine scleroderma, 190
  defined, 737
Single-blinded study, 707
  defined, 703
Sinoatrial node, defined, 737
Sinus headaches, 319
Sinusotomy, balloon
  defined, 714
  for sinusitis, 457
Sitz bath
  defined, 737
  for prostatitis, 649
Sjögren syndrome
  defined, 737
  scleroderma and, 190
Skeletal muscle relaxants
  centrally acting, 697
  peripherally acting, 697
Skin, 23–83
  cancer of, 66–74, 672. *See also* Skin cancer
  conditions of, relevance for massage therapists, 24–25
  construction of, 24, 25f
  cross-section of, 25f
  functions of, 23–24
  injuries to, 74–81. *See also specific types, e.g.,* Burn(s)
    burns, 74–77, 75f, 76f
    decubitus ulcers, 77–79, 78f
    scar tissue, 79–81, 80f
  pigmentations of, 71
  purpose of, 23
Skin disorders, 25–74
  lice
    body, 44
    head, 42–44, 42f
    pubic, 44–45, 45f
      mites, 40–42, 40f, 41f
      warts, 47–50, 47f, 49f
  neoplastic, 62–74
    actinic keratosis, 66–67, 67f, 74
    basal cell carcinoma, 67–69, 68f, 74
    malignant melanoma, 70–74, 72f
    psoriasis, 62–65, 63f
    skin cancer, 66–74
    squamous cell carcinoma, 69–70, 70f, 74
  noncontagious, 50–62
    acne rosacea, 50–52, 51f
    acne vulgaris, 52–55, 54f
    dermatitis, 56–60, 57f–59f
    eczema, 56–60, 57f–59f
    hives, 60–62, 61f
Skin lesions, candidiasis and, 549
Skull fracture, TBI due to, 308
SLE. *See* Systemic lupus erythematosus (SLE)
Sleep, stages of, 327
Sleep apnea
  central, 328
  obstructive, 328
Sleep disorders, 326–330
  causes of, 326–327
  complications of, 329
  defined, 326
  demographics of, 326
  diagnosis of, 329–330
  fibromyalgia and, 91
  massage for, 326, 330
  Parkinson disease and, 241
  signs and symptoms of, 329
  treatment of, 330
  types of, 327–329
Sleep paralysis, 329
  defined, 737
Sleeping pills, dependency issues related to, 267
Small cell lung cancer, 476
Smog, asthma and, case example, 464
Smoking
  aortic aneurysm due to, 369
  atherosclerosis due to, 374
  cessation, in chronic bronchitis management, 467
  GERD and, 502
  lung cancer due to, 475
  peptic ulcers due to, 506
  stroke due to, 304
Smooth muscle, compromised, aortic aneurysm due to, 369
SNRIs. *See* Serotonin norepinephrine reuptake inhibitors (SNRIs)
Soap(s)
  antimicrobial, defined, 10
  plain, defined, 10
Social anxiety disorder, 257
Social phobia, 257
Sodium urate, defined, 737
Solar keratosis, 66–67, 67f, 74
Solitary myeloma, 359
Somatomedin C, defined, 737
Somatotrophin, 89
  defined, 737
Sonogram, defined, 737
Sore(s)
  canker, 37
  mouth, 37
  pressure, 77–79, 78f
Southern tick-associated rash illness (STARI), 136
Spasmodic torticollis, 237
Spastic cerebral palsy, 287
Spastic paralysis, defined, 298, 737
Spasticity
  defined, 298, 737
  SCI and, 298–299, 300
Specific immunity, defined, 737
Specific muscle weakness, defined, 737
Speech, changes in, Parkinson disease and, 241
Spermicide(s), UTIs due to, 604
Sphincter, defined, 737
Sphygmomanometer, 379
  defined, 737
Spigelian hernia, 180
  defined, 737
Spina bifida meningocele, 294
  defined, 737
Spina bifida myelomeningocele, 294
  defined, 737
Spina bifida occulta, 293
  defined, 737
Spinal cord pressure, spondylosis and, 150
Spindle(s), muscle, defined, 729
Spine, spreading problems in, spondylosis and, 149–150
Spiral fractures, 114f
Spirochete(s), 7, 8f
Spirometry
  in asthma diagnosis, 463
  defined, 737
Spleen, enlarged, cirrhosis and, 527
Splenomegaly, 416
  anemia and, 342
  cirrhosis and, 527
  defined, 737
Splinting, cramps and, 107
Splint(s)s, shin, 102–105, 103f. *See also* Shin splints
Spondylitis, 64
  ankylosing. *See* Ankylosing spondylitis
  rheumatoid, 125
    defined, 735
Spondyloarthropathy
  defined, 737
  seronegative, 125
Spondylolisthesis, 162
  defined, 150, 737
Spondylolysis, defined, 150, 737
Spontaneous abortion
  causes of, 611
  defined, 610, 611
Spontaneous peritonitis, 552
Sporadic, defined, 737
Sports injuries, SCI due to, 298
Spriochete, defined, 737
Sprue
  celiac, 486–489
    defined, 716
  nontropical, 486–489
    defined, 731
Sputum, defined, 737
Squamous, defined, 737
Squamous cell carcinoma, 69–70, 70f, 74
  causes of, 69
  defined, 69
  esophageal cancer due to, 494
  location of, 69
  massage for, 70, 74
  mortality rate associated with, 69
  prevalence of, 69
  signs and symptoms of, 69, 70f
  treatment of, 69–70
SSRIs. *See* Selective serotonin reuptake inhibitors (SSRIs)
St. Anthony's fire, defined, 737

St. John's wort, for depression, 275
Stable angina, heart attack and, 389–390
Staghorn calculus, 589, 589f
  defined, 737
Staging, defined, 737
Stain(s), port wine, 71
Stapedius, defined, 737
Staphylococcus(i), 7, 7f
  defined, 737
Staphylococcus aureus, 26
  methicillin-resistant
    boils due to, 26
    defined, 729
STARI. *See* Southern tick-associated rash illness (STARI)
Starling equilibrium, 404
  defined, 737
Stasis dermatitis, 58
Static seizures, 325
Status epilepticus, 325
  defined, 737
STDs. *See* Sexually transmitted diseases (STDs)
Steatohepatitis, nonalcoholic, 526
  defined, 738
Steatorrhea, 546
  defined, 738
Stein-Leventhal syndrome, 638, 639f
  defined, 738
Stem cell implantation, in cancer management, 678, 679
Stenosis(es)
  defined, 6t, 150, 376, 738
  described, 490
Stent(s), defined, 738
Stereotactic radiosurgery, in Cushing syndrome, 566
Sterilization, defined, 10
Steroid(s), 558
  defined, 789
  for eczema, 59
  for psoriasis, 65
Stoma, 600
  defined, 789
Stomach, cardia of, defined, 716
Stomach emptying, delayed, GERD and, 502
Stomatitis
  angular, 37
  defined, 738
Strabismus
  cerebral palsy and, 288
  defined, 738
Stratum basale, defined, 738
Streptococcus(i), 7, 8f
  defined, 738
Streptococcus pneumoniae
  defined, 738
  sinusitis due to, 456
Stress. *See also* Hypothalmus-Pituitary-Adrenal Axis
  acne vulgaris due to, 53
  allergies and, 59
  cortisol and, 59
  Crohn disease and, 491
  peptic ulcers due to, 504–505
  stroke due to, 305
Stress fractures, 104, 113
Stress injury, repetitive, defined, 735
Stress response system, 271
Stretching, 18. *See also* PNF/MET/ stretching
Striatonigral degeneration, defined, 738
Stricture(s), GERD and, 501, 501f
Stritonigral degeneration, 243
Stroma, 627
  defined, 738
Stromal cell tumors, 650
  defined, 738
Stromal sarcoma, 624
Structural problems, sinusitis due to, 456
Struvite, defined, 738
Struvite stones, 590
Student's elbow, 172
Subacute, defined, 6t, 738
Subacute cutaneous lupus, defined, 738
Subacute stage of healing, 15
Subarachnoid hemorrhage, stroke due to, 304
Subcutaneous, defined, 738
Subluxation
  carpal tunnel syndrome due to, 201
  defined, 738
Substance P, 92
  defined, 738
Substantia nigra, 239
  defined, 738
Sudeck atrophy, 289–292, 291f. *See also* Complex regional pain syndrome (CRPS)
  defined, 738
Sun exposure, squamous cell carcinoma due to, 69
Superficial fascia, defined, 738
Superficial spreading melanoma, 71, 72f
Superior vena cava syndrome, 477
  defined, 738
Surface(s), care of, 11–13
Swedish massage, 20–21
Sycosis, herpetic, 37
Symmetric arthritis, 64
Sympathectomy
  for CRPS, 292
  defined, 738
  for Raynaud syndrome, 384
Symptom, defined, 6t
Synarthrosis(es), 87
  defined, 738
Syncytial, defined, 738
Syndesmophyte(s), 125
  defined, 738
Syndrome, defined, 6t
Syndrome X, 579–581
  defined, 738
Synkinesis, 284
  defined, 738
Synovectomy, defined, 738
Synovial joint, 128, 128f
  defined, 738
Synovial sheaths, 193–194, 194f
Syphilis, 663–664
  untreated, aortic aneurysm due to, 369
Systemic lupus erythematosus (SLE), 434, 435f
  defined, 738
Systemic scleroderma, 189
  limited, 189
    defined, 728
Systole, defined, 379, 738

T

T cells, 405–406
  imbalance and dysfunction of, eczema due to, 56
Table(s), care of, 12
Tachycardia
  anemia and, 344
  defined, 738
Tamiflu, for influenza, 449
Tamoxifen
  defined, 739
  uterine cancer due to, 625
Tangle, neurofibrillary, defined, 730
Target(s), 220
Tau, 223
  defined, 739
TCAs. *See* Tricyclic antidepressants (TCAs)
Tear(s), meniscus, 152
Teeth, grinding, 155
  TMJ disorders and, 156
Telangiectasia(s), 388
  defined, 739
  scleroderma and, 190
Temperature, regulation of, circulatory system in, 338
Tender points
  defined, 739
  fibromyalgia and, 92, 92f
Tendinitis, 192
  patellar, 143, 152
    defined, 781
Tendinosis, 192
  defined, 739
Tendon injuries, 152
Tennis elbow, defined, 739
TENS. *See* Transcutaneous electrical nerve stimulation (TENS)
Tension headaches, 316–318, 317f
Teratoma(s), 638, 650
  defined, 739
Terminal ileitis, 491
  defined, 739
Testosterone, 559
  defined, 739
  production of, acne vulgaris due to, 53
Tetraplegia
  defined, 739
  spastic, 298
Thalassemia, defined, 739
The great immitator, 230–234, 234t. *See also* Multiple sclerosis (MS)
Thenar, defined, 739
Thermal capsulorrhaphy
  defined, 739
  for dislocations, 129
Thermography, defined, 739
Third-degree burn, 76, 76f
Thrombocyte(s), 338–339
  atherosclerosis due to, 373
  defined, 714, 739
  inflammation and, 14
Thrombocytopenia, 354

defined, 739
Thromboembolism, pregnancy and, 656
Thrombosis(es)
cerebral, stroke due to, 303
deep vein, 364–368, 366f. *See also* Thrombophlebitis/deep vein thrombosis
cancer-related, 680
SCI and, 300
defined, 739
Thrombus, 345–348, 345f, 346f. *See also* Embolism/thrombus
defined, 345
Thrush, defined, 739
Thymoma(s), 210
defined, 739
Thymosin, 559
defined, 739
Thyroid, diffuse toxic, 573
Thyroid hormones, 558
Thyroid lymphoma, 583
Thyroid storm, 575
Thyroid supplement drugs, 698–699
Thyroiditis, Hashimoto
defined, 724
hypothyroidism and, 577
Thyroid-stimulating immunoglobulins, 573
Thyroxin, defined, 739
TIAs. *See* Transient ischemic attacks (TIAs)
Tibial tuberosity apophysitis, defined, 739
Tibialis anterior/tibialis posterior injury, 104
Tic douloureux, defined, 739
Tick(s), 8, 9f
deer, Lyme disease spread by, 134, 134f, 135
Tinea, 30
defined, 739
Tinea barbae, 33
defined, 739
Tinea capitis, 32, 32f
defined, 739
Tinea corporis, 31, 31f
defined, 739
Tinea cruris, 33, 33f
defined, 739
Tinea manus, 32
defined, 739
Tinea pedis, 32, 32f
defined, 739
Tinea unguium, 32
defined, 739
Tinea versicolor, 33
defined, 739
Tinel sign
in carpal tunnel syndrome diagnosis, 202
defined, 739
Tinnitus
defined, 740
Ménière disease and, 322
TINs. *See* Topical immunomodulators (TINs)
Tissue(s)
connective, types of, 87–90, 88f
granulation, defined, 723
scar, 79–81, 80f. *See also* Scar tissue
Tissue plasminogen activator (tPA), defined, 740
Titer, defined, 740
TMJ disorders. *See* Temporomandibular joint (TMJ) disorders
TNF blockers. *See* Tumor necrosis factor (TNF) blockers
Tobacco use, stomach cancer due to, 509
Tonic spasm, defined, 740
Tonic-clonic seizures, 325
defined, 740
Tooth enamel, decay of, GERD and, 501
Tophus(i), defined, 740
Topical immunomodulators (TINs)
defined, 740
for eczema, 59
Torsion, defined, 740
Torticollis
congenital, 238
defined, 740
infant, 238
spasmodic, 237
types of, 238
Toxic megacolon, 524
defined, 740
Toxic nodular goiter, 573
Toxoplasma gondii, defined, 740
tPA. *See* Tissue plasminogen activator (tPA)
Traction-inflammatory headaches, 316, 319–320
Transcranial magnet stimulation, for depression, 275
Transcriptase, 428
defined, 740
Transcutaneous, defined, 740
Transcutaneous discectomy, for disc disease, 208–209
Transcutaneous electrical nerve stimulation (TENS)
defined, 740
for peripheral neuropathy, 235–236
Transection, spinal cord effects of, 297
Transient ischemic attacks (TIAs)
described, 303
permanent memory loss due to, 225
Transitional cell carcinoma, 597–600. *See also* Bladder cancer
Transplant(s)
allogenic, defined, 712
autogenic, defined, 714
autologous, defined, 714
bone marrow
autologous, in cancer management, 678
for leukemia, 355
Transsphenoidal adenectomy, in Cushing syndrome, 566
Transverse fractures, 114f
Trauma
aortic aneurysm due to, 369
birth-related, cerebral palsy due to, 287
defined, 6t
physical, thrombophlebitis/deep vein thrombosis due to, 364
Treponema pallidum, defined, 740
Trichomoniasis, 665
Trichophyton
defined, 740
T. mentagrophytes, 32
T. rubrum, 32
T. tonsurans, 32
Tricyclic antidepressants (TCAs), 686
for anxiety disorders, 248
defined, 740
for depression, 274
Trigeminal nerve, 310, 311f
Trigger point(s) (TrPs), 97–98, 98f
active, 98
attachment, 97
central, 97
defined, 792
latent, 98
whiplash and, 197
Trigger point (TrP) therapy, 21–22
Triglyceride(s), described, 375
Triiodothyronine, defined, 740
Trimesters, of pregnancy, massage for, 657–658, 658f
Trophic, defined, 740
Trophic ulcers, 77–79, 78f
defined, 740
TrP. *See* Trigger point (TrP)
Tubercle(s), defined, 458, 740
Tuberous sclerosis, 262
Tubule(s), seminiferous, 608, 609f
defined, 736
Tumor(s). *See also specific types, e.g.*, Adenocarcinoma(s)
adrenal, 565
defined, 740
epithelial, of ovaries, 635
fibroid, 621–623, 622f
Tumor(s)—*continued*
germ cell, 650
Leydig cell, 650
defined, 727
malignant mixed mesodermal, 625
neuroendocrine, 543
phyllodes
of breast, 630
defined, 733
Sertoli cell, 650
defined, 736
stromal cell, 650
defined, 738
yolk sac, 650
defined, 741
Tumor necrosis factor (TNF), defined, 792
Tumor necrosis factor (TNF) blockers, for psoriasis, 65
Tunica intima, 370
defined, 740
Tunica media, 370
defined, 740
Turcot syndrome
colorectal cancer due to, 513
defined, 740
Tyrosine, 558
defined, 740

U

Ulcer(s)
anemia and, 343
decubitus, 77–79, 78f. *See also* Decubitus ulcers
diabetes mellitus and, 570, 571f

Hunner, 601
defined, 725
peptic, 504–508, 505f, 506f.
rodent, defined, 735
trophic, 77–79, 78f
defined, 740
Ulcerative proctitis, defined, 524
Umbilical hernia, 180
Undifferentiated thyroid cancer, 582–583
Unilateral, defined, 740
Universal and standard precautions, defined, 10
Unstable angina, heart attack and, 390
Urate, sodium, defined, 737
Ureaplasma urealyticum, defined, 740
Uremia, defined, 740
Ureterolithiasis, defined, 740
Ureteroscopic stone removal
defined, 740
for kidney stones, 592
Urethra, mechanical pressure on, BPH and, 641, 642f
Urethritis, nongonococcal, 665
defined, 731
Uric acid stones, 590
Urinary disorders, 588–606
Urinary retention, acute, 642
Urinary system, 587–606. *See also* Urinary disorders
components of, 587–588, 588f
function and structure of, 587–588, 588f
lupus effects on, 436
overview of, 587–588, 588f
Urogram, defined, 740
Urologic dysfunction, MS and, 232
Urothelial carcinoma, 597–600. *See also* Bladder cancer
Urticaria, 60–62, 61f. *See also* Hive(s)
defined, 740
Urushiol, 420
U.S. Department of Health, in tuberculosis, 460
Uterine artery embolization, 623
Uterine hyperplasia, 620
Uterine sarcoma, 623–626. *See also* Uterine cancer
Uterus, disorders of, 610–626
abortion, 610–612
cervical cancer, 612–615
dysmenorrhea, 616–618
endometriosis, 618–621, 619f
fibroid tumors, 621–623, 622f
uterine cancer, 623–626
UTIs. *See* Urinary tract infections (UTIs)
Uveitis, defined, 740

V

Vaccine(s)
Haemophilus influenzae type B, for meningitis, 251
Salk, 254
tuberculosis, 460
Vaginal infection, candidiasis and, 549
Vagotomy, defined, 740
Vagus nerve stimulation, for depression, 275
Valgus, defined, 740
Validity, defined, 703
Valley fever, 452
Vapocoolant, defined, 740
Varicocele, defined, 740
Varix(ces)
defined, 741
internal, cirrhosis and, 528
Varus, defined, 741
Vas deferens, 610
defined, 741
Vascular activity, inflammation and, 13, 14f
Vascular dementia, permanent memory loss due to, 225
Vascular disorders, 368–388
Vascular Ehlers-Danlos syndrome, 159
Vascular headaches, 316, 318
Vascular rosacea, acne rosacea and, 51
Vasculitis, defined, 741
Vasodilation, inflammation and, 13, 14f
Vein(s), 339
varicose, 385–388, 385f, 386f.
Venography
defined, 741
in thrombophlebitis/deep vein thrombosis diagnosis, 366
Venous insufficiency, chronic
defined, 717
thrombophlebitis/deep vein thrombosis and, 366
Ventricle(s)
defined, 741
left, heart attacks affecting, 388, 390f
Ventricular fibrillations, 389
heart attack and, 391
Venule(s), 339
defined, 741
Verbal communication, nervous system problems with, 222
Vermiform appendix, defined, 2
Verruca, defined, 741
Verrucous carcinoma, 48
Vertebra(ae), cervical
chronic misalignment of, TMJ disorders and, 157
misaligned, whiplash and, 197
Vertigo
benign paroxysmal positional, 331
defined, 715
rotational, Mèniére disease and, 322
Vesicle(s), defined, 741
Vesicoureteral reflux, 593
defined, 741
Vestibular neuronitis, acute, 331
Villus(i), defined, 741
Viral meningitis, 249
Virchow triad, 364
defined, 741
Viremia
defined, 741
herpes zoster and, 248
Virulent, defined, 741
Virus(es), 6
cancer due to, 673–674
gastroenteritis due to, 498
pneumonia due to, 451
primer for, 428
sinusitis due to, 456
Vision
impaired, diabetes mellitus and, 570
problems associated with, hypertension and, 380
Vision loss, sickle cell disease and, 363
Visual analog scales, 703, 704f
defined, 703
Vitamin D
in bone density maintenance, 119
for psoriasis, 64
von Willebrand disease, 351
defined, 741

W

Walking, MS effects on, 232
Waste products, removal of, circulatory system in, 338
Wasting, muscle, cirrhosis and, 528
Weakness
MS and, 232
muscle
disc disease and vocal dysphonia, 237
specific, defined, 737
Parkinson disease and, 240
Weaver's bottom, 172
Weight loss, rapid, cholesterol stones due to, 532
Wernicke-Korsakoff syndrome, defined, 7, 93
West Nile encephalitis, 245
Wheal, defined, 741
White blood cells (leukocytes), 338, 339f
functions of, 405
inflammation and, 14
Whiteheads, acne vulgaris and, 54
WHO-REAL, 413
Wolff law, defined, 741
Women's Health Initiative, in HRT, 654
World Health Organization (WHO)
in stomach cancer, 509
in tuberculosis, 458
WHO-REAL of, 413
Wound(s), gunshot, SCI due to, 297–298
Wright hyperabduction test
defined, 741
in thoracic outlet syndrome diagnosis, 214
Writer's cramp, 237
Wryneck, 238

X

Xeroderma, defined, 741
Xeroderma pigmentosum, 67
defined, 741
X-linked inheritance, 162

Y

Yolk sac tumors, 650
defined, 741
Yuppie flu, defined, 741

Z

Zoloft, for depression, 274
Zoster sine herpete, 247
Zygapophyseal joints, 213
defined, 74